8TH EDITION

INTRODUCTION TO
CRITICAL CARE
NURSING

EDITORS

MARY LOU SOLE
PhD, RN, CCNS, CNL, FAAN, FCCM

Dean and Professor, Orlando Health Endowed Chair in
   Nursing, University of Central Florida College of Nursing
Nurse Scientist, Orlando Health, Orlando, Florida

DEBORAH G. KLEIN
MSN, APRN, ACNS-BC, CCRN, FAHA, FAAN

Clinical Nurse Specialist, Coronary ICU, Heart Failure ICU,
   and Cardiac Short Stay/PACU/CARU, Cleveland Clinic
Clinical Preceptor, Frances Payne Bolton School of Nursing,
   Case Western Reserve University, Cleveland, Ohio
Adjunct Faculty, College of Nursing, Kent State University,
   Kent, Ohio

MARTHE J. MOSELEY
PhD, RN, CCRN-K, CCNS

Director, Inpatient Evaluation Center (IPEC), Office of
   Reporting, Analytics, Performance, Improvement and
   Deployment (RAPID), Veterans Health Administration,
   Washington, DC

ASSOCIATE EDITORS

MARY BETH FLYNN MAKIC
PhD, RN, CCNS, CCRN-K, FAAN, FNAP, FCNS

Professor, University of Colorado College of Nursing,
   Aurora, Colorado
Nurse Scientist, Denver Health, Denver, Colorado

LAUREN T. MORATA
DNP, APRN-CNS, CCRN, CCNS

Clinical Nurse Specialist, Clinical Quality, Lakeland Regional
   Health Medical Center, Lakeland, Florida

ELSEVIER

Elsevier
3251 Riverport Lane
St. Louis, Missouri 63043

INTRODUCTION TO CRITICAL CARE NURSING, EIGHTH EDITION   978-0-323-64193-7

Previous editions copyrighted 2017, 2013, 2009, 2005, 2001, 1997, 1993.

Library of Congress Control Number: 2020935150

Executive Content Strategist: Lee Henderson
Senior Content Development Specialist: Heather Bays
Publishing Services Manager: Julie Eddy
Senior Project Manager: Tracey Schriefer
Design Direction: Brian Salisbury

Printed in Canada

Last digit is the print number: 9 8 7 6 5 4 3 2

Working together
to grow libraries in
developing countries

www.elsevier.com • www.bookaid.org

*Since the first edition of this text published in 1991, it has become my life's work to provide
an easy-to-read text for students, novice nurses, and experienced nurses
who want a resource for practice. This book is dedicated to all acute
and critical care nurses who care for the lives of our sickest patients
at their most vulnerable times. Thank you for all that you do!
And to my amazing family for supporting me through this textbook
journey for 30 years!*

MLS

*To the acute and critical care nurses, patients, and their families, who guide the content of this book.
To my husband, Ron, and my sons, David and Seth, for their support in all that I do.
To my parents, Rena Sasson Goldenberg, RN, BSN, and Ira Goldenberg, MD,
for their guidance and inspiration.*

DGK

*To acute and critical care nurses who care for veteran patients and families across the United States.
In memory of my mom (a retired emergency department RN), Violet Halvorson; to my sister, Heidi Halvorson;
and son, Nicholas Moseley, both are faithful care receivers and givers.
And for my lifelong influential mentor, Marjory Olson.*

MJM

*To my acute and critical care nursing colleagues, patients, and families, who taught me the importance
of excellence in critical care practice. To my parents, sisters, husband, and children,
whose unconditional love and support are ever-present
and add true meaning to my life.*

MBFM

*For the acute and critical care clinicians who open this book, I hope the contents within
help answer your clinical queries and guide you to provide the best care to our patients.
In memory of my father, Tommy Yon and to my mother, Jackie Yon, who were my first nursing mentors;
my husband, Chris, who provides me with steadfast support; and finally, :
who should know all the contents of this book via osmosi
thank you.*

LTM

ABOUT THE EDITORS

MARY LOU SOLE

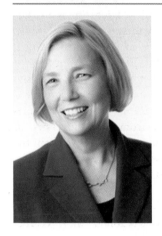

Mary Lou Sole, PhD, RN, CCNS, CNL, FAAN, FCCM, has extensive experience in critical care practice, education, consultation, and research. She is dean and professor and the Orlando Health Endowed Chair at the University of Central Florida (UCF) College of Nursing in Orlando, Florida. She also holds a per diem appointment as a Research Scientist at Orlando Health. Her research focus is on airway management of the critically ill. Dr. Sole began her career as a diploma graduate from the Ohio Valley General Hospital School of Nursing in Wheeling, West Virginia. She received a BSN from Ohio University, a master's degree in nursing from The Ohio State University, and a PhD in nursing from The University of Texas at Austin. Dr. Sole has published extensively and serves on many editorial boards. She has been active locally and nationally in many professional organizations, including the American Association of Critical-Care Nurses (AACN), the Society of Critical Care Medicine, and the American Academy of Nursing. She has received numerous local, state, and national awards for clinical practice, teaching, and research. Dr. Sole has been inducted as a fellow in both the American Academy of Nursing and the American College of Critical Care Medicine. She has been recognized for her research as the AACN Distinguished Research Lecturer and as an inductee into the Sigma Theta Tau International Researcher Hall of Fame.

DEBORAH G. KLEIN

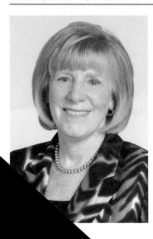

Deborah G. Klein, MSN, APRN, ACNS-BC, CCRN, FAHA, FAAN, has more than 40 years of experience in critical care practice, education, consultation, and research. She is currently Clinical Nurse Specialist for the Coronary ICU, Heart Failure ICU, and Cardiac Short Stay/PACU/CARU at the Cleveland Clinic in Cleveland, Ohio. She is a Clinical Preceptor at Frances Payne Bolton School of Nursing, Case Western Reserve University; and Adjunct Faculty at Kent State University College of Nursing. She received her BSN and MSN from Frances Payne Bolton School of Nursing, Case Western Reserve University, in Cleveland, Ohio. She is active both locally and nationally in professional organizations, including the American Heart Association and the American Association of Critical-Care Nurses, where she has served on the Board of Directors and on the Certification Corporation Board of Directors. She has served on editorial boards of several critical care nursing journals and has published extensively on critical care topics in peer-reviewed journals. Mrs. Klein has received local and national awards for clinical practice and teaching. She has been inducted as a Fellow in the American Heart Association and as a Fellow in the American Academy of Nursing.

MARTHE J. MOSELEY

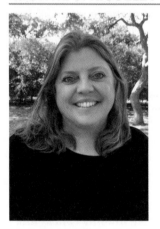

Marthe J. Moseley, PhD, RN, CCRN-K, CCNS, has more than 35 years of experience in critical care practice, education, consultation, and research. She is currently Director of the Inpatient Evaluation Center (IPEC) with the Veterans Health Administration in Washington, DC, and a Clinical Nurse Specialist for Acute and Critical Care. Dr. Moseley received a BA degree in nursing from Jamestown College in Jamestown, North Dakota, following the completion of a BA degree in health, physical education, and biology from Concordia College in Moorhead, Minnesota. She completed her MSN and PhD at The University of Texas Health Science Center at San Antonio. She has been active locally and nationally in professional organizations, including the American Association of Critical-Care Nurses. She is on the editorial boards of several critical care journals and has published in peer-reviewed journals on critical care topics. Dr. Moseley has received local and national awards for both clinical practice and teaching.

MARY BETH FLYNN MAKIC

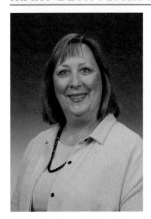

Mary Beth Flynn Makic, PhD, RN, CCNS, CCRN-K, FAAN, FNAP, FCNS, has more than 30 years of critical care experience, research, evidence-based practice, and clinical education. She is a Professor at the University of Colorado College of Nursing and program director for the Adult-Gerontology Clinical Nurse Specialist graduate program. She is also a research scientist at a level I trauma center, in Denver Colorado. Dr. Makic achieved her BSN from the University of Wisconsin, Madison, WI. She completed her Masters of Science at the University of Maryland at Baltimore with a focus on trauma patient populations and the advance practice role of a clinical nurse specialist. Her PhD was confirmed in 2007 from the University of Colorado Health Sciences Center, Denver, CO. She is active locally and nationally in several professional organizations. She was recently on the Board of Directors for the American Association of Critical Care Nurses. She also serves on the editorial board of several critical care journals and has published extensively in peer reviewer journals. Dr. Makic is well known for her passion of improving patient outcomes and nursing practice through evidence-based practice.

LAUREN T. MORATA

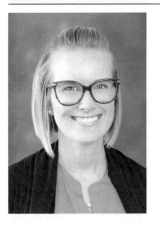

Lauren T. Morata, DNP, APRN, CCNS, is an experienced critical care and trauma nurse with a passion for evidence-based practice and research. She is a Clinical Nurse Specialist for Clinical Quality at Lakeland Regional Health. Dr. Morata graduated with her BS from the University of Central Florida. She received her MSN as clinical nurse specialist from the University of Cincinnati, and a DNP from the University of Central Florida. She is involved in professional organizations both locally and nationally, including the American Association of Critical-Care Nurses and the Society of Critical Care Medicine. She has been honored with awards both locally and nationally, most recently the AACN's Circle of Excellence.

CONTRIBUTORS

Katherine F. Alford, PhD, RN, CPHQ, CPPS
Quality, Risk, and Readiness Clinician
Quality Management
South Texas Veterans Health Care System
San Antonio, Texas

Christina Amidei, PhD, RN, CNRN, FAAN
Director of Clinical Research
Neurological Surgery
Northwestern University
Chicago, Illinois

Mamoona Arif Rahu, PhD, RN, CCRN
Trauma Clinical Educator
Trauma Services
Inova Fairfax Medical Campus
Fairfax, Virginia

Kathleen Black, MSN, RN, NE-BC
Chief Nursing Executive
Nursing
Bon Secours St. Francis Health System
Greenville, South Carolina

Christina Marie Canfield, MSN, RN
ICU Telemedicine Program Manager
Medical Operations
Cleveland Clinic
Cleveland, Ohio

Sandra J. Dotson-Kirn, PhD, RN
Adjunct Faculty
Nursing
Duquesne University
Pittsburgh, Pennsylvania

Nikki Dotson-Lorello, RN, CCRN, CPTC
Organ Recovery Coordinator
Organ Procurement
LifeShare of the Carolinas;
Clinical Nurse Supervisor
Immunotherapy
Levine Cancer Institute
Atrium Health
Charlotte, North Carolina

Douglas Houghton, DNP, APRN, ACNPC, CCRN, FAANP
Director of Advanced Practice Providers
Advanced Practice
Jackson Health System
Miami, Florida

Kathleen G. Kerber, MSN, APRN-CNS, CCRN, CNRN
Clinical Nurse Specialist
Nursing
The MetroHealth System
Cleveland, Ohio

Charly Murphree, MSN, RN
Nurse Manager
SICU/CVICU
Birmingham VA Medical Center
Birmingham, Alabama

Lynelle N.B. Pierce, MS, RN, CCRN, CCNS, FAAN
Clinical Assistant Professor
Nursing
University of Kansas School of Nursing;
Clinical Specialist, Critical Care
Nursing
The University of Kansas Hospital
Kansas City, Kansas

Jenny Lynn Sauls, PhD, MSN, RN
Professor and Director
Nursing
Middle Tennessee State University
Murfreesboro, Tennessee

Karen Baker Sovern, MSN, RN
Clinical Program Manager
Inpatient Evaluation Center (IPEC)
Veterans Health Administration
Mason, Ohio

Linda Staubli, MSN, RN, CCRN-K, ACCNS-AG
Clinical Nurse Specialist
Emergency Department
University of Colorado Hospital
Aurora, Colorado

Sarah Taylor, MSN, RN, ACNS-BC
Clinical Nurse Specialist
Trauma Burn Center
Michigan Medicine
Ann Arbor, Michigan

Megan Walsh, BS, RD/N, LD
Diabetes Educator
Diabetes Education
Sharecare
Tampa, Florida

Colleen Walsh-Irwin, DNP, RN, ANP-BC, AACC, FAANP
Program Manager, Evidence-Based Practice
Office of Nursing Services
Department of Veterans Affairs
Washington, DC;
Clinical Assistant Professor
School of Nursing
Stony Brook University
Stony Brook, New York;
Nurse Practitioner
Cardiology
Northport VA Medical Center
Northport, New York

Sharon Watts, DNP, FNP-BC, CDE
Diabetes Field Advisor
Office of Nursing
Veterans Health Administration
Cleveland, Ohio

John Whitcomb, PhD, RN, CCRN-K, FCCM
Professor and Director Undergraduate
    Nursing Programs
Nursing
Clemson University
Clemson, South Carolina

Jayne M. Willis, MSN, RN, NEA-BC, CENP
Chief Nurse Executive, Vice President
Nursing
Orlando Health
Orlando, Florida

Chris Winkleman, PhD, RN, ACNP, FAANP, FCCM, CCRN, CNE
Associate Professor;
Lead Faculty
Adult-Gerontology Acute Care Nurse
    Practitioner Program
Frances Payne Bolton School of Nursing
Case Western Reserve University
Cleveland, Ohio

Critical care nursing deals with human responses to life-threatening health problems. Critically ill patients continue to have high levels of acuity and complex care needs. These patients are cared for in critical care units, intermediate care units, outpatient settings, and at home. The critical care nurse is challenged to provide comprehensive care for these patients and their family members. The demand for critical care nurses who can work across the continuum of care continues to increase.

A solid knowledge foundation in concepts of critical care nursing is essential for practice. Nurses must also learn the assessment and technical skills associated with management of the critically ill patient.

The goal of this eighth edition of *Introduction to Critical Care Nursing* is to facilitate attainment of this foundation for care of the acutely and critically ill patient. The book continues to provide essential information in an easy-to-learn format. The textbook is targeted to both undergraduate nursing students and experienced nurses who are new to critical care. Both groups have found past editions of the book beneficial. In fact, undergraduate students who have taken a critical care course based on this textbook have easily passed critical care courses offered in their first nursing position!

ORGANIZATION

Introduction to Critical Care Nursing is organized into three sections. *Part I, Fundamental Concepts,* introduces the reader to critical care nursing; psychosocial concepts related to patients, families, and nurses; and legal, ethical, and end-of-life issues related to critical care nursing practice. *Part II, Tools for the Critical Care Nurse,* remains a unique feature of this text. Chapters in this section provide vital information on comfort and sedation, nutrition, recognition of dysrhythmias, hemodynamic monitoring, airway management and mechanical ventilation, management of life-threatening emergencies, and organ donation. These chapters provide information related to the many treatments and technologies that acutely and critically ill patients receive.

The final chapters of the book complete *Part III, Nursing Care During Critical Illness.* The nursing process is used as an organizing framework for each chapter. Nursing care plans continue to be included so that nurses new to critical care become familiar with patient problems and interventions common to many critically ill patients. A summary of anatomy and physiology is provided, as are pathophysiology diagrams for common problems seen in critical care.

Several features have been incorporated into each chapter to develop clinical reasoning and judgment skills. As the nursing licensure examination moves to a new model, *Next Generation NCLEX,* that evaluates nurses' ability to recognize changes in patient's clinical condition and determine appropriate interventions, practice in translating knowledge into actions is needed. Multiple features within each chapter are designed to develop the nurse's ability to recognize clues that suggest changes in a patient's condition and to develop an evidence-based, patient-centered plan of care to ensure safe delivery of care.

To develop clinical reasoning the nurse must use critical thinking within a specific patient context. Clinical judgment requires the recognition and analysis of cues, developing and prioritizing hypotheses, generating solutions, taking action, and evaluating outcomes. Key features such as pathophysiology flow charts, clinical and laboratory alerts, pharmacology tables, along with lifespan and genetics boxes, facilitate understanding of patient-specific cues that require interventions. Evidence-based practice boxes and QSEN exemplars facilitate understanding of opportunities to generate solutions and implement safe-care. The case studies and collaborative plan of care for critically ill patients allow for a deeper understanding of how to apply or translate knowledge into practice to optimize care of the acute and critically ill patients. Critical thinking questions in each chapter allow the reader to self-evaluate knowledge and the critical reasoning activities are designed to hone both clinical reasoning and judgment skills.

Features of each chapter include pharmacology tables, evidence-based practice boxes, clinical and laboratory alerts, lifespan considerations, critical reasoning activities, case studies, genetics, and Quality and Safety Education for Nurses (QSEN) competencies. Additions and revisions have been made based on reader feedback and current trends.

SPECIAL FEATURES

This edition features a full-color design with updated full-color figures to enhance reader understanding. Many new and revised learning aids appear in the eighth edition to highlight chapter content:

- A **Collaborative Plan of Care for the Critically Ill Patient** is introduced in Chapter 1. It can be individualized to meet specific needs of the patient.
- **Evidence-Based Practice** boxes identify problems in patient care, ask pertinent questions related to the problems, supply evidence addressing the questions, and offer implications for nursing practice. Most boxes provide references to systematic reviews and meta-analyses that provide a greater synthesis of the research evidence related to a problem.
- **QSEN Exemplars** present examples of quality and safety competencies in critical care.
- **Genetics** boxes discuss disorders with a genetic component, including diabetes, Marfan syndrome, and cystic fibrosis.
- **Clinical Alerts** highlight particular concerns, significance, and procedures to help students understand the potential problems encountered in that setting for selected disorders and disease states.

- **Laboratory Alerts** detail both common and cutting-edge tests and procedures to alert students to the importance of laboratory results.
- **Lifespan Considerations** alert the user to the special needs of select populations across the lifespan, such as pregnant patients and older adults, as they relate to critical illness.
- **Transplant Consideration** boxes have been incorporated into several chapters. These boxes include criteria for transplantation, patient management, and strategies for preventing rejection.
- Client-specific **Case Studies** with accompanying questions help students apply the chapter's content to real-life situations while also testing their critical-thinking abilities. Answers for these questions and the **Critical Reasoning Activities** found throughout each chapter are included on the companion Evolve website, which is free to instructors upon adoption.
- **Nursing Care Plans** describe patient problems, outcomes, nursing interventions, and rationales.
- **Pathophysiology Flow Charts** expand analysis of the course and outcomes of particular injuries and disorders.
- **Pharmacology Tables** reflect the most current and most commonly used critical care medications.

EVOLVE RESOURCES

We are pleased to offer additional content and learning aids to both instructors and students on our Evolve companion website, which has been customized for the new edition and is available at http://evolve.elsevier.com/Sole/.

For Students

Student resources on the Evolve site include the following:
- **Review Questions,** consisting of multiple-choice and multiple-response questions and answer rationales for each chapter.
- **Animations and Video Clips,** which feature innovative content from supplemental materials.
- **15 Procedures from** *Mosby's Clinical Skills: Critical Care Collection,* which demonstrate many of the primary procedures important in critical care nursing.

For Instructors

Instructor resources on the Evolve site include the following materials:
- A **TEACH for Nurses Lesson Plan,** which provides the following for each chapter:
  - Objectives and teaching focus.
  - Nursing curriculum standards, including QSEN, concept-based curricula, BSN Essentials, Adult CCRN, and PCCN.
  - Teaching and learning activities related to the chapter content outline.
  - Case study with questions and answers.
- **Answer Keys** to the Critical Reasoning Activities and Case Studies presented in the textbook.
- A **PowerPoint Presentation** collection of more than 700 slides offers a presentation for every chapter. The presentation includes chapter images, lecture notes, and audience response questions, and a few select chapters include a progressive case study.
- An electronic **Test Bank** of more than 650 questions.
- An **Image Collection** including all the images from the text.

Instructors have access to the student resources as well. Evolve can also be used to do the following:
- Publish your class syllabus, outline, and lecture notes.
- Set up "virtual office hours" and email communication.
- Share important dates and information through the online class calendar.
- Encourage student participation through chat rooms and discussion boards.

Critical care nursing is an exciting and challenging field. Healthcare organizations need critical care nurses who are knowledgeable about basic concepts as well as research-based practice, are technologically competent, and are caring toward patients and families. Our hope is that this edition of *Introduction to Critical Care Nursing* will provide the foundation for critical care nursing practice.

MLS
DGK
MJM
MBFM
LTM

CONTENTS

PART I

Fundamental Concepts

Overview of Critical Care Nursing

Mary Lou Sole, PhD, RN, CCNS, CNL, FAAN, FCCM
John Whitcomb, PhD, RN, CCRN-K, FCCM
Lauren Morata, DNP, APRN-CNS, CCRN, CCNS

Many additional resources, including self-assessment exercises, are located on the Evolve companion website at http://evolve.elsevier.com/Sole/.
- Animations
- Clinical Skills: Critical Care Collections
- Student Review Questions
- Video Clips

Consider working in a care setting where the patients have life-threatening conditions and need intense, round-the-clock care by a team of multiprofessionals. The nurse/patient ratio is low, sometimes 1:1, to ensure that care delivery is timely and that response to treatment is continuously assessed. Technology is abundant and readily available to assist in managing these complex, acutely ill patients. Treatment varies but often includes mechanical ventilation, multiple invasive lines, hemodynamic monitoring, and administration of many medications and fluids. This scenario depicts the essence of critical care. Many nurses choose to work in critical care settings because they enjoy working in a fast-paced environment that provides much contact with patients, families, and their multiprofessional colleagues. They constantly are learning new concepts in treatment and technology. Although not a career for every nurse, critical care nursing provides an exciting opportunity for those who thrive on working in such an environment.

DEFINITION OF CRITICAL CARE NURSING

Critical care nursing is concerned with human responses to life-threatening problems, such as trauma, major surgery, or complications of illness. The human response can be a physiological or psychological phenomenon. The focus of the critical care nurse includes both the patient's and the family's responses to illness and involves prevention as well as cure. Because patients' medical needs have become increasingly complex, critical care nursing encompasses care of both acutely ill and critically ill patients.

EVOLUTION OF CRITICAL CARE

The specialty of critical care has its roots in the 1950s, when patients with polio were cared for in specialized units. In the 1960s, recovery rooms were established for the care of patients who had undergone surgery, and coronary care units were instituted for the care of patients with cardiac problems. The patients who received care in these units had improved outcomes. Fig. 1.1 depicts an early cardiac surgical unit. Critical care nursing evolved as a specialty in the 1970s with the development of general critical care units. Since that time, critical care nursing has become increasingly specialized. Examples of specialized critical care units are cardiovascular, surgical, neurological, trauma, transplantation, burn, pediatric, and neonatal units. Fig. 1.2 shows a modern critical care unit.

Critical care nursing has expanded beyond the walls of traditional critical care units. For example, critically ill patients are cared for in emergency departments; postanesthesia units; step-down, intermediate care, and progressive care units; and interventional radiology and cardiology units. Critical care is also delivered during transport of critically ill patients from the field to the acute care hospital and during interfacility transport. With advances in technology, the electronic intensive care unit (eICU) has emerged as another setting for critical care nursing. In an eICU, patients are monitored remotely by critical care nurses and physicians.[14,47] Implementation of the eICU model has reduced hospital and critical care unit lengths of stay and has reduced mortality.[36] Acutely ill patients with high-technology requirements or complex problems, such as patients who are ventilator dependent, may be cared for in medical-surgical units, in long-term acute care hospitals, or at home.

Acute and critical care nurses practice in varied settings to manage and coordinate care for patients who require in-depth assessment, high-intensity therapies and interventions, and continuous nursing vigilance. They also function in various roles and levels, such as staff nurse, educator, and advanced practice nurse. Competencies for critical care nursing practice are listed in Box 1.1.

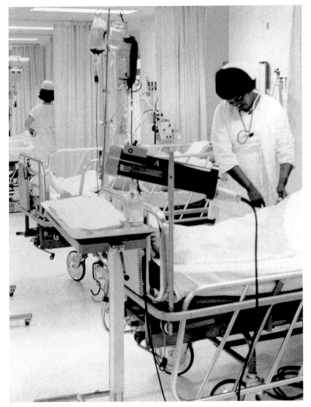

Fig. 1.1 Early cardiac critical care unit circa 1967, called the *cardiac constant care unit*. Note the open-bay concept of care delivery, large cardiac monitor at foot of bed, and absence of multiple pumps. (Reprinted with permission, Cleveland Clinic Center for Medical Arts & Photography © 2011–2019. All rights reserved.)

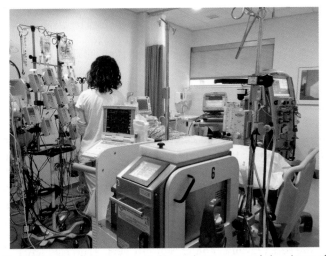

Fig. 1.2 Modern critical care unit. Note private room and abundance of electronic equipment supporting patient care management. (Reprinted with permission, Cleveland Clinic Center for Medical Arts & Photography © 2011–2019. All rights reserved.)

? CRITICAL REASONING ACTIVITY

Compare perceptions of critical care from the viewpoints of the student, nurse, multiprofessional healthcare team, patient, and family. What are the similarities and differences?

BOX 1.1 Competencies of Nurses Caring for the Critically Ill

- Clinical judgment and clinical reasoning skills
- Advocacy and moral agency in identifying and resolving ethical issues
- Caring practices that are tailored to the uniqueness of the patient and family
- Collaboration with patients, family members, and healthcare team members
- Systems thinking that promotes holistic nursing care
- Response to diversity
- Facilitator of learning for patients and family members, team members, and the community
- Clinical inquiry and innovation to promote the best patient outcome

Data from American Association of Critical-Care Nurses. AACN Synergy Model for Patient Care. https://www.aacn.org/~/media/aacn-website/nursing-excellence/standards/aacnsynergymodelforpatientcare.pdf.

PROFESSIONAL ORGANIZATIONS

Several professional organizations support critical care practice. These include the American Association of Critical-Care Nurses (AACN) and the Society of Critical Care Medicine (SCCM).

American Association of Critical-Care Nurses

The AACN is a professional organization that was established in 1969 to represent critical care nurses. It is the largest nursing specialty organization in the world, with more than 100,000 members, dedicated to providing knowledge and resources to those caring for acutely and critically ill patients. In addition to the national organization, more than 240 chapters support critical care nurses at the local level. The mission of the organization is to drive excellence in patient care through knowledge and influence. The vision of the organization supports creating a healthcare system driven by the needs of patients and families in which nurses make their optimal contributions. Values of the organization include accountability, collaboration, leadership, and innovation.[3]

The benefits of AACN membership include continuing education offerings, educational advancement scholarships, research grants, awards, and several official publications including *Critical Care Nurse* and *American Journal of Critical Care.* The organization publishes *Practice Alerts,* which present succinct, evidence-based practices to be applied at the bedside. The AACN sponsors the Beacon Award for Excellence, which is given for exceptional care, improved outcomes, and greater satisfaction with care. The organization also pioneered the Clinical Scene Investigator (CSI) Academy to develop bedside nurses as leaders and change agents who improve patient and fiscal outcomes.[4] The AACN website (http://www.aacn.org) provides membership information and a wealth of information related to critical care nursing.

Society of Critical Care Medicine

The SCCM is a multiprofessional society whose mission is to ensure high-quality care for all critically ill patients. The vision of the SCCM is to have care to all critically ill patients provided by an integrated team of professionals directed by an intensivist (physician who has education, training, and board certification in managing critically ill and injured patients). These teams use knowledge, technology, and compassion to provide timely, safe, effective, efficient, and equitable patient care.[42] Membership in the SCCM is open to all providers in critical care, including physicians, nurses, respiratory therapists, and pharmacists. The SCCM publishes several journals, including *Critical Care Medicine*. Membership and other information are available online at http://www.sccm.org.

Other Professional Organizations

Several other professional organizations also focus on improving care of critically ill patients. Examples include the American College of Chest Physicians (http://www.chestnet. org), the American Thoracic Society (http://www.thoracic. org), and the professional scientific councils of the American Heart Association (http://www.americanheart.org). Nurses can apply for membership in these and other related professional organizations.

STUDY BREAK

1. Which professional organization's primary focus is to support critical care nursing?
   A. American Association of Critical-Care Nurses
   B. American Association of Heart Failure Nurses
   C. American Nurses Association
   D. Society of Critical Care Medicine

CERTIFICATION

Critical care nurses are eligible for certification through the AACN. Certification validates knowledge of critical care nursing, promotes professional excellence, and helps nurses to maintain a current knowledge base.[2] The AACN Certification Corporation oversees the critical care certification process.

The AACN certification credentials are based on a synergy model of practice, which states that the needs of patients and families influence and drive competencies of nurses[5] (Fig. 1.3 and see Box 1.1). Although the synergy model is more than 20 years old, it remains relevant. Each patient and family is unique, with a varying capacity for health and vulnerability to illness. Patients who are more severely compromised have more complex needs, and nursing practice is based on meeting those needs.[12]

The certifications for nurses in acute and critical care bedside practice are known as *CCRN* and *PCCN*. The CCRN certification is available for nurses who provide care of critically ill adult, pediatric, or neonatal populations. The CCRN-E credential is available for nurses who work in eICUs. The PCCN certification is for nurses who provide acute care in progressive care, telemetry, and similar units. Once nurses achieve the CCRN or PCCN credential, they may be eligible to sit for additional subspecialty certification in cardiac medicine or cardiac surgery.

Advanced practice certification for critical care nurses is also available. Acute and critical care clinical nurse specialists can seek the ACCNS credential, which is available for those working with adult, pediatric, and neonatal populations. Acute care nurse practitioners can become certified as ACNPC-AG. The AACN has partnered with the American Organization for Nursing Leadership to offer certification for nurse managers and leaders.

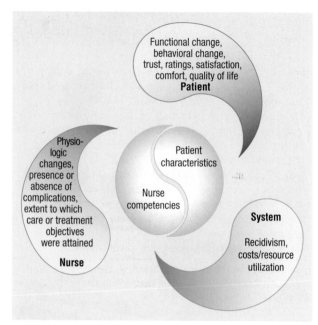

Fig. 1.3 The American Association of Critical-Care Nurses Synergy Model for Patient Care. (From Curley M. Patient-nurse synergy: Optimizing patients' outcomes. *Am J Crit Care.* 1998;7:69.)

All certifications have eligibility requirements to sit for the examination. Continuing education and ongoing care for acute or critically ill patients are required for recertification.

STUDY BREAK

2. A staff nurse states, "I'm a CCRN." What does CCRN mean?
   A. CCRN certification helps the hospital to maintain accreditation from The Joint Commission.
   B. CCRN certification means that the nurse has more knowledge than a noncertified nurse.
   C. CCRN is a registered trademark and stands for "Critical Care Registered Nurse."
   D. CCRN signifies that the nurse was eligible for certification in critical care and passed the CCRN examination.

STANDARDS

Standards serve as guidelines for clinical practice. They establish goals for patient care and provide mechanisms for nurses to assess the achievement of goals. Standards of practice delineate the nursing process: collect data, determine diagnoses, identify expected outcomes, develop a care plan, implement interventions, and evaluate progress toward goals. The standards of professional performance (Box 1.2) describe expectations of the acute and critical care nurse.

CRITICAL CARE NURSE CHARACTERISTICS

Essential nursing practices include monitoring and assessment; reassessment, interpreting information, and problem solving; evaluation of progress to outcomes; development of sustainable evidence-based practice; coordination of team activities and the care plan; patient and family education; and team skill development.

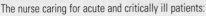

BOX 1.2 Standards of Professional Performance

The nurse caring for acute and critically ill patients:

- Systematically evaluates the quality and effectiveness of nursing practice
- Evaluates own practice in relation to professional practice standards, guidelines, statutes, rules, and regulations
- Acquires and maintains current knowledge and competency in patient care
- Contributes to the professional development of peers and other healthcare providers
- Acts ethically in all areas of practice
- Uses skilled communication to collaborate with the healthcare team to provide care in a safe, healing, humane, and caring environment
- Uses clinical inquiry and integrates research findings into practice
- Considers factors related to safety, effectiveness, cost, and effect in planning and delivering care
- Provides leadership in the practice setting for the profession

Data from Bell L. *AACN Scope and Standards for Acute and Critical Care Nursing Practice.* 2nd ed. Aliso Viejo, CA: American Association of Critical-Care Nurses; 2015.

The acuteness of patients' illnesses makes their care the top priority of critical care nurses. A missed detail in care could easily result in an adverse event or even death. Critical care nurses are very protective of their patients, wanting to make sure optimal outcomes are achieved. They typically are very busy and engrossed in their work. They are familiar with the noises, lights, and frequent interruptions of their patients' care. They know what to do and act quickly when doing so is indicated. A high level of organization is maintained to make sure that everything is done.

In addition to technical competence, critical care nurses establish relationships with patients and families. Chapter 2 details the importance of family-centered care in the busy critical care environment.

Juggling the patients' needs, the time available to care for them, and the nurse's needs makes the job particularly challenging yet rewarding at the same time. Compassion fatigue and moral distress are issues that critical care nurses face because of the fast-paced environment, critical nature of illness, and issues surrounding life and death of patients.[16,31,39] Critical care nurses often have job perfectionist tendencies and unrealistic expectations of self, further contributing to high stress levels. Support groups and debriefing conducted by professionals are strategies to help reduce stress, anxiety, and moral distress.

? CRITICAL REASONING ACTIVITY

Provide examples of strategies to improve communication and collaboration among the multiprofessional team members in critical care.

QUALITY AND SAFETY EMPHASIS

Quality and safety are essential components of patient care. Patients are at risk for a myriad of harms, which increase morbidity, mortality, length of hospital stay, and costs for care. The Quality and Safety Education for Nurses (QSEN) project,

sponsored by the American Association of Colleges of Nursing, provides a road map for integrating quality and safety principles into prelicensure nursing education (http://www.qsen.org).[9] The QSEN curriculum defines six core competencies that provide a foundation for quality care: patient-centered care, teamwork and collaboration, evidence-based practice, quality improvement, informatics, and safety. Applications of QSEN competencies to critical care nursing topics are integrated throughout this text.

Nurses and other healthcare professionals have been challenged to reduce medical errors and promote an environment that facilitates safe practices. The Joint Commission has identified *National Patient Safety Goals* to be addressed in hospitals, long-term care facilities, and other agencies that it accredits.[44] Examples are shown in Box 1.3; however, because goals are updated annually, it is important to regularly review The Joint Commission website (http://www.jointcommission.org).

Initiatives to promote a safe environment are being promoted by the government and other national groups, such as

BOX 1.3 Examples of Patient Safety Goals

Identify Patients Correctly
- Use at least two methods of patient identification
- Ensure correct patient identification for blood transfusions

Improve Communication Among Healthcare Providers
- Report important results of tests and diagnostic procedures on a timely basis

Use Medications Safely
- Label all medications and containers, including syringes and medicine cups
- Reduce harm associated with administration of anticoagulants
- Reconcile medications across the continuum of care

Use Alarms Safely
- Ensure that alarms are audible and respond to them in a timely manner

Prevent Infection
- Comply with guidelines for hand hygiene
- Implement evidence-based guidelines to prevent:
  - Infection with multidrug-resistant organisms
  - Central line–associated bloodstream infections
  - Surgical site infections
  - Catheter-associated urinary tract infections

Identify Safety Risks
- Assess patients for suicidal risk

Prevent Complications Associated With Surgery and Procedures
- Conduct a preprocedure verification process to ensure that surgery is done on the correct patient and site
- Mark the correct procedure site
- Perform a "time-out" before the procedure to ensure that the correct patient, site, and procedure are identified

Modified from The Joint Commission. National Patient Safety Goals. https://www.jointcommission.org/assets/1/6/2019_HAP_NPSGs_final2.pdf. Published January 1, 2019. Accessed March 31, 2019.

the Institute for Healthcare Improvement (IHI). The federal government published an action plan for reducing healthcare-associated infections and preventing infections with multidrug-resistant organisms.[46] The IHI introduced the concept of *bundles* of care to reduce harms, such as infections. Bundles are described as evidence-based best practices that are done as a whole to improve outcomes, and research is being done to evaluate their effectiveness.[29]

Another strategy to improve patient safety is the implementation of rapid response teams or medical emergency teams to address changes in patients' conditions. These teams bring critical care expertise to the bedside to assess and manage patients whose conditions are deteriorating and to provide early intervention and improve outcomes (see Chapter 11).[30] Although most rapid response calls are initiated by healthcare team members, patients and family members are often empowered to activate the team if needed. Many institutions are also piloting automated surveillance algorithms to identify high-risk patients from electronic health record data.[25,27] Ongoing research is underway to assess short-term and long-term outcomes of rapid response teams.

EVIDENCE-BASED PRACTICE

Nurses are encouraged to implement care that is evidence based and to challenge practices that have "always been done" but are not supported by clinical evidence. Research studies are graded by the quality of evidence, and many different rating scales are used. The AACN scale for rating evidence (Table 1.1) is a simple-to-use method for evaluating research studies.[37] Meta-analysis of many related research studies is considered to be the highest level of evidence; the next highest is derived from the randomized controlled trial. After evidence is rated, recommendations for practice are provided. Nurses can get involved in research in many ways, including participating in unit-based journal clubs to review studies and rate their quality.

Clinical practice guidelines are being implemented to ensure that care is appropriate and based on research. Relevant guidelines, such as nutrition and sedation, are discussed throughout the textbook. Many guidelines are available online, such as from the Agency for Healthcare Research and Quality (https://www.ahrq.gov/research/findings/evidence-based-reports/index.html).

HEALTHY WORK ENVIRONMENT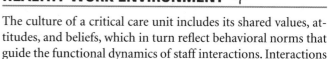

The culture of a critical care unit includes its shared values, attitudes, and beliefs, which in turn reflect behavioral norms that guide the functional dynamics of staff interactions. Interactions among providers, especially nurses and physicians, affect patient safety, clinical outcomes, and the recruitment and retention of nurses.

The AACN initiated a campaign to create work environments that are safe, healing, and humane.[7] Essential components of healthy work environments include respect, responsibility, and acknowledgment of the unique contributions of patients, families, nurses, and healthcare team members (Fig. 1.4).[6] Other aspects of a healthy work environment include effective decision making, appropriate staffing, meaningful recognition, and authentic leadership. Communication and collaboration provide the foundation for achieving a healthy work environment. A healthy work environment promotes nurse retention and job satisfaction.[48]

TABLE 1.1	American Association of Critical-Care Nurses' Levels of Research Evidence	
Level	**Description**	
A	Meta-analysis of multiple controlled studies or meta-synthesis of qualitative studies with results that consistently support a specific action, intervention, or treatment	
B	Well-designed controlled studies, both randomized and nonrandomized, with results that consistently support a specific action, intervention, or treatment	
C	Qualitative, descriptive, or correlational studies; integrative reviews; systematic reviews; or randomized controlled trials with inconsistent results	
D	Peer-reviewed professional organizational standards, with clinical studies to support recommendations	
E	Theory-based evidence from expert opinion or multiple case reports	
M	Manufacturer's recommendation only	

From Peterson M, Barnason S, Donnelly B, et al. Choosing the best evidence to guide clinical practice: Application of AACN levels of evidence. *Crit Care Nurse.* 2014;34(2):58–68.

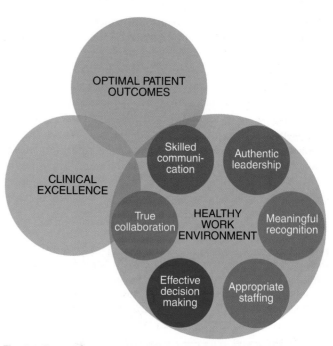

Fig. 1.4 Essential components of a healthy work environment. Interdependence of healthy work environment, clinical excellence, and optimal patient outcomes. (From American Association of Critical-Care Nurses. AACN standards for establishing and sustaining healthy work environments: A journey to excellence. *Am J Crit Care.* 2005;14[3]:189.)

Communication

Patient-centered communication is a strategy to improve the patient experience, a focus in today's healthcare delivery.[33] The goal is to elicit more information from patients and to better assess their understanding. Standardized approaches are helpful and are easily learned.[22] Approaches include *Ask-Tell-Ask*, a strategy for encouraging nurses to assess concerns before providing more information, especially when discussing stressful issues with patients and families.[40] *Tell Me More* is a tool that encourages information sharing in challenging situations.

Effective communication is also essential for delivering safe patient care. Many adverse events are directly attributable to faulty communication. Communication breakdowns often occur during *handoff* situations, when patient information is being transferred or exchanged. Common handoff situations include nursing and physician shift reports and patient transfers. Barriers to effective handoffs are noted in Box 1.4. Formal training in handoff communication with both nurses and other team members assists in improving communication and reducing errors, and tools are also available to enhance and evaluate handoffs.[1,13]

The *situation*, *background*, *assessment*, *recommendation* (SBAR) approach is useful in communication, especially with physicians (Box 1.5).[21] The SBAR technique delivers information in a way that is brief and action oriented. The QSEN

BOX 1.4 Barriers to Effective Handoff Communication

- **Physical setting:** background noise, lack of privacy, interruptions
- **Social setting:** organizational hierarchy and status issues
- **Language:** differences between people of varying racial and ethnic backgrounds or geographic areas
- **Communication medium:** limitations of communications via telephone, email, paper, or computerized records versus face to face

---

BOX 1.5 SBAR Approach

S—Situation: State what is happening at the present time that has warranted the SBAR communication

B—Background: Explain circumstances leading up to this situation. Put the situation in context for the reader or listener

A—Assessment: State what you think is the problem

R—Recommendation: State your recommendation to correct the problem

---

Exemplar box illustrates an example of SBAR communication for a patient handoff. Other strategies to improve handoff communication include standardizing processes for the handoff situation, using checklists to prompt and document essential information, and training all personnel in effective communication techniques.

✳ QSEN EXEMPLAR

SBAR for Teamwork and Collaboration

Best Practice Tool: The situation, background, assessment, recommendation (SBAR) report methodology may be particularly helpful in the critical care setting as a method of improving interdepartmental and shift-to-shift information transfer. A sample transfer SBAR report is illustrated.

Situation

My name is (caregiver) Mary Smith, RN, from the (unit) emergency department. I will be transferring (patient name) John Jones, a (age) 34-year-old (gender) man admitted (time/date) 3 hours ago with (diagnosis) diabetic ketoacidosis, to (receiving department) medical critical care unit. Attending physician is Dr. Michael Miller.

Background

Pertinent history—type 1 diabetes for 20 years; on insulin pump; managed pump failure 24 hours ago inappropriately; renal insufficiency. Summary of episode of care:

- Admitting glucose 648 mg/dL; positive ketones; pH 7.27; PaO_2 90 mm Hg; $PaCO_2$ 20 mm Hg; HCO_3^- 12 mEq/L; K^+ 3.4 mEq/L; BUN 40 mg/dL; creatinine 1.8 mg/dL; admitting weight 65 kg; lethargic
- Received 1 L normal saline in field. Normal saline now infusing at 200 mL/h
- Received IV bolus of 6.5 units regular insulin at 1300. Insulin infusion of 100 units regular in 100 mL normal saline infusing at 7.5 units per hour (7.5 mL/h). 1400 repeat glucose 502 mg/dL
- 20 mEq potassium chloride infused in emergency department
- 200 mL urine output last hour—hourly intake and output
- Hemoglobin A1c level 6 weeks ago was 9.2% (patient report)

Assessment

- Vital signs: BP 102/60 mm Hg; pulse 106 beats/min; respirations 30 breaths/min; temperature 37.5°C
- Intake: 1400 mL; output: 450 mL
- Pain level: 0/10
- Neurological: Lethargic but responsive to stimuli
- Respirations: Deep with acetone odor noted; lungs clear
- Cardiac: S_1/S_2; no murmurs
- Cardiac rhythm: Sinus tachycardia
- Code status: Full
- GI: Abdomen soft/slightly distended; hypoactive bowel sounds
- GU: Voiding frequently; urine concentrated
- Skin: Skin dry with poor turgor; intact
- IV: (Location) right forearm (catheter size) 18 G (condition) no redness/edema
- Assessment: Diabetic ketoacidosis secondary to poorly managed insulin pump failure with gradual improvement of glucose over past 2 hours

Recommendations

- Obtain hourly vital signs
- Repeat glucose, K^+, arterial blood gas due at 1600 today
- Continue normal saline at 200 mL/h for 4 hours
- IV insulin infusion at 7.5 units (7.5 mL) per hour—bedside glucose monitoring hourly and adjust per protocol
- Monitor urine output hourly
- Contact Dr. Miller with 1600 lab work for further orders
- Refer to diabetes educator and clinical dietitian
- Repeat renal profile in AM

Communication techniques and protocols from other high-risk industries have been implemented in healthcare settings to improve patient safety. One technique comes from the aviation industry crew resource management (CRM), which was developed to promote and improve communication and accountability among team members, a culture of safety, and stress recognition.[8,20]

In a CRM environment, everyone from the captain of the aircraft to the baggage handlers on the ground shares responsibility for safe flight operations. Differences in training are acknowledged, but each member of the team is empowered and has the autonomy to address problems without fear of retaliation or ridicule. Several components of CRM are pertinent to critical care nursing: monitor others' actions by double-checking, verifying, and when necessary correcting inaccurate or ambiguous information; and situational awareness.[8] If something seems wrong, individuals should trust their "gut instinct" and speak up to correct the situation.[17]

Collaboration

The ultimate goal of true collaboration in critical care is to create a *culture of safety*, defined as a nonhierarchical culture in which all members have the opportunity and the duty to ensure safe and effective care. Collaboration is founded on mutual respect and the recognition that each discipline involved in patient care brings distinct skills and perspectives to the table.

One strategy for collaboration is the implementation of multiprofessional bedside rounds one or two times per shift. Intensivist-led rounds and daily goal setting are recommended to address patient care issues and adherence to recommended guidelines and bundles of care. Such rounds improve communication, collaboration, and patient outcomes.[41] Examples of items to be addressed are noted in Box 1.6. It is important to include family members in patient rounds to facilitate communication and involvement. Some teams schedule regular afternoon rounds focused on communication with the family, whereas others include family in routine rounds.

Visualization of goals via standardized data on whiteboards or glass doors of the patient's room is helpful in facilitating communication among the healthcare team and with family members.[24,49]

Conducting morning briefings before interdisciplinary rounds is another strategy to improve communication, collaboration, and patient safety. Suggested content of the morning briefings includes answers to three questions: (1) *What happened during the night that the team needs to know* (e.g., adverse events, admissions)? (2) *Where should rounds begin* (e.g., the sickest patient who needs the most attention)? and (3) *What potential problems have been identified for the day* (e.g., staffing, procedures)?[45]

BOX 1.6 Items to Consider in Daily Multiprofessional Rounds

- Discharge needs
- Greatest safety risk
- Implementation of critical care "bundles"
- Assessment and recommended follow-up
- Cardiac and hemodynamic status
- Volume status
- Neurological status
- Pain, agitation, and delirium
- Sedation needs
- Gastrointestinal status, including bowel management
- Nutrition
- Skin issues
- Activity
- Infection status (culture results/therapeutic levels of antibiotics)
- Laboratory results
- Radiology test results
- Need for all ordered medications
- Whether central lines and invasive catheters and tubes can be removed
- Whether indwelling urinary catheter can be removed
- Issues that need to be addressed
- Family needs—educational, psychosocial, spiritual
- Code status
- Advance directives
- Parameters for calling the physician
- Treatment goals and strategies to achieve them
- Plans for discussing care and needs with families

STUDY BREAK

3. The strategy developed by the airline industry to improve communication and safety is:
   A. Ask-Tell-Ask
   B. Crew resource management
   C. Situation, background, assessment, and recommendation (SBAR)
   D. Teachback

COLLABORATIVE PLAN OF CARE FOR THE CRITICALLY ILL PATIENT

Critically ill patients have many similarities and needs for patient care. Therefore a collaborative plan of care for these patients is presented to prevent the need for duplication of many of these common nursing assessments and interventions throughout the textbook. As with any care plan, it must be individualized to the patient because some problems and nursing diagnoses may not be relevant.

◎ COLLABORATIVE PLAN OF CARE

The Critically Ill Patient

Patient Problem
Acute and/or Chronic Pain. Risk factors include underlying physical condition, chronic disorders, and/or treatment.

Desired Outcomes
- Prevention and/or relief of pain.
- Assessment of pain based on validated pain scale is reduced or at a target level.

Nursing Assessments/Interventions	Rationales
• Assess pain using a standardized approach: numeric rating scale for verbal patients; Behavioral Pain Scale (BPS) or Critical-Care Pain Observation Tool (CPOT) for nonverbal patients. *[handwritten:] If intubated*	• Establish baseline to assess for changes and responses to treatments and intervention using standardized approach.
• In collaboration with the team, develop a consistent plan to address the patient's pain; incorporate both pharmacological and nonpharmacological approaches, such as repositioning, music, guided imagery, and animal-assisted therapy.	• Provide a standardized approach to treatment that can be followed by all team members; nonpharmacological approaches effective and may reduce the need for and/or dose of medications.
• Explain procedure(s) and expected outcomes.	• Knowledge of expectations may reduce pain associated with procedure(s).

Patient Problem
Anxiety and Decreased Ability to Cope. Risk factors include the stressful critical care environment, sensory overload and deprivation, fear of the unknown, inability to communicate, and many other factors associated with critical illness.

Desired Outcomes
- Prevention and/or relief of anxiety.
- Assessment of agitation based on validated sedation scale is reduced or at a target level.
- Patient verbalizes reduced fear and anxiety, if able.
- Patient demonstrates positive coping mechanisms.

Nursing Assessments/Interventions	Rationales
• Assess patient's fear and anxiety on admission and every 4 hours; administer sedation per protocol using standardized scales, such as Richmond Agitation-Sedation Scale (RASS) or Sedation-Agitation Scale (SAS).	• Establish baseline to assess for changes and responses to treatments and intervention; standardized tools facilitate communication, assessment of intervention, and trending.
• In collaboration with the team, develop a consistent plan to address the patient's anxiety; include spiritual support services as requested by the patient and/or family.	• Provide a standardized approach to treatment that can be followed by all team members.
• Communicate with patient; explain procedures; provide calm and reassuring presence; provide information about family and current events.	• Demonstrate concern for the patient; educate about condition.
• Ask simple questions that can be responded to by nodding, eye blinking, communication boards, speaking devices, and similar strategies; expect frustration.	• Promote effective communication; strategies must be appropriate to culture and physical ability.
• Support family presence; encourage family members to communicate with the patient.	• Promote a sense of well-being.
• Use complementary approaches such as music therapy, guided imagery, and animal-assisted therapy.	• Reduce anxiety.
• Promote regular sleep-wake cycle, daytime activity, and scheduled rest periods; reduce external noise and stimuli as possible.	• Promote rest, healing, and recovery.

Patient Problem
Delirium. Risk factors include critical illness, treatment, and underlying condition.

Desired Outcomes
- Acute confusion is either prevented or decreased.
- No evidence of injury or harm due to delirium.
- Delirium treated properly if diagnosed.

Continued

◎ COLLABORATIVE PLAN OF CARE—cont'd

The Critically Ill Patient

Nursing Assessments/Interventions	Rationales
• Assess delirium using a validated screening tool: Confusion Assessment Method for the ICU (CAM-ICU) or Intensive Care Delirium Screening Checklist (ICDSC).	• Establish baseline to assess for changes and responses to intervention using a standardized approach.

• Implement the ABCDEF bundle (see http://www.icudelirium.org):
  • Assess for and manage pain
  • Both spontaneous awakening trials (SATs) and spontaneous breathing trials (SBTs) for ventilated patients
  • Choice of sedation and analgesia; incorporate goal-directed sedation
  • Delirium monitoring and management
  • Early mobility
  • Family engagement
	• Prevent delirium using evidence-based interventions; improve cognitive and functional outcomes.

• Speak slowly using simple sentences and nonmedical terminology.	• Promote effective communication with patients with delirium or cognitive impairment.

Family Problem

Potential for Dysfunctional Family Dynamics. Risk factors include crisis of critical illness, fear of the unknown, inability to effectively communicate with patient, altered family functioning, stress associated with balancing home needs and visitation. (Note: Family includes those self-identified as family members to the patient, including significant others or partners.)

Desired Outcomes
- Family experiences effective communication with the patient and healthcare team.
- Family can identify and discuss dysfunctional behavioral dynamics.
- Effective family coping.
- Reduction of anxiety.
- Able to provide support to patient.

Nursing Assessments/Interventions	Rationales
• Assess family structure; social, environmental, cultural, and spiritual needs; and communication patterns within the family and with the healthcare team.	• Establish baseline to assess family functioning and response to the patient's illness.
• Identify family spokesperson and document contact information.	• Establish primary contact for communication.
• Establish open, honest communication; provide information; offer support and realistic hope.	• Facilitate communication; meet family's need for information.
• Promote visitation according to patient's condition and family's need for presence. Unrestricted visitation is encouraged.	• Meet common need of family members.
• Assess family's knowledge of the patient's condition, treatment, and prognosis; allow time for questions.	• Identify knowledge deficits and provide opportunities for family education.
• Promote family/significant other's participation in patient care.	• Meet family's need for meaningful contributions to patient care.
• Promote family's communication with the healthcare team, such as participation in multidisciplinary rounds, family rounds, or appointments with key members of the healthcare team.	• Promote open communication and decision making; reduce family frustration of not being able to discuss the patient's condition.
• Provide opportunities to discuss the patient's condition and share concerns in a private setting.	• Foster communication in a caring and calm environment.
• Encourage family members to get adequate sleep and rest; provide strategies for communication of changes and updates in conditions should family members go home.	• Promote physical well-being of family members; provide strategies for communication of updates.
• Assess for ineffective coping (i.e., depression, withdrawal, anger, substance use).	• Identify the need for additional communication, support services, intervention, or referral.

Patient Problem

Potential for Pressure Injury. Risk factors include bed rest and physiological alterations associated with critical illness.

Desired Outcomes
- Intact skin and mucous membranes.
- Prevention of pressure injury.
- Patient and family participate in preventive measures.
- Patient and family verbalize understanding of interventions to prevent pressure injury.

COLLABORATIVE PLAN OF CARE—cont'd

The Critically Ill Patient

Nursing Assessments/Interventions	Rationales
• Assess skin and mucous membranes every shift for alterations and disruption. Pay special attention to bony prominences and areas of pressure associated with devices (e.g., nose, ears); take photos (per hospital policy) of actual and potential skin breakdown.	• Obtain baseline and ongoing assessment of potential skin breakdown or problems in pressure-prone areas; document photos to facilitate assessment.
• Use standardized tools for assessment: Braden or Norton scale.	• Provide a standardized measure for trending skin assessment; score may indicate need for consultation or specialized devices.
• Implement preventive strategies per hospital policy and consultation with wound, ostomy, and continence nurses (WOCNs): mattress overlays, specialized beds, barrier creams, or other strategies.	• Prevent skin breakdown in collaboration with WOCNs.
• Turn and reposition the patient on a regular basis and assess skin during the procedure; prevent shearing when pulling patient up in bed and during turning; use pillows and foam wedges when positioning.	• Relieve pressure and promote circulation; reduce risk for shearing; prevent pressure-related injury associated with positioning.
• Promote adequate nutrition; consult with dietitian and pharmacists to develop nutritional care plan.	• Promote skin integrity and wound healing.
• Prevent and/or treat incontinence. Use external collection devices as appropriate, such as external catheters. Protect skin with barrier cream.	• Reduce risk for skin breakdown associated with incontinence.
• Promote mobility, including chair rest and ambulation as tolerated by the patient; assess skin integrity on return to bed.	• Promote increased circulation and decrease risk for skin breakdown.

Patient Problem

Decreased Mobility. Risk factors include patient condition and treatment modalities.

Desired Outcomes

- Intact skin and mucous membranes.
- Prevention of loss of muscle mass.
- Stable cardiovascular and pulmonary responses to activity.
- Patient achieves optimum mobility considering illness severity and diagnosis.

Nursing Assessments/Interventions	Rationales
• Collaborate with physical therapist, occupational therapist, and other healthcare team members to determine a treatment plan.	• Develop treatment plan using experts.
• Ensure that active and passive range of motion (ROM) is done on a regular basis; use commercial ROM devices if available.	• Promote ROM and functional mobility.
• Promote progressive mobility, including chair rest and ambulation as tolerated; assess responses to activity (cardiopulmonary, neurological); use lifting devices and specialized equipment as indicated.	• Maintain muscle mass and ROM; prevent delirium; promote gradual increases in activity while assessing physiological responses; use lift devices to prevent injury to both patient and caregivers.
• Ensure that patient is receiving pharmacological and/or mechanical treatment to prevent venous thromboembolism (VTE).	• Prevent VTE, which is especially common in immobile patients.

Patient Problem

Potential for Insufficient Secretion Removal and Decreased Gas Exchange. Risk factors include disease process/decreased respiratory drive and treatment.

Desired Outcomes

- Airway maintained.
- Decreased work of breathing.
- Oxygen saturation at target level.
- Adequate gas exchange (normal arterial blood gases [ABGs], respiratory rate, lung sounds, level of consciousness).
- Airway free of excessive secretions, edema, or obstruction.
- Lung sounds clear.

Nursing Assessments/Interventions	Rationales
• Assess respiratory rate, depth, and rhythm; monitor ABGs, SpO_2, and $ETCO_2$.	• Assess adequacy of respiration and detect abnormalities.
• Assess for signs of hypoxemia (restlessness, confusion, agitation, irritability).	• Identify need for treatment to promote oxygenation.
• Auscultate breath sounds.	• Identify adventitious sounds, potentially indicating need for intervention.
• Unless the patient is intubated, encourage to cough and deep breathe on regular basis; use incentive spirometer and positive expiratory pressure, if indicated.	• Promote alveolar expansion and prevent atelectasis; assess cough ability.

Continued

⊚ COLLABORATIVE PLAN OF CARE—cont'd

The Critically Ill Patient

Nursing Assessments/Interventions	Rationales
• Suction (nasotracheal or endotracheal) as indicated by patient assessment; hyperoxygenate before suctioning.	• Maintain airway; prevent tissue/mucosal damage from excess suction; provide adequate oxygenation to promote tissue and cerebral perfusion.
• Assess amount, color, and consistency of secretions.	• Identify need for humidification; assess for possible infection.
• Turn and reposition on a regular basis; encourage mobility.	• Prevent atelectasis; promote alveolar function; mobilize secretions.

Patient Problem

Potential for Fluid, Electrolyte, and Acid-Base Imbalances. Risk factors include the disease process, inability to achieve biochemical hemostasis, and critical illness.

Desired Outcomes

• Recognition and early treatment of imbalances.
• Patient is free of musculoskeletal and cardiac changes.
• Patient and family understand the signs and symptoms associated with fluid and electrolyte imbalances.

Nursing Assessments/Interventions	Rationales
• Assess for indicators of alterations in fluid, electrolyte, and acid-base balance.	• Use baseline data to assess risks and gauge changes.
• Weigh patient daily.	• Assess changes in fluid status.
• Maintain adequate nutritional intake.	• If nutrition is inadequate, protein stores will be used for energy, resulting in nitrogen balance changes.
	• Muscle wasting may also increase.
• Administer medications as prescribed (i.e., diuretics, IV fluids, electrolyte replacement).	• Depending on the medication prescribed, the mechanisms may lead to increased fluid, retained fluid, or electrolyte shifts.

Patient Problem

Potential for Impaired Nutrition. Risk factors include "nothing by mouth" status and hypermetabolic state in some disease or illness states.

Desired Outcomes

• Adequate nutrition to promote resolution of illness, wound healing, and physical strength.
• Maintenance of baseline body weight.
• Nitrogen state is balanced or positive.

Nursing Assessments/Interventions	Rationales
• Obtain baseline height, weight, body mass index (BMI), and laboratory values; assess nutritional risk with standardized measures.	• Use baseline data to assess risks and gauge changes.
• Weigh patient daily.	• Assess changes in caloric intake and fluid status.
• Consult with dietitian, clinical pharmacist, and other team members to generate a nutrition care plan.	• Dietitian and clinical pharmacist are most knowledgeable on strategies to meet nutritional needs of patients.
• Implement guideline-based approaches to nutritional support.	• Develop optimal nutrition plan.
• Assess bowel sounds, abdominal distension, and intake/output on regular basis.	• Assess for complications such as ileus, impaired feeding tolerance, fluid overload, diarrhea, and constipation.
• If patient is receiving enteral nutrition, ensure proper tube placement, keep the head of bed elevated at least 30 degrees, avoid interruptions of feeding.	• Prevent aspiration associated with improper tube placement, poor absorption, or gastric regurgitation; ensure adequate input if feedings prescribed.

Patient Problem

Potential for Decreased Multisystem Tissue Perfusion. Risk factors include decreased cardiac output, cardiac dysrhythmias, hemodynamic instability, treatments such as positive end-expiratory pressure (PEEP), and cardiac abnormalities.

Desired Outcomes

• Adequate cardiac output.
• Oriented to person, time, and place.
• Systolic BP within 20 mm Hg of baseline.
• Heart rate 60 to 100 beats/min.
• Urine output at least 0.5 mL/kg.
• Regular respiratory rate.
• Lung sounds clear.
• Strong peripheral pulses.
• Warm, dry skin.

◎ COLLABORATIVE PLAN OF CARE—cont'd

The Critically Ill Patient

Nursing Assessments/Interventions	Rationales
• Assess level of consciousness.	• Assess for symptoms of decreased cerebral perfusion.
• Assess heart rate and blood pressure.	• Low cardiac output is associated with abnormally low or high heart rate and manifested by lower blood pressure.
• Assess skin color, moisture, and temperature.	• Assess for perfusion to the periphery manifested by cool, moist skin and possible cyanosis.
• Assess peripheral pulses, including capillary refill.	• Low cardiac output is associated with weak pulses and slow capillary refill.
• Assess urine output hourly.	• Assess for renal perfusion.
• Assess respiratory rate and lung sounds.	• Assess for impaired perfusion to the lungs.
• Assess for chest pain.	• Decreased perfusion to coronary arteries may result in pain, especially in those with underlying cardiac disease.

Patient Problem

Potential for Infection. Risk factors include invasive devices: ventilator-associated events (VAE), central line–associated bloodstream infections (CLABSI), catheter-associated urinary tract infections (CAUTI), and devices such as traction and intracranial monitoring.

Desired Outcome
• Prevention of infection.

Nursing Assessments/Interventions	Rationales
• Assess for presence of devices that increase the risk for infection.	• Devices interfere with the body's first line of defense.
• Monitor white blood cell (WBC) count.	• Assess for elevation associated with infection.
• Assess for signs of infection (depending on device): fever; redness, swelling, pain; color of drainage, secretions, urine.	• Changes often indicate infection.
• Practice meticulous hand hygiene.	• Prevent transmission of organisms.
• Remove devices as soon as they are no longer indicated.	• Decrease risk for infection.
• For the ventilated patient:	• Use evidence-based strategies to reduce infection.
• Elevate head of bed at least 30 degrees.	
• Interrupt sedation and assess for readiness to wean from ventilator daily.	
• Provide regular antiseptic oral care.	
• Administer prophylaxis for VTE.	
• Administer prophylaxis for peptic ulcer disease.	
• If available, use an endotracheal tube with port for removal of subglottic secretions.	
• To prevent CAUTI:	• Use evidence-based strategies to reduce infection.
• Insert indwelling urinary catheter only if indicated.	
• Insertion should be done only by a properly trained individual using strict aseptic technique.	
• Maintain a closed drainage system with unobstructed urine flow.	
• Remove catheter as soon as possible.	
• Consider external collection devices.	
• Provide regular perineal care.	
• Prevent fecal contamination.	
• To prevent CLABSI:	• Use evidence-based strategies to reduce infection.
• Ensure that strict aseptic technique is followed during insertion, including full barrier precautions.	
• Access devices by scrubbing the port or hub with appropriate antiseptic.	
• Perform dressing changes using strict aseptic technique.	
• Change dressings when wet or soiled.	
• Consider chlorhexidine-impregnated dressings and regular chlorhexidine bathing.	

Patient/Family Problem

Need for Health Teaching (Patient and Family). Risk factors include lack of knowledge about disease process and treatment plan.

Patient/Family Outcomes
• Patient and family verbalize adequate information related to condition and treatment plan.
• Patient and family able to make informed decisions regarding care.

Continued

◎ **COLLABORATIVE PLAN OF CARE—cont'd**

The Critically Ill Patient

Nursing Assessments/Interventions	Rationales
• Assess patient and family's understanding of condition and treatment plan.	• Establish baseline knowledge and need for instruction.
• Encourage all team members to be involved in patient and family education.	• Provide expertise of healthcare team in patient education.
• Provide specific, factual information on condition and treatment plan; reinforce teaching after rounds; effectively and consistently communicate the plan of care with members of the healthcare team.	• Provide accurate information to promote continuity of education; facilitate decision making regarding treatment options.
• Encourage patient and family members to ask questions.	• Ensure accurate information and facilitate understanding of information provided.

BP, Blood pressure; *ETCO₂,* end-tidal carbon dioxide; *SpO₂,* saturation of oxygen in pulsatile blood (by pulse oximetry).
Adapted from Gulanick M, Myers JL. *Nursing Care Plans: Diagnoses, Interventions, and Outcomes.* 9th ed. St. Louis, MO: Elsevier; 2017; Swearingen PL, Wright J. *All-in-One Nursing Care Planning Resource.* 5th ed. St. Louis, MO: Elsevier; 2019; Centers for Disease Control and Prevention. Healthcare-Associated Infections (HAIs). http://www.cdc.gov/hai/index.html. Published 2019. Accessed April 7, 2019.

 CRITICAL REASONING ACTIVITY

Identify and debate strategies for reducing stress and anxiety of critical care nurses.

TRENDS AND ISSUES IN CARE DELIVERY

The acuity of patients hospitalized in critical care units is high. Contributing to this trend is the increasingly aging population. Older adults have more chronic illnesses that contribute to the complexity of their care than do younger patients. They also tend to develop multisystem organ failure, which requires longer hospital stays, increases cost, and increases the need for intensive nursing care.

Healthcare costs continue to escalate while reimbursement rates are reduced. Hospitals are usually reimbursed based on performance and do not receive reimbursement to treat complications that may result from treatment. Evidence-based protocols are being incorporated into order sets to standardize care and reduce complications and their associated costs. Readmission rates for certain conditions also affect reimbursement. Both aging and chronic illness increase the likelihood of hospital readmissions. Strategies are being implemented to improve care transitions, especially to the home setting. Collaboration among hospitals, community organizations, caregivers, and patients is essential to achieve seamless care among multiple providers and sites. Changing nurse/patient ratios and employing unlicensed assistive personnel are also strategies being implemented to reduce costs. However, outcomes associated with changes in staffing need to be monitored and evaluated to ensure that patient outcomes and patient safety are not compromised.

Technology that assists in patient care continues to grow rapidly. Invasive and noninvasive monitoring systems are used to facilitate patient assessment and to evaluate responses to treatment. Many technological interventions have been introduced to improve patient safety. Point-of-care laboratory testing is done at the bedside to provide immediate values to expedite treatment. Computerized physician order entry and nursing documentation are expected. In many institutions, data from monitoring equipment are automatically downloaded into the computerized medical record. Sophisticated computer programs are being developed and tested to analyze physiological data for signs of patient deterioration, such as sepsis, and provide earlier alerts to caregivers. Nurses must become increasingly comfortable with applying the technology, troubleshooting equipment, and evaluating the accuracy of values. The use of technology must be balanced with delivering compassionate care.

As more technological advances become available to sustain and support life, ethical issues have skyrocketed. Termination of life support, organ and cell transplantation, and quality of life are just a few issues that nurses must address in everyday practice. Decisions are regularly made regarding applying technology to sustain life or withdrawing technology in futile situations. Nurses must be comfortable addressing ethical issues as they arise in the critical care setting. Increased attention to end-of-life care in the critical care unit is also needed. Palliative care that includes spiritual care is an important intervention that must be embraced by those working in critical care units (see Chapters 3 and 4).

Using telemedicine or eICUs to manage critically ill patients is another emerging trend. Data from monitors and robotics are transferred for evaluation, and the expert conducts an assessment from a distant location.[47] These virtual critical care consultations have improved patient outcomes. Nurses consult with those providing the telemedicine service based on established protocols and parameters, and then they identify changes in a patient's condition that need to be addressed. These telemedicine strategies do not replace the high-touch, hands-on care delivered by nurses in the critical care unit, but they assist healthcare workers at remote sites in decision making and treatment.

 CRITICAL REASONING ACTIVITY

Debate the pros and cons of hiring new graduates to work in a critical care unit.

The critical care environment itself is changing. Units are being redesigned with the interests of both patients and nurses in mind. Equipment is becoming more portable, thus making the transfer of patients for diagnostic testing or to other units easier and safer. In addition, portable equipment can be brought to the bedside for diagnostic testing, preventing the need to transfer unstable patients from the critical care unit. Some institutions have adopted a universal care model, or *acuity-adaptable* rooms. In this setting, patients remain in one unit throughout their hospitalization. The level of nursing care is adjusted to meet the needs of the patient. The universal care model eliminates the need to transfer patients to other units and promotes continuity of care.[11,28]

Patients are being transferred from critical care units much earlier than before. A high level of knowledge and skill is required by nurses who care for patients on stepdown units. Patients are discharged from the hospital often while they are still acutely ill. Nurses must ensure that patients and their family members have the knowledge and skills needed for home care and that adequate resources, such as home healthcare services, are available. Both critical care and advanced practice nurses may provide care to these high-acuity patients in the home, often through telehealth technology.

Implications of the opioid crisis in the critical care setting are widespread. Opioids are commonly administered in the critical care setting. Appropriate prescribing needs to be addressed through education of those ordering medication and collaboration with the critical care pharmacist.[19,35] Patients may have an opioid addition and require higher doses of routine sedative and pain medications.[18] Last, more patients with an opioid overdose are being treated in critical care settings.[43]

Medication and fluid shortages are recent issues that affect care delivery and potentially affect patient safety. Most shortages are for medications used in the critical care setting, such as medications used to treat high-acuity conditions and parenteral preparations.[32] During shortages, substitutions are often required, which may be less effective or associated with a greater risk for administration errors and adverse effects.

Antibiotic stewardship in the critical care setting is advocated to reduce the risk for antibiotic resistance. Strategies to promote proper administration of antibiotics include regular audits and feedback, antibiotic time-outs, rapid diagnostic tests, and computerized decision support tools.[38] Regular collaboration with critical care pharmacists is also essential.

ISSUES RELATED TO THE CRITICAL CARE NURSE

Many issues relate to the critical care nurse. Like the population in general, critical care nurses are growing older. To accommodate this growing workforce, hospitals are focusing attention on redesigning the environment with a focus on ergonomics, ease of use, and safety. Innovative staffing models are being developed to continue tapping into the wealth of clinical knowledge and expertise of older nurses who may no longer desire or be able to work full time or 12-hour shifts. Having adequate staffing with paraprofessionals who can assume responsibility for nonnursing tasks is another strategy to facilitate practice.

❓ CRITICAL REASONING ACTIVITY

Envision the critical care unit of the future. Describe the environment and how care could be delivered.

Critical care nurses are in demand; therefore priorities for recruiting, educating, and retaining nurses to work in critical care settings are essential. Many new graduates want to specialize in critical care, yet they are often told that they need to have 1 year of medical-surgical nursing experience. New graduates can be successful in the critical care setting with adequate supervision, orientation, and mentorship.[15] A critical care course, which often includes simulation, assists the nurse in gaining requisite knowledge and skills. Adequate time in orientation, under the guidance of a supportive preceptor to develop and learn the critical care nursing role, facilitates clinical skill acquisition. Starting employment in a stepdown or intermediate care unit is another strategy for gaining experience prior to working in a high-acuity critical care unit. Many institutions have implemented nurse residency programs to facilitate the transition from the student to staff nurse role.

Bullying and incivility occur in the workforce, especially in high-acuity settings. An environment where these behaviors are tolerated affects nurses, patients, and the organization.[34] A healthy work environment that promotes collaboration, respect, decision making, and communication helps to prevent these behaviors.[10]

Nurses who work in critical care settings are at risk for compassion fatigue, which consists of burnout and secondary traumatic stress. Burnout is a feeling of being ineffective and hopeless when work demands are intense and traumatic stress stems from exposure to patients with acuity illness and trauma.[26] Nurses with less experience are at a higher risk for compassion fatigue.[23] Again, a healthy work environment assists in reducing compassion fatigue in the critical care setting.[26]

STUDY BREAK

4. Communication, collaboration, and respect are exhibited in:
   A. Burnout
   B. Compassion fatigue
   C. Healthy work environments
   D. Incivility

Critical care nurses must be aware of current and emerging trends that affect their practice and patient care. Involvement in professional organizations, reading professional journals, participating in journal clubs, becoming involved in unit-based nurse practice councils, and attending local and national professional meetings are strategies for nurses to maintain currency in the ever-changing critical care environment.

REFERENCES

1. Abraham J, Kannampallil T, Patel VL. A systematic review of the literature on the evaluation of handoff tools: Implications for research and practice. *J Am Med Inform Assoc.* 2014;21(1): 154–162.
2. American Association of Critical-Care Nurses (AACN). Value of Certification. https://www.aacn.org/certification/value-of-certification-resource-center. Published 2019. Accessed April 7, 2019.
3. American Association of Critical-Care Nurses (AACN). About AACN. https://www.aacn.org/about-aacn. Published 2019. Accessed April 7, 2019.
4. American Association of Critical-Care Nurses (AACN). AACN Clinical Scene Investigator (CSI) Academy. https://www.aacn.org/nursing-excellence/csi-academy?tab=Nurses%20Leading%20Innovation. Published 2019. Accessed April 7, 2019.

5. American Association of Critical-Care Nurses (AACN). AACN Synergy Model for Patient Care. https://www.aacn.org/nursing-excellence/aacn-standards/synergy-model. Published 2019. Accessed April 7, 2019.

6. Barden C. *AACN Standards for Establishing and Sustaining Healthy Work Environments*. 2nd ed. Aliso Viejo, CA: AACN; 2015.

7. Barden C, Distrito C. Toward a healthy work environment. *Health Prog*. 2005;86(6):16–20.

8. Barton G, Bruce A, Schreiber R. Teaching nurses teamwork: Integrative review of competency-based team training in nursing education. *Nurse Educ Pract*. 2018;32:129–137.

9. Bednash GP, Cronenwett L, Dolansky MA. QSEN transforming education. *J Prof Nurs*. 2013;29(2):66–67.

10. Blake N. Building respect and reducing incivility in the workplace: Professional standards and recommendations to improve the work environment for nurses. *AACN Adv Crit Care*. 2016;27(4):368–371.

11. Bonuel N, Cesario S. Review of the literature: Acuity-adaptable patient room. *Crit Care Nurs Q*. 2013;36(2):251–271.

12. Curley MA. Patient-nurse synergy: Optimizing patients' outcomes. *Am J Crit Care*. 1998;7(1):64–72.

13. Davis J, Roach C, Elliott C, et al. Feedback and assessment tools for handoffs: A systematic review. *J Grad Med Educ*. 2017;9(1):18–32.

14. Davis TM, Barden C, Dean S, et al. American Telemedicine Association guidelines for TeleICU operations. *Telemed J E Health*. 2016;22(12):971–980.

15. DeGrande H, Liu F, Greene P, Stankus JA. The experiences of new graduate nurses hired and retained in adult intensive care units. *Intensive Crit Care Nurs*. 2018;49:72–78.

16. Dodek PM, Norena M, Ayas N, Wong H. Moral distress is associated with general workplace distress in intensive care unit personnel. *J Crit Care*. 2019;50:122–125.

17. Doucette JN. View from the cockpit: What the airline industry can teach us about patient safety. *Nursing*. 2006;36(11):50–53.

18. Goodwin AJ. Critical care outcomes among opioid users: Hidden sequelae of a growing crisis? *Crit Care Med*. 2018;46(6):1005–1006.

19. Gross JL, Perate AR, Elkassabany NM. Pain management in trauma in the age of the opioid crisis. *Anesthesiol Clin*. 2019;37(1):79–91.

20. Haerkens M, Kox M, Noe PM, Van Der Hoeven JG, Pickkers P. Crew resource management in the trauma room: A prospective 3-year cohort study. *Eur J Emerg Med*. 2018;25(4):281–287.

21. Haig KM, Sutton S, Whittington J. SBAR: A shared mental model for improving communication between clinicians. *Jt Comm J Qual Patient Saf*. 2006;32(3):167–175.

22. Hashim MJ. Patient-centered communication: Basic skills. *Am Fam Physician*. 2017;95(1):29–34.

23. Jakimowicz S, Perry L, Lewis J. Compassion satisfaction and fatigue: A cross-sectional survey of Australian intensive care nurses. *Aust Crit Care*. 2018;31(6):396–405.

24. Justice LB, Cooper DS, Henderson C, et al. Improving communication during cardiac ICU multidisciplinary rounds through visual display of patient daily goals. *Pediatr Crit Care Med*. 2016;17(7):677–683.

25. Kang MA, Churpek MM, Zadravecz FJ, et al. Real-time risk prediction on the wards: A feasibility study. *Crit Care Med*. 2016;44(8):1468–1473.

26. Kelly L, Todd M. Compassion fatigue and the healthy work environment. *AACN Adv Crit Care*. 2017;28(4):351–358.

27. Kipnis P, Turk BJ, Wulf DA, et al. Development and validation of an electronic medical record-based alert score for detection of inpatient deterioration outside the ICU. *J Biomed Inform*. 2016;64:10–19.

28. Kitchens JL, Fulton JS, Maze L. Patient and family description of receiving care in acuity adaptable care model. *J Nurs Manag*. 2018;26(7):874–880.

29. Lavallee JF, Gray TA, Dumville J, et al. The effects of care bundles on patient outcomes: A systematic review and meta-analysis. *Implement Sci*. 2017;12(1):142.

30. Lyons PG, Edelson DP, Churpek MM. Rapid response systems. *Resuscitation*. 2018;128:191–197.

31. Mason VM, Leslie G, Clark K, et al. Compassion fatigue, moral distress, and work engagement in surgical intensive care unit trauma nurses: A pilot study. *Dimens Crit Care Nurs*. 2014;33(4):215–225.

32. Mazer-Amirshahi M, Goyal M, Umar SA, et al. U.S. drug shortages for medications used in adult critical care (2001–2016). *J Crit Care*. 2017;41:283–288.

33. Newell S, Jordan Z. The patient experience of patient-centered communication with nurses in the hospital setting: A qualitative systematic review protocol. *JBI Database System Rev Implement Rep*. 2015;13(1):76–87.

34. Oja KJ. Incivility and professional comportment in critical care nurses. *AACN Adv Crit Care*. 2017;28(4):345–350.

35. Overton HN, Hanna MN, Bruhn WE, et al. Opioid-prescribing guidelines for common surgical procedures: An expert panel consensus. *J Am Coll Surg*. 2018;227(4):411–418.

36. Panlaqui OM, Broadfield E, Champion R, et al. Outcomes of telemedicine intervention in a regional intensive care unit: A before and after study. *Anaesth Intensive Care*. 2017;45(5):605–610.

37. Peterson MH, Barnason S, Donnelly B, et al. Choosing the best evidence to guide clinical practice: Application of AACN levels of evidence. *Crit Care Nurse*. 2014;34(2):58–68.

38. Pickens CI, Wunderink RG. Principles and practice of antibiotic stewardship in the ICU. *Chest*. 2019;156(1):163–171.

39. Prentice T, Janvier A, Gillam L, Davis PG. Moral distress within neonatal and paediatric intensive care units: A systematic review. *Arch Dis Child*. 2016;101(8):701–708.

40. Shapiro J, Robins L, Galowitz P, et al. Disclosure coaching: An ask-tell-ask model to support clinicians in disclosure conversations. *J Patient Saf*. 2018.

41. Sharma S, Friede R. Multidisciplinary rounds in the ICU. *StatPearls*. https://www.ncbi.nlm.nih.gov/books/NBK507776/ 2019.

42. Society of Critical Care Medicine (SCCM). About SCCM. https://www.sccm.org/About-SCCM. Published 2019. Accessed April 7, 2019.

43. Stevens JP, Wall MJ, Novack L, et al. The critical care crisis of opioid overdoses in the United States. *Ann Am Thorac Soc*. 2017;14(12):1803–1809.

44. The Joint Commission. National Patient Safety Goals. https://www.jointcommission.org/hap_2017_npsgs/. Published 2019. Accessed April 7, 2019.

45. Thompson D, Holzmueller C, Hunt D, et al. A morning briefing: Setting the stage for a clinically and operationally good day. *Jt Comm J Qual Patient Saf*. 2005;31(8):476–479.

46. U.S. Department of Health and Human Services (DHHS). National Action Plan to Prevent Health Care–Associated Infections: Road Map to Elimination. https://health.gov/hcq/prevent-hai-action-plan.asp. Published 2016. Accessed April 9, 2019.

47. Udeh C, Udeh B, Rahman N, et al. Telemedicine/virtual ICU: Where are we and where are we going? *Methodist Debakey Cardiovasc J*. 2018;14(2):126–133.

48. Ulrich B, Barden C, Cassidy L, Varn-Davis N. Critical care nurse work environments 2018: Findings and implications. *Crit Care Nurse*. 2019;39(2):67–84.

49. Wessman BT, Sona C, Schallom M. A novel ICU hand-over tool: The glass door of the patient room. *J Intensive Care Med*. 2017;32(8):514–519.

Patient and Family Response to the Critical Care Experience

Sandra J. Dotson-Kirn, PhD, MSN, BSN
Mary Lou Sole, PhD, RN, CCNS, CNL, FAAN, FCCM

Many additional resources, including self-assessment exercises, are located on the Evolve companion website at http://evolve.elsevier.com/Sole/.
- Animations
- Clinical Skills: Critical Care Collections
- Student Review Questions
- Video Clips

INTRODUCTION

Although any hospitalization is stressful, the critical care experience is especially challenging. This situation presents patients and families with issues beyond those directly related to the illness. The personal lives of the patients and those who care about them are affected in many ways. Being in an environment that is foreign to most and dealing with an undesirable health state creates apprehension that is displayed as being overwhelmed, traumatized, uncertain, and anguished.[46] Anxiety, depression, sleep deprivation, and acute stress disorder syndrome are experienced by many. Emotional responses are manifested in many ways, such as concern, fear, nervousness, anger, frustration, anticipatory grief, and impaired problem solving.[11,24,65] Healthcare teams are often so involved with the care of patients that they may neglect the concerns of families. Although attitudes are changing, some staff members believe that the presence of family members increases their workloads, makes their work difficult, and is stressful for them.[57]

Ongoing research into the experiences of critically ill patients and their families consistently supports the premise that nurses must consider the patient and the patient's family when providing care.[15,35] Nurses play a unique role in addressing the needs of both patients and their families in a busy and complex environment. In the past 2 decades, visitation policies in critical care units have changed from being rigid and restricted to open and relaxed, resulting in family needs being met and a higher satisfaction with care given.[32]

Advances in life-sustaining procedures and treatments present complicated ethical considerations in caring for the seriously ill, and it is often family members who weigh the efficacy and ethics of extending life versus the potential loss of quality of life (see Chapter 3). In addition, social and demographic changes such as an aging population and changes in family structure have altered the traditional definition of what constitutes *family*. Critical care nurses assume an advocacy role in caring for patients and their family members who have life-threatening illnesses and problems. The purpose of this chapter is to describe the critical illness experience and its effects on patients and their families.

THE CRITICAL CARE ENVIRONMENT

The *built environment,* or physical layout, of a critical care unit has a subtle but profound effect on patients, families, and the critical care team. Amid an apparent confusion of wires, tubes, and machinery, a critical care unit is designed for efficient and expeditious life-sustaining interventions. Patients and their family members are cared for in this environment with little or no advance preparation, often causing stress and anxiety. The resultant high stress levels are compounded by the often unrelenting sensory stimulation of light and noise, loss of privacy, lack of nonclinical physical contact, and emotional and physical pain. Issues related to the environment include sensory overload, noise, and sensory deprivation.

❓ CRITICAL REASONING ACTIVITY

You are bringing family members to the critical care unit to see the patient for the first time. The patient has been involved in a motor vehicle crash, and the environment is similar to that depicted in Fig. 2.1. What strategies do you use to explain the patient's condition and the environment to the family members?

TABLE 2.1   Noise Levels Associated With Patient Care Devices and Activities

Activity	Sound Level (dB[a])
Call-bell activation	48-63
Oxygen or chest tube bubbling	49-70
Conversations (staff, patients, and family)	59-90
Voice over intercom	60-70
Telephone ringing	60-75
Television (normal volume at 12 feet)	65
Raising or lowering head of bed	68-78
Cardiac monitor	72-77
Infusion pump	73-78
Ventilator sounds	76
Pneumatic tube arrival	88

Many studies have documented the detrimental effects of the sensory overload found in a typical critical care unit. Noise and light are listed among the stimuli that patients, families, and nurses view as stressors.[43] The noise level alone is enough stimulation to cause patient discomfort and sleep deprivation, and it is a major factor contributing to sensory overload. Both sleep disruption and delirium in the critically ill are related to noise levels.[66] Phlebotomy procedures are another sensory disturbance frequently encountered by patients in critical care units given the acuity of their situation.[19]

The World Health Organization established guidelines for hospital noise levels that recommend levels no greater than 30 dB in daytime and 40 dB at night.[7] Yet noise levels in hospitals routinely exceed those recommended, and efforts to reduce noise are not extremely successful due to the variety of noise sources. Table 2.1 provides a list of noise levels associated with patient care and discloses just how much noise is emitted with each device or activity.

Sensory disturbances also affect nurses, often leading to increased stress, emotional exhaustion, burnout, and fatigue, as well as to difficult communication and distractions, which may contribute to medical errors.[8,61] In addition, loud conversations may compromise patient confidentiality.

Several strategies can reduce noise within the acute care environment: reducing the volume of technical equipment, adjusting alarm volume when possible, organizing workflow to promote efficiency rather than multiple interruptions, closing patient doors, placing patients in private rooms, and installing sound-absorbing textiles.[33] Designate a private place for communication with family members and close the door during conversations that may be overheard by others. Avoid excessive or loud talking, answer phones quickly, and readily assess alarms on medical devices. Alarm sounds can be lowered, staff can use lower voices, and doors can sometimes be closed, but these interventions have limited effect on the noise level in the critical care unit.[25] The layout of the unit and transport of patients to and from the unit are examples of sources of noise that often cannot be altered.

Providing "sedative" music is another strategy to reduce anxiety and discomfort associated with increased noise levels.[4] Music is an inexpensive and easy-to-use therapy that reduces stress as indicated by lower cortisol levels, heart rate, and blood pressure in patients receiving the therapy rather than the control.[39]

Despite the potential for sensory overload, patients can also experience sensory deprivation in an environment that is very different from their usual surroundings. Sensory deprivation is associated with an increase in perceptual disturbances such as hallucinations, especially in older adults.[7] Provide stimulation by interacting with and orienting the patient, and encourage visitation of friends and family. Post family photos within the patient's sight, and provide music or television that the patient usually enjoys.

Lighting is another issue in the critical care environment. Adequate and appropriate exposure to light is a therapeutic modality for the health of both patients and staff. Inadequate or poorly placed lighting makes it more difficult to read medical records and medication labels and complicates accurate physical assessment of patients. In addition, the constant artificial lighting present in most critical care units tends to override patients' natural circadian rhythms. Constant artificial lighting has detrimental effects on healthy individuals and has even more of an impact on critically ill patients.[16] Simple measures such as designing rooms to take advantage of natural light can reduce depression, improve sleep quality, and enhance pain management.

The design of the critical care unit can affect delivery of care as well as the responses of patients and their families. New hospital construction or renovation of existing facilities provides an opportunity to design hospitals to best meet the needs of patients, families, and staff members. It is important for members of the healthcare team to work with architects and other planners to design a safe and healing environment. Best practices for design of critical care units include private rooms with items such as natural light, views of nature, adequate room for visitors, and noise-reducing features.[64] It is also important when designing or adapting a unit to meet the comfort needs of family members and promote rest should they wish to remain in a patient's room. Physical design of the critical care unit has received much attention over the past 2 decades, resulting in many units that are ideal for staff, patients, and their families.[56]

STUDY BREAK

1. Which of the following is associated with an increase in perceptual disturbances such as hallucinations, especially in older adults?
   A. Music therapy
   B. Scheduled rest periods
   C. Communication by family members
   D. The frequent sound of bedside alarms

THE CRITICALLY ILL PATIENT

Many factors influence an individual's response to critical illness. Factors include age and developmental stage, experiences

BOX 2.1 Patients' Recollection of the Critical Care Experience

- Anxiety
- Depression
- Difficulty communicating
- Difficulty sleeping
- Difficulty swallowing
- Fear
- Feelings of dread
- Inability to get comfortable
- Lack of control
- Lack of family or friends
- Loneliness
- Pain
- Physical restraint
- Thirst
- Thoughts of death and dying

with illness and hospitalization, family relationships and social support, other stressful experiences and coping mechanisms, and personal philosophies about life, death, and spirituality. Stressors related to treatment and the critical care environment can lead to anxiety, fear, insecurity, isolation, and loneliness.[1,5] Stressors that have been identified by patients when recalling their critical care experience are listed in Box 2.1. The cumulative effect of these stressors can promote anxiety and agitation, and in some cases it leads to the development of delirium and posttraumatic stress disorder (PTSD).[6,54,70] Nursing interventions to reduce stress are to ensure safety, reduce sleep deprivation, and minimize noxious sensory overload. One effective intervention is to group together nursing activities and medical procedures to maximize resting periods. Chapter 6 further discusses interventions to promote comfort and reduce anxiety.

Even if patients are sedated or unconscious, it is important to remember that many patients can still hear, understand, and respond emotionally to what is being said. Make every effort to talk to patients, regardless of their ability to interact. Reorient patients to time and place, update them on their progress, and remind them that they are safe and have family and people nearby who care about their well-being.

Increase pleasant sensory input by encouraging family members to speak to and touch the patient. Reorient the patient every 2 to 4 hours, and address the patient directly to minimize disorientation. Instead of repeatedly questioning the patient (e.g., "Do you know what day it is? Do you know where you are?"), incorporate this content into normal conversation (e.g., "It's 8 o'clock in the morning on the fifth of September. You are still in the critical care unit. Your family will be here to see you in about 10 minutes."). Do not discuss other patients and personnel in the patient's room because such information can increase confusion and contribute to sensory overload. Place objects that facilitate orientation, such as a clock or a calendar, within the patient's visual field. Ask family members to bring personal and meaningful items from home to assist in reorienting the patient. These items

also humanize the patient and help staff to recognize that the patient has a unique personality and should be treated accordingly.

Promoting rest and sleep are other important nursing interventions. Sleep is frequently interrupted by such activities as blood draws, physician visits, medication administration, and frequent assessment. A retrospective analysis of interactions that potentially disrupt sleep documented an average of 43 interactions during the 12-hour night shift, peaking at midnight. Uninterrupted sleep periods lasting 2 to 3 hours were documented only 6% of the time.[51] Multiple healthcare providers are involved in patient care, and their interventions are often determined by when staff are available rather than when the timing is ideal for the patient. Bundling nonpharmacological interventions such as removing noxious stimuli and increasing comfort are effective ways to promote rest and sleep.[20,53] Simply asking the patient or family about sleep preferences is another intervention.[30] Promote day-night cycles by positioning the patient near natural light during the day and reducing light levels in the patient's room at night. Reduce noise during the nighttime hours.

Stress and anxiety for the critically ill patient are caused by pain, discomfort, and many other factors. Critical care nurses are in the position to pinpoint exactly what stresses their patients, and they can minimize many of these stresses. Provide high-quality nursing care, offered with humanity and delivered professionally. Explain procedures or interventions before they are performed, plan care so that the patient has quality time with family members, encourage decision making, and facilitate communication.

STUDY BREAK

2. Which of the following statements is true regarding the sedated or unconscious patient?
   A. Cannot hear anything, so does not respond to noise
   B. Is not affected by music therapy or familiar voices
   C. Can still hear, understand, and respond emotionally to what is being said
   D. Will always be able to follow the most basic commands

? CRITICAL REASONING ACTIVITY

You are in charge of coordinating a family conference to discuss a patient's condition and goals for care and treatment. All family members are Haitian and speak Creole. What strategies do you incorporate when planning the family conference?

Discharge From Critical Care and Quality of Life After Critical Care

Many critically ill patients survive critical illnesses and injuries. Although discharge from a critical care unit represents progress toward recovery, many patients are discharged "quicker and sicker" to units that care for patients with lesser acuity, to long-term acute care hospitals, or to home. Transfer or discharge from the critical care unit is stressful for both patient and family. As a result of transfer from the critical care unit to another unit or area, patients and families may experience physiological or psychological disturbances, referred to as *relocation stress*.[27,52] They may also feel a sense of abandonment and fear losing the security of the higher level of care afforded in the critical care unit. Anticipate the stress associated with transfer and provide interventions that reduce these stressors.[14]

Survivors of critical illness experience many problems, but the three reported most often are disability and weakness, psychiatric pathologies, and cognitive dysfunction.[26] Collectively, these symptoms are deemed post-intensive care syndrome, or PICS.[17,44] Postdischarge therapy may be required to address PICS. Both patients and family members also have an increased risk of developing PTSD after a critical care experience.[34,63,70] Once home, the demands of follow-up care place an enormous burden on family members, who may be ill-prepared or unwilling to shoulder such a burden. Discharge planning and patient teaching are essential nursing interventions to improve patient and family outcomes. Ongoing family involvement and teaching, beginning at admission and continuing throughout the hospital stay, are crucial interventions. Initiate patient education early and continue it throughout the patient's hospitalization. With the healthcare team, develop a comprehensive discharge plan that includes scheduled follow-up phone calls for ongoing assessment, reevaluation, and support. One technique used to facilitate teaching and learning is the *teach-back method*, in which patients and family members are asked to repeat the information and instructions they have been given.[55,59]

Influences on Patients' and Families' Responses

Response to critical illness is influenced by various factors, including age and developmental stage; prior experiences with illness and hospitalization; family relationships and social support; prior stressful experiences and coping mechanisms; and personal philosophies about life, death, and spirituality. Patients who have survived a prior critical illness generally have less anxiety during subsequent admissions. For other patients, their only prior experience with critical illness may have ended with the death of a family member. This scenario can add considerably to the patient's fears and anxiety. Older adults have more negative outcomes (see Lifespan Considerations box).

🕮 LIFESPAN CONSIDERATIONS

Older Adults

- Some older adult patients have a diminished ability to adapt and cope with the major physical and psychosocial stressors of critical illness. This is often the result of multiple losses over the years, including loss of physical function, loss of family members, and loss of resources, such as homes and income.
- Some older adults with chronic illnesses who have endured multiple critical illnesses demonstrate amazing resilience.
- Older adults have a high risk of negative outcomes. Among older adult critical care survivors, health-related quality of life (HRQOL) worsened significantly, and most did not regain their baseline status after 1 year.[67] HRQOL is inversely related to both the severity of the illness and the length of stay.[45]
- Increased mortality, functional decline, and a decrease in HRQOL are common among older critical care survivors, especially after a prolonged length of stay in critical care, and among those older than 80 years.[3,29]

❓ CRITICAL REASONING ACTIVITY

You are leading a work group charged with championing the recently revised critical care visitation policy, specifically with regard to open visitation. Most staff members are resistant and feel that the new policy is not working. What are some of the objections you might encounter, and how would you address them?

FAMILY MEMBERS OF THE CRITICALLY ILL PATIENT

Critical care hospitalization is a crisis situation that affects the patient and the family. The stress experienced by the family may be detected by the patient, and the patient can suffer as a result of a family member's stress. The family is an integral part of the patient's healing process; therefore critical care nursing interventions must also focus on the family.

Patient and family-centered care recognizes the importance of the collaboration of both patients and families with the healthcare team in decision making. This paradigm shift in patient care is widely recognized as an integral part of care in all specialties, including critical care.[12,35,47] Centers for Medicare and Medicaid Services (CMS), the Agency for Healthcare Research and Quality (AHRQ), and many other organizations that are influential in health care acknowledge the importance of patient- and family-centered care.[3,10]

The nurse must recognize and acknowledge the importance of care that includes both patients and family members. Families are in a vulnerable state because of the stress they are experiencing and the fact that they are in foreign surroundings. For many families, both the hospital and the critical care unit are "alien" environments. Most family members have never or only rarely see a critical care unit. The machines and monitors that are commonplace to nurses can be frightening and overwhelming to them. Fig. 2.1 depicts what a family member sees when entering

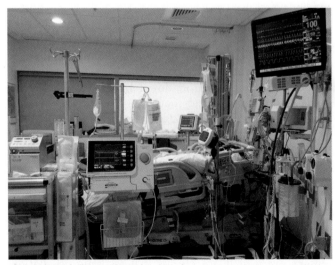

Fig. 2.1 If you were the family member and your loved one was this patient, how would you feel when you saw this situation? (Reprinted with permission, Cleveland Clinic Center for Art & Photography © 2019. All rights reserved.)

the room of a critically ill loved one. Imagine your thoughts and feelings if you were to encounter this situation.

Family Assessment

Once the patient has been admitted to the critical care unit, an assessment of the family provides valuable information for development of the plan of care. Obtain essential information during the admission assessment, and gather additional information throughout the hospital stay. Structured tools are available to assess the family but are not consistently used in everyday practice; however, concepts incorporated into tools can guide the nursing assessment. The structural, developmental, and functional categories described in the Calgary Family Assessment Model provide a useful way to gather information about the family.[69] *Structural assessment* is done on admission, and it identifies immediate family, extended family, and the decision makers. Other aspects of family structure include ethnicity, race, religion, and spirituality. Designating a spokesperson for primary communication with the family members is beneficial. The *developmental assessment* includes information related to the family's developmental stages and tasks. The *functional assessment* reveals how family members function and behave in relation to one another.[69]

In today's diverse society, it is important to assess the influence of culture and spirituality on both the patient and family. Especially important are beliefs about health and healing, cultural and spiritual practices, personal space and touch preferences, social organization, and the role of the family. Identify the primary language used for verbal and written communication. Use hospital-designated language interpreters when communicating with non-English speakers. Interpreters also serve as cultural guides to facilitate communication and understanding of the critical care experience.

A simple approach to cultural and spiritual assessment is to ask three questions that can easily be adapted for most situations: (1) What are your specific religious and spiritual practices? (2) What are your beliefs about illness (and death)? (3) What is most important to you and your family at this time?

An early, proactive approach is advised when assessing a patient's family. Observe the family; interact with them; and note significant facts such as the patient's role, family coping strategies, and socioeconomic issues. The family assessment may reveal whether the family members are angry, feeling guilty, or have unaddressed concerns regarding the patient's condition and care. An illness within the family may also uncover underlying conflicts among family members, especially when family members are estranged or have other unresolved issues. Once an assessment is completed, concisely record the collected data to identify key information related to family assessment that is shared among all healthcare team members caring for the patient.

Family Needs

Molter published a groundbreaking study of family needs in 1979; six of the top 10 needs of relatives of the critically ill related directly to receiving information.[48] Globally, many researchers have conducted follow-up studies using the Critical Care Family Needs Inventory[49] and have identified a predictable set of needs of the family members of critically ill patients: receiving information, receiving assurance, remaining near the patient, being comfortable, and having support available.[4,40,41,51] Family members report that they need assurance and stress reduction.[71] They also report being fatigued, stressed, and needing frequent updates on patient status.[11]

Addressing stress and coping of family members is important. If family members perceive stress, it may increase the workload of the nurse to address that stress. Knowledge of interventions that are known to be effective in reducing stress and promoting coping of family members enables the critical care nurse to create a plan of care that assists both patients and their families.

Some family members may be demanding or disruptive, or they may insist on constant vigilance from the nursing staff. These behaviors may reflect a sense of loss of control or possibly memories of an adverse outcome during a previous hospitalization. Recognize these factors as the reason for observed behaviors and determine the best way to communicate and intervene.

Family members often want confirmation that everything is being done for the patient, which may be challenging. Establish a partnership with the family built on mutual respect as well as credibility, competence, and compassion. One strategy is to encourage family members to assist in patient assessment (e.g., identify changes) and participate in selected aspects of the patient's care. Depending on institutional policy, it may be possible to enlist family members to help with tasks such as oral care, hygiene, range-of-motion exercises, or repositioning the patient. These activities give family members a sense of purpose and control, as well as potentially providing an additional layer of safety when the nurse is unavailable.

Research has been conducted regarding family-centered interventions and their effectiveness.[2,9,68] Structured methods for providing family assistance have been developed; however, a single and standardized method to ensure that families receive the care they need has not been accepted into everyday critical care practice. *The Clinical Practice Guidelines for Support of the Family in the Patient-Centered Intensive Care Unit* were developed by a multiprofessional group of the American College of Critical Care Medicine. The group made

---

BOX 2.2   Evidence-Based Recommendations for Supporting Family Members of Critically Ill Patients

Decision Making
- Make decisions based on a partnership among the patient, family, and the healthcare team
- Communicate the patient's status and prognosis to family members and explain options for treatment
- Hold family meetings with the healthcare team within 24 to 48 hours after critical care unit admission and repeat as often as needed
- Train critical care unit staff in communication, conflict management, and facilitation skills

Family Coping
- Train critical care unit staff in assessment of family needs, stress, and anxiety levels
- Assign consistent nursing and physician staff to each patient if possible
- Update family members in a language they can understand
- Provide information to family members in a variety of formats
- Provide family support using a team effort, including social workers, clergy, nursing and medical staff, and support groups

Staff Stress
- Keep all healthcare team members informed of treatment goals to ensure that messages given to the family are consistent
- Develop a mechanism for staff members to request a debriefing to voice concerns with the treatment plan, decompress, share feelings, or grieve

Cultural Support of Family
- If possible, match the provider's culture to that of the patient
- Educate staff on culturally competent care

Spiritual and Religious Support
- Assess spiritual needs and incorporate them into the plan of care
- Educate staff in spiritual and religious issues that facilitate patient assessment

Family Visitation
- Facilitate open visitation in the adult critical care environment, if possible
- Determine personalized visitation schedules in collaboration with the patient, family, and nurse; consider the best interest of the patient
- Provide open visitation in the pediatric critical care unit and neonatal critical care unit 24 hours a day
- Allow siblings to visit in the pediatric critical care unit and neonatal critical care unit (with parental approval) after participation in a previsit education program
- Do not restrict pets that are clean and properly immunized from visiting the critical care unit
- Develop guidelines for animal-assisted therapy

Family Environment of Care
- Build new critical care units with single-bed rooms to improve patient confidentiality, privacy, and social support
- Develop signage (e.g., easy-to-follow directions) to reduce stress on visitors

Family Presence During Rounds
- Allow parents or guardians of children in the critical care unit to participate in rounds
- Allow adult patients and family members to participate in rounds

Family Presence During Resuscitation
- Develop a process to allow the presence of family members during cardiopulmonary resuscitation

Palliative Care
- Educate staff in palliative care during formal critical care education

Modified from Davidson JE, Powers K, Hedayat KM, et al. Clinical practice guidelines for support of the family in the patient-centered intensive care unit: American College of Critical Care Medicine Task Force 2004–2005. *Crit Care Med.* 2007;35(2):605–622.

---

43 recommendations based on the best available evidence. Recommendations that received a grade of C (based on some evidence) or better are listed in Box 2.2.[18] The guidelines remain relevant today.[15,62]

In addition to guidelines, other interventions have been successfully used to assist families. A "family bundle" to provide a structure for planning and carrying out family care was developed and tested with positive results (Fig. 2.2).[36] Multiple studies have found that specific sets of interventions known to all nurses providing care may lower stress, improve coping, or increase comfort for families of critically ill patients.[52,54]

Communication

Receiving information and feeling safe are predominant, complementary needs of critically ill patients and their family members. Of all the members of the critical care team, nurses spend the most time at the bedside and as such are usually the first to hear about any perceived unmet needs of family members. Frequent updates on the patient's condition, anticipated therapies or procedures, and goals of the critical care team are an easy and effective way to allay anxiety while building a relationship of mutual trust.

Lack of communication is a principal complaint when families are dissatisfied with care.[21,22] Facilitate communication by providing a simple, honest report of the patient's condition, free of medical jargon. A follow-up assessment to gauge the family's level of understanding helps to tailor the care plan accordingly.

Scheduled rounds between the healthcare team and the family assist in maintaining open communication. A predetermined routine for these rounds provides an opportunity for the team to update the family on the patient's condition and answer questions posed by the family. It also provides time to identify goals for care and treatment to facilitate shared decision making. Scheduled family conferences provide a similar opportunity to facilitate communication. Family conferences may be held at the bedside or in a conference room, depending on space available and family needs. If possible, hold a preconference among team members to ensure that consistent messages are delivered during the family conference.

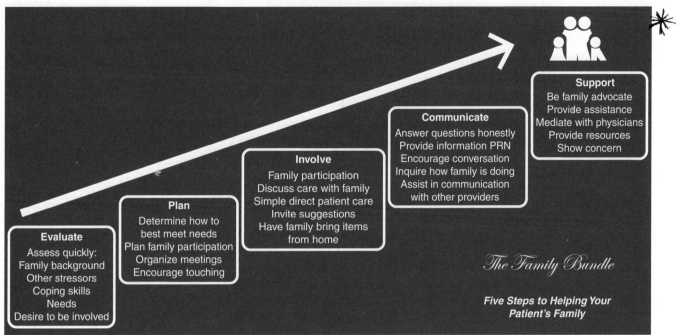

Fig. 2.2 EPICS family bundle. (From Knapp S. *Effects of an Evidence-Based Intervention on Stress and Coping of Family Members of Critically Ill Trauma Patients* [unpublished dissertation]. Orlando: University of Central Florida; 2009.)

BOX 2.3 Enhancing Communication With Family Members: Value Principles

V—Value what the family tells you
A—Acknowledge family emotions
L—Listen to the family members
U—Understand the patient as a person
E—Elicit (ask) questions of family members

From Lautrette A, Darmon M, Megarbane B, et al. A communication strategy and brochure for relatives of patients dying in the ICU. *N Engl J Med*. 2007;356(5):469–478.

Empathetic communication is important during rounds and family conferences. The VALUE mnemonic (Box 2.3) is a useful tool to enhance communication with family members of critically ill patients.[22]

Visitation

Visitation is among the most contentious and widely researched issues in nursing. Based on this research, great advancements have been made in visitation practices. Many critical care units have relaxed or eliminated restrictions on visiting hours. This greatly improves patient and family satisfaction, although some nurses remain reluctant to change. Nurses may view family-centered care and open or expanded visitation as challenging or stressful; however, administrative support can help nurses to adjust and improve their job satisfaction.[13,50]

Reasons cited for opposition to liberal visitation include the presumed increased physiological stress for the patient, family interference with the provision of care, and physical and mental exhaustion of family and friends.[58] An additional concern is that family members will be intrusive, creating burdens for

nurses; however, concerns about negative outcomes of liberalized visitation are unfounded.[64] Contrary to traditional thinking, it was well documented more than 30 years ago that family presence frequently has no effect on the patient's condition and at times the effect is positive, such as decreased intracranial pressures or blood pressures, or an increased heart rate in a bradycardic patient.[23,28,60] The QSEN Exemplar box illustrates an example of family-centered care.

✳ QSEN EXEMPLAR

Family-Centered Care

Mr. K. is a 34-year-old man who suffered a C7 spinal cord injury 10 years ago as a result of a diving accident. His primary caregiver is his mother. Mr. K. has been admitted to the critical care unit with respiratory failure secondary to pneumonia three times in the past year. A unit nurse reports that his mother obstructs care and is uncooperative with nursing staff. During the admission process, Mr. K.'s mother requests permission to stay with him throughout his hospitalization. She states that he developed a stage 3 pressure injury during his last admission, and she feels the need to oversee his physical care. The pressure injury took months to heal and significantly limited Mr. K.'s activities. Citing concerns related to the privacy of other patients and prior poor family relations, the staff ask management to deny the family's request. The clinical nurse specialist is consulted and meets with unit management and nursing staff to formalize a plan that will promote family involvement. Mr. K.'s mother is permitted to spend as much time at the bedside as desired but is also told that there are some specific times when the nurse may request that she leave the room for brief periods. After several days, the staff become comfortable with her presence, and team members actively engage her in tasks such as bathing, turning, and feeding. During a follow-up unit meeting, the staff suggest establishment of a facility-wide policy that provides specific guidelines to promote inclusion of family members as active partners in care.

Although practice is changing and research is limited, many institutions prohibit visitation by children. The American Association of Critical-Care Nurses (AACN) recommends welcoming children who are supervised by an adult family member. A unit culture change may need to occur to make child visitation a reality. Nurses need to be engaged, and the visiting child needs individual guidance and follow-up.[37] Visitation provides children with an opportunity to learn about their loved one and provides support during times of uncertainty.

Animal-assisted therapy may also be beneficial to a patient's recovery. Some critical care units have extended visitation to include pet therapy. These institutions have policies that permit the family pet or designated therapy animals to visit the patient.[31,38]

Nurses can assist in promoting policy changes to affect open-visitation policies. Unit-based councils and staff-led research are helpful to create change in the visitation policies. A significant benefit of a liberal visitation policy is its positive effect on the opinions of both patients and families regarding the quality of nursing care. When combined with family support, as demonstrated by the nurses' caring behaviors and interactions, liberal visitation is influential in shaping the critical care experience for both patients and families.

Family Presence During Resuscitation and Invasive Procedures

In conjunction with more liberal visitation policies, many institutions have implemented policies to allow families to be present during cardiopulmonary resuscitation and invasive procedures. Factors cited for limiting family members' presence include limited space at the bedside, violations of patient confidentiality, not enough staff members available to assist family members, increased stress on healthcare staff members (e.g., performance anxiety, risk for litigation), and increased stress and anxiety for family members; however, these factors have not been substantiated by research. Studies found that allowing family members to observe resuscitation and invasive procedures has positive effects, and the efforts promote increased knowledge of the patient's condition.[42] Box 2.4 presents the benefits of family presence.

> **BOX 2.4** **Benefits of Family Presence**
>
> **Being Present Helps Family Members to:**
> - Remove doubt about the patient's condition
> - Witness that everything possible is done
> - Decrease their anxiety and fear about what is happening to their loved one
>
> **Being Present Facilitates Family Members':**
> - Need to be together with their loved one
> - Need to help and support their loved one
> - Sense of closure and grieving should death occur

> **STUDY BREAK**
> 4. Health-related quality of life (HRQOL) is inversely related to:
>   A. Inadequate diet and insufficient exercise
>   B. Amount of family visitation
>   C. The severity of illness and the length of stay
>   D. The amount of noise to which the patient is exposed

Practice Alerts

The AACN has issued Practice Alerts to guide the critical care nurse in implementing open visitation and family presence during resuscitation and invasive procedures. Expected nursing practices are highlighted in Box 2.5.

> **BOX 2.5** **Family Presence During Resuscitation and Invasive Procedures**
>
> **Expected Practice**
> - Family members of all patients undergoing resuscitation and invasive procedures should be given the opportunity to be present at the bedside per the patient's wishes
> - All patient-care units should have an approved written practice document
>
> **Actions for Nursing Practice**
> - Ensure the health care facility has supportive written policies and procedures
> - Make certain that policies, procedures, and educational programs include components that include topics such as benefits, criteria, contraindications, and role of the family presence facilitator
> - Develop proficiency standards for all staff
> - Determine the unit's rate of compliance and re-educate staff if compliance is less than 90%
> - Develop documentation standards for family presence
>
> From American Association of Critical-Care Nurses. Practice Alert: Family Presence During Resuscitation and Invasive Procedures. https://www.aacn.org/~/media/aacn-website/clincial-resources/practice-alerts/fampres-resuscpafeb2016ccnpages.pdf. Published 2016. Accessed March 9, 2019.

> **CASE STUDY**
>
> Mr. D., a 40-year-old man, was involved in a head-on motor vehicle collision. His main injuries are a closed head injury with fractures to the right femur and left tibia and fibula. He also has a minor liver laceration. He was unresponsive and hemodynamically unstable on arrival to the emergency department and was admitted to the surgical critical care unit after a ventriculostomy was placed to reduce and monitor intracranial pressure (ICP). Surgery on the femur fracture is delayed until Mr. D.'s ICP is under control. He is married and has two small children: a 5-year-old boy and a 3-year-old girl. Mr. D. has multiple bandages, casts on his legs, and an ICP monitoring device. He is intubated and dependent on a ventilator.
>
> His wife is at the bedside and expresses a feeling of "helplessness." She cries frequently and expresses great concern every time one of the alarms in the room sounds. She watches the monitor almost constantly and repeatedly asks what each waveform and number means. The nurses notice that she asks the same questions repeatedly, as if she does not remember having asked them before.
>
> She states that she wants to be able to help in any way she can. She says that Mr. D. is a hard worker and he loves his children very much. She also mentions that she does not work outside of the home because the cost of day care is more than the income she would produce if she did have a job. A friend who comes to visit tells Mrs. D. to "be strong for the children."
>
> **Questions**
> 1. Mr. D.'s ICP increases to unsatisfactory levels when Mrs. D. enters the room and talks to him. Should she be discouraged from talking to him? Should visitation be suspended? Why or why not?
> 2. Are Mrs. D.'s concerns about the monitor and alarms appropriate? What measures would likely help her to manage her fears regarding them?
> 3. What are some things Mrs. D. could be encouraged to do to make her feel less helpless?
> 4. Should the children be allowed to visit their father? Why or why not?

? CRITICAL REASONING ACTIVITY

You are caring for a patient whose family members include other medical professionals (e.g., staff nurse, nurse practitioner, physician). The family is frequently critical of the patient's management and is constantly making suggestions regarding nursing care. How do you respond?

REFERENCES

1. Abrão F, Santos EF, Araújo R, Oliveira R, Costa A. Feelings of patients while staying in intensive care unit. *J Nurs UFPE/Revista de Enfermagem UFPE*. 2014;8(3):523–529.
2. Adams JA, Anderson RA, Docherty SL, et al. Nursing strategies to support family members of ICU patients at high risk of dying. *Heart Lung*. 2014;43(5):406–415.
3. Agency for Healthcare Research and Quality. Guide to Patient and Family Engagement in Hospital Quality and Safety. http://www.ahrq.gov/professionals/systems/hospital/engagingfamilies/guide.html. Published 2017. Accessed February 2019.
4. Batista VC, Coutinho Monteschio LV, de Godoy FJ, et al. Needs of the relatives of patients hospitalized in an intensive therapy unit. *Rev Saude Publica: Cuidado e Fundamental*. 2019;11(2):540–546.
5. Baumgarten M, Poulsen I. Patients' experiences of being mechanically ventilated in an ICU: A qualitative metasynthesis. *Scand J Caring Sci*. 2015;29(2):205–214.
6. Baxter A. Posttraumatic stress disorder and the intensive care unit patient: Implications for staff and advanced practice critical care nurses. *Dimen Criti Care Nurs*. 2004;23(4):145–152.
7. Berglund B, Lindvall T, Schwela DH, eds. *Guidelines for Community Noise*. Geneva, Switzerland: World Health Organization; 1999.
8. Blake N. The effect of alarm fatigue on the work environment. *AACN Adv Criti Care*. 2014;25(1):18–19.
9. Breisinger L, Bires AM, Cline TW. Stress reduction in postcardiac surgery family members: Implementation of a postcardiac surgery tool kit. *Crit Care Nurs Q*. 2018;41(2):186–196.
10. Centers for Medicare and Medicaid Services. HCAHPS: Patients' Perspectives of Care Survey. https://www.cms.gov/Medicare/Quality-Initiatives-Patient-Assessment-Instruments/Hospital-QualityInits/HospitalHCAHPS.html. Published 2017. Accessed February 7, 2019.
11. Chang P-Y, Wang H-P, Chang T-H, et al. Stress, stress-related symptoms and social support among Taiwanese primary family caregivers in intensive care units. *Intensive Crit Care Nurs*. 2018;49:37–43.
12. Clark AP. *A Paradigm Shift for Patient/Family-Centered Care in Intensive Care Units: Bring in the Family*. Vol 37. Alisa Veijo, CA: American Association of Critical-Care Nurses; 2017:96–99.
13. Coats H, Bourget E, Starks H, et al. Nurses' reflections on benefits and challenges of implementing family-centered care in pediatric intensive care units. *Am J Crit Care*. 2018;27(1):52–58.
14. Cognet S, Coyer F. Discharge practices for the intensive care patient: A qualitative exploration in the general ward setting. *Intensive Crit Care Nurs*. 2014;30(5):292–300.
15. Coombs M, Puntillo KA, Franck LS, et al. Implementing the SCCM family-centered care guidelines in critical care nursing practice. *AACN Adv Crit Care*. 2017;28(2):138–147.
16. Danielson SJ, Rappaport CA, Loher MK, Gehlbach BK. Looking for light in the din: An examination of the circadian-disrupting properties of a medical intensive care unit. *Intensive Crit Care Nurs*. 2018;46:57–63.
17. Davidson JE, Hopkins RO, Louis D, Ikwashyna TJ. Post-Intensive Care Syndrome. https://www.sccm.org/MyICUCare/THRIVE/Post-intensive-Care-Syndrome. Published 2013. Accessed March 8, 2019.
18. Davidson JE, Powers K, Hedayat KM, et al. Clinical practice guidelines for support of the family in the patient-centered intensive care unit: American College of Critical Care Medicine Task Force 2004–2005. *Crit Care Med*. 2007;35(2):605–622.
19. Dragonetti A, D'Orazio A, Garripoli G. La qualità del sonno in Area critica. Studio prospettico...Sleep quality in ICUs. Prospective study. *SCENARIO: Official Italian Journal of ANIARTI*. 2017;34(3):4–11.
20. Du C, Trinks H, Simons T, Glanzer L. Evaluating sleep in a surgical trauma burn intensive care unit: An elusive dilemma. *Am J Crit Care*. 2017;26(3):e32–e33.
21. Gadepalli SK, Canvasser J, Eskenazi Y, et al. Roles and experiences of parents in necrotizing enterocolitis: An international survey of parental perspectives of communication in the NICU. *Adv Neonatal Care*. 2017;17(6):489–498.
22. Garrouste-Orgeas M, Flahault C, Fasse L, et al. The ICU-Diary study: Prospective, multicenter comparative study of the impact of an ICU diary on the wellbeing of patients and families in French ICUs. *Trials*. 2017;18(1):542.
23. Giuliano K, Giuliano A. Cardiovascular (CV) responses to family visitation and nurse-physician rounds. *Heart Lung*. 1992;21(3):290.
24. Glick DR, Motta M, Wiegand DL, et al. Anticipatory grief and impaired problem solving among surrogate decision makers of critically ill patients: A cross-sectional study. *Intensive Crit Care Nurs*. 2018;49:1–5.
25. Goeren D, John S, Meskill K, et al. Quiet time: A noise reduction initiative in a neurosurgical intensive care unit. *Crit Care Nurs*. 2018;38(4):38–44.
26. Govindan S, Iwashyna TJ, Watson SR, et al. Issues of survivorship are rarely addressed during intensive care unit stays. Baseline results from a statewide quality improvement collaborative. *Ann Am Thorac Soc*. 2014;11(4):587–591.
27. Guest M. Patient transfer from the intensive care unit to a general ward. *Nurs Stand*. 2017;32(10):45–51.
28. Hepworth JT, Hendrickson SG, Lopez J. Time series analysis of physiological response during ICU visitation. *West J Nurs Res*. 1994;16(6):704–717.
29. Heyland D, Garland A, Bagshaw S, et al. Recovery after critical illness in patients aged 80 years or older: A multi-center prospective observational cohort study. *Intensive Care Med*. 2015;41(11):1911–1920.
30. Hofhuis JGM, Rose L, Blackwood B, et al. Clinical practices to promote sleep in the ICU: A multinational survey. *Int J Nurs Stud*. 2018;81:107–114.
31. Hosey MM, Jaskulski J, Wegener ST, et al. Animal-assisted intervention in the ICU: A tool for humanization. *Crit Care*. 2018;22(1):22.
32. Jacob M. Needs of patients' family members in an intensive care unit with continuous visitation. *Am J Crit Care*. 2016;25(2):118–125.
33. Johansson L, Knutsson S, Bergbom I, Lindahl B. Noise in the ICU patient room: Staff knowledge and clinical improvements. *Intensive Crit Care Nurs*. 2016;35:1–9.
34. Kiernan F. Care of ICU survivors in the community: A guide GPs. *Br J Gen Pract*. 2017;67(663):477–478.
35. Kleinpell R, Buchman TG, Harmon L, Nielsen M. Pr patient- and family-centered care in the intensive dissemination project. *AACN Adv Crit Care*. 2017;.

36. Knapp SJ, Sole ML, Byers JF. The EPICS Family Bundle and its effects on stress and coping of families of critically ill trauma patients. *App Nurs Res*. 2013;26(2):51–57.

37. Knutsson S, Enskär K, Golsäter M. Nurses' experiences of what constitutes the encounter with children visiting a sick parent at an adult ICU. *Intensive Crit Care Nurs*. 2017;39:9–17.

38. Kramlich D. Complementary health practitioners in the acute and critical care setting: Nursing considerations. *Crit Care Nurse*. 2017;37(3):60–65.

39. Lee C-H, Lee C-Y, Hsu M-Y, et al. Effects of music intervention on state anxiety and physiological indices in patients undergoing mechanical ventilation in the intensive care unit. *Biol Res Nurs*. 2017;19(2):137–144.

40. Leske JS. Overview of family needs after critical illness: From assessment to intervention. *AACN Clin Issues Crit Care Nurs*. 1991;2(2):220–228.

41. Leske JS. Needs of adult family members after critical illness: Prescriptions for interventions. *Crit Care Nurs Clin N Am*. 1992;4(4):587–596.

42. Leske JS. Family presence during resuscitation after trauma. *J Trauma Nurs*. 2017;24(2):85–96.

43. Locihová H, Axmann K, Padyšáková H, Pončíková V. Perception of intensive care stressors by patients, nurses and family. *Central Eur J Nurs Midwif*. 2018;9(1):758–766.

44. Marra A, Pandharipande PP, Girard TD, et al. Co-occurrence of post-intensive care syndrome problems among 406 survivors of critical illness. *Crit Care Med*. 2018;46(9):1393–1401.

45. McKinley S, Fien M, Elliott R, Elliott D. Health related quality of life and associated factors in ICU survivors six months after discharge. *Aus Crit Care*. 2015;28(1):39.

46. Minton C, Batten L, Huntington A. A multicase study of prolonged critical illness in the intensive care unit: Families' experiences. *Intensive Crit Care Nurs*. 2019;50:21–27.

47. Millenson ML, Shapiro E, Greenhouse PK, DiGioia AM III. Patient- and family-centered care: A systematic approach to better ethics and care. *AMA J Ethics*. 2016;18(1):49–55.

48. Molter N. Needs of relatives of critically ill patients: A descriptive study. *Heart Lung*. 1979;8:332–339.

49. Molter N. Family-centered critical care: An interview with Nancy C. Molter, MS, RN, CCRN. Interview by Jane Stover Leske. *AACN Clin Issues Crit Care Nurs*. 1991;2:185–187.

50. Monroe M, Wofford L. Open visitation and nurse job satisfaction: An integrative review. *J Clin Nurs*. 2017;26(23–24):4868–4876.

51. Mousavi SS, Chaman R, Khosravi A, et al. The needs of parents of preterm infants in Iran and a comparison with those in other countries: A systematic review and meta-analysis. *Iran J Pediatr*. 2016;26(5):1–18.

52. Oh H, Lee S, Kim J, et al. Clinical validity of a relocation stress scale for the families of patients transferred from intensive care units. *J Clin Nurs*. 2015;24(13–14):1805–1814.

53. Patel J, Baldwin J, Bunting P, Laha S. The effect of a multicomponent multidisciplinary bundle of interventions on sleep and delirium in medical and surgical intensive care patients. *Anaesthesia*. 2014;69(6):540–549.

54. Patel MB, Jackson JC, Morandi A, et al. Incidence and risk factors for intensive care unit–related post-traumatic stress disorder in veterans and civilians. *Am J Respirat Crit Care Med*. 2016;193(12):1373–1381.

55. Peter D, Robinson P, Jordan M, Lawrence S, Casey K, Salas-Lopez D. Reducing readmissions using teach-back. *J Nurs Adm*. 2015;45(1):35–42.

56. Rashid M. Two decades (1993–2012) of adult intensive care unit design. *Crit Care Nurs Q*. 2014;37(1):3–32.

57. Ribeiro Chaves RG, Macedo de Sousa FG, Oliveira Silva AC, et al. Importance of the family in the care process: Attitudes of nurses in the context of intensive therapy. *J Nurs UFPE/Revista de Enfermagem UFPE*. 2017;11(12):4989–4998.

58. Riley BH, White J, Graham S, Alexandrov A. Traditional/restrictive vs patient-centered intensive care unit visitation: Perceptions of patients' family members, physicians, and nurses. *Am J Crit Care*. 2014;23(4):316–324.

59. Ryan-Madonna M, Levin RF, Lauder B. Effectiveness of the teach-back method for improving caregivers' confidence in caring for hospice patients and decreasing hospitalizations. *J Hosp Palliat Nurs*. 2019;21(1):61–70.

60. Stannard D. Ask the experts. I'm familiar with the research on family and patient needs regarding visitation, but what does the research say regarding the physiological effect of visitation? *Crit Care Nurse*. 1997;17(1):94.

61. Thomas L, Donohue-Porter P. The impact of cognitive load, interruptions, and distractions on procedural failures and medication administration errors. *Nurs Res*. 2016;65(2):e63–e64.

62. Torbey MT, Brophy GM, Varelas PN, et al. Guidelines for family-centered care in neuro-ICU populations: Caveats for routine palliative care. *Crit Care Med*. 2017;45(6):e620–e621.

63. Trevick S, Lord A, Trevick SA, Lord AS. Post-traumatic stress disorder and complicated grief are common in caregivers of neuro-ICU patients. *Neurocrit Care*. 2017;26(3):436–443.

64. Trochelman K, Albert N, Spence J, Murray T, Slifcak E. Patients and their families weigh in on evidence-based hospital design. *Crit Care Nurse*. 2012;32(1):e1–e11.

65. Turner-Cobb JM, Smith PC, Ramchandani P, et al. The acute psychobiological impact of the intensive care experience on relatives. *Psychol Health Med*. 2016;21(1):20–26.

66. van de Pol I, van Iterson M, Maaskant J. Effect of nocturnal sound reduction on the incidence of delirium in intensive care unit patients: An interrupted time series analysis. *Intensive Crit Care Nurs*. 2017;41:18–25.

67. Villa P, Pintado MC, Luján J, et al. Functional status and quality of life in elderly intensive care unit survivors. *J Am Geriatr Soc*. 2016;64(3):536–542.

68. White DB, Angus DC, Shields AM, et al. A randomized trial of a family-support intervention in intensive care units. *N Eng J Med*. 2018;378(25):2365–2375.

69. Wright L, Leahey M. *A Guide to Family Assessment & Intervention*. 2nd ed. Philadelphia, PA: F.A. Davis; 1984.

70. Wu KK, Cho VW, Chow FL, Tsang APY. Posttraumatic stress after treatment in an intensive care unit. *East Asian Arch Psychiat*. 2018;28(2):39–44.

71. Zaken ZB. Needs of relatives of surgical patients: Perceptions of relatives and medical staff. *MEDSURG Nurs*. 2018;27(2):110–116.

Ethical and Legal Issues in Critical Care Nursing

Jayne M. Willis, MSN, RN, NEA-BC, CENP
Kathleen Black, MSN, RN, NE-BC

Many additional resources, including self-assessment exercises, are located on the Evolve companion website at http://evolve.elsevier.com/Sole/.
- Animations
- Clinical Skills: Critical Care Collections
- Student Review Questions
- Video Clips

INTRODUCTION

Critical care nurses are often confronted with ethical and legal dilemmas related to informed consent, withholding or withdrawing life-sustaining treatment, organ and tissue transplantation, confidentiality, and increasingly, justice in the distribution of healthcare resources. Many dilemmas are byproducts of advanced medical technologies and therapies developed over the past several decades. Although technology provides substantial benefits to critically ill patients, extensive public and professional debate occurs over the appropriate use of these technologies, especially those that are life sustaining. One of the primary concerns in critical care is whether a patient's values and beliefs about treatment can be overridden by the technological imperative, or the strong tendency to use technology because it is available.

Although many ethical dilemmas are not unique to critical care, they occur with greater frequency in critical care settings. Therefore it is crucial that critical care nurses examine the nature and scope of their ethical and legal obligations to patients.

The ethical and legal issues that frequently arise in the nursing care of acute and critically ill patients are examined in this chapter. The discussion includes problems that surround patients' rights and nurses' obligations, informed consent, and withholding and withdrawing treatment. The elements of ethical decision making and the involvement of the nurse are discussed.

ETHICAL OBLIGATIONS AND NURSE ADVOCACY

Critical care nurses' ethical and legal responsibilities for patient care have increased dramatically since the early 1990s. Evolving case law and current concepts of nurse advocacy and accountability indicate that nurses have substantial ethical and legal obligations to promote and protect the welfare of their patients.

The duty to practice ethically and to serve as an ethical agent on behalf of patients is an integral part of nurses' professional practice. The nurse's duty is stated in the *Code of Ethics for Nurses With Interpretive Statements,* which was adopted by the American Nurses Association (ANA) in 1976 and last revised in 2015 in response to the complexities of modern nursing and in anticipation of healthcare advances.[6] The document describes the moral principles that guide professional nursing practice and serves the following purposes: (1) it delineates the ethical obligations and duties of every individual who enters the profession; (2) it is the profession's nonnegotiable ethical standard; and (3) it is the expression of nursing's own understanding of its commitment to society.[5]

The Code of Ethics consists of nine provision statements. The first three describe fundamental values and commitments of the nurse, the next three describe the boundaries of duty and loyalty, and the final three describe duties beyond individual patient encounters. The interpretive statements of the Code provide specific guidance in applying each provision to current nursing practice. Nurses in all practice arenas, including critical care, must be knowledgeable about the provisions of the code and incorporate its basic tenets into their clinical practice.[13] The Code is a powerful tool that shapes and evaluates individual practice and the nursing profession. However, situations may arise in which the Code provides only limited direction. Critical care nurses must remain knowledgeable and abreast of ethical issues and changes in the literature so that they may make appropriate decisions when difficult clinical situations arise. Additional ANA position statements related to human rights and ethics are available on the ANA website (http://www.nursingworld.org).

Ethics are an important part of everyday nursing practice. Critical care nurses must have the knowledge, skills, and tools to uphold their professional values. Fifty nursing leaders came together to strongly support basic ethical values and principles and more effectively enable nurses' ethical practice. The meeting resulted in the release of *A Blueprint for 21st Century Nursing Ethics: Report of the National Nursing Summit.* This blueprint covers issues including weighing personal risk with professional responsibilities and moral courage to expose deficiencies in care. The report makes both overarching and specific recommendations in four key areas: clinical practice, nursing education, nursing research, and nursing policy. The blueprint can be accessed at http://www.bioethicsinstitute.org/nursing-ethics-summit-report.[25]

Nurses' ethical obligation to serve as advocates for their patients is derived from the unique nature of the nurse-patient relationship. Critical care nurses assume a significant caregiving role that is characterized by intimate, extended contact with persons who are often the most physiologically and psychologically vulnerable and with their families. Critical care nurses have a moral and professional responsibility to act as advocates on their patients' behalf because of their unique relationship with their patients and their specialized nursing knowledge. The American Association of Critical-Care Nurses (AACN) mission, vision, and values are framed within an ethic of care and ethical principles.[1] An ethic of care is a moral orientation that acknowledges the interrelatedness and interdependence of individuals, systems, and society. When ethical care is practiced, individual uniqueness, personal relationships, and the dynamic nature of life are respected. Compassion, collaboration, accountability, and trust are essential characteristics of ethical nursing practice.[1]

AACN ethics resources are available on the organization's website (https://www.aacn.org/clinical-resources/ethics-moral-distress#).

> **❓ CRITICAL REASONING ACTIVITY**
>
> You are taking care of Mrs. H., a 90-year-old patient with gastrointestinal bleeding. She has developed numerous complications and requires mechanical ventilation. She is unresponsive to nurses and family members. She has been in the hospital for 2 weeks and requires a transfusion nearly every day to sustain adequate hemoglobin and hematocrit levels. Her prognosis is poor. Before this hospitalization, she lived independently in her own home. Her children tell you they are tired of seeing their mother suffer. How do you respond to the family, and what follow-up do you perform?

ETHICAL DECISION MAKING

As reflected in the ANA Code of Ethics, one of the primary ethical obligations of professional nurses is protection of their patients' basic rights. This obligation requires nurses to recognize ethical dilemmas that actually or potentially threaten patients' rights and to participate in the resolution of those dilemmas.

An ethical dilemma is a difficult problem or situation in which conflicts arise during the process of making morally justifiable decisions. In the critical care setting, ethical principles may have competing priorities. For example, *autonomy*–respect for individual decision making may be in direct conflict with *maleficence*–do no harm or beneficence–do good. When these conflicts occur, ethical dilemmas can arise for the healthcare team.[22] In identifying a situation as an ethical dilemma, certain criteria must be met. More than one solution must exist, and there is no clear "right" or "wrong." Each solution must carry equal weight and must be ethically defensible. Whether to give the one available critical care bed to a patient with cancer who is experiencing hypotension after chemotherapy or to a patient in the emergency department who has an acute myocardial infarction is an example of an ethical dilemma. The conflicting issue in this example is which patient should be given the bed, based on the moral allocation of limited resources.

Several warning signs can assist the critical care nurse in recognizing an ethical dilemma. If these warning signs occur, the critical care nurse must reassess the situation and determine whether an ethical dilemma exists and what additional actions are needed.[26]

- Is the situation emotionally charged?
- Has the patient's condition changed significantly?
- Is there confusion or conflict about the facts?
- Is there increased hesitancy about the right course of action?
- Is the proposed action a deviation from customary practice?
- Is there a perceived need for secrecy around the proposed action?

Arriving at a morally justifiable decision when an ethical dilemma exists can be difficult for patients, families, and health professionals. Critical care nurses must be careful not to impose their own value system on that of the patient. Each patient and family has a set of personal values that are influenced by their environment and culture.

One helpful way to approach ethical decision making is to use a systematic, structured process, such as the one depicted in Fig. 3.1. This model provides a framework for evaluating the related ethical principles and the potential outcomes, as well as relevant facts concerning the contextual factors and the patient's physiological and personal factors. Using this approach, the patient, family, and healthcare team members evaluate choices and identify the option that promotes the patient's best interests.

Ethical decision making includes implementing the decision and evaluating the short-term and long-term outcomes. Evaluation provides meaningful feedback about decisions and actions in specific instances, as well as about the effectiveness of the decision-making process. The final stage in the decision-making process is assessing whether the decision in a specific case can be applied to other dilemmas in similar circumstances. In other words, is this decision useful in similar cases? A systematic approach to decision making does not guarantee that morally justifiable decisions are reached or that the outcome is beneficial to the patient. However, it ensures that all applicable information is considered in the decision.

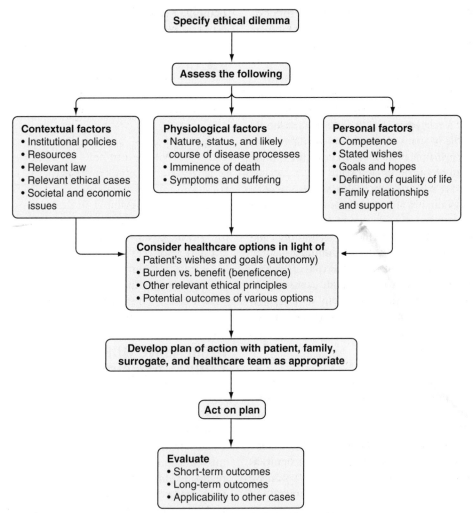

Fig. 3.1 The process of ethical decision making.

STUDY BREAK

1. Which of the following statements regarding the American Nurses Association (ANA) *Code of Ethics for Nurses With Interpretive Statements* is TRUE?
   A. The Code of Ethics delineates the ethical obligation of every nurse who enters the profession.
   B. The Code of Ethics expresses nurses' understanding of their commitment to society.
   C. One of the primary ethical obligations for nurses is to protect patients' basic rights.
   D. All the above.

❓ CRITICAL REASONING ACTIVITY

You are taking care of Mr. J., a 23-year-old man with a closed head injury. During the night shift, you note a change in the level of consciousness at 3:00 AM. You call the physician, who tells you to watch Mr. J. until the physician attends rounds the next morning. He tells you not to call him again. Mr. J.'s neurological status continues to deteriorate. What actions do you take? What is the rationale for your actions?

ETHICAL PRINCIPLES

As reflected in the decision-making model, relevant ethical principles are considered when a moral dilemma exists

(Box 3.1). These principles are intended to provide respect and dignity for all persons.

Principlism is a widely applied ethical approach based on four fundamental moral principles related to contemporary ethical dilemmas: respect for autonomy, beneficence, nonmaleficence, and justice.[9] The principle of *autonomy* states that all persons should be free to govern their lives to the greatest degree possible. The autonomy principle implies a strong sense of

BOX 3.1 Ethical Principles

- **Autonomy:** Respect for the individual and the ability of individuals to make decisions about their own health and future (the basis for the practice of informed consent)
- **Beneficence:** Actions intended to benefit the patients or others
- **Nonmaleficence:** Actions intended not to harm or bring harm to others
- **Justice:** Being fair or just to the wider community in terms of the consequences of an action; in health care, justice is described as the fair allocation or distribution of healthcare resources
- **Veracity:** The obligation to tell the truth
- **Fidelity:** The moral duty to be faithful to the commitments that one makes to others
- **Confidentiality:** Respect for an individual's autonomy and the right of individuals to control the information relating to their own health

self-determination and an acceptance of responsibility for one's own choices and actions. To respect the autonomy of others means to respect their freedom of choice and to allow them to make their own decisions.

The principle of *beneficence* is the duty to provide benefits to others when in a position to do so and to help balance harms and benefits. In other words, the benefits of an action should outweigh the burdens. A related concept is *futility*. Care should not be given if it is futile in terms of improving comfort or the medical outcome. The principle of *nonmaleficence* is the explicit duty not to inflict harm on others intentionally.

The principle of *justice* requires that healthcare resources be distributed fairly and equitably among groups of people. The principle of justice is particularly relevant to critical care because most healthcare resources, including technology and pharmaceuticals, are expended in this practice setting.

Other principles are also relevant. The principle of *veracity* states that persons are obligated to tell the truth in their communication with others. The principle of *fidelity* requires that one has a moral duty to be faithful to the commitments made to others. These two principles, along with *confidentiality*, are key to the nurse-patient relationship.

Creating an Ethical Environment

Critical care nurses and their leadership focus on nursing initiatives at the unit, service line, and organizational levels to improve quality, patient satisfaction, and nursing retention. The AACN's Healthy Work Environment Initiative and the American Nurses Credentialing Center (ANCC) Magnet Recognition Program assist critical care nursing teams to create a positive and fulfilling organizational culture through engagement and empowerment.[3,7] Both programs allow nurses to promote, plan, and develop an ethical environment in which to practice.

Addressing ethical problems and participating in ethical decision making are key to improving quality of care. Interdisciplinary collaboration and collegial working relationships that generate mutual respect are important elements of a successful critical care team. Hospitals that are pursuing or achieve Magnet certification must demonstrate evidence of creating ethical work environments by meeting specific criteria. Box 3.2 lists

---

BOX 3.2   Examples of Evidence to Support ANCC Magnet Recognition Criteria

- Evidence that nurses are educated through ongoing education in:
  - Application of ethical principles
  - ANA Bill of Rights for Registered Nurses
  - Professional organization standards
  - State nurse practice act
  - ANA Code of Ethics for Nurses
- Policies and procedures that address how nurses respond to ethical issues
- Descriptions of how nurses lead in development of and participation in ethics programs
- Evidence that nurses have been educated in research and protection of human subjects and in patient privacy, security, and confidentiality
- Evidence of direct care nurses' participation on the ethics committees

ANA, American Nurses Association; *ANCC,* American Nurses Credentialing Center.

---

examples of evidence required to support ANCC Magnet criteria related to ethical work environments.[7]

? CRITICAL REASONING ACTIVITY

It is 2 days later, and Mr. J., described earlier, now has a herniated brainstem and is declared brain dead but remains on life support. His wife is at the bedside and is fully aware of the situation. You do not know whether Mr. J. signed an organ donor card. What are your ethical and legal obligations regarding organ donation at this point? How would you approach the situation?

STUDY BREAK

2. The ethical principle that refers to the patient's right to informed consent is:
   - A. Autonomy
   - B. Veracity
   - C. Justice
   - D. Beneficence

INCREASING NURSES' INVOLVEMENT IN ETHICAL DECISION MAKING

Although nurses play a significant role in the care of patients, they often report limited involvement in the formal processes of ethical decision making. Nurses' perception of this limited involvement may be related to many factors, such as lack of formal education in ethics, lack of institutional mechanisms for review of dilemmas, perceived lack of administrative or peer support for involvement in decision making, concern about reprisals, and perceived lack of decision-making authority. Research has shown that ethics education has a significant positive influence on moral confidence, moral action, and use of ethics resources by nurses.[15] If nurses are to fulfill their advocacy obligations to patients, they must become active in the process of ethical decision making at all levels.

Moral Distress and Moral Resilience

Ethical dilemmas are among the many issues that can lead to *moral distress* for critical care nurses. Moral distress occurs when the nurse knows the ethically appropriate action to take but is unable to act on it or when the nurse acts in a manner contrary to personal and professional values.[20] Moral distress is one of the key issues affecting the workplace environment. Healthy, thriving work environments are eroded when critical care nurses experience unanswered moral distress. Consequences of moral distress are well documented. Nurses with moral distress are sick more often, suffer burnout, and disengage from their work environment, leading to increased turnover and even career changes.[19] Professional nursing and healthcare organizations are addressing the challenges of ethical incongruency by building moral resilience. *Moral resilience* is defined as the ability of nurses to rebalance and resolve ethical incongruency both personally and organizationally when faced with ethical dilemmas.[24] Personal and organizational strategies are needed to assist critical care nurses to address ethical situations in their practice.[27] Box 3.3 lists personal strategies to nurture and grow moral resilience in nursing practice.[27]

Mechanisms to Address Ethical Concerns

A critical element for true collaboration is that healthcare organizations ensure unrestricted access to structured forums such as ethics committees and allow time to resolve disputes among critical participants, including patients, families, and the healthcare team.[3] Actively addressing ethical dilemmas and avoiding moral distress are crucial factors in creating a healthy workplace in which critical care nurses can make optimal contributions to patients and their families.

The Joint Commission requires that a formal mechanism be in place to address patients' ethical concerns. Bioethics committees are one way to address this need. Typical membership of a bioethics committee includes physicians, nurses, chaplains, social workers, and, if available, bioethicists. A multiprofessional committee can serve as an educational and policy-making body and, in some cases, provide ethics consultation on a case-by-case basis. The purpose of ethics consultation is to improve the process and outcomes of patient care by helping to identify, analyze, and resolve ethical problems. This service should be used when the issues cannot be resolved among the healthcare team, patient, and family. Box 3.4 lists examples of situations in which an ethics consultation may be considered.

Nurses can become more involved with ethical decision making through participation in institutional ethics committees, multiprofessional ethics forums and roundtables, peer review and quality improvement committees, and institutional research review boards. Nurses can also improve and update their knowledge through formal and continuing education courses on bioethics, as well as through telephone and computerized electronic consultation and reference services. Educational programs and ethics consultation services are available through several ethics and law centers in the United States. Three important ethical consultation services are listed in Box 3.5. Additional online educational resources are listed in Box 3.6.

❓ CRITICAL REASONING ACTIVITY

You are caring for Mrs. M., a 68-year-old woman with an acute myocardial infarction. She is in the critical care unit after a successful angioplasty. Her husband brought in her living will, which states that Mrs. M. does not desire resuscitation. Mrs. M. is pain free and alert. As you start your beginning-of-shift assessment, Mrs. M. says, "You know, now that I've made it through the angioplasty, I realize that tubes and machines may not be so bad after all. I haven't made it this far to give up now. If I go into cardiac arrest, I want you to do all that you can for me." What ethical principle is Mrs. M. using? As her nurse, what actions should you take and why?

BOX 3.3 Critical Care Nurse Strategies to Promote and Sustain Moral Resilience

- Advocate with courage for patients
- Trust your personal value system
- Foster your spirituality
- Show self-confidence in your knowledge
- Cultivate your own moral compass and practice it
- Practice reflective review of moral decisions and actions
- Champion and support colleagues facing ethical dilemmas
- Seek assistance from colleagues for ethical dilemmas
- Develop personal care strategies to promote mental health
- Build communication skills
- Know and live the ANA Code of Ethics
- Know organizational resources
- Embrace mentorship

Modified from Stutzer K, Bylone M. Building moral resilience. *Crit Care Nurse.* 2018;38(1):77–89.

BOX 3.4 Situations in Which Ethics Consultation May Be Considered

- Disagreement or conflict exists on whether to pursue aggressive life-sustaining treatment, such as cardiopulmonary resuscitation, in a seriously ill patient or to emphasize comfort and palliative care
- The family demands life-sustaining treatment, such as mechanical ventilation or tube feeding, which the physician and nurses consider futile
- Competing family members are present and want to make critical decisions on behalf of the patient
- A seriously ill patient is incapacitated and does not have a surrogate decision maker or an advance directive

---

BOX 3.5 Ethics Consultation Services

American Nurses Association Center for Ethics and Human Rights
8515 Georgia Avenue, Suite 400
Silver Spring, MD 20910
http://nursingworld.org/ethics/

Johns Hopkins Berman Institute of Bioethics
Deering Hall
1809 Ashland Avenue
Baltimore, MD 21205
http://www.bioethics.jhu.edu

Kennedy Institute of Ethics
Georgetown University
3700 O Street NW
Washington, DC 20057-1212
https://kennedyinstitute.georgetown.edu/

BOX 3.6 Internet Resources for Bioethics

- *American Journal of Bioethics:* http://www.bioethics.net
- American Society for Bioethics and Humanities: http://www.asbh.org
- Department of Medical Ethics & Health Policy–University of Pennsylvania: http://www.bioethics.upenn.edu
- National Institutes of Health Department of Bioethics: http://www.bioethics.nih.gov

SELECTED ETHICAL TOPICS IN CRITICAL CARE

Informed Consent

Many complex dilemmas in critical care nursing concern informed consent. Consent problems arise because patients are experiencing acute, life-threatening illnesses that interfere with their ability to make decisions about treatment or participation in a clinical research study. The doctrine of informed consent is based on the principle of autonomy; competent adults have the right to self-determination or to make decisions regarding their acceptance or rejection of treatment.

Elements of Informed Consent. Three primary elements must be present for a person's consent or decline of medical treatment or research participation to be considered valid: competence, voluntariness, and disclosure of information. Competence (or *capacity*) refers to a person's ability to understand information regarding a proposed medical or nursing treatment. *Competence* is a legal term and is determined in court. Healthcare providers evaluate mental capacity. The ability of patients to understand relevant information is an essential prerequisite to their participation in the decision-making process and should be carefully evaluated as part of the informed consent process. Patients providing informed consent should be free from severe pain and depression. Critically ill patients usually do not have the mental capacity to provide informed consent because of the severe nature of their illness or their treatment (e.g., sedation). If the patient is not mentally capable of providing consent, informed consent is obtained from the designated healthcare surrogate or legal authorized representative (proxy). State law governs consent issues, and legal counsel should be consulted for specific questions.

Consent must be given voluntarily, without coercion or fraud, for the consent to be legally binding. This includes freedom from pressure from family members, healthcare providers, and payers. Persons who consent should base their decision on sufficient knowledge. Basic information considered necessary for decision making includes the following:

- A diagnosis of the patient's specific health problem and condition
- The nature, duration, and purpose of the proposed treatment or procedures
- The probable outcome of any medical or nursing intervention
- The benefits of medical or nursing interventions
- The potential risks that are generally considered common or hazardous
- Alternative treatments and their feasibility
- Short-term and long-term prognoses if the proposed treatment or treatments are not provided

Informed consent is not a form. It is a *process* that entails the exchange of information between the healthcare provider and the patient or patient's proxy. Frequently, critical care nurses are asked to witness the consent process for procedures and tests. Critical care nurses should serve as advocates for the patient and ensure that the informed consent process has been completed per legal standards and institutional policy. Critical care nurses may provide additional patient education to support decision making, but the process of obtaining informed consent is a physician obligation.

Decisions Regarding Life-Sustaining Treatment

Care of persons who are terminally ill or in a persistent vegetative state raises profound questions about the constitutional rights of persons or surrogates to make decisions related to death or life-sustaining care, as well as the rights of the state to intervene in treatment decisions. Table 3.1 reviews three landmark legal cases—Quinlan, Cruzan, and Schiavo—that have influenced legal and ethical precedents in the right-to-die debate. Table 3.2 lists definitions for some terms pertinent to these issues.

The issue of treatment for persons whose quality of life is severely compromised, as in irreversible coma or brain death, is often a result of advanced biomedical technology. Technology frequently sustains life in persons who would have previously died of their illnesses. The widespread use of advanced life-support systems and cardiopulmonary resuscitation (CPR) has changed the nature and context of dying. A "natural death" in the traditional sense is rare; most patients who die in healthcare facilities undergo resuscitation efforts.

The benefits derived from aggressive technological management often outweigh the negative effects, but the use of life-sustaining technologies for persons with severely impaired quality of life, or for those who are terminally ill, has stimulated intensive debate and litigation. Two key issues in this debate are the appropriate use of technology and the ability of the seriously ill person to retain decision-making rights. These issues are based on the ethical principles of beneficence and autonomy.

At the heart of the technology controversy are conflicting beliefs about the morality and legality of allowing persons who are terminally ill or severely debilitated to request withdrawing or withholding medical treatment. In these situations, two levels of treatment must be considered: ordinary care and extraordinary care. These levels of care are at two ends of a continuum of potential treatment options. Based on one's beliefs, some therapies fit either category; however, this distinction is still helpful from a legal and ethical perspective. Ethicists believe that any treatment can become extraordinary whenever the patient decides that the burdens outweigh the benefits.

The concept of medical futility is moving to the forefront of the end-of-life debate. Judgment regarding futility in the critical care setting is difficult because it differs greatly among cultures and disciplines. Each goal is then evaluated based on what is achievable or deemed "futile." Debate over futility of specific treatments is essentially a debate on quality of life and which treatments are worthwhile to assist patients in achieving their goals. The cost of health care and the push toward major healthcare reform are generating public discussion regarding the financial effect of medical treatments at the end-of-life. Discussion on the economics of treatments is as uncomfortable in the United States as talking about death. This topic has not played a major role in end-of-life decision making in the past,

TABLE 3.1 Landmark Legal Cases in the Right-to-Die Debate

Case	Events	Impact
Karen Quinlan	Karen Ann Quinlan was the first modern icon of the right-to-die debate. The 21-year-old Quinlan collapsed at a party after swallowing alcohol and the tranquilizer diazepam (Valium) on April 14, 1975. Doctors saved her life, but she suffered brain damage and lapsed into a "persistent vegetative state." Her family waged a much-publicized legal battle for the right to remove her life-support machinery. They succeeded, but in a final twist, Quinlan kept breathing after the respirator was unplugged. She remained in a coma for almost 10 years in a New Jersey nursing home until her death in 1985.	In finding for the Quinlan family, the courts identified a right to decline life-saving medical treatment under the general right of privacy. According to the court, Quinlan's right to privacy outweighed the state's interest in preserving her life, and her father, as her surrogate, could exercise that right for her.
Nancy Cruzan	Nancy Cruzan became a public figure after a 1983 auto accident left her permanently unconscious and without any higher brain function. She was kept alive only by a feeding tube and steady medical care. Cruzan's family waged a legal battle to have her feeding tube removed. The case went all the way to the U.S. Supreme Court, which ruled that the Cruzans had not provided "clear and convincing evidence" that Nancy Cruzan did not wish to have her life artificially preserved. The Cruzans later presented such evidence to the Missouri courts, which ruled in their favor in late 1990. The Cruzans stopped feeding Nancy in December 1990, and she died later the same month.	The Cruzan case had a significant effect on end-of-life decision making across the country. After the Cruzan decision, the Patient Self-Determination Act was passed by Congress to allow individuals to make their own decisions about end-of-life care and routine care, should they be unable to make decisions for themselves. The case prompted the development of hospital ethics councils and increased the number of advance directives.
Theresa Schiavo	Theresa Marie "Terri" Schiavo was a Florida woman who sustained brain damage and became dependent on a feeding tube. She collapsed in her home in 1990 and experienced respiratory and cardiac arrest, leading to 15 years of institutionalization and a diagnosis of persistent vegetative state. In 1998 her husband, who was her guardian, petitioned the court to remove her feeding tube. Terri Schiavo's parents opposed the removal, arguing that Terri was conscious. The court determined that Terri would not wish to continue life-prolonging measures. Subsequently a 7-year battle occurred that included involvement by politicians and advocacy groups. Before the court's decision was carried out on March 18, 2005, the Florida legislature and the United States Congress had passed laws to prevent removal of Schiavo's feeding tube. These laws were later overturned by the Supreme Courts of Florida and the United States. On March 31, 2005, after a complex legal history in the courts, Terri Schiavo died at a Florida hospice at the age of 41.	This case received national and international media attention with public debate regarding the moral consequences of withdrawing life support. The movement to challenge the decisions made for Schiavo threatened to destabilize end-of-life law that had developed principally through the cases of Quinlan and Cruzan. Although the Schiavo case had little effect on right-to-die jurisprudence, it illustrated the range of difficulties that can complicate decision making concerning the termination of treatment in incapacitated persons and the importance of having written advance directives.

but experts agree it is moving up the line of priorities in medical futility debates.[18]

Traditionally, extraordinary care includes complex, invasive, and experimental treatments such as resuscitation efforts by CPR or emergency cardiac care, maintenance of life support through invasive means, or renal dialysis. Experimental treatments such as gene therapy also are extraordinary therapies.

Ordinary care involves common, noninvasive, tested treatments such as providing nutrition, hydration, or antibiotic therapy. In the critical care setting the noninvasive criterion does not apply; *ordinary care* is defined as usual and customary for the patient's condition. Maintenance of hydration and nutrition through a tube feeding is an example of a treatment that falls somewhere between ordinary and extraordinary care and is a debatable issue. Therefore it is important for individuals to document their wishes rather than rely on the members of the healthcare team to assist in the decision-making process related to nutrition and hydration.

Cardiopulmonary Resuscitation Decisions. The goals of resuscitation are to preserve life, restore health, relieve suffering, limit disability, and respect the individual's decision, rights, and privacy.[4] Frequently, ethical questions arise about the use of CPR and emergency cardiac care because such treatment may conflict with a patient's desires or best interests. The critical care nurse should be guided by scientifically proven data, patient preferences, and ethical and cultural norms.

The American Heart Association has developed guidelines to assist practitioners in making the difficult decision to provide or withhold emergency cardiovascular care.[4] The generally accepted position is that resuscitation should cease if the physician determines that efforts are futile or hopeless. Futility constitutes sufficient reason for either withholding or ceasing extraordinary treatments.

Withholding or stopping extraordinary resuscitation efforts is ethically and legally appropriate if patients or surrogates have previously made their preferences known through *advance directives*. It is also acceptable if the physician determines that resuscitation is futile or has discussed the situation with the patient, family, or surrogate as appropriate and there is mutual agreement not to resuscitate in the event of cardiopulmonary arrest. For the nurse not to initiate the resuscitation, a *do not resuscitate* (DNR) order must be written. Most physicians also write supporting documentation regarding the order

TABLE 3.2   Definitions in Critical Care Decision Making

Concept	Definition
Advance directive	Witnessed written document or oral statement in which instructions are given by a person to express desires related to healthcare decisions. The directive may include, but is not limited to, the designation of a healthcare surrogate, a living will, or an anatomical gift.
Living will	A witnessed written document or oral statement voluntarily executed by a person that expresses the person's instructions concerning life-prolonging procedures.
Healthcare decision	Informed consent, refusal of consent, or withdrawal of consent for health care, unless stated in the advance directive.
Incapacity or incompetent decision	Patient is physically or mentally unable to communicate a willful and knowing healthcare decision.
Informed consent	Consent voluntarily given after a sufficient explanation and disclosure of information.
Proxy	A competent adult who has not been expressly designated to make healthcare decisions for an incapacitated person but is authorized by state statute to make healthcare decisions for the person.
Surrogate	A competent adult designated by a person to make healthcare decisions should that person become incapacitated.
Terminal condition	A condition in which there is no reasonable medical probability of recovery and that can be expected to cause death without treatment.
Persistent vegetative state	A permanent, irreversible unconsciousness condition that demonstrates an absence of voluntary action or cognitive behavior or an inability to communicate or interact purposefully with the environment.
Brain death	Complete and irreversible cessation of brain function.
Clinical death or cardiac death	Irreversible cessation of spontaneous ventilation and circulation.
Life-prolonging procedure	Any medical procedure or treatment, including sustenance and hydration, that sustains, restores, or supplants a spontaneous vital function. Does not include the administration of medications or treatments deemed necessary to provide comfort care or to alleviate pain.
Resuscitation	Intervention with the intent of preserving life, restoring health, or reversing clinical death.
Do not resuscitate (DNR) order	A medical order that prohibits the use of cardiopulmonary resuscitation and emergency cardiac care to reverse signs of clinical death. The DNR order may or may not be specified in patients' advance directives.
Physician Orders for Life-Sustaining Treatment (POLST)	The POLST form is a medical order indicating a patient's wishes regarding treatments that are commonly used in a medical crisis. The POLST complements the advance directive; it is not intended to replace it.
Allow natural death	An alternate term with less negative connotations but essentially meaning DNR.

Adapted from The Florida Senate. 2018 Florida Statutes, 765.101, http://www.flsenate.gov/Laws/Statutes/. Published August 2018. Accessed March 3, 2019.

in the progress notes, such as conversations held with the patient and family members. Additional information is provided in Chapter 4.

Family presence during resuscitation and invasive procedures has been a debated topic for the last decade. There is growing evidence that family presence during resuscitation and invasive procedures helps not only families but also the healthcare team.[2,12] Family presence during resuscitation and invasive procedures is supported by professional organizations, including the Emergency Nurses Association, the AACN, and the American Heart Association. A large, multisite, descripted study found no differences in implementation of resuscitation events with and without the family present.[14] Current recommendations are for institutions to establish a process for allowing families who wish to be present to do so. This includes designating a trained clinician or chaplain to support the family throughout the process.

Withholding or Withdrawing Life Support. Withholding life support, withdrawing life support, or both can range from not initiating hemodialysis (withholding) to terminal weaning from mechanical ventilation (withdrawing). Decisions are made based on consideration of all factors in the ethical decision-making model. In all instances of withholding and

withdrawing life support, comfort measures are maintained, including management of pain, pulmonary secretions, and other symptoms as needed.

Most decisions regarding withdrawing and withholding of life support are not made in the courts. They are made based on open communication with the patient, family, and surrogate, as appropriate. An ethical decision-making approach is used to decide on the best actions to take or not take in the situation. If ethical or legal questions arise, ethics consultation services, ethics committees, and risk managers can provide assistance. The value of clearly stating in writing one's end-of-life issues before becoming critically ill (advance directive) is key to avoiding having treatment given or not given against one's wishes.

End-of-Life Issues

Patient Self-Determination Act. In response to public concern about end-of-life decisions and the overall lack of consistent hospital policies, the United States Congress enacted the Patient Self-Determination Act.[21] This Act requires that all healthcare facilities that receive Medicare and Medicaid funding inform their patients about their right to initiate an advance directive and the right to consent to or refuse medical treatment.

Discussions regarding advance directives and end-of-life wishes should be made as early as possible, preferably before death is imminent. The ideal time to discuss advance directives is when a person is relatively healthy, not in the critical care or hospital setting. This allows more time for discussion, processing, and decision making. Assess patients regarding their perceptions of quality of life and end-of-life wishes in a caring and culturally sensitive way and document the patient's wishes in the medical record. Encourage patients to complete advance directives, including living wills and durable power of attorney, to ensure that their wishes will be followed if they are terminally ill or in a persistent vegetative state.

Advance Directives. An *advance directive* is a communication that specifies a person's preference about medical treatment should that person become incapacitated. Several types of advance directives exist, including DNR orders, allow-a-natural-death orders, living wills, healthcare proxies, and other legal documents (see Table 3.2). It is important for nurses to know whether a patient has an advance directive and that the directive be followed. To enhance advance directives and ensure common conversation and language, the Physician Orders for Life-Sustaining Treatment (POLST) has been promoted in many states. The POLST form is a medical order indicating a patient's wishes regarding treatments that are commonly used in a medical crisis. The POLST complements the advance directive and is not intended to replace it. The goal of POLST is a conversation with an emphasis on advanced care planning, shared decision making, and ensuring that a patient's end-of-life wishes are honored. Not all states participate in the POLST initiative. More information can be found in Chapter 4 and at http://www.POLST.org.

The *living will* provides a mechanism by which individuals can authorize the withholding of specific treatments if they become incapacitated. Although living wills provide direction to caregivers, in some states living wills are not legally binding and are advisory. When completing a living will, individuals can add special instructions about end-of-life wishes. Individuals can change their directive at any time.

The *durable power of attorney for health care* is more protective of patients' interests regarding medical treatment than is the living will. With a durable power of attorney for health care, patients legally designate an agent whom they trust, such as a family member or friend, to make decisions on their behalf should they become incapacitated. This person is called the *healthcare surrogate* or proxy. A durable power of attorney for health care allows the surrogate to make decisions whenever the patient is incapacitated, not just at the time of terminal illness. Some legal commentators recommend the joint use of a living will and a durable power of attorney to give added protection to a person's preferences about medical treatment.

Ultimately, if self-determination and informed consent are to have real value, patients or their surrogates must be given an opportunity to consider options and to shape decisions that affect their life or death. Communication and shared decision making among the patient, family, and healthcare team regarding end-of-life issues are key.[16] Unfortunately, this frequently does not happen before admission to a critical care unit. The critical care nurse must be part of the team that educates the patient and family so that they can determine and communicate end-of-life wishes.

Some situations may result in moral distress for the nurse. A nurse who is unable to follow these legal documents because of personal or religious beliefs must ask to have the client reassigned to another nurse. For instance, some advance directives may call for withdrawing life support when certain conditions are met, and this may conflict with the nurse's personal or religious beliefs. Nurses who frequently ask to be reassigned to another client may need to consider another nursing specialty in which their beliefs do not conflict with advance directives.

The nurse must also be cognizant of the facility's policies regarding advance directives. For example, if a DNR order is on the chart, does it meet all requirements for a legal document per facility policy? Is it signed by the physician? Is the chart notated properly? Is there a healthcare proxy? Are the forms proper? Is there a living will? All critical care nurses should review key policies and documents related to DNR and withdrawing and withholding life support, because these situations occur frequently. Knowledge of institutional policies will facilitate honoring the patients' and families' wishes in a compassionate and caring environment.

? CRITICAL REASONING ACTIVITY

You are the charge nurse of a nine-bed critical care unit. You have one open bed. The house supervisor calls and tells you that there are two patients who need a critical care bed. The first is a 23-year-old woman currently in the operating room after multiple trauma. The second patient is a 78-year-old man who is in the emergency department with severe septic shock. According to the supervisor, both patients are going to need mechanical ventilation and inotropic therapy. What are your decisions and actions at this point? On what ethical principles are your actions based?

STUDY BREAK
3. Which of the following is NOT an example of a patient's healthcare advance directive?
   A. A living will
   B. Determination of a healthcare surrogate
   C. Organ donation designation
   D. Physicians Orders for Life-Sustaining Treatment (POLST)

Aid in Dying. *Aid in dying* (AID) is a term used to describe allowing qualified terminally ill patients who have the capacity to make decisions to take a lethal dose of oral medication to end their own lives.[11] *Physician-assisted suicide, death with dignity,* and *assisted death* are other terms used to refer to competent patients intentionally choosing the time and circumstances of their death. As of 2018, AID is legal in eight jurisdictions in the United States. Critical care nurses must know the intricacies of the nurse's role in AID and differentiate this from removal of nonbeneficial treatments. The key difference between withdrawal of nonbeneficial treatments and AID is that AID is intended to cause death, whereas withdrawal of nonbeneficial treatments and the accompanying sedation are intended to relieve suffering and to allow natural death. It is within the scope of practice for critical care nurses to administer medications to terminally ill patients (or authorized surrogates) who have chosen compassionate extubation. Titrating pain medications and sedatives to ease suffering during removal of the endotracheal tube is not considered euthanasia if the patient stops breathing and is considered ethical and legal in that context.[23] This is an example of the doctrine of double effect, which states that if a planned action has a known, negative adverse effect, it is ethical to act as long as the adverse effect is not the intended goal of the planned action.[28] Administering medications in this context is different from AID.

In states where AID is legal, the patient must have decision-making capacity and must initiate the process of AID. The surrogate is not authorized to make the decision on the patient's behalf, and the nurse cannot administer the prescribed medications with the intent to expedite death. The patient must prepare and self-administer the lethal medications. The ANA adopted a position paper that advocates against nurse involvement in assisted suicide and euthanasia, citing that these practices are in direct conflict with the Code of Ethics.[6] It is illegal and outside the scope of practice for a nurse to administer medications with the intent to hasten death. Critical care nurses in states where AID is legal should be well informed of the state laws and their organization's policies in anticipation of patients asking questions about AID. Healthcare providers may not start conversations about AID and may only respond to questions if the terminally ill patient requests information.

STUDY BREAK

4. The family of a patient who is at the end-of-life has requested pain medication because the patient is grimacing and appears to be in pain. The patient has a do not resuscitate (DNR) status. The nurse assesses the patient and notes the grimacing and an increased heart rate. The patient has orders for IV pain medication, but the nurse is concerned that the medication may affect the patient's breathing and hasten death. What is the appropriate action to take?

A. Hold the medication and inform the patient's family that giving pain medication can lead to the patient's death and that this would be considered euthanasia.

B. Inform the patient's family that the patient most likely cannot feel pain because the patient is so close to death.

C. The patient is suffering; administer the IV pain medication to hasten death.

D. Administer the IV pain medication as ordered, with the intent to relieve pain.

Organ and Tissue Transplantation

Improved surgical methods and increasingly effective immunosuppressive drug therapy have increased the number and the types of successfully transplanted organs and tissues.

Despite the successes in transplantation, there is a severe shortage of organs to meet the growing demand. Under the National Organ Transplant Act of 1984, the United States Congress established the Organ Procurement and Transplantation Network to facilitate fair allocation of organs and tissues for transplantation. This system is administered by the United Network for Organ Sharing, a group that maintains a list of patients who are awaiting organ and tissue transplantation and helps to coordinate the procurement of organs. In 2019 more than 113,000 people were on the organ transplantation waiting list in the United States.[29] The organ shortage has motivated multiple efforts to increase the organ supply. These efforts include creating registries for donors and designating organ donor status on driver's licenses. There are legal mandates for *required request* and mandatory organ procurement organization notification when a patient's death is imminent. In some situations, removal of the organ to be transplanted is not life-threatening and can be accomplished without causing significant harm to a living donor (e.g., kidney and bone marrow). Other types of organ and tissue removal (e.g., heart) are performed only in donors who meet the legal definition for brain death.

Since the 1968 Harvard Medical School Ad Hoc Committee's *brain death* definition, organs have primarily been removed from patients with cardiac function who have been pronounced dead based on neurological criteria but continue to receive mechanical ventilation. The concept of brain death is distinct from the concept of persistent vegetative state or irreversible coma. In brain death, complete and irreversible cessation of brain function occurs, whereas in irreversible coma or persistent vegetative state, some brain function remains intact. If a patient is a designated organ donor and brain death is determined, the patient is pronounced to be dead; however, perfusion and oxygenation of organs are maintained until the organs can be removed in the operating room. Even with optimal artificial perfusion and oxygenation, organs intended for transplantation must be removed and transplanted quickly.

The rate of organ recovery from deceased persons has increased in the category of donation after cardiac death—that is, a death declared on the basis of cardiopulmonary criteria (irreversible cessation of circulatory and respiratory function) rather than brain death.[8] Most commonly, the kidneys, liver, and pancreas are recovered after cardiac death because of the length of time in which these organs can be deprived of oxygen and still be transplanted successfully. It is an ethically acceptable practice to retrieve organs after cardiac death to increase the number of organs available for transplantation.[10] Nonetheless, the practice remains controversial. Critical care societies have collaborated on a consensus document to provide evidence-based information and recommendations related to organ donation.[17]

Critical care professionals must ensure that the decision to withdraw care is made separately from the decision to donate organs. In addition, donation after cardiac death is often performed in the operating room. Critical care personnel need to create a plan of care should the patient not die as expected. Donors must be dead according to specified hospital policy before organ procurement. The process of organ procurement cannot be the proximate cause of death.

Everyone in the United States has the legal right to donate organs. To uphold that right, family members or significant others must be given the opportunity to donate organs or tissues on behalf of their loved ones if there is no advance directive. Local organ procurement organizations have *designated requestors* whose role is to seek consent for organ donation. The role of the critical care nurse is to refer potential organ donors to the organ procurement organization. Because the consent rate for organ donation is only approximately 50%, it is important to approach potential donors sensitively and with awareness of cultural and religious implications. Designated requestors are trained to address donation with regard to such issues.

Ethical Concerns Surrounding Organ and Tissue Transplantation. Organ and tissue transplantation involve numerous and complex ethical issues. The first consideration is given to the rights and privileges of all moral agents involved: the donor, the recipient, the family or surrogate, and all other recipients and donors. Three of the most controversial issues in transplantation are the moral value that should be placed on the human body part, the just distribution of a human body part, and the complex problems inherent in applying the concept of brain death to clinical situations. Additional information on organ donation and transplantation is provided in Chapter 5.

CASE STUDY

Mr. W. is a 67-year-old patient in the coronary care unit who has severe heart failure and chronic obstructive pulmonary disease. Mr. W. has been in and out of the hospital for 3 years and requires oxygen therapy at night. He has severe, chronic chest pain and dyspnea. He had a respiratory arrest and was put on the ventilator last night. He awakens after the resuscitation and communicates that the breathing tube be removed and that he be allowed to die. He is tired of the pain and dyspnea. He asks for medication to make him comfortable after the tube is removed. His family agrees with the plan of care.

Mr. W.'s wishes are followed. He is extubated and is given morphine for sedation and comfort. Mr. W.'s family members all remain at the bedside, taking turns holding his hand and talking to him.

Questions

1. Apply the ethical decision-making model discussed in this chapter to this case. What are the relevant ethical principles? Are there other areas that must be assessed before proceeding?
2. As the critical care nurse caring for Mr. W., what are your priorities at this point? On what ethical principles are these priorities based?
3. Suppose that you have strong religious beliefs about withdrawal of life support. If you were assigned to Mr. W., what actions should you take?

REFERENCES

1. American Association of Critical-Care Nurses. AACN Mission, Vision, Values and Ethics of Care. http://www.aacn.org. Published 2019. Accessed February 19, 2019.
2. American Association of Critical-Care Nurses. AACN Practice Alert: Family Presence During Resuscitation and Invasive Procedures. http://www.aacn.org/clinical-resources/practice-alerts/family-presence-during-resusitation-and-invasive procedures. Published 2016. Accessed February 18, 2019.
3. American Association of Critical-Care Nurses. *AACN Standards for Establishing and Sustaining Healthy Work Environments: A Journey to Excellence.* 2nd ed. Aliso Vieja, CA: American Association of Critical-Care Nurses; 2016.
4. American Heart Association. American Heart Association 2015 Guidelines for Cardiopulmonary Resuscitation and Emergency Cardiopulmonary Care. https://www.heart.org. Published 2015. Accessed February 22, 2019.
5. American Nurses Association. *Code of Ethics for Nurses With Interpretive Statements.* Silver Spring, MD: American Nurses Association; 2015.
6. American Nurses Association. American Nurses Association Position Statement Euthanasia, Assisted Suicide, and Aid in Dying Date. https://www.nursingworld.org/~4ae33e/globalassets/docs/ana/euthanasia-assisted-suicideaid-in-dying_ps042513.pdf. Published 2013. Accessed March 2, 2019.
7. American Nurses Credentialing Center. *Magnet Recognition Program: Application Manual.* Silver Spring, MD: American Nurses Credentialing Center; 2019.
8. Bastami S, Matthes O, Krones T, Biller-Andorno N. Systematic review of attitudes toward donation after cardiac death among healthcare providers and the general public. *Crit Care Med.* 2013;41(3):897–905.
9. Beauchamp T, Childress J. *Principles of Biomedical Ethics.* 7th ed. Oxford, England: Oxford University Press; 2012.
10. Bernat JL, D'Alessandro AM, Port FK, et al. Report of a national conference on donation after cardiac death. *Am J Trans.* 2006;6:281–291.
11. Davidson JE, Hooper FG. Aid in dying: The role of the critical care nurse. *AACN Adv Crit Care.* 2017;28(2):218–222.
12. Flanders SA, Strasen JH. Review of evidence about family presence during resuscitation. *Crit Care Nurs Clin North Am.* 2014;26:533–550.
13. Fowler M. *Guide to the Code of Ethics for Nurses: Development, Application and Interpretation.* 2nd ed. Silver Spring, MD: American Nurses Association; 2015.
14. Goldberger ZD, Nallamothu BK, Nichol G, et al. Policies allowing family presence during resuscitation and patterns of care during in-hospital cardiac arrest. *Circ Cardiovasc Qual Outcomes.* 2015;8:226–234.
15. Grady C, Danis M, Soeken KL, et al. Does ethics education influence the moral action of practicing nurses and social workers? *Am J Bioethics.* 2008;8(4):2–14.
16. Heyland DK, Tranmer J, Feldman-Steward D. End-of-life decision making in the seriously ill hospitalized patient: An organizing framework and results of a preliminary study. *J Pall Care.* 2000;16:S31–S39.
17. Kotloff RM, Blosser S, Fulda GJ, et al. Management of the potential organ donor in the ICU: Society of Critical Care Medicine/American College of Chest Physicians, Association of Organ Procurement Organizations consensus statement. *Crit Care Med.* 2015;43:1291–1325.
18. Kummer HB, Thompson DR. *Critical Care Ethics: A Practice Guide.* 3rd ed. Mount Prospect, IL: Society of Critical Care Medicine; 2009.
19. Lamiani G, Borghi L, Argentero P. When health professionals cannot do the right thing: A systematic review of moral distress and its correlates. *J Health Psychol.* 2017;22(1):51–67.
20. McAndrew NS, Leske J, Schroeter K. Moral distress in critical care nursing: The state of the science. *Nurs Ethics.* 2018;25(5):552–570.
21. Public Law No. 101-508, 4206, 104 Stat. 291 The Self-Determination Act amends the Social Security Act's provisions on Medicare and Medicaid. *Social Security Act.* 1927;42(1990):L U.S.C. 1396.
22. Rainer J, Schneider JK, Lorenz RA. Ethical dilemmas in nursing: An integrative review. *J Clin Nurs.* 2018;27(19–20):3446–3461.

23. Rose TF. Physician assisted suicide: Development, status, and nursing perspectives. *J Nurs Law.* 2007;11(3):141–151.

24. Rushton CH. Cultivating moral resilience. *Am J Nursing.* 2017;117(2):S11–S15.

25. Rushton CH, Broome M. The Nursing Ethics Summit Group: Blueprint for 21st Century Nursing Ethics: Report of the National Nursing Ethics Summit. http://www.bioethicsinstitute.org/nursing-ethics-summit-report. Accessed February 2019.

26. Rushton CH, Scanlon C. A road map for negotiating end-of-life care. *Medsurg Nurs.* 1998;6(1):59–62.

27. Stutzer K, Bylone M. Building moral resilience. *Crit Care Nurs.* 2018;38(1):77–89.

28. Wholihan D, Olson E. The doctrine of double effect: A review for the bedside nurse providing end-of-life care. *J Hospice Palliative Nurs.* 2017;19(3):205.

29. United Network for Organ Sharing. Data. http://www.unos.org. Published 2019. Accessed March 2, 2019.

Palliative and End-of-Life Care

Douglas Houghton, DNP, APRN, ACNPC, CCRN, FAANP

Many additional resources, including self-assessment exercises, are located on the Evolve companion website at http://evolve.elsevier.com/Sole/.

- Animations
- Clinical Skills: Critical Care Collections
- Student Review Questions
- Video Clips

INTRODUCTION

Advances in technology during the past several decades have vastly improved the ability of healthcare providers to care for critically ill patients, at least in terms of survival rates. Interventions such as extracorporeal membrane oxygenation (ECMO) are increasingly used in the sickest patients, saving many lives but prolonging the dying of others.[41] Left ventricular assist devices (LVADs), once only a bridge to heart transplantation, are now used as "destination" therapy for patients with severe heart failure who are not candidates for transplantation.[49] The appropriate use of these invasive and expensive resources is a matter of much debate, leading to complex ethical issues and decision making in the care of persons with a critical or chronic illness. There is significant variation by hospital and region in critical care unit admissions for common medical conditions, demonstrating a lack of agreement on the appropriate intensity of care for many critically ill persons. Interestingly, in a study of 156,842 hospitalizations, the use of more invasive interventions did not ensure increased survival.[15] In 2014 the Institute of Medicine published *Dying in America,* a comprehensive review of the current state of the issue with recommendations for improvement. This important study revealed areas of progress in recent years, such as significant increases in healthcare providers' education in end-of-life and palliative care. It also identified significant opportunities for improvement, citing fragmentation of care, increasing healthcare costs, and little translation of end-of-life education to those providers who may need it most.[31] These problems affect more than 2.7 million Americans who die every year, the vast majority from progression of chronic or long-term illnesses such as heart failure, chronic lung disease, and complications of diabetes.[14] Although this is a large number, the death rate per 100,000 people in the United States has decreased by more than 40% between 1969 and 2013.[14] It can be concluded from these data that more Americans are living with chronic disease processes prior to their deaths and that many may benefit from palliative care. Early

identification of those patients who are in the dying process is warranted to ensure that they receive care that is consistent with their wishes and do not needlessly suffer from nonbeneficial aggressive care interventions.

Many critical care units remain a relatively hostile, often uncomfortable and impersonal place for dying patients and their families. The landmark Study to Understand Prognoses and Preferences for Outcomes and Risks of Treatment (SUPPORT) revealed many disparities between patients' care preferences and the care they received. The most significant findings from the study included a lack of clear communication between patients and healthcare providers, a high frequency of aggressive care, and widespread pain and suffering among inpatients.[64] Although improvements have been made in the years since the study's publication, proxy-reported pain in inpatients increased from 54.3% to 60.8% between 1998 and 2010.[62]

The United States has the highest use of critical care units in the last 180 days of life (40.3%) when compared to other Western nations (18%), with 27.2% of Americans admitted to a critical care unit in the last 30 days of life; however, the United States has the *lowest* proportion of patients dying in the hospital (22.2%).[6] This fact is encouraging, because family members of dying patients report higher-quality end-of-life care when dying occurs outside the hospital setting.[69] Increased national attention to the issue has stimulated funding for research and development of care guidelines for the dying patient in the critical care setting. The American Association of Critical-Care Nurses (AACN) has compiled relevant nursing publications and research on its website (see online resources in Box 4.1).

A large percentage of deaths in the critical care unit are preceded by decisions to withhold or withdraw aggressive support. The percentages vary based on patient population, culture, and unit type.[37,39] Many of these decisions are made by surrogate decision makers because most patients in the critical care unit are unable to make decisions about their own care.[21] Surrogate decision makers frequently rely on factors other than the prognosis relayed to them by the physician, increasing the likelihood

---

BOX 4.1 End-of-Life Online Resources

- American Academy of Hospice and Palliative Medicine: http://www.aahpm.org
- American Association of Colleges of Nursing: https://www.aacnnursing.org/ELNEC/Resources
- American Association of Critical-Care Nurses: https://www.aacn.org/clinical-resources/palliative-end-of-life
- Center to Advance Palliative Care: https://www.capc.org/toolkits/integrating-palliative-care-practices-in-the-icu/
- Institute of Medicine, *Dying in America: Improving Quality and Honoring Individual Preferences Near the End-of-Life:* http://www.nap.edu.org/hmd/Reports/2014/Dying-In-America-Improving-Quality-and-Honoring-Individual-Preferences-Near-the-End-of-Life.aspx
- National Hospice and Palliative Care Organization: http://www.nhpco.org
- National Library of Medicine: http://www.nlm.nih.gov/medlineplus/endoflifeissues.html
- Northwestern University, Education in Palliative and End-of-Life Care Program: https://www.bioethics.northwestern.edu/education/epec.html
- University of Washington, End-of-Life Care Research Program: http://depts.washington.edu/eolcare/

BOX 4.2 Medically Futile Versus Potentially Inappropriate Interventions

Medically Futile Interventions

Interventions that simply cannot accomplish the intended physiologic goal.

Potentially Inappropriate Interventions

Interventions that have at least some chance of the effect sought by the patient, but clinicians believe that competing ethical considerations justify not providing them (i.e., providing dialysis to a patient with permanent anoxic encephalopathy).

From Bosslet GT, Pope TM, Rubenfeld GD, et al. An official ATS/AACN/ACCP/ESICM/SCCM policy statement: Responding to requests for potentially inappropriate treatments in intensive care units. *Am J Resp Crit Care Med.* 2015;191(11):1318–1330.

---

of conflict situations.[36] Often these surrogates experience high stress and anxiety levels, which may negatively affect their ability to make informed decisions for their loved one.[36,50]

Multiple factors influence the continuation of aggressive care in the face of a poor prognosis, including religious beliefs and ethnicity.[28,47,66] The failure of clinicians, family members, and patients to openly and honestly discuss prognosis, end-of-life issues, and preferences is one of the most significant factors preventing early identification of patients who are unlikely to benefit from aggressive care. Patients and surrogates often do not understand the explanations of providers, nor the ramifications of their choices.[30,67] As patient advocates, nurses can and must play a key role in ensuring that choices are understood and goals of care are clear.[4] The terms *nonbeneficial care, inappropriate care,* and *potentially inappropriate care* have largely replaced *futile care,* with the latter term reserved only for interventions that are not achievable. Nonbeneficial treatment is defined as care provided to patients that would result in a quality of life the patient would not want or that is inconsistent with the patient's stated goals of care.[25] The term *inappropriate care* is commonly used and refers to critical care unit interventions with no reasonable expectation of achieving patient survival outside the acute care setting or in situations in which the patient's neurological condition is such that the patient cannot perceive the benefits.[35,48] Multiple studies have been conducted to provide data to support this complex decision-making process.

In 2015 five major medical and nursing critical care organizations produced a consensus document based on available evidence, providing guidance to clinicians on how to respond to requests for potentially inappropriate treatment in the critical care unit.[9] Few valid assessment tools exist to accurately predict or determine when an intervention is unlikely to achieve its desired goal, further contributing to conflict at the end-of-life (Box 4.2). The identification of the dying patient is often subjective and based on the healthcare providers' opinions and interpretations of patient response and results.[22] This makes the determination of the appropriate intensity of care for patients near the end-of-life extremely difficult. Mounting evidence demonstrates that high-intensity or aggressive care near the end-of-life is associated with a decreased quality of life, increased costs, and little to no improvement in duration of life.[69]

Societal values and those of healthcare providers also play a significant role in how end-of-life care in the United States is provided. These values often include a commonly held belief that patients die of distinct illnesses, which implies that such illnesses are potentially curable. Dying is often viewed as failure on the part of the system or providers. The purpose of the healthcare system in the United States is to treat illness, disease, and injury, and this "life-saving" culture often continues to drive aggressive care even when it becomes obvious that the ultimate outcome will be the death of the individual. Fortunately, significant progress has been made in the medical-legal arena in establishing the rights of patients and surrogates to decide for themselves the intensity and duration of care.[68]

Effects on Nurses and the Healthcare Team

Many clinicians experience personal ethical conflicts when providing interventions and aggressive care to patients that they perceive to be futile or inappropriate, causing significant moral distress that can lead to burnout.[1,29,54,59] Care choices made by patients or surrogates often differ from those that clinicians might make personally, causing further strain in remaining nonjudgmental in such situations. Recurrent moral distress is often cited as the cause for leaving a job, as well as being a significant cause of job dissatisfaction and stress. Though moral distress is most common and studied among nurses, it is reported in physicians and other care providers as well.[29] Interventions to alleviate moral distress through the development of

---

STUDY BREAK

1. Which of the following is NOT typically a reason why aggressive medical care is continued for patients who are unlikely to survive?
   A. Religious and/or cultural beliefs
   B. Financial or payor status
   C. Lack of discussion of patient and family goals of care
   D. Lack of clear communication of prognosis by providers

moral resilience include self-care, mindfulness, seeking support from colleagues, ethics education, clarifying goals of care, organizational support, and striving to accept differing values in our patients and families.[55-57]

Patients' dignity is often compromised during a critical care unit stay,[23] and their preferences and wishes may not be elicited by providers in goals of care conferences.[18] Such situations contradict basic nursing ethical principles, causing further moral distress.[4] At times, healthcare providers do not clearly communicate a poor prognosis to patients or the family members, denying them the ability to make informed choices.[17,34,38] When life support is withdrawn and patients die, caregivers often experience a sense of loss or grief, especially if the patient's stay was lengthy. Attendance at funerals or unit debriefing sessions after a death may help to resolve emotional strain. Finding a balance between maintaining a professional, healthy distance and being authentic and humane is a difficult task.

 CRITICAL REASONING ACTIVITY

When educating a family about the process of withdrawal of life support, such as mechanical ventilation, the nurse must convey what concepts?

DIMENSIONS OF END-OF-LIFE CARE

Nursing care in the critical care setting at the end-of-life is focused on five dimensions: (1) alleviation of distressing symptoms (palliation); (2) communication and conflict resolution; (3) withdrawing, limiting, or withholding therapy; (4) emotional and psychological care of the patient and family; and (5) caregiver organizational support.

Palliative Care

Palliation is the provision of care interventions that are designed to relieve symptoms of illness or injury that negatively affect the quality of life. Common distressing symptoms that may occur with multiple disease states include pain, anxiety, hunger, thirst, dyspnea, diarrhea, nausea, confusion, agitation, and disturbance in sleep patterns.[7,36] Distressing symptoms are common among patients in the critical care unit, and every effort should be made to identify and aggressively treat those symptoms.

Palliative care is often confused with hospice care, which is reserved for the terminally ill. Palliative care is *not* a substitute for aggressive, life-saving care but rather a complementary supplement to care. In contrast, hospice care is generally reserved for those with a prognosis of less than 6 months to live and is usually *in place of* aggressive life-sustaining or restorative care.[44] There is growing consensus that palliative care should be an integral part of every ill or injured patient's care and should not be reserved only for the dying patient.[5,27,43,44] Relief of distressing symptoms should always be provided whenever possible, even when the primary focus of care is life-saving or aggressive treatment. An important part of palliative care consists of "simple" nursing interventions such as frequent repositioning, good hygiene and skin care, and creation of a peaceful environment to the extent possible in the critical care setting.

For those patients with recognized life-limiting illness or injury, palliative care consultations with experts in symptom management can provide significant benefits to the patients and their families. The use of palliative care experts to assist in managing patients' care decreases critical care unit admissions and lengths of stay and has the potential to achieve significant cost savings if palliative care consultations became the standard for all patients with serious or chronic illness.[32,33] Improved communication with patients and families and better symptom management are additional benefits noted.[5,19] Palliative care may be provided through a consultative model or via an integrative approach, in which palliative care principles are integrated into the daily medical and nursing practice in the critical care unit. Some institutions have implemented pathways to assist in patient care management at the end-of-life. Although randomized trials have not yet been completed to evaluate the outcomes of these pathways, increased accessibility to palliative care has multiple benefits for critical and terminally ill patients.[16,61]

Earlier identification of patients unlikely to benefit from further aggressive care, improved communication between patients and families and the medical team, and better management of pain and other symptoms are effective strategies to improve end-of-life care. These strategies may be better achieved when guided by palliative care experts.[5,31]

STUDY BREAK

2. The focus of palliative care includes all of the following EXCEPT:
   A. Aggressive symptom management
   B. Getting the patient off of life support as soon as possible
   C. Improving communication between the healthcare team and the patient and family
   D. Decreasing patient and family anxiety and distress

Pain management is a major focus of palliative care and begins with proper identification; therefore frequent nursing assessment is necessary. When assessing pain, the nurse must consider that the expression of pain varies based on cultural and individual characteristics.[52] Different nonpharmacological and pharmacological approaches may be necessary to ensure proper pain management. Medications to control pain and relieve anxiety in the critically ill patient are described in Chapter 6.

Communication and Conflict Resolution

Clear, ongoing, and honest communication among the members of the healthcare team, the patient, and the family is a key factor in improving the quality of care for the dying patient in the critical care unit.[17] Communication is also incredibly challenging, in part because of the complex nature of predicting prognosis with accuracy in a critically ill person. Significant differences in perception of the patient's prognosis for recovery have been identified among surrogates, physicians, and nurses. The most accurate prognostication occurs when physicians and nurses work together, emphasizing the need for a multiprofessional team approach.[45] A shared decision-making model with clinicians and patients or their surrogates collaborating to determine patient prognosis and goals of care is recommended by

BOX 4.3 Guidelines for Effective Communication to Facilitate End-of-Life Care

- **Present a clear and consistent message** to the family. Mixed messages confuse families and patients, as do unfamiliar medical terms. The multiprofessional team needs to communicate and strive to reach agreement on goals of care and prognosis.
- **Allow ample time** for family members to express themselves during family conferences. Ask about previous discussions or feelings of the patient regarding life-sustaining treatments. Aim for all (healthcare providers, patients, and families) to *agree on the plan of treatment*. The plan should be based on the known or perceived preferences of the patient. Arriving at such a plan through communication minimizes legal actions against providers, relieves patient and family anxiety, and provides an environment in which the patient is the focus of concern.

- **Emphasize that the patient will not be abandoned** if the goals of care shift from aggressive therapy to "comfort" care (palliation) only. Let the patient and family know who is responsible for the care and that they can rely on those individuals to be present and available when needed.
- **Facilitate continuity of care.** If a transfer to an alternative level of care, such as a hospice unit or ventilator unit, is required, ensure that all pertinent information is conveyed to the new providers. Details of the history, prognosis, care requirements, palliative interventions, and psychosocial needs should be part of the information transfer.

Data from Bosslet GT, Pope TM, Rubenfeld GD, et al. An official ATS/AACN/ACCP/ESICM/SCCM policy statement: Responding to requests for potentially inappropriate treatments in intensive care units. *Am J Resp Crit Care Med.* 2015;191(11):1318–1330; Downar J, Delaney JW, Hawryluck L, Kenny L. Guidelines for the withdrawal of life-sustaining measures. *Intensive Care Med.* 2016;42:1003–1017.

critical care guidelines.[35] A process-based method for resolving disputes between care teams and patients or their surrogates has been described and is supported by major nursing and critical care societies.[9,48] Guidelines for effective communication are described in Box 4.3.

Schedule regular conferences with the patient and family to facilitate communication and identify goals of care. During the conference, make the family feel comfortable talking about death and dying issues, focusing on how the patient likely would decide in the given situation if unable to communicate his or her wishes. Clarify what the family understands and answer any questions, allowing them to talk about the family member's life and medical history. Provide honest information about the patient's prognosis. Discuss goals for palliative care, emphasizing that patient comfort will be maintained. Use skills of effective communication such as reflection, empathy, and silence. Conclude with a plan and follow-up communication.

Withholding, Limiting, or Withdrawing Therapy

Most deaths in the critical care unit are preceded by some manner of withholding, withdrawing, or limiting medical treatments, with significant variation among different patient populations.[28,37,40,51] Decisions to withdraw, withhold, or limit treatment should be made with multiprofessional team and family participation using a shared decision-making model.[35] Appropriate withdrawal, limiting, or withholding of therapy

EVIDENCE-BASED PRACTICE

Critical Care Nurses' Experiences With Spiritual Care

Problem

Nurses receive little education on spiritual care in most nursing programs. Little knowledge exists about how chaplains and spiritual care interact with critical care nurses when caring for patients at the end-of-life.

Clinical Questions

When caring for patients at the end-of-life, how do chaplains interact with and support critical care nurses, patients, and families in the critical care unit? What do critical care nurses understand about the role of spiritual care in practice?

Evidence

Participants: Twenty-five critical care nurses with at least 5 years of experience who had cared for at least five patients who had died on their shift, in which a spiritual referral was initiated.

Methods: A semistructured interview format was used to collect data about the experience of the critical care nurses working with a spiritual care provider while caring for a patient at the end-of-life.

Results: Three main themes were identified:

1. The value and role of chaplain presence: Nurses identified how chaplains supported the patient, family, and the nurse through their presence and expressed gratitude and relief at having support from spiritual care providers.

2. The nurses' experience of working with spiritual care providers on the unit: Nurses felt that it was a measure of their caring to initiate spiritual referrals and that they worked in cooperation with the spiritual care provider to comfort the patient and family.

3. Critical care nurses' provision of spiritual care through their practice: Nurse participants expressed that their role of caring for patients in critical care near the end-of-life included positive intentions for the patient, presence, and providing compassion through their work.

Implications for Nursing

This study demonstrated the beneficial effects of spiritual care referrals for critically ill patients, especially those near the end-of-life. The spiritual care providers supported the nurses, the patient, and the family through their presence and worked with the nurses to provide compassionate end-of-life care. Nurses felt that the provision of spiritual care to the patient added value to the provision of patient- and family-centered care.

Level of Evidence

C—Descriptive study

Reference

Bone N, Swinton M, Hoad H, et al. Critical care nurses' experiences with spiritual care: The SPIRIT study. *Am J Crit Care.* 2018;27(3):212–219.

does not constitute euthanasia or assisted suicide, both of which are illegal in the United States (except in California, the District of Columbia, Oregon, Hawaii, Vermont, and Washington, where assisted suicide is permitted in select instances).[20] Minimal moral distress on the part of the healthcare team, patients, and families should result if generally accepted ethical and legal principles are followed during this process.[1,48]

A growing number of states have endorsed the use of a standardized end-of-life order set for inpatient or outpatient use, known as Physician (or Provider) Orders for Life-Sustaining Treatment (POLST). This form is designed to be mutually agreed on between the provider and patient or surrogate and clearly specifies the kind of care the patient prefers at the end-of-life. POLST has become a strong national movement and represents growing public sentiment in support of having control over personal end-of-life care (http://www.polst.org). An example of this order set is shown in Fig. 4.1, where Oregon refers to POLST as Portable Orders for Life-Sustaining Treatment. Oregon has invested in public education initiatives on end-of-life care and coordination of patient preferences across care settings. These efforts have clearly been worthwhile, as demonstrated by the fact that only 18.2% of Oregonians enter a critical care unit in the last 30 days of life, compared with 28.5% in the rest of the United States.[65]

Preparing patients (if conscious) and families for what will likely occur during the withdrawal process is key to alleviating anxiety and undue distress. Anticipate patient symptoms, such as dyspnea during ventilator withdrawal, and medicate to alleviate such symptoms even if high doses of medications are required. Assess pain using a validated pain scale such as the Critical-Care Pain Observation Tool (CPOT) and assess agitation using either the Sedation-Agitation Scale (SAS) or the Richmond Agitation-Sedation Scale (RASS) (see Chapter 6). Assess the patient's response (e.g., comfort) to determine how much medication is appropriate in a given situation and titrate therapy as needed to relieve emotional and physical distress, even if such dosing hastens the death of the patient as a secondary effect. Commonly used medication regimens include morphine sulfate or other opioids for pain or dyspnea and IV benzodiazepines for anxiolysis.[24] Pharmacological management of life support withdrawal is critical in ensuring a peaceful death for both patient and family (see Box 4.4 for expert recommendations on medication use). An actively engaged critical care nurse is vital in ensuring that patients die in comfort during the withdrawal process.

Ventilator Withdrawal. The most commonly withheld or withdrawn medical intervention in the critical care setting is mechanical ventilation. This process is known as *terminal weaning* (see the Clinical Alert box) and can consist of titration of ventilator support to minimal levels, removal of the ventilator but not the artificial airway, or extubation. Assess the patient's response using the Respiratory Distress Observation Scale to determine how much medication is appropriate in a given situation and titrate therapy as needed to relieve emotional and physical distress, even if such dosing hastens the death of the patient as a secondary effect.[13] Some debate and regional practice variations exist, but excellent practice resources

for end-of-life care and ventilator withdrawal are available from the AACN website (see Box 4.1). Consult your institution's policy and procedure manual for specific requirements or variations related to withdrawal of care.

> ### ! CLINICAL ALERT
> #### Terminal Weaning
> During terminal weaning of ventilatory support, patients may exhibit symptoms of respiratory distress, such as tachypnea, dyspnea, or use of accessory muscles. Titrate pain medication and sedation as needed to relieve such symptoms.

Other Commonly Withheld Therapies. Vasopressors, antibiotics, blood and blood products, dialysis, and nutritional support are other common therapies that may be ethically withheld when goals of treatment shift to palliation instead of cure. Because of the increase in the use of cardiovascular implantable electronic devices, such as cardioverter-defibrillators, address the deactivation of these devices as appropriate before withdrawing or withholding ventilation or other therapies that may result in cardiac arrest.[10] Again, the primary nursing responsibility is to assess and ensure patient comfort during the withdrawal or withholding process.

Hospice Referral. When it has been determined that aggressive medical care interventions will be withheld or withdrawn, it may be appropriate to initiate a referral to a hospice care provider. Hospice is a model of care that emphasizes comfort rather than cure and views dying as a normal human process. It is a philosophy of care rather than a specific place and can be provided in various care settings, as dictated by patient needs. Referrals are increasingly being made to improve the quality of end-of-life care, regardless of diagnosis (see the QSEN Exemplar box).

> ### ✳ QSEN EXEMPLAR
> #### Patient-Centered Care, Teamwork, and Collaboration
> Mr. J., a 68-year-old man with end-stage chronic obstructive pulmonary disease, was hospitalized for exacerbation of his condition. He was hypoxemic and dyspneic and was being treated with bilevel positive airway pressure (BiPAP). He was alert, oriented, and able to make his own decisions. His wife, Mrs. J., was at the bedside and stated that she did not like to see her husband suffering. She also noted how uncomfortable Mr. J. was with BiPAP treatment. Mr. J. acknowledged his discomfort. During multiprofessional rounds led by the intensivist, Mrs. J. was in the room. The nurse conveyed to the physician Mr. J.'s discomfort and low oxygen saturation (85%) despite the BiPAP. This communication created the opportunity for shared decision making and goal setting. The physician noted that the BiPAP was not effective and asked, "What are the goals of care: comfort or more aggressive treatment?" Both Mr. and Mrs. J. acknowledged that comfort was most important. A shared decision was made to place Mr. J. on high-flow oxygen rather than BiPAP. The respiratory therapist replaced the BiPAP with high-flow oxygen. Mr. J. immediately noted increased comfort. His oxygen saturation improved, and he was able to clear his airway better. This example demonstrates the importance of multiprofessional rounds, family participation during such rounds, and the complementary roles of team members.

Oregon POLST™
Portable Orders for Life-Sustaining Treatment*

Follow these medical orders until orders change. Any section not completed implies full treatment for that section.

Patient Last Name:	Suffix:	Patient First Name:	Patient Middle Name:

Preferred Name:	Date of Birth: (mm/dd/yyyy) ____ / ____ / ____	Gender: ☐M ☐F ☐X	MRN (optional)

Address: (street / city / state zip):

A
Check One

CARDIOPULMONARY RESUSCITATION (CPR): *Unresponsive, pulseless, & not breathing.*

☐ **Attempt Resuscitation/CPR**   ☐ **Do Not Attempt Resuscitation/DNR**

If patient not in cardiopulmonary arrest, follow orders in B.

B
Check One

MEDICAL INTERVENTIONS: *If patient has pulse and is breathing.*

☐ **Comfort Measures Only.** Provide treatments to relieve pain and suffering through the use of any medication by any route, positioning, wound care and other measures. Use oxygen, suction and manual treatment of airway obstruction as needed for comfort. *Patient prefers no transfer to hospital for life-sustaining treatments. Transfer if comfort needs cannot be met in current location.* **Treatment Plan: Provide treatments for comfort through symptom management.**

☐ **Limited Treatment.** In addition to care described in Comfort Measures Only, use medical treatment, antibiotics, IV fluids and cardiac monitor as indicated. No intubation, advanced airway interventions, or mechanical ventilation. May consider less invasive airway support (e.g. CPAP, BiPAP). *Transfer to hospital if indicated. Generally avoid the intensive care unit.* **Treatment Plan: Provide basic medical treatments.**

☐ **Full Treatment.** In addition to care described in Comfort Measures Only and Limited Treatment, use intubation, advanced airway interventions, and mechanical ventilation as indicated. *Transfer to hospital and/or intensive care unit if indicated.* **Treatment Plan: All treatments including breathing machine.**

Additional Orders: _____

C
Check All That Apply

DOCUMENTATION OF WHO WAS PRESENT FOR DISCUSSION *See reverse side for add'l info.*

☐ Patient
☐ Parent of minor
☐ Person appointed on advance directive
☐ Court-appointed guardian

☐ Surrogate for patient with developmental disabilities or significant mental health condition (Note: Special requirements for completion - see reverse side)
☐ Relative or friend (without written appointment)

Discussed with (list all names and relationship): _____

D

PATIENT OR SURROGATE SIGNATURE

Signature: *recommended*	Name (print):	Relationship (write "self" if patient):

This form will be sent to the POLST Registry unless the patient wishes to opt out, if so check opt out box ☐

E
Must Print Name, Sign & Date

ATTESTATION OF MD / DO / NP / PA / ND   (REQUIRED)

By signing below, I attest that these medical orders are, to the best of my knowledge, consistent with the patient's **current** medical condition and preferences.

Print Signing MD / DO / NP / PA / ND Name: *required*	Signer Phone Number:	Signer License Number: *(optional)*
MD / DO / NP / PA / ND Signature: *required*	Date: *required*	"Signed" means a physical signature, electronic signature or verbal order documented per standard medical practice. Refer to OAR 333-270-0030

SEND FORM WITH PATIENT WHENEVER TRANSFERRED OR DISCHARGED
SUBMIT COPY OF BOTH SIDES OF FORM TO REGISTRY IF PATIENT DID NOT OPT OUT IN SECTION D

* Also known as Physician Orders for Life-Sustaining Treatment

Fig. 4.1 Portable Orders for Life-Sustaining Treatment (POLST). (From Center for Ethics in Health Care, Oregon Health and Science University, Portland, OR.)

Also known as Physician Orders for Life-Sustaining Treatment

HIPAA PERMITS DISCLOSURE TO HEALTH CARE PROFESSIONALS & ELECTRONIC REGISTRY AS NECESSARY FOR TREATMENT

| Information Regarding POLST | PATIENT'S NAME: _____ |

The POLST form is:
- **Always voluntary and cannot be required**
- **A medical order for people with a serious illness or frailty**
- An expression of wishes for emergency treatment in one's current state of health (if something happened today)
- A form that can be changed at any time, with a health care professional, to reflect new treatment wishes
- **Not an advance directive,** which is ALSO recommended (an advance directive is the appropriate legal document to appoint a surrogate/health care decision maker)

Contact Information (Optional)

| Emergency Contact: | Relationship: | Phone Number: |

Health Care Professional Information

| Preparer Name: | Preparer Title: | Phone Number: | Date Prepared: |

PA's Supervising Physician: | Phone Number:

Primary Care Professional:

Directions for Health Care Professionals

Completing Oregon POLST™

- Discussion and attestation should be accompanied by a note in the medical record.
- Any section not completed implies full treatment for that section.
- An order of CPR in Section A is incompatible with an order for Comfort Measures Only in Section B (will not be accepted in Registry).
- Photocopies, faxes, and electronically-signed forms are legal and valid.
- Verbal / phone orders from MD/DO/NP/PA/ND in accordance with facility/community policy can be submitted to the Registry.
- For information on determining the legal decision maker(s) for incapacitated patients, refer to ORS 127.505 - 127.660.
- A person with developmental disabilities or significant mental health condition requires additional consideration before completing the POLST form; refer to *Guidance for Health Care Professionals* at www.oregonpolst.org.

Oregon POLST Registry Information

Health Care Professionals:
(1) Send a copy of <u>both</u> sides of this POLST form to the Oregon POLST Registry unless the patient opts out.
(2) The following must be completed:
- Patient's full name
- Date of birth
- MD / DO / NP / ND signature
- Date signed

Registry Contact Information:

Toll Free: 1-877-367-7657
Fax or eFAX: 503-418-2161
www.orpolstregistry.org
polstreg@ohsu.edu

Oregon POLST Registry
3181 SW Sam Jackson Park Rd.
Mail Code: BTE 234
Portland, OR 97239

Patients:
If address is listed on front page, mailed confirmation packets from Registry may take four weeks for delivery.

MAY PUT REGISTRY ID STICKER HERE:

Updating POLST: A POLST Form only needs to be revised if patient treatment preferences have changed.

This POLST should be reviewed periodically, including when:
- The patient is transferred from one care setting or care level to another (including upon admission or at discharge), or
- There is a substantial change in the patient's health status.

If patient wishes haven't changed, the POLST Form does not need to be revised, updated, rewritten or resent to the Registry.

Voiding POLST: A copy of the voided POLST <u>must</u> be sent to the Registry unless patient has opted-out.

- A person with capacity, or the valid surrogate of a person without capacity, can void the form and request alternative treatment.
- For paper forms, draw line through sections A through E and write "VOID" in large letters if POLST is replaced or becomes invalid.
- If included in an electronic medical record, follow your systems ePOLST voiding procedures.
- Regardless of paper or ePOLST form, send a copy of the voided form to the POLST Registry (required unless patient has opted out).

For permission to use the copyrighted form contact the OHSU Center for Ethics in Health Care at polst@ohsu.edu or (503) 494-3965. Information on the Oregon POLST Program is available online at **www.oregonpolst.org or at polst@ohsu.edu.**

SEND FORM WITH PATIENT WHENEVER TRANSFERRED OR DISCHARGED, SUBMIT COPY TO REGISTRY

Fig. 4.1 cont'd

BOX 4.4   Expert Recommendations for Pharmacological Management of Life Support Withdrawal

Key Points

Medications can be used to treat evident symptoms OR in anticipation of symptoms that are not yet present.

Effects of neuromuscular blocking agents should be allowed to wear off prior to withdrawal.

Choice of Opioid and Sedative Medications

Patients who are comfortable on stable doses of opioid should be continued on that opioid at that dose when starting withdrawal.

Morphine is the opioid of choice to treat pain or dyspnea in an opioid-naive patient.

Barbiturates or propofol can be second-line medications for sedation during withdrawal when benzodiazepines are ineffective.

Titration of Opioids

Opioids should be titrated to symptoms, with no dose limit.

Opioid-naive patients can be started on bolus doses of 2 mg IV morphine, titrated to effect.

Pain or respiratory distress should be treated with a bolus dose of opioid followed by an infusion.

Titration of Sedatives

Sedatives should be used only once pain and dyspnea are treated with opioids.

Combinations of opioids and benzodiazepines can be used during withdrawal.

Sedatives should be titrated to symptoms, with no dose limit.

Benzodiazepine-naive patients can be started on bolus doses of 2 mg IV midazolam, followed by an infusion of 1 mg/h.

Propofol can be used as an alternative to benzodiazepines.

Other Medications

Inhaled epinephrine should be used to treat postextubation stridor in conscious patients.

Antinauseants should be ordered as needed (PRN) with opioids.

Consider anticholinergic medication to prevent upper airway secretions.

Consider furosemide to prevent congestive heart failure symptoms postextubation.

Adapted from Downar J, Delaney JW, Hawryluck L, Kenny L. Guidelines for the withdrawal of life-sustaining measures. *Intensive Care Med.* 2016;42:1003–1017.

Hospice care for the critically ill patient is usually provided in an inpatient setting and can include withdrawal of ventilator support or other therapies. For patients who are less dependent on technologies for survival, the dying process occasionally may be managed in the patient's home with multiprofessional team support. Referral to hospice may provide a more supportive and tranquil environment for the patient during the dying process. Should such a transfer occur, it is crucial to ensure a smooth transition and good communication between the critical care staff, the receiving hospice provider, the patient, and the family.

 CRITICAL REASONING ACTIVITY

What is palliative care, and does it apply only to patients with a terminal illness?

Emotional and Psychological Care of the Patient and Family

One of the most challenging aspects of end-of-life care is addressing the emotional and psychological needs of the patient and family. Needs are as variable as family situations, so carefully assess what the patient's and family's needs *are* instead of making assumptions about what they *ought* to be. Use nonjudgmental assessment, being keenly aware of the patient's and family's personal feelings or values about the situation. The results of this assessment determine priorities in this dimension of care. Keep in mind that "family" can consist of many different persons in an individual's life. It may include unmarried life partners (same or opposite sex), close friends, and "aunts," "uncles," or "cousins" who may have no legal relationship to the patient.

For some families, spiritual counseling from pastoral care services might be a priority. For others, the need may be for statistics documenting their loved one's chances of survival with a particular diagnosis. One common need is receiving clear, consistent, and accurate information about the patient's condition, what to expect during the withdrawal and dying process (if applicable), and reassurance that the patient will not suffer during the dying process.[24,68] Coordinating the communication process between the patient, the family, and the healthcare team contributes to building family resilience in the critical care setting and is a key nursing role. Other nursing activities that promote family resilience include managing expectations to ensure a realistic understanding of condition and prognosis and supporting the patient's or surrogate's decision-making process.[26,42,46] Many institutions have bereavement counselors with extensive training in assisting patients and families through the dying process and its aftermath. Social workers, spiritual care providers, and licensed mental health professionals frequently can assist in meeting the needs of families. Spiritual care providers can be an essential element of end-of-life care, and their presence is valued by nurses, patients, and families.[8]

Maintaining the patient's dignity during the dying process is of the utmost importance. Make time to listen to family accounts of the patient's life before the illness or injury and acknowledge the patient's individuality and humanity. Use a calm manner and voice, maintain a quiet and private environment, and allow unrestricted family presence with the patient before, during, and after the patient's death. Provide items for family comfort, such as tissues, refreshments, and chairs. When no words seem appropriate, maintain a respectful, conscious presence. The patient's death may be a relatively routine part of

BOX 4.5 Nursing Interventions to Support Care at the End-of-Life

- Assess patient's and family members' understanding of the condition and prognosis to address educational needs
- Educate family members about what will happen when life support is withdrawn to decrease their fear of the unknown
- Assure family members that the patient will not suffer
- Assure family members that the patient will not be abandoned
- Provide for any needed emotional support and spiritual care resources, such as grief counselors and spiritual care providers
- Facilitate physician communication with the family
- Provide for visitation and presence of family and extended family; most family members do not want the patient to die alone

your work experience, but keep in mind that family members will likely remember the situation, your actions, and those of the healthcare team for many years. Nursing interventions to support the family at the end-of-life are summarized in Box 4.5.

Caregiver Organizational Support

Providing end-of-life care requires much time, and inadequate staffing patterns may be a barrier to providing optimal care. Nursing administrators should keep this in mind when staffing to allow nurses time to adequately care for the dying patient. Should staffing ratios be less than adequate, assistance from colleagues can help to relieve the nurse who is caring for a dying patient of other responsibilities.

In addition to providing adequate staffing resources, helpful organizational behaviors include bereavement programs for families and assistance or guidance in making funeral arrangements. For situations in which the nurse and the patient or family do not speak the same language, interpreter services are essential to providing excellent end-of-life care. Debriefing or support sessions for staff members may be helpful in easing the stress of caring for dying patients.

Critical care nurses have expressed the need for provider and public education concerning end-of-life issues.[58] Efforts to educate the public on various end-of-life issues are vital to improving care through promotion of advance directives and conversations with loved ones concerning life-support options.[65]

Nurses have also identified the need for professional end-of-life education.[11,58] The AACN first developed the *End-of-Life Competency Statements for a Peaceful Death* in 2002, which spurred the improvement of end-of-life education in undergraduate nursing curricula.[2] Training is also available to prepare nurse educators to teach bedside nurses about delivering competent and compassionate care to the dying patient.[3] Empowered nurses and an ethical organizational climate are correlated with lower levels of moral distress.[1]

❓ CRITICAL REASONING ACTIVITY

The nurse assesses that there is significant disagreement among family members about what course of treatment is best for the patient. What action would be most effective in improving the situation?

CASE STUDY

Mr. M. is a 26-year-old Hispanic man who sustained severe injuries in a high-speed motorcycle accident, requiring admission to the critical care unit. According to his mother, he had previously been in perfect health, other than having mild asthma as a child. His most significant injuries are a cervical spine fracture and quadriplegia at the C2 level and a devastating traumatic brain injury consisting of a subarachnoid hemorrhage and diffuse axonal injury. He has subsequently developed acute respiratory distress syndrome, requiring high levels of mechanical ventilation support during the first 3 days of his hospitalization. His prognosis for functional recovery from his brain injury is deemed "poor" by the neurosurgeon, and because of his high quadriplegia, he will remain ventilator dependent for life. Mr. M.'s family is Cuban, very close-knit, and religious (Catholic), consisting of two sisters, his father and mother, and a grandmother who lives with them. Many of them do not speak English well, including his mother, who is his designated legal surrogate. All are very tearful and devastated by his injuries but remain hopeful that "God will help him recover and move again." His 20-year-old sister, in a private conversation with the nurse, states that her brother told her before he would prefer to die if he were ever paralyzed "from the neck down." She is afraid to verbalize these feelings with the rest of the family because she thinks her mother will accuse her of not loving her brother or of wanting to kill him.

Questions

1. What should the nurse say to Mr. M.'s sister? What course of action could the nurse recommend?
2. What resources in the institution would be most helpful to this family at this time? Why?
3. How does the family's cultural and religious background influence their perspective on this situation?
4. What learning needs does this family have? How could these be most appropriately met?

CULTURALLY COMPETENT END-OF-LIFE CARE

Many clinicians believe they lack the skills and preparation to guide difficult end-of-life discussions with patients and families of critically ill patients. This discomfort may be magnified when clinicians assist patients and families who are from a cultural or ethnic background that differs from their own. Cultural influences on care at the end-of-life are highly variable, even by region.[40,47,51]

The United States is well recognized as a nation of people from increasingly diverse cultural backgrounds and ethnicities. Therefore it is necessary to understand how cultural and ethnic differences affect crucial end-of-life decision-making processes and communication preferences in diverse groups, especially during stressful situations. Caring for persons of diverse cultural backgrounds can be difficult and frustrating for nurses, especially when institutional resources to support culturally diverse care are lacking. Better understanding and institutional support of these cultural differences in end-of-life care preferences will lead to more effective and satisfying care and communication with patients and families.[11,24]

Religious doctrine and beliefs profoundly influence patients' and families' choices for end-of-life care.[47,53] Significant differences in perspective may exist between and *within* many major religious groups, and these values are often deeply and subtly ingrained in belief systems underpinning care choices, including those of healthcare providers.[12]

Research on end-of-life care preferences in various cultural, ethnic, and religious groups has grown rapidly, although it is scarce in smaller cultural groups. In general, whites prefer less invasive and aggressive options near the end-of-life, whereas black and Hispanic ethnic groups tend to choose more aggressive care options.[60,63] Remember that research findings apply to groups in general and *may not apply to individual preferences or situations*. Become familiar with the values and beliefs of common cultural groups in your practice setting and try to recognize the influences of your personal religious and cultural contexts.

SUMMARY

Palliative and end-of-life issues are evolving rapidly as an integral part of high-quality, personalized critical care. The critical care nurse has a vital role in ensuring that patient and family needs for communication, information, support, and comfort are met in a reliable manner. Ongoing nursing education on palliative and end-of-life topics is important in ensuring that nurses are empowered to act as patient and family advocates, contributing to an ethical climate for practice.

REFERENCES

1. Altaker KW, Howie-Esquivel J, Cataldo JK. Relationships among palliative care, ethical climate, empowerment, and moral distress in intensive care unit nurses. *Am J Crit Care.* 2018;27(4):295–302.
2. American Association of Colleges of Nursing. *End-of-Life Competency Statements for a Peaceful Death.* Washington, DC: American Association of Colleges of Nursing; 2002.
3. American Association of Colleges of Nursing. End of Life Nursing Education Consortium (ELNEC). https://www.aacnnursing.org/ELNEC. Accessed October 28, 2018.
4. American Nurses Association. *Code of Ethics With Interpretive Statements.* Silver Spring, MD: American Nurses Association; 2015.
5. Aslakson RA, Curtis JR, Nelson JE. The changing role of palliative care in the ICU. *Crit Care Med.* 2014;42(11):2418–2428.
6. Bekelman JE, Halpern SD, Blankart CR, et al. Comparison of site of death, health care utilization, and hospital expenditures for patients dying with cancer in 7 developed countries. *JAMA.* 2016;315(3):272–283.
7. Blinderman CD, Billings JA. Comfort care for patients dying in the hospital. *New Engl J Med.* 2015;373(26):2549–2561.
8. Bone N, Swinton M, Hoad H, et al. Critical care nurses' experiences with spiritual care: The spirit study. *Am J Crit Care.* 2018;27(3):212–219.
9. Bosslet GT, Pope TM, Rubenfeld GD, et al. An official ATS/AACN/ACCP/ESICM/SCCM policy statement: Responding to requests for potentially inappropriate treatments in intensive care units. *Am J Resp Crit Care Med.* 2015;191(11):1318–1330.
10. Brady DR. Planning for deactivation of implantable cardioverter defibrillators at the end of life in patients with heart failure. *Crit Care Nurse.* 2016;36(3):24–32.
11. Brooks LA, Manias E, Nicholson P. Communication and decision-making about end-of-life care in the intensive care unit. *Am J Crit Care.* 2017;26(4):336–341.
12. Bülow HH, Sprung CL, Reinhart K, et al. The world's major religions' points of view on end-of-life decisions in the intensive care unit. *Intensive Care Med.* 2008;34(3):423–430.
13. Campbell ML, Templin T, Walch, J. A Respiratory Distress Observation Scale for patients unable to self-report dyspnea. *J Palliative Med* 2010:13(3), 285–290.
14. Centers for Disease Control and Prevention. Number of Deaths for Leading Causes of Death. https://www.cdc.gov/nchs/fastats/deaths.htm. Updated 2017. Accessed February 10, 2019.
15. Chang DW, Shapiro MF. Association between intensive care unit utilization during hospitalization and costs, use of invasive procedures, and mortality. *JAMA Int Med.* 2016;176(10):1492–1499.
16. Chatterjee K, Goyal A, Kakkera K, et al. National trends (2009–2013) for palliative care utilization for patients receiving prolonged mechanical ventilation. *Crit Care Med.* 2018;46(8):1230–1237.
17. Chiarchiaro J, Buddadhumaruk P, Arnold RM, et al. Quality of communication in the ICU and surrogate's understanding of prognosis. *Crit Care Med.* 2015;43(3):542–548.
18. Chiarchiaro J, Ernecoff NC, Scheunemann LP, Hough CL. Physicians rarely elicit critically ill patients' previously expressed treatment preferences in intensive care units. *Am J Resp Crit Care Med.* 2017;196(2):242–245.
19. Chiarchiaro J, White DB, Ernecoff NC, et al. Conflict management strategies in the ICU differ between palliative care specialists and intensivists. *Crit Care Med.* 2016;44(5):934–942.
20. Death With Dignity. Current Death With Dignity Laws. https://www.deathwithdignity.org/learn/death-with-dignity-acts/. Accessed November 11, 2018.
21. DeMartino ES, Dudzinski DM, Doyle CK, et al. Who decides when a patient can't? Statutes on alternate decision makers. *N Eng J Med.* 2017;376(15):1478–1482.
22. Detsky ME, Harhay MO, Bayard DF, et al. Discriminative accuracy of physician and nurse predictions for survival and functional outcomes 6 months after an ICU admission. *JAMA.* 2017;317(21):2187–2195.
23. Douglas SL, Daly BJ, Lipson AR. Differences in predictions for survival and expectations for goals of care between physicians and family surrogate decision makers of chronically critically ill adults. *Res Rev J Nurse Health Sci.* 2017;3(3):74–84.
24. Downar J, Delaney JW, Hawryluck L, Kenny L. Guidelines for the withdrawal of life-sustaining measures. *Intensive Care Med.* 2016;42:1003–1017.
25. Downar J, You JJ, Bagshaw SM, et al; Canadian Critical Care Trials Group. Nonbeneficial treatment Canada: Definitions, causes and potential solutions from the perspective of healthcare practitioners. *Crit Care Med.* 2015;43(2):270–281.
26. Ellis L, Gergen J, Wohlgemuth, et al. Empowering the "cheerers": Role of the surgical intensive care unit nurses in enhancing family resilience. *Am J Crit Care.* 2016;25(1):39–45.
27. Frontera JA, Curtis JR, Nelson JE, et al. Integrating palliative care into the care of neurocritically ill patients: A report from the Improving Palliative Care in the ICU Project Advisory Board and the Center to Advance Palliative Care. *Crit Care Med.* 2015;43(9):1964–1977.

28. Hart JL, Harhay MO, Gabler NB, et al. Variability among US intensive care units in managing the care of patients admitted with preexisting limits on life-sustaining therapies. *JAMA Intern Med.* 2015;175(6):1019–1026.

29. Henrich NJ, Dodek PM, Gladstone E, et al. Consequences of moral distress in the intensive care unit: A qualitative study. *Am J Crit Care.* 2017;26(4):e48–e57.

30. Hoffman TC, Del Mar C. Patients' expectations of the benefits and harms of treatments, screening, and tests: A systematic review. *JAMA Intern Med.* 2015;175(2):274–286.

31. Institute of Medicine, Committee on Approaching Death. *Dying in America: Improving Quality and Honoring Individual Preferences Near the End of Life.* Washington, DC: National Academies Press; 2014.

32. Khandelwal N, Bensker DC, Coe NB, et al. Potential influence of advance care planning and palliative care consultation on ICU costs for patients with chronic and serious illness. *Crit Care Med.* 2016;44(8):1474–1481.

33. Khandelwal N, Kross EK, Engelberg RA, et al. Estimating the effect of palliative care interventions and advance care planning on ICU utilization: A systematic review. *Crit Care Med.* 2015;43(5):1102–1111.

34. Kon AA, Davidson JE. Retiring the term futility in value-laden decisions regarding potentially inappropriate medical treatment. *Crit Care Nurse.* 2017;37(1):9–11.

35. Kon AA, Shepard EK, Sederstrom NO, et al. Defining futile and potentially inappropriate interventions: A policy statement from the Society of Critical Care Medicine Ethics Committee. *Crit Care Med.* 2016;44(9):1769–1774.

36. Li L, Nelson JE, Hanson LC, et al. How surrogate decision-makers for patients with chronic illness perceive and carry out their role. *Crit Care Med.* 2018;46(5):699–704.

37. Lobo SM, De Simoni FHB, Jakob SM, et al. Decision-making on withholding or withdrawing life support in the ICU. *Chest.* 2017;152(2):321–329.

38. Ma J, Ward EM, Siegel RL, Jernal A. Temporal trends in mortality in the United States, 1969–2013. *JAMA.* 2015;314(16):1731–1739.

39. Mark NM, Rayner SG, Lee NJ, Curtis JR. Global variability in withholding and withdrawal of life-sustaining treatment in the intensive care unit: A systematic review. *Intensive Care Med.* 2015;41:1572–1585.

40. Mark NM, Rayner SG, Lee NJ, Curtis JR. Global variability in withholding and withdrawal of life-sustaining treatment in the intensive care unit: A systematic review. *Int Care Med.* 2015;41(9):1572–1585.

41. McCarthy FH, McDermott KM, Kini V, et al. Trends in U.S. extracorporeal membrane oxygenation use and outcomes: 2002–2012. *Semin Thorac Cardiovasc Surg.* 2015;27(2):81–88.

42. Mullen JE, Reynolds MR, Larson JS. Caring for pediatric patients' families at the child's end of life. *Crit Care Nurse.* 2015;35(6):46–56.

43. Munro CL, Savel RH. Aggressive care AND palliative care. *Am J Crit Care.* 2018;26(5):84–86.

44. National Hospice and Palliative Care Organization. Hospice Care. http://www.nhpco.org/about/hospice-care. Accessed October 28, 2018.

45. Neville TH, Wiley JF, Yamamoto MC, et al. Concordance of nurses and physicians on whether critical care patients are receiving futile treatment. *Am J Crit Care.* 2015;24(5):403–411.

46. Nunez ER, Schenker Y, Joel ID, et al. Acutely bereaved surrogates' stories about the decision to limit life support in the ICU. *Crit Care Med.* 2015;43(11):2387–2393.

47. Ohr S, Jeong S, Saul P. Cultural and religious beliefs and values, and their impact on preferences for end-of-life care among four ethnic groups of community-dwelling older persons. *J Clin Nursing.* 2016;26:1681–1689.

48. Olmstead JA, Dahnke MD. The need for an effective process to resolve conflicts over medical futility: A case study and analysis. *Crit Care Nurse.* 2016;36(6):13–23.

49. O'Neill BJ, Kazer MW. Destination to nowhere: A new look at aggressive treatment for heart failure—A case study. *Crit Care Nurse.* 2014;34(2):47–56.

50. Petrinec AB, Mazanec PM, Burant CJ. Coping strategies and posttraumatic stress symptoms in post-ICU family decision makers. *Crit Care Med.* 2015;43(6):1205–1212.

51. Phua J, Joynt GM, Nishimura M, et al. Withholding and withdrawal of life-sustaining treatments in intensive care units in Asia. *JAMA Intern Med.* 2015;175(3):363–371.

52. Pillay T, Adriaan van Zyl H, Blackbeard D. Chronic pain perception and cultural experience. *Procedia Soc Behav Sci.* 2014;113:151–160.

53. Rhodes RL, Elwood B, Lee SC, et al. The desires of their hearts: The multidisciplinary perspectives of African Americans on end-of-life care in the African American community. *Am J Hospice Pall Med.* 2017;34(6):510–517.

54. Rodney PA. What we know about moral distress. *AJN.* 2017;117(2):S7–S10.

55. Rushton CH. Moral resilience: A capacity for navigating moral distress in critical care. *AACN Adv Crit Care.* 2016;27(1):111–119.

56. Rushton CH. Cultivating moral resilience. *AJN.* 2017;117(2):S11–S15.

57. Rushton CH, Schoonover-Shoffner K, Kennedy MS. A collaborative state of the science initiative: Transforming moral distress into moral resilience in nursing. *AJN.* 2017;117(2):S2–S6.

58. Sauerland J, Marotta K, Peinemann MA, et al. Assessing and addressing moral distress and ethical climate part II. *Dimens Crit Care Nurs.* 2015;34(1):33–46.

59. Savel RH, Munro CL. Moral distress, moral courage. *Am J Crit Care.* 2015;24(4):276–278.

60. Sharma RK, Freedman VA, Mor V, et al. Association of racial differences with end-of-life care quality in the United States. *JAMA Intern Med.* 2017;177(22):1858–1860.

61. Shorr C, Angelo M. Trends for palliative care use in the prolonged mechanically ventilated patient: Are we moving toward a proactive approach? *Crit Care Med.* 2018;46(8):1374–1375.

62. Singer AE, Meeker D, Teno JM, et al. Symptom trends in the last year of life from 1998–2010. *Ann Intern Med.* 2015;162:175–183.

63. Solloway B. Racial differences persist in end-of-life care. *NEJM Journal Watch.* https://www.jwatch.org/na43011/2016/12/29/racial-differences-persist-end-life-care. Published December 29, 2016. Accessed 2018.

64. SUPPORT Principal Investigators. A controlled trial to improve care for seriously ill hospitalized patients: The study to understand prognoses and preferences for outcomes and risks of treatments (SUPPORT). *JAMA.* 2005;274(20):1591–1598.

65. Tolle SW, Teno JM. Lessons from Oregon in embracing complexity in end-of-life care. *N Eng J Med.* 2017;376(11):1078–1082.

66. White DB, Ernecoff N, Buddadhumaruk P, et al. Prevalence of and factors related to discordance about prognosis between physicians and surrogate decision makers of critically ill patients. *JAMA.* 2016;315(19):2086–2094.

67. Wilson ME, Krupa A, Hinds RF. A video to improve patient and surrogate understanding of cardiopulmonary resuscitation choices in the ICU: A randomized controlled trial. *Crit Care Med.* 2015;43(3):621–629.

68. Wolf SM, Berlinger N, Jennings B. Forty years of work on end-of-life care—From patients' rights to systemic reform. *N Engl J Med.* 2015;327(7):678–682.

69. Wright AA, Keating NL, Ayanian JZ, et al. Family perspectives on aggressive cancer care near the end of life. *JAMA.* 2016;315(3):284–292.

Organ Donation

Nikki Dotson-Lorello, BSN, RN, CCRN, CPTC
Deborah G. Klein, MSN, APRN, ACNS-BC, CCRN, FAHA, FAAN

Many additional resources, including self-assessment exercises, are located on the Evolve companion website at http://evolve.elsevier.com/Sole/.
- Animations
- Clinical Skills: Critical Care Collections
- Student Review Questions
- Video Clips

INTRODUCTION

For more than 50 years, solid organ transplantation has been the only definitive treatment option for patients living with end-stage organ failure; however, organ transplantation is associated with many challenges. A scarcity of organs reduces the likelihood of transplantation for many individuals. On average, 22 people die daily while waiting for an organ transplant. More than 114,000 people in the United States are active on organ transplant waiting lists. In 2018 there were 17,562 organ donations and 36,529 organ transplants (Figs. 5.1 and 5.2).[23] Of these transplants, 29,680 were from deceased donors and 6894 were from living donors.[23] The number of patients active on transplant waiting lists fluctuates due to multiple factors, including death while awaiting transplant or being inactive on the waiting list as a result of infection or high acuity.

Cause of death for the organ donor is an important consideration in organ availability and is a significant part of donor evaluation (Box 5.1). One example is donor death resulting from massive brain trauma. In massive brain trauma there is rapid progression from initial injury to brain death and concurrent massive surges in blood pressure and blood vessel tone. These surges can cause cardiac and lung damage and end-organ ischemia affecting viability of organs for transplant. A second example is donor death resulting from drug overdose. This potential donor may be classified as an "increased-risk" donor due to the risk for transmitting bloodborne infections. Measures to maximize organ donation and recovery from the limited pool of donors is a recognized goal in critical care practice.[15]

Critical care nurses work collaboratively with organ procurement organizations (OPOs) and transplant teams throughout the continuum of care from identification of a potential organ donor, assisting with brain death testing, providing emotional support for the donor families, donor management, organ procurement process, and emotional support for multiprofessional team members.[2] This chapter provides an overview of the organ donation process throughout all phases of care: evaluation, referral, brain death testing, donor management, and management criteria for specific organs. Management of the solid organ recipient is not discussed in this chapter, as care for these patients is highly specialized.

ORGAN DONATION

Organ donation has developed into a separate entity from organ transplantation. Critical care nurses are often the first to identify a potential organ donor. Nurses must understand clinical triggers associated with actual and impending brain death to initiate a referral to the OPO.

Throughout history, death had been defined as the cessation of blood flow when the heart permanently stops beating in response to catastrophic illness or injury. The ability to care for patients after brain injuries previously considered fatal, and the ability to recover organs for transplantation, led to exploration of the concept of *brain death*. This concept dates to 1959 with the introduction of "coma dépassé," a state beyond coma indicating loss of life functions such as reflexes, consciousness, and mobility. In 1968 an Ad Hoc Committee of Harvard Medical School described "irreversible coma" (what is now considered brain death), incorporating most clinical testing.[1] The "Harvard criteria" have been the foundation for current brain death testing.

Criteria for brain death are defined as absent cerebral and brainstem function associated with a nonsurvivable head injury.[1,15] The head injury may be structural, such as catastrophic brain trauma, or caused by intracerebral hemorrhage.[15] Injuries may also be metabolic, as occurs in profound and prolonged hypoxemia or prolonged cardiopulmonary arrest.[15] An individual is determined to be dead based on neurological criteria *(brain*

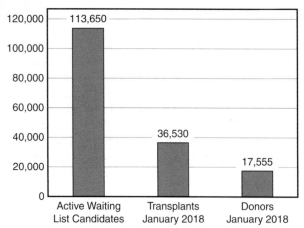

Fig. 5.1 Illustration of the great imbalance between organ supply and demand. (From Organ Procurement and Transplantation Network. OPTN National Data Reports. https://optn.transplant.hrsa.gov/data/view-data-reports/. Accessed February 28, 2019.)

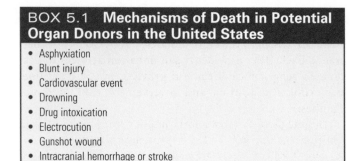

BOX 5.1   Mechanisms of Death in Potential Organ Donors in the United States

- Asphyxiation
- Blunt injury
- Cardiovascular event
- Drowning
- Drug intoxication
- Electrocution
- Gunshot wound
- Intracranial hemorrhage or stroke
- Seizure
- Stab wound

death) when these clinical requirements are met and not when the heart stops beating *(circulatory death)*. This formerly controversial concept is still not completely understood by healthcare professionals and the general public. For example, a patient who is dead by neurological criteria may appear to be "alive" only because the ventilator is moving air in and out of the lungs, artificially causing the chest to rise and fall. The patient will have a pulse and warm skin because artificial support is being provided, such as mechanical ventilation, vasoactive and inotropic medications, and IV fluids. Any discussion of death touches on cultural, personal, and religious perspectives and must be addressed carefully. The concept of brain death also requires careful, sensitive communication with patients' families when brain death testing is a consideration, as well as consistent messages from multiprofessional team members.[15]

In 1968 the Uniform Anatomical Gift Act (UAGA) was passed in the United States. This law established a legal framework for individuals to authorize an anatomical gift of their organs, tissues, and eyes following death.[26] It also prohibited the trafficking of human organs. Individual states have adopted the UAGA, which was revised in 1987 and 2006.[26]

The National Organ Transplant Act of 1984 called for an Organ Procurement and Transplantation Network (OPTN) to be created and run by a private, nonprofit organization under federal contract.[24] This Act established the OPTN to provide oversight for transplantation and organ donation, as well as to develop and maintain a national registry for organ sharing and matching.[23] The United Network for Organ Sharing (UNOS) was first awarded the national OPTN contract in 1986, and UNOS continues as the only organization to operate the OPTN. Multiple resources are available from UNOS for healthcare providers, transplant professionals, and members of the public seeking information on organ donation and transplantation. This information and access is taxpayer funded and available at http://www.unos.org.

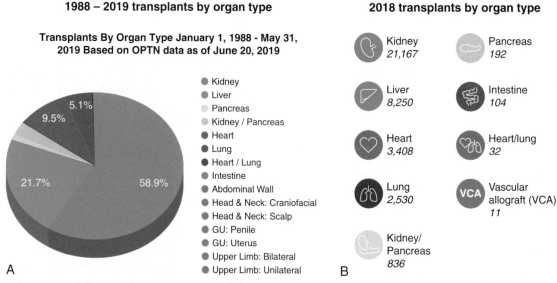

Fig. 5.2 **A,** Transplants in 1988 to 2019 by organ type. **B,** Transplants in 2018 by organ type. *GU,* Genitourinary. (From United Network for Organ Sharing. Transplant Trend. https://unos.org/data/transplant-trends/. Published 2019. Accessed June 30, 2019.)

The Health Care Financing Administration was given the authority to certify OPOs. Today, 58 nonprofit OPOs serve donation needs in the United States, Puerto Rico, and Bermuda. Each OPO provides organ donation services to designated geographical areas and provides public education, professional education, and bereavement care to donor families.[23]

Despite these national efforts, donor organs remain scarce, limiting the availability of transplantation. In 1998 the Centers for Medicare and Medicaid Services imposed requirements for hospital reporting in an effort to increase organ donation. Any hospital that receives Medicare or Medicaid reimbursement must notify the local OPO in all cases of impending death.[6,18] It is the responsibility of the OPO to have a trained staff member obtain consent for organ or tissue donation from the family of the deceased patient. Many hospitals have developed clinical criteria or triggers to ensure the appropriate referral of potential organ donors to the OPO.[6] Such clinical triggers include a Glasgow Coma Scale score less than 5; stroke; anoxia; and/or brain trauma with a declining neurological examination, including decrease in or loss of one or more brainstem reflexes. Impending withdrawal of mechanical ventilation for a dying patient is also an appropriate trigger if family members initiate a discussion about donation.[15]

Organ donation saves lives. Tissue donation, although not life-saving, improves quality of life. One tissue donor can enhance the lives of more than 75 people.[9] Tissue donation includes skin, corneas, veins, heart valves, bone, cartilage, and tendons. A corneal donation may give the gift of sight. Skin donation provides skin grafting to treat severe burns or extensive wounds. Research protocols for donation are now available for organ donors with HIV to recipients with HIV and vascularized composite allografts (VCAs) for hand and face transplants. Hospitals are required to have a formal arrangement with a tissue bank for the referral of potential donors.[9,19,24]

❓ CRITICAL REASONING ACTIVITY

A 52-year-old woman with a history of diabetes mellitus, hypertension, and uterine fibroids experiences a catastrophic intracranial hemorrhage. She is admitted to a tertiary care center following activation of the emergency medical services system by her family who witnessed the event, including her loss of consciousness. She had been independent with activities of daily living and worked full time as an accountant. Following stabilization in the emergency department, including intubation and mechanical ventilation, her emergent head computed tomography (CT) scan shows massive intracranial hemorrhage, significant midline shift, brain edema, and blood within the ventricles. Her neurological examination is declining despite aggressive care to maximize recovery.

1. At what point is it appropriate to initiate a referral to the local organ procurement organization?

2. She continues to experience decline in her neurological assessment to the point that her pupils become fixed, dilated, and midpoint, and she has lost all brainstem reflexes. What is the optimal strategy to communicate this change with the patient's family?

TYPES OF ORGAN DONATION

Organ donation may occur in three options: living donor, brain death, or circulatory death. A *living donor*, who is otherwise healthy, may donate an organ such as a kidney, a lobe of a lung or liver, part of a pancreas, or a segment of the intestine. Living donation is done only after clinical evaluation identifies an appropriate match between the donor and recipient and that the donor is healthy enough to tolerate surgery and has no psychosocial contraindications. A living donor does not have to be biologically related to the recipient. In fact, 1 in 4 living donors are not biologically related.[13,15]

A *brain dead donor* may donate following consent from self, such as through donor designation on a driver's license or organ donor card, or from the legally authorized representative. Thoughtful, caring, and compassionate communication must occur among the healthcare providers, OPO staff members, and the patient's family. A patient may become an organ donor following *circulatory death*; after clinical criteria are met, organs are recovered following withdrawal of life-sustaining therapies and subsequent asystole within a protocol-directed time frame.

Organ donors can also be described in many ways: standard donors, nondirected/altruistic living donors, paired donors, increased-risk donors, and expanded criteria donors. Table 5.1 describes the types of organ donors and the most common organs donated.[9,15,25]

STUDY BREAK

1. A patient determined to be brain dead may be considered an organ donor by:
   A. First-person consent
   B. Consent from the patient's fiancée
   C. This patient cannot be an organ donor
   D. No consent is required, as the patient is brain dead

Living Donor and Kidney Paired Exchange Donation

To qualify as a living donor, the person must meet several criteria:

- Be at least 18 years old and willing to donate
- Have good physical and mental health
- Be well informed regarding risks, benefits, and potential outcomes, both good and bad, for donor and recipient
- Have a good support system
- Be able to take time off from work or school for diagnostic workup
- Be able to take 2 to 3 weeks off work or school after the surgery
- Be free from diabetes, cancer, and kidney and heart disease; have normal blood pressure or controlled hypertension; and be free from hepatitis C or HIV
- Have a body mass index (BMI) less than 35
- Have no drug or alcohol problems

Policies are provided by OPTN to advocate for, screen, and care for the living donor. Every living donor is assigned an independent living donor advocate (ILDA) who functions independent of the transplant team to avoid any conflict of interest.

TABLE 5.1 Types of Organ Donors in the United States

Donor Type	Description	Organs Donated
Standard criteria donor	Under 50 years of age Declared brain dead from traumatic injuries or stroke	Kidney, pancreas, liver, intestine, heart, lung, tissues
Deceased, heart-beating donors	Declared brain dead because of nonsurvivable head injuries or neurological events such as prolonged cardiopulmonary arrest, severe stroke, or intracranial hemorrhage	Kidney, pancreas, liver, intestine, heart, lung, abdominal wall, face, penis, uterus, upper limb
Donation after circulatory death (formerly donation after cardiac death and non–heart-beating donors)	Donation after withdrawal of life-sustaining therapy. The patient must become asystolic within a prescribed period following withdrawal of controlled ventilation and vasoactive medications.	Kidney, liver, lung
Living donor	An organ or part of an organ is offered by a healthy individual to a patient with end-organ disease. Living donors may be related or unrelated.	Kidney, one or two lobes of the liver, a lung or part of a lung, part of a pancreas, part of the intestine
Nondirected/altruistic living donor	An individual who donates an organ or part of an organ to a stranger.	Kidney (most common), liver lobe (rare)
Increased-risk donor	Decision to transplant an increased-risk donor organ is based on the critical state of the recipient in whom the risk of not transplanting an organ is greater than the risk of disease transmission from a donor. Patient and family must consent to accept an increased-risk donor CDC definition includes but is not limited to: • People who have had sex with a person known to have HIV, HBV, or HCV in the preceding 12 months • Men who have had sex with men in the preceding 12 months • Women who have had sex with a man who had sex with men in the preceding 12 months • People who have had sex in exchange for money in the preceding 12 months • People who have had sex with a person who has injected drugs by IV, intramuscular, or subcutaneous route for nonmedical reasons in the preceding 12 months • A child who is ≤18 months of age, born to a mother known to be infected with or at increased risk for HIV, HBV, or HCV • A child who has been breastfed within the preceding 12 months whose mother is known to be infected with or at increased risk for HIV • People who have injected drugs by IV, intramuscular, or subcutaneous route for nonmedical reasons in the preceding 12 months • People who have been in lockup, jail, prison, or a juvenile correctional facility for more than 72 hours in the preceding 12 months • People who have been newly diagnosed with or have been treated for syphilis, gonorrhea, *Chlamydia*, or genital ulcers in the preceding 12 months • People who test positive for Epstein-Barr virus (EBV), cytomegalovirus (CMV), or toxoplasmosis • People who have been on hemodialysis in the preceding 12 months • Donor at increased risk for HIV, HBV, or HCV infection when medical and behavioral history cannot be obtained or risk factors cannot be determined	Heart, lung, kidney, pancreas, liver, islet cells, small bowel, stomach, uterus, face, appendages, skin
Expanded criteria donor	Deceased donor Donor >50 years of age with two of the following: high blood pressure, creatinine ≥1.5 mg/dL, or death from stroke Donor >60 years of age	Kidney, liver, heart, pancreas, lung, intestine
Hepatitis C core antibody–positive donor	A donor who has a positive serological finding for hepatitis C core antibody. The donor may have been successfully treated for hepatitis C or had prior exposure to the point at which he or she developed antibodies to the virus. Active hepatitis C precludes donation.	Kidney, liver, heart, lung

CDC, Centers for Disease Control and Prevention; *HBV,* hepatitis B virus: *HCV,* hepatitis C virus.
Data from Organ Procurement and Transplantation Network. Data and Policy. https://optn.transplant.hrsa.gov/. Accessed November 17, 2018.

Evaluation for a living donor typically begins after the intended recipient is active on the transplant waiting list and includes medical and psychosocial evaluation. Evaluation of motivation to donate is performed to determine if any coercion or financial incentives are present. The evaluation process also determines that the donor is healthy and at low enough risk for organ recovery surgery. Individual transplant centers may allow flexibility in age and screening of the living donor criteria acceptance. Gender and race are not factors in determining a successful match, but donors must have a blood type compatible with the intended recipient. After evaluation, living donor donation is coordinated by the transplant team.

Kidney paired exchange donation is an option for candidates who have a living donor who is medically able but cannot donate a kidney to their intended candidate because they are incompatible. This is a pilot program, governed by OPTN. UNOS works with transplant centers in the United States to ensure that the donor in each pair is compatible with recipients in another pair (or multiple pairs).[25] Living donor exchange is then arranged through the OPTN, ensuring a compatible match for both recipients.

Brain Dead Donor

A *brain dead donor* is one who is pronounced dead according to neurological criteria. Evaluation of brain death includes clinical evaluation and neurodiagnostic studies. Revised guidelines for brain death testing were published in 2010 and define brain death as complete, irreversible cessation of function of the brain and brainstem.[15,28] Cardiopulmonary function and end-organ perfusion may be maintained artificially by mechanical ventilation, infusion of inotropic or vasoactive medications, maintenance of intravascular volume, and treatment of fluid and electrolyte derangements. Brain death is diagnosed by physical examination, usually by a neurologist or neurosurgeon. Determination of brain death consists of these steps: (1) prerequisites for the clinical evaluation (Table 5.2); (2) the clinical evaluation (neurological assessment) (Table 5.3); (3) neurodiagnostic testing, including electroencephalogram, cerebral angiography, or radionuclide cerebral perfusion scan (Table 5.4); and (4) identification of potential confounding factors. Confounding factors must be evaluated before imaging because equivocal results can confuse clinicians and family members regarding status of brain death testing (Table 5.5).[15,16,28] Hypothermia, high-dose central nervous system depressants, and massive drug or toxin ingestion may severely depress consciousness and interfere with valid brain death testing.[15,16] Thus these conditions must be reversed prior to brain death testing.

Once the following conditions are met, the patient may be pronounced dead by neurological criteria: (1) documentation of the cause of catastrophic brain injury (metabolic or structural), (2) elimination of possible reversible causes for the significantly depressed neurological examination, (3) clinical evaluation consistent with brain death (including carbon dioxide unresponsiveness at the brainstem documented by apnea testing [see Table 5.3]), and (4) clinically appropriate neurodiagnostic testing within a brain death protocol consistent with brain death.[15,16] When these tests are completed, the time of concluded brain death testing becomes the documented time of death. Federal and state laws require the physician to contact the OPO following determination of brain death.[6] However, the OPO is usually contacted before brain death declaration in response to clinical triggers and initiates evaluation of the potential donor before brain death declaration.

Once the patient is considered medically suitable for organ donation and the family has a clear understanding that death has in fact occurred by neurological criteria, an OPO staff member approaches the family to obtain consent for organ donation. In addition, the primary team caring for the patient discusses brain death and reassures families that death has been determined. This discussion should occur separate from discussions by the OPO staff member regarding consent for organ donation. Separating these discussions is considered best practice and is correlated with significantly higher organ donation consent rates.[15]

TABLE 5.2	Prerequisites for Clinical Evaluation of Brain Death
Steps	**Clinical Evaluation**
1. Establish irreversible coma and cause of coma	Established by patient history, physical examination, neuroimaging, and laboratory tests. The clinician: • Excludes the effect of CNS depressant medication. • Recognizes that prior use of targeted temperature management may delay drug metabolism. • Verifies no recent administration of neuromuscular blockade medications. • Verifies no severe electrolyte, acid-base, or endocrine disturbance. • Verifies no confounding factors present that may "mimic" brain death, such as locked-in syndrome, fulminant Guillain-Barré syndrome, severe hypothermia, post–cardiac arrest syndrome, massive baclofen/anticholinergic overdose, severe overdose of CNS depressants, massive overdose of valproic acid or tricyclic antidepressants, or severe snake envenomation.
2. Achieve normal core temperature	Warming blanket is often needed to maintain normothermia. Vasodilation following catecholamine depletion leads to additional heat loss as blood flow increases to the periphery and causes additional heat loss after final brainstem herniation.
3. Achieve normal systolic blood pressure	Hypovolemia and loss of peripheral vascular tone are often present, which may be corrected with IV fluids, vasopressors, or inotropic medications. Neurological examination is most reliable with a systolic blood pressure ≥100 mm Hg.
4. Perform neurological examination	One neurological exam, although controversial, is now considered sufficient for diagnosing brain death in most states. Brain death must be pronounced and documented by a physician. When two clinical examinations are used, one of the examinations is completed by a neurologist or neurosurgeon.

CNS, Central nervous system.

Modified from Wijdicks EF, Varelas PN, Gronseth GS, et al. Evidence-based guideline update: Determining brain death in adults: Report of the Quality Standards Subcommittee of the American Academy of Neurology. *Neurology.* 2010;74(23):1911–1918.

TABLE 5.3 Clinical Evaluation for Brain Death

Neurological Assessment	Clinical Evaluation
Coma	• Patient lacks all evidence of responsiveness. • Noxious stimuli should not produce a motor response other than spinally mediated reflexes.
Absence of brainstem reflexes	• Absence of pupillary response to bright light: Usually the pupils are fixed with midsize or dilated position (4-9 mm). Constricted pupils suggest the possibility of drug intoxication. • Absence of ocular movements using oculocephalic testing and oculovestibular reflex testing. • Oculocephalic testing: Once the integrity of the cervical spine is ensured, the head is briskly rotated horizontally and vertically. There should be no movement of the eyes relative to head movement. • Oculovestibular reflex testing (caloric testing): After the patency of both external auditory canals is confirmed, the patient's head is elevated to 30 degrees. The external auditory canal of each ear is irrigated (one ear at a time) with approximately 50 mL of ice water. Movement of the eyes should be absent during 1 minute of observation. • Absence of corneal reflex: Demonstrated by touching the cornea with a piece of tissue paper, a cotton swab, or squirts of water. No eyelid movement should be seen. • Absence of facial muscle movement to a noxious stimulus: Deep pressure on the condyles at the level of the temporomandibular joints and deep pressure at the supraorbital ridge should produce no grimacing or facial muscle movement. • Absence of the pharyngeal and tracheal reflexes: The pharyngeal or gag reflex is tested after stimulation of the posterior pharynx with a tongue blade or suction device. The tracheal reflex is tested by examining the cough response to tracheal suctioning. The catheter should be inserted into the trachea and advanced to the level of the carina followed by one or two suctioning passes.
Apnea	• Absence of a breathing drive is tested with a CO_2 challenge with documentation of an increase in $PaCO_2$ above normal levels. • Prerequisites: (1) normotension, (2) normothermia, (3) euvolemia, (4) eucapnia ($PaCO_2$ 35-45 mm Hg), (5) absence of hypoxia, and (6) no prior evidence of CO_2 retention (i.e., chronic obstructive pulmonary disease, severe obesity). **Procedure:** 1. Adjust vasopressors to a systolic blood pressure ≥100 mm Hg. 2. Preoxygenate for at least 10 minutes with 100% oxygen to a PaO_2 >200 mm Hg. 3. Reduce ventilation frequency to 10 breaths/min to eucapnia. 4. Reduce positive end-expiratory pressure (PEEP) to 5 cm H_2O (oxygen desaturation with decreasing PEEP may suggest difficulty with apnea testing). 5. If pulse oximetry oxygen saturation remains >95%, obtain a baseline blood gas (PaO_2, $PaCO_2$, pH, bicarbonate, base excess). 6. Disconnect the patient from the ventilator. 7. Preserve oxygenation (e.g., place an insufflation catheter through the endotracheal tube and close to the level of the carina and deliver 100% O_2 at 6 L/min). 8. Look closely for respiratory movements for 8-10 minutes. Respiration is defined as abdominal or chest excursions and may include a brief gasp. 9. Abort if systolic blood pressure decreases to <90 mm Hg. 10. Abort if oxygen saturation measured by pulse oximetry is <85% for >30 seconds. 11. If no respiratory drive is observed, repeat arterial blood gas (PaO_2, $PaCO_2$, pH, bicarbonate, base excess) after approximately 8 minutes. 12. If respiratory movements are absent and arterial $PaCO_2$ is ≥60 mm Hg (or 20 mm Hg increase in arterial $PaCO_2$ over a baseline normal arterial $PaCO_2$), the apnea test result is positive (i.e., supports the clinical diagnosis of brain death). 13. If the test is inconclusive but the patient is hemodynamically stable during the procedure, it may be repeated for a longer period (10-15 minutes) after the patient is again adequately preoxygenated.

CO_2, Carbon dioxide; $PaCO_2$, partial pressure of carbon dioxide; PaO_2, partial pressure of oxygen.
Modified from Wijdicks EF, Varelas PN, Gronseth GS, et al. Evidence-based guideline update: Determining brain death in adults: Report of the Quality Standards Subcommittee of the American Academy of Neurology. *Neurology.* 2010;74(23):1911–1918.

Consent for any organ donation may be obtained from the legal authorized representative (usually a family member) through donor designation. If first-person consent (donor designation) exists, the OPO holds an informative discussion with the family, as family consent is not absolutely necessary. If family consent is required, the OPO staff member starts the conversation by asking the family about the patient's character. Organ donation is presented as an opportunity for something good to come out of tragedy and a way for a loved one to "live on." The benefits to the family are the initial focus of the conversation.

The relationship between the critical care unit staff and the family is an important factor in a family's decision to donate organs of a loved one.[15] Developing trust between the multiprofessional team and the patient's family is important throughout the critical care hospitalization. Trust is also important when brain death and organ donation are discussed. Families often have many questions, concerns, or fears about

TABLE 5.4 Neurodiagnostic Testing in Brain Death Determination

Test	Description	Advantages	Disadvantages	Normal Findings	Findings in Brain Death
Four-vessel cerebral angiography	Injection of radiopaque contrast into blood supply to the brain	Short time to obtain results; easy to read; definitive when consistent with brain death clinical criteria	Invasive; radiopaque contrast may compromise kidney function. Blood flow may persist after clinical evidence of brain death if terminal injury not associated with ICP elevation (hypoxic injury, craniectomy).	Blood flow into all areas of brain, contrast documented in large blood vessels of brain	No blood flow into the brain
Radionuclide cerebral perfusion scanning	IV injection of radioisotope tracer	Less invasive; rapid interpretation; no radiopaque contrast load on kidneys	Requires transport of unstable patient. May yield radiographic evidence of flow in clinical examination consistent with brain death (craniotomy defect, absence of significant ICP elevation).	Images show uptake of radioisotope tracer in viable brain tissue	Absence of radioisotope tracer uptake in brain tissue (Fig. 5.3)
Diagnostic EEG	Performed at bedside using multiple scalp electrodes; EEG tracing evaluated over at least 30 minutes and in response to stimulation	Easy to perform at bedside; noninvasive; results available quickly	Electrical interference in critical care unit (infusion pumps, beds, ventilators, personnel) may be reflected in EEG and be difficult to explain to family. EEG can be affected by hypothermia and residual CNS depressant effects.	Consistent waveforms on EEG tracing including variability in response to stimulation	Absence of cerebral electrical activity and no variability in response to stimulation

CNS, Central nervous system; EEG, electroencephalogram; ICP, intracranial pressure.
Adapted from Arbour R. Brain death: Assessment, controversy and confounding factors. Crit Care Nurs. 2013;33(6):27–46; Wijdicks EF, Varelas PN, Gronseth GS, et al. Evidence-based guideline update: Determining brain death in adults: Report of the Quality Standards Subcommittee of the American Academy of Neurology. Neurology. 2010;74(23):1911–1918.

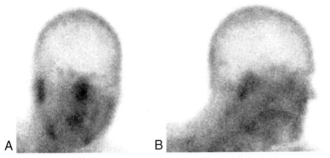

Fig. 5.3 Radionuclide brain perfusion study consistent with brain death. **A,** Anterior posterior view. **B,** Lateral view. Lighter color indicates absence of isotope uptake and absence of perfusion. Darker color indicates isotope uptake and presence of perfusion to the neck and face (nose).

organ donation that may affect willingness to consent.[15] Common concerns include disfigurement of the donor that will not allow for an open casket at the funeral, that the potential donor will receive inferior medical care, that the potential donor may not really be dead, and that the family will have to pay for the donation process. All members of the multiprofessional team should provide information, support, and clarity. They must project caring and compassion and ensure that families have easy access to their loved one so that they can say goodbye.[7,15]

Organ Donation After Circulatory Death

In 2007 the OPTN established guidelines for donation after circulatory death (DCD), also known as *donation after cardiac death* or *donation after circulatory determination of death*.[10] In this type of donation, the patient has an illness from which no recovery is expected, does not meet brain death criteria, and depends on life-sustaining medical and mechanical interventions, such as mechanical ventilation, vasoactive medications, or inotropic medications. Once the family begins discussion about withdrawal of life support or a decision to withdraw life support is imminent, the OPO is notified. If the patient meets age and medical criteria for organ donation, the OPO coordinator (not the OPO staff member) conducts further clinical and respiratory drive assessments. Clinical assessment determines organ viability and cardiopulmonary status and includes dosing requirements for vasoactive and inotropic medications for blood pressure support. Respiratory drive assessment is done collaboratively with the physician, nurse, respiratory therapist, and OPO coordinator and includes degree of ventilator assistance required to maintain oxygenation, oxygen requirements, and assessment of intrinsic respiratory drive. These data help determine the likelihood of patient death within the appropriate time limit (protocol directed) following

TABLE 5.5   Potential Confounding Factors Affecting Brain Death Testing

Confounding Factor	Clinical Implications in Brain Death Testing
High cervical spinal cord injury	Cough and gag reflexes, motor responses to noxious stimulation, intrinsic respiratory drive and valid apnea testing require intact spinal cord function. High spinal cord injury can yield absent responses to brainstem testing with preserved brain or brainstem function.
Complex spinal reflex movements	Arm adduction or elbow flexion may resemble purposeful movement. Muscle stretch reflexes, abdominal muscle movements, facial twitching, persistent Babinski reflexes, and toe flexion from plantar stimulation may be elicited by mechanical stimulation of the spinal cord or sensory nerve roots. "Lazarus sign" (shoulder adduction, elbow flexion, arm lifting, possible crossing of hands) may also occur.
Muscle fasciculations	Fasciculations of extremities, chest, and abdomen may occur, beginning shortly after terminal brainstem herniation with duration up to 2-3 days. May falsely imply brain or brainstem function.
Ventilator auto-triggering: Overbreathing of ventilator set rate in absence of intrinsic respiratory drive	May falsely imply residual brainstem function and preservation of intrinsic respiratory drive. May delay or abort formal brain death protocols.
Interventions for suspected cardiogenic ventilator auto-triggering	Identify or rule out indications of intrinsic respiratory drive on clinical evaluation and ventilator waveform analysis. Analyze ventilator flow and pressure waveforms concurrently with clinical evaluation. Adjust ventilator trigger settings to eliminate auto-triggering. Match precordial motion with cardiac cycle, pulse palpation, auditory tone (beep), and QRS on bedside monitor, as well as corresponding oscillations on ventilator flow and pressure waveforms (done collaboratively at the bedside by critical care nurse, respiratory therapist, and physician).
Targeted temperature management (TTM)	TTM slows neuronal impulse generation and conduction. Drug metabolism and elimination are prolonged, including CNS depressant and NMB medications. EEG, pupillary light response, and brainstem reflexes are altered by TTM. Absent motor and pupillary light responses 72 hours following arrest are not reliable predictors of outcome. Waiting 72 hours after rewarming (4-5 days after cardiac arrest) may be appropriate to account for prolonged effects of CNS depressants and NMB used during TTM.

CNS, Central nervous system; *EEG,* electroencephalogram; *NMB,* neuromuscular blockade.
Adapted from Arbour R. Brain death: Assessment, controversy and confounding factors. *Crit Care Nurs.* 2013;33(6):27–46; Wijdicks EF, Varelas PN, Gronseth GS, et al. Evidence-based guideline update: Determining brain death in adults: Report of the Quality Standards Subcommittee of the American Academy of Neurology. *Neurology.* 2010;74(23):1911–1918.

withdrawal of physiological support. The option to donate organs after circulatory death is presented by the OPO coordinator or staff member to the family. The decision to withdraw life support is made first and is independent of the decision to donate. The legal next of kin must consent to organ donation.[6,7,9]

CARE OF THE FAMILY

Care of the grieving family is an integral part of the donation process. These families have special needs that result from both their decision to donate and the death of a loved one. The critical care nurse and the OPO staff member establish a unique relationship with the grieving family as part of the donation process. Working collaboratively, all multiprofessional team members can deliver optimal care for the patient as a potential donor, as well as for the patient's family.

Advocacy, honesty, and empathy help to develop trust between the patient's family and the multiprofessional team. Encourage family members to speak and ask questions during family meetings. Facilitate early visiting and communicate honestly about the patient's prognosis. Start family discussion with a thorough explanation of the patient's grave condition and include definitions of terms, including *brain death.* This helps ensure the family's understanding of death before organ donation and is vital to avoid later misunderstandings. Assess and acknowledge the family's cultural, ethnic, and religious beliefs regarding death. Understanding the religious perspectives of the family of a potential donor better prepares healthcare providers for discussions about brain death and organ donation, as can careful choice of words and use of the same terminology when discussing brain death.[7,9] See Evidence-Based Practice: Interventions to Increase Organ Donation.

EVIDENCE-BASED PRACTICE

Interventions to Increase Organ Donation

Problem
Over the last decade, there have been many initiatives worldwide to increase the number of organ donors. However, it is not clear which initiatives are most effective. The aim of this study was to provide an overview of interventions aimed at healthcare professionals in order to increase the number of organ donors.

Clinical Question
Which initiatives aimed at healthcare professionals are most effective in increasing the number of organ donors?

Evidence
The authors searched PubMed, EMBASE, CINAHL, PsycINFO, and the Cochrane Library for English-language studies published before April 24, 2019. Studies that were included described interventions in hospitals aimed at healthcare professionals who are involved in the identification, referral, and care of a family of potential organ donors. After the title abstract and full-text selection, two reviewers independently assessed each study's quality and extracted data.

From the 18,854 records initially extracted from 5 databases, 22 studies were included in the review. Of these 22 studies, 14 showed statistically significant effects on identification rate, family consent rate, and/or donation rate. Interventions that positively influenced one or more of these outcomes were training of emergency personnel in organ donation, an electronic support system to identify and/or refer potential donors, a collaborative care pathway, donation request by a trained professional, and additional family support in the critical care unit by a trained nurse. The methodological quality of the studies was relatively low, mainly because of the study designs.

Implication for Nursing
Although data may be limited, collaboration between the critical care unit and other departments (neurology, emergency medicine, neurosurgery) to identify triggers facilitates identification of potential organ donors. Training of healthcare professionals and additional support for families of potential donors may increase the number of organ donors. Nursing knowledge of the organ donation process, including support for families of potential donors, is an important component of increasing consent for organ donation.

Level of Evidence
A—Systematic review

Reference
Witjes M, Jansen NE, van der Hoeven JG, Abdo WF. Interventions aimed at healthcare professionals to increase the number of organ donors: A systematic review. *Crit Care.* 2019;23(1):227.

EVALUATION OF THE POTENTIAL ORGAN DONOR

As part of the donor evaluation process, the OPO coordinator completes a thorough physical examination and obtains an extensive medical and social history from the patient's medical records and family. A medical history screening includes the presence or absence of diabetes mellitus, hypertension, risk factors exposing the donor to potential infections, and malignancy, as well as the mechanism of brain death. Although active cancer does not disqualify a potential donor, consideration may be given to when and how long the potential donor had a cancer-free interval, the tumor type, treatment, and follow-up.[20] A social history of cigarette use, heavy alcohol use, IV drug use, and any risk factors for potential transmission of bloodborne illnesses establishes a donor risk profile. These factors are evaluated by the recipient transplant center and potential recipient when considering an organ offer.

Laboratory tests include basic metabolic panel, hepatic panel, coagulopathy survey, complete blood count, urinalysis, and blood cultures. The potential donor is screened for ABO typing and subtyping and human leukocyte antigen (HLA) histocompatibility, which is useful in predicting organ rejection in the recipient. Serological testing screens the potential donor for transmissible diseases, including HIV; hepatitis A, B, and C; Epstein-Barr virus (EBV); cytomegalovirus (CMV); toxoplasmosis; and sexually transmitted infections.[15]

The use of antiviral medications to treat hepatitis C virus (HCV) has raised the possibility of increasing the donor pool by enabling heart and lung transplantation from donors with HCV infection into recipients without HCV infection. A recent study demonstrated in patients without HCV infection who received a heart or lung transplant from a donor with HCV infection that treatment with an antiviral regimen for 4 weeks, initiated within a few hours of transplantation, prevented the HCV infection.[29]

The OPO coordinator evaluates the potential donor's medical and social history in the context of the circumstances of the terminal brain injury, as well as laboratory results, in determining the type of donor. Types of donors include the Centers for Disease Control and Prevention (CDC) increased-risk, standard criteria, or expanded criteria donors. *An increased-risk donor* is defined as one who, according to medical and social history, has documented risk of disease transmission. Risk indicators include IV drug use, incarceration, high-risk sexual behaviors, and poor historian. A *standard criteria donor* is a patient younger than 50 years of age who is declared brain dead and has no significant comorbidities affecting organ function. An *expanded criteria donor* includes donors older than 60 years of age or donors older than 50 years of age with two of the following: a history of high blood pressure, a creatinine greater than or equal to 1.5 mg/dL, or death resulting from a stroke (see Table 5.1). Recipients and families ultimately decide on acceptance of organs from expanded criteria donors.[4]

> **! CLINICAL ALERT**
> All major religions, including Islam, Christianity, Judaism, and Hinduism, support organ donation as a charitable helping act.

> **STUDY BREAK**
> 2. An increased-risk donor is defined as one who:
>   A. Is older than 65 years of age
>   B. Has a history of measles
>   C. Is an active cigarette smoker
>   D. Has a documented risk of disease transmission

Serial laboratory studies are obtained during donor evaluation, donor management, and organ matching to assess donor stability and effectiveness of donor management in resolving acid-base, fluid, and electrolyte imbalances. This process is vital to organ recovery, organ matching, and recipient outcomes.[15,16]

The OPO coordinator identifies potential recipients for organs that can be donated through a computerized system called *UNet,* which is operated by UNOS and matches organs to potential recipients. When a potential donor organ becomes available, the OPO coordinator enters demographic and medical data on the UNet site to match the organ to the most appropriate recipient. The OPO coordinator then electronically sends offers to the transplant centers contacting the designated representative on call for the potential recipient.

CRITICAL REASONING ACTIVITY

The same 52-year-old patient becomes increasingly hypoxemic and hemodynamically unstable. Brain death testing has not yet been completed, and the family has not been approached about organ donation. The multiprofessional team provides aggressive ventilator management to maintain adequate oxygenation. In addition, hemodynamic stability continues to decline, and the addition of four vasoactive and inotropic medications is only marginally effective at maintaining a mean arterial pressure of 50 mm Hg.

What would be appropriate treatment decisions by the team to support blood pressure and tissue perfusion?

DONOR MANAGEMENT

To avoid conflict of interest, the OPO staff member has no direct involvement in management of the patient until brain death is formally declared and consent has been obtained for organ donation. Once consent is obtained, the OPO coordinator directs management of the patient in collaboration with the multiprofessional team (Box 5.2).

Consequences of brain death include autoregulatory loss resulting in intense vasoconstriction from catecholamine release, followed by vasodilation from catecholamine depletion, resulting in a relative hypovolemia and a potential for cardiac dysrhythmias. Loss of hypothalamus function causes a loss of temperature regulation. Loss of pituitary function results in decreased antidiuretic hormone secretion, causing diabetes insipidus with massive volume loss and electrolyte imbalances, and depletion of cortisol, thyroid-stimulating hormone, and thyroid hormones. Concurrent with the significant inflammatory

BOX 5.2 Focus of Donor Management

- Maintain blood pressure
- Maintain normal serum glucose level
- Maintain normothermia
- Treat anemia
- Treat coagulopathy and thrombocytopenia
- Provide appropriate mechanical ventilation
- Maintain optimal fluid and electrolyte levels
- Treat polyuria
- Maintain normal acid-base balance

state from massive hypotension, bradycardia and poor gas exchange occur. Decreased insulin levels or increased insulin resistance occurs and further contributes to acid-base imbalance and fluid and electrolyte depletion. Optimal donor management effectively replaces neurohormonal regulation, modulates the proinflammatory state, replaces intravascular volume, and supports vasomotor tone as well as the ability of the heart muscle to contract.[14-16] Table 5.6 outlines medications used in donor management.

CLINICAL ALERT

To avoid conflict of interest, the OPO staff member has no direct involvement in the management of a potential organ donor patient until brain death is formally declared and consent has been obtained for organ donation.

Care is focused on preserving organ function and viability: maintaining hemodynamic and pulmonary stability, normothermia, and normal laboratory parameters. Standardized order sets can be used, focusing on optimizing fluid, electrolyte, and acid-base balance and oxygenation.[14-16] A pulmonary artery catheter or central venous catheter can provide volume-responsive hemodynamic parameters, including central venous pressure and pulmonary artery occlusion pressure, and determine cardiac output and cardiac index. Provide frequent assessments and guide interventions until the organs are recovered.

Organ Recovery

Organ recovery occurs in the operating room (OR) and can take 12 to 36 hours to complete. If the facility where the donor is located (donor facility) is near the transplant facility, the local transplant team will go on site for organ recovery. If the transplant team is not local, the OPO coordinator collaborates with the transplant team to allocate resources for transportation of the transplant team to the donor facility. Once all organs have been accepted, the OPO coordinator sets an OR time.

In the OR, the transplant team optimizes recovery of vascular structures and carefully inspects the donor organs before starting any invasive procedure on the recipient. During organ recovery from the brain dead organ donor, the anesthesiologist monitors vital signs and mechanical support to ensure hemodynamic stability. Once all organs are recovered, the OPO coordinator updates the family if requested, updates all administrative personnel in the donor facility as directed, and communicates with the nursing unit regarding the outcome.

The surgical recovery for a donor organ varies based on the organ being procured, type of donor such as DCD versus brain dead organ donor, as well as needs identified by the transplant teams and their recipients. Surgical recovery represents the end point of donor recognition, donor management, and organ matching.

The next step for the recovered donor organs is life-saving implantation within the transplant recipient(s). To illustrate this process, recovery of a donor liver is described. Patient

TABLE 5.6 PHARMACOLOGY

Medications Commonly Used in Donor Management

Medication	Action/Use	Dose/Route	Side Effects	Nursing Implications
Esmolol (Brevibloc)	Beta-blocker used to control tachycardia and decrease myocardial oxygen consumption from catecholamine release Protects heart muscle from ischemia	*IV loading dose:* 500 mcg/kg/min over 1 min *IV infusion:* 50 mcg/kg/min for 4h and titrate up to 200 mcg/kg/min	Decreased cardiac output Hypotension Bradycardia Heart block	Rapid onset Short acting, well tolerated Careful titration to avoid decreased cardiac output and hypotension as catecholamine stores depleted
Nitroprusside (Nipride)	Causes arterial vasodilation Used to control severe blood pressure elevations from massive catecholamine release May protect end organs from volume shifts into lungs from vasoconstriction	*IV infusion:* 0.5-10 mcg/kg/min	Hypotension Hypotension may occur rapidly in hypovolemic patients	Rapid onset Careful titration to avoid hypotension as catecholamine stores depleted
Nicardipine	Calcium channel blocker that causes arterial vasodilation Used to control severe blood pressure elevations and vasoconstriction from catecholamine release	*IV infusion:* 2.5-10 mg/h and titrate Maximum dose: 15 mg/h	Hypotension Heart blocks (higher risk with concurrent beta-blocker infusion)	Rapid onset Has negative inotropic effect at higher doses Administer through central line if possible to avoid extravasation
Isotonic crystalloid/volume resuscitation (e.g., 0.9% NS or Lactated Ringer's solution)	Provides intravascular volume replacement to treat hypovolemia Used as continuous infusion or rapid bolus administration	May infuse as much as 3-4 L IV bolus initially Titrated based on volume replacement needs	Risk of pulmonary edema Dilution of clotting factors Dilution of platelets/cellular components Hypothermia	Rapid administration and correction of circulating volume deficit Monitor platelets, clotting factors, and signs of bleeding Monitor body temperature
Dopamine	Catecholamine agent with alpha and beta actions *Moderate doses (2-10 mcg/kg/min):* stimulates beta receptors to increase cardiac contractility and heart rate *High doses (10-20 mcg/kg/min):* stimulates alpha receptors to increase blood pressure through vasoconstriction	*IV infusion:* 1-10 mcg/kg/min up to 50 mcg/kg/min	Tachycardia Dysrhythmias	Administer through central line if possible to avoid extravasation
Dobutamine	Stimulates beta$_1$ receptors to increase contractility and heart rate to increase cardiac output	*IV infusion:* 1-10 mcg/kg/min and titrated	Dysrhythmias Tachycardia Hypotension	Rapid acting Monitor heart rate, blood pressure, cardiac output/index, and clinical signs of tissue perfusion
Norepinephrine (Levophed)	Stimulates alpha receptors to cause vasoconstriction to increase blood pressure Stimulates beta receptors to increase contractility, heart rate, and coronary blood flow	*IV infusion:* 0.5-20 mcg/min; higher doses possible	Dysrhythmias Tachycardia	Rapid acting Monitor heart rate and blood pressure Administer through central line if possible to avoid extravasation
Phenylephrine (Neo-Synephrine)	Stimulates alpha receptors to cause vasoconstriction to increase blood pressure	*IV infusion:* 20-300 mcg/min	Reflex bradycardia Hypertension Ventricular dysrhythmias	Rapid acting Monitor heart rate and blood pressure Administer through central line if possible to avoid extravasation
Vasopressin	Potent vasoconstrictor that augments effects of other vasopressor medications Replacement therapy for ADH depletion in treatment of DI to control urine output and preserve circulating blood volume	*IV infusion:* 0.01-0.04 units/min	Excessive vasoconstriction Risk of ischemia at high doses	Monitor urine output, serum electrolytes, and serum/urine osmolality Monitor urine specific gravity in response to therapy

Continued

TABLE 5.6 PHARMACOLOGY—cont'd

Medications Commonly Used in Donor Management

Medication	Action/Use	Dose/Route	Side Effects	Nursing Implications
Desmopressin acetate (DDAVP)	Synthetic ADH used to replace ADH depletion Controls urine output in setting of DI	*IV dose:* 1-4 mcg IV push over 1 min *IV infusion:* 0.01-0.04 units/min	Hyponatremia Hypertension from hypervolemia	Monitor urine output, urine specific gravity, serum sodium, and serum/urine osmolality Repeat bolus dosing or upward titration may be required
Levothyroxine (T$_4$)	Used to replace thyroid hormone depletion following loss of pituitary function and thyroid-stimulating hormone Augments metabolism at cellular and tissue level, improving cardiovascular and acid-base balance	*IV bolus:* 20 mcg IV *IV infusion:* 10-20 mcg/h and titrated	Dysrhythmias Hypertension	With peripheral hypoperfusion and decreased cardiac output, T$_4$ may not be as readily converted to active T$_3$ Potentially longer time to onset, less effective Monitor blood pressure and tissue perfusion Be prepared to decrease dose of vasopressor agents and medications that strengthen heart muscle contraction
Methylprednisolone	Decreases inflammatory state after brainstem herniation Used to replace stress hormone depletion	*IV dose:* 250 mg IV	Hyperglycemia	Ease of administration Monitor arterial blood gases and blood pressure Titrate vasoactive medications in response to therapy
Insulin	Used to treat hyperglycemia from the stress response and high-dose steroid administration	*IV infusion:* Typically protocol directed-titrated to point-of-care blood glucose levels	Hypoglycemia	Ease of administration and titration Decreased risk of osmotic diuresis, volume depletion, and electrolyte imbalances Monitor blood glucose levels and titrate infusion dose per protocol

ADH, Antidiuretic hormone; *DI,* diabetes insipidus; *NS,* normal saline; *T$_3$,* triiodothyronine.

Data from Korte C, Garber JL, Descourouez JL, et al. Pharmacist's guide to management of organ donors after brain death. *Am J Health Syst Pharm.* 2016;72(22):1829–1839; Kotloff RM, Blosser S, Fulda G, et al. Management of the potential organ donor in the ICU: Society of Critical Care Medicine/American College of Chest Physicians/Association of Organ Procurement Organizations consensus statement. *Crit Care Med.* 2015;43(6):1291–1325.

identification and appropriate positioning on the OR table after brain death and consent for donation are established. The chest and abdomen are prepped, followed by an incision from the sternum to the pubis. The liver is mobilized by dissecting connective tissue, celiac and hepatic arteries, and veins. Careful dissection and irrigation of the gallbladder and biliary system are performed. Cold solution selected by the transplant surgical team is infused through the portal system, and the liver is placed into "slush" for transport to the recipient hospital for implantation. At the recipient hospital, excess tissue is dissected away and optimal sizing of vessels is established. The liver is assessed for injury, and vascular structures are assessed to ensure that no leaks are present. After ascertaining that no injuries are present, the liver is ready for implantation.

In cases involving DCD, the patient is prepared for organ donation over several hours. The surgical team is notified and the OPO coordinator sets the time of organ recovery based on when the family chooses the time to withdraw life support. The patient is transferred to the OR, where life-sustaining measures are withdrawn (e.g., extubation, stopping of IV medications). The patient is then pronounced dead by a hospital physician. The time from onset of asystole to the declaration of death is generally 90 seconds to 5 minutes, at which time a separate transplant surgical team starts the organ recovery process. Current recommendations are to recover the liver in less than 30 minutes after withdrawal of life-sustaining measures; kidneys may be recovered up to 90 minutes after withdrawal of life-sustaining measures.[26] If the patient does not die quickly enough to permit the recovery of organs, he or she may be moved back to the critical care unit or a designated palliative care bed, where the planned organ donation process stops and end-of-life care continues, including family support.[5,15,21]

CRITICAL REASONING ACTIVITY

A 56-year-old patient is admitted to the critical care unit following cardiopulmonary arrest. He receives advanced life support efforts with a return of spontaneous circulation after 25 minutes. Targeted temperature management (TTM) is initiated to optimize chances for neurological recovery. During TTM the patient receives central nervous system (CNS) depressants, including fentanyl (opioid analgesia), midazolam (sedative-hypnotic) in high doses, and vecuronium for neuromuscular blockade (NMB) to prevent shivering. He is maintained at a core body temperature of 33.4°C for 24 hours. Following rewarming over 16 hours, his baseline body temperature is 36.8°C. The CNS depressants and NMB are discontinued during rewarming. Twelve hours after rewarming is completed, the patient exhibits no brainstem reflexes and has flaccid trunk and extremities.

1. What is the most appropriate response when discussion of brain death testing is initiated?
2. What are some possible confounding factors the nurse may identify in this case that affect validity of brain death testing?

TRANSPLANT CANDIDATE EVALUATION

Comprehensive evaluation of each potential transplant candidate is performed to ensure that transplantation is the best option, determine other medical or surgical alternatives, and determine the best matching criteria for a potential donor offer. For example, a potential recipient with cirrhosis and hepatitis C may be a good match with a donor who is hepatitis C core antibody–positive. In this respect, both donor and recipient evaluation mirror one another. Acuity of the potential recipient is a significant issue. For example, liver transplant candidates who have severe, acute liver failure with multisystem complications may be higher on the waiting list. Their transplant team may consider a wider pool of potential donors if the risk of death is high.[5,24]

Donor-derived infections are another challenge for transplant recipients. Although potential donors who are febrile are carefully screened for potential infections that could be transmitted, infections can be missed if the donor's history is incomplete. Donor-derived infections that have been transmitted to recipients include CMV, EBV, HIV, lymphocytic choriomeningitis virus, West Nile virus, hepatitis B and C, herpes simplex, and Chagas disease.[4,11] It is mandatory to report any donor-derived infections to the OPO, UNOS, and ultimately to the CDC.

 QSEN EXEMPLAR

Quality Improvement

A 21-year-old patient was admitted to the critical care unit on the previous evening at 2100 with a traumatic brain injury after falling from a cliff. The patient was declared brain dead the next morning at 0900, and mechanical ventilation was removed. The family arrived from out of town after brain death was declared. The family inquires about organ donation. The nurse contacts the organ procurement organization (OPO), and after sharing the sequence of events, the nurse learns that organ donation is not an option due to the patient being off mechanical ventilation. The nurse requests a meeting to identify strategies to avoid this from occurring in the future. The OPO staff member conducts a retrospective review of the medical records and the OPO database and discovers that the hospital never called in a referral. A meeting was arranged with the OPO staff member and the critical care unit team to review this case, Centers for Medicaid and Medicare Services (CMS) regulations, and best practices for timely referrals of potential organ donors. Protocols and policies on brain death and OPO notification are reviewed and revised and unit-based education is completed.

Lung Transplant

Lung transplantation is the treatment of choice for patients with end-stage lung disease when no other treatment options are available. The most common indications are chronic obstructive pulmonary disease, idiopathic pulmonary fibrosis, pulmonary hypertension, emphysema caused by alpha-1 antitrypsin deficiency, sarcoidosis, non–cystic fibrosis bronchiectasis, and lymphangioleiomyomatosis cystic fibrosis, as well as urgent retransplantation for graft failure.

Efforts to increase the number of lung transplant recipients have resulted in a variety of lung transplantation options, including heart-lung transplantation, single lung transplantation, double lung en bloc, and living donor lobar transplant. Considerations in selecting the type of lung transplantation include the specific disease process, the need for cardiac transplantation, and donor availability.[8]

Approximately 1500 patients are on the national waiting list for lung transplantation. In 2018, 2530 lung transplants were performed, with a projected 1-year survival of 88% and a 3-year survival of 72%. More than 80% of transplant recipients had no restrictions at 1, 3, 5, and 10 years after transplantation.[12,23]

Lung donors can be living or deceased. Donors must be ABO compatible with the recipient, and the donor's size must match the recipient's. The ideal donor meets the following criteria[15]:

- Age less than 55 years
- Smoking history less than 20 pack-years
- Clear chest radiograph
- PaO_2 greater than 300 mm Hg on 100% oxygen and 5 cm H_2O of positive end-expiratory pressure (PEEP)
- No history of significant chronic lung disease, infection, or aspiration; no significant chest trauma; no prior cardiopulmonary surgery
- No organisms on donor Gram stain
- Clear and anatomically normal findings on bronchoscopy

Few donors fit the ideal criteria; therefore transplant centers have expanded their criteria in an effort to expand the donor pool.[3,4,22] Donor evaluation, history, and management are crucial for identifying risk factors for lung dysfunction. These risk factors include any donor smoking history, elevated oxygen requirements, history of cardiopulmonary bypass, large-volume blood transfusion, and obesity in the recipient. Identification of risk factors can optimize recipient selection, evaluation, and donor management.[22]

Kidney Transplant

Kidney transplantation is the therapeutic choice for patients in end-stage renal disease (ESRD). After successful kidney transplantation, the patient is free from the restrictions of dialysis and free from the manifestations of uremia.[27] More than 100,000 patients are on the national waiting list for kidney transplantation. In 2018, 21,167 kidney transplants were performed, with a projected 1-year survival of 93.4%, 3-year survival of 90.1%, and 5-year survival of 84.6%.[23]

Attempts to increase the donor pool have resulted in two types of donation: living donor or cadaver donor. Living donors can be related or unrelated to the potential recipient. The most desirable source of an organ is a living, related donor who matches the recipient closely. If a potential living donor does not match the recipient, the two may enter into a paired exchange program. A paired exchange program allows a living donor to be matched to another potential recipient whose living donor also does not match with either blood types or preformed antibodies against a donor.[25]

Prospective living donors undergo physical and psychological evaluation and are screened for ABO blood group, tissue-specific antigen, and HLA histocompatibility. They must also be screened for any contraindications to surgery and be determined as healthy enough to tolerate donor kidney recovery. Living donors are also screened to determine if coercion or financial incentives are potentially driving the donation decision. The number of living donors is slowly increasing because of the limited supply of cadaver donors and public outreach education, as well as the development and refinement of living donor programs within active transplant centers. Of the 21,167 kidney transplants performed in 2018, 6442 came from living donors.[23]

Heart Transplant

Heart transplantation is the primary therapeutic choice for many patients with advanced heart failure who have not responded successfully to maximal medical therapy. Indications for heart transplant evaluation include (1) severe cardiovascular disease leading to severe, progressive ventricular dysfunction; (2) severe hypertensive or viral cardiomyopathy; and (3) congenital heart disease following multiple procedures in childhood where an end point is reached in that further reparative procedures offer no benefit with increased risk. Previously, the upper age limit for heart transplant candidacy was 65 years of age, but that number continues to increase. Nearly 4000 candidates are on the national waiting list for heart transplantation. In 2018, 3408 heart transplants were performed. The projected 1-year survival exceeds 85% for adults and 90% for pediatric patients, and the 5-year survival is 72.6%.[17,23]

Because of the significant imbalance between the number of patients who may benefit from heart transplantation and the number of available donors, an additional focus of care is optimal management of end-stage heart failure. Optimal management is multifaceted, including pharmacological therapies and mechanical assist devices to maximize cardiac output and tissue perfusion. Mechanical assist devices include cardiac resynchronization therapy with biventricular pacing to increase efficiency of the cardiac cycle, intraaortic balloon pump therapy, and implanted right- and left-ventricular assist devices. These interventions support the heart and augment regional blood flow and tissue perfusion. Surgical interventions such as ventricular volume reduction surgery achieved by removing akinetic or dyskinetic myocardium after myocardial infarction may improve symptoms.

Criteria used to determine suitability of a potential donor heart include age; cause of donor death; clinical factors such as smoking, drug use, laboratory values (troponin, creatine kinase MB), vasoactive medications, and echocardiography results; and timing and use of hormonal resuscitation protocols. Donors must be ABO compatible, and most programs prefer that there be no history of smoking, diabetes, dyslipidemia, or

hypertension. The potential donor's family history of cardiac disease is reviewed when evaluating extended criteria. If the potential organ donor suffered a cardiac arrest, evaluation of heart function, donor management, and downtime are all considered.

A significant mismatch remains between donor heart availability and potential recipients on heart transplant waiting lists. As a result, donor heart criteria have expanded to include older hearts (>55 years), donor hearts with an ischemic time of more than 4 hours, and the creation of an alternative list to match excluded potential recipients with donor hearts that otherwise would not be used. Donor heart criteria have also expanded to include hearts recovered from DCD. In some cases, hearts from DCD donors have been preserved outside the body by machine perfusion with good recipient outcomes and cardiac indices. In the past, donor hearts with wall motion abnormalities requiring high doses of inotropic medications, refractory shock, or ventricular dysrhythmias were declined. However, because of the significant shortage of transplantable organs, donor hearts previously thought to be unacceptable have been used with good recipient outcomes.

STUDY BREAK

3. Most organ procurement programs prefer a negative patient history for all of the following EXCEPT:
   A. Smoking
   B. Low levels of low density lipoprotein (LDL)
   C. Diabetes
   D. Hypertension

Liver Transplant

Liver transplantation is the standard treatment for patients with progressive, irreversible acute or chronic liver disease for which there are no other medical or surgical options. Leading indications for liver transplantation include hepatocellular carcinoma (within specific criteria), hepatitis C, cirrhosis, fulminant hepatic failure from acute hepatitis, drug toxicity (e.g., significant acetaminophen ingestion), and many others. Nearly 14,000 candidates are on the national waiting list for liver transplantation. In 2018, 8250 liver transplants were performed. Of this total, 7849 were from deceased donors and 401 were from living donors. The incidence of graft failure at 1 year has decreased to 9.8% for recipients of deceased donor livers. The 5-year survival for recipients of living donor livers is projected at 74.6%.[5,23]

Screening of potential donors by the OPO coordinator includes blood type, body size, and the presence or absence of active infection or metastatic disease, as these can be transmitted to the recipient.[6,15,17] Human leukocyte antigen tissue typing is not used because it has not been known to significantly affect outcomes. Liver function studies, donor nutritional state, age, and donor medical and social history are evaluated not only to determine donor suitability but also to identify the best recipient match. For example, a liver from an individual weighing 250 pounds may be potentially too large to transplant into a recipient weighing 100 pounds.

With the increase in success rates for liver transplantation, finding suitable donors has become challenging. Living and extended criteria donors are more widely accepted as potential options for patients in need of a liver transplant. The largest group of extended criteria donors is individuals older than 65 years, and long-term outcomes are being evaluated. Outcomes of living liver donors in adult-to-adult liver transplantation are similar to those of deceased donor liver transplants, with 1-year survival at 91% and 5-year survival higher at 83% (living) and 75% (deceased).[17,23] Some transplant programs report comparable outcomes between DCD and brain dead, heart-beating donors.[10] Other efforts to increase the number of liver transplant recipients include reduced-size liver transplants (living donor left lobe of liver transplanted to a recipient) and split-liver transplantation (one liver divided between an adult and a child).

Depending on the donor's medical and social history, including illicit drug use or drug overdose as mechanism of death, a donor may be classified as increased risk to transmit blood-borne illnesses. Expanded criteria donors, such as those older than 65 years of age with comorbidities, provide an additional option for organ transplantation. Definitions of expanded criteria donors vary between transplant centers. At the time of the organ offer, the potential recipient is apprised of the donor information.

CASE STUDY

Mr. G. is a 36-year-old man who sustained prolonged cardiopulmonary arrest while shopping in a department store. After immediate life-support measures, return of spontaneous circulation was achieved. He was unconscious and required IV access, endotracheal intubation, and mechanical ventilation. He was transported to the emergency department (ED). Neurological assessment revealed pupils dilated at 5 mm and sluggish in response to light; myoclonic movements; and preserved but decreased cough, gag, and corneal reflexes. Urgent head computed tomography (CT) was significant for severe, diffuse cerebral edema and compression of the ventricles.

Mr. G. was not considered a candidate for targeted temperature management and was transferred to the critical care unit. On admission his blood pressure (BP) was 192/94 mm Hg and his heart rate (HR) was 155 beats/min. Critical care management included administration of antihypertensive agents.

Over the next several hours, his HR decreased to 46 beats/min and BP decreased to 60/44 mm Hg. His respiratory rate was 24 breaths/min, above the ventilator set rate. Aggressive vasoactive and inotropic medication support was initiated with increasing dosages of epinephrine, norepinephrine, and phenylephrine. Ventilator management was adjusted to maximize oxygenation and ventilation. Despite aggressive resuscitation and physiological support, neurological status did not improve.

During the late evening hours of day 2 in the hospital, his BP dropped precipitously to a mean arterial pressure of 58 mm Hg despite maximal dosing of vasopressors. Neurological evaluation revealed pupils fixed and dilated and absent cough, gag, and corneal reflexes. The critical nature of the patient's condition was discussed with the family, and the concept of potential brain death was introduced by the multiprofessional team. The family had many questions about Mr. G.'s treatment, injury, and prognosis, as well as the meaning of "brain death." The OPO coordinator was contacted.

Formal brain death testing, including radionuclide brain flow study, and clinical examination were performed on day 3 in the hospital. Fig. 5.3 illustrates a radionuclide brain perfusion study consistent with brain death. Clinical examination findings were consistent with brain death, and Mr. G. was pronounced dead according to neurological criteria at that time. The multiprofessional team communicated with the family throughout the testing process.

The OPO coordinator initiated preliminary evaluation of Mr. G.'s suitability as an organ donor. Once the family members understood what brain death meant, the OPO staff member discussed the option of organ donation. Mr. G.'s family consented to organ donation, seeing it as a way to have something positive come from this painful tragedy. Following donation consent, the OPO coordinator placed Mr. G.'s donor information into the UNOS database. Both kidneys were matched with recipients, enabling two patients to be liberated from dialysis. His pancreas was recovered and transplanted, effectively treating severe diabetes in one patient. His liver was transplanted, saving the life of a patient with end-stage liver disease.

Questions

1. When catastrophic, nonsurvivable brain injury is refractory to aggressive care and progresses to terminal brainstem herniation, what interventions are a priority to maintain cardiovascular stability following terminal brainstem herniation?
2. With a deteriorating neurological examination, what are three indications that it is appropriate to begin formal brain death testing?
3. What are the benefits of separating discussions of brain death from conversations about organ donation?

REFERENCES

1. Ad Hoc Committee of Harvard Medical School. A definition of irreversible coma: Report of the Ad Hoc Committee of Harvard Medical School. *JAMA*. 1968;205(6):337–340.
2. Association of Organ Procurement. About OPOs. http://www.aopo.org/about-opos/. Accessed June 22, 2019.
3. Bazan VM, Zwischenberger JB. ECMO in lung transplantation: A review. *Clin Surg*. 2018;3:2016.
4. Bittle GJ, Sanchez PG, Kon ZN, et al. The use of lung donors older than 55 years: A review of the United Network of Organ Sharing database. *J Heart Lung Transplant*. 2013;32(8):760–768.
5. Bloom MB, Raza S, Bhakra A, et al. Impact of deceased donor demographics and critical care end points on liver transplantation and graft survival rates. *J Am Coll Surg*. 2015;220:38–47.
6. Centers for Medicare and Medicaid Services. CFR 482.45: Condition of Participation: Organ, Tissue, and Eye Procurement. https://www.govinfo.gov/content/pkg/CFR-2011-title42-vol5/pdf/CFR-2011-title42-vol5-sec482-45.pdf. Published 2011. Accessed June 22, 2019.
7. Chandler JA, Connors M, Holland G, Shemie SD. Effective requesting: A scoping review of literature on asking families to consent to organ and tissue donation. *Transplantation*. 2017;101(5S):S1–S16.
8. Costa J, Benvenuto LJ, Sonnett JR, et al. Long-term outcomes and management of lung transplant recipients. *Best Pract Res Clin Anaesthesiol*. 2017;31(2):285–297.
9. Donate Life America. General Public Education. https://www.donatelife.net. Accessed June 22, 2019.
10. Eren EA, Latchana N, Beal E, et al. Donations after circulatory death in liver transplant. *Exp Clin Transplant*. 2016;14(5):463–470.
11. Fishman J. Infection in organ transplantation. *Am J Transplant*. 2017;17(4):856–879.

12. INOVA Health System. Survival Statistics: Lung Transplant. https://www.inova.org/healthcare-services/lung-transplant/transplantation-and-beyond/survival-statistics/index.jsp. Accessed June 22, 2019.

13. Irving MJ, Jan S, Tong A, et al. What factors influence people's decisions to register for organ donation? The results of a nominal group study. *Transplant Int.* 2014;27:617–624.

14. Korte C, Garber JL, Descourouez JL, et al. Pharmacist's guide to management of organ donors after brain death. *Am J Health Sys Pharm.* 2016;72(22):1829–1839.

15. Kotloff RM, Blosser S, Fulda G, et al. Management of the potential organ donor in the ICU: Society of Critical Care Medicine/American College of Chest Physicians/Association of Organ Procurement Organizations consensus statement. *Crit Care Med.* 2015;43(6):1291–1325.

16. Lakshmi K. Brain death and care of the organ donor. *J Anaesthesiol Clin Pharmacol.* 2016;32(2):146–152.

17. Organ Procurement and Transplant Network. Transplant by Donor Type. https://optn.transplant.hrsa.gov/data/view-data-reports/. Accessed June 22, 2019.

18. Public Law 98-507. http://www.history.nih.gov/research/downloads/PL98-507.pdf. Published October 19, 1984. Accessed June 22, 2019.

19. Razdan M, Degenholtz HB, Kahn JM, Driessen J. Breakdown in the organ donation process and its effect on organ availability. *J Transplant.* 2015;831501.

20. Shanzhou H, Yunhun T, et al. Outcomes of organ transplantation from donors with a cancer history. *Med Sci Monti.* 2018;24:997–1007.

21. Shemie SD, Robertson A, Beitel J, et al. End of life conversations with families of potential donors: Leading practices in offering the opportunity for organ donation. *Transplantation.* 2017;101(5S):S17–S26.

22. Snell GI, Levvey BJ, Westall GP. The changing landscape of lung donation for transplantation. *Am J Transplant.* 2015;15:859–860.

23. U.S. Department of Health and Human Services. Data Rep. https://optn.transplant.hrsa.gov/data/. Accessed June 22, 2019.

24. U.S. Department of Health and Human Services. Governance. https://optn.transplant.hrsa.gov/governance/. Accessed June 22, 2019.

25. United Network for Organ Sharing (UNOS). Living Donor. https://transplantliving.org/living-donation/being-a-living-donor/qualifications/. Accessed June 22, 2019.

26. Verheijde JL, Rady MY, McGregor JL. The United States Revised Uniform Anatomical Gift Act (2006): New challenges to balancing patient rights and physician responsibilities. *Philos Ethics Humanit Med.* 2007;2:19.

27. Wang JH, Skeans MA, Israni AK. Current status of kidney transplant outcomes: Dying to survive. *Adv Chronic Kidney Dis.* 2016;23(5):281–286.

28. Wijdicks EF, Varelas PN, Gronseth GS, et al. Evidence-based guideline update: Determining brain death in adults: Report of the Quality Standards Subcommittee of the American Academy of Neurology. *Neurology.* 2010;74(23):1911–1918.

29. Woolley AE, Singh SK, Goldberg HJ, et al. Heart and lung transplantation from HCV-infected donors to uninfected recipients. *NEJM.* 2019;380(17):1606–1617.

Comfort and Sedation

Mamoona Arif Rahu, PhD, RN, CCRN

Many additional resources, including self-assessment exercises, are located on the Evolve companion website at http://evolve.elsevier.com/Sole/.
- Animations
- Clinical Skills: Critical Care Collections
- Student Review Questions
- Video Clips

INTRODUCTION

Maintaining an optimal level of comfort for the critically ill patient is a universal goal for physicians and nurses.[22] Patients in the critical care unit experience pain from preexisting diseases, invasive procedures, or trauma. Pain can also be caused by monitoring devices (catheters, drains), noninvasive ventilating devices, endotracheal tubes, routine nursing care (airway suctioning, dressing changes, patient positioning), and prolonged immobility.

Unrelieved pain may contribute to inadequate sleep, which may lead to exhaustion, anxiety, disorientation, and agitation. The effects of a critical care unit stay may persist long after discharge, and many patients develop posttraumatic stress disorder (PTSD) or post-intensive care syndrome (PICS) as a result of their experience in a critical care unit.[9,53]

The patient's perception, expression, and tolerance of pain and anxiety vary because of different psychological, social, and cultural influences. Therefore it is important for healthcare providers to assess and manage pain and anxiety appropriately. Pain and anxiety are major contributors to patient morbidity and length of stay. This chapter focuses on the assessment and management strategies for the critically ill patient experiencing acute pain, anxiety, or both.

DEFINITIONS OF PAIN AND ANXIETY

The International Association for the Study of Pain defines pain as an unpleasant sensory and emotional experience associated with actual or potential tissue damage.[40] Pain is a subjective experience leading to variable tolerability. The patient is the true authority on the pain that is being experienced, and the patient's pain should be managed accordingly. Many theoretical bases for the development of pain have been proposed. The gate control theory is the most widely used in research and therapy (Box 6.1).[39]

Anxiety is a state marked by apprehension, agitation, autonomic arousal, fearful withdrawal, or any combination of these.[68]

It is a prolonged state of apprehension in response to a real or perceived fear. Anxiety must be assessed in the same way as pain: the patient's level of anxiety is whatever the patient reports.

Pain and anxiety are often interrelated and may be difficult to differentiate because the physiological and behavioral findings are similar for each. The relationship between pain and anxiety is cyclical, with each exacerbating the other.[54] Pain that is inadequately treated leads to greater anxiety, and anxiety is associated with higher pain intensity. Anxiety contributes to pain perception by activating pain pathways, altering the cognitive evaluation of pain, increasing aversion to pain, and increasing the report of pain. If pain and anxiety are unresolved and escalate, the patient often experiences feelings of powerlessness, suffering, and psychological changes such as agitation and delirium. Anxiety is not a benign state, and unrelieved anxiety leads to greater morbidity and mortality, especially in patients with cardiovascular disease.[20,71]

PREDISPOSING FACTORS TO PAIN AND ANXIETY

Many factors inherent to the critical care environment place patients at risk of developing pain and anxiety. Pain perception occurs as a result of preexisting diseases, invasive procedures, monitoring devices, nursing care, or trauma. The perception of pain may also be influenced by the expectation of pain, prior pain experiences and levels of tolerability, and a patient's emotional state and cognitive processes.

Patients who are mechanically ventilated experience vulnerability, consisting of anxiety, fear, and loneliness.[7] Anxiety is further escalated by the continuous noise of alarms, equipment, and personnel; bright ambient lighting; and excessive stimulation from inadequate analgesia, frequent assessments, repositioning, lack of mobility, and uncomfortable room temperature. Sleep deprivation and the circumstances that resulted in an admission to the critical care unit also increase patient anxiety.

PHYSIOLOGY OF PAIN AND ANXIETY

Pain

All pain results from a signal cascade within the body's neurological network. Pain is initiated by signals that travel through the peripheral nervous system to the central nervous system (CNS) for processing.[33] Pain is classified as *acute, chronic,* or *acute on chronic; malignant* or *nonmalignant;* and *nociceptive* or *neuropathic.* In all forms of acute pain, the sympathetic nervous system (SNS) is activated quickly, and several physiological responses occur (Box 6.2). In contrast, some forms of chronic pain may result in less activation of the SNS and a different clinical presentation.

The sensation of pain is carried to the CNS by activation of two separate pathways (Fig. 6.1). The fast (sharp) pain signals are transmitted to the spinal cord by slowly conducting, thinly myelinated A-delta afferent fibers. A-delta fibers are activated by high-intensity physical (hot and cold) stimuli that are important in initiating rapid reactions. Conversely, slow (burning; chronic) pain is transmitted by the unmyelinated, polymodal C fibers, which are activated by a variety of high-intensity mechanical, chemical, hot, and cold stimuli.

The most abundant receptors in the nervous system for pain recognition are nociceptors whose cell bodies are in the dorsal root ganglia. The sensation of pain received by peripheral endings of sensory neurons is called *nociception.* The nociceptive pain is divided into somatic and visceral. Nociceptive pain is

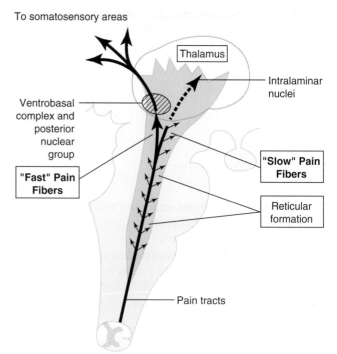

Fig. 6.1 Transmission of pain signals into the brainstem, thalamus, and cerebral cortex by way of the "fast" pain pathway and "slow" pain pathway. (From Guyton A, Hall J. *Textbook of Medical Physiology.* 13th ed. Philadelphia, PA: Saunders; 2015.)

detected by specialized transducers attached to A-delta and C fibers. *Somatic pain* results from irritation or damage to the nervous system. *Visceral pain* is diffuse, poorly localized, and often referred.

Nociceptors differ from other nerve receptors in the body in that they adapt very little to the pain response. If the stimulus for pain is not removed, the body continues to experience pain until the stimulus is discontinued or other interventions (e.g., analgesic agents) are initiated. This is a protective mechanism so that the body tissues being damaged will be removed from harm. Identifying the correct pain-inducing stimulus is important in the effective management of pain. Removal of the stimulus should always precede other treatment measures in managing pain.

BOX 6.2   Physiological Responses to Pain and Anxiety

- Constipation
- Cool extremities
- Diaphoresis
- Hypertension
- Increased cardiac output
- Increased glucose production (gluconeogenesis)
- Mydriasis (pupillary dilation)
- Nausea
- Pallor and flushing
- Sleep disturbance
- Tachycardia
- Tachypnea
- Urinary retention

STUDY BREAK
1. Pain that is diffuse and poorly localized is:
   A. Visceral pain
   B. Somatic pain
   C. Acute postoperative pain
   D. A-delta pain

Anxiety

The physiology of anxiety is less clearly understood than that of pain and is a more complex process because no actual tissue injury is thought to occur. Anxiety stimulates the SNS response.

Anxiety has been linked to the reward and punishment centers within the limbic system of the brain. Stimulation in the punishment centers frequently inhibits the reward centers completely.[33] The punishment center is also responsible for helping a person to escape from potentially harmful situations. The punishment center has dominance over the reward center for the person to escape harm.

 CRITICAL REASONING ACTIVITY

Describe factors that increase the risk for pain and anxiety in critically ill patients.

POSITIVE EFFECTS OF PAIN AND ANXIETY

In the healthy person, pain and anxiety are adaptive mechanisms used to increase mental and physical performance levels to allow a person to move away from potential harm. When the SNS is activated, the person becomes more vigilant of the environment, especially to potential dangers. Once dangers are recognized, the person makes a choice whether to flee the situation or combat the possible threat. For this reason, SNS activation is known as the "fight-or-flight" response.

NEGATIVE EFFECTS OF PAIN AND ANXIETY

Physical Effects

Both pain and anxiety activate the SNS. Catecholamine levels increase, which may place a significant burden on the cardiovascular system, especially in a critically ill patient. Activation of the SNS results in tachycardia and hypertension, which leads to increased myocardial oxygen demand.

In patients with a history of cardiovascular disease, anxiety is associated with recurrent cardiac events and increased mortality.[71] Anxiety at baseline was associated with an increased 10-year mortality rate after percutaneous coronary intervention (PCI) in patients with heart disease.[20]

Hyperventilation (tachypnea) secondary to pain and anxiety can be stressful to the patient because rapid breathing requires significant effort with the use of accessory muscles. Hyperventilation may cause respiratory alkalosis, resulting in impaired tissue perfusion.

If the patient is mechanically ventilated, an increased respiratory rate leads to feelings of breathlessness. As the patient "fights" the mechanical ventilator (dyssynchrony), further alveolar damage ensues, and the endotracheal or tracheostomy tube creates a "choking" sensation and increased anxiety. Dyspnea is a frequent issue in mechanically ventilated patients and is often unrecognized and undertreated by healthcare providers.[10,11] Dyspnea is highly associated with anxiety and pain and may be improved by managing the underlying condition, adjusting the ventilator settings, and administering bronchodilators or opioids.[10,11,21]

Psychological Effects

Many critically ill patients report feelings of panic and fear. Pain and anxiety exacerbate reports of lack of sleep; nightmares; and feelings of bewilderment, isolation, and loneliness. Approximately half of critically ill patients recall having pain, anxiety, and fear as stressful experiences during their hospitalization in the critical care unit.[25,36] In a study of patient experience, patients on mechanical ventilation and light sedation expressed feelings of fear and difficulty in communication.[62]

During 2-year follow-up, 59% of patients still experienced general anxiety, depression, and PTSD.[9] In a prospective observational study of long-term survivors of acute lung injury (ALI) requiring prolonged mechanical ventilation, 35% of patients had PTSD symptoms during follow-up, 50% had taken psychiatric medications, and 40% had required psychiatric treatment since hospital discharge.[9]

Extreme anxiety, moderate to severe pain, delirium, mechanical ventilation, and smoking habits are independent risk factors to developing agitation. Agitation increases ventilator dyssynchrony and increases ventilator days.[3]

Delirium has also been associated with sleep disturbances, abnormal psychomotor activity, and emotional disturbances (i.e., fear, anxiety, anger, depression, apathy, euphoria).[5,22,37] Unrecognized and untreated delirium is a predictor of negative clinical outcomes in critically ill patients, including increased mortality, critical care unit and hospital length of stay, cost of care, and long-term cognitive impairment consistent with a dementia-like state.[37]

STUDY BREAK

2. Which of the following may be associated with anxiety?
   A. Drowsiness
   B. Increased heart rate
   C. Decreased respiratory rate
   D. Vertigo

PREVENTING AND TREATING PAIN AND ANXIETY

The American College of Critical Care Medicine/Society of Critical Care Medicine (SCCM) has updated comprehensive guidelines for integrated, evidence-based, and patient-centered protocols for preventing and treating pain, agitation/sedation, delirium, immobility, and sleep disruption (PADIS) in critically-ill adult patients.[22] The committee recommends the use of validated monitoring instruments, nonpharmacological and pharmacological therapies, and coordinating care that aligns patient's goals (Box 6.3).

The PADIS guidelines have been successfully integrated into the elements of the care bundle to facilitate awakening and breathing coordination, delirium monitoring and management, early exercise and mobility (rehabilitation), sleep, and family engagement, commonly known as the *ABCDEF bundle* (Table 6.1).[22] Implementation of the ABCDEF bundle has resulted in patients spending less time on mechanical ventilation, less delirium, early mobilization, decreased critical care unit length of stay, and decreased hospital length of stay.[22,26] With well-developed nurse-driven analgesia and sedation protocols (ASPs), patients experience more ventilator-free days and less use of benzodiazepines and opioids.[44] The ABCDEF bundle resources can be found at http://www.aacn.org and https://www.sccm.org/ICULiberation/.

BOX 6.3 Guidelines for Pain, Agitation, and Delirium

- Integrate a multiprofessional approach to manage pain, agitation, and delirium to achieve significant, synergistic benefits
- Implement an assessment-driven, protocol-based, stepwise approach for pain and sedation management
- Use valid and reliable assessment tools for pain, sedation, and delirium to target appropriate treatment strategies
- Assess and treat pain promptly in all patients
- Preemptively treat patients with analgesics first and an adjunct to an opioid to decrease pain intensity and opioid use
- Decrease levels of sedation, while ensuring adequate pain control and delirium management, to allow patients active participation in ventilator weaning trials along with early mobility activities
- Institute prevention strategies to avoid complications and improve clinical outcomes
- Actively engage patients in the pain management plan
- Offer nonpharmacologic interventions such as music, relaxation, massage, and cold therapy for procedural pain
- Regularly reassess pain and adjust the treatment accordingly
- Establish a comprehensive quality improvement program that monitors both health care provider practice and patient outcomes related to pain management

From Devlin JW, Skrobik Y, Gélinas C, et al. Clinical practice guidelines for the prevention and management of pain, agitation/sedation, delirium, immobility, and sleep disruption in adult patients in the ICU. *Crit Care Med.* 2018;46(9):e825–e873.

TABLE 6.1 ABCDEF Bundle

Assess, prevent, and manage pain	- Use standardized tools to assess and manage pain:
	  - Behavioral Pain Scale (BPS)
	  - Critical-Care Pain Observation Tool (CPOT)
	- Pain should be treated before a sedative agent is considered.
	- Use pharmacological and nonpharmacological measures to achieve pain management goals.

Both spontaneous awakening trial (SAT) and spontaneous breathing trial (SBT)	- The coordination of SAT and SBT requires a collaborative approach among physicians, nurses, respiratory therapists, and pharmacists to assess the patient and administer the appropriate type and amount of sedation, safely allow the patient to wake up daily, and evaluate the patient's ability to breathe independently of the ventilator. - Decrease sedatives until the patient is responsive. - Complete the SAT screen. If the patient passes the screening, perform the SAT. - Complete the SBT safety screen. If the patient passes the screening, perform the SBT. - If the patient passes the SBT, consider extubation.

Choice of analgesia and sedation	- Treat pain first. Use standardized tools to assess and manage pain.
	- Use standardized tools to assess and manage sedation:
	  - Richmond Agitation-Sedation Scale (RASS)
	  - Sedation-Agitation Scale (SAS)
	- Promote comfort by ensuring adequate pain control, anxiolysis, and prevention and treatment of delirium.
	- Use both pharmacological and nonpharmacological interventions. Identify target goals for analgesia and sedation.

Delirium assessment and management	- Monitor patient throughout the day (before and after SAT) for the presence of delirium.
	- Use validated tools to assess for delirium:
	  - Confusion Assessment Method for the ICU
	  - Intensive Care Delirium Screening Checklist
	- Identify and treat cause(s) of delirium or altered mental status:
	  - Infection or sepsis
	  - Dehydration, hypoglycemia
	  - Sleep deprivation
	  - Alcohol, benzodiazepine, or home medication withdrawal
	  - Medications: anticholinergics, benzodiazepines, opiates, steroids
	- Treat with nonpharmacological measures first:
	  - Decrease nighttime disturbances to enhance sleep.
	  - Increase mobility efforts (physical-occupational therapy).
	  - Allow patient to use eyeglasses and hearing aids.
	  - Encourage interactions with family and friends.

Early mobility and exercise	- Collaborate with respiratory, physical, and occupational therapists to develop a mobility protocol.
	- Evaluate and assess all patients for progressive mobility needs.
	  - RASS −5/−4: Passive ROM
	  - RASS −3/−2: Passive ROM and sit
	  - RASS −1 to +1: Active ROM, sit, stand, walk
	  - Progress activity as tolerated
	- Use available assist devices as needed.

Family engagement and empowerment	- Engage the family early and often in the patient's plan of care.

ROM, Range of motion.

Adapted from Devlin JW, Skrobik Y, Gelinas C, et al. Clinical practice guidelines for the prevention and management of pain, agitation/sedation, delirium, immobility, and sleep disruption in adult patients in the ICU. *Crit Care Med.* 2018;46:e825–e873.

CRITICAL REASONING ACTIVITY

Differentiate between subjective and objective tools when assessing pain and provide examples of each.

Pain Assessment

Quality pain management begins with a thorough assessment, ongoing reassessment, and documentation to facilitate treatment and communication among healthcare providers.

Pain assessment is challenging in patients who cannot communicate; these patients represent most critically ill patients. Factors that alter verbal communication in critically ill patients include endotracheal intubation, altered level of consciousness, restraints, sedation, and therapeutic paralysis.

The PADIS guidelines mandate evaluation of both physiological and behavioral response to pain in patients who are unable to communicate.[22] Optimal pain assessment in adult critical care settings is essential because nurses often underrate and undermedicate the patient's pain. Inaccurate pain assessments and resulting inadequate treatment of pain in critically ill adults can lead to significant physiological consequences.

Assessment involves the collection of the patient's self-report of the pain experience as well as behavioral markers. If a patient can respond, ask the patient to describe the pain or anxiety being experienced or to provide a numeric score to indicate the level of pain or anxiety. Observe behavioral or physiological cues of pain. Typical physiological responses related to pain are detailed in Box 6.2. In the healthy person, these responses are adaptive mechanisms and result from activation of the SNS.

As part of the assessment of pain and anxiety, note what procedures cause pain and evaluate the effectiveness of interventions to prevent or relieve pain and anxiety. When patients exhibit signs of anxiety or agitation, identify and treat the potential cause, such as hypoxemia, hypoglycemia, hypotension, pain, and withdrawal from alcohol and drugs. When possible, ask patients about any herbal remedies they use as complementary and alternative medical therapies and whether they take them along with prescription or over-the-counter medications. These products may lead to adverse herb-drug interactions, especially in older adults who are more likely to be taking multiple drugs.

Pain Measurement Tools for Patients Who Can Communicate.

To assess pain, ask the patient to identify several characteristics associated with the pain: precipitating cause, severity, location (including radiation to other sites), duration, and any alleviating or aggravating factors. Patients with chronic pain conditions, such as arthritis, may be able to provide a detailed list of effective pain remedies that may be useful to implement.

Several tools are available to ensure that the appropriate pain assessment questions are asked. One tool used in assessing the patient with chest pain is the PQRST method. The PQRST method is a mnemonic the nurse can use to ensure that all chest pain characteristics are documented.

P—*Provocation or position.* What precipitated the chest pain symptoms, and where in the chest area is the pain located?

Q—*Quality.* Is the pain sharp, dull, crushing?

R—*Radiation.* Does the pain travel to other parts of the body?

S—*Severity or symptoms associated with the pain.* The patient is asked to rate the pain on a numeric scale and to describe what other symptoms are present.

T—*Timing or triggers for the pain.* Is the pain constant or intermittent, and does it occur with certain activities?

One of the most common methods used to determine pain severity is to ask patients to rate their pain on a numbered scale such as 0 to 10 (administered either verbally or visually). A score of 0 indicates no pain, and a score of 10 indicates the worst pain the patient could possibly imagine. Reassess the pain score after medications or other pain-relieving measures have been provided. Institutional policies provide guidelines for the method and frequency of pain assessment. Some institutions require nurses to intervene for a pain score greater than a predesignated number. Use the pain rating method only with patients who are cognitively aware of their surroundings and can follow simple commands. It is possible for patients with mild to moderate dementia to self-report pain, but this ability decreases with progression of the disease. Numeric rating is not an appropriate method to assess pain in patients who are disoriented or have severe cognitive impairment.

Another widely used subjective pain measurement tool is the Visual Analog Scale (VAS). The VAS is a 10-cm line that looks similar to a timeline. The scale may be drawn horizontally or vertically, and it may or may not be numbered. If numbered, 0 indicates no pain, whereas 10 indicates the most pain (Fig. 6.2). To use the VAS, hold up the scale and ask the patient to point to the level of pain on the line. If the patient is able to communicate in writing, the patient can place an "X" on the VAS with a pencil. The VAS can also be used to evaluate a patient's level of anxiety, with 0 representing no anxiety and 10 representing the most anxiety. The VAS is used only with patients who are alert and able to follow directions.

It is imperative to identify ways to communicate effectively with patients who have limited communication abilities. Several writing tablets and computer applications (app) are available for patients to use to communicate their pain level.

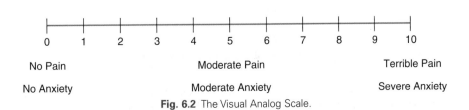

Fig. 6.2 The Visual Analog Scale.

The ICU Patient Communicator app by the SCCM[66] was designed to assist critical care providers to communicate with patients who are unable to speak because of mechanical ventilation, hearing loss, or speech limitations. The ICU Patient Communicator app allows patients to identify where on the body they are feeling sensations, as well as the severity of those sensations. Pain, itching, and nausea can be identified in exact locations on the body and rated on a scale of 0 to 10 for severity.

Pain Measurement Tools for Patients Unable to Communicate.

Assessment of pain in the noncommunicative patient requires identification of an optimal pain scale using the behavioral-physiological tools. The PADIS guidelines recommend use of behavioral assessment tools in critically ill adults unable to self-report pain and in whom behaviors are observable. Vital signs are not valid indicators for pain and should be used only as cues to initiate further assessment.

Observe behaviors using either the Behavioral Pain Scale in intubated (BPS)[55] or nonintubated (BPS-NI)[13] patients or the Critical-Care Pain Observation Tool (CPOT).[29,60] Both tools demonstrate the greatest validity and reliability for monitoring pain in noncommunicative patients.[22] As appropriate, involve the family in the pain assessment process.

Widely used and validated, the BPS was developed to assess pain in the critically ill adult who is nonverbal and unable to communicate (Table 6.2). The BPS, comprising the original BPS and the BPS-NI, includes three behavioral indicators: facial expression, movement of upper limbs, and compliance with ventilation for intubated patients, or vocalization for nonintubated patients. Each indicator is rated from 1 to 4, with a total BPS score ranging from 3 to 12.

The CPOT (Table 6.3) includes four behavioral categories: facial expression, body movements, muscle tension, and compliance with the ventilator for intubated patients or vocalization for extubated patients. Items in each category are scored from 0 to 2, with a total CPOT score ranging from 0 to 8 (see QSEN Exemplar box).

TABLE 6.2 The Behavioral Pain Scale (BPS) for Intubated and Nonintubated Patients

Item	Description	Score
Facial expression	Relaxed	1
	Partially tightened (e.g., brow lowering)	2
	Fully tightened (e.g., eyelid closing)	3
	Grimacing	4
Upper limbs	No movement	1
	Partially bent	2
	Fully bent with finger flexion	3
	Permanently retracted	4
Compliance with mechanical ventilation (intubated)	Tolerating movement	1
	Coughing but tolerating ventilation most of the time	2
	Fighting ventilator	3
	Unable to control ventilation	4
	OR	
Vocalization (nonintubated)	No pain vocalization	1
	Infrequent moaning ($\leq$3/mn) and not prolonged ($\leq$3 s)	2
	Frequent moaning ($>$3/mn) or prolonged ($>$3 s)	3
	Howling or verbal complaints including Ow!, Ouch! or breath-holding	4

From Payen JF, Bru O, Bosson JL, et al. Assessing pain in critically ill sedated patients by using a behavioral pain scale. *Crit Care Med.* 2001;29:2258–2263.

STUDY BREAK

3. Which of the following is a validated tool for assessing pain in critically ill, nonverbal patients?
   A. Critical-Care Pain Observation Tool
   B. FACES Scale
   C. Visual Analog Scale
   D. Confusion Assessment Method (CAM)

⚹ QSEN EXEMPLAR

Patient-Centered Care; Evidence-Based Practice

Pain assessment is challenging in the critical care setting because of the physical and cognitive impairments of many critically ill patients and impediments to communication such as intubation. Critical care nurses commonly use behavioral observations and vital signs as primary assessment data when developing pain relief strategies and comfort-promoting interventions. The Behavioral Pain Scale (BPS) and Critical-Care Pain Observation Tool (CPOT) are behavioral pain assessment tools for noncommunicative and sedated patients in the critical care unit. A prospective, observational study included 72 consecutive intubated and mechanically ventilated patients after cardiac surgery who were not able to self-report pain. Two nurses assessed the BPS and CPOT simultaneously and independently at the following four moments: rest, a nonpainful procedure (oral care), rest, and a painful procedure (turning). Both scores showed a significant increase of 2 points between rest and turning. Discriminant validation of the BPS and CPOT was demonstrated by a significant increase in scores during a painful procedure (turning) ($p = 0.001$). However, the CPOT score remained unchanged when comparing a nonpainful procedure (oral care) with rest, whereas the BPS score significantly increased during a nonpainful (oral care) procedure. The authors suggest that the increase in BPS pain score during mouth care was the result of changes in facial expression and movements of the upper limbs. Both tools showed a fair to good interrater reliability, 0.74 for all assessments. Internal consistency of the BPS and the CPOT was acceptable during the painful procedure (turning) of 0.75 and 0.62, respectively. The authors recommend using an objective pain scale in daily practice to optimize pain treatment and use of analgesics and sedatives in critically ill patients. They also recommended use of the CPOT for ventilated patients because of its better ability to distinguish painful from nonpainful interventions.

Reference

Rijkenberg S, Stilma W, Bosman RJ, et al. Pain measurement in mechanically ventilated patients after cardiac surgery: Comparison of the Behavioral Pain Scale (BPS) and the Critical-Care Pain Observation Tool (CPOT). *J Cardiothorac Vasc Anesth.* 2017;31(4):1227–1234.

TABLE 6.3 Critical-Care Pain Observation Tool

Indicator	Score
Facial Expression	
• Relaxed, no muscle tension	0
• Tense facial muscles (brow lowering, orbit tightening, and levator contraction)	1
• Grimacing with tense facial muscles	2
Body Movements	
• Absence of movements	0
• Protection	1
• Restlessness	2
Muscle Tension in Upper Extremities	
• Relaxed	0
• Tense, rigid	1
• Very tense or rigid	2
Compliance With the Ventilator	
• Tolerating ventilator or movement	0
• Coughing but tolerating ventilator	1
• Fighting ventilator	2
OR	
Nonventilator, Vocalization	
• No sound	0
• Sighing, moaning	1
• Crying out, sobbing	2
Total Score	_____

Data from Gelinas C, Fillion L, Puntillo KA, et al. Validation of critical-care pain observation tool in adult patients. *Am J Crit Care.* 2006;15:420–427.

TABLE 6.4 Richmond Agitation-Sedation Scale (RASS)

Term	Score
Combative—Overtly combative or violent; immediate danger to staff	+4
Very agitated—Pulls on or removes tubes or catheters or has aggressive behavior toward staff	+3
Agitated—Frequent nonpurposeful movements; fights ventilator	+2
Restless—Anxious or apprehensive but movements are not aggressive or vigorous	+1
Alert and calm	0
Drowsy—Not fully alert, but has sustained (>10 sec) awakening, with eye contact, to voice[a]	−1
Light sedation—Briefly awakens (<10 sec) with eye contact, to voice[a]	−2
Moderate sedation—Any movement (but no eye contact) to voice[a]	−3
Deep sedation—No response to voice, but any movement to physical stimulation[a]	−4
Unarousable—No response to voice or physical stimulation	−5

[a]In a loud voice, state patient's name and direct patient to open eyes and look at speaker.
From Sessler CN, Gosnell MS, Grap MJ, et al. The Richmond Agitation-Sedation Scale: Validity and reliability in adult intensive care unit patients. *Am J Respir Crit Care Med.* 2002;166:1338–1344.

Assessment of Agitation and Sedation

Agitation typically produces hyperactive psychomotor functions, including tachycardia, hypertension, and movement. Patients are usually sedated to limit this hyperactivity. The goal is to maintain light levels of sedation, which is associated with shorter duration of mechanical ventilation and shorter critical care unit length of stay.[22] By using lower doses of medications, the patient is less likely to experience medication accumulation or adverse effects. These adverse effects include increased hospital stay, delayed ventilator weaning, immobility, and increased rates of ventilator-associated pneumonia. Conversely, not enough sedation may lead to agitation, inappropriate use of paralytics, increased metabolic demand, and an increased risk of myocardial ischemia. The level of sedation can be measured using objective tools or scales to monitor depth of sedation and brain function. An ideal sedation scale provides data that are simple to compute and record, accurately describe the degree of sedation or agitation within well-defined categories, guide the titration of therapy, and are valid and reliable in critically ill patients.

Sedation Measurement Tools. The PADIS guidelines recommend two valid and reliable sedation scales for targeting sedation, maintaining light levels of sedation, or using daily awakening trials to reduce sedative exposure: the Richmond Agitation-Sedation Scale (RASS)[64] and the Sedation-Agitation Scale (SAS).[61] The appropriate target level of sedation depends on the patient's disease process and the therapeutic or support interventions required.

The RASS is a 10-point scale, ranging from 4 (combative) through 0 (calm, alert) to −5 (unarousable). The patient is assessed for 30 to 60 seconds in three steps, using discrete criteria (Table 6.4). The RASS has strong interrater reliability and internal consistency, is useful in detecting changes in sedation status over consecutive days of hospitalization, and correlates with the administered dose of sedative and analgesic medications.[59,64] Light sedation is defined as a RASS score of −2 to +1 (or its equivalent using other scales).

The SAS (Table 6.5) describes patient behaviors seen in the continuum of sedation to agitation. Scores range from 1 (unarousable) to 7 (dangerously agitated).

Continuous Monitoring of Sedation. No technological device provides the bedside nurse with an absolute measurement of the patient's pain or anxiety. Although various devices that assess the patient's brain activity are available, the PADIS guidelines recommend that objective measures of brain function (i.e., electroencephalography [EEG] and Bispectral Index Score [BIS]) not be used as the primary method to monitor pain and depth of sedation in noncomatose, nonparalyzed, critically ill adult patients.[22,30]

Continuous EEG monitoring may be used to assess levels of sedation in nonconvulsive seizure or patients with an elevated intracranial pressure (ICP). The EEG records spontaneous brain activity that originates from the cortical pyramidal cells

TABLE 6.5   Sedation-Agitation Scale

Score	Characteristic	Examples of Patient's Behavior
7	Dangerously agitated	Pulls at endotracheal tube, tries to remove catheters, climbs over bed rail, strikes at staff, thrashes from side to side
6	Very agitated	Does not calm despite frequent verbal reminding of limits, requires physical restraints, bites endotracheal tube
5	Agitated	Anxious or mildly agitated, attempts to sit up, calms down in response to verbal instructions
4	Calm and cooperative	Calm, awakens easily, follows commands
3	Sedated	Difficult to arouse, awakens to verbal stimuli or gentle shaking but drifts off again, follows simple commands
2	Very sedated	Arouses to physical stimuli but does not communicate or follow commands, may move spontaneously
1	Unarousable	Minimal or no response to noxious stimuli, does not communicate or follow commands

From Riker RR, Fraser GL, Simmons LE, et al. Validating the Sedation-Agitation Scale with the Bispectral Index and Visual Analog Scale in adult ICU patients after cardiac surgery. *Intensive Care Med.* 2001;27:853–858.

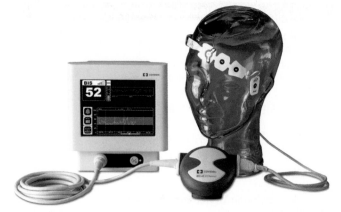

Fig. 6.3 The Bispectral Index Score (BIS) monitor and electrode. (Image used by permission of Nellcor Puritan Bennett LLC, Boulder, CO, doing business as Covidien.)

on the surface of the brain by placing electrodes on the patient's head. These devices digitize the raw EEG signal and apply a complex algorithm that results in a numeric score ranging from 0 (isoelectric EEG) to 100 (fully awake).[28] The EEG generally changes from a low-amplitude, high-frequency signal while the patient is awake to a high-amplitude, low-frequency signal when the patient is deeply anesthetized.

The BIS monitor (Aspect Medical Systems, Boulder, CO) and the Patient State Index (PSI) Analyzer (Physiometrix, North Billerica, MA) may be used as an adjunct to subjective sedation assessments in adult patients in the critical care unit who are receiving neuromuscular blocking agents. These devices provide a noninvasive, objective analysis of the level of wakefulness. To obtain a signal, an electrode is placed across the patient's forehead and attached to a monitor. The monitor displays the raw EEG and the BIS or PSI value, which ranges from 0 (no cortical activity) to 100 (completely awake).[17]

The BIS monitor and electrode are shown in Fig. 6.3. A value greater than 90 typically indicates full consciousness, a score of 40 to 60 represents deep sedation, and a score of 0 represents complete EEG suppression. A BIS value greater than 60 is associated with patient awareness and recollection. A BIS value less than 60 is the goal in critically ill patients who require sedation.[45,76] There is a strong correlation with BIS and RASS scores in assessment of sedation level in the critical care unit.[57,73] For adequate sedation (RASS value of 0 to −3), the median BIS value was found to be 56 (range 42 to 89),[45] and for inadequate sedation (RASS value ≥1), the BIS value was 80 and above.[57]

Pupillary Reflex Measurement. Pupillometry is the measurement of pupil size and reactivity to light. The Pupillometer (Neuroptics, Laguna Hills, CA) is a noninvasive monitoring device that allows dynamic pupillary diameter measurement by an infrared camera. Specifically, it measures the pupillary dilatation reflex (PDR), a sympathetic reflex that dilates the pupil in response to noxious stimuli. Portable pupillometry is useful in the management of pain because it allows for assessments of the effect of opioids.[52] With administration of opioid, the PDR is decreased. When patients experience ongoing pain, combined with diminished PDR (indicating significant central opioid effect), additional administration of opioids is not beneficial. Therefore patients with ongoing pain but diminished PDR may be ideal candidates for regional block, ketamine, or other nonopioid therapy.[47,52]

Assessment of Delirium

Delirium (acute brain dysfunction) is characterized by an acutely changing or fluctuating mental status, inattention, disorganized thinking, and altered levels of consciousness. Acute delirium is common in critically ill patients; incidence ranges between 45% and 87%.[41] Untreated delirium may result in longer duration of mechanical ventilation and longer critical care unit stay than experienced by patients without delirium.

Delirium is categorized according to the level of alertness and level of psychomotor activity. It is divided into three clinical subtypes: hyperactive, hypoactive, and mixed (Table 6.6). Patients with *hyperactive delirium* are agitated, combative, and disoriented.[12] These patients place themselves or others at risk for injury because of their altered thought processes and resultant behaviors. Psychotic features such as hallucinations, delusions, and paranoia may be seen. Patients may believe that members of the nursing or medical staff are attempting to harm them.

Hypoactive delirium is often referred to as quiet delirium and often goes undiagnosed and underestimated when there is no active monitoring with a validated clinical instrument. It is also the most prevalent subtype, occurring in more than 50% of hospitalized patients.[12]

TABLE 6.6 Clinical Subtypes of Delirium

Subtype	Characteristics
Hyperactive	Agitation Restlessness Attempts to remove catheters or tubes Hitting Biting Emotional lability
Hypoactive	Withdrawal Flat affect Apathy Lethargy Decreased responsiveness
Mixed	Concurrent or sequential appearance of some features of both hyperactive and hypoactive delirium

The *mixed subtype* describes the fluctuating nature of delirium. Some agitated patients with hyperactive delirium may receive sedatives to calm them and then may emerge from sedation in a hypoactive state. This hyperactive delirium occurs in approximately 45% of hospitalized patients.[12]

The exact pathophysiological mechanisms involved in the development and progression of delirium are unknown. Risk factors for the development of delirium in the critical care unit include coma, preexisting dementia, history of hypertension or alcoholism, and a high severity of illness at admission (hypoxemia, metabolic disturbances, electrolyte imbalances, head trauma). Older patients are especially at risk for delirium.[12] Neurotransmitter levels are affected by medications with anticholinergic properties. Benzodiazepines, opioids, and other psychotropic medications are associated with an increased risk of developing delirium, yet these medications are commonly given to critically ill patients.

❓ CRITICAL REASONING ACTIVITY

What is delirium? What are some of the behaviors seen in the hyperactive subtype?

Delirium Measurement Tools. Because delirium occurs in many patients who are receiving mechanical ventilation and is associated with negative outcomes, assess all critically ill patients for delirium. Two of the most frequently used and validated instruments are the Confusion Assessment Method for the ICU (CAM-ICU)[24] and the Intensive Care Delirium Screening Checklist (ICDSC).[8] The CAM-ICU (Box 6.4) is designed to be a serial assessment tool for use by bedside nurses and physicians. It is easy to use, takes only 2 minutes to complete, and requires minimal training. The first step is to assess consciousness using a validated sedation scale. A patient is considered delirium positive on the CAM-ICU if the following are present: criteria 1 (acute mental status change) and 2 (inattention), and either 3 (disorganized thinking) or 4 (altered level of consciousness).

BOX 6.4 The Confusion Assessment Method for the Critical Care Unit

Step 1. Level of Consciousness: RASS
Assess RASS. If RASS is ≥ −3 proceed to CAM-ICU; otherwise, "unable to assess"

Step 2. Content of Consciousness: CAM-ICU
Feature 1: Acute Change or Fluctuating Course of Mental Status
Is the mental status different from baseline?
OR
  Has mental status fluctuated in the past 24 hours as evidenced by scores on a sedation/level of consciousness scale (i.e., RASS/SAS), GCS, or previous delirium assessment?
AND

Feature 2: Inattention
Conduct the Letters Attention Test (or Picture Test available in training manual). Say to the patient, "I am going to read you a series of 10 letters. Whenever you hear the letter 'A,' indicate by squeezing my hand." Read letters 3 seconds apart from one of the following sequences. Count errors when patient does not squeeze on the letter "A" or squeezes on any other letter. More than 2 errors is considered present.

S A V E A H A A R T or **C A S A B L A N C A** or **A B A D B A D A A Y**
AND

Feature 3: Altered Level of Consciousness
Considered present if the RASS score is anything other than 0, alert and calm
OR

Feature 4: Disorganized Thinking
Ask a series of yes/no questions:
1. Will a stone float on water?
2. Are there fish in the sea?
3. Does one pound weigh more than two pounds?
4. Can you use a hammer to pound a nail?
  Count the number of wrong answers.
  Ask patient to follow a two-part simple command:
1. "Hold up this many fingers" (Hold 2 fingers in front of patient).
2. "Now do the same thing with the other hand." If patient is unable to complete entire command, it is considered an error.
  Considered present if more than one error noted.
  Patient considered positive for delirium when Features 1 and 2 present along with either Feature 3 or 4.

GCS, Glasgow Coma Scale; *RASS*, Richmond Agitation Sedation Scale; *SAS*, Sedation-Agitation Scale.
Additional resources can be found at https://www.icudelirium.org/medical-professionals/delirium/monitoring-delirium-in-the-icu

The ICDSC is a screening checklist of eight items based on *Diagnostic and Statistical Manual of Mental Disorders* (DSM) criteria (Table 6.7). After consciousness is assessed and rated on a scale of A through E, the patient is assessed for seven indicators of delirium. One point is given for each positive sign of delirium identified. The scores range from 0 to 8 points, and a patient with more than 4 points is defined as *delirium positive.*

TABLE 6.7   Intensive Care Delirium Screening Checklist[a]

Screening	Score

1. **Altered level of consciousness**
  a. Deep sedation/coma entire shift (SAS 1, 2; RASS –4, –5) = unable to assess
  b. Agitation at any time (SAS 5, 6; RASS 1-4) = 1 point
  c. Normal wakefulness entire shift (SAS 4; RASS 0) = 0 points
  d. Light sedation (SAS 3; RASS –1, –2, –3) = 1 point (no sedatives) = 0 points (recent sedatives)
	___

2. **Inattention.** Difficulty following instructions, easily distracts, does not reliably squeeze hands to spoken letter A (e.g., SAVEAHAART)	___
3. **Disorientation.** Disoriented to person, place, time, situation, caregivers	___
4. **Hallucination-delusion-psychosis.** Responds positively to having hallucinations or is afraid of people or things in surroundings	___
5. **Psychomotor agitation or retardation.** Exhibits hyperactivity requiring sedatives or restraints to prevent harm or hypoactive behaviors	___
6. **Inappropriate speech or mood.** Exhibits inappropriate emotions or interactions, incoherent speech, apathy, or overly demanding behavior	___
7. **Sleep-wake cycle disturbance.** Awakens frequently from or less than 4h sleep at night; or sleeping much of the day	___
8. **Symptom fluctuation.** Any of the above symptoms of delirium (items 2-6) fluctuate over a 24h period	___
Total Score (0-8)	___

[a]Assess the patient over the entire shift, as not all behaviors may be present at the same time. Assess level of consciousness first. If the patient is deeply sedated or comatose, the patient is unable to be screened for delirium. Items 1 to 4 required a focused assessment, whereas items 5 to 8 are based on observations throughout the shift. A score of 4 to 8 is positive for delirium.
RASS, Richmond Agitation-Sedation Score; *SAS,* Sedation-Agitation Score.
Adapted from Bergeron N, Dubois MJ, Dumont M, et al. Intensive Care Delirium Screening Checklist: Evaluation of a new screening tool. *Intensive Care Med.* 2001;27:859–864; and screening tools at http://www.icudelirium.org.

Management of delirium focuses on keeping the patient safe. The PADIS guidelines recommend using a multicomponent, nonpharmacological intervention that is focused on reducing modifiable risk factors for delirium; improving cognition; and optimizing sleep, mobility, hearing, and vision.[22] Use the least restrictive measures because unnecessary use of restraints or medication may precipitate or exacerbate delirium.

Apply splints or binders to restrict movement if the patient is pulling at catheters, drains, or dressings. Remove any type of tubing as soon as possible, particularly nasogastric tubes, which are irritating to agitated patients. Avoid routine use of haloperidol, an atypical antipsychotic, or a 3-hydroxy-3-methylglutaryl coenzyme A reductase inhibitor (i.e., a statin) to treat delirium.[22] If these measures are not successful, medication may be necessary to improve cognition, not to sedate the patient.

STUDY BREAK

4. Which of the following is a validated tool for assessing delirium in critically ill patients?
A. Visual Analog Scale
B. Behavioral Pain Scale
C. FACES Scale
D. Confusion Assessment Method

MANAGEMENT OF PAIN AND ANXIETY

Nonpharmacological Management

Nonpharmacological approaches to manage pain and anxiety are early strategies because many medications used for analgesia or sedation have potentially negative hemodynamic effects. Efforts to reduce anxiety include frequent reorientation, providing patient comfort, and optimizing the environment. For example, explain the different types of alarms to the patient and family to lessen anxiety levels. Many nonpharmacological approaches are categorized as complementary and alternative therapies. The most commonly used complementary therapies in the critical care unit are environmental manipulation and complementary and alternative therapies.

Environmental Manipulation

Decrease patient anxiety and pain by changing the environment so that it appears less hostile. Provide ongoing reorientation and repetition of explanations and information. Place calendars and clocks within sight to assist in reorientation.

Family engagement is one of the most important strategies to decrease the patient's anxiety or pain. Family members often benefit from role modeling, as nursing staff members support and reassure patients while avoiding arguments with patients who have irrational ideas or misperceptions (see Chapter 2). The patient's family is often able to interpret patient behaviors to the nursing staff, especially those associated with pain or anxiety. Encourage family members to participate in the care whenever the patient's condition allows it. Examples of family participation include coaching during breathing exercises, assisting with passive and active range of motion, and providing hygiene measures.

Another effective strategy is altering the patient's room. Ask family members to bring in pictures of family members and other small keepsakes to provide diversions from the stressful critical care environment. Technology, such as tablet computers, can provide another mechanism for sharing photos and music. Depending on a unit's design, position the bed so that it faces a window. There are also critical care units in which the monitoring equipment is concealed behind cabinetry to provide a homelike atmosphere. Some patients may benefit from being moved to a different room. Physically moving the patient to a different location prevents the patient from becoming tired of the surroundings, and it may provide some sense of clinical improvement for the patient and family.

Complementary and Alternative Therapy

Three complementary therapies that critical care nurse can independently initiate, are inexpensive, and are within the scope of nursing practice are guided imagery, music, and essential oils and aromatherapy.

Guided Imagery. Guided imagery is a mind-body intervention intended to relieve stress and to promote a sense of peace and tranquility. It involves a form of directed daydreaming that provides relaxation and distraction and refocuses pain perception. It is a way of purposefully diverting and focusing thoughts. Guided imagery is a simple and inexpensive strategy that all nurses can easily incorporate into their daily practice during most procedures and interventions, such as painful procedures and ventilator weaning. For example, when performing a needlestick puncture, instruct the patient to imagine walking on a beach or other pleasant sensation. Box 6.5 provides directions on using guided imagery. Combine guided imagery with gentle touch or light massage to decrease pain and tension.[27] Benefits of the guided imagery program include reduced stress and anxiety, decreased pain and narcotic consumption, decreased length of stay, enhanced sleep, and increased patient satisfaction.[34]

Music Therapy. Similar to guided imagery, a music therapy program offers patients a diversionary technique for pain and anxiety relief. Some institutions have staff members dedicated solely to music therapy. When appropriate, a music therapist comes to the patient's bedside in the critical care unit and offers one-on-one therapy.

Music therapy may be effective in reducing pain and anxiety if patients are able to participate.[31,32] Music therapy is an ideal intervention for patients with low-energy states who fatigue easily, such as those who require ventilatory support, because it does not require the focused concentration necessary for guided imagery. When patients can select their own music, there is a significant reduction in anxiety and sedative exposure during ventilator support.[6,15,50]

Musical selections without lyrics that contain slow, flowing rhythms that duplicate pulses of 60 to 80 beats/min decrease anxiety in the listener.[9] Music can also provide an alternative focus on a pleasant, comforting stimulus, rather than on stressful environmental stimuli or thoughts.

Careful scrutiny of musical selections and of personal preferences of what is considered relaxing is important for success (see Evidence-Based Practice box).

EVIDENCE-BASED PRACTICE

Problem
Mechanical ventilation often causes major distress and anxiety in patients, putting them at greater risk for complications. Side effects of analgesia and sedation may lead to the prolongation of mechanical ventilation and, subsequently, to a longer length of hospitalization and increased cost.

Clinical Question
What is the effect of music interventions compared with standard care on anxiety and other outcomes in mechanically ventilated patients?

Evidence
Music has been used to heal for centuries. Current scientific evidence identifies neurochemical changes that occur when listening to music. Music listening may have a beneficial effect on reducing anxiety, reducing respiratory rate and systolic blood pressure, and reducing consumption of sedatives and analgesics in mechanically ventilated patients. Implementation of a patient-directed music protocol empowered patients in their own anxiety management.

Implication for Nursing
Music therapy may be effective in reducing pain and anxiety if patients are able to participate. Allow patients to select their own music because music preference plays an important part in the effectiveness of music relaxation. The anxiety-reducing effect of music is that music can help patients focus their attention away from stressful events to something pleasant and soothing. The use of a professional music therapist helps to engage patients who may be distressed, frustrated, fearful, or isolated to select music they may enjoy. For patients in the critical care unit who are receiving sedation and mechanical ventilation, passive listening to prerecorded music incorporated into daily care is also beneficial.

Level of Evidence
A—Systematic review

Reference
Mofredj A, Alaya S, Tassaioust K, et al. Music therapy, a review of the potential therapeutic benefits for the critically ill. *J Crit Care*. 2016;35:195–199.

BOX 6.5 Practicing Guided Imagery

Have the patients imagine a scenario of themselves on a warm beach, in their favorite place, or with their favorite person, in which they can hear, smell, feel, taste, and touch.

1. **Get Comfortable**—get into a relaxed position.
2. **Breathe From Your Belly**—use diaphragmic deep breathing and close your eyes, focusing on "breathing in peace and breathing out stress." This means letting your belly expand and contract with your breath.
3. **Choose a Scene**—and imagine yourself there.
4. **Immerse Yourself in Sensory Details**—involve all of your senses. What does it look like? How does it feel? What special scents are involved?
5. **Relax**—enjoy your "surroundings" and let yourself be far from what stresses you. When you're ready to come back to reality, count back from 10 or 20 and tell yourself that when you get to 1, you'll feel serene and alert and enjoy the rest of your day. When you return, you'll feel calmer and refreshed, like returning from a mini-vacation, but you won't have left the room!

Essential Oils and Aromatherapy. Creating a calm and soothing environment is an independent nursing intervention to decrease anxiety of critically ill patients. Essential oils and aromatherapy are effective when used as an adjunctive therapy for pain management.[2,16,43] When the aroma of essential oils stimulates cilia of the nasal passages, an electrical signal is sent to the olfactory bulb causing serotonin, endorphin, and noradrenaline release.[35] In a study of critically ill patients undergoing percutaneous coronary intervention, use of essential oils with lavender, Roman chamomile, and neroli with a 6:2:0.5 ratio before and after the procedure resulted in a significant decrease in anxiety and improvement in quality of sleep.[16] Essential oils that assist with pain management include lavender, German chamomile, sweet marjoram, dwarf pine, rosemary, and ginger.[1] Essential oil and aromatherapy are noninvasive and individualized to the patient's preference. However, ensure that patients do not have allergies or other adverse reactions to scents before using aromatherapy.

Animal-Assisted Therapy. Animal-assisted therapy (AAT) involves interaction between patients and trained animals (as therapist) accompanied by human owners or handlers. Some units allow personal pets to be brought into the patient's room. Dogs and cats are commonly used animals in the hospital setting.[38,56] AAT improves the patient's physiological and emotional well-being, builds motivation, reduces anxiety levels, and eases suffering.[38]

Pharmacological Management

Many critically ill patients require medications to relieve pain, anxiety, or both. The appropriate management of pain and anxiety may result in improved pulmonary function, earlier ambulation and mobilization, decreased stress response with lower catecholamine concentrations, and lower oxygen consumption, leading to improved outcomes. According to the PADIS guidelines, an assessment-driven protocol should include clear guidance on medication choice and dosing and make treating pain a priority over providing sedatives.[22] Table 6.8 summarizes pharmacological therapies used in managing pain and anxiety, and Table 6.9 illustrates an order set for pain, agitation, and delirium.

Opioids. Medications for managing pain include opioids and nonsteroidal antiinflammatory drugs (NSAIDs). Prior to opioid administration, determine the patient's history of ever receiving an opioid. Opioid-naive patients are at higher risk for oversedation and aspiration, especially if they receive opioids in inappropriate dosages (Box 6.6). The selection of an opioid is based on its pharmacological effects and potential for adverse effects. The benefits of opioids include rapid onset, ease of titration, lack of accumulation, and low cost. IV opioids are considered as the first-line medication class of choice to treat non-neuropathic pain in critically ill patients.[22] In addition, use nonopioid analgesics to decrease the number of opioids and their side effects.

The most commonly used opioids in critically ill patients are fentanyl, morphine, and hydromorphone. Fentanyl has the fastest onset and the shortest duration, but repeated dosing may cause accumulation and prolonged effects. Morphine has a longer duration of action, and intermittent dosing may be given. However, hypotension may result from vasodilation, and its active metabolite may cause prolonged sedation in patients with renal insufficiency. Hydromorphone is similar to morphine in its duration of action.

Fentanyl may also be administered by a transdermal patch in hemodynamically stable patients with chronic pain. The patch provides consistent medication delivery, but the extent of absorption varies depending on permeability, temperature, perfusion, and thickness of the skin. Fentanyl patches are not recommended for acute analgesia because it takes 12 to 24 hours to achieve peak effect and, once the patch is removed, another 12 to 24 hours until the medication is no longer present in the body.

Adverse effects of opioids are common. Respiratory depression is a concern in nonintubated patients or those on minimal ventilator settings. Hypotension may occur in hemodynamically unstable patients or in hypovolemic patients. A depressed level of consciousness and hallucinations leading to increased agitation is seen in some patients. Gastric retention and ileus may occur as well.

Renal or hepatic insufficiency may alter opioid and metabolite elimination. Titration to the desired response and assessment of prolonged effects are necessary. Older adult patients may have reduced opioid requirements. Administration of a reversal agent such as naloxone is not recommended after prolonged analgesia. It can induce withdrawal and may cause nausea, cardiac stress, and dysrhythmias.

Preventing pain is more effective than treating established pain. When patients are administered opioids on an "as-needed" basis, they may receive less than the prescribed dose, and delays in treatment may occur. Administer analgesics on a continuous or scheduled intermittent basis, with supplemental bolus doses as required. IV administration usually requires lower and more frequent doses than intramuscular administration to achieve patient comfort. Intramuscular administration is not recommended in hemodynamically unstable patients because of altered perfusion and variable absorption. Establish a pain management plan for each patient and reevaluate the plan as the patient's clinical condition changes.

Adjuvants to Opioid Therapy. A "multimodal analgesia" approach is essential in the management of mild to moderate procedural pain in the critical care unit. Nonopioid analgesics such as acetaminophen, nefopam, ketamine, neuropathic agents, and NSAIDs decrease pain intensity and opioid consumption for pain management in critically ill adults.[22]

Acetaminophen. The most commonly used pain reliever is *acetaminophen,* which belongs to a class of medications called *analgesics* (pain relievers) and *antipyretics* (fever reducers). The exact mechanism of action of acetaminophen is not known. It may reduce the production of prostaglandins in the brain. Acetaminophen is used to treat mild to moderate pain, such as pain associated with prolonged bed rest. In combination with an opioid, acetaminophen has a greater analgesic effect than higher doses of an opioid alone. The IV form of acetaminophen (Ofirmev) is used for the treatment of acute pain and fever in adults and children.[72] Administer acetaminophen cautiously in patients with hepatic dysfunction.

TABLE 6.8 PHARMACOLOGY

Medications Frequently Used in the Treatment of Pain, Agitation, Delirium, and Neuromuscular Blockade[a]

Medication	Action/Use	Dose/Route	Side Effects	Nursing Implications
Opioids				
Fentanyl (Sublimaze [IV], Duragesic [patch])	Opioid; inhibits ascending pain pathway in CNS; increases pain threshold; alters pain perception	*IV bolus*: 50-100 mcg q1-2h *Infusion*: 25-50 mcg/h; titrate to desired effect; maximum 700 mcg/h (unlabeled dosage) *TD*: 12.5 mcg/h; higher dose may be required	Bradycardia Hypotension Respiratory depression Decreased gastric motility Constipation Muscle rigidity Itching	Titrate infusion slowly in increments. Monitor BP, heart rate, and respiratory status. Administer fluids as indicated. Give as an infusion for extended therapy. *Patch*: Apply to upper torso. Avoid direct heat (e.g., heating blanket), which accelerates fentanyl release. Change patch q72h and apply to a new site. *Antidote*: Naloxone.
Hydromorphone (Dilaudid)	Opioid; inhibits ascending pain pathway in CNS; increases pain threshold; alters pain perception	*PO tablet*: 2-4 mg q4-6h *PO solution*: 2.5-10 mg q3-6h *SC/IM*: 1-2 mg q4-6h PRN *IV initial dose*: 0.2-1 mg q2-3h (given slowly over 2-3 min)	Hypotension Respiratory depression Decreased gastric motility Constipation Seizures	Titrate infusion slowly in increments. Monitor BP, heart rate, and respiratory status. Administer fluids as indicated. The estimated relative potency of hydromorphone to morphine is 7:1. Monitor liver function. Administer lower doses in the older patient. Hydromorphone HP injection should never be administered to opioid-naive patients. *Antidote*: Naloxone.
Morphine (Duramorph, MS Contin, Roxanol)	Opioid; depresses pain impulse transmission at spinal cord level by interacting with opioid receptors	Moderate to severe pain: *SC/IM*: 2.5-15 mg q2-6h PRN *PO*: 10-30 mg q3-4h PRN *Immediate-release tablets or oral solution*: 10-30 mg q3-4h PRN *Extended-release tablets*: 15–30 mg q12h *Rectal*: 10-20 mg q4h PRN *IV bolus*: 2-10 mg/70 kg of body weight q3-4h PRN; give slowly over 4-5 min *Continuous infusion*: 0.8-10 mg/h *Epidural*: initial injection of 5 mg in lumbar region; may give 1-2 mg more after 1h to a maximum of 10 mg *Continuous epidural*: 2-4 mg/24h *Intrathecal*: 0.2-1 mg one time; repeat doses not recommended Chest pain: *Initial*: 4-8 mg IV repeat PRN *Maintenance*: 2-8 mg q5-15 min PRN	Hypotension Respiratory depression Nausea and vomiting Decreased gastric motility Constipation Urinary retention Itching or rash	Titrate infusion slowly in increments. Monitor BP, heart rate, and respiratory status. Administer fluids as indicated. Administer lower doses in older adults. Gradually taper to avoid withdrawals. *Antidote*: Naloxone.

Continued

TABLE 6.8 PHARMACOLOGY—cont'd

Medications Frequently Used in the Treatment of Pain, Agitation, Delirium, and Neuromuscular Blockade[a]

Medication	Action/Use	Dose/Route	Side Effects	Nursing Implications
Nonopioids Adjuvant				
Acetaminophen (Tylenol) IV (Ofirmev)	Nonnarcotic analgesic; blocks pain impulses peripherally that occur in response to prostaglandin synthesis; no antiinflammatory properties	*PO/PR:* 325-650 mg q4-6h PRN, not to exceed 4 g/day *IV bolus:* Patient ≥50 kg: 650 mg IV q4h *or* 1000 mg IV q6h, not to exceed 4 g/day; patient <50 kg: 12.5 mg/kg IV q4h *or* 15 mg/kg IV q6h, not to exceed 75 mg/kg in 24h or 3.75 g/day; infuse IV over at least 15 min	Renal failure with prolonged high dosage Blood dyscrasias Hepatic toxicity	Schedule 1000-mg doses at least q6h. Monitor renal and liver function. Assess other medications for acetaminophen content (e.g., Percocet). Treat overdose with acetylcysteine.
N-methyl-D-aspartate (NMDA) Receptor Antagonist				
Ketamine (Ketalar)	Nonbarbiturate general anesthetic; interrupts association pathways of the brain selectively; produces a somatesthetic sensory blockade	Acute pain: *Bolus IV:* 0.2-0.3 mg/kg; maximum 0.35 mg/kg *Continuous infusion:* 0.1-0.5 mg/kg/h to reduce pain while avoiding adverse effects; maximum 1 mg/kg/h Rapid sequence intubation: *Bolus IV:* 2 mg/kg Procedural: *Induction IV:* 1-4.5 mg/kg one time *Induction IM:* 6.5-13 mg/kg one time *Maintenance:* Repeat half or all of the induction dose	Emergence reactions Hypertension Respiratory depression Apnea Nausea and vomiting Anaphylaxis	Monitor BP, heart rate, and respiratory status. Protect the patient's airway, as vomiting is a common side effect. Increases intracranial pressure, so should be used cautiously in head-injured patients. Psychological manifestations vary and may involve unpleasant hallucinations, confusion, and excitement.
Nonsteroidal Antiinflammatory Drugs (NSAIDs)				
Aspirin (Ecotrin, Bayer)	Blocks pain impulses in the CNS; decreases inflammation by inhibition of prostaglandin synthesis	Pain: *PO:* 325-1000 mg q4-6h PRN; maximum 4 g/day *Rectal:* 1 suppository (300–600 mg) q4h PRN; maximum 4 g/day	Bleeding Gastrointestinal ulcers Tinnitus Thrombocytopenia	Administer with food if taking PO. Do not exceed recommended doses. Monitor complete blood count and renal function.
Ibuprofen (Advil, Motrin) (IV: Caldolor)	Inhibits COX-1, COX-2 by blocking arachidonate; used to treat pain and reduce inflammation	Mild to moderate pain: *PO:* 200-400 mg q4-6h PRN; doses >400 mg have not been proven to provide greater efficacy; maximum 3200 mg/day *IV:* 400-800 mg IV over at least 30 min q6h PRN; do not exceed 3200 mg/day	Bleeding Gastrointestinal ulcers Tinnitus Thrombocytopenia Thrombotic events	Do not exceed recommended doses. Monitor complete blood count. Monitor renal and liver function. Patients should be well hydrated before IV ibuprofen administration.
Ketorolac (Toradol)	Inhibits prostaglandin synthesis; used to treat pain and inflammation	*IV/IM:* 30 mg q6h; maximum 120 mg/day *Patients ≥65 years of age, renal impairment, or patient <50 kg:* 15 mg q6h; maximum 60 mg/day	Headache Dyspepsia Nausea Acute renal failure	Monitor complete blood count. Monitor renal and liver function. Do not use to treat perioperative pain associated with cardiac surgery. Do not administer epidural or intrathecal route because solution contains alcohol. Duration should not exceed 5 days. Infuse over 1-2 min, no less than 15 sec.

TABLE 6.8 PHARMACOLOGY—cont'd

Medications Frequently Used in the Treatment of Pain, Agitation, Delirium, and Neuromuscular Blockade[a]

Medication	Action/Use	Dose/Route	Side Effects	Nursing Implications
Naproxen (Aleve)	Inhibits COX-1, COX-2; used to treat pain, inflammation, and fever	Pain: *PO (tablets/oral suspension):* 250-500 mg q12h PRN; maximum 1500 mg/day	Edema Ecchymosis Dyspnea Dyspepsia Abdominal pain	Monitor complete blood count. Monitor for allergic reactions and angioedema. Administer with food. Black box warning: avoid aspirin, alcohol, steroid; increased risk of GI bleeding.
Celecoxib (Celebrex)	Inhibits prostaglandin synthesis via inhibition of COX-2; used to treat pain and inflammation	Pain: *PO:* initial, 400 mg once, plus one additional 200-mg dose if needed on the first day; maintenance, 200 mg bid PRN	Headache Hypertension Diarrhea Nausea	Patient should be on the lowest effective dose. Avoid use in older adults. Black box warning: contraindicated in GI bleeding, peptic ulcer disease, myocardial infarction, stroke.
Neuropathics Gabapentin	Mechanism unknown	*PO:* 900 mg; 3.6 g/day in divided doses tid	Somnolence Confusion Changes in BP Changes in vision	Ongoing research needed as to effectiveness in the critically ill.
Pregabalin (Lyrica)	GABA analog; strongly binds to the alpha 2 delta site in CNS tissues; effects noradrenergic and serotonergic pathways in the brainstem, modulating pain transmission in the spinal cord	*PO:* initial, 75 mg orally bid; maintenance, may increase to 150 mg bid within 1 wk based on efficacy and tolerability; may further increase to 300 mg bid for insufficient pain relief after 2-3 wk of treatment	Angioedema Somnolence Dizziness	Monitor for signs and symptoms of depression, mood changes, or suicidal thoughts. Assess for allergic reactions. Wean slowly.
Epidural Analgesias Bupivacaine	Local anesthetic/analgesic; blocks generation and conduction of nerve impulses	Concentration of 0.25%-0.75% (25-150 mg) provides partial to complete motor block	Hypotension Respiratory paralysis Nausea and vomiting Itching Urinary retention	Assess dermatomes for sensation and movement. Monitor renal and liver function. Ensure medication is preservative free.
Ropivacaine	Local anesthetic/analgesic; blocks generation and conduction of nerve impulses; used for postoperative pain management	Dosing varies based on location. Concentration of 0.2% (2-5 mg/mL) Lumbar/thoracic epidural for continuous infusion (12-28 mg/h)	Hypotension Bradycardia Paresthesia Pruritus Rigors	Assess dermatomes for sensation and movement. Monitor renal and liver function.
Treatment of Agitation Midazolam (Versed)	Benzodiazepine; depresses subcortical levels in the CNS; used to reduce anxiety and provide sedation	*Continuous infusion:* loading dose (IV bolus), 0.01-0.05 mg/kg (usually 1-5 mg) over 2-3 min, q10-15 min PRN *Maintenance dose:* 0.02-0.1 mg/kg/h by continuous infusion	CNS depression Hypotension Respiratory depression Paradoxical agitation	Use a valid sedation scale to monitor effect. Titrate infusion up or down by 25%-50% of the initial infusion rate to ensure adequate titration of sedation level and to prevent tolerance development. Use the lowest dose to achieve desired effect. Monitor BP and respiratory status. Administer fluids as indicated. Slowly wean medication after prolonged therapy (decrease by 10%-25% every few hours). Lower doses may be needed for patients >65 years. *Antidote:* Flumazenil.

Continued

TABLE 6.8 PHARMACOLOGY—cont'd

Medications Frequently Used in the Treatment of Pain, Agitation, Delirium, and Neuromuscular Blockade[a]

Medication	Action/Use	Dose/Route	Side Effects	Nursing Implications
Lorazepam (Ativan)	Benzodiazepine; potentiates the actions of GABA; used to reduce anxiety and provide sedation	**Critical Care Unit Agitation** *PO:* initially 2-3 mg/day given bid-tid; maximum dose 10 mg/day *IM:* 0.05 mg/kg; 4 mg maximum *IV, intermittent:* initial dose: 0.02-0.04 mg/kg; maximum dose 2 mg; maintenance dose: 0.02-0.06 mg/kg IV q2-6h; inject no faster than 2 mg/min *IV, continuous infusion:* 0.01-0.1 mg/kg/h IV to maintain desired level of sedation	Hypotension (less than midazolam) Respiratory depression Paradoxical agitation Hyperosmolar metabolic acidosis (IV prolonged infusion)	Administer lower doses in older adults. Monitor BP and respiratory status. Assess acid-base status with prolonged infusion. Avoid smaller veins to prevent thrombophlebitis. Higher than recommended doses infusions have been associated with tubular necrosis, lactic acidosis, and hyperosmolar states because of the polyethylene glycol and propylene glycol solvents.
Propofol (Diprivan)	Nonbenzodiazepine; depresses the CNS by activation of GABA receptor; used to reduce anxiety and provide sedation and anesthesia	*Initial IV infusion:* 5 mcg/kg/min for 5 min; increase dose in 5-10 mcg/kg/min increments over 5-10 min until sedation target achieved *Maintenance:* infusion rate of 5-50 mcg/kg/min (or higher) Administration should not exceed 4 mg/kg/h unless the benefits outweigh the risks	Hypotension Respiratory depression CNS depression Fever Sepsis Hyperlipidemia	Patient should be intubated and mechanically ventilated. Avoid rapid bolus administration to reduce respiratory depression. Monitor BP and hemodynamic status. Change infusion set q12h. Emulsion is preservative free and may support growth of microorganisms. Monitor plasma lipid levels.
Dexmedetomidine (Precedex)	Selective alpha$_2$-adrenoreceptor agonist; used to reduce anxiety and provide sedation	*IV, loading dose:* 1 mcg/kg over 10 min (must dilute) *IV, continuous infusion:* 0.2-0.7 mcg/kg/h	Bradycardia Hypotension Nausea	Give only by continuous infusion. Monitor heart rate. Evaluate hepatic and renal function.
Delirium Haloperidol (Haldol)	Neuroleptic; depresses cerebral cortex, hypothalamus, and limbic system; used to treat delirium and alcohol withdrawal	*PO:* 0.25-5 mg bid or tid; maximum 30 mg/day *IM:* 2-5 mg q1-8h PRN *IV, intermittent:* 0.03-0.15 mg/kg IV (2-10 mg) q30 min to 6h. Mild agitation: 0.5-2 mg. Moderate agitation: 5 mg. Severe agitation: 10 mg; may require dosing q30 min (maximum single dose, 40 mg) *IV, continuous infusion:* 3-25 mg/h by continuous infusion has been used for ventilator patients with agitation and delirium	Drowsiness Tachycardia Prolonged QT interval Extrapyramidal symptoms Euphoria/agitation, paradoxical agitation Neuroleptic malignant syndrome	Measure QT interval at start of therapy and periodically. Obtain 12-lead ECG. Monitor BP with initial treatment or adjustments in dose. Use with caution when patient is receiving other proarrhythmic agents. Administer anticholinergic for extrapyramidal symptoms.
Quetiapine (Seroquel)	Antagonist to multiple neurotransmitter receptors in the brain; used to treat agitation and acute psychosis (unlabeled uses), schizophrenia, bipolar affective disorder	*PO/NG:* 25 mg q8h or at bedtime; hold for oversedation (RASS −3 to −5) unless otherwise specified	Drowsiness Dizziness Increased risk of suicidal thoughts	Give at bedtime. This is not a home medication. Check potassium and magnesium levels. Monitor QT intervals.

TABLE 6.8 PHARMACOLOGY—cont'd

Medications Frequently Used in the Treatment of Pain, Agitation, Delirium, and Neuromuscular Blockade[a]

Medication	Action/Use	Dose/Route	Side Effects	Nursing Implications
Risperidone (Risperdal)	Action unknown; used to treat anxiety, schizophrenia, bipolar disorders; unlabeled use for acute psychosis and agitation	*PO/NG:* 2 mg/day as single dose or in divided doses. Increase dose to maximum 4-8 mg/day Recommended range for risperidone 0.5-2.0 mg q12h	Drowsiness Fast, pounding, or irregular heartbeat Upset stomach Blurred vision Fainting Dizziness Seizures	Often given at bedtime. Hold for oversedation (RASS −3 to −5) unless otherwise specified. This is not a home medication.
Therapeutic Paralysis Atracurium (Tracrium)	Neuromuscular blockade	*IV:* loading dose, 0.4-0.5 mg/kg *IV, continuous maintenance infusion:* 5-10 mcg/kg/min to a maximum of 17.5 mcg/kg/min	Hypotension Tachycardia Rash	Ensure adequate airway. Safer than other paralytic agents in patients with hepatic or renal failure. Conduct train-of-four assessment to monitor level of paralysis.
Succinylcholine	Neuromuscular blockade; short-term use	*IV:* loading dose, 0.3-1.1 mg/kg; maximum dose 150 mg	Hyperkalemia	Secure airway. Avoid in patients with elevated serum potassium.
Reversal Agent Naloxone	Opioid antagonist; treat opioid-induced respiratory depression and opioid overdose	*IV, IM, SC:* 0.4-2.0 mg; repeat q2-3 min to maximum of 10 mg *Nasal:* one spray q2-3 min	Seizures Opioid withdrawal Tachycardia, dysrhythmias Nausea/vomiting Pulmonary edema, dyspnea	Assess respiratory status. Anticipate withdrawal symptoms within 2h for those with dependence or addiction.

[a]All dosages are for adult patients; this table does not account for typical dose adjustments used with older adults or those undergoing alcohol withdrawal.

bid, Two times per day; *BP,* blood pressure; *CNS,* central nervous system; *ECG,* electrocardiogram; *GABA,* gamma-aminobutyric acid; *HP,* high potency; *IM,* intramuscular; *NG,* nasogastric; *PO,* by mouth; *PR,* per rectum; *PRN,* as needed; *q,* every; *RASS,* Richmond Agitation-Sedation Scale; *SC,* subcutaneous; *TD,* transdermal; *tid,* three times per day.

Data from CELEBREX (celecoxib) [package insert]. New York, NY: GD Searle LLC; 2016; Gahart BL, Nazareno AR, Ortega MQ. *Gahart's 2019 Intravenous Medications: A Handbook for Nurses and Health Professionals.* 32nd ed. St. Louis, MO: Elsevier, Inc.; 2019; Ketalar (ketamine hydrochloride) [package insert]. Lake Forest, IL: Hospira, Inc.; 2018; Lee EN, Lee JH. The effects of low dose ketamine on acute pain in emergency setting: A systematic review and meta-analysis. *PLoS One.* 2016;11(10):e0165461; LYRICA (pregabalin) [package insert]. New York, NY: Pfizer, Inc.; 2019; NAPROSYN(R) (naproxen) oral tablets [package insert]. Alpharetta, GA: Canton Laboratories, LLC; 2017; Naproxen oral suspension [package insert]. Naples, FL: Key Therapeutics, LLC; 2016; Schwenk ES, Viscusi ER, Buvanendran A, et al. Consensus guidelines on the use of intravenous ketamine infusions for acute pain management from the American Society of Regional Anesthesia and Pain Medicine, the American Academy of Pain Medicine, and the American Society of Anesthesiologists. *Reg Anesth Pain Med.* 2018;43(5):456–466; Skidmore-Roth L. *Mosby's 2019 Nursing Drug Reference.* 35th ed. St. Louis, MO: Elsevier; 2019.

Nefopam. *Nefopam* is a centrally acting nonopioid analgesic used as an alternative to opioids developed in the early 1970s. It was introduced as having morphine-sparing effects following surgery. Nefopam inhibits the reuptake of serotonin, norepinephrine, and dopamine, the three most important substances in the transmission of pain, and has supraspinal and spinal sites of action.[42] A single and slow infusion of nefopam is effective in critically ill patients who have moderate to severe pain. Administer cautiously to critically ill patients with hemodynamic instability. A 20-mL dose has an analgesic effect comparable to 6 mL of IV morphine. Although not available in the United States or Canada, nefopam is a low-cost medication that is available in nearly 30 countries. In cardiac surgery patients, nefopam's analgesic effect resembles IV fentanyl with less nausea when delivered as patient-controlled analgesia.[46]

Ketamine. Ketamine is classified as an anesthetic agent but at subanesthetic dose is used for pain management. Low-dose ketamine (1 to 2 mL/kg/h) as an adjunct to opioid therapy controls moderate to severe pain and reduces the risk of sedation or respiratory depression compared to opioids and other CNS depressants. It has a wide safety margin with minimal cardiopulmonary depression and can concomitantly be administered with opioids and other pain medications. Patients might appear awake with preserved airway reflexes and respiratory drive, but they are unable to respond to sensory input.[58]

Neuropathic Medications. The PADIS guidelines also recommend using neuropathic pain medication (e.g., gabapentin,

TABLE 6.9 Pain, Agitation, and Delirium Order Set

Sedation Orders: Ventilated Patient in Critical Care Unit
- Assess level of sedation q4h
- Target RASS Score _____
- SAT protocol twice daily, or as directed by provider
- SBT safety screen twice daily, or as directed by provider

Pain Management
- Pain assessment clinically or by scale
- Rule out and correct reversible causes
- Opioids are the agents of choice for treatment of nonneuropathic pain
- Medications
  - Fentanyl
  - Morphine
  - Hydromorphone

Agitation Management
- Agitation assessment by RASS
- Minimize benzodiazepine usage
- Nonbenzodiazepine agents (propofol, dexmedetomidine) are preferred
- Medications
  - Midazolam
  - Lorazepam
  - Propofol
  - Dexmedetomidine

Delirium Management
- Nonpharmacological therapy
  - Mobility protocol
  - Maximize sleep-wake conditions (sleep protocol)
  - Minimize benzodiazepine use
  - Eyeglasses and hearing aids
  - Encourage family participation in patient orientation
- PT evaluation and treatment
- OT evaluation and treatment
- Medications
  - Haloperidol
  - Quetiapine
  - Risperidone

Diagnostic Tests
- In patients prescribed antipsychotics for delirium control, 12-lead ECG at baseline to assess QT-interval.

ECG, Electrocardiogram; *OT,* occupational therapy; *PT,* physical therapy; *RASS,* Richmond Agitation-Sedation Scale; *SAT,* spontaneous awakening trial; *SBT,* spontaneous breathing trial.

BOX 6.6 Definitions of Opioid-Naive and Opioid-Tolerant

Opioid-naive—patients who have received opiates for less than 1 week, are not chronically receiving opioid analgesics on a daily basis, and have not received opioid doses at least as much as those listed below for 1 week or longer

Opioid-tolerant—patients who have received at least the following for 1 week or longer:
- 60 mg oral morphine/day
- 25 mcg transdermal fentanyl/hour
- 30 mg oral oxycodone/day
- 8 mg oral hydromorphone/day
- 25 mg oral oxymorphone/day
- An equianalgesic dose of another opioid

insufficiency is higher in patients with hypovolemia or renal hypoperfusion, in older adults, and in patients with preexisting renal impairment. Do not administer NSAIDs to patients with asthma and aspirin sensitivity.

NSAIDs are available in oral, liquid, and IV forms (i.e., aspirin, ibuprofen, and ketorolac). An IV preparation of ibuprofen (Caldolor) is available to treat mild to moderate pain, providing more options for the critically ill patient.[67] IV administration may reduce opioid requirements. NSAIDs are active ingredients in many other preparations; therefore it is important to ensure that the maximum daily dosage is not exceeded. When these medications are given, patients are at an increased risk for renal damage (ibuprofen). Laboratory results must be used to guide therapy and monitor effects of treatment. Results will also assist in determining the most appropriate NSAID for the patient. Collaboration with the clinical pharmacist is essential.

Patient-Controlled Analgesia. Patient-controlled analgesia (PCA) is a medication delivery system in which the patient is able to control when medication is given. PCA involves a special type of infusion pump (Fig. 6.4) that has a "locked" supply of opioid medication. When the patient feels pain or just before any pain-inducing therapy, the patient can depress a button on the pump that delivers a prescribed bolus of medication. Opioids delivered by PCA pump result in stable drug concentrations, good quality of analgesia, less sedation, less opioid consumption, and potentially fewer side effects. PCA is a safe and effective method of pain management.[65]

PCA is rarely appropriate for critically ill patients because most are unable to depress the button, or they are too ill to manage their pain effectively. However, some patients may benefit from PCA therapy to manage postoperative incisional pain.[65] Typical patient criteria for PCA therapy are listed in Box 6.7.

Elastomeric Infusion Pump. An elastomeric infusion pump catheter is indicated for the delivery of medication (such as local anesthetics like 0.2% ropivacaine) to or around surgical wound sites for preoperative, perioperative, and postoperative

carbamazepine, pregabalin) with opioids for neuropathic pain management in critically ill adults, Guillain-Barré syndrome, or recent cardiac surgery patients. These medications reduce opioid consumption within 24 hours of their initiation, are readily available, but require patients to swallow or have an enteral feeding tube.[22]

Nonsteroidal Antiinflammatory Drugs. NSAIDs provide analgesia by inhibiting cyclooxygenase, a critical enzyme in the inflammatory cascade. NSAIDs have the potential to cause significant adverse effects, including gastrointestinal bleeding, bleeding secondary to platelet inhibition, and renal insufficiency. The risk of developing NSAID-induced renal

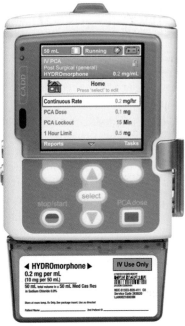

Fig. 6.4 A patient-controlled analgesia infusion pump. (Courtesy Smiths Medical ASD, Inc., St. Paul, MN.)

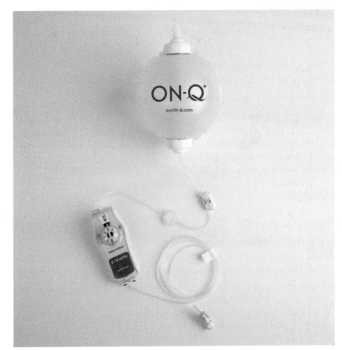

Fig. 6.5 ON-Q pain pump. (Courtesy Avanos, Irvine, CA.)

BOX 6.7 Criteria for Patient-Controlled Analgesia Therapy

- An elective surgical procedure
- Large surgical wounds likely to result in pain (e.g., thoracotomy incisions)
- Large traumatic wounds
- Normal cognitive function
- Normal motor skills (able to depress the medication delivery button)

---

pain management. The ON-Q pain pump (I-Flow Corporation, Lake Forest, CA) is an elastomeric infusion pump that delivers medication at a flow rate determined by the pressure in the elastomeric reservoir, the flow restriction in the infusion circuit, and the viscosity of the fluid (Fig. 6.5). These elastomeric devices are currently used in the extrathoracic, paraspinous space to create a continuous intercostal nerve block. ON-Q has been used on adult patients with blunt trauma and three or more unilateral rib fractures and has shown significantly improved pulmonary function, pain control, and shortened length of stay in patients with rib fractures.

Epidural Analgesia. Opioids, dilute local anesthetic agents, or both can also be delivered through a catheter placed in the epidural, intrathecal caudal space or via nerve blockade to interrupt the transmission of pain. The discovery of opioid receptors in the spinal cord is considered a major breakthrough in the management of pain associated with traumatic injury of the chest and abdomen. Patients with such injuries do not want to cough, breathe deeply, ambulate, or participate in pulmonary exercises because these activities are too painful. Eventually, atelectasis, hypoxemia, respiratory failure, and pneumonia result. Epidural analgesia provides great relief for patients with multiple rib fractures and improves pulmonary function.[48]

The administration of epidural agents has many benefits in addition to pain relief (Table 6.10). Some of the most commonly used epidural local anesthetics are bupivacaine, levobupivacaine, and ropivacaine.

Patients receiving epidural analgesia are carefully assessed to determine the appropriateness of spinal analgesia. Contraindications include coagulopathies, cardiovascular instability, sepsis, spine injury, infection or injury to the skin at the proposed insertion site, patient refusal, inability to lie still during catheter insertion, and alcohol or drug intoxication. In addition, it is

TABLE 6.10 Potential Benefits of Epidural Analgesia

System	Response
Pulmonary	↑ Vital capacity ↑ Functional residual capacity Improved airway resistance
Cardiac	Coronary artery vasodilation ↓ Blood pressure, heart rate
Gastrointestinal	Less nausea and vomiting Faster return of gastrointestinal function
Neurological	↓ Total opioid requirement ↓ Sedation
Activity	Earlier extubation Earlier mobilization ↓ Length of stay

difficult to place an epidural catheter in patients who are obese or have compression fractures of the lumbar spine. Because of issues associated with spinal analgesia, research is being conducted to assess outcomes of caudal epidural analgesia or paravertebral blockade as an alternative to spinal epidural analgesia.

Potential side effects of spinal analgesia with opioids include respiratory depression, sedation, nausea and vomiting, and urinary retention. Potential side effects of spinal analgesia with local anesthetics include sympathetic blockade (hypotension, venous pooling), motor weakness, sensory block, and urinary retention.

Sedative Agents. Anxiety in the critical care setting is treated with benzodiazepines, propofol, or dexmedetomidine. Both pain and anxiety may exist with evidence of psychotic features (as manifested in delirium). In this situation, neuroleptic agents, antidepressants, and anesthetic agents are administered.

Benzodiazepines are sedatives and hypnotics that block new information and potentially unpleasant experiences at that moment. Although they are not considered analgesics, they do moderate the anticipatory pain response. Benzodiazepines vary in their potency, onset and duration of action, distribution, and metabolism. The patient's age, prior alcohol abuse, concurrent medication therapy, and current medical condition affect the intensity and duration of medication activity. Older adult patients and patients with renal or hepatic insufficiency may exhibit slower clearance of benzodiazepines, which may contribute to a significant delay in elimination.

Titrate benzodiazepines to a predefined end point—for example, a specific level of sedation using either the RASS or SAS. Sedation may be maintained with intermittent doses of lorazepam, diazepam, or midazolam; however, patients requiring frequent doses to maintain the desired effect may benefit from a continuous infusion by using the lowest effective dose. Monitor patients receiving continuous infusions for oversedation.

Propofol is a preferred sedative over benzodiazepines to improve clinical outcomes in mechanically ventilated patients.[22] Propofol is an IV general anesthetic; however, sedative and hypnotic effects are achieved at lower doses. Propofol has no analgesic properties. It has a rapid onset and short duration of sedation once it is discontinued. Adverse effects include hypotension, bradycardia, and pain when the medication is infused through a peripheral IV site. Propofol is available as an emulsion in a phospholipid substance, which provides 1.1 kcal/mL from fat, and it should be counted as a caloric source. Long-term or high-dose infusions may result in high triglyceride levels, metabolic acidosis, or dysrhythmias; therefore monitor triglyceride levels after 2 days of infusion. Propofol requires a dedicated IV catheter for continuous infusion because of the risk of incompatibility and infection. The infusion should not hang for more than 12 hours.

Dexmedetomidine is also preferred over benzodiazepines for mechanically ventilated patients. Dexmedetomidine is a potent anesthetic agent with selective alpha-2 agonist properties that is approved for short-term use (less than 24 hours) as a sedative in patients receiving mechanical ventilation.[14] It is recommended not to exceed 24 hours of use; however, its use has widened over the past few years.[75]

Dexmedetomidine has mild analgesic properties, reduces concurrent analgesic and sedative requirements, and produces anxiolytic effects comparable to those of the benzodiazepines. Transient elevations in blood pressure may be seen with rapid administration. Bradycardia and hypotension may develop, especially in the presence of hypovolemia, in patients with severe ventricular dysfunction, and in older adults. Evidence shows that dexmedetomidine reduces duration of mechanical ventilation by 1.85 days and length of stay in the critical care unit by 1.26 days[18] and significantly decreases postoperative delirium.[70] Overall, administration of dexmedetomidine or propofol, rather than a benzodiazepine regimen, in critically ill adults has shown to reduce critical care unit length of stay and duration of mechanical ventilation.

Neuromuscular Blockade. Neuromuscular blockade (NMB) agents, historically used in the operating room, are used in critically ill patients to facilitate endotracheal intubation and mechanical ventilation, to control increases in ICP, and to facilitate procedures at the bedside (e.g., bronchoscopy, tracheostomy). The goal of NMB is complete chemical paralysis.

During a difficult endotracheal intubation, the use of a rapidly acting NMB agent (rapid-sequence intubation) allows the airway to be secured quickly and without trauma. Following intubation, some patients are unable to tolerate mechanical ventilation despite adequate sedation, especially nontraditional modes such as inverse ratio and pressure control.[19] Long-acting NMB agents may improve chest wall compliance, reduce peak airway pressures, and prevent the patient from ventilator dyssynchrony.[74] The result is improved gas exchange with increased oxygen delivery and decreased oxygen consumption. In patients with elevated ICP, suctioning, coughing, and agitation can provoke dangerous elevations in ICP. NMB agents diminish ICP elevations during these activities. In some patients, complete immobility may be required for a short period for minor surgical and diagnostic procedures performed at the bedside.

NMB agents do not possess any sedative or analgesic properties. Any patient who receives effective NMB is not able to communicate nor to produce any voluntary muscle movement, including breathing. Therefore ensure that any patient receiving these agents receives sedation. Healthcare staff at many institutions start continuous infusions of sedative medications before they administer an NMB agent.

If the patient is receiving NMB therapy, closely monitor for respiratory problems, skin breakdown, corneal abrasions, and the development of venous thrombi. Assess for nonverbal cues of pain and anxiety, such as an increase in heart rate or blood pressure. Nursing care for patients receiving NMB therapy is presented in Box 6.8.

Assess the level or degree of paralysis by using a peripheral nerve stimulator to determine a train-of-four (TOF) response. The TOF procedure evaluates the level of NMB to ensure that the greatest amount of NMB is achieved with the lowest dose of

BOX 6.8 Nursing Care of the Patient Receiving Neuromuscular Blockade

- Perform train-of-four testing before initiation, 15 minutes after dosage change, then every 4 hours, to monitor the degree of paralysis
- Ensure appropriate sedation
- Lubricate eyes to prevent corneal abrasions
- Ensure prophylaxis for deep vein thrombosis
- Reposition the patient every 2 hours as tolerated
- Monitor skin integrity
- Provide oral hygiene
- Maintain mechanical ventilation
- Monitor breath sounds; suction airway as needed
- Provide passive range of motion
- Monitor heart rate, respiratory rate, blood pressure, and oxygen saturation
- Place indwelling urinary catheter to monitor urine output
- Monitor bowel sounds; monitor for abdominal distention

NMB medication. The ulnar nerve and the facial nerve are the most frequently used sites for peripheral nerve stimulation. The peripheral nerve stimulator delivers four low-energy impulses, and the number of muscular twitches is assessed. Four twitches of the thumb or facial muscle indicate incomplete NMB. The absence of twitches indicates complete NMB. The TOF goal is two out of four twitches. An example of a peripheral nerve stimulator is shown in Fig. 6.6.

No tools or devices can adequately assess pain and sedation in patients receiving NMB agents. The patient is monitored for physiological changes (see Box 6.2), and if changes occur, the nurse must determine whether pain or anxiety is the potential cause. The BIS or PSI system may assist in monitoring in these patients.

Several NMB agents are available; those most frequently used are outlined in Table 6.8. Succinylcholine (paralytic), when administered with etomidate (sedative), is frequently used for rapid-sequence intubation because of its short half-life. However, do not administer succinylcholine in the presence of hyperkalemia because ventricular dysrhythmias and cardiac arrest may occur. Pancuronium is a long-acting NMB agent. When it is given in bolus doses, tachycardia and hypertension may result. The effects of pancuronium are prolonged in patients with liver disease and renal failure. Newer NMB agents such as atracurium and cisatracurium are used in critically ill patients because they are associated with fewer side effects and can be used safely in patients with liver or renal failure. Short-term infusion of cisatracurium reduces hospital mortality and barotrauma and minimizes neuromuscular weakness for critically ill adults with acute respiratory distress syndrome (ARDS) who are receiving mechanical ventilation.[51]

Tolerance and Withdrawal. Patients who require high-dose opioid or sedative therapy to maintain sedation may develop physiological dependence and tolerance to the medication. Collaborate with the clinical pharmacist and physician to develop a plan for tapering the medications slowly and systematically and consider other medications. Stopping these medications abruptly may lead to withdrawal symptoms. Opioid withdrawal symptoms include pupillary dilation, sweating, rhinorrhea, tachycardia, hypertension, tachypnea, vomiting, diarrhea, increased sensitivity to pain, restlessness, and anxiety. Signs of benzodiazepine withdrawal include tremor, headache, nausea, sweating, fatigue, anxiety, agitation, increased sensitivity to light and sound, muscle cramps, sleep disturbances, and seizures.

MANAGEMENT CHALLENGES

Invasive Procedures

Many invasive procedures, including nasogastric tube insertion; tracheal suctioning; central venous catheter insertion; chest tube insertion; wound care; and removal of tubes, lines, and sheaths take place in the critical care unit. All of these invasive procedures have the likelihood of inducing pain or anxiety. If pain or anxiety occurs during a procedure, the length and difficulty of the procedure may be increased, inaccurate data may be obtained, and physical harm can result.[22] To avoid negative outcomes, assess and manage the patient's comfort and anxiety before, during, and after such procedures. Many times, the patient is kept in a conscious state during the procedure to avoid the risk of complications such as respiratory depression and hypotension. Therefore sedative or analgesic agents, or both, are given in a way that the patient appears sedate yet is able to verbalize. This type of sedation has been referred to as procedural sedation or conscious sedation.

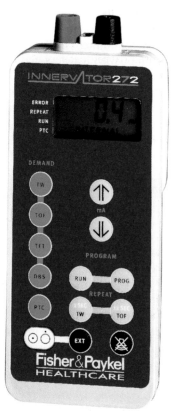

Fig. 6.6 A train-of-four peripheral nerve stimulator. (Courtesy Fisher and Paykel Healthcare, Auckland, New Zealand.)

Typical nursing care during these procedures involves monitoring vital signs including pulse oximetry, ensuring a patent airway, and observing for the adverse effects of medications. With the advent of the electronic medical record, customized pain assessment forms can be developed to improve clinical efficiency and documentation.

Substance Abuse

Critically ill patients who have a history of substance abuse or drug use disorders pose special challenges. Drug use disorder combined with alcohol has been associated with increased need for mechanical ventilation and a longer critical care stay.[63] A history of alcoholism alone also increases development of septic shock, critical care unit mortality, and hospital mortality.[49] Over the years, there has been a substantial increase in opioid-associated overdose and mortality rate in critical care units.[69] The pharmacological management of critically ill patients typically involves the administration of sedative and hypnotic medications. Patients with a history of alcoholism and substance abuse often have a higher-than-normal dosage threshold to achieve therapeutic actions with many analgesics, sedatives, and hypnotic medications.

Assess all patients with a history of alcohol use for symptoms of alcohol withdrawal syndrome (AWS), particularly in the first 24 to 48 hours. AWS usually presents within 72 to 96 hours after the patient's last alcohol intake. The initial symptoms, such as disorientation, agitation, tachycardia, and delirium tremens (shaking of the extremities or digits), may be mild. If untreated, symptoms can progress to severe confusion, paranoid-like behavior, seizures, convulsions, and even death. AWS assessment tools, such as the Clinical Institute Withdrawal Assessment for Alcohol, Revised (CIWA-Ar), are available.[4] The CIWA-Ar is used to determine the severity of the withdrawal symptoms as they are actively experienced but does not predict which patients are at risk for withdrawal. This tool relies on patient communication for information on nausea and vomiting, anxiety, tactile and auditory disturbances, and headache. Therefore in mechanically ventilated patients who are noncommunicative, this tool may not be applicable. Assess agitation symptoms using RASS or SAS, and whenever feasible with CIWA-Ar, to match medication dosing and symptom severity and improve outcomes. The most important treatment of AWS is prevention, which has been shown to improve morbidity and mortality and decrease hospital and critical care unit lengths of stay. Fluid resuscitation; correction of electrolyte deficiencies; and parenteral administration of thiamine, multivitamin, and folate are usually performed daily to alleviate AWS symptoms, prevent symptom progression, and treat underlying comorbidities. Benzodiazepines and/or dexmedetomidine and ethanol infusion have shown to reduce the duration and severity of AWS.[23]

Lifespan Considerations

Evaluate lifespan issues when managing pain and anxiety. Older adult patients often have a high prevalence of pain, and they might experience many painful conditions (neoplasms, injuries and other external causes, and diseases of the musculoskeletal and connective tissues systems). Patients older than 65 years of age pose special concerns because of their physiological characteristics, many comorbid conditions, use of multiple medications, physical frailty, and cognitive and sensory deficits. Older adults are also more vulnerable to alcohol abuse and substance abuse, and they may be more vulnerable to toxicity from analgesics. Older adults often have decreased renal function with a reduced creatinine clearance rate, resulting in a longer elimination half-life of analgesic medications.

Some older adult patients believe that pain is a normal process of aging and is something they must learn to accept as normal. Older adults often believe that if they complain of pain, nursing staff will label them as "problem" patients. Finally, older adults may comment to their family and friends that the nurse is too busy to listen to their complaints, and they do not want to be a "bother."

Treatment of pain and anxiety in pregnant women requires consultation with the clinical pharmacist to consider both the mother and baby. Refer to the Lifespan Considerations box for additional strategies related to management of pain and anxiety.

LIFESPAN CONSIDERATIONS

Older Adults

- Speak slowly and clearly when evaluating pain and anxiety.
- Verify any underlying cognitive deficits (e.g., dementia, Alzheimer's disease, cerebrovascular accident).
- Ensure that scales or other assessment tools have a large font.
- Stoic behavior may be the patient's normal baseline; therefore assess for nonverbal cues to pain (facial grimace or withdrawal).
- Observe for changes in behavior, such as confusion or agitation. Older adult patients are at risk of developing delirium.
- Older adult patients may be resistant to taking additional medications; therefore offer nonpharmacological strategies to manage anxiety or pain.
- Older adult patients may not ask for as-needed medications in a timely fashion. Collaborate with the clinical pharmacist to identify the need for routine scheduling of medications.
- Assess renal and liver function and collaborate with clinical pharmacist and physician to adjust medication dosages.
- Assess for paradoxical effects of medications in older adults; for example, benzodiazepines often cause agitation.

Pregnant Women

- Collaborate with the clinical pharmacist regarding the safety of medications for managing sedation and anxiety in pregnant women and to identify benefits versus risks.
- If opioids are administered during pregnancy, the infant must be assessed and monitored for neonatal abstinence syndrome. Collaborate with the obstetrician and neonatologist.

CASE STUDY

Mr. B. is a 52-year-old man in the surgical critical care unit after liver transplantation on the previous day. He has a 15-year history of hepatic cirrhosis secondary to alcohol abuse. He is intubated and is receiving multiple vasopressor medications for hypotension. At 6:30 AM he follows simple commands and denies pain or anxiety with simple head nods. At 7:00 AM Mr. B. is kicking his legs and places his arms outside the side rails. Attempts by the nurse to reorient him result in his pulling at his endotracheal tube. His wrists are restrained with soft restraints. At this time, he does not follow any simple commands. He continually shakes his head back and forth. Facial grimacing is noted, and he is biting down on the endotracheal tube, which is causing the ventilator to sound the high-pressure alarm. His blood pressure is 185/110 mm Hg, with a mean arterial pressure of 135 mm Hg. The monitor displays sinus tachycardia at a rate of 140 beats/min. Medication infusions include epinephrine (3 mcg/min), norepinephrine (15 mcg/min), dopamine (2 mcg/kg/min), and fentanyl (100 mcg/h). His only other medications are his immunosuppressive medication regimen.

Questions

1. Score Mr. B.'s pain, agitation/sedation, and delirium using the following objective tools:

Tool	Score
Behavioral Pain Scale (BPS)	
Critical-Care Pain Observation Tool (CPOT)	
Richmond Agitation-Sedation Scale (RASS)	
Sedation-Agitation Scale (SAS)	
Confusion Assessment Method for the Intensive Care Unit (CAM-ICU)	

2. Would complementary or alternative medicine therapies be appropriate at this time? If not, what therapies would be appropriate?
3. What type of medication is Mr. B. receiving for pain?
4. Is this an appropriate dose of pain medication for Mr. B.?
5. What other medications could be given to manage his agitated state?

REFERENCES

1. Ali B, Al-Wabel A, Shams S, et al. Essential oils used in aromatherapy: A systemic review. *Asian Pac J Trop Biomed*. 2015;5(8):601–611.
2. Allard ME, Katseres J. Using essential oils to enhance nursing practice and for self-care. *Am J Nurs*. 2016;116(2):42–49.
3. Almeida TM, Azevedo LC, Nosé PM, et al. Risk factors for agitation in critically ill patients. *Rev Bras Ter Intensiva*. 2016;28(4):413–419.
4. Bakhla AK, Khess CR, Verma V, et al. Factor structure of CIWA-Ar in alcohol withdrawal. *J Addict*. 2014;1–7.
5. Balas MC, Weinhouse GL, Denehy L, et al. Interpreting and implementing the 2018 pain, agitation/sedation, delirium, immobility, and sleep disruption clinical practice guidelines. *Crit Care Med*. 2018;46(9):1464–1470.
6. Bamikole PO, Theriault BM, Caldwell SL, Schlesinger JJ. Patient-directed music therapy in the ICU. *Crit Care Med*. 2018;46(11): e1085.
7. Baumgarten M, Poulsen I. Patients' experiences of being mechanically ventilated in an ICU: A qualitative metasynthesis. *Scand J Caring Sci*. 2015;29(2):205–214.
8. Bergeron N, Dubois MJ, Dumont M, et al. Intensive Care Delirium Screening Checklist: Evaluation of a new screening tool. *Intensive Care Med*. 2001;27:859–864.
9. Bienvenu OJ, Colantuoni E, Mendez-Tellez PA, et al. Cooccurrence of and remission from general anxiety, depression, and posttraumatic stress disorder symptoms after acute lung injury: A 2-year longitudinal study. *Crit Care Med*. 2015;43(3):642–653.
10. Binks AP, Desjardin S, Riker R. ICU clinicians underestimate breathing discomfort in ventilated subjects. *Respir Care*. 2017;62(2):150–155.
11. Campbell M. Dyspnea. *Crit Care Nurs Clin North Am*. 2017;29(4):461–470.
12. Canet E, Amjad S, Robbins R, et al. Differential clinical characteristics, management, and outcome of delirium among ward compared with ICU patients. *Intern Med J*. 2019.
13. Chanques G, Payen JF, Mercier G, et al. Assessing pain in nonintubated critically ill patients unable to self report: An adaptation of the Behavioral Pain Scale. *Intensive Care Med*. 2009;35: 2060–2067.
14. Chen K, Lu Z, Xin YC, et al. Alpha-2 agonists for long-term sedation during mechanical ventilation in critically ill patients. *Cochrane Database Syst Rev*. 2015;6(1):1–94.
15. Chlan LL, Heidenscheit A, Skaar DJ, Neidecker MV. Economic evaluation of a patient-directed music intervention for ICU patients receiving mechanical ventilatory support. *Crit Care Med*. 2018;46(9):1430–1435.
16. Cho MY, Min ES, Hur MH. Effects of aromatherapy on the anxiety, vital signs, and sleep quality of percutaneous coronary intervention patients in intensive care units. *Evid Based Complement Alternat Med*. 2013;1–6.
17. Coleman RM, Tousignant-Laflamme Y, Ouellet P, et al. The use of the bispectral index in the detection of pain in mechanically ventilated adults in the intensive care unit: A review of the literature. *Pain Res Manag*. 2015;20(1):e33–e37.
18. Cruickshank M, Henderson L, MacLennan G, et al. Alpha-2 agonists for sedation of mechanically ventilated adults in intensive care units: A systematic review. *Health Technol Assess*. 2016;20(25):v–xx, 1–117.
19. deBacker J, Hart N, Fan E. Neuromuscular blockade in the 21st century management of the critically ill patient. *Chest*. 2017;151(3):697–706.
20. de Jager TAJ, Dulfer K, Radhoe S, et al. Predictive value of depression and anxiety for long-term mortality: Differences in outcome between acute coronary syndrome and stable angina pectoris. *Int J Cardiol*. 2018;1(250):43–48.
21. Demoule A, Similowski T. Respiratory suffering in the ICU: Time for our next great cause. *Am J Respir Crit Care Med*. 2019;199(11):1302–1304.
22. Devlin JW, Skrobik Y, Gelinas C, et al. Clinical practice guidelines for the prevention and management of pain, agitation/sedation, delirium, immobility, and sleep disruption in adult patients in the ICU. *Crit Care Med*. 2018;46:e825–e873.
23. Dixit D, Endicott J, Burry L, et al. Management of acute alcohol withdrawal syndrome in critically ill patients. *Pharmacotherapy*. 2016;36(7):797–822.
24. Ely EW, Margolin R, Francis J, et al. Evaluation of delirium in critically ill patients: Validation of the Confusion Assessment Method for the Intensive Care Unit (CAM-ICU). *Crit Care Med*. 2001;29(7):1370–1379.

25. Fink RM, Makic MB, Poteet AW, Oman KS. The ventilated patient's experience. *Dimens Crit Care Nurs.* 2015;34(5):301–308.

26. Fish J, Baxa J, Willenborg M, et al. Five-year outcomes after implementing a pain, agitation, and delirium guideline in a mixed ICU. *Crit Care Med.* 2019;47(1):18.

27. Forward JB, Greuter NE, Crisall SJ, Lester HF. Effect of structured touch and guided imagery for pain and anxiety in elective joint replacement patients—A randomized controlled trial: M-TIJRP. *Perm J.* 2015;19(4):18–28.

28. Fraser GL, Riker RR. Bispectral index monitoring in the intensive care unit provides more signal than noise. *Pharmacotherapy.* 2005;25:19S–27S.

29. Gelinas C, Fillion L, Puntillo KA, et al. Validation of the Critical-Care Pain Observation Tool in adult patients. *Am J Crit Care.* 2006;15:420–427.

30. Gelinas C. Pain assessment in the critically ill adult: Recent evidence and new trends. *Intensive Crit Care Nurs.* 2016;34:1–11.

31. Golino AJ, Leone R, Gollenberg A, et al. Impact of an active music therapy intervention on intensive care patients. *Am J Crit Care.* 2019;28(1):48–55.

32. Gullick JG, Kwan XX. Patient-directed music therapy reduces anxiety and sedation exposure in mechanically-ventilated patients: A research critique. *Aust Crit Care.* 2015;28(2):103–105.

33. Guyton A, Hall J. *Textbook of Medical Physiology.* 13th ed. Philadelphia, PA: Saunders; 2016.

34. Hadjibalassi M, Lambrinou E, Papastavrou E, Papathanassoglou E. The effect of guided imagery on physiological and psychological outcomes of adult ICU patients: A systematic literature review and methodological implications. *Aust Crit Care.* 2018;31(2):73–86.

35. Hamlin AS, Robertson TM. Pain and complementary therapies. *Crit Care Nurs Clin North Am.* 2017;29(4):449–460.

36. Haugdahl HS, Storli SL, Meland B, et al. Underestimation of patient breathlessness by nurses and physicians during a spontaneous breathing trial. *Am J Respir Crit Care Med.* 2015;192(12):1440–1448.

37. Herling SF, Greve IE, Vasilevskis EE, et al. Interventions for preventing intensive care unit delirium in adults. *Cochrane Database Syst Rev.* 2018;23:11.

38. Hosey MM, Jaskulski J, Wegener ST, et al. Animal-assisted intervention in the ICU: A tool for humanization. *Crit Care.* 2018;22(1):22.

39. Huether SE. Pain, temperature regulation, sleep, and sensory function. In: McCance KL, Huether SE, eds. *Pathophysiology: The Biologic Basis for Disease in Adults and Children.* 8th ed. St. Louis, MO: Mosby; 2019: 468–503.

40. International Association for the Study of Pain (IASP). Part III. Pain Terms, a Current List With Definitions and Notes on Usage. https://www.iasp-pain.org/terminology?navItemNumber=576#Pain. Updated December 14, 2017. Accessed June 18, 2019.

41. Jackson P, Khan A. Delirium in critically ill patients. *Crit Care Clin.* 2015;31(3):589–603.

42. Jin HS, Kim YC, Yoo Y, et al. Opioid sparing effect and safety of nefopam in patient controlled analgesia after laparotomy: A randomized, double blind study. *J Int Med Res.* 2016;44(4):844–854.

43. Jopke K, Sanders H, White-Traut R. Use of essential oils following traumatic burn injury: A case study. *J Pediatr Nurs.* 2017;34:72–77.

44. Kaplan JB, Eifermanb DS, Porter K, MacDermott J, et al. Impact of a nursing-driven sedation protocol with criteria for infusion initiation in the surgical intensive care unit. *J Crit Care.* 2019;50:195–200.

45. Karamchandani K, Rewari V, Trikha A, et al. Bispectral index correlates well with Richmond agitation sedation scale in mechanically ventilated critically ill patients. *J Anesthes.* 2010;24:394–398.

46. Kim K, Kim WJ, Choi DK, et al. The analgesic efficacy and safety of nefopam in patient-controlled analgesia after cardiac surgery: A randomized, double-blind, prospective study. *J Int Med Res.* 2014;42(3):684–692.

47. Lukaszewicz AC, Dereu D, Gayat E, Payen D. The relevance of pupillometry for evaluation of analgesia before noxious procedures in the intensive care unit. *Anesth Analg.* 2015;120(6):1297–1300.

48. Lynch N, Salottolo K, Foster K, et al. Comparative effectiveness analysis of two regional analgesia techniques for the pain management of isolated multiple rib fractures. *J Pain Res.* 2019;24(12):1701–1708.

49. McPeake JM, Shaw M, O'Neill A, et al. Do alcohol use disorders impact on long term outcomes from intensive care? *Crit Care.* 2015;19:185.

50. Mofredj A, Alaya S, Tassaioust K, et al. Music therapy: A review of the potential therapeutic benefits for the critically ill. *J Crit Care.* 2016;35:195–199.

51. National Heart, Lung, and Blood Institute PETAL Clinical Trials Network, Moss M, Huang DT, Brower RG, et al. Early neuromuscular blockade in the acute respiratory distress syndrome. *N Engl J Med.* 2019;380(21):1997–2008.

52. Neice AE, Behrends M, Bokoch MP, et al. Prediction of opioid analgesic efficacy by measurement of pupillary unrest. *Anesth Analg.* 2017;124(3):915–921.

53. Parker AM, Sricharoenchai T, Raparla S. Posttraumatic stress disorder in critical illness survivors: A metaanalysis. *Crit Care Med.* 2015;43(5):1121–1129.

54. Park S, Na SH, Oh J, et al. Pain and anxiety and their relationship with medication doses in the intensive care unit. *J Crit Care.* 2018;47:65–69.

55. Payen JF, Bru O, Bosson JL, et al. Assessing pain in critically ill sedated patients by using a behavioral pain scale. *Crit Care Med.* 2001;29:2258–2263.

56. Pérez-Camargo G, Creagan ET. The design of visitation facilities to engage patients with their own cats and dogs. *Complement Ther Clin Pract.* 2018;31:193–199.

57. Prottengeier J, Moritz A, Heinrich S, et al. Sedation assessment in a mobile intensive care unit: A prospective pilot-study on the relation of clinical sedation scales and the bispectral index. *Crit Care.* 2014;18(6):615.

58. Pruskowski KA, Harbourt K, Pajoumand M, et al. Impact of ketamine use on adjunctive analgesic and sedative medications in critically ill trauma patients. *Pharmacotherapy.* 2017;37(12):1537–1544.

59. Rasheed AM, Amirah MF, Abdallah M, et al. Ramsay Sedation Scale and Richmond Agitation Sedation Scale: A cross-sectional study. *Dimens Crit Care Nurs.* 2019;38(2):90–95.

60. Rijkenberg S, Stilma W, Bosman RJ, et al. Pain measurement in mechanically ventilated patients after cardiac surgery: Comparison of the Behavioral Pain Scale (BPS) and the Critical-Care Pain Observation Tool (CPOT). *J Cardiothorac Vasc Anesth.* 2017;31(4):1227–1234.

61. Riker RR, Fraser GL, Simmons LE, et al. Validating the Sedation-Agitation Scale with the bispectral index and Visual Analog Scale in adult ICU patients after cardiac surgery. *Intensive Care Med.* 2001;27:853–858.

62. Roberts M, Bortolotto SJ, Weyant RA, et al. The experience of acute mechanical ventilation from the patient's perspective. *Dimens Crit Care Nurs.* 2019;38(4):201–212.

63. Secombe PJ, Stewart PC. The impact of alcohol-related admissions on resource use in critically ill patients from 2009 to 2015: An observational study. *Anaesth Intensive Care.* 2018;46(1): 58–66.

64. Sessler CN, Gosnell MS, Grap MJ, et al. The Richmond Agitation-Sedation Scale: Validity and reliability in adult intensive care unit patients. *Am J Respir Crit Care Med.* 2002;166:1338–1344.

65. Sinatra RS, Viscusi ER, Ding L, et al. Meta-analysis of the efficacy of the fentanyl iontophoretic transdermal system versus intravenous patient-controlled analgesia in postoperative pain management. *Expert Opin Pharmacother.* 2015;16(11):1607–1613.

66. Society of Critical Care Medicine. ICU Patient Communicator Application. https://www.sccm.org/MyICUCare/THRIVE/Patient-and-Family-Resources/Patient-and-Family. Accessed May 19, 2019.

67. Southworth SR, Woodward EJ, Peng A, Rock AD. An integrated safety analysis of intravenous ibuprofen (Caldolor®) in adults. *J Pain Res.* 2015;8:753–765.

68. Spielberger CD. *Manual for the State-Trait Anxiety Inventory (Form Y).* Palo Alto, CA: Mind Garden; 1983.

69. Stevens JP, Wall MJ, Novack L, et al. The critical care crisis of opioid overdoses in the United States. *Ann Am Thorac Soc.* 2017; 14(12):1803–1809.

70. Subramaniam B, Shankar P, Shaefi S, et al. Effect of intravenous acetaminophen vs placebo combined with propofol or dexmedetomidine on postoperative delirium among older patients following cardiac surgery: The DEXACET randomized clinical trial. *JAMA.* 2019;321(7):686–696.

71. Tully PJ, Winefield HR, Baker RA, et al. Depression, anxiety and major adverse cardiovascular and cerebrovascular events in patients following coronary artery bypass graft surgery: A five year longitudinal cohort study. *Biopsychosoc Med.* 2015;9:14.

72. Turkoski BB. Acetaminophen by infusion. *Orthop Nurs.* 2015;34(3): 166–169.

73. Wang ZH, Chen H, Yang YL, et al. Bispectral index can reliably detect deep sedation in mechanically ventilated patients: A prospective multicenter validation study. *Anesth Analg.* 2017;125(1):176–183.

74. Warr J, Thiboutot Z, Rose L, et al. Current therapeutic uses, pharmacology, and clinical considerations of neuromuscular blocking agents for critically ill adults. *Ann Pharmacother.* 2011;45(9):1116–1126.

75. Weerink MAS, Struys MMRF, Hannivoort LN, et al. Clinical pharmacokinetics and pharmacodynamics of dexmedetomidine. *Clin Pharmacokinet.* 2017;56(8):893–913.

76. Young GB, Mantia J. Continuous EEG monitoring in the intensive care unit. *Handb Clin Neurol.* 2017;140:107–116.

PART II

Tools for the Critical Care Nurse

Nutritional Therapy

Lauren Morata, DNP, APRN-CNS, CCRN, CCNS
Megan Walsh, RD/N, LD

Many additional resources, including self-assessment exercises, are located on the Evolve companion website at http://evolve.elsevier.com/Sole/.
- Animations
- Clinical Skills: Critical Care Collections
- Student Review Questions
- Video Clips

INTRODUCTION

The approach to nutrition has evolved from a secondary and supportive treatment focused on preservation of lean mass to a therapeutic intervention that prevents harm and facilitates healing.[21] The critical care nurse and multiprofessional team members are responsible for optimizing the patient's nutritional status in an effort to reduce the risks of adverse outcomes and malnutrition. The true prevalence of malnutrition in hospitalized patients is unknown; however, studies have cited rates ranging from 20% to 68%.[9] Nosocomial malnutrition, or a declining nutritional status during the hospital stay, occurs in approximately 70% of inpatient adults regardless of their prehospital nutritional status.[9] Malnutrition is associated with increasing readmission rates, length of stay, healthcare costs, and mortality.[9] Critically ill patients have an increased risk of malnutrition and related complications due to alterations in protein and energy metabolism. Trauma, burns, sepsis, or other critical illnesses are often exacerbated by a frequent inability to tolerate oral nutrition.[21]

This chapter reviews the gastrointestinal (GI) system's function related to nutrition and the basic assessment of a patient's nutritional status. Nutrient formulas and supplements, goals of therapy, practice guidelines for enteral nutrition (EN) and parenteral nutrition (PN), and complications related to nutritional therapy are also discussed.

ANATOMY AND PHYSIOLOGY OF THE ALIMENTARY TRACT

The main organs of digestion form the alimentary tract, which extends from the mouth to the anus (Fig. 7.1). The GI tract, though often used to reference the entire alimentary tract, refers only to the stomach and intestines.[15] The alimentary tract facilitates the acquisition of nutrients through a combination of mechanical and chemical digestive processes starting in the mouth. Mastication, the process of chewing, creates a bolus of food that is then broken down via enzymatic reactions.[7] The average person secretes approximately 1 liter of saliva daily, which facilitates the digestion of starches and lubrication of masticated food.[7] Upon swallowing, or deglutition, the food bolus travels from the pharynx via voluntary and involuntary movements to the esophagus and through the esophageal sphincter to the stomach. Through peristalsis, and the concurrent secretions of gastrin, hydrochloric acid, mucus, and pepsinogen, the stomach creates a semifluid mixture of food, secretions, and water, called chyme. Chyme is then slowly released into the small intestine at a rate that facilitates digestion and absorption.[7] Most absorption occurs in the small intestine through the epithelium via enzymatic breakdown: peptides are split into amino acids, disaccharides into monosaccharides, and fats into glycerol and fatty acids.[7] The large intestine uses large circular movements to propel the chyme forward, while absorbing most water and electrolytes in the proximal half of the colon.[7] The distal half of the colon stores feces until excretion occurs through the anus.

Multiple accessory organs also participate in absorption, digestion, and excretion. These accessory organs include the parotid, submandibular, and sublingual salivary glands; tongue; teeth; liver; gallbladder; pancreas; and vermiform appendix. The salivary glands, tongue, and teeth assist in the production of saliva, mastication, and deglutition. These processes aid in the digestion and absorption of nutrients.

The liver regulates the appetite center in the brain, secretes bile, and aids in the metabolism of macronutrients. Hepatocytes, or liver cells, form bile, which flows through multiple ducts in the liver that eventually join with the cystic duct of the gallbladder, forming the common bile duct. Bile backs up into the gallbladder, where it is stored and concentrated. When chyme enters the small intestine, the gallbladder contracts, releasing bile into the duodenum. Bile aids in fat digestion and absorption. In addition, the

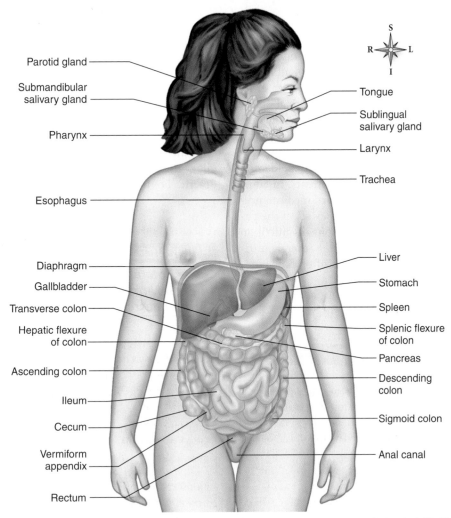

Fig. 7.1 Alimentary tract. (From Patton KT, Thibodeau GA. *Anatomy and Physiology.* 10th ed. St. Louis, MO: Elsevier; 2019.)

Labels:
- Parotid gland
- Submandibular salivary gland
- Pharynx
- Esophagus
- Diaphragm
- Gallbladder
- Transverse colon
- Hepatic flexure of colon
- Ascending colon
- Ileum
- Cecum
- Vermiform appendix
- Rectum
- Tongue
- Sublingual salivary gland
- Larynx
- Trachea
- Liver
- Stomach
- Spleen
- Splenic flexure of colon
- Pancreas
- Descending colon
- Sigmoid colon
- Anal canal

liver stores iron and vitamins B$_{12}$, A, and D. Glycogen, a storage form of carbohydrate in the liver, is broken down, releasing glucose into the bloodstream. The pancreas also contributes to carbohydrate digestion and glycemic control.[15]

The acinar cells of the pancreas secrete the digestive enzymes amylase, lipase, and protease, which aid in the breakdown of the macronutrients carbohydrate, fat, and protein, respectively. After release from the acinar cells, the digestive enzymes enter the pancreatic duct. The pancreatic duct joins with the common bile duct, and pancreatic secretions empty into the duodenum. The pancreas secretes bicarbonate to neutralize the acidity of gastric juices entering the duodenum.[15]

The pancreatic islets are made up of beta cells, which secrete insulin, and alpha cells, which secrete glucagon. Insulin is the hormone that controls carbohydrate metabolism by allowing glucose to enter cells and be used as energy, lowering the serum blood glucose level. Glucagon is a hormone that increases the serum blood glucose level by stimulating gluconeogenesis, the production of glucose from fat or protein sources, as well as the breakdown of glycogen. The pancreas also secretes the hormones somatostatin, ghrelin, and pancreatic polypeptide, which

contribute to digestion due to their effects on endocrine secretions of the pancreas; gastrointestinal motility; and appetite, hunger, and satiety cues.[15]

The vermiform appendix has often been classified as an organ that no longer serves a functional purpose in the body; however, it is still considered an accessory organ to the digestive system due to its communication with the cecum. It functions as a storage and reproduction site for nonpathogenic bacteria, contributing to the normal flora of the large intestine. In digesting insoluble fiber, these bacteria release gases, contributing to the production of flatus. Of concern for the critical care nurse, bacteria stored in the appendix can migrate to the large intestine in response to disruptions in normal flora due to illness or antibiotic use.[15]

The alimentary tract and its accessory organs are essential to the use of nutrients from foods ingested. During critical illness, function of the alimentary tract may be compromised due to insults from injury, inability to consume food orally, and concomitant medications and interventions. Due to the inherent risks of critical illness, the nutrition status of patients must be continually assessed and monitored.

ASSESSMENT

Critical illness causes a catabolic stress state, increasing the inflammatory response and metabolic demands of the patient.[21] An initial nutrition screening is required of all hospitalized patients within 48 hours of admission; however, critically ill patients are at a higher risk for nutritional status deterioration, necessitating a full nutritional assessment.[21] The objective of the nutrition assessment in the critically ill patient is to document baseline subjective and objective nutrition parameters, determine nutrition risk factors, identify deficits, and establish estimated needs for patients. In addition, the nutrition assessment serves to discern medical, psychosocial, and socioeconomic factors that may affect the patient's nutrition status and administration of nutrition therapy (see Lifespan Considerations box).[4,3] Several nutrition screening tools exist, but the adoption of each depends on the healthcare facility.

Additional considerations must be taken in evaluating disease states that may affect nutrition needs, affect onset of nutrition support, and contribute to intolerance. Some conditions may increase nutrient needs, alter the route and method of administration, and contribute to providers delaying initiation of nutrition support. Often these delays in nutrition support are based on inconclusive or insufficient evidence. For example, research demonstrates the benefits of EN compared with PN in patients with acute pancreatitis; however, the optimal timing of initiation was debated until the publication of a recent meta-analysis (see Evidence-Based Practice box).[18]

LIFESPAN CONSIDERATIONS

Older Adults
- Decreased intake caused by poor dentition and ill-fitting dentures
- Chronic diseases that decrease the appetite or the ability to obtain and prepare appropriate and adequate meals (e.g., dementia, chronic obstructive pulmonary disease, osteoarthritis, heart failure, loss of functional mobility)
- Food insecurity, defined as limited access to a reliable source of nutritious, affordable food in sufficient quantity:
  - Fixed and/or decreased income level
  - Social isolation (e.g., living alone, limited mobility)
  - Barriers to access to food (e.g., lack of transportation, minimal availability of meal delivery services)
- Medication side effects and/or interactions that may affect intake by altering appetite, flavor, taste, and/or odor perceptions

Pregnant Women
- Hyperemesis gravidarum may require:
  - Administration of total parenteral nutrition (TPN) to meet nutritional needs
  - IV fluid hydration
- Increasing nutritional needs based on trimester:
  - First trimester: does not require additional caloric intake
  - Second trimester: additional 340 calories per day
  - Third trimester: additional 450 calories per day
  - First 20 weeks: no additional protein required; second 20 weeks: additional 25 g per day
- Glycemic control:
  - Critical illness increases the risk for hyperglycemia, with a higher demand on insulin in pregnant women; monitor blood glucose frequently
  - Evaluate for gestational diabetes as indicated
- Increased risk for foodborne illnesses secondary to a weakened immune system
- Encourage patient to consume a balanced diet as well as to initiate or continue prenatal vitamins to facilitate fetal health and development

References
American College of Obstetricians and Gynecologists. *Your Pregnancy and Childbirth: Month to Month.* 6th ed. Washington, DC: American College of Obstetricians and Gynecologists; 2016.

Anarya S, Singh K, Sabharwal M. Changes during aging and their association with malnutrition. *J Clin Gerontol Geriatr.* 2015;6:78–84.

EVIDENCE-BASED PRACTICE

Early Enteral Nutrition Compared With Late Enteral Nutrition or Parenteral Nutrition in Acute Pancreatitis

Problem
Patients with acute pancreatitis are often kept NPO (nothing by mouth) for several days before nutrition is initiated. Research has demonstrated a reduction in complications with the use of enteral nutrition (EN) instead of parenteral nutrition (PN) in patients with acute pancreatitis; however, the optimal timing of initiation of EN has not been established.

Clinical Question
Should EN begin early (within 24 hours of admission) in patients with acute pancreatitis?

Evidence
A meta-analysis of 8 randomized controlled trials was conducted, analyzing the outcomes of 727 patients who had acute pancreatitis. Patients with predicted severe or severe acute pancreatitis who received early EN had reduced rates of multiple organ failure. A decreasing trend in mortality, infections, pancreatic infections, and adverse events was observed in patients with predicted or confirmed severe acute pancreatitis who received early EN.

Conclusions
In predicted severe or severe acute pancreatitis, patients should receive EN within 24 to 48 hours of admission. The analysis finds that patients who receive early EN have a significant reduction in multiple organ failure and pancreatic infections. The results of this analysis did not produce the same benefits for mild to moderate acute pancreatitis. Failure to start EN for 72 to 96 hours in severe acute pancreatitis may affect the patients' nutrition status negatively and increase the risk of complications.

Implications for Nursing
When caring for patients with severe acute pancreatitis, advocate for early EN to decrease the patients' risk of multiple organ failure and pancreatic infections. During multiprofessional rounds, address nutrition support and recommend early initiation of EN in patients with severe pancreatitis.

Level of Evidence
A—Meta-analysis

Reference
Qi D, Yu B, Huang J, Peng M. Meta-analysis of early enteral nutrition provided within 24 hours of admission on clinical outcomes in acute pancreatitis. *J Parenter Enteral Nutr.* 2018;42(7):1139–1147.

Auscultate the abdomen to assess contractility of the GI tract. Although reduced or absent bowel sounds may indicate a worse prognosis, initiation of EN should not be withheld, as bowel sounds alone do not provide information on mucosal and barrier integrity nor on absorption.[21] Palpate the abdomen last to avoid affecting auscultation of bowel sounds. Assessment of the alimentary tract requires the nurse to evaluate the cardiovascular and neurological functions of the patient. Patients with inadequate perfusion on vasopressors or an altered level of consciousness require different nutrition therapy than does the awake, alert patient.

Determining nutrient needs for patients is a pivotal part of the nutrition assessment. Calculation of caloric, protein, and fluid requirements is standard when completing a nutrition assessment. Reference standards for the intake of vitamins, minerals, and trace elements are published. Enteral formulas are designed to provide the recommended daily intake for vitamins and minerals when infusing at goal rate. Supplemental vitamins and minerals are given to critically ill patients to facilitate healing, improve skin integrity, and address real or potential deficiencies.

Indirect calorimetry is considered the most accurate method of determining energy expenditure. Calorie requirements are determined by measuring an individual's oxygen consumption and carbon dioxide production over a period of time. Oxygen consumption is then converted into resting energy expenditure using the Weir formula and a standardized constant respiratory quotient.[12] Collaborative guidelines from the American Society for Parenteral and Enteral Nutrition (ASPEN) and the Society of Critical Care Medicine (SCCM) recommend the use of indirect calorimetry to predict a patient's estimated energy requirements; however, the quality of evidence is low. Furthermore, the availability of indirect calorimetry is often limited by cost and access to the equipment, as well as adequate training on how to use the equipment effectively.[21]

In the absence of indirect calorimetry, ASPEN recommends using a published predictive equation or a simplistic weight-based equation to provide a range of calories per kilogram (kcal/kg) to meet the patient's energy requirements (Table 7.1).[12] More than 200 equations have been published, but the accuracy of these equations ranges from 40% to 75% when compared with indirect calorimetry. Research has not yet identified a superior equation, as multiple factors affect the reliability of each equation in the critical care setting. For example, predictive equations are less accurate in patients who are overweight or obese when compared to patients with a normal body weight. Regardless of the method used to determine energy requirements, weekly monitoring and reassessment of estimated needs to optimize protein and energy requirements is recommended in the critically ill patient.[21]

Protein needs are increased due to illness and other factors, such as wounds and interventional therapies; therefore 1.2 g/kg or greater of protein daily is recommended for critically ill patients (see Table 7.1).[21,12] Evaluate the calorie and protein status of a patient by monitoring skin integrity, weight, and physical signs of muscle and fat wasting. The serum protein markers (albumin, prealbumin, total protein, and transferrin) are not validated methods for assessing nutrition adequacy and should not be used to evaluate nutrition status in the critical care unit.[21]

OVERVIEW OF NUTRITIONAL THERAPY

Preferred Route of Nutrition

A recent Cochrane review found that evidence was insufficient to determine if one route of nutrition was superior to another when evaluating impact on mortality, ventilator-free days, and adverse

TABLE 7.1 Estimated Nutrition Needs		
Caloric Requirements	**Protein Requirements**	**Considerations**
Low BMI (<18.5) 30-45 kcal/kg/day (based on actual body weight)	1.2-2 g/kg/day	While energy requirements are higher, in the intubated patient it is not recommended to exceed 30 kcal/kg of body weight in daily nutrition support
Normal BMI (18.5-24.9) 25-30 kcal/kg/day (based on actual body weight)	1.2-2 g/kg/day	Protein requirement increased during critical illness
Overweight (BMI 25-29.9) 25-30 kcal/kg/day (based on actual body weight)	1.2-2 g/kg/day	Protein requirement increased during critical illness
Obesity (BMI 30-50) 11-14 kcal/kg/day (based on actual body weight)	1.5-2 g/kg/day (when BMI 30-40) 2-2.5 g/kg/day (when BMI >40)	Hypocaloric, high-protein feedings to preserve lean body mass in the patient in a critical care unit
Morbid Obesity (BMI >50) 22-25 kcal/kg/day (based on ideal body weight)	2-2.5 g/kg/day	Hypocaloric, high-protein feedings to preserve lean body mass in the patient in a critical care unit

BMI, Body mass index.

events.[11] EN preserves immune function and health of the alimentary tract and lowers the risk of infection due to oral access versus central venous access; therefore EN remains the preferred route per critical care guidelines for nutritional therapy.[21]

Enteral Nutrition

Optimizing. Most critically ill patients may safely receive and should begin EN within 24 to 48 hours of admission.[21] Studies evaluating early EN (within 24 hours) when compared to delayed EN found benefits associated with decreasing pneumonia, mortality, and critical care unit length of stay and maintaining the integrity of the GI tract.[21,22] Exclusions to initiating early EN include diagnoses such as bowel obstruction, hemodynamic instability, GI bleeding, bowel ischemia, or intraabdominal hypertension.[19]

Many facilities have protocols to begin EN as early as medically feasible with interdisciplinary consults implemented as needed to maximize therapy. Nursing supports early initiation of EN by querying the physician daily if the patient is appropriate to start EN. In addition, nursing can promote optimal nutrition intake by advocating for decreased fasting times for procedures.

Traditionally, patients are kept NPO (nothing by mouth) from midnight prior to surgery until, at times, multiple days postoperatively. This is often due to waiting for the return of bowel function or resolution of postoperative ileus prior to beginning nutrition. Research suggests that reducing fasting times for procedures is associated with improvement in patient outcomes and nutrition status. Current recommendations support reduced fasting times, and enhanced recovery after surgery (ERAS) protocols have been developed; however, there is a disconnect in the implementation into current practice.[10]

Evidence has shown that a 2-hour fast for liquids and a 6-hour fast for solids is adequate time for gastric emptying to avoid pulmonary aspiration during general anesthesia. Research finds that resuming oral or enteral nutrition within 24 hours postoperatively not only is safe and tolerated but also improves recovery. Early initiation of gastric feeding may improve ileus and expedite the return of bowel function.[10]

EN can be delivered by three methods: trophic, targeted hourly rate, and volume-based feeding (VBF). Trophic feeding provides patients with less than their estimated nutrition needs due to an actual or perceived risk of intolerance. In some cases, patients are started on trophic feeds and advanced to a goal volume or rate as tolerated. Trophic feeding rates are most often between 10 and 30 mL/h.

In the targeted hourly rate method, a goal *rate* for EN administration is calculated based on the daily estimated nutritional need. Initiation of EN either occurs at a trophic rate and advances

to the hourly goal or is initiated at the hourly goal rate. The rate is set and remains at the specified hourly volume (e.g., 45 mL/h). This method does not typically account for missed EN secondary to procedures, nursing care, or diagnostic tests; therefore the patient is at risk for suboptimal nutrition therapy. Certain tests or procedures may not require fasting; clarify with the practitioner who is ordering or performing procedures how long to hold EN or whether holding EN is necessary. Upon procedure completion, resume nutrition support promptly. Compensating for missed EN via VBF can help optimize the patient's nutrition status.

Upon implementing the VBF method, the practitioner orders the appropriate EN as a goal *volume* to be infused over 24 hours. Increases in the hourly rate occur in response to interruptions in EN therapy, with the goal of compensating for gaps in EN therapy. For example, if the goal volume is 1200 mL and the patient's EN is held for 12 hours for a procedure, the patient has 12 hours remaining in the day to achieve the goal volume. Recalculate the rate of administration based on the remaining hours (1200 mL divided by 12 hours) and run the EN at 100 mL/h for the remainder of the day. In this method, patients receive more prescribed calories and protein when compared to the target hourly rate method (see QSEN Exemplar box).[8]

✳ **QSEN EXEMPLAR**

Evidence-Based Practice

The Society of Critical Care Medicine (SCCM) and American Society for Parenteral and Enteral Nutrition (ASPEN) guidelines recommend providing greater than 80% of prescribed nutrition needs to critically ill patients. Audits across critical care units show that 50% to 70% of prescribed nutrition is administered on average. Heyland and colleagues conducted a prospective, multicenter, quality improvement collaborative with an evaluation component to assess the efficacy of a novel enteral feeding protocol, known as the PEP uP protocol (enhanced protein-energy provision via the enteral route feeding protocol). The protocol was implemented in seven distinct critical care units within five hospitals with a focus on optimizing nutrition in the critical care setting by (1) using a 24-hour volume goal (i.e., volume-based feeding [VBF]) instead of a targeted hourly goal rate; (2) using semidigested formulas; (3) using prophylactic protein supplements and motility agents; and (4) increasing the threshold for gastric residual volume (GRV) to greater than 300 mL. The evaluation data were collected from a large international, multicenter observational study of nutrition practices in the critical care unit—the International Nutrition Survey (INS 2014). The INS surveyed 50 critical care units in the United States, 7 of which participated in the PEP uP protocol. The other 43 critical care units were used as controls in the evaluation of the PEP uP protocol. A total of 1108 patients were included: 126 from PEP uP sites, and the remainder from control critical care units. In the PEP uP sites, enteral nutrition (EN) was started earlier, at an average of 31 hours from admission compared to 51 hours from admission in the control sites. Over the first 5 days of critical care unit stay, the PEP uP sites provided 35% of prescribed energy compared to 24% in the control sites and 42% of prescribed protein compared to 25% in the control sites. Nurses can optimize nutrition support in the critical care unit by advocating for early initiation of EN and implementing a VBF protocol. Management of GRV according to guidelines may also help decrease interruptions in delivery of EN.

Reference

Heyland DK, Lemuix M, Shu L, et al. What is "best achievable" practice in implementing the enhanced protein-energy provision via the enteral route feeding protocol in intensive care units in the United States? Results of a multicenter, quality improvement collaborative. *J Parenter Enteral Nutr.* 2018;42(2):308–317.

? CRITICAL REASONING ACTIVITY

What strategies can you use to reduce interruptions in the delivery of enteral feeding?

Delivery Route. Enteral nutrition can be administered through a number of options, with the optimal access depending on the patient's acute and long-term nutrition support needs. Often the intubated patient receives an orogastric tube (OGT) for stomach decompression after intubation. The OGT can easily be transitioned from a decompressive device to EN access. Nasogastric tubes (NGTs) are another gastric tube option; however, NGTs increase the risk of sinusitis by 200% in intubated patients.[13] The placement of all blindly inserted gastric tubes should be confirmed via radiographic study prior to use, then checked every 4 hours during continuous feeding based on external tube length (see Clinical Alert box).[2,5]

! CLINICAL ALERT

Assessment of Feeding Tube Placement

Misplaced feeding tubes increase the risk of complications, including nutrition delays, aspiration pneumonia, and pneumothorax. Radiographic confirmation of correct tube placement is expected before initiation of tube feedings or administration of medications. Tube placement must also be verified if the tube becomes dislodged and requires reinsertion. Auscultatory or pH testing methods alone for assessing tube placement are unreliable. Patients with the highest risk of placement complications are intubated patients and those with an altered level of consciousness or an impaired gag reflex.

Patients at high risk for aspiration should have their feeding tube placed postpyloric in the small bowel given the reduction in aspiration and regurgitation.[21] Small bowel feeding tubes (SBFTs) are safe and do not increase the likelihood of complications when compared to the gastric route.[1] Use of SBFTs requires additional training to safely achieve postpyloric placement. Some institutions use a bedside electromagnetic placement device (EMPD) to assist with accurate placement. The EMPD tracks the location of the SBFT through the use of a stylet that emits an electromagnetic signal from its distal tip.[17] The signal is then transformed to a tracing on the screen of the EMPD, which allows the nurse to determine the location and trajectory of the SBFT.[17] The accuracy of EMPD-placed SBFTs by skilled nurses is upward of 97%, with some institutions eliminating radiographic confirmation; however, radiographic studies are still recommended for SBFT confirmation.[2,17]

Long-term (typically longer than 4 to 5 weeks) nutritional access is considered based on the patient's swallowing ability, aspiration risks, goals of care or wishes, and ability to meet nutritional requirements. Feeding tubes can be inserted externally through the stomach or jejunum. A percutaneous endoscopic gastrostomy (PEG) tube is inserted under local to moderate sedation, allowing enteral feedings to begin within 4 hours after placement.[5] If a patient does not tolerate gastric feedings, a percutaneous endoscopic gastrojejunostomy (PEGJ) tube can

be placed, allowing jejunal feeding and bypassing the stomach. The PEG portion is often used for medication administration to facilitate adequate absorption, and the PEGJ portion is used for continuous EN. Another postpyloric long-term feeding tube option is the surgically placed percutaneous endoscopic jejunostomy (PEJ) tube; however, endoscopic placement is available to certain patients based on clinical disposition. PEJ tubes have significantly better long-term patency than PEGJ tubes, which tend to recoil back into the stomach.

Nursing Considerations. During administration of EN, elevate the patient's head of bed to 30 degrees or higher to prevent aspiration. Placing the head of bed higher than 30 degrees requires frequent integumentary assessments and patient repositioning to reduce the risk of pressure injury. Whenever medications are administered via an enteral feeding tube, flush the tube with 30 mL of water before and after each medication is administered. Patients requiring fluid restriction may receive 15 mL for flush. If the patient's EN is to be placed on hold, flush the feeding tube to prevent a buildup of residue in the tube and reduce the risk of clogging.[5]

Liquid medication formulations are preferred for administration via the enteral feeding tube; however, they increase the risk of diarrhea, as many liquid medications use sorbitol as an excipient. If enough sorbitol is consumed, the sugar alcohol can have a laxative effect. Sustained-release medications must not be crushed and given via a feeding tube because of the potential for overdose. When administering EN via a feeding tube, collaborate with the pharmacist to ensure safe and effective medication administration. Bioavailability of some medications may be reduced when administered with enteral feedings. EN may require temporary discontinuation before and after medication administration. For example, current recommendations for administration of phenytoin are to stop enteral feedings 1 to 2 hours before and after dosing.[23] This method may not always be optimal, especially for malnourished patients. Other options include monitoring and adjusting phenytoin dosages based on serum drug levels while the patient is receiving EN or transitioning the patient to IV therapy during continuous EN administration. Once EN is discontinued, the drug dosage or route of administration is readjusted.

The location of enteral access in the alimentary tract may also affect bioavailability of some medications. In patients receiving medications via a small bowel or jejunostomy tube, care should be given to ensure that all medications are effectively absorbed in the small bowel. For example, antacid medications such as pantoprazole or famotidine are ineffective when administered directly into the small intestine given their mechanism of action. The administration of rivaroxaban distal to the stomach is not recommended, as this may decrease the patient's exposure to the medication.[9] Open communication with the pharmacist and multiprofessional team to effectively reconcile the medication administration record will facilitate safe and effective therapy.

? CRITICAL REASONING ACTIVITY

What types of enteral nutrition–drug interactions can cause complications?

Tolerance. Upon initiating EN, intolerance to therapy is evaluated. Intolerance is often defined as abdominal distension, constipation, emesis, or nausea. In years past, gastric residual volumes (GRVs) were used to evaluate intolerance; however, recent guidelines do not recommend routine monitoring of GRVs. Research found that GRVs greater than 250 mL did not increase the patient's risk for either aspiration or pneumonia. Monitoring GRVs compromised EN delivery, increased nursing workload, and led to an increase in enteral devices clogging.[21] In patients with postpyloric enteral access, GRVs should not be assessed given the location, pliability, and small bore of the tube.

Critically ill patients are often on medications that decrease motility, such as narcotics and sedatives, increasing the risk of EN intolerance. To reduce the risk of intolerance in this population, a proactive bowel regimen should accompany the initiation of EN unless contraindicated. If patients become constipated or demonstrate signs and symptoms of intolerance, promotility medications may be considered. Common medications used for motility and bowel regimens are outlined in Table 7.2.[21,12,20,16,14]

 CRITICAL REASONING ACTIVITY

What assessment findings are indicative of a patient's intolerance to enteral nutrition (EN)?

Types. In addition to the method and route of EN administration, the formula and supplements prescribed can also affect

nutrition therapy. Various formulas and supplements for enteral nutrition exist and can be tailored to specific disease states. Tables 7.3 and 7.4 discuss the common formulas and supplements used in critical care.

STUDY BREAK

2. Which of the following is a sign or symptom of enteral nutrition (EN) intolerance?
   A. Gas and flatus
   B. Gastric residual volumes (GRVs) of 250 mL
   C. Abdominal distension and pain
   D. Absent bowel sounds

Parenteral Nutrition

Optimizing. PN is a form of nutrition that supplies protein, fat, minerals, electrolytes, and carbohydrates via the IV route. In patients where EN is contraindicated due to the structure or function of the alimentary tract (e.g., discontinuity, obstruction, hyperemesis gravidarum), assess patients early for the provision of PN. A multiprofessional approach to PN implementation may reduce the associated risks, including hyperglycemia, electrolyte imbalances, immune suppression, increased oxidative stress, and potential infectious morbidity.

PN should be withheld for the first 7 days of a critical care admission if the patient is at low nutrition risk and EN is not feasible.[21] If the patient cannot receive EN and is found to be severely malnourished or have a high nutritional risk, initiate

---

TABLE 7.2 Pharmacology
Medications Frequently Used for Motility and Bowel Regimens

Medication	Action/Use	Dose/Route	Side Effects	Nursing Implications
Bisacodyl	Laxative; stimulant	5-15 mg qAM or qHS/PO 10 mg single dose/rectal	Nausea, vomiting, diarrhea, cramping, rectal burning, tetany	Educate patient on avoiding long-term use (>1 wk); ensure patient hydration
Docusate sodium	Laxative; stool softener	50-300 mg daily/PO 4 mL/enema	Nausea, cramps, anorexia, diarrhea	Product may take up to 3 days to soften stool; ensure patient hydration
Erythromycin	Prokinetic	250-500 mg tid/PO	Tachyphylaxis, cardiac toxicity	Monitor for allergic reactions; response may decline with prolonged therapy
Metoclopramide	Prokinetic	10 mg q6h/IV 5 mg q6h/IV if CrCl <40	Sedation, fatigue, dystonia, tardive dyskinesia, suicidal ideation, seizures, neuroleptic malignant syndrome, neutropenia, hypotension, diarrhea	Increased risk of hypertension if combined with MAOIs; EPS risk increases with prolonged and high-dose use; nurse must monitor for QT prolongation; avoid in combination with haloperidol as this increases the risk for tardive dyskinesia, EPS, and prolonged QT intervals; may require dosage adjustments in renal failure
Polyethylene glycol	Laxative	17 g daily/PO	Diarrhea, nausea, stomach cramping, abdominal distension	Should be dissolved in 4-8 ounces of a beverage; do not continue for >2 wk
Senna	Laxative; stimulant	17.2 mg daily–17.2 mg bid/PO	Electrolyte abnormalities, diarrhea, nausea, abdominal cramping	Ensure patient hydration; evaluate for other signs of constipation such as impaction

bid, Two times a day; *CrCl,* creatinine clearance; *EPS,* extrapyramidal symptoms; *MAOI,* monoamine oxidase inhibitors; *PO,* by mouth; *qAM,* every morning; *qHS,* every hour of sleep; *tid,* three times a day.
Data from Chapman MJ, Fraser RJ, Kluger MT, et al. Erythromycin improves gastric emptying in critically ill patients intolerant of nasogastric feeding. *Crit Care Med.* 2000;28:2334–2337; Skidmore-Roth L. *Mosby's 2019 Nursing Drug Reference.* 32nd ed. St. Louis, MO: Elsevier, Inc.; 2019; Polyethylene glycol [package insert]. Braintree, MA: Braintree Laboratories, Inc.; 2001.

TABLE 7.3 Common Formulas

Type	Description	Calories (kcal/mL)	Disease States
Standard (Jevity, Nutren, Fibersouce HN, Isosource)	Fiber containing, average osmolality	1; 1.2; 1.5; 2	Patient with minimal, or no comorbid conditions
Low residue (Osmolite, Nutren, Isosource HN)	No fiber, low osmolality	1; 1.2; 1.5	Surgical patients, GI conditions
Elemental (Vital, Vivonex, Peptamen)	Fully hydrolyzed protein	1.2; 1.5	Patients with intolerance, GI surgery, or trauma
Peptide based (Pivot, Impact)	Partially hydrolyzed protein	1.5	SIRS, ARDS, improves protein absorption
Diabetes specific (Glucerna, Diabetisource)	Lower carbohydrate content, higher protein	1; 1.2; 1.5	Improves glucose control for diabetics or patients with hyperglycemia
Renal specific (Suplena, Nepro)	Lower in sodium, phosphorus, and potassium; high and low protein formulations available, carbohydrate controlled	1.8	Chronic kidney disease or end-stage renal disease; high-protein formula used for patients on dialysis and low-protein formula used for patients not requiring dialysis.

ARDS, Acute respiratory distress syndrome; *GI,* gastrointestinal; *SIRS,* systemic inflammatory response syndrome.

TABLE 7.4 Common Supplements

Supplement	Details
Protein	Whole grams of protein provided as a powder, gel, or liquid to increase protein content of enteral nutrition (EN) Often provide 10-20 g protein/serving
Insoluble fiber	Added to EN to provide prebiotics, or insoluble fiber, which can add bulk to stool Decreased incidence of loose bowel movements or diarrhea
Arginine/glutamine	Added to promote wound and pressure injury healing

PN as soon as possible after admission. In patients receiving EN, consider PN after 7 to 10 days of EN therapy if nutritional goals are not being met. Do not use PN unnecessarily, as its initiation and the treatment itself are not without risks. However, if PN is indicated, initiate the nutrition early to maximize benefits. If possible, consider trophic feeds to reduce the risk of sepsis and wean the patient from PN as soon as possible.[11]

Delivery Route and Types. There are two types of PN, total and peripheral, with total parenteral nutrition (TPN) being more common given the concentrated dosing and lower fluid volume. Peripheral parenteral nutrition (PPN) is not indicated for use in the adult population. PPN does not provide full nutrition support to patients and has the risk of compromising peripheral veins.

TPN involves the administration of a highly concentrated dextrose solution ($\geq$10%) with a high osmolarity (>900 mOsm/L).[6] Due to the high concentration of dextrose, patients receiving TPN have an increased risk of hyperglycemia and require frequent glucose monitoring and management. The caustic nature of the hyperosmolar fluid requires central venous access through a peripherally inserted central catheter (PICC), port, or central venous access located in the subclavian, jugular, or femoral veins. Central venous access increases the patient's risk for a nosocomial infection (i.e., central line–associated bloodstream infection [CLABSI]). Decrease risk to the patient by implementing CLABSI prevention bundles and adhering to hand hygiene practices (see Chapter 1).

Lipids. Lipids or fatty acids are infused with TPN to prevent essential fatty acid deficiency. Provision of lipids should not exceed 30% of a patient's total calorie intake from TPN. In patients receiving lipids, monitor triglyceride levels and withhold lipids if levels are elevated. Some medications use lipids as an emulsifier (e.g., the sedative propofol), and lipids are often held until discontinuation of these medications to prevent hypertriglyceridemia. Lipids can be infused concurrently with TPN or separately.

> **STUDY BREAK**
> 3. When is total parenteral nutrition (TPN) indicated?
>   A. After a failed swallow assessment
>   B. Immediately after intubation
>   C. After 7 days without nutrition
>   D. When a patient has a low oral intake

Nursing Considerations. Use a dedicated port in the central venous access device to administer TPN and lipids. Preferably, do not administer other medications via the same port as TPN.

Monitor and evaluate electrolytes closely in patients receiving TPN, as these patients' high nutrition risk predisposes them to refeeding syndrome. Refeeding syndrome is a potentially life-threatening electrolyte fluctuation in response to aggressive administration of nutrition therapy in a previously malnourished patient.[12] The guidelines recommend a slow titration of TPN to feeding goal over a 3- to 4-day period in at-risk patients.[21] Electrolyte monitoring and repletion is especially important, and in severe cases of refeeding, nutrition support has to be reduced to allow adequate electrolyte repletion.

If TPN is discontinued abruptly, monitor for signs and symptoms of hypoglycemia. Ideally, a patient who has been receiving TPN is transitioned to EN. Upon initiation of EN, ensure that the patient is receiving more than 80% of estimated caloric needs from EN or an oral diet prior to discontinuing TPN.[5]

❓ CRITICAL REASONING ACTIVITY

What factors would you consider when selecting a type of nutrition support?

Monitoring and Evaluating the Nutrition Care Plan

An interdisciplinary approach is essential when developing and reviewing the nutrition plan of care to ensure that best practices and evidence-based therapies are implemented (see Evidence-Based Practice box).[21] Laboratory and diagnostic studies can be useful in the assessment and administration of nutrition therapy (see Laboratory Alert box).[14] In addition, assessment of daily weights, fluid balance, and functional status can assist in evaluating the adequacy of energy and protein provision. If goals are not being met, reassessment of the plan is necessary to help the patient achieve optimal nutrition outcomes. Assessment of weight loss, abnormal laboratory values, and the appearance of dehydration or fluid overload are indicators that the nutritional care plan may need to be adjusted.

EVIDENCE-BASED PRACTICE

Nutritional Support in Critical Illness

Problem

Critically ill patients are at high risk for malnutrition secondary to the catabolic stress state associated with critical illness. Nutrition therapy is essential to attenuate the metabolic response to stress, prevent cellular injury, and modulate immune responses.

Clinical Question

What are recommended practices to optimize nutrition therapy in critically ill patients?

Evidence

The Society of Critical Care Medicine (SCCM) and the American Society for Parenteral and Enteral Nutrition (ASPEN) convened an expert panel to review available evidence related to nutrition therapy in critically ill patients. They evaluated primarily randomized controlled trials and meta-analyses to rate the evidence; however, they also included cohort trials, observational studies, and retrospective studies. If data were limited, the group achieved consensus on the best clinical practice recommendations. Evidence thus varied for each of the many recommendations. Recommendations relevant to the majority of critically ill patients are noted below.

- Nutrition assessment
  - Determine risk using valid assessment tools (NRS 2002 or NUTRiC).
  - Adjust assessment based on comorbid conditions.
  - Determine energy requirements.
    - Indirect calorimetry
    - Predictive equations
    - Simplistic formula of 25 to 30 kcal/kg
  - Ensure adequate protein intake.
- Enteral nutrition (EN)
  - Start EN within 24 to 48 hours if patient unable to maintain oral intake.
  - The presence of bowel sounds is not required to start EN.
  - Gastric feedings can be safely administered to most patients.
  - Consider postpyloric feedings in those at high risk for aspiration or those who have a history of intolerance to gastric feedings.
  - Those at low nutritional risk do not require specialized nutrition therapy.
  - Advance nutrition for those at high risk to target goal as tolerated over 24 to 48 hours.
- Monitor tolerance to EN
  - Avoid stopping feeding inappropriately.
  - Gastric residual volumes (GRVs) should not be used to assess aspiration risk.
  - If GRV is assessed, avoid holding EN for volumes less than 500 mL.
  - Assess for aspiration risk and implement interventions to reduce aspiration.
  - Do not interrupt EN for diarrhea; assess and treat potential causes of diarrhea.
- Selection of EN formula
  - Use standard polymeric formulas.
  - Avoid routine use of specialty formulas in medical patients.
  - Avoid routine use of disease-specific formulas in the surgical patient.
  - Consider formulas containing fiber or peptides for persistent diarrhea.
- Parenteral nutrition (PN)
  - Avoid administration for the first 7 days of admission in low-risk patients.
  - Start PN as soon as possible when EN is contraindicated in patients at high nutritional risk.
  - Consider supplemental PN if the patient is unable to meet at least 60% of energy and protein requirements after 7 to 10 days of EN.
  - Use a nutrition therapy team to manage PN.
- Obesity
  - Start early EN within 24 to 48 hours.
  - Administer high-protein, hypocaloric feedings to preserve lean muscle mass.

Implications for Nursing

These guidelines provide a broad range of recommendations for the critically ill patient. Collaborate with members of the multiprofessional team to implement the recommendations according to patient assessment. In addition, implement the recommended nutrition bundle in critically ill patients:

- Assess critically ill patients on admission for nutrition risk; calculate energy and protein requirements to determine goals of therapy.
- Start EN within 24 to 48 hours after admission; increase goals over the first week.
- Initiate interventions to reduce aspiration risk and improve tolerance of EN.
- Implement EN protocols.
- Do not use GRVs as part of routine monitoring.
- Initiate PN early when EN is not feasible or is insufficient in meeting nutrition goals.
- Maintain head of bed elevation at 30 to 45 degrees, unless contraindicated.

Level of Evidence

D—Professional standards developed from evidence

Reference

Taylor BE, McClave SA, Martindale RG, et al. Guidelines for the provision and assessment of nutrition support therapy in the adult critically ill patient: Society of Critical Care Medicine (SCCM) and American Society for Parenteral and Enteral Nutrition (ASPEN). *Crit Care Med.* 2016;44(2):159–211.

! LABORATORY ALERT

Laboratory Test	Normal Range	General Critical Valuesª	Significance
Prealbumin	15-36 mg/dL	<10.7 mg/dL	Serum levels fluctuate quickly: 1.9-day half-life. More reliable indication of protein synthesis and catabolism than albumin.
			Affected by inflammatory process; not a validated method for evaluating nutrition status.
Albumin	3.5-5 g/dL	<3.5 g/dL	Half-life between 18 and 21 days.
			Not a reliable indication of protein synthesis and catabolism.
			Many disease states decrease serum albumin levels, including inflammatory processes, liver disease, acute reaction, and nephrotic syndrome.
Triglycerides (TGs)	Male: 40-160 mg/dL	>400 mg/dL	TGs act as a storage form of energy, and when excess builds up in the bloodstream, it is deposited into tissue.
	Female: 35-135 mg/dL		Hypertriglyceridemia: may consider withholding lipids from TPN; implement alternative sedative regimens as indicated (i.e., propofol is suspended in lipids).
Sodium	136-145 mEq/L	<120 mEq/L	Many factors and disease states affect serum sodium levels.
		>160 mEq/L	Hyponatremia: may affect neurological function; indicative of the syndrome of inappropriate antidiuretic hormone secretion (SIADH); may be caused by excessive free water or inadequate dietary provision of sodium.
			Hypernatremia: may affect neurological function; sign of dehydration, inadequate free water intake, excessive sodium in IV fluids.
Potassium	3.5-5 mEq/L	<3.0 mEq/L	Levels are affected by acid-base balance, sodium resorption, and aldosterone.
		>6.1 mEq/L	Hypokalemia: caused by GI losses, medications, or inadequate dietary intake/IV supplementation when NPO, hypothermia.
			Hyperkalemia: due to dehydration, certain medications, renal impairment.
Magnesium	1.3-2.1 mEq/L	<0.5 mEq/L	Most organ functions depend on magnesium, and levels must be closely monitored in cardiac patients.
		>3.0 mEq/L	Hypomagnesemia: due to malnutrition.
			Hypermagnesemia: most often caused by renal disease or excessive intake of magnesium.
Phosphate	3-4.5 mg/dL	<1.0 mg/dL	Hypophosphatemia: caused by phosphate shifting from extracellular to intracellular, renal phosphate wasting, GI losses, or intracellular losses.
			Hyperphosphatemia: caused by renal disease or excessive dietary intake.
Glucose	74-106 mg/dL (fasting)	Male: <50 mg/dL >450 mg/dL Female: <40 mg/dL >450 mg/dL	Hyperglycemia: true elevation indicates diabetes; however, there are many causes. Can be elevated due to stress, pregnancy, IV fluids containing dextrose, and/or medications.
			Hypoglycemia: often a result of insulin overdose, concomitant medications, or starvation.

ªCritical values vary by facility and laboratory.
GI, Gastrointestinal; *NPO*, nothing by mouth; *TPN*, total parenteral nutrition.
Data from Pagana KD, Pagana TJ. *Mosby's Manual of Diagnostic and Laboratory Tests*. 6th ed. St. Louis, MO: Elsevier, Inc.; 2018.

CASE STUDY

Mrs. A. is a 50-year-old female who was admitted after an out-of-hospital cardiac arrest with return of spontaneous circulation and intubation in the field. Targeted temperature management (TTM) was initiated, her blood pressure was being supported by vasopressors, and an analgosedation regimen was initiated to control shivering. On hospital day 3, TTM was discontinued and vasopressors were weaned. She is neurologically intact. Objective data include the following: height, 164 cm; weight, 92 kg; body mass index (BMI), 34.2; history of stable nutrition intake at home per the family. Laboratory data include a potassium level of 4.1 mEq/L, magnesium level of 2.5 mEq/L, and prealbumin level of 8 mg/dL. Urine output has been approximately 50 mL/h, and bowel sounds are hypoactive. During multiprofessional rounds, the nurse advocates for enteral nutrition (EN) via the orogastric tube (OGT), given Mrs. A's inability to wean from the ventilator. The dietitian recommends a polymeric formula with hypocaloric and high-protein content, which is ordered at a targeted hourly rate by the physician. Two days later, on hospital day 5, the nursing assessment reveals bloating and distension. Based on discussions with the family and chart review, the nurse determines that the patient has not had a bowel movement in 6 days.

Questions
1. What combination of assessment findings determines the patient's nutritional status and EN tolerance?
2. Given the patient's gastrointestinal (GI) signs and symptoms, what should the nurse recommend during multiprofessional rounds?
3. How do you justify the preferred route of intake in the critically ill patient?
4. What is the overall goal of nutritional therapy?

REFERENCES

1. Alkhawaja S, Martin C, Butler RJ, Gwadry-Sridhar F. Post-pyloric versus gastric tube feeding for critically ill adult patients. *Cochrane Database Syst Rev.* https://www.cochrane.org/CD008875/ANAESTH_post-pyloric-versus-gastric-tube-feeding-critically-ill-adult-patients. Published August 4, 2015. Accessed December 15, 2018.

2. American Association of Critical-Care Nurses. AACN practice alert: Initial and ongoing verification of feeding tube placement in adults. *Crit Care Nurs.* 2016;36(2):e8–e13.

3. American College of Obstetricians and Gynecologists. *Your Pregnancy and Childbirth: Month to Month.* 6th ed. Washington, DC: American College of Obstetricians and Gynecologists; 2016.

4. Anarya S, Singh K, Sabharwal M. Changes during aging and their association with malnutrition. *J Clin Gerontol Geriatr.* 2015;6: 78–84.

5. Boullata JI, Carrera AL, Harvey L, et al. ASPEN safe practices for enteral nutrition therapy. *JPEN J Parenter Enteral Nutr.* 2017;41(1):15–103.

6. Boullata JI, Gilbert K, Sacks G, et al. ASPEN clinical guidelines: Parenteral nutrition ordering, order review, compounding, labeling and dispensing. *JPEN J Parenter Enteral Nutr.* 2014;1–44.

7. Hall JE, Guyton AC. *Guyton and Hall Textbook of Medical Physiology.* 13th ed. Philadelphia, PA: Elsevier; 2016.

8. Heyland DK, Lemuix M, Shu L, et al. What is "best achievable" practice in implementing the enhanced protein-energy provision via the enteral route feeding protocol in intensive care units in the United States? Results of a multicenter, quality improvement collaborative. *JPEN J Parenter Enteral Nutr.* 2018;42(2):308–317.

9. Kirkland LL, Shaughnessy E. Recognition and prevention of nosocomial malnutrition: A review and a call to action. *Am J Med.* 2017;130(12):1345–1350.

10. Lambert E, Carey S. Practice guideline recommendations on perioperative fasting: A systemic review. *JPEN J Parenter Enteral Nutr.* 2016;40(8):1158–1165.

11. Lewis S, Schofield-Robinson O, Alderson P, Smith A. Enteral versus parenteral nutrition and enteral versus a combination of enteral and parenteral nutrition for adults in the intensive care unit. *Cochrane Database Syst Rev.* https://www.cochranelibrary.com/cdsr/doi/10.1002/14651858.CD012276.pub2/full 2018. Published June 8, 2018. Accessed December 21, 2018.

12. Mahan LK, Raymond JL. *Krause's Food and the Nutrition Care Process.* 14th ed. St. Louis, MO: Elsevier, Inc.; 2017.

13. Metheny NA, Hinyard LJ, Mohammed KA. Incidence of sinusitis associated with endotracheal and nasogastric tubes: NIS database. *Am J Crit Care.* 2018;27(1):24–31.

14. Pagana KD, Pagana TJ. *Mosby's Manual of Diagnostic and Laboratory Tests.* 6th ed. St. Louis, MO: Elsevier, Inc.; 2018.

15. Patton KT, Thibodeau GA. *Anatomy and Physiology.* 10th ed. St. Louis, MO: Elsevier; 2019.

16. Polyethylene glycol [package insert]. Braintree, MA: Braintree Laboratories, Inc.; 2001.

17. Powers J, Luebbenhusen M, Spitzer T, et al. Verification of an electromagnetic placement device compared with abdominal radiograph to predict accuracy of feeding tube placement. *JPEN J Parenter Enteral Nutr.* 2011;35(4):535–539.

18. Qi D, Yu B, Huang J, Peng M. Meta-analysis of early enteral nutrition provided within 24 hours of admission on clinical outcomes in acute pancreatitis. *JPEN J Parenter Enteral Nutr.* 2018; 42(7):1139–1147.

19. Reintam BA, Starkopf J, Alhazzani W, et al. Early enteral nutrition in critically ill patients: ESICM clinical practice guidelines. *Intensive Care Med.* 2017;43(3):380–398.

20. Rivaroxaban [package insert]. Titusville, NJ: Janssen Pharmaceuticals, Inc.; 2015.

21. Taylor BE, McClave SA, Martindale RG, et al. Guidelines for the provision and assessment of nutrition support therapy in the adult critically ill patient: Society of Critical Care Medicine (SCCM) and American Society for Parenteral and Enteral Nutrition (ASPEN). *Crit Care Med.* 2016;44(2):159–211.

22. Tian F, Heighes PT, Allingstrup MJ, et al. Early nutrition provided within 24 hours of ICU admission: A meta-analysis of randomized controlled trials. *Crit Care Med.* 2018;46(7):1049–1056.

23. Williams NT. Medication administration through enteral feeding tubes. *Am J Health Syst Pharm.* 2008;65(24):2347–2357.

Dysrhythmia Interpretation and Management

Marthe J. Moseley, PhD, RN, CCRN-K, CCNS

Many additional resources, including self-assessment exercises, are located on the Evolve companion website at http://evolve.elsevier.com/Sole/.
- Animations
- Clinical Skills: Critical Care Collections
- Student Review Questions
- Video Clips

INTRODUCTION

The interpretation of cardiac rhythm disturbances or dysrhythmias is an essential skill for nurses employed in patient care areas where electrocardiographic monitoring occurs. The ability to rapidly analyze a rhythm disturbance and initiate appropriate treatment improves patient safety and optimizes successful outcomes. The critical care nurse is often the healthcare professional responsible for the continuous monitoring of the patient's cardiac rhythm and has the opportunity to provide early intervention that can prevent an adverse clinical situation. This responsibility requires not only a mastery of interpreting dysrhythmias, but also the ability to identify the unique monitoring needs of each patient. This chapter reviews basic cardiac dysrhythmias, etiological factors, clinical significance, and appropriate treatments to aid the novice critical care nurse in mastering dysrhythmia recognition.

The terms *dysrhythmia* and *cardiac arrhythmia* refer to an abnormal cardiac rhythm that deviates from normal sinus rhythm (NSR). The term *dysrhythmia* is used throughout this text.

The goal of this chapter is to provide an essential understanding of electrocardiography for analyzing and interpreting cardiac dysrhythmias. Electrocardiography is the process of creating a visual tracing of the electrical activity of the cells in the heart. This tracing is called the *electrocardiogram* (ECG). The critical care nurse understands the need for cardiac monitoring, lead selection, and rhythm interpretation. Part of the difficulty in learning rhythm interpretation is that many of the terms used are synonymous. Throughout this chapter, these terms are clarified within the discussion of general concepts of dysrhythmia interpretation.

OVERVIEW OF ELECTROCARDIOGRAM MONITORING

The first ECG was recorded in 1887 by British physiologist Augustus Waller via a capillary electrometer.[4] The electrocardiogram was subsequently named. The PQRST complex was described by Dr. Willem Einthoven, who proceeded to commercially produce a string galvanometer that was popularized in the early 1900s. Dr. Einthoven won the Nobel Prize in Physiology for Medicine in 1924 for inventing the electrocardiograph. The first electrical ECG machine weighed 50 pounds and was powered by a 6-volt automobile battery. Today, the 12-lead ECG machine is an essential mainstay of health care as a diagnostic tool.

Continuous ECG monitoring did not become common practice until the 1960s, when the first coronary care units were developed. Early cardiac monitoring consisted of monitoring for a heart rate that was too fast or too slow and for life-threatening dysrhythmias, including ventricular tachycardia (VT), ventricular fibrillation (VF), and asystole.[4] Today, cardiac monitoring is increasingly sophisticated. Technologies allow for continuous monitoring of 12 leads, and trending of many physiological variables can be performed over any time frame. Cardiac monitoring is also performed outside the critical care unit, including in the home setting. Box 8.1 lists priority patient populations for dysrhythmia monitoring.

CARDIAC PHYSIOLOGY REVIEW

The ECG detects a summation of electrical signals generated by specialized cells of the heart called *pacemaker cells*. Pacemaker cells have the property of *automaticity*, meaning that these cells can generate a stimulus or an action potential without outside

BOX 8.1   Indications for Cardiac Dysrhythmia Monitoring

- Immediate recognition of sudden cardiac arrest
- Recognition of deteriorating conditions
- Facilitate the management of dysrhythmias if not immediately life-threatening
- Syncope and palpitations (to guide appropriate management)
- Early recognition of ischemia
- Chest pain or coronary artery disease
- Major cardiac interventions
- Atrial tachyarrhythmias
- Chronic atrial fibrillation
- Sinus bradycardias
- Atrioventricular block
- After electrophysiology procedures or ablations
- After pacemaker or implantable cardioverter-defibrillator (ICD) implantation
- Arrhythmic syndromes: Wolff-Parkinson-White syndrome
- Preexisting rhythm devices
- Moderate to severe imbalance of potassium or magnesium
- Drug overdose
- Intraaortic balloon counterpulsation
- Acute decompensated heart failure or infective endocarditis
- Stroke
- Conditions requiring critical care admission
- Procedures that require moderate sedation or anesthesia

Data from American Heart Association. 2017 Update to practice standards for electrocardiographic monitoring in hospital settings: A scientific statement from the American Heart Association. *Circulation.* 2017;136:e273–e344.

stimulation. This electrical signal is conducted through specialized fibers of the conduction system to the mechanical or muscle cells of the heart where a cardiac contraction is generated. Thus there must be an electrical signal for the mechanical event of contraction to occur. The coordinated electrical activity followed by a synchronous mechanical event constitutes the *cardiac cycle.*

The heart's conduction system (Fig. 8.1) is responsible for the *cardiac cycle* (Fig. 8.2), which begins with an impulse that is generated from a small, concentrated area of pacemaker cells high in the right atrium called the *sinoatrial* (SA) *node* or *sinus node.* The SA node has the fastest rate of discharge and thus is the dominant pacemaker of the heart. The sinus node impulse quickly passes through the internodal conduction tracts and the Bachmann's bundle, conductive fibers in the right and left atria.

The impulse quickly reaches the atrioventricular (AV) node located in the area called the *AV junction,* between the atria and the ventricles. Here the impulse is slowed to allow time for ventricular filling during relaxation or ventricular *diastole.* The AV node has pacemaker properties and can discharge an impulse if the SA node fails. The electrical impulse is then rapidly conducted through the bundle of His to the ventricles via the left and right bundle branches. The left bundle branch further divides into the left anterior fascicle and the left posterior fascicle. The bundle branches divide into smaller and smaller branches, finally terminating in tiny fibers called *Purkinje fibers* that reach the myocardial muscle cells or myocytes. The bundle of His, the right and left bundle branches, and the Purkinje fibers are also known as the *His-Purkinje system.* The ventricles have pacemaker capabilities if the sinus or AV nodes cease to generate impulses.

The electrical signal stimulates the atrial muscle, called atrial *systole,* and causes the atria to contract simultaneously and eject their blood volume into the ventricles. Simultaneously, the ventricles fill with blood during ventricular diastole. During atrial systole, a bolus of atrial blood is ejected into the ventricles. This step is called the *atrial kick,* and it contributes approximately 30% more blood to the cardiac output of the ventricles. The inflow or AV valves (tricuspid and mitral) close because of the increasing pressure of the blood volume in the ventricles. By this time the electrical impulse reaches the Purkinje fibers, and the muscle cells have become stimulated and cause ventricular contraction. The outflow valves (aortic and pulmonic) open because of increased pressure and volume in the ventricles, allowing for ejection of the ventricular blood, called *ventricular systole.* At the same time ventricular systole is occurring, atrial diastole, or filling, is occurring. The atria are relaxed and filling with blood from the periphery (deoxygenated) and the lungs (oxygenated). Then, because of the rhythmic pacing of the heart, the muscle cells are again stimulated, the atria contract, and atrial blood is ejected once again into the ventricles. This process of electrical stimulation and mechanical response occurs rhythmically 60 to 100 times per minute in the normal heart. The coordination of the electrical and mechanical events in the upper and lower chambers of the heart results in the emptying and filling of these chambers, and the valves open and close because of pressure changes. These physiological actions result in what is known as *cardiac output,* which continually adjusts to the needs of the body's tissues (see Fig. 8.2).

Cardiac Electrophysiology

Specialized cardiac pacemaker cells possess the property of *automaticity* and can generate an electrical impulse on their own. Nonpacemaker or muscle cells must receive an outside stimulus in normal circumstances to generate a response. The response generated by either the pacemaker or the muscle cells once stimulated is called the *action potential.* The cardiac action potential consists of phases related to depolarization, repolarization, and the resting or polarized state of the cell. Although this summary describes the action potential of a single cell, imagine that this is occurring in millions of cardiac cells almost simultaneously, resulting in coordinated contractions of the atria and ventricles.

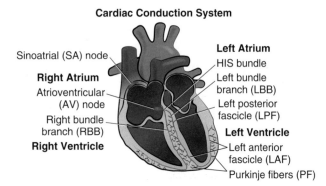

Cardiac Conduction System

Sinoatrial (SA) node
Right Atrium
Atrioventricular (AV) node
Right bundle branch (RBB)
Right Ventricle

Left Atrium
HIS bundle
Left bundle branch (LBB)
Left posterior fascicle (LPF)
Left Ventricle
Left anterior fascicle (LAF)
Purkinje fibers (PF)

Fig. 8.1 The electrical conduction system of the heart.

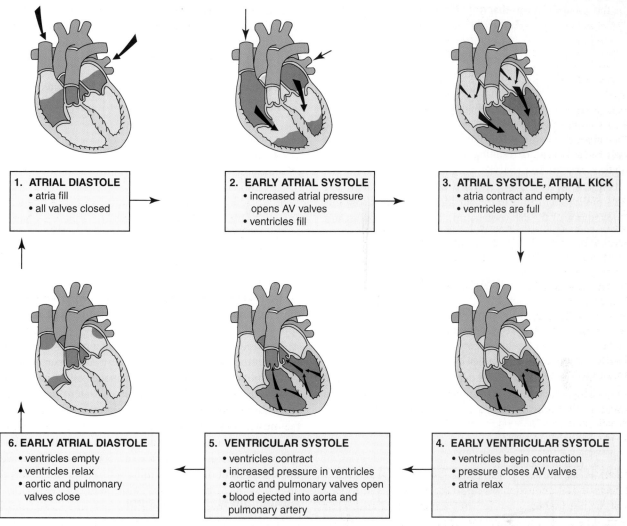

Fig. 8.2 The cardiac cycle. *AV,* Atrioventricular. (Modified from Hubert RJ, VanMeter KC. *Gould's Pathophysiology for Health Professions.* 6th ed. St. Louis, MO: Elsevier; 2018.)

During the resting state of the cell, there is a difference in polarity, or charge, between the extracellular and intracellular environments that is maintained by the cell membrane. Specialized pumps prevent ions from passing through the cell membrane by diffusion. The inside of the cell is predominantly negatively charged, whereas the outside is positively charged. The resting membrane potential occurs when the cell is in the polarized or resting state. The polarized cell has a higher concentration of positive ions, including sodium outside the cell, causing the extracellular environment to be positive. The interior of the cell is more negative, and the concentration of potassium is higher. The voltage in the interior of the cardiac muscle cell during resting membrane potential is −90 mV, whereas that of the pacemaker cells in the SA and AV nodes is −65 mV.

The stimulation of a cardiac muscle cell by an electrical impulse changes the permeability of the myocardial cell membrane. Sodium ions rush into the cell via sodium channels in the cell membrane, and potassium ions flow out of the cell, resulting in a more positively charged cell interior (Fig. 8.3). The action potential describes the flow of ions inside and outside the cell, as

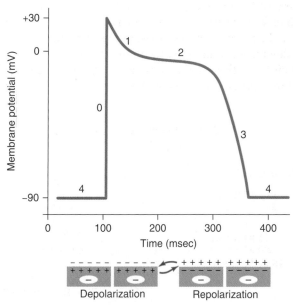

Fig. 8.3 Cardiac action potential.

well as the voltage changes that occur. The first phase of the action potential occurs when the cell membrane becomes permeable to sodium molecules. When the membrane potential reaches −65 mV, also known as *threshold,* more channels in the cell membrane open up and allow sodium ions to rush into the cell; the cell interior quickly reaches +30 mV, resulting in *depolarization.* Following this fast phase in sodium influx, the plateau phase of the action potential occurs when calcium channels open and calcium flows into the cell. This slower phase allows for a longer period of depolarization, resulting in sustained muscle contraction. The next event of the action potential occurs when the cell returns to resting state. This process is called *repolarization* and results from ions returning to the outside (calcium and sodium) and the interior of the cell (potassium). Sodium and potassium pumps within the cell membrane maintain this concentration gradient across the cell membrane when the cell is polarized. These pumps require energy in the form of adenosine triphosphate (ATP). Now the cell has returned to its resting state with a polarity of −90 mV once again. Depolarization of adjacent cells occurs simultaneously as the stimulus moves across the cardiac muscle, allowing for almost instantaneous depolarization of the entire muscle mass and resultant contraction (Fig. 8.4).

Pacemaker cells exhibit the property of *automaticity,* enabling these cells to reach threshold and depolarize without an outside stimulus. The cell membrane becomes suddenly permeable to sodium during the resting state and reaches threshold, resulting

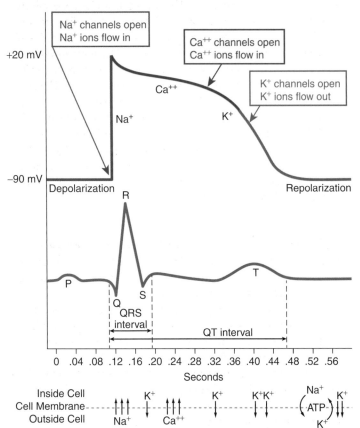

Fig. 8.4 Cardiac action potential with the electrocardiogram and movement of electrolytes. *ATP,* Adenosine triphosphate; *Ca,* calcium; *K,* potassium; *Na,* sodium.

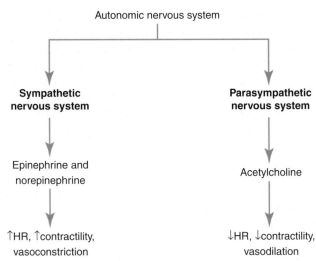

Fig. 8.5 Autonomic nervous system. *HR,* Heart rate.

in spontaneous depolarization. Resting membrane potential for these automatic cells is −65 mV, and threshold is reached at approximately −50 mV.

The sinus node reaches threshold at a rate of 60 to 100 times per minute. Because this is the fastest pacemaker in the heart, the SA node is the dominant pacemaker of the heart. The AV node and His-Purkinje pacemakers are latent pacemakers that reach threshold at a slower rate but can take over if the SA node fails or if sinus impulse conduction is blocked. The AV node has an inherent rate of 40 to 60 beats/min, and the His-Purkinje system can fire at a lower rate of 15 to 20 beats/min with an upper rate limit of 40 beats/min.

Autonomic Nervous System

The rate of spontaneous depolarization of the pacemaker cells is influenced by the autonomic nervous system. The sympathetic nervous system releases catecholamines, causing the SA node to fire more quickly in response to epinephrine and norepinephrine. The parasympathetic nervous system releases acetylcholine, which slows the heart rate. During normal circumstances these substances modulate each other, and the cardiac response allows for appropriate changes in cardiac output to meet the varying demands of the body (Fig. 8.5).

STUDY BREAK

1. What are two significant considerations when a patient's heart rate increases, manifesting with symptoms?
   A. Venous return diminishes and cardiac filling increases
   B. Venous return increases and cardiac filling decreases
   C. Ventricular filling decreases and coronary perfusion is reduced
   D. Ventricular filling increases and coronary perfusion is increased

---

THE 12-LEAD ELECTROCARDIOGRAM

The 12-lead ECG is an important diagnostic tool that provides information about myocardial ischemia, injury, cell necrosis, electrolyte disturbances, increased cardiac muscle mass (hypertrophy), conduction abnormalities, and abnormal heart rhythms.

Electrodes applied to the skin transmit the electrical signals of the movement of the cardiac impulse through the conduction system. This signal passes through skin, muscle, and bone on the patient end and finally through electrodes and wires outside of the patient's body to be amplified by the ECG machine and either transcribed to ECG paper or displayed digitally. The ECG machine records the summation of the waves of depolarization and repolarization occurring during the cardiac cycle. During the polarized or resting state, a flat, or *isoelectric,* line is inscribed that means that no current or electrical activity is occurring.

The 12-lead ECG provides a view of the electrical activity of the heart from 12 different views, both frontally and horizontally. Cardiac electrical activity is not one-dimensional; thus observation in two planes provides a more complete view in the horizontal and vertical planes. When assessing the 12-lead ECG or a rhythm strip, it is helpful to understand that the electrical activity is viewed in relation to the positive electrode of that particular lead. The positive electrode is the "viewing eye" of the camera. When an electrical signal is aimed directly at the positive electrode, an upright inflection off the isoelectric line is visualized. If the impulse is moving away from the positive electrode, a negative deflection off the isoelectric line is seen. If the signal is perpendicular to the imaginary line between the positive and negative poles of the lead, the tracing is equiphasic, with equally positive and negative deflection (Fig. 8.6). A tracing may be observed on a monitor, displayed digitally on a computer screen, or recorded on paper.

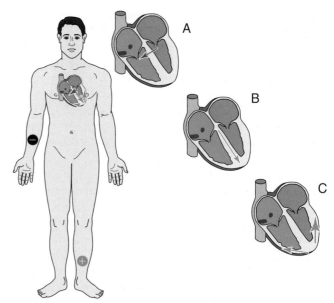

Fig. 8.7 Direction of normal current flow through the ventricles. **A,** Activation of the septum beginning on the left side of the septum moving across toward the right side of the septum. **B,** Activation moves down and to the left within the septum between both of the ventricular chambers. **C,** Activation throughout the Purkinje system.

The electrical activity of normal conduction occurs downward between the right arm and the left leg, called the *mean cardiac vector* or direction of current flow. Thus the positive electrode reflects this electrical activity by an upright inflection if the flow of current is directed at that positive electrode or a negative deflection if moving away from that positive electrode. The wave of current flow of the cardiac cycle or the vector is inscribed on the ECG paper in relation to the lead vector that is being viewed. The lead reflects the magnitude and the direction of current flow (Fig. 8.7).

The 12-lead ECG consists of three standard bipolar limb leads (I, II, and III), three augmented unipolar limb leads (aV_R, aV_L, and aV_F), and six precordial unipolar leads (V_1, V_2, V_3, V_4, V_5, and V_6). Bipolar leads consist of a positive and a negative lead, whereas the unipolar leads consist of a positive electrode and the ECG machine itself.

Standard Limb Leads

The standard three limb leads are I, II, and III. Limb leads are placed on the arms and legs. These leads are bipolar, meaning that a positive lead perspective is on one limb and a negative lead perspective is on another limb.

Lead I records the magnitude and direction of current flow between the negative lead on the right arm and the positive lead on the left arm. Lead II records activity between the negative lead on the right arm and the positive lead on the left leg. Lead III records activity from the negative lead on the left arm to the positive lead on the left leg (Fig. 8.8). The normal ECG waveforms are upright in these leads, with lead II often producing the most upright waveforms.

The bipolar limb leads form Einthoven's triangle (Fig. 8.9). This is an equilateral upside-down triangle with the heart in the center.

Three Basic Laws of Electrocardiography

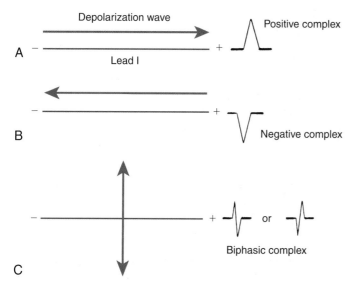

Fig. 8.6 A, A positive complex is seen in any lead if the wave of depolarization spreads toward the positive pole of the lead. **B,** A negative complex is seen if the depolarization wave spreads toward the negative pole (away from the positive pole) of the lead. **C,** A biphasic (partly positive, partly negative) complex is seen if the mean direction of the wave is at right angles. These apply to the P wave, QRS complex, and T wave. (From Goldberger AL, Goldberger ZD, Shvilkin A. *Goldberger's Clinical Electrocardiography: A Simplified Approach.* 9th ed. St. Louis, MO: Elsevier; 2018.)

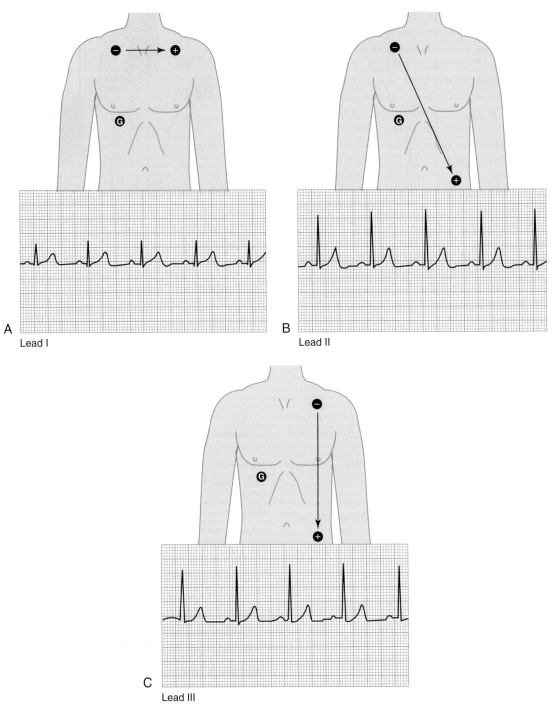

A
Lead I

B
Lead II

C
Lead III

Fig. 8.8 Standard bipolar limb leads. **A,** Lead I. **B,** Lead II. **C,** Lead III.

Augmented Limb Leads

The augmented limb leads are unipolar, meaning that they record electrical flow in only one direction. A reference point is established in the ECG machine, and electrical flow is recorded from that reference point toward the right arm (aV$_R$), the left arm (aV$_L$), and the left foot (aV$_F$) (see Fig. 8.9A–C). The *a* in the names of these leads means *augmented*; because these leads produce small ECG complexes, they must be augmented or enlarged. The *V* means *voltage* and the subscripts *R, L,* and *F* stand for *right arm, left arm,* and *left foot,* where the positive electrode is located. The augmented limb leads are displayed by using the electrodes already in place for the limb leads.

The addition of the augmented limb leads to the Einthoven's triangle form a hexaxial reference figure when the six frontal plane leads are intersected in the center of each lead (see Fig. 8.9D). The figure is used to determine the exact direction of current flow, called *axis determination,* a requisite skill of 12-lead ECG analysis. Assessment of axis deviation is an advanced skill and not addressed in this chapter. Fig. 8.9 demonstrates that leads I and aV$_L$ are in proximity, as are leads II, III, and aV$_F$.

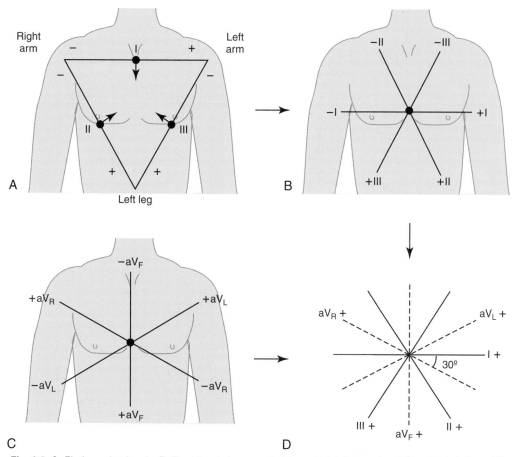

Fig. 8.9 A, Einthoven's triangle. **B,** The triangle is converted to a triaxial diagram by shifting leads I, II, and III so that they intersect at a common point. **C,** Triaxial lead diagram showing the relationship of the three augmented (unipolar) leads, aV$_R$, aV$_L$, and aV$_F$. Notice that each lead is represented by an axis with a positive and negative pole. **D,** The hexaxial reference figure combining the three axis leads from part B with the three axis leads from part C, producing the hexaxial reference.

Therefore the QRS patterns of leads that are close together usually appear similar. Because current flow is directed between the left arm and left foot, leads I, II, III, aV$_L$, and aV$_F$, the waveforms are usually positive if conduction is normal.

Precordial Leads

The six precordial leads (also called *chest leads*) are positioned on the chest wall directly over the heart. These leads provide a view of cardiac electrical activity from a horizontal plane rather than the frontal plane view of the limb leads. Precise placement of these leads is crucial for providing an accurate representation and for comparing with previous and future ECG tracings. A misplaced V lead can result in erroneous or missed diagnoses of acute coronary syndrome and lethal dysrhythmias as well as incorrect interpretation of ST segment changes. The precordial leads are unipolar, with a positive electrode and the AV node as a center reference (Fig. 8.10). Landmarks for placement of these leads are the intercostal spaces, the sternum, and the clavicular and axillary lines.

Grouping of Leads

Each lead provides a view of the electrical activity of the heart from a different angle. Leads that view the current flow in the heart from the same angle can be grouped together. Anatomical regions are described as *septal, anterior, lateral,* and *inferior.* Septal leads are V$_1$ and V$_2$; anterior leads are V$_3$ and V$_4$; lateral leads are V$_5$, V$_6$, I, and aV$_L$; and inferior leads are II, III, and aV$_F$.[3] Assessing leads that localize these regions of the heart assists in identifying the location of myocardial ischemia, injury, and infarct. Posterior and right ventricular electrodes are not commonly part of the standard 12-lead ECG; however, if indicated, newer ECG machines can record tracings from these areas. The 15-lead ECG is an additional assessment that is warranted if the patient is suspected of having an inferior myocardial infarction, because right ventricular and posterior involvement are common with this type of infarct (Fig. 8.11).

Continuous Cardiac Monitoring

Continuous cardiac monitoring is conducted in a variety of patient care settings, including the emergency department, ambulances, high-risk obstetric units, cardiac catheterization and electrophysiology laboratories, critical care units, operating rooms, postanesthesia care units, endoscopy suites, progressive care units, and outpatient settings. Depending on the sophistication of the monitoring system, any of the 12 leads can be

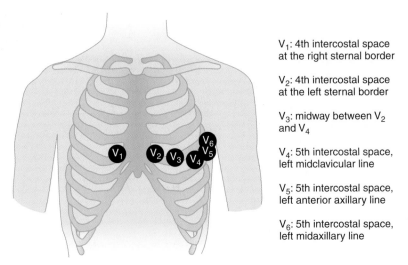

V₁: 4th intercostal space at the right sternal border

V₂: 4th intercostal space at the left sternal border

V₃: midway between V₂ and V₄

V₄: 5th intercostal space, left midclavicular line

V₅: 5th intercostal space, left anterior axillary line

V₆: 5th intercostal space, left midaxillary line

Fig. 8.10 Precordial chest leads.

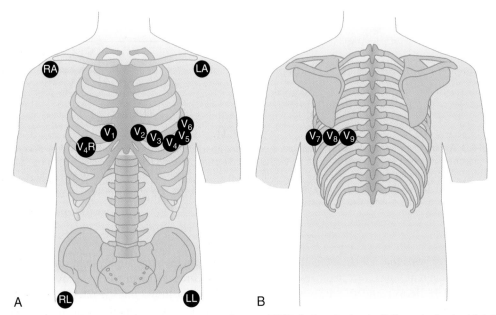

Fig. 8.11 Lead placement for a 15-lead electrocardiogram (ECG). **A,** Anterior leads. **B,** Posterior leads. *LA,* left arm; *LL,* left leg; *RA,* right arm; *RL,* right leg; *V₁–V₉,* chest leads for 15-lead ECG.

monitored continuously. The most critical elements of cardiac monitoring are in skin preparation, lead placement, and appropriate lead selection.

Skin Preparation and Lead Placement

Adequate skin preparation of electrode sites requires clipping the hair, cleansing the skin, and drying the skin. Cleansing includes washing with soap and water, or alcohol, to remove skin debris and oils.

The three-lead monitoring system depicts only the standard limb leads. These leads are marked as *RA, LA,* and *LL.* The right and left arm leads (RA and LA) are placed just above the right and left clavicles, and the leg lead (LL) is placed on the left abdominal area below the level of the umbilicus (Fig. 8.12A).

Five-lead monitoring systems that monitor all of the limb leads and one chest lead are commonly available. Instead of placing the limb leads on the arms and legs, these leads are placed just above the right and left clavicles and on the right and left abdomen below the level of the umbilicus. The precordial or chest lead is placed in the selected V lead position, usually V₁ (see Fig. 8.12B). Some five-lead systems can derive a 12-lead tracing (Fig. 8.13).

Before application, check the electrodes to ensure that the gel is moist. Attach the electrode to the lead wire and place it in the designated location. Following electrode placement, assess the signal to ensure that the waveform is clear and not disrupted by artifact. At the beginning of each shift, assess that electrodes are placed in the correct anatomical positions. Change electrodes based on institutional policy.

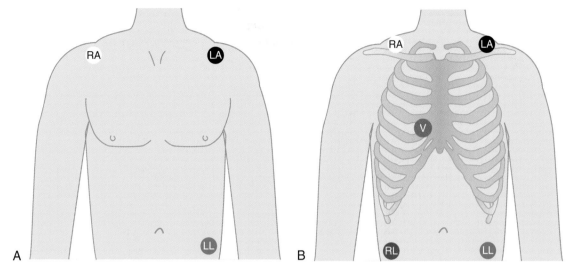

Fig. 8.12 A, Three-lead electrocardiographic (ECG) monitoring system. **B,** Five-lead monitoring system with V lead placed in V₁ position. *LA,* Left arm; *LL,* left leg; *RA,* right arm; *RL,* right leg; *V,* chest lead.

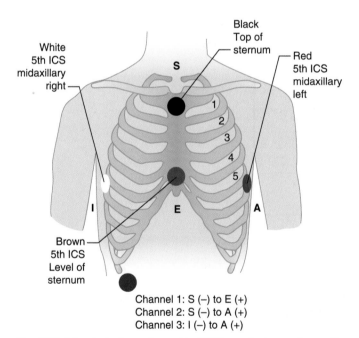

Fig. 8.13 5-Lead electrocardiographic (ECG) monitoring system with 12-lead capability. *ICS,* Intercostal space.

Determine lead selection by the patient's diagnosis and the risk for an ischemic cardiac event, dysrhythmia, or other factors. Typically, the first lead selected is V₁ for dysrhythmia monitoring. If the system is able to simultaneously monitor a second lead, selection of this lead is based on the patient's diagnosis and individual needs. A limb lead is usually selected, such as III, because of the easy visualization of P waves; however, if the patient has a history of ischemia, the second lead can be based on the patient's 12-lead ECG, identifying the lead showing the greatest ischemic change. For dysrhythmia monitoring in a system that provides continuous monitoring of two leads, V₁ and III are the standard recommendations.[1,8]

In most settings, a 6-second strip of the patient's rhythm is obtained and documented in the patient's chart at intervals from every 4 to 8 hours, based on the patient acuity level and institutional policy. In addition, it is essential to document a rhythm strip any time a change in rhythm is noted. If the patient experiences chest discomfort or other signs of myocardial ischemia or a dysrhythmia, obtain a 12-lead ECG. Many ECG machines can print a continuous 12-lead rhythm recording, allowing for assessment of a dysrhythmia from 12 different views. This is a helpful tool when diagnosing heart block, atrial dysrhythmia, or wide QRS complex tachycardia.

ST-segment monitoring allows for continuous monitoring for changes in the ST segment that may reflect myocardial ischemia.[2] The decision about which lead is selected is based on the "ST-segment fingerprint" noted on the 12-lead ECG. The lead that demonstrates the ST change warrants the lead that is monitored.[8] ST-segment monitoring is warranted in patients with acute coronary syndrome, those at risk for silent ischemia, and those who have undergone cardiac interventions such as angioplasty and stent placement.

BASICS OF DYSRHYTHMIA ANALYSIS

Measurements

ECG paper contains a standardized grid where the horizontal axis measures time and the vertical axis measures voltage or amplitude (Fig. 8.14). Larger boxes are circumscribed by darker lines and smaller boxes by lighter lines. The larger boxes contain 5 smaller boxes on the horizontal line and 5 on the vertical line, for a total of 25 per large box. Horizontally, the smaller boxes denote 0.04 second each, or 40 milliseconds (ms); the larger box contains 5 smaller horizontal boxes and thus equals 0.20 second, or 200 ms. Along the uppermost aspect of the ECG paper are vertical hash marks that occur every 15 large boxes. The area

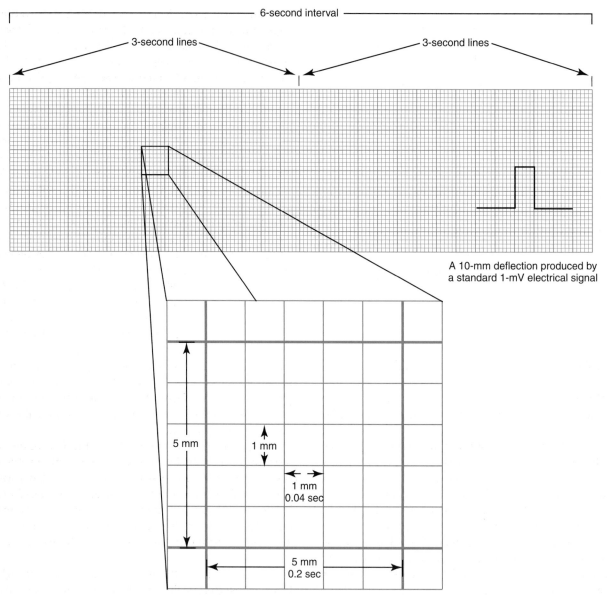

Fig. 8.14 Electrocardiogram paper records time horizontally in seconds or milliseconds. Each large box contains 25 smaller boxes, with 5 on the horizontal axis and 5 on the vertical axis. Each small horizontal box is 0.04 second, whereas each large box is 0.20 second in duration. Vertically, the graph depicts size or voltage in millivolts and in millimeters. Fifteen large boxes equal 3 seconds, and 30 large boxes equal 6 seconds used in calculating heart rate. (From Wesley K. *Huszar's ECG and 12-lead interpretation.* 5th ed. St. Louis, MO: Elsevier; 2017.)

between these marks equals 3 seconds. Some ECG paper has markings every second.

The monitoring standard is to use a 6-second rhythm strip for analysis and documentation of cardiac rhythms. A 6-second strip consists of two 3-second intervals or a span of three hash marks. The measurement of time on the ECG tracing represents the speed of depolarization and repolarization in the atria and ventricles and is printed at 25 mm/sec.

Amplitude is measured on the vertical axis of the ECG paper (see Fig. 8.14). Each small box is equal to 0.1 mV in amplitude. Waveform amplitude indicates the amount of electrical voltage generated in the various areas of the heart. Low-voltage and small waveforms are expected from the small muscle mass of

the atria. Large-voltage and large waveforms are expected from the larger muscle mass of the ventricles.

Waveforms and Intervals

The normal ECG tracing is composed of P, Q, R, S, and T waves (Fig. 8.15). These waveforms rise from a flat baseline called the *isoelectric line.*

P Wave. The P wave represents atrial depolarization. It is usually upright in leads I and II and has a rounded, symmetrical shape. The amplitude of the P wave is measured at the center of the waveform and normally does not exceed three boxes, or 3 mm, in height.

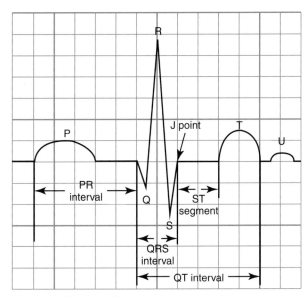

Fig. 8.15 Electrocardiogram waveforms.

Normally a P wave indicates that the SA node initiated the impulse that depolarized the atrium. However, a change in the shape of the intrinsic or baseline P wave may indicate that the impulse arose from a site in the atria other than the SA node.

PR Interval. The downslope of the P wave returns to the iso-electric line for a short time before the beginning of the QRS complex. The interval from the beginning of the P wave to the next deflection from the baseline is called the *PR interval*. The PR interval measures the time it takes for the electrical impulse to depolarize the atria, travel to the AV node, and dwell there briefly before entering the bundle of His. The normal PR interval is 0.12 to 0.20 second, three to five small boxes wide (see Fig. 8.15). When the PR interval is longer than normal, the speed of conduction is delayed in the AV node. When the PR interval is shorter than normal, the speed of conduction is abnormally fast.

QRS Complex. The QRS complex represents ventricular depolarization (see Fig. 8.15). Atrial repolarization also occurs simultaneously to ventricular depolarization, but because of the larger muscle mass of the ventricles, visualization of atrial repolarization is obscured by the QRS complex. The classic QRS complex begins with a negative, or downward, deflection immediately after the PR interval. The first negative deflection after the P wave is called the *Q wave.*

A Q wave may or may not be present before the R wave. If the first deflection from the isoelectric line is positive, or upright, the waveform is called an *R wave*. The size of the R wave varies across leads. The R wave is positive and tall in those leads where the direction of current is going toward the positive electrode lead. All limb leads, except for aV_R, normally have tall R waves. In the precordial leads, the R wave begins small and progressively becomes taller and more positive, going from small in V_1 to a maximal size in V_5. This change in size is called *R wave progression* and occurs because the direction of current flow is moving more directly toward the positive electrode of V_5 (Fig. 8.16).

The S wave is a negative waveform that follows the R wave. The S wave deflects below the isoelectric line. Some patients may have a second positive waveform in their QRS complex. If so, then that second positive waveform is called *R prime* (R′).

The term *QRS complex* is a generic term designating the waveforms representing ventricular depolarization. In reality, the complex may be an R wave, a QS wave, or other wave, depending on the lead viewed or any abnormalities that are present. Fig. 8.17 depicts the various shapes of the QRS complex and their nomenclature.

If a Q wave is present on the 12-lead ECG (not the cardiac monitor), it must be determined if it represents a pathological condition or is normal. A pathological Q wave has a width of 0.04 seconds and a depth that is greater than one-fourth the height of the R wave amplitude. Pathological Q waves are found on ECGs of individuals who have had myocardial infarctions, and they represent myocardial muscle death (Fig. 8.18).

QRS Interval. The QRS interval is measured from where it leaves the isoelectric line of the PR interval to the end of the QRS complex (see Fig. 8.15). The waveform that initiates the QRS complex (whether it is a Q wave or an R wave) marks the beginning of the interval. The normal width of the QRS complex is 0.06 to 0.10 second. This width equals 1.5 to 2.5 small boxes.

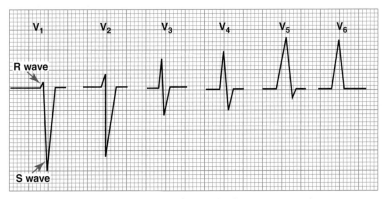

Fig. 8.16 The normal 12-lead precordial R wave progression.

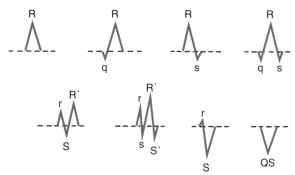

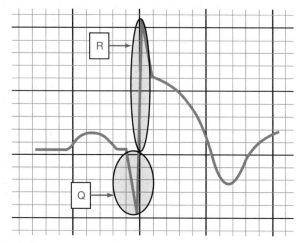

Fig. 8.17 Nomenclature for QRS complexes of various shapes: Different types of QRS complexes. An R wave is a positive waveform. A negative deflection before the R wave is a Q wave. The S wave is a negative deflection after the R wave. If the waveform is tall or deep, the letter naming the waveform is a capital letter. If the waveform is small in either direction, the waveform is labeled with a lowercase letter.

Fig. 8.18 Pathological Q wave is greater than one-fourth the height of the R wave.

A QRS width greater than 0.10 second may signify a delay in conduction through the ventricles potentially caused by a variety of factors, including myocardial infarction, atherosclerosis of the aging conduction system, or cardiomyopathy.

T Wave. The T wave represents ventricular repolarization (see Fig. 8.15). T-wave amplitude is measured at the center of the waveform and is usually no higher than five small boxes, or 5 mm. In contrast to P waves, which are usually symmetrical, T waves are usually asymmetrical. Changes in T-wave amplitude or direction can indicate electrical disturbances resulting from an electrolyte imbalance or from myocardial ischemia or injury. For example, hyperkalemia can cause tall, peaked T waves, and ischemia may cause a flattened T wave or an inverted or upside-down T wave.

Some students who are novices in dysrhythmia interpretation have difficulty differentiating the P wave and the T wave. Understanding that the P wave normally precedes the QRS complex and the T wave normally follows the QRS complex aids in identification of these waveforms. In addition, the T wave usually has greater width and amplitude than the P wave

because the atria are smaller muscle masses and therefore produce smaller waveforms than do the larger ventricles.

ST Segment. The ST segment connects the QRS complex to the T wave and is usually isoelectric, or flat. However, in some conditions the segment may be depressed (falling below baseline) or elevated (rising above baseline). The point at which the QRS complex ends and the ST segment begins is called the J (junction) *point.* ST-segment change is measured 0.04 second after the J point. To identify ST-segment elevation, use the isoelectric portion of the PR segment as a reference for baseline. Next, note whether the ST segment is level with the PR segment (see Fig. 8.15). If the ST segment is above or below the baseline, count the number of small boxes above or below at 60 ms after the J point.[2,8] A displacement in the ST segment can indicate myocardial ischemia or injury. If ST displacement is noted and is a new finding, obtain a 12-lead ECG and notify the provider. Assess the patient for signs and symptoms of myocardial ischemia.

QT Interval. The QT interval is measured from the beginning of the QRS complex to the end of the T wave (see Fig. 8.15). This interval measures the total time taken for ventricular depolarization and repolarization. Abnormal prolongation of the QT interval increases vulnerability to lethal dysrhythmias, such as VT and ventricular fibrillation. Normally, the QT interval becomes longer with slower heart rates and shortens with faster heart rates, thus requiring a correction of the value. Generally, the QT interval is less than half the R to R interval.

A preferred calculation that corrects for varying heart rates is a calculated QT interval, or *QTc,* which is based on the QT interval divided by the square root of the R to R interval. QT and QTc are routinely measured when analyzing a rhythm strip. Normal QTc is less than 0.47 second in males and 0.48 second in females. Many monitoring systems can calculate the QTc if the R to R interval is measured. QTc accuracy is based on a regular rhythm. In irregular rhythms such as atrial fibrillation, an average QTc may be necessary because the QT interval varies from beat to beat.

Risk of a lethal heart rhythm called *torsades de pointes* occurs if QTc is prolonged greater than 0.50 second.[7,8] Observe for prolonged QT intervals when medications that prolong the QT interval are started, doses are increased, or in the case of overdose.

U Wave. A final waveform that is occasionally noted on the ECG is the U wave. If present, this waveform follows the T wave, and it represents repolarization of a small segment of the ventricles or delayed repolarization. The U wave is usually small, rounded, and less than 2 mm in height (see Fig. 8.15). Larger U waves may be present in patients with hypokalemia, cardiomyopathy, and digoxin toxicity.

CAUSES OF DYSRHYTHMIAS

Dysrhythmias may occur when automaticity of the normal pacemaker cells of the heart is either stimulated or suppressed. For example, if the SA node fails to fire, latent pacemakers from the AV node or ventricles may fire as a backup safety mechanism. The SA node may fire more rapidly because of the influence of circulating catecholamines. Cells, either within or outside the normal conduction system, may take on characteristics of pacemaker cells and begin firing because of electrolyte imbalances, ischemia, injury, necrosis, and myocardial stretch caused by hypertrophy. *Ectopic beats* or *ectopic rhythms* arise from cells that normally do not have pacemaker capabilities. Slowed conduction can create alternative conductive pathways that produce abnormally fast heart rhythms. If conduction is sufficiently decreased, latent pacemakers may take over this function.

EVIDENCE-BASED PRACTICE

Implementation of Practice Standards for Electrocardiographic Monitoring

Problem

Electrocardiographic (ECG) monitoring of patients in hospitals is not often validated beyond initial competency assessment. Implementation of the American Heart Association (AHA) practice standards is influenced by the nurses' knowledge and affects quality of care and patient outcomes.

Clinical Question

What are the recommendations regarding ECG monitoring and sustained nurses' knowledge that influence quality of care and patient outcomes?

Evidence

The Practical Use of the Latest Standards of Electrocardiography (PULSE) randomized clinical trial was conducted over 6 years in 65 cardiac units at 17 hospitals. Baseline data were assessed, and outcomes were measured at time 2 after group 1 hospitals received the intervention and at time 3 after group 2 hospitals received the intervention. Measurement periods were 15 months apart. The two-part intervention consisted of an online ECG monitoring education program, including strategies to sustain practice change. Nursing knowledge was measured by a validated online test in 3013 nurses. Quality of care related to ECG monitoring was assessed by 4587 patients through on-site observation, and patient outcomes were determined by mortality, in-hospital myocardial infarction, and not surviving a cardiac arrest in 95,884 hospital admissions. Nurses' knowledge in both groups improved significantly immediately after intervention but did not demonstrate a sustained effect at 15 months. Accurate electrode placement, accurate rhythm interpretation, appropriate monitoring, and ST-segment monitoring when indicated were the indicators of quality of care and were associated with significant improvement and sustained at 15 months. In addition, in-hospital myocardial infarction declined significantly and was sustained after intervention.

Implications for Nursing

Education courses to enhance nursing knowledge and strategies to improve the quality of care and patient outcomes using standards of ECG monitoring can aid in making practice changes. Further research is needed to identify the best strategies to influence sustained change beyond 15 months.

Level of Evidence

B—Randomized clinical trial

Reference

Funk M, Fennie KP, Stephens KE, et al. Association of implementation of practice standards for electrocardiographic monitoring with nurses' knowledge, quality of care, and patient outcomes: Findings from the Practice Use of the Latest Standards of Electrocardiography (PULSE) trial. *Circ Cardiovasc Qual Outcomes.* 2017;10:e003132.

DYSRHYTHMIA ANALYSIS

Analysis of a cardiac rhythm must be conducted systematically to correctly interpret the rhythm. Proper dysrhythmia analysis includes assessment of the following:

- Atrial and ventricular rates
- Regularity of rhythm
- Measurement of PR, QRS, and QT/QTc intervals
- Shape or morphological characteristics of waveforms and their consistency
- Identification of the underlying rhythm and any noted dysrhythmia in addition to the underlying rhythm
- Patient tolerance of the rhythm
- Clinical implications of the rhythm

Rate

The rate represents how fast the heart is depolarizing. Under normal conditions, the atria and the ventricles depolarize in a regular sequence. However, each can depolarize at a different rate. P waves are used to calculate the atrial rate, and QRS waves or R waves are used to calculate the ventricular rate. Rate can be assessed in various ways that are described as follows.

Six-second method: A quick and easy estimate of heart rate can be accomplished by counting the number of P waves or QRS waves within a 6-second strip to obtain atrial and ventricular heart rates per minute. This is the optimal method for irregular rhythms. Identify the lines above the ECG paper that represent 6 seconds, and count the number of P waves within the lines; then add a zero to identify the atrial heart rate estimate for 1 minute. Next, identify the number of QRS waves in the 6-second strip and again add a zero to identify the ventricular rate (Fig. 8.19).

Large box method: In this method, two consecutive P and QRS waves are located. Count the number of large boxes between the highest points of two consecutive P waves; divide that number of large boxes into 300 to determine the atrial rate. Count the number of large boxes between the highest points of two consecutive QRS waves; divide that number of large boxes into 300 to determine the ventricular rate (Fig. 8.20). This method is accurate only if the rhythm is regular. If one large box is between the two QRS waves, the rate is 300 beats/min ($300 \div 1 = 300$); two large boxes equal 150 ($300/2 = 300$) and so on. A mnemonic can be used to simplify this method. Memorize *300-150-100-75-60-50-42-38*.

Small box method: The small box method is used to calculate a more exact rate of a regular rhythm. In this method, locate two consecutive P and QRS waves. Count the number of small boxes between the highest points of these consecutive P waves; divide that number into 1500 to determine the atrial rate. Count the number of small boxes between the highest points of two consecutive QRS waves; divide that number into 1500 to determine the ventricular rate (Fig. 8.21). This method is accurate only if the rhythm is regular. Charts are available to calculate heart rate based on the rule of 1500.

Cardiac monitors continuously display heart rates. However, always verify the accuracy of the displayed rate using one of the rate calculation methods described.

Lead II

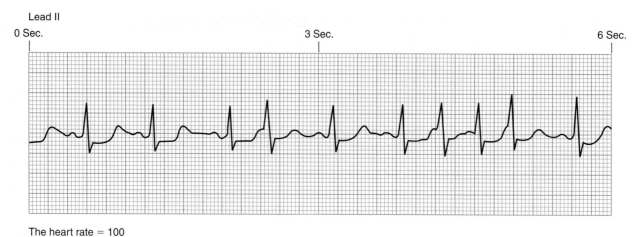

The heart rate = 100

Fig. 8.19 Six-second method of rate calculation.

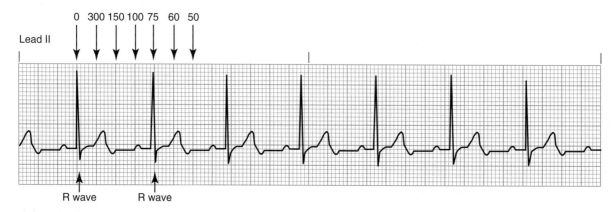

Big Box Method of Heart Rate Calculation

- Identify an R wave on a solid vertical line.
- Count the number of big boxes between the first and the following R waves.
- Divide 300 by the number of big boxes between R waves or count the cadence (300...150...100...75...60) representing the big boxes between R waves.

NOTE: Since the position of the second R wave occurs with the arrow reading 75, the heart rate in this example is approximately 75 beats/min.

Fig. 8.20 Large box method of heart rate calculation.

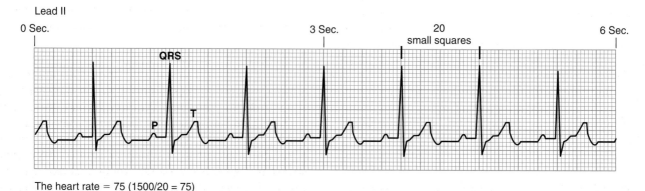

The heart rate = 75 (1500/20 = 75)

Fig. 8.21 Small box method of heart rate calculation.

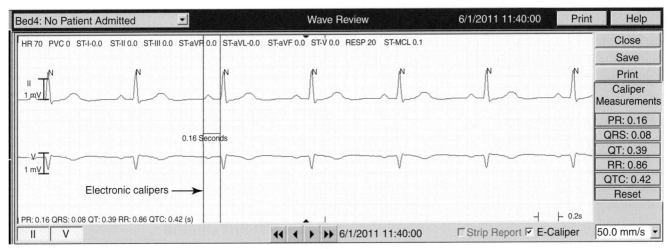

Fig. 8.22 Electronic calipers. (Courtesy Philips Healthcare, Andover, MA.)

Regularity

Regularity is assessed by using electronic or physical calipers, or a piece of paper and pencil. To determine atrial regularity, identify the P wave and place one caliper point on the peak of the P wave. Locate the next P wave and place the second caliper point on its peak. The second point is left stationary, and the calipers are flipped over. If the first caliper point lands exactly on the next P wave, the atrial rhythm is regular. If the point lands one small box or less away from the next P wave, the rhythm is essentially regular. If the point lands more than one small box away, the rhythm is considered irregular. Electronic calipers on some monitoring systems are used in the same way. For example, Fig. 8.22 depicts use of electronic calipers in measuring the PR interval.

The same process can be performed with a simple piece of paper. Place the paper parallel and below the rhythm line, make a hash mark below the first and second P waves, then move the paper over to determine if the distance between the second and third P waves is equal to that between the first and second P waves. When an atrial rhythm is regular, each P wave is an equal distance from the next P wave.

This process is also used to assess ventricular regularity, except that a line marking the peak of two consecutive R waves is used. One pencil line is placed under one R wave, and the other pencil line is placed under the next R wave. Then the paper is moved to the second and third R waves to determine if the R wave comes as expected. Then the paper is moved down the rhythm strip to determine if the subsequent R waves land on the hash mark. If the hash mark is more than one small box away from the next R wave, the rhythm is irregular (Fig. 8.23).

Irregular rhythms can be regularly irregular or irregularly irregular. Regularly irregular rhythms have a pattern. Irregularly irregular rhythms have no pattern and no predictability. Atrial fibrillation is an example of an irregularly irregular rhythm.

Measurement of PR, QRS, and QT/QTc Intervals

PR, QRS, and QT/QTc intervals are measured and documented as part of rhythm analysis. In some dysrhythmias, intervals such

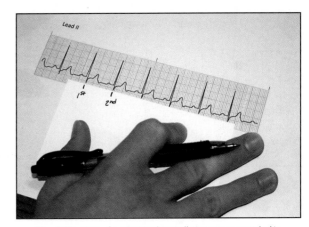

Fig. 8.23 Use of paper and pencil to assess regularity.

as the PR interval may change; thus all PR intervals are measured to ensure that they are consistent. QRS intervals can lengthen in response to new bundle branch blocks or with ventricular dysrhythmias. QT/QTc intervals can lengthen in response to certain medications as well as electrolyte imbalances. Intervals are measured with calipers or paper and pencil as previously described by identifying the number of small boxes and multiplying by 0.04 second. If the end of the interval being measured falls between boxes, add 0.02 to the measurement, as this is the time allowed for half of a box of measurement.

Morphological Characteristics of Waveforms

Assess the P, QRS, and T waves of the rhythm strip for shape and consistency. All waveforms should look alike in the normal ECG. Abnormal shapes may indicate that the stimulus that caused the waveform came from an ectopic focus, or that there is a delay or block in conduction creating a bundle branch block. It is important to also confirm that a P wave precedes the QRS complex and that the T wave follows the QRS complex. Several dysrhythmias are characterized by abnormal location or sequencing of waveforms, such as the P waves in complete heart block.

Identification of Underlying Rhythm and Any Noted Dysrhythmia

Identify the underlying rhythm first. After this step, determine the dysrhythmia that disrupts the underlying rhythm.

Patient Tolerance of the Rhythm and Clinical Implications of the Rhythm

Once an abnormal heart rhythm is identified, the priority is to assess the patient for any symptoms that may be related to the dysrhythmia (Box 8.2). Assess for hemodynamic deterioration: obtain vital signs, assess for alterations in level of consciousness, auscultate lung sounds, and ask the patient if dyspnea or chest discomfort are present. Instability is manifested by any of the following: hypotension, acutely altered mental status, signs of shock, ischemic chest discomfort, or acute heart failure. In addition, obtain a 12-lead ECG to aid in identifying the dysrhythmia.

The next step is to determine if there are causes of the dysrhythmia that can be treated immediately. An example is a patient with a fast, wide complex tachycardia who has a pulse but low blood pressure. The immediate priority is to treat the patient's fast heart rhythm with a therapy such as emergent cardioversion, but the next critical step is to identify potential causes of the dysrhythmia, such as hypokalemia, hypomagnesemia, hypoxemia, or ischemia.

BASIC DYSRHYTHMIAS

The basic dysrhythmias are classified based on their site of origin, including:
- SA node
- Atrial
- AV node or junctional
- Ventricular
- Heart blocks of the AV node

The following discussion reviews the ECG characteristics and provides examples of each dysrhythmia. Specific criteria that can be used to recognize and identify dysrhythmias are presented systematically for each one. The discussion includes typical causes, patient responses, and appropriate treatment. Medications used to treat common dysrhythmias are described in Table 8.1.

BOX 8.2   Symptoms of Decreased Cardiac Output

- Change in level of consciousness
- Chest discomfort
- Hypotension
- Shortness of breath; respiratory distress
- Pulmonary congestion; crackles
- Rapid, slow, or weak pulse
- Dizziness
- Syncope
- Fatigue
- Restlessness

TABLE 8.1   Pharmacology

Antidysrhythmic Medication Classifications

Class[a]	Description	Examples
IA	Inhibits the fast sodium channel	Quinidine, procainamide, disopyramide, ajmaline
	Prolongs repolarization time	
	Used to treat atrial and ventricular dysrhythmias	
IB	Inhibits the fast sodium channel	Lidocaine, mexiletine
	Shortens the action potential duration	
	Used to treat ventricular dysrhythmias only	
IC	Inhibits the fast sodium channel	Flecainide, propafenone
	Shortens the action potential duration of only Purkinje fibers	
	Controls ventricular tachydysrhythmias resistant to other medication therapies	
	Has proarrhythmic effects	
II	Causes beta-adrenergic blockade	Metoprolol, esmolol, propranolol, atenolol, timolol, carvedilol, sotalol
III	Lengthens the action potential	Amiodarone, dronedarone, sotalol, bretylium, ibutilide, dofetilide
	Acts on the repolarization phase	
IV	Blocks the slow inward movement of calcium to slow impulse conduction, especially in the atrioventricular node	Diltiazem, verapamil, nifedipine
	Used for treatment of supraventricular tachycardias	
V	Opens the potassium channel	Adenosine, digoxin, magnesium sulfate

[a]Class I, sodium channel blockers; Class II, beta-adrenergic blockers; Class III, potassium channel blockers; Class IV, calcium channel blockers; Class V, antiarrhythmics.

Adapted from Gahart B, Nazareno A, Ortega MQ. *Gahart's 2019 Intravenous Medications.* 35th ed. St. Louis, MO: Elsevier; 2019.

The learner who is new to identification of dysrhythmias will benefit from extensive practice in reading rhythm strips and collaborating with experienced colleagues who are adept at rhythm interpretation. Maintaining a pocket notebook (or using handheld devices with cardiac rhythm applications) with ECG criteria for each rhythm helps the learner memorize the criteria specific for common dysrhythmias. Other suggested learning aids are to complete a classroom or online course in basic rhythm interpretation. Finally, mastering the identification of dysrhythmias requires practice, practice, and more practice. Another essential assessment skill is recognition of hemodynamic instability related to decreased cardiac output associated with some dysrhythmias (see Box 8.2).

Normal Sinus Rhythm

Normal sinus rhythm (NSR) reflects normal conduction of the sinus impulse through the atria and ventricles. Any deviation from sinus rhythm is a dysrhythmia; thus it is critical to remember and understand the criteria that determine NSR.

Sinus rhythm is initiated by an impulse in the sinus node. The generated impulse propagates through the conductive fibers of the atria, reaches the AV node where there is a slight pause, and then spreads throughout the ventricles, causing depolarization and resultant cardiac contraction in a timely and organized manner (Fig. 8.24).

Rhythm Analysis

- *Rate:* Atrial and ventricular rates are the same and range from 60 to 100 beats/min.
- *Regularity:* Rhythm is regular or essentially regular.
- *Interval measurements:* PR interval is 0.12 to 0.20 second. QRS interval is 0.06 to 0.10 second.
- *Shape and sequence:* P and QRS waves are consistent in shape. P waves are small and rounded. A P wave precedes every QRS complex, which is then followed by a T wave.
- *Hemodynamic effect:* Patient is hemodynamically stable.

Dysrhythmias of the Sinoatrial Node

Sinus Tachycardia. Tachycardia is defined as a heart rate greater than 100 beats/min. Sinus tachycardia results when the SA node fires faster than 100 beats/min (Fig. 8.25). Sinus tachycardia is a normal response to stimulation of the sympathetic nervous system. Sinus tachycardia is also a normal finding in children younger than 6 years of age.

Rhythm analysis.
- *Rate:* Both atrial and ventricular rates are greater than 100 beats/min, up to 160 beats/min, but may be as high as 180 beats/min.
- *Regularity:* Onset is gradual rather than abrupt. Sinus tachycardia is regular or essentially regular.
- *Interval measurements:* PR interval is 0.12 to 0.20 second (at higher rates, the P wave may not be readily visible). QRS interval is 0.06 to 0.10 second. QT may shorten.
- *Shape and sequence:* P and QRS waves are consistent in shape. P waves are small and rounded. A P wave precedes every QRS complex, which is then followed by a T wave.
- *Patient response:* The fast heart rhythm may cause a decrease in cardiac output because of the shorter filling time for the ventricles. Vulnerable populations are those with ischemic heart disease who are adversely affected by the shorter time for coronary filling during diastole.

Lead II

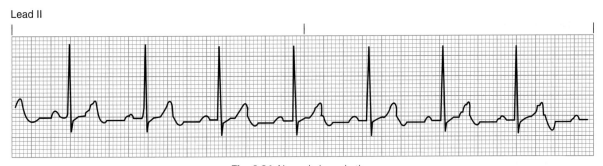

Fig. 8.24 Normal sinus rhythm.

Lead II

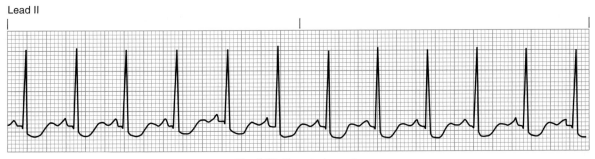

Fig. 8.25 Sinus tachycardia.

Lead II

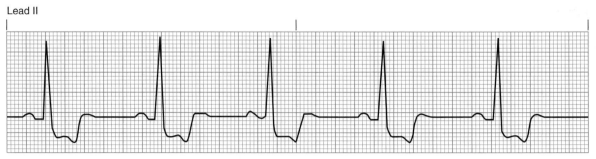

Fig. 8.26 Sinus bradycardia.

- *Causes:* Hyperthyroidism, hypovolemia, heart failure, anemia, exercise, use of stimulants, fever, and sympathetic response to fear or pain and anxiety may each cause sinus tachycardia.
- *Care and treatment:* The dysrhythmia itself is not treated, but the cause is identified and treated appropriately. For example, pain medications are administered to treat pain, or antipyretics are given to treat fever.

Sinus Bradycardia. Bradycardia is defined as a heart rate less than 60 beats/min. Sinus bradycardia may be a normal heart rhythm for some individuals such as athletes, or it may occur during sleep. Although sinus bradycardia may be asymptomatic, it may cause instability if it results in a decrease in cardiac output. The key is to assess the patient and determine if the bradycardia is accompanied by signs of instability (Fig. 8.26).

Rhythm analysis.
- *Rate:* Both atrial and ventricular rates are less than 60 beats/min.
- *Regularity:* Rhythm is regular or essentially regular.
- *Interval measurements:* Measurements are normal, but QT may be prolonged.
- *Shape and sequence:* P and QRS waves are consistent in shape. P waves are small and rounded. A P wave precedes every QRS complex, which is then followed by a T wave.
- *Patient response:* The slowed heart rhythm may cause a decrease in cardiac output, resulting in hypotension and decreased organ perfusion.
- *Causes:* Vasovagal response; medications such as digoxin or AV nodal blocking agents, including calcium channel blockers and beta blockers; myocardial infarction; normal physiological variant in the athlete; disease of the sinus node; increased intracranial pressure; hypoxemia; and hypothermia may cause sinus bradycardia.
- *Care and treatment:* Assess for hemodynamic instability related to the bradycardia. If the patient is symptomatic, interventions include administration of atropine. If atropine is not effective in increasing heart rate, then transcutaneous pacing, dopamine infusion, or epinephrine infusion may be administered.[3,6] Atropine is avoided for treatment of bradycardia associated with hypothermia.

> **! CLINICAL ALERT**
>
> ***Clinical Indications Suggesting Symptomatic Findings***
>
> - Anxiety
> - Chest pain or pressure
> - Dizziness
> - Fainting or near-fainting
> - Fatigue
> - Lightheadedness
> - Pounding in the chest
> - Shortness of breath
> - Weakness

Sinus Arrhythmia. Sinus arrhythmia is a cyclical change in heart rate that is associated with respiration. The heart rate slightly increases during inspiration and slightly slows during exhalation because of changes in vagal tone. The ECG tracing demonstrates an alternating pattern of faster and slower heart rate that changes with the respiratory cycle (Fig. 8.27).

Rhythm analysis.
- *Rate:* Atrial and ventricular rates are between 60 and 100 beats/min.
- *Regularity:* This rhythm is cyclically irregular, slowing with exhalation and increasing with inspiration.
- *Interval measurements:* Measurements are normal.
- *Shape and sequence:* P and QRS waves are consistent in shape. P waves are small and rounded. A P wave precedes every QRS complex, which is then followed by a T wave.
- *Patient response:* This rhythm is tolerated well.
- *Care and treatment:* No treatment is required.

Sinus Pauses. Sinus pauses occur when the SA node either fails to generate an impulse (sinus arrest) or the impulse is blocked and does not exit from the SA node (sinus exit block). The result of the sinus node not firing is a pause without any electrical activity.

Lead V1

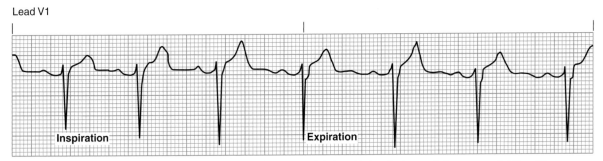

Fig. 8.27 Sinus arrhythmia. The heart rate increases slightly with inspiration and decreases slightly with expiration.

| Lead II

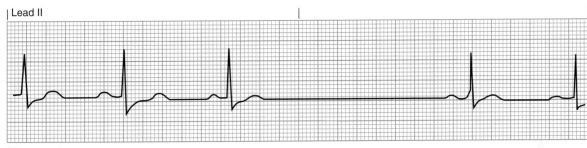

A Sinus arrest

| Lead II

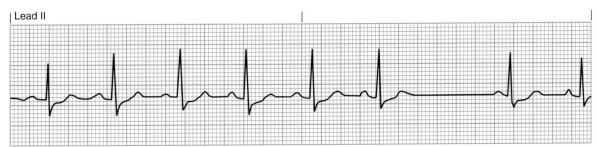

B Sinus exit block   **Fig. 8.28 A,** Sinus arrest. **B,** Sinus exit block.

Sinus arrest. Failure of the SA node to generate an impulse is called *sinus arrest.* The arrest results from a lack of stimulus from the SA node. The sinus beat following the arrest is not on time because the sinus node has been reset and the next sinus impulse begins a new rhythm. The result is that no atrial or ventricular depolarization occurs for one heartbeat or more (Fig. 8.28A).

If the pause is long enough, the AV node or ventricular backup pacemaker may fire, resulting in escape beats. These beats are called *junctional escape* or *ventricular escape beats.* Typically, the sinus node resumes normal generation of impulses following the pause.

Sinus exit block. Sinus exit block also results in a pause, but the P wave following the pause in rhythm is on time or regular because the sinus node does not reset. The sinus impulse simply fails to "exit" the sinus node (see Fig. 8.28B).

Rhythm analysis.
- *Rate:* Atrial and ventricular rates are usually between 60 and 100 beats/min, but any pause may result in a heart rate less than 60 beats/min.
- *Regularity:* The rhythm is irregular for the period of the pause but regular when sinus rhythm resumes. In SA exit

block, the P wave following the pause occurs on time. In sinus arrest, the P wave following the pause is not on time.
- *Interval measurements:* Measurements of conducted beats are normal.
- *Shape and sequence:* P and QRS waves are consistent in shape. P waves are small and rounded. A P wave precedes every QRS complex, which is then followed by a T wave.
- *Patient response:* Single pauses in rhythm may not be significant, but frequent pauses may result in a severe bradycardia. The patient with multiple pauses may experience signs and symptoms of decreased cardiac output (see Box 8.2).
- *Causes:* Hypoxemia; ischemia or damage of the sinus node related to myocardial infarction; AV nodal blocking medications such as beta blockers, calcium channel blockers, and digoxin; and increased vagal tone may cause sinus exit block.
- *Care and treatment:* If the patient is symptomatic, treatment may be needed, including temporary and permanent insertion of a pacemaker. Collaborate with the provider and pharmacist to explore causes, and discuss the need to adjust medications.

Dysrhythmias of the Atria

Normally, the SA node is the dominant pacemaker initiating the heart rhythm; however, cells outside the SA node within the atria can create an ectopic focus that can cause a dysrhythmia. An ectopic focus is an abnormal beat or a rhythm that occurs outside the normal conduction system. In this case, atrial dysrhythmias arise in the atrial tissue.

> ### ❓ CRITICAL REASONING ACTIVITY
>
> You are working in the critical care unit and a patient's heart rate suddenly decreases from 88 to 50 beats/min. What are potential reasons for the decreased heart rate? What assessments will you make?

Premature Atrial Contractions. A premature atrial contraction (PAC) is a single ectopic beat arising from atrial tissue, not the sinus node. The PAC occurs earlier than the next normal beat and interrupts the regularity of the underlying rhythm. The P wave of the PAC has a different shape than the sinus P wave because it arises from a different area in the atria; it may follow or be in the T wave of the preceding normal beat. If the early P wave is in the T wave, this T wave will look different from the T wave of a normal beat. Following the PAC, a pause occurs and then the underlying rhythm typically resumes. The pause is noncompensatory, which means that when measuring the P to P intervals for atrial regularity, the P wave following the pause does not occur on time. Box 8.3 discusses how to distinguish compensatory and noncompensatory pauses. PACs are common but denote an irritable area in the atria that has developed the property of automaticity (Fig. 8.29A).

Nonconducted PACs are beats that create an early P wave but are not followed by a QRS complex. The ventricles are unable to depolarize in response to this early stimulus because they are not fully repolarized from the normally conducted beat preceding the PAC (see Fig. 8.29B). This creates a pause, but a P wave occurs either in or after the T wave. This is why comparing the shapes of the normal PQRST is a critical requirement in rhythm analysis. The frequency of occurrence of PACs varies (Box 8.4).

BOX 8.3 Compensatory Versus Noncompensatory Pause

- Analyze a rhythm strip with a premature beat using calipers or paper and pencil.
- Locate two consecutive normal beats just before the premature beat and place the caliper points or pencil marks on the R wave of each normal beat.
- Flip the calipers (or paper) over, to where the next normal beat should have occurred. The premature beat occurs early.
- Avoid losing placement and flip the calipers (or paper) over one more time. If the point of the calipers or the mark on the paper lands exactly on the next normal beat's R wave, the sinus node compensated for the one premature beat and kept its normal rhythm (see figure).
- If the caliper point or pencil mark does not land on the next normal beat's R wave, the sinus node did not compensate and had to establish a new rhythm, resulting in a noncompensatory pause.

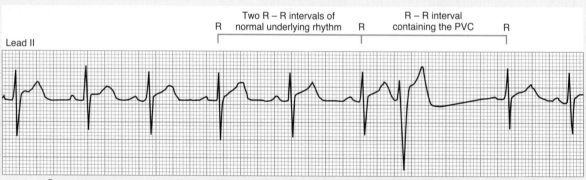

Compensatory pause; sinus rhythm with premature ventricular contraction (PVC). The pause following the PVC is compensatory. (From Paul S, Hebra JD. *The nurse's guide to cardiac rhythm interpretation: implications for patient care.* Philadelphia: Saunders; 1998.)

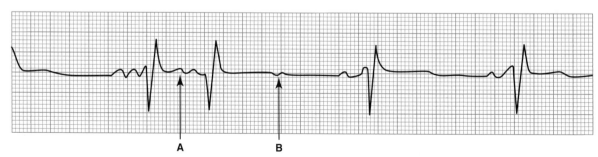

Fig. 8.29 A, Premature atrial contractions (PACs) shown in the third beat. **B,** A nonconducted PAC.

Rhythm analysis.

- *Rate:* The rate matches that of the underlying rhythm.
- *Regularity:* The PAC interrupts the regularity of the underlying rhythm for a single beat. The PAC is followed by a noncompensatory pause (see Box 8.3).
- *Interval measurements:* The PAC may have a different PR interval than the normal sinus beat, usually shorter.
- *Shape and sequence:* The P wave of the PAC is typically a different shape than the sinus P wave. The T wave of the preceding beat may be distorted if the P wave of the PAC lies within it.
- *Patient response:* Premature atrial contractions are usually well tolerated, although the patient may complain of palpitations.
- *Causes:* Stimulants such as caffeine or tobacco, myocardial hypertrophy or dilation, ischemia, lung disease, hypokalemia, and hypomagnesemia may cause PACs. It may also be a normal variant.
- *Care and treatment:* Increasing numbers of PACs may occur before atrial fibrillation or atrial flutter. No treatment is indicated for PACs.

STUDY BREAK

2. You are asked to look at a patient's rhythm strip and notice that there are no P waves in the rhythm. Your understanding of the rhythm is that the patient may have:

A. Sinus rhythm
B. Sinus arrhythmia
C. Junctional rhythm
D. Premature atrial contractions

Atrial Tachycardia. Atrial tachycardia is a rapid rhythm that arises from an ectopic focus in the atria. Because of the fast rate, atrial tachycardia can be life-threatening. The ectopic atrial focus generates impulses more rapidly than the AV node can conduct while still in the refractory phase from the previous impulse, and these impulses are not transmitted to the ventricles. Therefore more P waves may be seen than QRS complexes and T waves. This refractoriness serves as a safety mechanism to prevent the ventricles from contracting too rapidly. The AV node may block impulses in a set pattern, such as every second, third, or fourth beat. However, if the ventricles respond to every ectopic atrial impulse, it is called 1:1 conduction, one P wave for each QRS complex. Because the P wave arises outside the sinus node, the shape is different from the sinus P wave (Fig. 8.30).

If an abnormal P wave cannot be visualized on the ECG but the QRS complex is narrow, the term *supraventricular tachycardia (SVT)* is often used. This is a generic term that describes any tachycardia that is not ventricular in origin; it is also used when the source above the ventricles cannot be identified, usually because the rate is too fast.

Rhythm analysis.

- *Rate:* The rate ranges from 150 to 250 beats/min.
- *Regularity:* The rhythm is regular if all P waves are conducted.
- *Interval measurements:* The PR interval is different from the sinus PR interval. If the ectopic P wave arises near the junction, the PR interval may be shortened. If close to the sinus node, it is nearer the normal PR interval in duration.
- *Shape and sequence:* The P wave shape is different from that of the sinus P wave. The QRS complex is narrow unless there is a bundle branch block. If the P wave of the ectopic rhythm occurs in the T wave, this may alter the shape.
- *Patient response:* The faster the tachycardia, the more symptomatic the patient may become. This arises from decreased cardiac output (see Box 8.2) and resultant decreased organ perfusion.
- *Causes:* Atrial tachycardia can occur in patients with normal hearts as well as those with cardiac disease. Causes include digitalis toxicity, electrolyte imbalances, lung disease, ischemic heart disease, and cardiac valvular abnormalities.
- *Care and treatment:* Assess the patient's tolerance of the tachycardia. If the rate is greater than 150 beats/min and the patient is symptomatic, emergent cardioversion is considered. *Cardioversion* is the delivery of a synchronized electrical shock to the heart by an external defibrillator (see Chapter 11). Medications that may be used include adenosine, beta-blockers, calcium channel blockers, and amiodarone.[3,7]

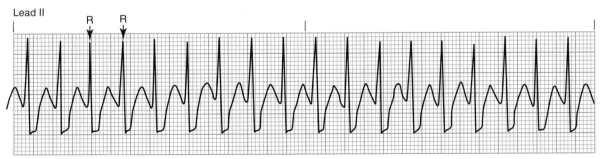

Lead II   R   R

Fig. 8.30 Atrial tachycardia with 1:1 conduction. *R,* R wave of the QRS complex.

Wandering Atrial Pacemaker. Wandering atrial pacemaker is a dysrhythmia characterized by at least three different ectopic atrial foci followed by a QRS complex at a rate less than 100 beats/min. At least three different P wave shapes are noted. P waves in wandering atrial pacemaker can be upright, inverted, flat, pointed, notched, or slanted in different directions. The PR interval varies because the impulses originate from different locations within the atria, taking various times to reach the AV node (Fig. 8.31).

Rhythm analysis.
- *Rate:* Rate is less than 100 beats/min.
- *Regularity:* The rate may be slightly irregular.
- *Interval measurements:* PR intervals vary based on the sites of the ectopic foci.
- *Shape and sequence:* At least three different P shapes are noted. The QRS complex is narrow and followed by a T wave.
- *Patient response:* Patients usually tolerate this rhythm unless the rate increases.
- *Causes:* May occur in lung disease, such as chronic obstructive pulmonary disease, or be a normal variant in the young and in older adults.
- *Care and treatment:* No treatment is usually indicated.

Multifocal Atrial Tachycardia. Multifocal atrial tachycardia is essentially the same as wandering atrial pacemaker, except the heart rate exceeds 100 beats/min (Fig. 8.32). At least three ectopic P waves are noted. This dysrhythmia is found almost exclusively in the patient with chronic obstructive pulmonary disease. Pulmonary hypertension occurs and results in increased atrial pressure and dilation, creating irritable atrial foci.

Rhythm analysis.
- *Rate:* The heart rate is greater than 100 beats/min.
- *Regularity:* The rhythm is slightly irregular.
- *Interval measurements:* PR intervals vary.
- *Shape and sequence:* P waves differ in shape. A P wave precedes every QRS complex, which is followed by a T wave.
- *Patient response:* The response varies and is determined by the patient's tolerance of the tachycardia.
- *Causes:* Chronic obstructive pulmonary disease causes dilation of the atria with resultant ectopic foci from the stretched tissue.
- *Care and treatment:* The treatment goal is to optimize the patient's pulmonary status.

Atrial Flutter. Atrial flutter arises from a single irritable focus in the atria. The atrial focus fires at an extremely rapid, regular rate, between 240 and 320 beats/min. An ECG tracing with a rate faster than 340 beats/min is designated as *type II flutter;* the mechanism remains undefined. The P waves are called *flutter waves* and have a sawtooth appearance (Fig. 8.33A). The ventricular response may be regular or irregular based on how many flutter waves are conducted through the AV node. The number of flutter waves to each QRS complex is called the conduction ratio. The conduction ratio may remain the same or vary depending on the number of flutter waves that are conducted to the ventricles. The description of atrial flutter might be constant at 2:1, 3:1, 4:1, 5:1, and so forth, or it may be variable. Flutter waves occur through the QRS complex and the T wave and often alter their appearance (see Fig. 8.33A). It is helpful to identify the best lead for visualizing the flutter waves in atrial flutter and use this as the second monitor lead.

Lead II

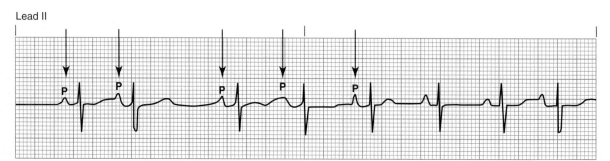

Fig. 8.31 Wandering atrial pacemaker. *Arrows* indicate different shapes of P waves.

Lead II

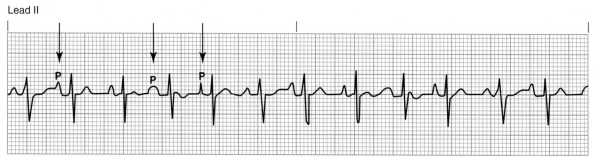

Fig. 8.32 Multifocal atrial tachycardia. *Arrows* indicate different shapes of P waves.

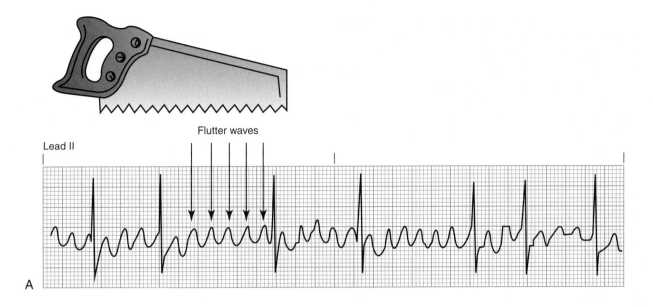

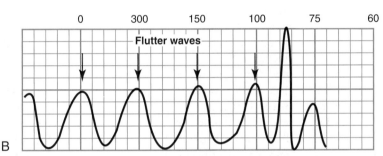

Fig. 8.33 Atrial flutter. **A,** Flutter waves show a sawtooth pattern at an atrial rate of 250 to 350 beats/min. **B,** Enlarged view shows one large box between flutter waves.

Rhythm analysis.

- *Rate:* Atrial rate is between 240 and 320 beats/min but is typically 300 beats/min (one large box between flutter waves; see Fig. 8.33B). Ventricular rate is determined by the conduction ratio of the flutter waves.
- *Regularity:* Flutter waves are regular, but the QRS complex and T waves may not be regular depending on the conduction ratio of the atrial flutter.
- *Interval measurements:* No PR interval is present. QRS and QT intervals are normal unless distorted by a flutter wave.
- *Shape and sequence:* P or flutter waves are consistent in shape and look like teeth on a saw blade. QRST waves are altered in shape by the flutter waves.
- *Patient response:* Usually the patient is asymptomatic unless atrial flutter results in a tachycardia called rapid ventricular response (RVR). Atrial flutter with RVR occurs when atrial impulses cause a ventricular response greater than 100 beats/min.
- *Causes:* Lung disease, ischemic heart disease, hyperthyroidism, hypoxemia, heart failure, and alcoholism can cause atrial flutter.
- *Care and treatment:* Alterations in atrial blood flow leading to blood stasis can cause clot formation. Patients identified with atrial flutter usually receive chronic antithrombotic

therapy unless contraindicated. Rate control is accomplished with medications that block the AV node. Elective cardioversion may be performed once the patient has been taking anticoagulants for approximately 3 weeks before and 4 weeks after cardioversion.[5] Interventional electrophysiological treatments, including ablation of the irritable focus, may be indicated.[5]

Atrial Fibrillation. Atrial fibrillation is the most common dysrhythmia observed in clinical practice. Atrial fibrillation arises from multiple ectopic foci in the atria, causing chaotic quivering of the atria and ineffectual atrial contraction. The AV node is bombarded with hundreds of atrial impulses and conducts these impulses in an unpredictable manner to the ventricles. The atrial rate may be as high 700 and no discernible P waves can be identified, resulting in a wavy baseline and an extremely irregular ventricular response. This irregularity is called *irregularly irregular* (Fig. 8.34). The ineffectual contraction of the atria results in loss of atrial kick. If too many impulses conduct to the ventricles, atrial fibrillation with RVR may result and compromise cardiac output. When atrial fibrillation occurs sporadically, it is called *paroxysmal atrial fibrillation.*

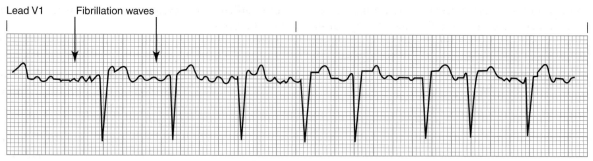

Fig. 8.34 Atrial fibrillation.

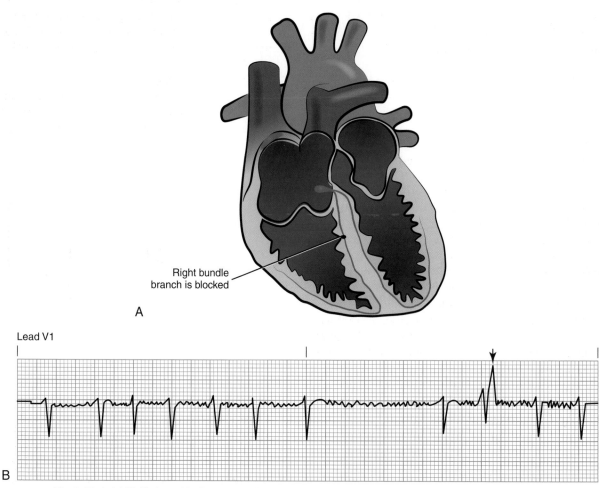

Fig. 8.35 Atrial fibrillation with aberrant conduction. **A,** The site in the right bundle branch that has not repolarized in time. **B,** The manifestation of the QRS complex (aberrantly conducted beat) in the ninth beat *(arrow)* caused by the nonrepolarized tissue.

If the atrial impulse is conducted through the ventricles in a normal fashion, the QRS complex is narrow and appears normal, although the rhythm is irregularly irregular. However, if the impulse reaches one of the bundle branches before full repolarization, the QRS complex is widened in classic bundle branch block morphological finding. The widened QRS is due to the delay caused by the bundle branch block and results in slowed conduction through either the right or the left ventricle, depending on which bundle branch has not fully repolarized.

When this event occurs, the impulse is said to be aberrantly conducted (Fig. 8.35).

In atrial fibrillation, aberrantly conducted beats are referred to as Ashman beats. Ashman beats are more likely to occur when an atrial impulse arrives at the AV node just after a previously conducted impulse (see Fig. 8.35; note that the ninth beat has this appearance). Ashman beats are often seen when the rate changes from slower to faster, referred to as a long-short cycle. Ashman beats are not clinically significant.

One complication of atrial fibrillation is thromboembolism. The blood that collects in the atria is agitated by fibrillation, and normal clotting is accelerated. Small thrombi, called *mural thrombi,* begin to form along the walls of the atria. These clots may dislodge, resulting in pulmonary embolism or stroke.

Rhythm analysis.

- *Rate:* Atrial rate is uncountable; ventricular rate may vary widely.
- *Regularity:* Ventricular response is irregularly irregular.
- *Interval measurements:* PR interval is absent. The QRS complex and QT interval are normal in duration unless a bundle branch block exists.
- *Shape and sequence:* No recognizable or discernible P waves are present. The isoelectric line is wavy. QRS waves are consistent in shape unless aberrantly conducted. The QRS complex is followed by a T wave.
- *Patient response:* The patient may or may not be aware of the atrial fibrillation. If the ventricular response is rapid, the patient may show signs of decreased cardiac output or worsening of heart failure symptoms.
- *Causes:* Ischemic heart disease, valvular heart disease, hyperthyroidism, lung disease, heart failure, and aging may cause atrial fibrillation.
- *Care and treatment:* As with atrial flutter, alterations in blood flow and hemostasis may predispose the patient to clot formation. If there are no contraindications, the patient is prescribed anticoagulants. After at least 3 weeks of antithrombotic therapy, elective cardioversion can be considered followed by 4 more weeks of antithrombotic therapy.[5] Anticoagulation with warfarin, a factor Xa inhibitor, or direct thrombin inhibitor are useful for cardioversion, provided that contraindications to the selected medication are absent. Ventricular rate control is attained by administration of AV nodal blocking agents. As with atrial flutter, ablation may be attempted. Symptomatic tachycardia is usually treated with medications because of the risk of thromboembolism. Emergent cardioversion is considered if the tachycardia is associated with hemodynamic instability.[5]

? CRITICAL REASONING ACTIVITY

Discuss why patients with pulmonary disease are prone to atrial dysrhythmias.

Dysrhythmias of the Atrioventricular Node

Dysrhythmias of the AV node are called *junctional rhythms,* which include junctional escape rhythm, premature junctional contractions (PJCs), accelerated junctional rhythm, junctional tachycardia, and paroxysmal SVT. Several ECG changes are common to all junctional dysrhythmias. These changes include P-wave abnormalities and PR-interval changes.

P-Wave Changes. Because of the location of the AV node—in the center of the heart—impulses generated may be conducted forward, backward, or both. With the potential of forward, backward, or bidirectional impulse conduction, three different P waveforms may be associated with junctional rhythms:

1. When the AV node impulse is conducted backward, the impulse enters the atria first. Conduction back toward the atria allows for at least partial depolarization of the atria. When depolarization occurs backward, an inverted P wave is created in leads where the P wave is usually upright. Once the atria have been depolarized, the impulse then moves down the bundle of His and depolarizes both ventricles normally (Fig. 8.36A). A short PR interval (<0.12 second) is noted.
2. When the impulse is conducted both forward and backward, *P waves may be present after the QRS complex.* In this type of conduction, the impulse first moves into the ventricles, depolarizing them and creating a QRS complex. Because the impulse is also conducted backward, some atrial depolarization occurs, and a late P wave is noted after the QRS complex (see Fig. 8.36B).
3. When the AV node impulse moves forward, P waves may be absent because the impulse enters the ventricle first. The atria receive the wave of depolarization at the same time as the ventricles; thus because of the larger muscle mass of the ventricles, there is no P wave (see Fig. 8.36C).

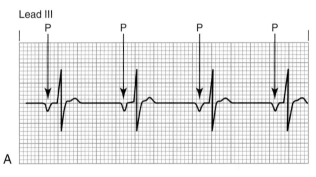

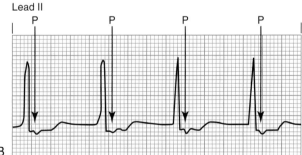

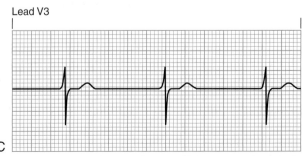

Fig. 8.36 P waves in junctional dysrhythmias. **A,** Backward conduction with inverted P wave. **B,** Forward and backward conduction with retrograde P wave. **C,** Forward conduction with absent P wave.

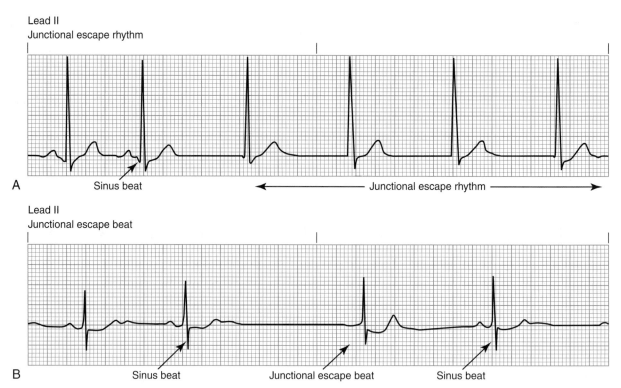

Lead II
Junctional escape rhythm

A   Sinus beat   ← Junctional escape rhythm →

Lead II
Junctional escape beat

B   Sinus beat   Junctional escape beat   Sinus beat

Fig. 8.37 A, Junctional escape rhythm. **B,** Junctional escape beat.

Junctional Escape Rhythm. Junctional escape rhythms occur when the dominant pacemaker, the SA node, fails to fire. A junctional escape rhythm has an inverted P wave and short PR interval preceding the QRS complex, a P wave that follows the QRS complex (retrograde), or no visible P wave. The escape rhythm may consist of many successive beats (Fig. 8.37A), or it may occur as a single escape beat that follows a pause, such as a sinus pause (see Fig. 8.37B).

   Rhythm analysis.
- *Rate:* Heart rate is 40 to 60 beats/min.
- *Regularity:* The rhythm is regular.
- *Interval measurements:* If a P wave is present before the QRS complex, the PR interval is shortened less than 0.12 ms. QRS complex is normal.
- *Shape and sequence:* P waves may be inverted, follow the QRS complex, or be absent.
- *Patient response:* The patient is assessed for tolerance of the bradycardia.
- *Causes:* The escape rhythm results from loss of sinus node activity.
- *Care and treatment:* Determine the patient's tolerance of the bradycardia. Alert the provider of the change in rhythm. If symptomatic, administer atropine; consider transcutaneous pacing, dopamine infusion, or epinephrine infusion.[3]

Accelerated Junctional Rhythm and Junctional Tachycardia. The normal intrinsic rate for the AV node and junctional tissue is 40 to 60 beats/min, but rates can accelerate. An accelerated junctional rhythm has a rate between 60 and 100 beats/min

(Fig. 8.38A), and the rate for junctional tachycardia is greater than 100 beats/min (see Fig. 8.38B).

   Rhythm analysis.
- *Rate:* Accelerated junctional rhythm is 60 to 100 beats/min. Junctional tachycardia rhythm is greater than 100 beats/min.
- *Regularity:* The rhythm is regular.
- *Interval measurements:* If a P wave is present before the QRS complex, the PR interval is shortened less than 0.12 ms. The QRS complex is followed by a T wave, and both are normal in shape.
- *Shape and sequence:* The P wave may have a variety of configurations: precede the QRS complex, be inverted, not visible, or follow the QRS complex.
- *Patient response:* A patient may have a decrease in cardiac output and hemodynamic instability, depending on the rate.
- *Causes:* Sinoatrial node disease, ischemic heart disease, electrolyte imbalances, digitalis toxicity, and hypoxemia can be causes.
- *Care and treatment:* Assess and treat the tachycardia if the patient is hemodynamically unstable. Alert the provider to the change in rhythm.

Premature Junctional Contractions. Irritable areas in the AV node and junctional tissue can generate premature beats that are earlier than the next expected beat (Fig. 8.39). These premature beats are similar to PACs but with characteristics of a junctional beat. The regularity of the underlying rhythm is interrupted by the premature junctional beat. The PJC is followed by a noncompensatory pause.

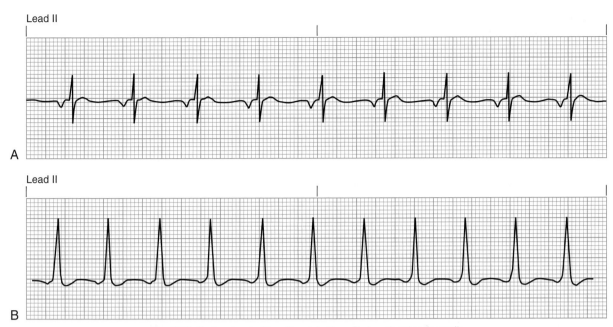

Fig. 8.38 A, Accelerated junctional rhythm. **B,** Junctional tachycardia.

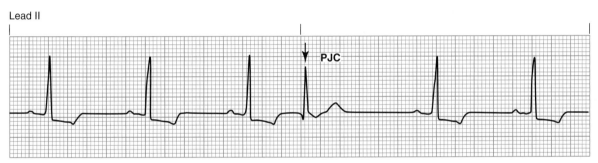

Fig. 8.39 Sinus rhythm with premature junctional contraction *(PJC)*.

Rhythm analysis.

- *Rate:* The rate is that of the underlying rhythm.
- *Regularity:* The underlying rhythm is interrupted by a premature beat that momentarily disrupts regularity.
- *Interval measurements:* The PJC is early; thus it is next to the T wave.
- *Shape and sequence:* The P wave may have a variety of configurations: precede the QRS complex, be inverted, not visible, or follow the QRS complex. The QRS complex is followed by the T wave, and both are normal in shape.
- *Patient response:* The rhythm is well tolerated, but the patient may experience palpitations if the PJCs occur frequently.
- *Causes:* PJCs may be a normal variant; may be caused by digitalis toxicity, ischemic or valvular heart disease, or heart failure; or may be a response to endogenous or exogenous catecholamines such as epinephrine.
- *Care and treatment:* No treatment is indicated.

Paroxysmal Supraventricular Tachycardia. Paroxysmal supraventricular tachycardia (PSVT) occurs above the ventricles, and it has an abrupt onset and cessation. It is initiated by either a PAC or a PJC. An abnormal conduction pathway through the AV node or an accessory pathway around the AV node results in extreme tachycardia. The QRS complex is typically narrow, and a P wave may or may not be present. The primary criteria are those of the abrupt onset and cessation of the dysrhythmia (Fig. 8.40).

Rhythm analysis.

- *Rate:* Heart rate is 150 to 250 beats/min.
- *Regularity:* The rhythm is regular.
- *Interval measurements:* If the P wave is present, the PR interval is shortened. Other intervals are normal.
- *Shape and sequence:* P wave (if present) and QRS complex are consistent in shape. The QRS complex is narrow and followed by a T wave.
- *Patient response:* The patient may be asymptomatic or symptomatic.
- *Causes:* PSVT often occurs in healthy, young adults without structural heart disease. It may be precipitated by increased catecholamines, stimulants, heart disease, electrolyte imbalances, and anatomical abnormality.
- *Care and treatment:* If the patient is asymptomatic, vagal maneuvers may be attempted. If the patient is symptomatic and the heart rate is greater than 150 beats/min, emergent

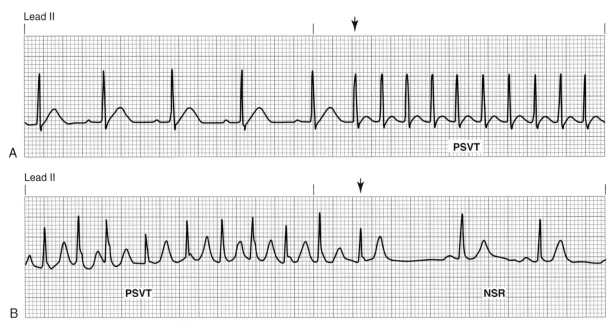

Fig. 8.40 Paroxysmal supraventricular tachycardia (PSVT). **A,** The abrupt onset initiated by a premature junctional contraction *(arrow).* **B,** The abrupt cessation of the PSVT *(arrow). NSR,* Normal sinus rhythm.

cardioversion is considered. Adenosine or AV nodal blocking agents are usually administered. Once stabilized, the patient is referred for further evaluation by an electrophysiologist.

STUDY BREAK

3. The patient's cardiac monitor is alarming. The heart rate is 200 beats/min, and the QRS complex is very narrow. The patient states that he feels lightheaded and his BP is 80/40 mm Hg. You understand that your priority is to:
   A. Continue to observe the patient
   B. Anticipate assisting to administer adenosine
   C. Get a complete set of vital signs
   D. Assess if it is time to change the IV access site

Dysrhythmias of the Ventricle

Ventricular dysrhythmias arise from ectopic foci in the ventricles. Because the stimulus depolarizes the ventricles in a slower, abnormal way, the QRS complex appears widened and has a bizarre shape. The QRS complex is wider than 0.12 second and often wider than 0.16 second. The polarity of the T wave can be opposite that of the QRS complex.

Depolarization from abnormal ventricular beats rarely activates the atria in a retrograde fashion. Therefore most ventricular dysrhythmias have no apparent P waves. However, if a P wave is present, it is usually seen in the T wave of the following beat or it has no relationship to the QRS complex and is dissociated from the ventricular rhythm. Ventricular dysrhythmias can be life-threatening; thus fast recognition and intervention are imperative.

Premature Ventricular Contractions. Premature ventricular contractions (PVCs) are a common ventricular dysrhythmia.

PVCs are early beats that interrupt the underlying rhythm; they can arise from a single ectopic focus or from multiple foci within the ventricles. A single ectopic focus produces PVC waveforms that look alike, called unifocal PVCs (Fig. 8.41A and C). Waveforms of PVCs arising from multiple foci are not identical and are called multifocal PVCs (see Fig. 8.41B). PVCs do not generally reset the sinus node, so the next sinus beat following the pause occurs on time. This is called a *compensatory pause.*

PVCs may occur in a predictable pattern, such as every other beat, every third beat, or every fourth beat. Box 8.4 lists the nomenclature for early beats. Bigeminal PVCs are noted in Fig. 8.41A. Premature ventricular contractions can also occur sequentially. Two PVCs in a row are called a *pair* (see Fig. 8.41C), and three or more in a row are called *nonsustained VT.*

The peak of the T wave through the downslope of the T wave is considered the vulnerable period, which coincides with partial repolarization of the ventricles. If a PVC occurs during the T wave, VT may occur. When the R wave of PVC falls on the T wave of a normal beat, it is referred to as the *R-on-T phenomenon* (Fig. 8.42).

PVCs may occur in healthy individuals and usually do not require treatment. The nurse must determine if PVCs are increasing in number by evaluating the trend. If PVCs are increasing, the nurse should evaluate for potential causes such as electrolyte imbalances, myocardial ischemia or injury, and hypoxemia. Runs of nonsustained VT may be a precursor to development of sustained VT.

Rhythm analysis.
- *Rate:* The rate matches the underlying rhythm.
- *Regularity:* The rhythm is interrupted by the premature beat.
- *Interval measurements:* There is no PR interval, and the QRS complex is greater than 0.12 second.

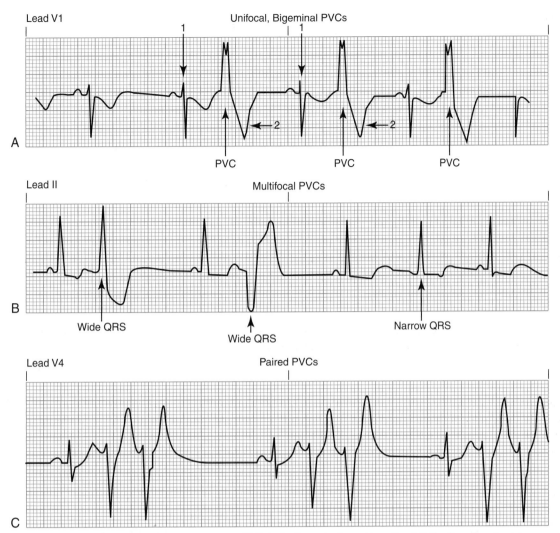

Fig. 8.41 Premature ventricular contractions (PVCs). **A,** Sinus rhythm with unifocal PVCs. The sinus beat is *1; 2* points to the presence of an inverted T wave. **B,** Sinus rhythm with multifocal PVCs; note the different configuration of the PVCs, indicating generation from more than one focus. **C,** The PVCs are in pairs and look the same, indicating that they are from the same foci.

- *Shape and sequence:* The QRS complex of the PVC is wide and bizarre looking. The T wave may be oriented opposite to the direction of the QRS complex of the PVC.
- *Patient response:* Patients may experience palpitations and may become symptomatic if the PVCs occur frequently.
- *Causes:* Hypoxemia, ischemic heart disease, hypokalemia, hypomagnesemia, acid-base imbalances, and increased catecholamine levels can cause PVCs.
- *Care and treatment:* Treat the cause if PVCs are increasing in frequency.

Ventricular Tachycardia. Ventricular tachycardia (VT) is a rapid, life-threatening dysrhythmia originating from a single ectopic focus in the ventricles. It is characterized by at least three PVCs in a row. VT occurs at a rate greater than 100 beats/min, but the rate is usually approximately 150 beats/min and may be up to 250 beats/min. Depolarization of the ventricles is abnormal and produces a widened QRS complex (Fig. 8.43). The patient may or may not have a pulse.

The wave of depolarization associated with VT rarely reaches the atria. Therefore P waves are usually absent. If P waves are present, they have no association with the QRS complex. The sinus node may continue to depolarize at its normal rate, independent of the ventricular ectopic focus. P waves may appear to be randomly scattered throughout the rhythm, but the P waves are actually fired at a consistent rate from the sinus node. This is called AV dissociation, another clue that the rhythm is VT. Occasionally a P wave will "capture" the ventricle because of the timing of atrial depolarization, interrupting the VT with a single capture beat that appears normal and narrow. Then the VT recurs. Capture beats are a diagnostic clue to differentiating wide complex tachycardias.

Torsades de pointes ("twisting about the point") is a type of VT caused by a prolonged QT interval, and it is often caused by magnesium deficiency.[3,5] Unlike VT, where the QRS complex waveforms have similar shapes, torsades de pointes is characterized by the presence of both positive and negative complexes that move above and below the isoelectric line.

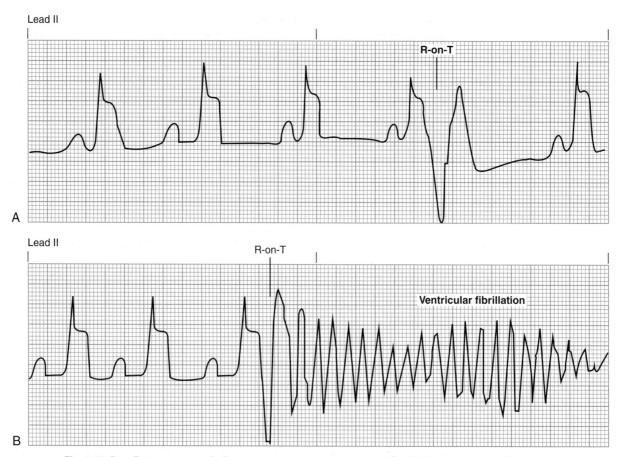

Fig. 8.42 R-on-T phenomenon. **A,** Single premature ventricular contraction (PVC) on T wave. **B,** PVC causing ventricular fibrillation.

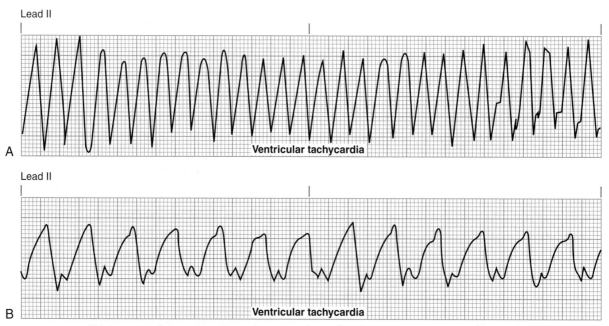

Fig. 8.43 Ventricular tachycardia (VT). **A,** One example of VT with a more narrow QRS complex. **B,** Another example of VT with a wider QRS complex.

This lethal dysrhythmia is treated as pulseless VT.[3,5] It can often be prevented by routine measurement of the QT/QTc intervals, especially if the patient is receiving medications that prolong the QT interval. Increases in QT/QTc intervals are reported to the provider, potential medication-related causes are explored, and magnesium levels are monitored and corrected (Fig. 8.44).

Rhythm analysis.
- *Rate:* The heart rate is 110 to 250 beats/min.
- *Regularity:* The rhythm is regular unless capture beats occur and momentarily interrupt the VT.
- *Interval measurements:* There is no PR interval. The QRS complex is greater than 0.12 second and often wider than 0.16 second.
- *Shape and sequence:* QRS waves are consistent in shape but appear wide and bizarre. The polarity of the T wave is opposite to that seen in the QRS complex.
- *Patient response:* If enough cardiac output is generated by the VT, a pulse and blood pressure are present. If cardiac output is impaired, the patient has signs and symptoms of low cardiac output and may experience a cardiac arrest.
- *Causes:* Hypoxemia, acid-base imbalance, exacerbation of heart failure, ischemic heart disease, cardiomyopathy, hypokalemia, hypomagnesemia, valvular heart disease, genetic abnormalities, and QT prolongation are all possible causes of VT.
- *Care and treatment:* Determine whether the patient has a pulse. If no pulse is present, provide emergent basic and advanced life-support interventions, including defibrillation.[3,5] If a pulse is present and the blood pressure is stable, the patient can be treated with IV amiodarone or lidocaine. Cardioversion is used as an emergency measure if the patient continues to have a pulse but becomes hemodynamically unstable.

Ventricular Fibrillation. Ventricular fibrillation (VF) is a chaotic rhythm characterized by a quivering of the ventricles, which results in total loss of cardiac output and pulse. VF is a life-threatening emergency, and the more immediate the treatment, the better the survival will be. VF produces a wavy baseline without a PQRST complex (Fig. 8.45).

Because a loose lead or electrical interference can produce a waveform similar to VF, it is always important to immediately assess the patient for pulse and consciousness.

Rhythm analysis.
- *Rate:* Heart rate is not discernible.
- *Regularity:* Heart rhythm is not discernible.
- *Interval measurements:* There are no waveforms.
- *Shape and sequence:* The baseline is wavy and chaotic, with no PQRST complexes.
- *Patient response:* The patient is in cardiac arrest.
- *Causes:* VF can be caused by ischemic and valvular heart disease, electrolyte and acid-base imbalances, and QT prolongation.
- *Care and treatment:* Begin immediate basic life support (BLS) and advanced cardiovascular life support (ACLS) interventions.

Idioventricular Rhythm or Ventricular Escape Rhythm. Idioventricular rhythm is an escape rhythm that is generated by the Purkinje fibers. This rhythm emerges only when the SA and AV nodes fail to initiate an impulse. The Purkinje fibers are capable of an intrinsic rate of 20 to 40 beats/min. Because this last pacemaker is in the ventricles, the QRS complex appears wide and bizarre with a slow rate (Fig. 8.46).

An idioventricular rhythm is considered a lethal dysrhythmia because the Purkinje fiber pacemakers may cease to fire, resulting in asystole. A single ventricular escape beat may occur following a pause if the junctional escape pacemaker does not fire (see Fig. 8.46).

If the rate is between 40 and 100 beats/min, this rhythm is called *accelerated idioventricular rhythm* (AIVR). This wide-complex rhythm is often seen following reperfusion of a coronary artery by thrombolytics; percutaneous coronary interventions, such as angioplasty or stent placement; and cardiac surgery (Fig. 8.47).

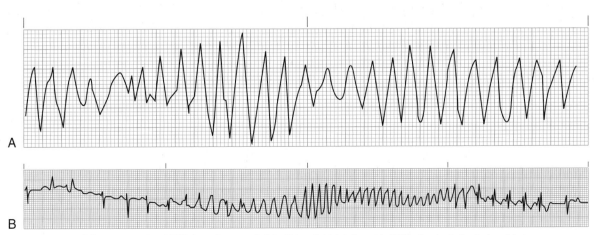

A is presented at 100% for a 6-second strip. **B** has been reduced to 55% of actual size to be able to see a longer waveform over 12 seconds, showing how a patient goes into and comes out of rhythm.

Fig. 8.44 Torsades de pointes.

Lead II

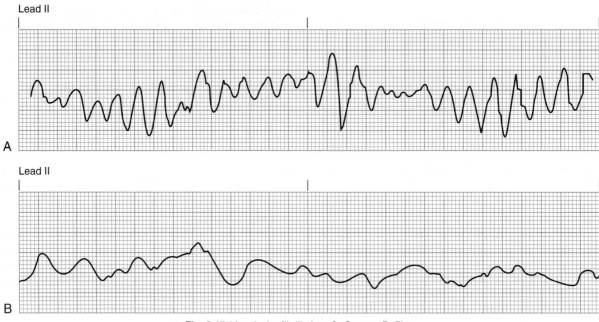

Lead II

A

B

Fig. 8.45 Ventricular fibrillation. **A,** Coarse. **B,** Fine.

Lead V1

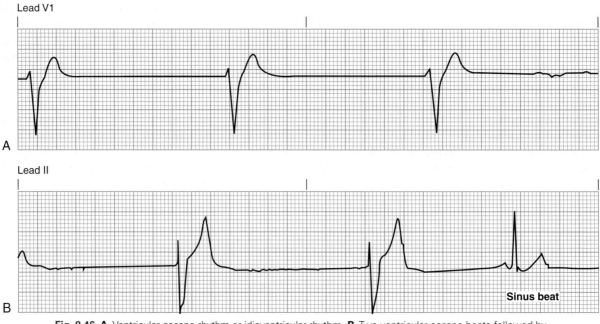

Lead II

A

B

Sinus beat

Fig. 8.46 **A,** Ventricular escape rhythm or idioventricular rhythm. **B,** Two ventricular escape beats followed by a sinus beat.

Lead V1

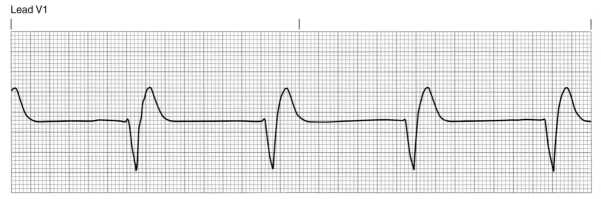

Fig. 8.47 Accelerated idioventricular rhythm (AIVR).

Rhythm analysis.
- *Rate:* The rate of idioventricular rhythm is 20 to 40 beats/min, and the rate of AIVR is 40 to 100 beats/min.
- *Regularity:* The rhythm is regular.
- *Interval measurements:* No P waves are present, and the QRS complex is greater than 0.12 second.
- *Shape and sequence:* QRS waves are wide and bizarre in shape. The QRS complex is followed by a T wave of opposite polarity.
- *Patient response:* The extreme bradycardia may cause the same symptoms as any severe bradycardia. This mechanism is the last backup pacemaker, and asystole may occur.
- *Causes:* Failure of the SA and AV nodal pacemakers causes idioventricular rhythm.
- *Care and treatment:* Initiate BLS and ACLS protocols. Consider emergent transcutaneous pacing.

Asystole. Asystole is characterized by complete cessation of electrical activity. A flat baseline is seen, without any evidence of P, QRS, or T waveforms. A pulse is absent and there is no cardiac output; cardiac arrest has occurred (Fig. 8.48A).

Asystole often occurs following VF or ventricular escape rhythm. Following a ventricular escape rhythm, this rhythm is referred to as ventricular standstill (see Fig. 8.48B). Pulse should be assessed immediately because a lead or electrode coming off may mimic this dysrhythmia. During cardiac arrest situations, if asystole occurs when another rhythm has been monitored, a check of two leads should occur to confirm asystole.

Rhythm analysis.
- *Rate:* Heart rate is absent.
- *Regularity:* Heart rhythm is absent.
- *Interval measurements:* PQRST waveforms are absent.
- *Shape and sequence:* Waveform presents as a flat or undulating line on the monitor.

- *Patient response:* The patient is in cardiac arrest.
- *Causes:* Asystole is usually preceded by another dysrhythmia such as VF or ventricular escape rhythm.
- *Care and treatment:* Initiate BLS and ACLS protocols.

Atrioventricular Blocks

Atrioventricular block, which is also known as *heart block,* refers to an inability of the AV node to conduct sinus impulses to the ventricles in a normal manner. Atrioventricular blocks can cause a delay in conduction from the SA node through the AV node or completely block conduction intermittently or continuously. Atrioventricular blocks may arise from normal aging of the conduction system or be caused by damage to the conduction system from ischemic heart disease.

Four types of AV block exist, each categorized in terms of degree. The four types of block are first degree, second degree type I, second degree type II, and third degree. The greater the degree of block, the more severe the consequences. First-degree block has minimal consequences, whereas third-degree block may be life-threatening.

First-Degree Atrioventricular Block. First-degree AV block describes consistent delayed conduction through the AV node or the atrial conductive tissue. It is represented on the ECG as a prolonged PR interval. It is a common dysrhythmia in older adults and in patients with cardiac disease. As the normal conduction pathway ages or becomes diseased, impulse conduction becomes slower than normal (Fig. 8.49).

Rhythm analysis.
- *Rate:* Heart rate is determined by the underlying rhythm.
- *Regularity:* The underlying rhythm determines regularity.
- *Interval measurements:* PR interval is prolonged and is greater than 0.20 second. QRS complex and QT/QTc measurements are normal.

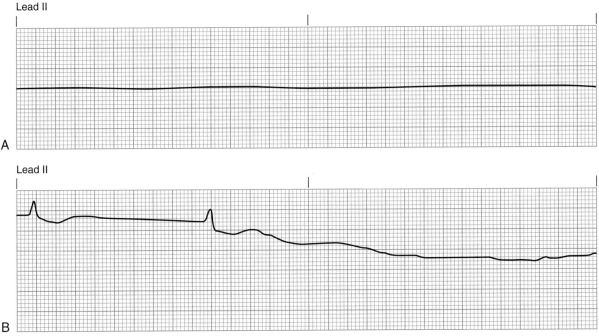

Lead II

A

Lead II

B

Fig. 8.48 A, Asystole. **B,** Ventricular standstill.

Lead III

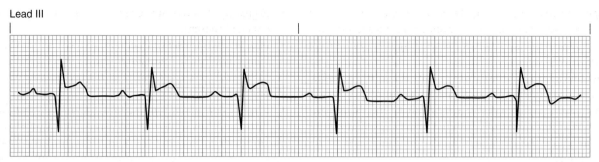

Fig. 8.49 First-degree atrioventricular block.

Lead II

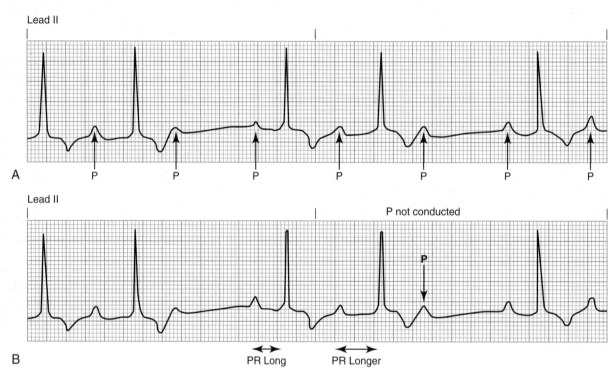

Fig. 8.50 Second-degree atrioventricular block type I (Mobitz I, Wenckebach). **A,** Shows every other P wave as a nonconducted beat, yet for the P waves that are conducted, the PR interval is prolonged. **B,** Shows how the PR interval is long on the labeled example, followed by a PR interval that is longer on the labeled example and then by a P wave that is not conducted.

- *Shape and sequence:* P and QRS waves are consistent in shape. P waves are small and rounded. A P wave precedes every QRS complex, which is followed by a T wave.
- *Patient response:* Atrioventricular block is well tolerated.
- *Causes:* Aging and ischemic and valvular heart disease can cause AV block.
- *Care and treatment:* No treatment is required.

Second-Degree Heart Block. *Second-degree heart block* refers to AV conduction that is intermittently blocked. Two types of second-degree block may occur, and each has specific diagnostic criteria for accurate diagnosis.

Second-degree atrioventricular block type I. Also called *Mobitz I* or *Wenckebach phenomenon,* second-degree AV block type I is represented on the ECG as a progressive lengthening of the PR interval until there is a P wave without a QRS complex. The AV node progressively delays conduction

to the ventricles, resulting in progressively longer PR intervals until finally a QRS complex is dropped. The PR interval following the dropped QRS complex is shorter than the PR interval preceding the dropped beat. By not conducting this one beat, the AV node recovers and is able to conduct the next atrial impulse (Fig. 8.50). If dropped beats occur frequently, it is useful to describe the conduction ratio, such as 2:1, 3:1, or 4:1.

Rhythm analysis.

- *Rate:* The rate is slower than the underlying rhythm because of the dropped beat.
- *Regularity:* P-P intervals stay the same, but R-R intervals shorten until the dropped beat.
- *Interval measurements:* The PR interval becomes progressively longer until a QRS complex is dropped. The PR interval before the dropped QRS complex is longer than the PR interval of the next conducted PQRST waveforms.

- *Shape and sequence:* P and QRS waves are consistent in shape. P waves are small and rounded. A P wave precedes every QRS complex, which is followed by a T wave, except for the dropped beats.
- *Patient response:* This rhythm is usually well tolerated unless there is an underlying bradycardia or frequent dropped beats.
- *Causes:* Aging, AV nodal blocking medications, acute inferior wall myocardial infarction or right ventricular infarction, ischemic heart disease, digitalis toxicity, and excess vagal response are all possible causes.
- *Care and treatment:* This type of block is usually well tolerated, and no treatment is indicated unless the dropped beats occur frequently. If the patient is symptomatic, medications that may contribute to the rhythm are discontinued. A permanent pacemaker may be indicated if the cause is not resolved.

Second-degree atrioventricular block type II. Second-degree AV block type II (Mobitz II) is a more critical type of heart block that requires early recognition and intervention. The conduction abnormality occurs below the AV node, either in the bundle of His or the bundle branches. A P wave is generated but is not conducted to the ventricles for one or more beats. The PR interval remains the same throughout, except for the dropped beat(s) (Fig. 8.51). Second-degree AV block type II is often associated with a bundle branch block and a corresponding widened QRS complex; however, narrow QRS complexes may be observed. Second-degree AV block type II can progress to the more clinically significant third-degree block and may cause the patient to be symptomatic.

Rhythm analysis.
- *Rate:* Heart rate is slower than the underlying rhythm because of the dropped beats.
- *Regularity:* P waves are regular, but QRS complexes are occasionally absent.
- *Interval measurements:* Intervals are constant for the underlying rhythm. PR intervals of the conducted beats do not change. QRS complexes may be widened because of a bundle branch block.
- *Shape and sequence:* P and QRS waves are consistent in shape. P waves are small and rounded. QRS complexes are missing.
- *Patient response:* The patient may tolerate one missed beat, but symptoms may occur if frequent beats are missed.
- *Causes:* Heart disease, increased vagal tone, conduction system disease, ablation of the AV node, and inferior and right ventricular myocardial infarctions are possible causes of second-degree AV block type II.
- *Care and treatment:* The patient may require emergent treatment with transcutaneous or transvenous pacing followed by insertion of a permanent pacemaker if the cause is not resolved.[3,6]

Third-Degree Block. Third-degree block is often called complete heart block because no atrial impulses are conducted through the AV node to the ventricles. The block in conduction can occur at the level of the AV node, the bundle of His, or the bundle branches.

In complete heart block, the atria and ventricles beat independently of each other because the AV node is completely blocked to the sinus impulse and it is not conducted to the ventricles. An escape rhythm arises from the junctional tissue or the ventricles. The atria beat at one rate, and the ventricles beat at a different rate. The atrial rate is dictated by the sinus node. The ventricular rate is slow, and usually only a ventricular or junctional escape rhythm is present. No communication

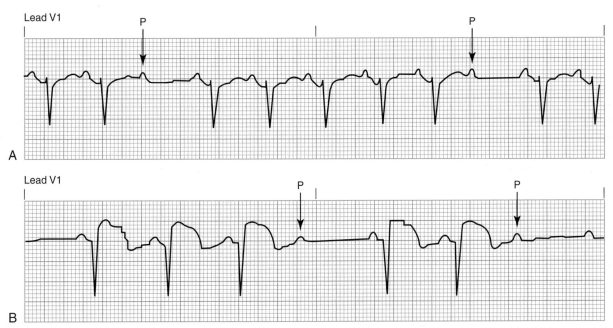

Fig. 8.51 Second-degree atrioventricular block type II (Mobitz II). **A,** The PR interval is constant; at the third and ninth P waves, there is no QRS complex following the P wave. **B,** No QRS complex follows the fourth and seventh P waves. Note for the P waves that are conducted, the PR interval is constant.

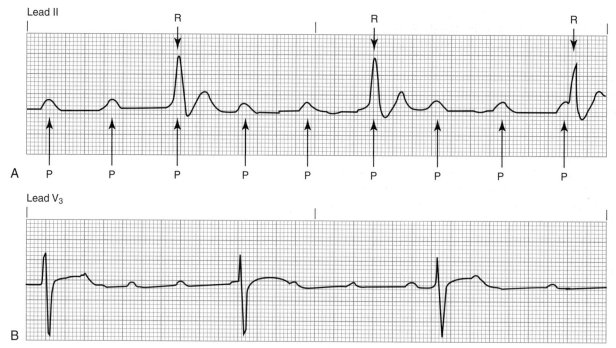

Fig. 8.52 Third-degree atrioventricular block (complete heart block). **A,** P waves regular and present throughout at an atrial rate of 94 beats/min and ventricular rhythm of 30 beats/min. The P waves are not associated with the QRS complexes. **B,** Similar tracing; atrial rate of 100 beats/min and ventricular rate of 30 beats/min.

exists between the atria and ventricles. Third-degree block is a type of AV dissociation (Fig. 8.52).

One hallmark of third-degree heart block is that the P waves have no association with the QRS complexes and appear throughout the QRS waveform. Both the P-P and R-R intervals are regular, but the rates for each are different because they have no relationship to each other. Whenever a rhythm strip appears to have no consistent, predictable relationship between P waves and QRS complexes, third-degree block is considered.

Rhythm analysis.
- *Rate:* The atrial rate is greater than the ventricular rate.
- *Regularity:* P-P intervals are regular and R-R intervals are regular, but they not associated with each other.
- *Interval measurements:* There is no PR interval in the absence of conduction. The QRS complex is often widened greater than 0.12 second with a ventricular escape rhythm.
- *Shape and sequence:* P and QRS waves are consistent in shape. P waves are small and rounded. The QRS complex is followed by a T wave. There is no relationship between the P waves and QRS complexes.
- *Patient response:* Patients may become symptomatic because of the bradycardia of the escape rhythm.
- *Causes:* Ischemic heart disease, acute myocardial infarction, and conduction system disease are possible causes of third-degree heart block.
- *Care and treatment:* Treatments include transcutaneous or transvenous pacing and implanting a permanent pacemaker.[6]

❓ CRITICAL REASONING ACTIVITY

A 65-year-old woman with type 2 diabetes presents to the emergency department; she is short of breath and complaining of neck and shoulder pain. Her blood pressure is 185/95 mm Hg, and her heart rate is 155 beats/min. How will you initially manage this patient? What medical intervention would you anticipate? List serious signs and symptoms of hemodynamic instability in a patient with a tachydysrhythmia.

CARDIAC PACEMAKERS

A cardiac pacemaker delivers electrical current to the myocardium to stimulate depolarization when the heart rate is too slow or the heart is unable to initiate or conduct a native beat. A pacemaker is often implanted to treat symptomatic bradycardia, which may occur from a number of different pathophysiological conditions. These include second-degree AV block type II, third-degree AV block, and sick sinus syndrome. The need for a pacemaker may be temporary (e.g., after an acute myocardial infarction or cardiac surgery) or permanent. Battery-operated external pulse generators are used to provide electrical energy for temporary transvenous pacemakers. Implanted permanent pacemakers are used to treat chronic conditions. These devices have a battery life of up to 10 years, which varies based on the manufacturer.

It is important that patients be assessed for the need for pacing. Unnecessary pacing may lead to worsened outcomes, including heart failure, rehospitalization, increased mortality, and new onset of atrial fibrillation.[5,6]

Temporary Pacemakers

Types of temporary pacemakers include the following[3,6]:

- *Transcutaneous:* Electrical stimulation is delivered through the skin via external electrode pads connected to an external pacemaker (a defibrillator with pacemaker functions; see Chapter 11).
- *Transvenous:* A pacing catheter (Fig. 8.53) is inserted percutaneously into the right ventricle, where it contacts the endocardium near the ventricular septum. It is connected to a small external pulse generator (Fig. 8.54) by electrode wires. Note the electrical ports on the pacing catheter, which are covered by black caps (see Fig. 8.53). These are connected to the pulse generator, whereupon pacing thresholds are set for each specific patient.
- *Epicardial:* Pacing wires are inserted into the epicardial wall of the heart during cardiac surgery (Fig. 8.55); wires are brought through the chest wall and can be connected to a pulse generator if needed (Fig. 8.56). Note that only two pacing wires are shown in Fig. 8.55; however, in cardiac bypass surgery patients, four wires are often placed through the chest wall of the patient, two wires from the atrium and two wires from the ventricles. These four wires are connected to the temporary pacemaker, and pacing thresholds are set for each patient.

Permanent Pacemakers

Permanent pacemakers have electrode wires that are typically placed transvenously through the cephalic or subclavian vein into the heart chambers (Fig. 8.57). The leads are attached to the pulse generator, placed in a surgically created pocket just below the left clavicle.[6]

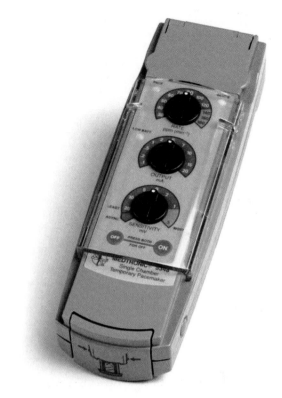

Fig. 8.54 Single-chamber temporary pulse generator. (Reproduced with permission of Medtronic, Inc., Minneapolis, MN.)

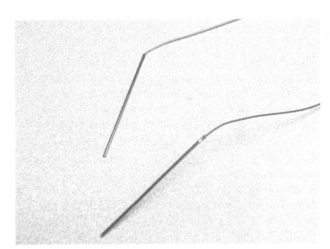

Fig. 8.55 Epicardial wires. (From Wiegand DLM. *AACN Procedure Manual for Critical Care.* 6th ed. St. Louis, MO: Elsevier; 2011.)

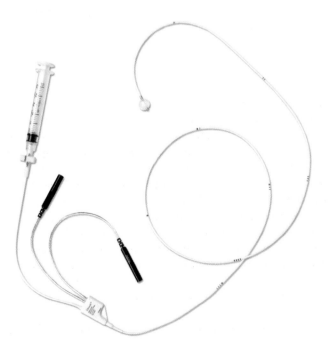

Fig. 8.53 Balloon-tipped bipolar lead wire for transvenous pacing. (From Wiegand DLM. *AACN Procedure Manual for Critical Care.* 6th ed. St. Louis, MO: Elsevier; 2011.)

Pacemakers may be used to stimulate the atrium, ventricle, or both chambers (dual-chamber pacemakers). Atrial pacing is used to mimic normal conduction and to produce atrial contraction, thus providing atrial kick. Ventricular pacing stimulates ventricular depolarization and is commonly used in emergency situations or when pacing is required infrequently. Dual-chamber pacing allows for stimulation of both atria and ventricles as needed to synchronize the chambers and mimic the normal cardiac cycle.

Permanent pacemakers may be programmed in a variety of ways, and a standardized code is used to determine the pacing

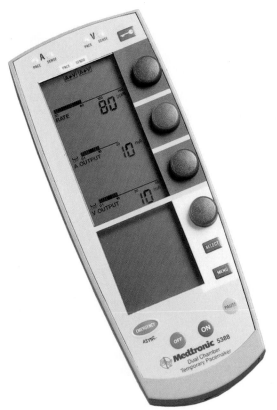

Fig. 8.56 Dual-chamber temporary pulse generator. (Reproduced with permission of Medtronic, Inc., Minneapolis, MN.)

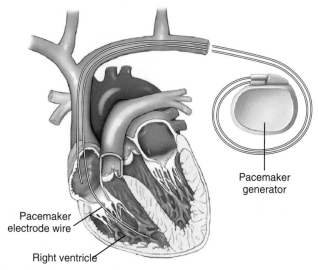

Fig. 8.57 Permanent dual-chamber (atrioventricular) pacemaker. (From Wesley K. *Huszar's ECG and 12-Lead Interpretation*. 5th ed. St. Louis, MO: Elsevier; 2017.)

mode that is programmed.[6] The North American Society of Pacing and Electrophysiology and the British Pacing and Electrophysiology Group have revised the standardized generic code for pacemakers; it is described in Chapter 13. It is important to know the programming information for the pacemaker to assess proper functioning on the rhythm strip.

Terms for Pacemaker Function. Other terms used in describing pacemaker function are mode, rate, electrical output, sensitivity, sense-pace indicator, and AV interval.

Mode. Pacemakers can be operated in a *demand* mode or *fixed rate (asynchronous)* mode. The demand mode paces the heart when no intrinsic or native beat is sensed. For example, if the rate control is set at 60 beats/min, the pacemaker will only pace if the patient's heart rate drops to less than 60 beats/min. The fixed rate mode paces the heart at a set rate, independent of any activity the patient's heart generates. The fixed rate mode may compete with the patient's own rhythm and deliver an impulse on the T wave (R on T), with the potential for producing VT or fibrillation. The demand mode is safer and is the mode of choice.

Rate. The rate control determines the number of impulses delivered per minute to the atrium, the ventricle, or both. The rate is set to produce effective cardiac output and to reduce symptoms.

Electrical output. The electrical output is the amount of electrical energy needed to stimulate depolarization. The output is measured in *milliamperes* (mA), which varies depending on the type of pacing. Transcutaneous pacing requires higher milliamperes than transvenous or epicardial pacing because the electrical energy must be delivered through the chest wall.

Sensitivity. The sensitivity is the ability of the pacemaker to recognize the body's intrinsic or native electrical activity. It is measured in *millivolts* (mV). Some temporary pacemakers have a sense-pace indicator. If the generator detects the patient's own beat, the "sense" indicator lights. When the generator delivers a paced beat, the "pace" light comes on. Temporary pacemakers have dials or keypads for adjusting sensitivity.

Atrioventricular interval. The AV interval indicator is used to determine the interval between atrial and ventricular stimulation. It is used only in dual-chamber pacemakers.

Pacemaker Rhythms. Pacemaker rhythms are usually easy to identify on the cardiac monitor or rhythm strip. The electrical stimulation is noted by an electrical artifact called the *pacer spike*. If the atrium is paced, the spike appears before the P wave (Fig. 8.58). If the ventricle is paced, the spike appears before the QRS complex (Fig. 8.59). If both the atrium and the ventricle are paced, spikes are noted before both the P wave and the QRS complex (Fig. 8.60). The heart rate is carefully assessed on the rhythm strip. The heart rate should not be lower than the rate set on the pacemaker.

The pacemaker spike is usually followed by a larger-than-normal P wave in atrial pacing or a widened QRS complex in ventricular pacing. Sometimes the P wave is not seen even though an atrial pacer spike is present. Because the heart is paced in an artificial or abnormal fashion, the path of depolarization is altered, resulting in waveforms and intervals that are also altered.

Pacemaker Malfunction. Three primary problems can occur with a pacemaker. These problems include failure to pace (also called *failure to fire*), failure to capture, and failure to sense. If troubleshooting does not resolve pacemaker malfunction, emergency transcutaneous pacing may be needed to ensure an adequate cardiac output.

Lead II

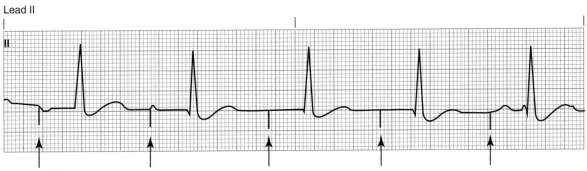

Fig. 8.58 Atrial paced rhythm.

Lead II

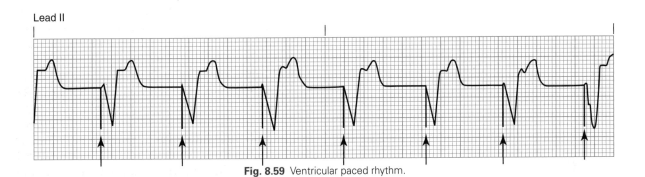

Fig. 8.59 Ventricular paced rhythm.

Lead II

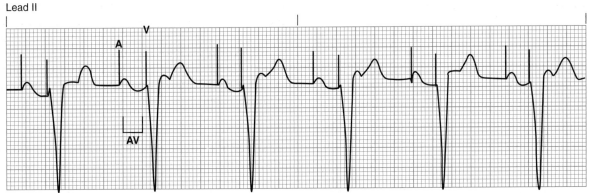

Fig. 8.60 Dual-chamber (atrioventricular) paced rhythm. *A,* Atrial pacer spike; *AV,* Atrioventricular pacer interval; *V,* ventricular pacer spike.

Failure to pace. *Failure to pace* or *failure to fire* occurs when the pacemaker fails to initiate an electrical stimulus when it should fire. The problem is noted by absence of pacer spikes on the rhythm strip. Causes of failure to pace include battery or pulse generator failure, fracture or displacement of a pacemaker wire, or loose connections (Fig. 8.61).

Failure to capture. When the pacemaker generates an electrical impulse (pacer spike) and no depolarization is noted, it is described as *failure to capture.* On the ECG, a pacer spike is noted, but it is not followed by a P wave (atrial pacemaker) or a QRS complex (ventricular pacemaker) (Fig. 8.62). Common causes of failure to capture include output (mA) set too low or displacement of the pacing lead wire from the myocardium (transvenous or epicardial leads). Other causes of failure to capture include battery failure, fracture of the pacemaker wire,

or increased pacing threshold as a result of medication or electrolyte imbalance. Adjusting the output if the patient has a temporary pacemaker and placing the patient on his or her left side are nursing interventions to treat failure to capture. Turning the patient onto the left side facilitates contact of a transvenous pacing wire with the endocardium and septum.

Failure to sense. When the pacemaker does not sense the patient's own cardiac rhythm and initiates an electrical impulse, it is called *failure to sense.* Failure to sense manifests as pacer spikes that fall too closely to the patient's own rhythm, earlier than the programmed rate (Fig. 8.63). The most common cause is displacement of the pacemaker electrode wire. Turning the patient to the left side and adjusting the sensitivity (temporary pacemaker) are nursing interventions to use when failure to sense occurs.

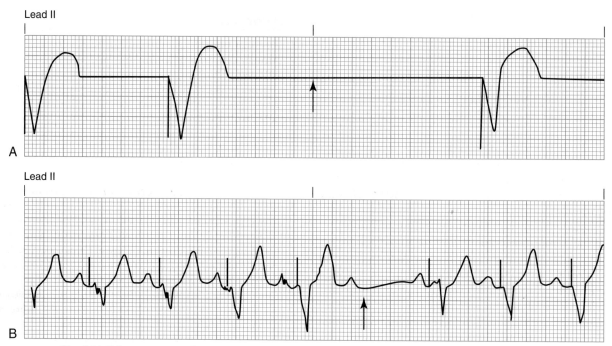

Fig. 8.61 Failure to pace or fire. **A,** Arrow indicates failure to pace from a ventricular pacemaker. **B,** Arrow indicates failure to pace from an atrial pacemaker.

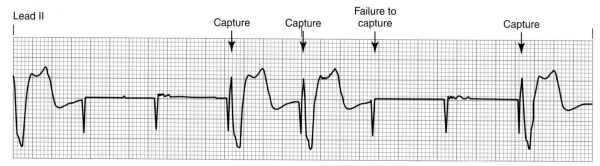

Fig. 8.62 Failure to capture: ventricular pacemaker.

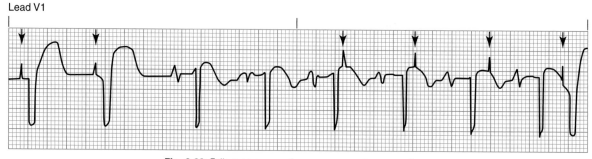

Fig. 8.63 Failure to sense. *Arrows* represent pacer spikes.

CRITICAL REASONING ACTIVITY

Why does tachycardia sometimes lead to heart failure?

OTHER DEVICES WITH PACEMAKER CAPABILITIES

Implantable cardioverter-defibrillators (ICDs) have pacemaker capabilities.[6] The pacemaker feature of these devices is used to treat fast heart rhythms, such as VT, with anti-tachycardia pacing, as well as slow heart rhythms that may occur following defibrillation. Anti-tachycardia pacing is a short, fast burst of pacing impulses that attempt to terminate the tachycardia.

Biventricular pacemakers and ICDs have an additional electrode wire placed through the coronary sinus into the left ventricle. Additional pacing wires are in the atria and the ventricle. Pacing both ventricles simultaneously improves heart function in a certain number of patients with heart failure. Synchronous depolarization of both ventricles improves cardiac output and ejection fraction. Many patients with ICDs benefit from telemonitoring technologies (see QSEN Exemplar box).

✳ QSEN EXEMPLAR

Safety

Use of the external temporary pacemaker is standard for patients who have symptomatic bradycardia. Before pacing is started, educate the patient about indications and potential complications. Once the pacemaker is initiated, evaluate the pacing threshold and set the pacemaker rate at a level to optimize hemodynamic status. Trend patient assessments to ensure hemodynamic stability.

Reference

Dalia T, Amr BS. Pacemaker indications. *StatPearls [Internet]*. https://www.ncbi.nlm.nih.gov/books/NBK507823/. Updated January 25, 2019.

CASE STUDY

Mr. P. is a 56-year-old man who was successfully extubated (endotracheal tube removed) 4 hours after coronary artery bypass graft surgery. However, 2 hours later, he complains of his heart racing, and it is determined that he has palpitations. The heart rate on the bedside monitor is 168 beats/min, blood pressure is 90/60 mm Hg, and respiratory rate is 26 breaths/min. The electrocardiogram (ECG) shows an irregularly irregular rhythm, a change from the sinus rhythm noted at the last assessment.

Questions

1. Based on this description, what is your interpretation of the rhythm?
2. What complications could occur as a result of this rhythm?
3. What clinical data would lead you to anticipate that this complication could occur?
4. What data are you going to communicate to the provider?
5. What orders do you expect to obtain?
6. What nursing actions do you need to take and why?
7. What are some of the etiological factors of this dysrhythmia?

REFERENCES

1. American Association of Critical-Care Nurses. Practice alert: Accurate dysrhythmia monitoring in adults. *Crit Care Nurse*. 2016;36(6):e26–e34.
2. American Association of Critical-Care Nurses. Practice alert: Ensuring accurate ST-segment monitoring. *Crit Care Nurse*. 2016;36(6):e18–e25.
3. American Heart Association (AHA). *Handbook of Emergency Cardiovascular Care for Healthcare Providers*. Dallas, TX: American Heart Association; 2015.
4. Hannibal G. It started with Einthoven: The history of the ECG and cardiac monitoring. *AACN Adv Crit Care*. 2011;64:1–76.
5. January CT, Wann LS, Calkins H, Chen LY, Cigarroa JE, Cleveland JC Jr, et al. AHA/ACC/HRS focused update of the 2014 AHA/ACC/HRS guideline for the management of patients with atrial fibrillation: A report of the American College of Cardiology/American Heart Association Task Force on Clinical Practice Guidelines and the Heart Rhythm Society. *Circulation*. 2019;139:1–49.
6. Kusumoto FM, Schoenfeld MH, Barrett C, Edgerton JR, Ellenbogen KA, Gold MR, et al. ACC/AHA/HRS guideline on the evaluation and management of patients with bradycardia and cardiac conduction delay: A report of the American College of Cardiology/American Heart Association Task Force on Clinical Practice Guidelines and the Heart Rhythm Society. *Heart Rhythm*. 2018;1–199.
7. Panchal AR, Berg KM, Rios MD, et al; American Heart Association (AHA). American Heart Association focused update on advanced cardiovascular life support use of antiarrhythmic medications during and immediately after cardiac arrest. *Circulation*. 2018;138:e740–e749.
8. Sandau KE, Funk M, Auerbach A, et al; American Heart Association (AHA). Update to practice standards for electrocardiographic monitoring in hospital settings: A scientific statement from the American Heart Association. *Circulation*. 2017;136:e273–e344.

Hemodynamic Monitoring

Charly Murphree, RN, MSN

Many additional resources, including self-assessment exercises, are located on the Evolve companion website at http://evolve.elsevier.com/Sole/.
- Animations
- Clinical Skills: Critical Care Collections
- Student Review Questions
- Video Clips

INTRODUCTION

A thorough understanding of hemodynamic monitoring is essential to care for the critically ill patient. The goal of hemodynamic monitoring is to accurately assess the patient and provide therapies to optimize oxygen delivery and tissue perfusion. This can be accomplished by monitoring the dynamic physiological relationship between many variables to determine whether oxygen delivery is adequate to meet the oxygen demands of the tissues and organs. Ensuring that the data are accurate and analyzed correctly to guide therapy and assess the outcome of interventions is a complex skill. This chapter reviews the basics of cardiovascular anatomy and physiology, the fundamentals of hemodynamic monitoring, and various modalities available to the clinician to assess and manage hemodynamic status.

REVIEW OF ANATOMY AND PHYSIOLOGY

Cardiovascular System

The cardiovascular system is a closed network of arteries, capillaries, and veins through which blood, oxygen, hormones, and nutrients are delivered to the tissues by the pumping action of the heart (Fig. 9.1). Metabolic wastes are removed from the circulating blood via the liver and kidneys. The major components of the cardiovascular system are described.

Heart. The heart is a four-chambered organ that weighs approximately 1 pound and lies obliquely in the thoracic cavity. The heart is responsible for pumping oxygenated blood forward through the arterial vasculature and receiving deoxygenated blood via the venous vasculature. Four one-way valves regulate blood flow through the heart. Two atrioventricular (AV) valves (tricuspid and mitral) open during ventricular diastole, allowing blood to flow from the atria into the ventricles. At end-diastole the atria contract and force the remaining atrial blood into the ventricles—this is commonly referred to as the "atrial kick" and contributes up to 30% of the cardiac output (CO). As the ventricles begin to contract in systole, the AV valves close and the semilunar valves (pulmonic and aortic) open, allowing blood to flow into the pulmonary and systemic vasculature. At the end of ventricular systole, the semilunar valves close and the cycle begins again (Fig. 9.2).

Arteries. Arteries are the tough, elastic vessels that carry blood away from the heart. Arteries consist of three layers: the adventitia, the media, and the intima. The adventitia is composed chiefly of longitudinally arranged collagen fibers, which make up the tough outer lining. The media consists of concentrically arranged smooth muscle. The intima consists of endothelial connective tissue that is continuous with that of the heart. The endothelial lining of the vessel is slick and smooth, allowing blood to flow freely. The elasticity of the vessels allows them to expand to accommodate volumetric changes that result with the contraction and relaxation of the heart. When the artery diameter is less than 0.5 mm, it is called an *arteriole*. The arterial system is a high-pressure, low-volume, high-resistance circuit responsible for delivering oxygen and nutrient-rich blood to the capillary system. Arteries have the ability to dilate or constrict in response to metabolic demand.

Capillaries. The capillaries are exchange vessels, composed of a network of low-pressure, thin-walled microscopic vessels allowing for easy passage of hormones, nutrients, and oxygen to the target tissues. They also receive metabolic wastes and carbon dioxide from the tissues and begin the process of returning deoxygenated blood to the venous portion of the cardiovascular system.

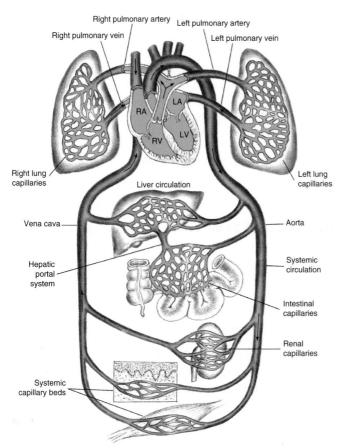

Fig. 9.1 Diagram of the cardiovascular system. *LA,* Left atrium; *LV,* left ventricle; *RA,* right atrium; *RV,* right ventricle. (From Patton K, Thibodeau S, eds. *Anthony's Textbook of Anatomy and Physiology.* 20th ed. St. Louis, MO: Elsevier; 2013.)

Veins. Compared with the arteries, veins are thin-walled, less elastic, fibrous, larger in diameter, and known as high-capacity, low-resistance vessels. The majority of the circulating blood volume is in the venous system. Veins of the extremities contain valves to assist with maintaining a one-way flow of deoxygenated blood returning to the heart. Eventually the veins connect to larger vessels and become the coronary sinus, which empties into the right atrium. The venous system has the ability to respond to metabolic needs by vasodilation or vasoconstriction, thereby increasing or decreasing venous return. Venous return is the flow of blood back to the heart. Approximately 70% of the circulating blood volume is located in the venous system at any given time. Several factors influence venous return, including muscle contraction, breathing, venous compliance, and gravity.

Blood. Blood accounts for approximately 7% of our body weight, which is approximately 5 L of blood. The fluid component, or plasma, makes up approximately 60% of the blood volume. The remaining 40% consists of the cellular components: erythrocytes (red blood cells), leukocytes (white blood cells), and platelets. The more viscous the blood, the greater the turbulence in blood flow, resulting in a reduction in flow in the microcirculation. The red blood cell component of blood is

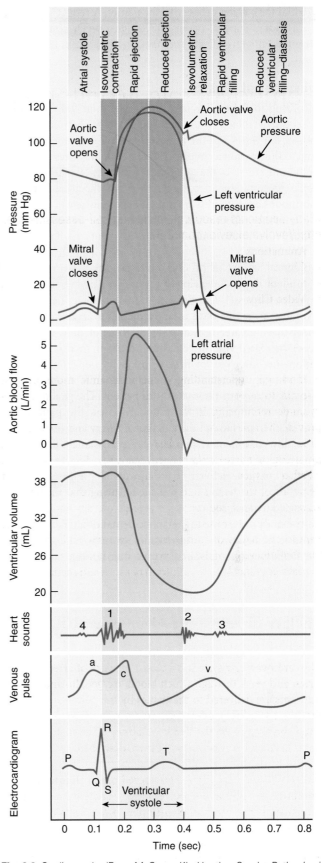

Fig. 9.2 Cardiac cycle. (From McCance KL, Huether S, eds. *Pathophysiology: The Biologic Basis for Disease in Adults and Children.* 8th ed. St. Louis, MO: Elsevier; 2019.)

essential for oxygen delivery to the tissues. A reduction in oxygen delivery (supply) or an increase in oxygen consumption (demand) directly affects the hemodynamic responses of the body.

Principles of Physics

According to Poiseuille's law, the rate of fluid flow through a vessel is determined by the pressure difference between the two ends of the vessel and the resistance within the lumen. For any fluid to flow within a circuit, a difference in pressures within the circuit must exist. In the cardiovascular system, the driving pressure is generated by the contractile force of the heart. There is a continuous drop in pressure from the left ventricle to the tissues and a further reduction in pressure from the tissue bed to the right atrium. Without these pressure gradients, no flow occurs.

Resistance is a measure of the ease with which the fluid flows through the lumen of a vessel. It is essentially a measure of friction, which depends on *viscosity* of the fluid and the radius and length of the vessel. A vessel with a small diameter has a greater resistance than one with a larger diameter (Fig. 9.3). Longer vessels have greater resistance to the flow of fluid within the vessel. Increased viscosity of a fluid results in increased friction within the fluid; rate of flow is inversely proportional to the fluid viscosity. Consider how much easier it is to drink water through a straw than it is to drink a milkshake (viscosity). How much more difficult is it to drink a milkshake through a long, thin straw than through a wide, shorter straw (resistance)?

Highly compliant systems have low resistance; therefore if resistance increases, compliance decreases. For example, an atherosclerotic vessel, with narrowing of the intima, has a reduced capacitance and compliance, leading to increased resistance and hypertension.

The body's response to metabolic demands alters the flow of blood to and from the target tissues. In response to increased metabolic demands, the circulatory system increases the volume of blood flow to the target tissues by increasing the diameter of the vessel (vasodilation), resulting in reduced resistance within the vessel.

Another determinant of flow rate is the degree of turbulence within a vessel. The rate of fluid movement in laminar flow is greater than the rate in turbulent flow. A vessel lining that has excess plaque accumulation or calcification results in more turbulence, reduced flow, and reduced tissue perfusion.

Components of Cardiac Output

Cardiac output (CO) is determined by multiplying heart rate by stroke volume (SV). *Stroke volume* is the amount of blood ejected by the heart with each beat. SV is affected by preload, afterload, and contractility (Fig. 9.4). Understanding hemodynamics requires a working knowledge of normal intracardiac pressures, as each chamber of the heart has a unique pressure (Fig. 9.5). In addition, a familiarity with the cardiac cycle (see Fig. 9.2) assists in understanding hemodynamic concepts. Relevant concepts are defined next.

Heart rate is a major determinant of CO. Slow heart rates can result in a decreased CO, particularly if the body cannot compensate with an increase in SV. Fast heart rates can also result in decreased CO because the ventricles have less diastolic time and can result in poor ventricular filling, decreasing SV. In addition, the coronary arteries fill during diastole. Fast heart rates can result in decreased coronary artery filling and subsequently in decreased coronary tissue perfusion.

Determinants of Stroke Volume. *Preload* is the degree of ventricular stretch before the next contraction. The degree of stretch is directly affected by the amount of blood volume present in the ventricles at end-diastole. In hemodynamic monitoring, preload is quantified by measuring ventricular end-diastolic pressures. Based on the Frank-Starling mechanism, when ventricular fibers are at maximal stretch, maximal CO results.

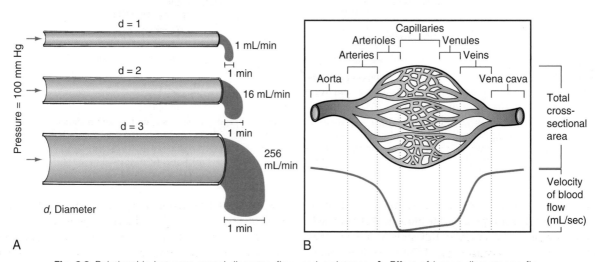

Fig. 9.3 Relationship between vessel diameter, flow, and resistance. **A,** Effect of lumen diameter on flow through vessel. **B,** Blood flows with great speed in the large arteries. However, branching of arterial vessels increases the total cross-sectional areas of the arterioles and capillaries, thus reducing the flow rate. (**A,** From McCance KL, Huether S, eds. *Pathophysiology: The Biologic Basis for Disease in Adults and Children.* 7th ed. St. Louis, MO: Elsevier; 2015. **B,** From Thibodeau G, Patton K. *Anatomy and Physiology.* 9th ed. St. Louis, MO: Mosby; 2016.)

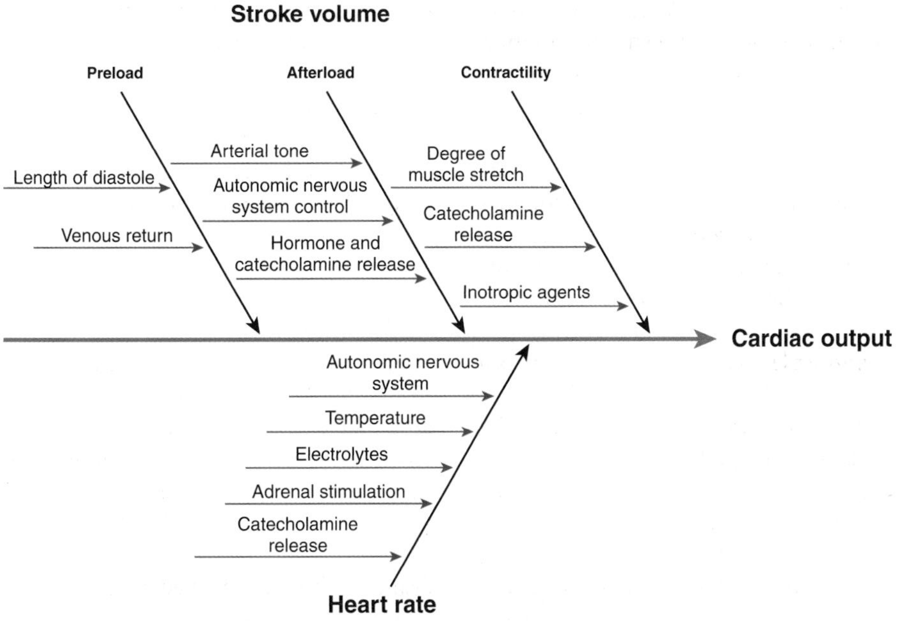

Stroke volume

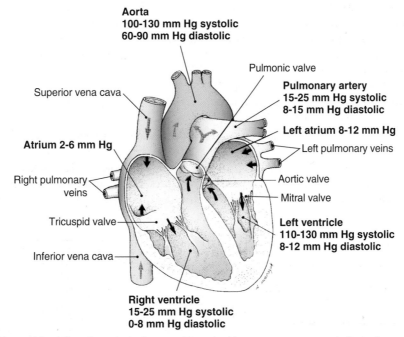

Fig. 9.4 Cardiac output components. Cardiac output is determined by heart rate and stroke volume.

Aorta
100-130 mm Hg systolic
60-90 mm Hg diastolic

Pulmonic valve

Superior vena cava

Pulmonary artery
15-25 mm Hg systolic
8-15 mm Hg diastolic

Left atrium 8-12 mm Hg

Atrium 2-6 mm Hg

Left pulmonary veins

Right pulmonary
veins

Aortic valve

Mitral valve

Tricuspid valve

Left ventricle
110-130 mm Hg systolic
8-12 mm Hg diastolic

Inferior vena cava

Right ventricle
15-25 mm Hg systolic
0-8 mm Hg diastolic

Fig. 9.5 Normal blood flow through the heart and intrachamber pressures; *arrows* indicate the normal direction of blood flow. This schematic representation of the heart shows all four chambers and valves visible in the anterior view to facilitate conceptualization of blood flow. (From Ralston SH, Penman ID, Strachan MWJ, Hobson RP. *Davidson's Principles and Practice of Medicine.* 23rd ed. Edinburgh, Scotland: Elsevier Ltd; 2018.)

Another way of explaining the mechanism is that within physiological limits, the heart pumps all of the blood that is returned by the venous system.[18] Too much end-diastolic volume in the right ventricle can result in congestion of the systemic vasculature, and too much end-diastolic volume in the left ventricle can cause fluid to back up into the pulmonary vasculature. Too little blood at end-diastolic volume results in a reduction in CO. Optimizing preload or ventricular filling is the goal of many therapeutic interventions in critical care.

Afterload is the amount of resistance the ventricles must overcome to deliver the SV into the receiving vasculature. The left ventricle during systole must create the force necessary to open the aortic valve and overcome the resistance in the systemic circulation. The right ventricle must create enough force to open the pulmonic valve and overcome the resistance in the pulmonary circulation. Arterial systemic tone, blood viscosity, flow patterns (laminar versus turbulent), and valve competency all affect the degree of afterload the ventricle must overcome (Fig. 9.6).

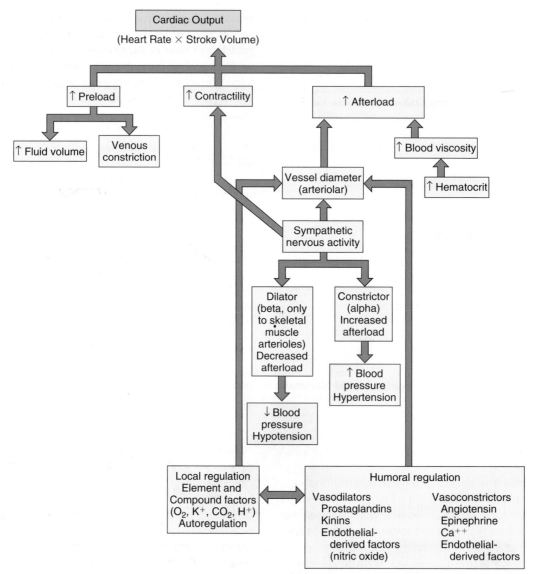

Fig. 9.6 Factors regulating blood flow. (Modified from McCance KL, Huether S, eds. *Pathophysiology: The Biologic Basis for Disease in Adults and Children.* 7th ed. St. Louis, MO: Elsevier; 2015.)

Contractility is the strength of myocardial muscle fiber shortening during the systolic phase of the cardiac cycle. It is the force with which the heart propels the SV forward into the vasculature. The preload influences contractility because optimizing the preload ensures maximal stretch of the myocardial fibers according to the Frank-Starling law. Contractility is not directly measured; however, it can be expressed by the calculated values of right or left ventricular stroke work index.

❓ CRITICAL REASONING ACTIVITY

How does stroke volume affect cardiac output?

Regulation of Cardiovascular Function

Cardiovascular anatomy and physiology are described in greater depth in Chapter 13. Function changes with aging (see Lifespan Considerations box). The autonomic nervous system has two branches that control the cardiovascular system: the sympathetic and the parasympathetic. Sympathetic nervous system

activity enhances myocardial performance by shortening the conduction time through the AV node, enhancing rhythmicity of the AV pacemaker cells and increased myocardial contractility. Parasympathetic nervous system activity via the vagus nerves results in blocking of cardiac action potentials initiated by the sinus node in the atria, thus decreasing heart rate.

The cardiovascular system is also regulated by hormonal influences to maintain adequate oxygen delivery to meet the demands of the tissues (see Fig. 9.6). Norepinephrine increases the heart rate and myocardial contractility and causes vasoconstriction. Epinephrine produces its effects by stimulating the alpha-adrenergic receptors located in the walls of the arteriole. In addition, epinephrine is a beta-adrenergic stimulator and may cause vasodilation of arterioles in skeletal muscle.

The right atrium secretes atrial natriuretic peptides (ANPs), and the ventricular myocardium secretes brain natriuretic peptides (BNPs) in response to stretch from the heart chambers. ANPs and BNPs cause vasodilation and diuresis and inhibit the sympathetic response and the renin-angiotensin-aldosterone system (RAAS) in an attempt to decrease circulating blood volume and decrease stress on the myocardium.

The RAAS is activated in the kidney in response to low blood pressure, low intravascular volume, or low sodium levels. Renin is released by the kidney and converts to angiotensin I. Angiotensin I converts to angiotensin II in the lungs. Angiotensin II is a potent vasoconstrictor, resulting in systemic arterial vasoconstriction in an attempt to increase blood pressure. Angiotensin II also activates aldosterone from the adrenal glands, resulting in retention of sodium and water at the distal convoluted tubule of the kidney in an attempt to increase blood pressure.

In addition to the systemic responses of the RAAS and the autonomic nervous system, several hormones (i.e., endothelin-1, serotonin, and thromboxane A_2) are released at the local tissue level and result in vasoconstriction of the vascular bed (see Fig. 9.6). Other hormones, such as nitric oxide, prostaglandins, bradykinin, and kallidin, have vasodilatory properties.[28]

HEMODYNAMIC MONITORING MODALITIES

Invasive and noninvasive hemodynamic monitoring is a major part of a comprehensive assessment of the critically ill patient. The goal in evaluating hemodynamic data is to determine if oxygen supply is meeting oxygen demands. The hemodynamic assessment aids in surveillance and early detection of oxygen imbalance, quantifying the severity of disease, and serves as a guide for assessing and adjusting therapies. Traditional hemodynamic monitoring uses specific end points to guide therapies (e.g., mean arterial pressure [MAP], CO, central venous pressure [CVP], pulmonary artery occlusion pressure [PAOP], urine output, pH, and lactate). Newer modalities, such as bedside echocardiography, mixed venous oxygen saturation (SvO_2) monitoring, central venous oxygen saturation ($ScvO_2$), and changes in the arterial pressure waveform, continually measure

ever-changing bodily responses. Normal hemodynamic values are described in Table 9.1; however, these values only provide a guideline to assist in interpretation of assessment findings. The primary goal of hemodynamic monitoring is to assess and trend adequacy of tissue oxygenation and perfusion, rather than to compare a patient's values to so-called normal parameters.

Noninvasive Monitoring

Some critically ill patients can be adequately assessed and managed with noninvasive hemodynamic monitoring. Noninvasive technologies include noninvasive blood pressure (NIBP) measurement, assessment of jugular venous pressure, and frequent assessments of laboratory tests, such as lactate.

Noninvasive Blood Pressure. For decades, clinicians have used NIBP monitoring to assess patients. Typically, NIBP is used for routine examinations and monitoring. Benefits of NIBP monitoring are ease of use, quick availability, and minimal patient complications.[47] To obtain accurate and reliable readings, an understanding of the science of pressure measurement is required. It is vitally important to select an appropriate cuff size. If the cuff size is too small for the patient, the pressures recorded will be falsely elevated; if the cuff size is too large, the resulting pressures will be falsely low. In addition, positioning the patient's arm at the level of the heart for measurements is also important for accurate readings.

Patients who are hemodynamically unstable, either profoundly hypotensive or profoundly hypertensive, cannot be adequately assessed using NIBP measurement.[47] In the obese patient with conically shaped upper arms, it is technically difficult to measure a NIBP because the cuff often does not fit appropriately or stay positioned. Blood pressure readings are also affected by the presence of cardiac dysrhythmias, respiratory variation, shivering, seizures, external cuff compression, decreased peripheral perfusion, peripheral vasoconstriction, and patient talking or movement during the measurement. Isolated blood pressure readings are not used to guide patient management; trending of values over time and assessing the response to interventions are crucial to maximize patient outcomes.

Jugular Venous Pressure. Assessment of the jugular veins provides an estimate of intravascular volume, and it is an indirect measure of CVP. Because the internal jugular vein directly communicates with the right atrium, it can serve as a manometer to provide an estimate of the CVP. Jugular venous distension occurs when the CVP is elevated, which can occur with fluid overload, right ventricular dysfunction, superior vena cava obstruction, and right heart failure. The technique for assessing jugular venous pressure is pictured in Fig. 9.7.

Lactate. Anything that deprives the tissues of oxygen disrupts the Krebs cycle, resulting in anaerobic metabolism and increased production of lactic acid. Normal arterial lactate levels range from 0.3 to 0.8 mmol/L (3 to 7 mg/dL), and venous values range from 0.6 to 2.2 mmol/L (5 to 20 mg/dL).[33] In lactic acidosis the lactate level is elevated, commonly above 4 mmol/L (0.5 to 1.6 mEq/L).[33] Lactate levels may be measured to

TABLE 9.1 Normal Hemodynamic Values[a]

Hemodynamic Parameter	Significance	Normal Range
Cardiac output (CO)	Amount of blood pumped out by a ventricle every minute	4-8 L/min
Cardiac index (CI)	CO individualized to patient body surface area (BSA; size)	2.5-4.2 L/min/m^2
Central venous pressure (CVP)	Pressure created by volume of blood in right heart at end-diastole; used to guide assessment of fluid balance and responsiveness to fluid administration	2-6 mm Hg
Right atrial pressure (RAP)	Used interchangeably with CVP; pressure created by volume of blood in right heart at end-diastole; measured with a pulmonary artery catheter	2-6 mm Hg
Left atrial pressure (LAP)	Pressure created by volume of blood in left heart at end-diastole	8-12 mm Hg
Pulmonary artery occlusion pressure (PAOP) *(wedge)*	Pressure created by volume of blood in left heart at end-diastole	8-12 mm Hg
Pulmonary artery pressure (PAP) (pulmonary artery systole [PAS] and pulmonary artery diastole [PAD])	Pulsatile pressure in the pulmonary artery	PAS 15-25 mm Hg PAD 8-15 mm Hg
Stroke volume (SV)	Amount of blood ejected from the ventricle with each contraction	60-130 mL/beat
Stroke index (SI)	SV individualized to BSA	30-65 mL/beat/m^2
Systemic vascular resistance (SVR)	Resistance that the left ventricle must overcome to open the aortic valve and eject a volume of blood into the systemic circulation; generally, as SVR increases, CO falls	770-1500 dynes/sec/cm^{-5}
Systemic vascular resistance index (SVRI)	SVR individualized to BSA	1680-2580 dynes/sec/cm^{-5}/m^2
Pulmonary vascular resistance (PVR)	Resistance that the right ventricle must overcome to open the pulmonic valve and eject a volume of blood in the pulmonary vasculature	<250 dynes/sec/cm^{-5}
Pulmonary vascular resistance index (PVRI)	PVR individualized to BSA	255-285 dynes/sec/cm^{-5}/m^2
Right cardiac work index (RCWI)	Amount of work the right ventricle performs each minute when ejecting blood; increases or decreases depending on changes in volume or pressure; used as a measure of contractility	0.54-0.66 kg-m/m^2
Right ventricular stroke work index (RVSWI)	Amount of work the right ventricle performs with each heartbeat; increases or decreases depending on changes in SV and PAP mean; used as a measure of contractility	7.9-9.7 g-m/beat/m^2
Left cardiac work index (LCWI)	Amount of work the left ventricle performs each minute when ejecting blood; increases or decreases depending on changes in CO and mean arterial pressure (MAP); used as a measure of contractility	3.4-4.2 kg-m/m^2
Left ventricular stroke work index (LVSWI)	Amount of work the left ventricle performs with each heartbeat; increases or decreases depending on changes in SV and MAP; used as a measure of contractility	50-62 g-m/beat/m^2
Right ventricular end-diastolic volume (RVEDV) and right ventricular end-diastolic pressure (RVEDP)	Measures right ventricular preload	0-8 mm Hg (RVEDP)
Left ventricular end-diastolic volume (LVEDV) and left ventricular end-diastolic pressure (LVEDP)	Measures left ventricular preload	4-12 mm Hg (LVEDP)
Mixed venous oxygen saturation (SvO$_2$)	Provides an assessment of balance between oxygen supply and demand. Measured in the pulmonary artery. Higher values indicate increased O$_2$ supply, decreased O$_2$ demand, or the inability to extract oxygen from blood; lower values indicate decreased O$_2$ supply from low hemoglobin, low CO, low SaO$_2$, and/or increased O$_2$ consumption	60%-75%
Central venous oxygen saturation (ScvO$_2$)	Similar to SvO$_2$ but measured in the distal portion of a central venous catheter proximal to the right atrium and before the point where the cardiac sinus returns deoxygenated blood from the myocardium, thus the reason for the discrepancy between SvO$_2$ and ScvO$_2$ normal ranges	65%-85%

[a]Note that normal values vary by various references.

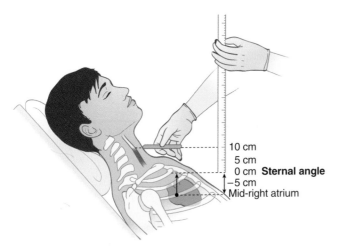

Fig. 9.7 Assessment of jugular venous pressure.

10 cm
5 cm
0 cm **Sternal angle**
−5 cm
Mid-right atrium

determine tissue hypoperfusion in shock, to establish adequacy of resuscitation, and to assist in diagnosis of patients who have metabolic acidosis of unknown cause.[21] The use of lactate levels to guide therapy with a goal of reducing levels 20% every 2 hours can be used in conjunction with other parameters such as MAP, heart rate, urine output, hemoglobin levels, arterial oxygen saturation (SaO_2), and $ScvO_2$ to manage patients and reduce critical care unit length of stay and critical care unit and hospital mortality.[21]

Invasive Hemodynamic Monitoring

Indications. Invasive methods of hemodynamic monitoring are used to obtain more detailed physiological information. Common indications for invasive monitoring are outlined in Box 9.1.

BOX 9.1 Indications for Invasive Hemodynamic Monitoring

Arterial Line
- Treat hemodynamic instability
- Assess efficacy of vasoactive medications
- Obtain frequent blood samples for arterial blood gas analysis or other laboratory tests
- Can be used in conjunction with a stroke volume measurement device

Central Venous Catheter
- Measure right heart filling pressures
- Estimate fluid status
- Guide volume resuscitation
- Assess central venous oxygen saturation ($ScvO_2$)
- Administer large-volume fluid resuscitation or medications
- Access to place transvenous pacemaker

Pulmonary Artery Catheter
- Assess left heart function with PAOP pressures
- Identify and treat cause of hemodynamic instability
- Assess pulmonary artery pressures
- Assess mixed venous oxygen saturation (SvO_2)
- Directly measure cardiac output

PAOP, Pulmonary artery occlusion pressure.

A comprehensive hemodynamic assessment is used to guide interventions in patients with the following diagnoses: shock, cardiac tamponade, ruptured ventricular septum, heart failure, and right ventricular infarction. In addition, hemodynamic monitoring is used with complex surgical patients to guide therapy and detect complications early.

The first step in a hemodynamic assessment is to determine the adequacy of tissue perfusion to determine whether the patient is in a state of shock that requires fluid resuscitation. Once preload is optimized, afterload and contractility are addressed.

Equipment Common to All Intravascular Monitoring. The basic hemodynamic monitoring system has five major components: (1) the invasive catheter, (2) high-pressure noncompliant tubing, (3) the transducer with a stopcock, (4) a pressurized flush system, and (5) the bedside monitoring system (Fig. 9.8).

The *invasive catheter* varies depending on the type of catheter, purpose, and location of insertion. The catheter can be placed into an artery, a vein, or the heart. An arterial catheter consists of a relatively small-gauge, short, pliable catheter that is placed over a guidewire or in a catheter-over-needle system. CVP or $ScvO_2$ monitoring is obtained through a central venous catheter (CVC), most commonly placed in the subclavian or internal jugular vein (Fig. 9.9). The femoral vein may be used when the thoracic veins are not available or in a trauma situation. Femoral catheters are associated with higher infection rates and should be removed as soon as possible. Pulmonary artery (PA) pressure and SvO_2 monitoring require a longer catheter that is placed into the PA (Fig. 9.10).

Noncompliant pressure tubing designed specifically for hemodynamic monitoring is used to minimize artifact and increase the accuracy of the data transmission. Noncompliant tubing allows for the efficient and accurate transfer of intravascular pressure changes to the transducer and monitoring system. To maintain the most accurate pressure readings, the tubing should be no longer than 36 to 48 inches, with a minimum number of additional stopcocks.

The *transducer* (Fig. 9.11) translates intravascular pressure changes into waveforms and numerical data. To ensure that the data are accurate, the system must be calibrated to atmospheric pressure by zeroing the transducer. A three-way stopcock attached to the transducer is generally used as the reference point for zeroing and leveling the system. This is referred to as the *air-fluid interface* or the zeroing stopcock.

The *flush system* maintains patency of the pressure tubing and catheter. The flush solution (usually 0.9% normal saline) is placed in a pressure bag that is inflated to 300 mm Hg to ensure a constant flow of fluid through the pressure tubing, usually 2 to 5 mL/h per lumen. A clinical review concluded that flush systems using heparin prolong catheter patency.[19] However, the use of heparin carries additional risks, including the development of heparin-induced thrombocytopenia. Consider the risk-to-benefit ratio when determining whether to use heparin or normal saline flush solutions.

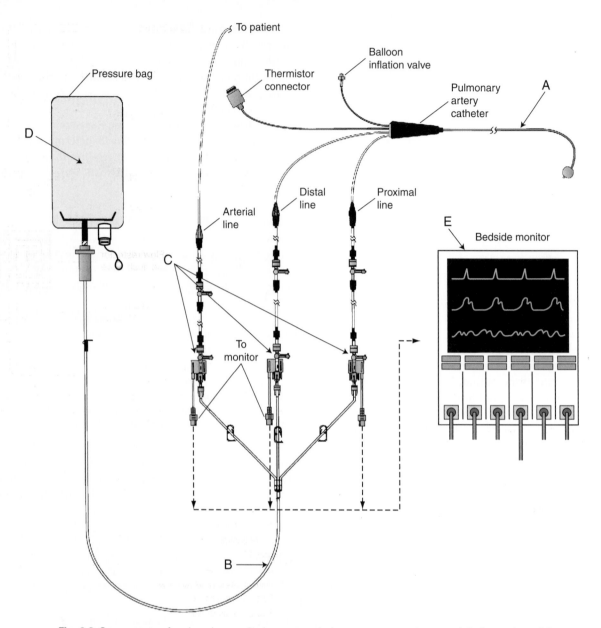

Fig. 9.8 Components of an invasive monitoring system (pulmonary artery catheter and designated arterial line) connected to one flush solution. **A,** Invasive catheter. **B,** Noncompliant pressure tubing. **C,** Transducer and zeroing stopcock. **D,** Pressurized flush system. **E,** Bedside monitoring system. (Not to scale.)

Bedside monitoring systems vary, but all have the same general function and purpose. They provide the visual display of waveforms and numerical information generated by the transducer and can store and record the data. The clinician interprets the data.

Nursing Implications. Accuracy in hemodynamic monitoring is essential for clinical decision making (see Clinical Alert box). Four major components for validating the accuracy of hemodynamic monitoring systems are (1) positioning the patient, (2) leveling the air-fluid interface (zeroing stopcock) to the phlebostatic axis, (3) zeroing the transducer, and (4) assessing dynamic responsiveness (performing the *square wave test*).[31] Preventing and assessing for complications

(Box 9.2) are also key nursing interventions for patients with invasive hemodynamic monitoring catheters.

! CLINICAL ALERT

Hemodynamic Monitoring

Keys to success in hemodynamic monitoring are ensuring that the data are accurate, conducting waveform analysis, and integrating the data with other assessment variables. Never base clinical decision making solely on one variable and do not interpret hemodynamic values in isolation. Integration of clinical data, patient presentation, and subjective assessment are crucial to making clinical decisions to improve patient outcomes. Hemodynamic data are most beneficial when directed by established protocols with specific end points of therapy.[1-3,22,26,27,32,38]

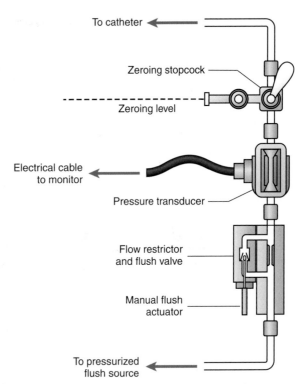

Fig. 9.11 A schematic of a typical pressure transducer. (From Kruse JA. Fast flush test. In: Kruse JA, Fink MP, Carlson RW, eds. *Saunders Manual of Critical Care.* Philadelphia, PA: Saunders; 2003.)

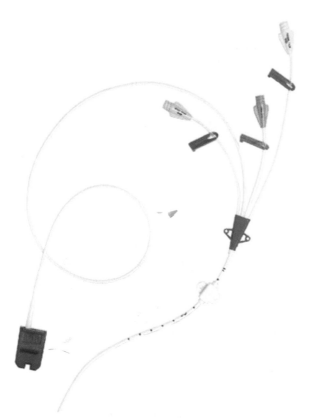

Fig. 9.9 Example of a triple-lumen central line to measure central venous pressure and oxygen saturation. (Courtesy Edwards Lifesciences, Irvine, CA.)

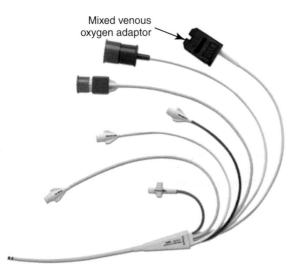

Fig. 9.10 Example of a pulmonary artery catheter with capability of monitoring mixed venous oxygenation. (Courtesy Edwards Lifesciences, Irvine, CA.)

Patient Positioning. Hemodynamic data can be accurately measured with the patient supine or lateral and with the head of the bed (HOB) flat or elevated as long as the air-fluid interface used to zero the transducer is level to the phlebostatic axis. HOB elevation to 30 degrees is a key factor in the prevention of complications, such as ventilator-associated pneumonia, and provides a comfortable position for most patients.[25-27,37]

BOX 9.2 Potential Complications of Invasive Hemodynamic Monitoring Devices

- Vascular complications
  - Thrombosis
  - Hematoma
- Infection
- Bleeding
- Pneumothorax or hemothorax
- Cardiac dysrhythmias
- Pericardial tamponade

✳ QSEN EXEMPLAR

Evidence-Based Practice

The American Association of Critical-Care Nurses 2016 Practice Alert summarized results of studies and determined that accurate hemodynamic data can be obtained in lateral positions from 30 to 90 degrees, although it is technically more difficult to level the transducer to the atria. In the 30-degree lateral position, the transducer is placed half the distance from the surface of the bed to the left sternal border. The patient must be positioned exactly at a 30-degree lateral position for this method to be accurate. If the patient is in a 90-degree right lateral position, the transducer is leveled to the fourth intercostal space, mid-sternum. If the patient is in a 90-degree left lateral position, the transducer is leveled to the fourth intercostal space, left parasternal border.

References

American Association of Critical-Care Nurses. Practice alert: Pulmonary artery/central venous pressure monitoring in adults. *Crit Care Nurse.* 2016;36:e2–e218.

Rajaram SS, Desai NK, Kalra A, et al. Pulmonary artery catheters for adult patients in intensive care. *Cochrane Database Syst Rev.* 2013;(2):CD003408.

Leveling the Air-Fluid Interface. Position the zeroing stopcock of the transducer system at the level of the atria for accurate readings. This external anatomical location is called the *phlebostatic axis,* and it is located by identifying the fourth intercostal space at the midway point of the anterior-posterior diameter of the chest wall (Fig. 9.12).[31] A permanent marker can be used to mark the location of the phlebostatic axis on the patient to ensure that future measurements are done using the same reference point.[30] Once the level of the phlebostatic axis is identified, secure the transducer and zeroing stopcock to the chest wall or to an IV pole positioned near the patient. The relationship of the air-fluid interface to the phlebostatic axis must be maintained so that the numerical readings transmitted to the monitor are accurate. When the transducer is affixed to the patient's chest wall, regularly assess skin integrity to prevent skin breakdown.

Because of the effects of hydrostatic pressure on the fluid-filled monitoring system, variations in the height of the transducer system by as little as 1 cm below the phlebostatic axis can result in a false elevation by as much as 0.73 mm Hg. Conversely, if the transducer is above the phlebostatic axis, a false low reading results. Therefore the location of the zeroing stopcock must be regularly monitored and releveled with each change in the patient's position.

Zero Referencing. The effects of atmospheric pressure on the fluid-filled hemodynamic monitoring system must be negated for accurate measurements. At sea level the atmospheric pressure exerts a force of 760 mm Hg on any object on the Earth's surface. To eliminate the effect of the atmospheric pressure on the physiological variables, the transducer system is "zeroed" at the level of the phlebostatic axis.[31] To accomplish this task, open the zeroing stopcock of the transducer to air (closed to the patient) and calibrate (zero) the monitoring system to read a pressure of 0 mm Hg. Each computer system has a zeroing function that is easy to perform. Zero referencing is done when the catheter is inserted, at the beginning of each shift, when repositioning the patient, and when there are significant changes in hemodynamic status.

Dynamic Response Testing. Fluid-filled monitoring systems rely on the ability of the transducer to translate the vascular pressure into waveforms and numerical data. To verify that the transducer system accurately represents cardiovascular pressures, perform the dynamic response, or *square wave,* test. This test is done by recording the pressure waveform while activating the fast-flush valve or actuator on the pressure tubing system for at least 1 second. The resulting graph should depict a rapid upstroke from the baseline with a plateau before returning to the baseline (i.e., a *square wave*).[11] When the pressure tracing returns to the baseline, a small undershoot should occur below the baseline, along with one or two oscillations within 0.12 second, before resuming the pressure waveform. If the dynamic response test meets these criteria, the system is optimally damped (Fig. 9.13A), and the resulting waveforms and numerical data can be interpreted as accurate. Perform the dynamic response test after catheter insertion, at least once per shift, after drawing blood from the line, and any time the system is opened. It is a simple but crucial test that must be incorporated into routine hemodynamic assessment to ensure accuracy.[11]

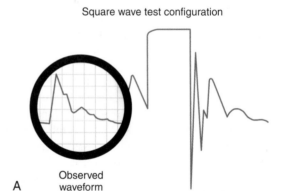

Square wave test configuration

Observed
waveform

A

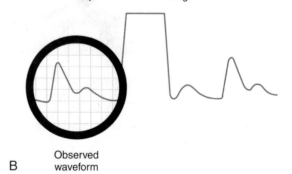

Square wave test configuration

Observed
waveform

B

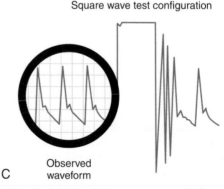

Square wave test configuration

Observed
waveform

C

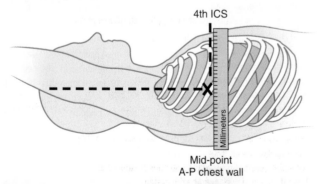

4th ICS

Millimeters

Mid-point
A-P chest wall

Fig. 9.12 Locating the phlebostatic axis in the supine position. *A-P,* Anterior-posterior; *ICS,* intercostal space.

Fig. 9.13 A, Optimal dynamic response test. **B,** Overdamped dynamic response test. **C,** Underdamped dynamic response test.

The system is overdamped if the dynamic response test results in no oscillations, the upstroke is slurred, or a small undershoot is not produced (see Fig. 9.13B). An overdamped system can result in a systolic pressure that is falsely low and a diastolic pressure that is falsely elevated.

Conversely, the system is underdamped if the dynamic response test results in excessive oscillations (see Fig. 9.13C). The displayed pressure waveform and numerical data will show erroneously high systolic pressures and low diastolic pressures. Box 9.3 describes the causes of abnormal dynamic response test results and interventions for troubleshooting systems that are overdamped or underdamped.

Preventing Infection. Central line–associated bloodstream infections (CLABSIs) result in thousands of deaths each year and billions of dollars in added costs. Invasive catheters are direct portals to the circulating blood; therefore strict infection control measures must be implemented to prevent CLABSI. To reduce the risk for CLABSI, a central line bundle was developed that emphasizes strict hand washing, strict sterile technique with maximal barrier precautions during placement, chlorhexidine skin antisepsis, optimal catheter site selection, and daily review of line necessity.[45,46] Maintaining the site properly, minimizing the number of times the system is opened, using sutureless securement devices, cleansing patients with chlorhexidine baths, changing the tubing system no more frequently than every 72 to 96 hours, aseptic treatment of tubing infusion ports, and aseptic treatment of medications and fluids given to the patient are recommended.[5,45,46] See the Evidence-Based Practice box for more discussion related to bathing. A decreased rate of CLABSI is associated with use of the subclavian vein site, although it has the highest rate of complications resulting from pneumothorax and phrenic nerve damage. In comparison, use of the internal jugular site has a lower complication rate than the subclavian but is associated with higher infection rates. The femoral site is the least preferred for cannulation among adult patients as a result of higher infection rates and patient mobility restrictions.[45,46] Box 9.4 describes general strategies for managing hemodynamic monitoring systems.

EVIDENCE-BASED PRACTICE

Problem

Central line–associated bloodstream infections (CLABSIs) are a major complication of invasive lines. Chlorhexidine dressings have been recommended in intervention bundles to reduce CLABSI. Bathing with chlorhexidine-impregnated washcloths is another strategy that has been tested.

Clinical Question

What is the effectiveness of chlorhexidine bathing on the risk of infection in adult critical care patients?

Evidence

The authors conducted a systematic review of 17 trials that evaluated outcomes of chlorhexidine bathing. It was estimated that the bathing reduced the risk of CLABSI by 56%. Bathing also reducing colonization with methicillin-resistant *Staphylococcus aureus* and bacteremia. The authors note that the effectiveness of the chlorhexidine bathing may be of greatest benefit in critical care unit populations with the highest risk for infection.

Implications for Nursing

Nurses are responsible for patient hygiene. Chlorhexidine bathing may be part of the standard of care at many critical care units. If used, nurses should monitor for any skin irritation that may be associated with the chlorhexidine.

Level of Evidence

A—Systematic review and meta-analysis

Reference

Frost SA, Alogso M, Metcalfe L, et al. Chlorhexidine bathing and health care–associated infections among adult intensive care patients: A systematic review and meta-analysis. *Crit Care*. 2016;20:379.

BOX 9.3 Abnormal Dynamic Response Test: Causes and Interventions

Overdamped System
- Blood clots, blood left in the catheter after obtaining a blood sample, air bubbles at any point between the catheter tip and transducer
  - Flush the system or aspirate, disconnecting from the patient, if needed, to adequately flush the system to remove clots or air bubbles
- Compliant tubing
  - Change to noncompliant tubing or commercially available tubing system
- Loose connections
  - Ensure that all connections are secure
- Kinks in the tubing system
  - Straighten tubing
- Flush system integrity
  - Ensure that there is an adequate amount of flush solution
  - Ensure that the pressure bag is at 300 mm Hg

Underdamped System
- Excessive tubing length (normal is <36 to 48 inches)
  - Remove extraneous tubing, stopcocks, or extensions
- Small-bore tubing
  - Replace small-bore tubing with a larger bore set
- Cause unknown
  - Add a damping device into the system to reduce artifact
  - Can be the result of patient anatomy and some diagnoses

BOX 9.4 General Nursing Strategies for Managing Hemodynamic Monitoring Systems

- Document insertion date
- Change occlusive dressings according to institutional policy
  - Assess for signs of infection
  - Date dressing changes
- Maintain patency of the flush system
  - Flush the system after each use of a port
  - Clear any blood from the tubing, ports, and stopcocks
  - Maintain a pressure of 300 mm Hg on the flush solution using a pressure bag
  - Ensure adequate amount of flush solution
- Ensure tightened connections in the tubing and flush system
- Keep tubing free of kinks
- Minimize excess tubing and the number of stopcocks
- Limit disconnecting or opening the system
- Ensure that alarm limits are set on the monitor and alarms are turned on

Arterial Pressure Monitoring

Arterial pressure monitoring is indicated for patients who are at risk for compromised tissue perfusion. Other indications include the need for frequent laboratory testing, hypotension or hypertension, and monitoring response to vasoactive medications. This common procedure involves cannulating an artery and recording pressures via the fluid-filled monitoring system. The radial artery is the site of choice because of its ready accessibility and collateral perfusion to the hand via the ulnar artery. Alternative sites include the femoral and brachial arteries. Before cannulation of the radial artery, assess collateral circulation by performing an Allen test or a modified Allen test (Box 9.5).[4] Cannulation can be facilitated by Doppler ultrasonography.

Invasive arterial pressure monitoring is the most accurate method of measuring the systemic blood pressure because it allows for continuous, beat-to-beat analysis of the arterial pressure. Arterial pressure monitoring is thus the method of choice in assessing blood pressure in the hemodynamically unstable patient.[40]

The normal arterial waveform (Fig. 9.14) consists of a sharp upstroke, the peak of which represents the systolic pressure. This pressure is a direct reflection of left ventricular function. Normal values for systolic pressures are less than 140 mm Hg. The lowest point on the arterial waveform represents the end-diastolic pressure and reflects systemic resistance. Normal values for diastolic pressure are less than 90 mm Hg.[11]

The downstroke of the arterial waveform consists of a small notch called the *dicrotic notch*, which represents aortic valve closure and the beginning of diastole. This is commonly considered the reference point between the systolic and diastolic phases of the cardiac system. The remainder of the downstroke is arterial distribution of blood flow through the arterial system.

Complications. The major complications of arterial pressure monitoring include thrombosis, embolism, blood loss, and

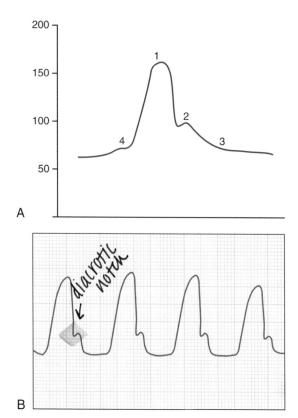

Fig. 9.14 A, Normal arterial pressure tracing. *1,* Peak systolic pressure; *2,* dicrotic notch; *3,* diastolic pressure; *4,* anacrotic notch. **B,** Arterial pressure waveform obtained from arterial line.

infection. Embolism may occur as a result of small clot formation around the tip of the catheter or from air entering the system. Thrombosis (clot) may occur if a continuous flush solution is not properly maintained. Rapid blood loss can result from sudden dislodgment of the catheter from the artery or from a disconnection in the tubing connections. Maintain monitoring alarms that are individualized to the patient's parameters at all times to decrease the risk of undetected bleeding or line disconnection. Although infection is a risk of intraarterial catheters, routine replacement of the catheter is not recommended unless an infection is suspected.[10]

Clinical Considerations. The invasive method of obtaining blood pressure is considered to be more accurate than noninvasive methods. In patients who are hypotensive, a serious discrepancy may exist between the blood pressures obtained by invasive and noninvasive means.[41,47] The cuff pressure may be significantly lower, leading to dangerous mistakes in the treatment of such a patient. Under normal circumstances, a difference of 10 to 20 mm Hg between invasive and noninvasive blood pressure is expected, with the invasive blood pressure generally higher than the noninvasive value.[43] When the noninvasive value is higher than the invasive number, suspect equipment malfunction or technical error. Check the intraarterial system. Zero reference and level the system, and perform a square wave test to evaluate accuracy. Box 9.6 lists the possible causes of inaccurate invasive blood pressure readings.

BOX 9.5   Allen and Modified Allen Test Procedure

Allen Test
- Ask the patient to form a tight fist with the wrist in a neutral position
- Occlude the radial artery by applying pressure with the thumb for approximately 10 seconds
- Ask the patient to open the fist while the clinician maintains thumb pressure on the radial artery
- Ulnar circulation is adequate if blanching resolves within 5 seconds and inadequate if the hand remains pale for more than 10 seconds

Modified Allen Test
- Ask the patient to form a tight fist with the wrist in a neutral position
- Occlude radial and ulnar arteries for approximately 10 seconds
- Ask the patient to open the fist, revealing a blanched hand
- Release pressure on the ulnar artery, maintaining pressure on the radial artery
- Ulnar circulation is adequate if blanching resolves within 5 seconds and inadequate if the hand remains pale for more than 10 seconds

BOX 9.6 Causes of Inaccurate Arterial Line Readings

- Air bubbles in the catheter system
- Failure to zero the transducer air-fluid interface
- Blood in the catheter system
- Blood clot at the catheter tip
- Kinking of the tubing system
- Catheter tip lodging against the arterial wall
- Soft, compliant tubing
- Long tubing (>48 inches)
- Too many stopcocks (>3)

Nursing Implications. Refer to Box 9.4 for standard management of all invasive hemodynamic systems. Additional interventions specific to management of the intraarterial catheter include the following:

- Document assessment of the extremity regularly for perfusion: color, temperature, sensation, pulse, and capillary refill (normal time to refill is <3 seconds).
- Keep the patient's wrist in a neutral position and if needed place it on an arm board (radial artery catheters).
- When the catheter is removed, ensure that adequate pressure is applied to the insertion site until hemostasis is obtained (for a minimum of 5 minutes for radial artery catheters). The time required varies depending on the type, size, and location of the catheter and on the patient's coagulation status.
- Never administer medications via an arterial line because of potential harmful complications.

Right Atrial Pressure/Central Venous Pressure Monitoring

In critically ill patients, the right atrial pressure (RAP) or CVP is used to estimate central venous blood volume and right heart function. The pressure is obtained from the right atrial port of a pulmonary artery catheter (PAC) and is also called the *RAP*. Because no valves are present between the venae cavae and right atrium, both the CVP and the RAP are essentially equal pressures. This measurement assesses preload of the right side of the heart. The term *RAP* is used most often in this textbook. Normal RAP/CVP ranges from 2 to 6 mm Hg.

The RAP is obtained from a central line inserted into the superior or inferior vena cava. The thoracic central veins (subclavian and internal jugular veins) are the most common insertion sites. Catheters used for RAP measurement are generally stiff and radiopaque, and they vary in length and diameter depending on the vein that is used. Shorter catheters are inserted into the subclavian and internal jugular veins, and longer catheters are used for insertion into the upper extremities or femoral vein. Central venous catheters often have multiple lumens that facilitate pressure monitoring, administration of fluids and medications, and blood sampling. If the placement of a PAC is anticipated, a catheter with an introducer may be used.

During insertion, place the patient's bed in the Trendelenburg position to promote venous filling in the upper body for easier insertion of the catheter, unless the patient has respiratory distress or increased intracranial pressure. This position also prevents air embolism during insertion. If the Trendelenburg position is contraindicated, place a blanket roll between the patient's shoulder blades to facilitate insertion. The provider cleans the skin with an antiseptic, drapes the patient, and injects a local anesthetic to reduce pain during insertion. A needled syringe is used to puncture the vessel and to confirm placement by backward flow of blood into the syringe. The syringe is removed, and a guidewire is threaded through the needle into the vessel. The needle is then removed so that the catheter may be passed over the guidewire. Once the catheter is in place, the provider will suture or use a sutureless device to secure the catheter and place a dressing per facility policy. After the procedure, obtain a chest radiograph to verify placement and assess for complications. Fig. 9.15 shows a position of a central venous catheter (CVC) in the right atrium along with the corresponding waveform.

The RAP, along with other measurements, is used to assess and guide fluid resuscitation and estimate right-sided cardiac function. The interpretation of the RAP should be compared with the stroke index (SI).[34] If both the RAP and the SI are low, hypovolemia is likely. If the RAP is high and the SI is low, right ventricular dysfunction is likely.

Because the normal RAP value is low and within a narrow range, it is important to obtain an accurate reading of the RAP. Level the system at the phlebostatic axis and zero the system, then verify an optimal dynamic response test.

Measure the RAP at end-expiration and at the end of ventricular diastole. Simultaneously, obtain a graph of the cardiac rhythm (electrocardiogram [ECG]), RAP, and respiratory

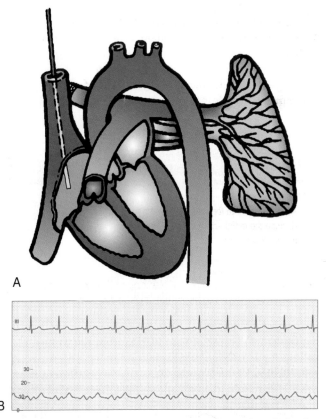

Fig. 9.15 A, Position of central venous catheter in right atrium. **B,** Cardiac rhythm and associated waveforms.

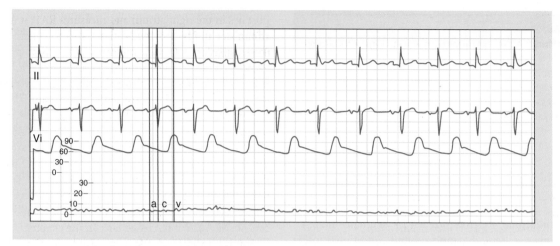

Fig. 9.16 Identifying the *a*, *c*, and *v* waveforms to determine right atrial pressure.

tracing (if available) to obtain an accurate measurement of RAP. The RAP tracing is composed of three major waveforms: *a*, *c*, and *v* waves (Fig. 9.16). The *a* wave is produced by atrial contraction and follows the P wave on the ECG tracing. The *c* wave is produced by closure of the tricuspid valve and follows the R wave. Finally, the *v* wave correlates with right atrial filling and right ventricular systole; it follows the T wave on the ECG.[29]

To measure the RAP, identify the *a*, *c*, and *v* waves of the RAP tracing at end-expiration (see Fig. 9.16). Measure the RAP at end-expiration to ensure that pleural pressure changes do not skew the numeric value. True RAP is best measured by locating the *c* wave and identifying the value immediately preceding the *c* wave (called the *pre-c measurement*). Alternatively, the average of the *a* wave may be computed, or the z-point method may be determined. The z-point method consists of identifying the RAP by locating the end of the QRS complex and using that as the reference point on the tracing. Box 9.7 outlines circumstances for using the different methods for determining RAP.

Complications. Maintain maximum sterile barrier precautions during insertion because CLABSIs are common, increasing the risk of sepsis.[45,46] Other complications may occur during insertion, including carotid puncture, pneumothorax, hemothorax, perforation of the right atrium or ventricle, and cardiac dysrhythmias. Obtain a chest radiograph after insertion to confirm placement and detect complications.

Clinical Considerations. Abnormalities in RAP are generally caused by any condition that alters venous tone, blood volume, or right ventricular contractility. For example, a patient with a low RAP may be hypovolemic because of dehydration or traumatic blood loss. Low pressures are also seen in relative hypovolemia because of vasodilation from rewarming, medications, or sepsis. In all of these conditions, a decreased RAP reflects blood return to the heart that is insufficient to meet the body's requirements. Confounding the interpretation of a low RAP is that the value may be negative in an individual in the upright position, even if cardiac function and volume status are normal.

BOX 9.7   Methods for Determining Accurate Right Atrial Pressure

Pre-*c* Method
- Most accurate measure of right-sided preload; method of choice for numerical assessment
- Represents the last atrial pressure before ventricular contraction
- Difficult to use because the *c* wave is often unidentifiable

Mean of the *a* Wave
- Clinically significant because the *a* wave results from atrial contraction
- Used if the *c* wave cannot be identified
- Obtain the numerical value for the top and bottom of the *a* wave; calculate the sum and divide by 2

Z-Point Method
- Used when atrial-ventricular synchrony is not present: atrial fibrillation, third-degree heart block
- Standardized approach results in the most reproducible value between clinicians
- Does not account for hemodynamic effects on kidneys or liver that result from the prominent *a* or *v* waves
- Locate the end of the QRS complex; use the numerical value associated with the exact point of intersection of the right atrial pressure waveform

---

A high RAP measurement indicates conditions that reduce the right ventricle's ability to eject blood, thereby increasing right ventricular pressure and RAP. Such conditions include hypervolemia (seen with aggressive administration of IV fluids), severe vasoconstriction, and mechanical ventilation (additional positive pressure increases RAP). Conditions causing RAP increase include pulmonary hypertension and heart failure.

Nursing Implications. The critical care nurse is responsible for collecting and recording patient data, ensuring the accuracy of the data, and reporting abnormal findings and trends to the provider. Analyzing the various hemodynamic parameters is a collaborative responsibility between physician and nurse to ensure prompt and appropriate treatment. Measurements of RAP are essential to compare with other physiological parameters and assessment findings.

Pulmonary Artery Pressure Monitoring

Pulmonary artery catheters are used to diagnose and manage a variety of conditions in critically ill patients. The ability to measure pressures in the PA and the left side of the heart became reality after a flow-directed PAC was invented by doctors Jeremy Swan and William Ganz in 1970.[42] Thermodilution PACs with the ability to obtain PA pressures and CO measurement became the gold standard to which all new hemodynamic monitoring methods are compared.[40] In the last 30 years, the PAC has been redesigned to obtain a variety of hemodynamic parameters, including measurements of continuous cardiac output (CCO), right ventricular end-diastolic volume, right ventricular ejection fraction, and SvO$_2$.

To determine pulmonary artery pressure (PAP), a specialized catheter is placed directly into the PA (Fig. 9.17). The PAC is a long, flexible, multilumen, balloon-tipped catheter that enables measurement of several hemodynamic parameters. The proximal port lies in the right atrium and measures RAP; it is also used to administer fluids and medications and to obtain intermittent thermodilution CO measurements. The distal port measures PAP and PAOP; mixed venous blood samples are also drawn from this port. The thermistor port incorporates a temperature-sensitive wire that allows computer calculation of CO with the thermodilution method. Many catheters have an additional proximal infusion port for fluid and medication administration. The balloon inflation lumen provides the ability to inflate and deflate the small-volume (approximately 1.5-mL) balloon at the distal tip of the catheter. The balloon is inflated to facilitate insertion of the catheter and to measure PAOP, which provides information about the function of the left side of the heart.[36] The concept of PAOP is discussed later in the chapter.

Several specialized PACs are available. One PAC enables transvenous pacing. This technique involves the insertion of a pacemaker wire through additional lumina in the PAC, which exits the catheter into the right ventricle to provide ventricular pacing. The CCO PAC provides continuous monitoring of CO. A PAC with a fiberoptic lumen at the tip of the catheter was developed for continuous measurement of SvO$_2$. The concepts of CCO and SvO$_2$ are discussed later in the chapter.

Nurses assist providers during PAC insertion. After the physician obtains informed consent, the nurse provides additional education on patient positioning and what the patient may feel or experience during the procedure. In addition, the nurse

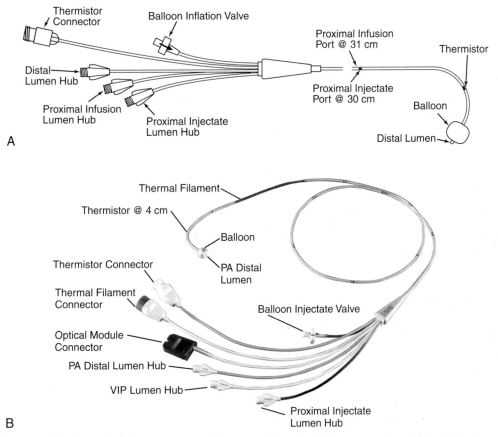

Fig. 9.17 A, A five-lumen pulmonary artery catheter containing the four-lumen components in addition to a second proximal lumen for infusion of fluid or medications. **B,** CCOmbo 777 catheter. (Courtesy Edwards Lifesciences, Irvine, CA.)

provides measures to alleviate the patient's anxiety before and during the procedure.

The method of PAC insertion is similar to that for the CVC.[30] Once the access port is in place, the PAC is passed freely into the vessel through the introducer. The provider inserting the catheter instructs the nurse (or other professional assisting with insertion) to inflate and deflate the balloon during the procedure to facilitate flow from the right atrium to the PA. The insertion technique may vary according to provider preference, brand of equipment used, and the patient's anatomy.[30]

During PAC insertion, monitor and record respiratory rate and effort and heart rate and rhythm, and assess for dysrhythmias. Monitor blood pressure and visualize and record waveforms while the catheter is advanced. Ventricular dysrhythmias may occur as the catheter passes into and then through the right ventricle into the PA. Assist with balloon inflation during the procedure. As the catheter passes through each chamber, observe the waveform characteristics and record pressure values: RAP, right ventricular pressure, PAP, and PAOP (Fig. 9.18). The PAOP

waveform signals the end of insertion, at which time the balloon is deflated. Once the balloon is deflated, the tip of the catheter settles back into the PA position. After the catheter is inserted and placement is verified, the balloon is inflated only to obtain periodic PAOP measurements; otherwise it remains deflated to prevent complications such as pulmonary infarction and PA rupture. Nursing priorities are to accurately interpret PAC waveforms, recognize the effect of respiratory variations, prevent complications, and document hemodynamic values. Graphing the pressure waveforms and ECG tracing is also recommended.[30]

As a patient advocate, it is essential to promote patient safety throughout the procedure. Ensure that sterility is maintained, monitor the patient, and assist with balloon inflation and deflation. Because PAC insertion involves certain risks, ensure that emergency medications and equipment are readily available. Complications of insertion include hemothorax, pneumothorax, perforation of the vein or cardiac chamber, and cardiac dysrhythmias, especially as the PAC passes through the right ventricle. After the procedure, obtain a chest radiograph to

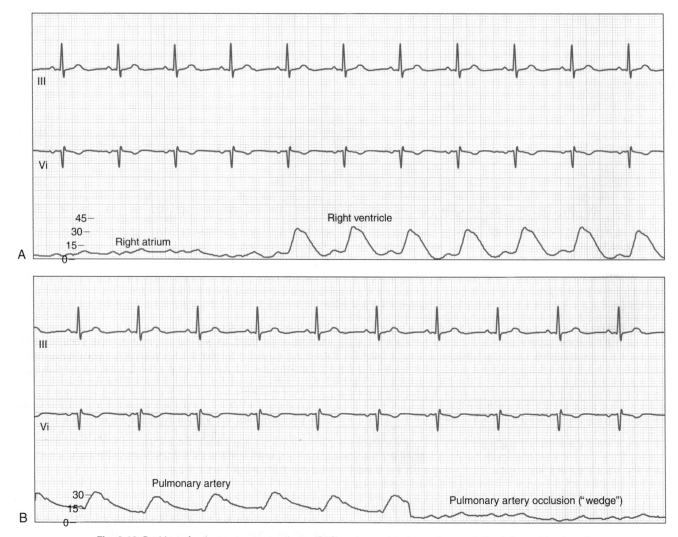

Fig. 9.18 Position of pulmonary artery catheter (PAC) and associated waveforms. **A,** Dual-channel tracing of cardiac rhythm with pressure waveforms obtained as the PAC is inserted into the right atrium and right ventricle. **B,** Dual-channel tracing of cardiac rhythm with the pulmonary artery, and pulmonary artery occlusion pressure waveforms as the catheter is floated into proper position.

verify placement and assess for complications. Once the position is verified, document the depth of catheter insertion at the insertion site; depth markings are noted on the PAC.

STUDY BREAK
2. Pulmonary artery catheters are used primarily to assess:
   A. Left ventricular function
   B. Pulmonary function
   C. Right atrial function
   D. Right ventricular function

Hemodynamic Parameters Monitored via the Pulmonary Artery Catheter. The PAC is designed to estimate left ventricular filling pressure. Several pressures and parameters are measured or calculated by the PAC: RAP, pulmonary artery systole (PAS), pulmonary artery diastole (PAD), mean pulmonary artery pressure (PAPm), PAOP, pulmonary and systemic vascular resistance; and CO. SvO_2 is measured if a fiberoptic catheter is inserted.

The PAS is the peak pressure as the right ventricle ejects its SV and reflects the amount of pressure needed to open the pulmonic valve to pump blood into the pulmonary vasculature. The PAD represents the resistance of the pulmonary vascular bed as measured when the pulmonic valve is closed and the tricuspid valve is opened. The PAPm is the average pressure exerted on the pulmonary vasculature. The normal PAP (PAS/PAD) is approximately 25/10 mm Hg, and the PAPm is 15 mm Hg.[29,30]

The PAOP is obtained when the balloon of the PAC is inflated to wedge the catheter from the PA into a small capillary. The resulting pressure reflects the left atrial pressure and left ventricular end-diastolic pressure (LVEDP) when the mitral valve is open. When properly assessed, the PAOP is a reliable indicator of left ventricular function. Normal PAOP is 8 to 12 mm Hg. The PAOP is measured at regular intervals as ordered by the provider or in accordance with unit protocols. To obtain the PAOP, inflate the balloon with no more than 1.5 mL of air using a PA-designated syringe, for no longer than 8 to 10 seconds, while noting the waveform change from the PAP to the PAOP. To obtain accurate measurement of the PAOP, print the PAOP waveform simultaneously with the ECG waveform and respiratory patterns. Similar to RAP, obtain PAP and PAOP measurements at end-expiration. In the patient who is spontaneously breathing, pressures are highest at end-expiration and decline with inhalation (Fig. 9.19A). Obtain measurements from the waveform just before pressures decline. In the mechanically ventilated patient, pressures increase with inhalation and decrease with exhalation (see Fig. 9.19B). In these patients, obtain the measurement just before the increase in pressures during inhalation. Many newer technology bedside monitors have built in screen profiles to aid in the process of appropriately obtaining measurements in correlation to waveforms.

Clinical Considerations. Trending of PAOP provides an indirect measure of LVEDP. The PAOP is used to estimate the preload of the left heart, just as RAP/CVP is used to measure

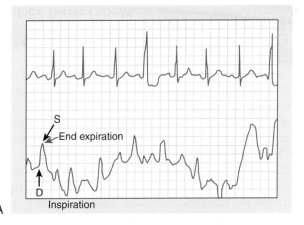

A

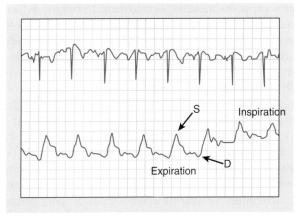

B

Fig. 9.19 Effect of respiration on pulmonary artery waveforms in patients. **A,** Spontaneous breathing. **B,** Mechanical ventilation. *D,* Diastolic pressure; *S,* systolic pressure.

preload of the right heart. In the absence of valvular disease and pulmonary vascular congestion, the PAD also closely approximates left ventricle function because the mitral valve is open during end-diastole. The PAD is often used as an indirect measurement of PAOP.

An increase in LVEDP (and therefore PAOP) indicates an increase in left ventricular blood volume to be ejected with the next systole. Increased PAOP may occur in patients who have fluid volume excess resulting from overzealous administration of IV fluid, as well as in patients with renal dysfunction. An increase in PAOP also provides information about impending left ventricular failure, as may be seen with myocardial infarction.

A decrease in LVEDP (and a subsequently low PAOP) signals a reduction in left ventricular blood volume available for the next contraction. Conditions causing a low PAOP include those that cause fluid volume deficit, such as dehydration, excessive diuretic therapy, and hemorrhage.

Nursing Implications. Routinely monitor RAP, PAP, and PAOP to identify trends and the clinical significance of the values. The catheter position must be maintained in the PA. Assess placement and review chest radiograph results, monitor for normal PA waveforms, and ensure that the balloon is deflated except during PAOP measurements.

Determine how much air is needed to obtain the PAOP (≤1.5 mL) and record this value. If the PAOP is obtained with a much smaller amount of air, the catheter may have migrated further into the PA. Do not inflate the balloon if this occurs. If the PAOP waveform is not seen with inflation of 1.5 mL of air, the catheter may be out of position or the balloon may have ruptured. In both of these situations, verify PAC position by a chest radiograph and observe the PAP waveform. For example, if the PAC has migrated into a small vessel, a PAOP waveform may be seen. If the PAC has migrated into the right ventricle, the waveform will show higher pressure, and ventricular dysrhythmias may be noted (see Fig. 9.18). If the PAD is used to estimate the PAOP, periodically compare the PAD and PAOP values to assess the accuracy of the PAD measurement, especially in patients experiencing acute hemodynamic changes. When it is determined that the PAC is no longer needed, nurses who are trained in removing the catheter often perform the procedure as outlined in the policy and procedure manual for the unit.

Cardiac Output Monitoring

The CO is the amount of blood ejected by the heart each minute and is calculated from the heart rate and SV. Cardiac index (CI) is the CO adjusted for an individual's size or body surface area. Monitoring of CO and CI is done to assess the heart's ability to pump oxygenated blood to the tissues. Cardiac output is a measure of blood flow and is considered a reliable parameter to determine whether interventions have been successful. Causes of low and high CO are outlined in Box 9.8. Two methods are commonly used to evaluate CO via the PAC: thermodilution cardiac output (TdCO) and CCO.

> ### ❓ CRITICAL REASONING ACTIVITY
>
> If a patient's mean arterial pressure continues to rise significantly, indicating an increase in resistance and an altered ability of the heart to eject blood, what parameters would also be affected as a result?

Thermodilution Cardiac Output. To measure the CO via the TdCO method, the thermistor connector on the PAC is attached to a CO module on the cardiac monitor. A set volume (5 to 10 mL) of room-temperature solution of 0.9% normal saline is injected quickly and smoothly via the proximal port. Many institutions use a closed injectate delivery system to facilitate the procedure (Fig. 9.20). As the fluid bolus passes from the right ventricle and subsequently the PA distal end, the difference in temperature is sensed by the thermistor located at the distal portion of the catheter (Fig. 9.21). The TdCO is calculated as the difference in temperature over time washout curve. Normal CO is represented by a smooth curve with a rapid upstroke and slow return to the baseline. The CO module calculates the area under this curve. The CO is inversely proportional to the area under the curve—patients with a high CO have a low calculated area under the curve.[17] Therefore the TdCO measurement is least accurate in patients with a low CO state and most accurate in a high CO state. Several steps must be taken to obtain accurate TdCO measurements. Box 9.9 describes these important points.

BOX 9.8 Interpretation of Abnormal Cardiac Output/Index Values

Low Cardiac Output/Index
- Heart rate that is too fast or too slow, leading to inadequate ventricular filling
- Stroke volume reduction as a result of:
  - **Decreased preload**
    - Hemorrhage
    - Hypovolemia from diuresis, dehydration, etc.
    - Vasodilation
    - Fluid shifts (i.e., third-spacing) outside the intravascular space
  - **Increased afterload**
    - Vasoconstriction
    - Increased blood viscosity
  - **Decreased contractility**
    - Myocardial infarction or ischemia
    - Heart failure
    - Cardiomyopathy
    - Cardiogenic shock
    - Cardiac tamponade

High Cardiac Output/Index
- Heart rate elevation secondary to:
  - Increased activity
  - Anemia
  - Metabolic demands
  - Adrenal disorders
  - Fever
  - Anxiety
- Stroke volume increase as a result of:
  - **Increased preload**
    - Fluid resuscitation
    - Alteration in ventricular compliance
  - **Decreased afterload**
    - Vasodilation in sepsis
    - Decreased blood viscosity (anemia)
    - Increased contractility
    - Hypermetabolic states
    - Medication therapy

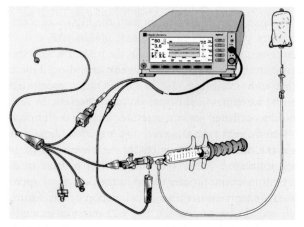

Fig. 9.20 Illustration of the closed injectate delivery system (room-temperature fluids) for thermodilution cardiac output measurement.

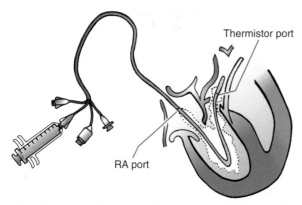

Fig. 9.21 Illustration of injection of fluid into the right atrium *(RA)* for cardiac output measurement.

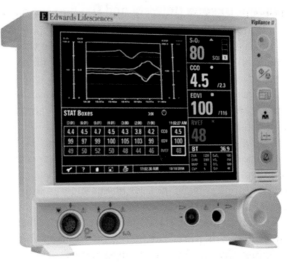

Fig. 9.22 A sample monitor interface displaying hemodynamic parameters and trends, including continuous cardiac output and mixed venous oxygen saturation. (Courtesy Edwards Lifesciences, Irvine, CA.)

BOX 9.9 Steps to Ensure Accurate Thermodilution Cardiac Output Measurements

- Before the procedure, assess the correct position of the PAC by verifying the waveform or measuring the PAOP.
- Enter the appropriate computation or calibration constant (per manufacturer's instruction) into the CO computer. The type and size of the PAC and the volume and temperature of the injectate solution are factors that determine this value.
- Assess the proximal port for patency.
- Do not infuse vasoactive drugs through the port used to obtain TdCO measurements. Rapid infusion of the injectate solution for the TdCO will result in delivery of these medications beyond the recommended dosage and cause potentially harmful side effects.
- Position the patient in the supine position with the backrest elevation at 0 to 30 degrees.
- Room-temperature injectate is acceptable as long as there is at least a 10°F difference between the temperature of the injectate and the patient's temperature.
- Inject the solution smoothly and rapidly (within 4 seconds) at the end of expiration to reduce the effect of chest wall motion and intrathoracic pressure changes.
- Obtain three CO measurements and calculate the average CO (a feature on the CO computer averages the measurements). Values should be within 10% of each other. Measurements outside of 10% agreement should be discarded and repeated before averaging the results. The first CO is usually the most variable.

CO, Cardiac output; *PAC,* pulmonary artery catheter; *PAOP,* pulmonary artery occlusion pressure; *TdCO,* thermodilution cardiac output.

Continuous Cardiac Output. Measurement of CCO is based on the same principles as TdCO. The CCO system uses a modified PA catheter and a CO computer specific to the device. The specialized catheter has a copper filament near the proximal port that delivers pulses of energy at prescribed time intervals and warms the blood as it enters the right ventricle. This temperature change is detected by the thermistor at the tip of the catheter approximately every 3 to 6 seconds. The computer interprets the temperature change and averages the CO measurements over the last 60 seconds. Fig. 9.22 shows an example of a computer interface for CCO and other hemodynamic parameters. CCO removes the potential for operator error associated

with intermittent TdCO measurement. Other advantages of CCO are that no extra fluid is administered to the patient, data are available for trending throughout the shift, and there is no need to change the computation constant in the CO module. Patients with a CCO device can be positioned supine with the HOB elevated up to 45 degrees. Drawbacks to CCO include that the device may not accurately sense the CCO in the patient whose body temperature is greater than 40°C to 43°C, because the thermal filament heats to a maximum of 44°C. Continuous cardiac output does not reflect acute changes in CO. Because the measurements provide an average of CO over time, a delay may be common in detecting acute changes in CO of 1 L/min.[39]

Controversy Surrounding the Pulmonary Artery Catheter

Use of the PAC has decreased since evidence suggested that its use was associated with increased mortality,[10] and less invasive monitoring has been developed. The PAC has limited ability to assess RAP and PAOP for preload status. PAC pressures are influenced by conditions that can increase the PAOP but do not reflect a change in preload. These include positive end-expiratory pressure and decreased ventricular compliance or a stiff ventricle. Studies have consistently shown that CVP, RAP, and PAOP are poor predictors of CO and fluid responsiveness, and that CVP should not be used as a basis for clinical decision making regarding fluid management.[25-27] Yet PAC pressures are widely used to guide fluid resuscitation. A Cochrane meta-analysis showed no difference in mortality, length of critical care unit stay, or length of hospital stay between patients managed with a PAC and those without a PAC.[38] Studies are needed to test protocols that guide therapy to determine whether the PAC can be used effectively.

Monitoring strategies are shifting to hemodynamic goal-directed therapy to guide interventions, such as administration of fluids. Many of the newer hemodynamic devices are designed to assess SV and changes in SV and other hemodynamic parameters.[2,3,8,9,14-19,22,42]

Balancing Oxygen Delivery and Oxygen Demand

The primary goal in caring for the critically ill is to determine whether oxygen delivery is meeting the oxygen and metabolic demands of the patient. Oxygen delivery is determined by CO and the arterial oxygen content of the blood. To determine if oxygen delivery is adequate, assess the CO, hemoglobin level, and SaO_2. Oxygenated arterial blood passes through the capillary network to deliver oxygen and nutrients to the tissues. However, not all of the oxygen is used by the tissues, and residual oxygen bound to hemoglobin in the venous circulation is returned to the right heart to be oxygenated again. Venous oxygen saturation is the percent of hemoglobin saturated in the central venous circulation and provides an assessment of the amount of oxygen extracted by the tissues. The oxygen saturation of this mixed venous blood from various organs and tissues that have different metabolic needs provides a global picture of both oxygen delivery and oxygen consumption, or oxygen demand. Factors that affect venous oxygen saturation include CO, hemoglobin, SaO_2, and tissue oxygen consumption.

Oxygen delivery and consumption can be calculated using a variety of formulas (Table 9.2). Two invasive techniques are also available for clinical determination of venous oxygen saturation: SvO_2 and $ScvO_2$. The SvO_2 is measured in the PA, and $ScvO_2$ is measured in the central venous system, usually the superior vena cava. Both SvO_2 and $ScvO_2$ methods use fiberoptic catheters that are connected to monitors and computers with an optical module (see Fig. 9.11). Calibration of the system is done at insertion and if the system becomes disconnected

from the optical module. To calibrate the equipment, a blood sample is obtained from either the PA (SvO_2) or the central venous catheter ($ScvO_2$), and a blood gas analysis is done. Oxygen saturation results are used for calibration. Fig. 9.22 shows an example of the clinical information provided by one monitoring device.

Monitoring SvO_2 and $ScvO_2$ is indicated for any critically ill or injured patient who has the potential to develop an imbalance between oxygen delivery and oxygen consumption or demand. Patients with trauma, acute respiratory distress syndrome, sepsis, and complex cardiac surgery may benefit from venous oxygen saturation monitoring (SvO_2).[7]

An SvO_2 between 60% and 75% indicates an adequate balance between supply and demand. The normal range for $ScvO_2$ (65% to 80%) is slightly higher because the measurement is from the blood in the central venous circulation versus the PA.

Many nursing interventions and clinical conditions affect the SvO_2 and $ScvO_2$. Table 9.3 highlights causes for alterations in SvO_2 values. Any changes in SaO_2, tissue metabolism, hemoglobin, or CO affect the values. For example, endotracheal suctioning may cause a transient decrease in the SvO_2 and $ScvO_2$ values if SaO_2 decreases during the procedure. Factors that increase the metabolic rate, such as shivering, fever, or an increase in physical activity, can also lead to a dramatic decrease in SvO_2 and $ScvO_2$. Values are high in sepsis because the cells are unable to use the available oxygen.

When interpreting values for SvO_2 and $ScvO_2$, integrate clinical data and patient assessment to ensure good clinical decision making. Decreased SvO_2 and $ScvO_2$ values result from

TABLE 9.2   Hemodynamic Calculations

Parameter	Calculation	Normal Values
Mean arterial pressure	[Systolic BP + (2 × Diastolic BP)] ÷ 3	70-105 mm Hg
Arterial oxygen content (CaO_2)	[1.34 × Hgb (g/dL) × SaO_2] + [0.003 × PaO_2]	19-20 mL/dL
Venous oxygen content (CvO_2)	[1.34 × Hgb (g/dL) × SvO_2] + [0.003 × PvO_2]	12-15 mL/dL
Oxygen delivery (DO_2)	CO × CaO_2 × 10	900-1100 mL/min
Oxygen consumption (VO_2)	$C(a\text{-}v)O_2$ × CO × 10	200-250 mL/min
Oxygen extraction ratio (O_2ER)	[(CaO_2 − CvO_2)/CaO_2] × 100	22%-30%

BP, Blood pressure; *CO,* cardiac output; *Hgb,* hemoglobin; *PaO_2,* partial pressure of arterial oxygen; *PvO_2,* partial pressure of venous oxygen; *SaO_2,* arterial oxygen saturation; *SvO_2,* mixed venous oxygen saturation.

TABLE 9.3   Alterations in Mixed Venous Oxygen Saturation

Alteration	Cause	Possible Etiology
Low SvO_2 (<60%)	Decreased O_2 delivery	Hypoxia or hemorrhage, anemic states, hypovolemia, cardiogenic shock, dysrhythmias, myocardial infarction, congestive heart failure, cardiac tamponade, massive transfusions of stored blood, restrictive lung disease, ventilation/perfusion abnormalities
	Increased O_2 consumption	Strenuous activity, fever, pain, anxiety or stress, hormonal imbalances, increased work of breathing, bathing, septic shock (late), seizures, shivering
High SvO_2 (>75%)	Increased O_2 delivery	Increase in FiO_2, hyperoxygenation
	Decreased O_2 consumption	Hypothermia, anesthesia, hypothyroidism, neuromuscular blockade, early stages of sepsis
High SvO_2 (>80%)	Technical error	PAC in wedged position, fibrin clot at end of catheter, computer needs to be recalibrated

FiO_2, Fraction of inspired oxygen; *O_2,* oxygen; *PAC,* pulmonary artery catheter; *SvO_2,* mixed venous oxygen saturation.

a failure to deliver adequate oxygen to the tissues or increased oxygen consumption. Elevated SvO_2 and $ScvO_2$ values can indicate that the tissues are not using the oxygen delivered, which is related to four physiological reasons:

1. Shunting, either intravascular or intracardiac, does not allow the tissues to be exposed to the oxygen being delivered to the tissue bed.
2. A shift of the oxyhemoglobin dissociation curve to the left results in an increased affinity of hemoglobin for oxygen.
3. An increased diffusion distance between the capillaries and cells is present because of interstitial edema.
4. Cells are unable to use the oxygen being delivered, a frequent phenomenon in sepsis.

❓ CRITICAL REASONING ACTIVITY

Describe how cardiac output affects the delivery of oxygen to tissues. What parameters would be the best to monitor in a patient to assess this influence?

STROKE VOLUME OPTIMIZATION

Clinicians have struggled to find a reliable and accurate method to evaluate clinical volume status.[11] Newer technologies have been developed to measure blood flow. SV assessment may be more reliable than static measures of pressure such as RAP, PAOP, and MAP to determine cardiac performance and the need for fluids and vasoactive medications. The first step in a hemodynamic assessment is to determine whether the patient requires fluid to optimize preload and allow the heart to pump more efficiently. Determining fluid responsiveness (also called *preload responsiveness*) means that with the administration of a fluid bolus the patient will respond with an increase in SV of 10% or greater.[2,22] The fundamental reason to give IV fluids is to increase SV. Fluid replacement, either colloid or crystalloid solutions, is essential to achieve and maintain adequate tissue perfusion. If fluid volume is inadequate, hypovolemia, hypotension, and inadequate perfusion of end organs will occur. Conversely, excess administration of fluids may precipitate heart failure, especially in patients with underlying cardiac disease.

Technologies allow for ongoing assessment of SV at the bedside. These include noninvasive Doppler imaging (Uscom, Sydney, Australia), esophageal Doppler imaging (Deltex Medical, Greenville, SC), endotracheally applied bioimpedance (ConMed Corporation, Lithia Springs, GA), bioreactance (Cheetah Medical, Newton Center, MA), and pulse contour methods (Edwards Lifesciences, Irvine, CA; LiDCO Ltd, Lake Villa, IL; and Pulsion Medical Systems, Feldkirchen, Germany).

❓ CRITICAL REASONING ACTIVITY

A patient who has undergone surgery has received a bed bath, requiring turning, and subsequent suctioning through the endotracheal tube. During these care activities, the patient experiences coughing and pain. What consequences will these activities and the experience of pain have on the patient's mixed venous oxygen saturation status?

Respiratory Variation to Assess Preload Responsiveness

Right Atrial Pressure Variation. Although the RAP is less predictive of responsiveness to fluid resuscitation, assessing the degree of change with respiration has the potential to be a useful indicator of responsiveness. A change of RAP greater than 1 mm Hg with inspiration is indicative of a positive responder, whereas a change of RAP of less than 1 mm Hg is likely to indicate a nonresponder.[25,26] Assessment of variation does not require specialized equipment to evaluate (other than a transduced central line) and can be used on the spontaneously breathing patient.

Systolic Pressure Variation. Patients receiving positive pressure ventilation have a decrease in SV with inspiration that ultimately leads to a decrease in systolic blood pressure. The normal systolic pressure variation is 8 to 10 mm Hg. A change of greater than 10 mm Hg indicates that a patient is preload responsive and fluid resuscitation is needed.[7] The limitation to this strategy is that it requires the patient to be mechanically ventilated in a strict volume control mode. In addition, the predictive capability may be affected if a patient has an alteration in the lung or chest wall compliance.

Arterial Pulse Pressure Variation. Changes in arterial pressure with inspiration and expiration can be used to gauge fluid responsiveness or preload responsiveness.[20] *Arterial pulse pressure* is defined as the difference between arterial systolic and diastolic pressure measurements. The arterial pulse pressure is affected by three variables: SV, resistance, and compliance. Because arterial resistance and compliance do not change significantly with each breath, the variation in pulse pressure is likely caused by variations in SV. A *pulse pressure variation* (PPV) of more than 10% to 12% is predictive of a patient's ability to respond to fluid resuscitation. Tidal volume must be adequate and constant, requiring the patient to be mechanically ventilated and sedated to suppress spontaneous ventilation. Studies evaluating PPV have been conducted using larger tidal volumes of 10 mL/kg, which is no longer the standard of care. Studies using lower tidal volumes are needed.

Stroke Volume Variation. Another way to assess volume status is analysis of the degree of variation in SV. The dividing line between responders and nonresponders with regard to fluid resuscitation is a *stroke volume variability* (SVV) of 9.5%.[18,19,30] Assessment of SVV requires an arterial line, a specialized transducer, and the use of a pulse contour device such as the FloTrac (discussed later in the chapter). This assessment is only predictive in the patient who is mechanically ventilated in a controlled mode with tidal volumes of more than 8 mL/kg with constant respiratory rates. Also, dysrhythmias, such as atrial fibrillation, dramatically affect SVV because the irregular rhythm results in SV changes that are independent of respiratory variability.

Bioimpedance (SonoSite, Highland Heights, OH), endotracheally applied bioimpedance (SonoSite, Highland Heights, OH), and bioreactance (Cheetah Medical, Newton Center, MA) technologies are also less invasive ways to measure hemodynamic parameters. These methods are completely noninvasive and use transcutaneous electrodes to measure parameters such as CO, blood pressure, SV, and SVV. Noninvasive devices are being used clinically to determine preload responsiveness and guide fluid resuscitation in postoperative and septic patients.[12,32]

STUDY BREAK

3. An increase in pulse pressure variation (PPV) of _____ indicates that the patient will likely respond to fluid resuscitation.

A. 2%

B. 5%

C. 8%

D. 10%

Doppler Technology Methods of Hemodynamic Assessment

Echocardiography that uses Doppler technology has been the most commonly used method to measure SV; however, it is expensive, requires technical expertise, and is usually a one-time measurement. Technology for bedside assessment of SV and fluid responsiveness in critically ill patients is rapidly evolving. Esophageal Doppler monitoring (EDM) uses a thin silicone probe placed in the distal esophagus, allowing the clinician to evaluate descending aortic blood flow, which provides real-time assessment of left ventricular performance (Fig. 9.23). The probe is easily placed in a manner similar to an orogastric or nasogastric tube. Some patients may require sedation to tolerate the procedure. The probe is lubricated and inserted either orally or nasally with the bevel facing upward until the depth of the catheter is approximately 35 to 40 cm. Focusing the probe

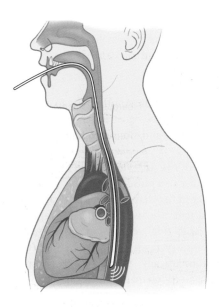

Fig. 9.23 Esophageal Doppler probe placement. (Courtesy Deltex Medical, Inc., Greenville, SC.)

BOX 9.10 **Esophageal Doppler Monitoring Contraindications**

Local Disease
- Esophageal stent
- Carcinoma of the esophagus or pharynx
- Previous esophageal surgery
- Esophageal stricture
- Esophageal varices
- Pharyngeal pouch

Aortic Abnormalities
- Intraaortic balloon pump
- Coarctation of the aorta

Systemic
- Severe coagulopathy

From King SL, Lim MST. The use of the oesophageal Doppler monitor in the intensive care unit. *Crit Care Resusc*. 2004;6:113–122.

entails rotating, advancing, or withdrawing the probe until the loudest sound is heard from the monitor. Box 9.10 outlines indications and contraindications for EDM.

The EDM monitor interface (Fig. 9.24) provides a variety of clinical parameters, including CO and SV derived from a

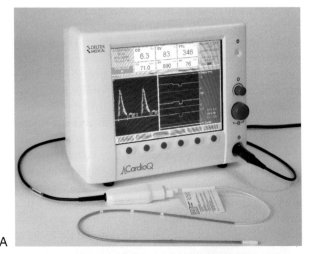

A

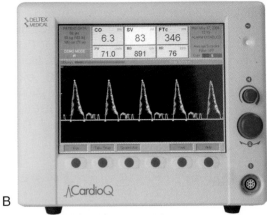

B

Fig. 9.24 A, CardioQ monitoring system for assessing cardiac output and function via the esophageal Doppler probe. **B,** Numerical and graphical data provided by the CardioQ device. (Courtesy Deltex Medical, Inc., Greenville, SC.)

proprietary algorithm. The corrected flow time (FTc), peak velocity (PV), and minute distance are obtained from the Doppler velocity measurements.[2,13] The base of the waveform depicts the FTc and is indicative of left ventricular preload. The height of the waveform represents PV and reflects contractility. Normal FTc is 330 to 360 milliseconds (ms). Normal PV varies by age: 90 to 120 cm/sec for a 20-year-old person, 70 to 100 cm/sec for a 50-year-old person, and 50 to 80 cm/sec for a 70-year-old person.[21] An FTc of less than 330 ms almost always represents an underfilled left ventricle. When both SV and PV are normal, this is indicative of hypovolemia. When FTc increases in response to a fluid challenge, hypovolemia is confirmed. If both SV and PV are low, the problem is most likely contractility or left ventricular dysfunction. In this situation the patient does not need fluids and may respond to medications to decrease preload, decrease afterload, or increase contractility. Table 9.4 provides interpretation guidelines for waveform and numerical variations. The EDM technology has been demonstrated to reduce critical care unit length of stay, hospital length of stay, and infectious complications when compared with those patients managed by invasive technologies.[10] Because EDM is minimally invasive, risk to the patient is significantly lower than with invasive monitoring. In addition, EDM is simple to use and provides a vast amount of clinical information to guide therapy in the critical care environment.[16]

Pulse Contour Methods of Hemodynamic Assessment

Several devices are available that use pulse contour analysis to determine various hemodynamic parameters, including SV and CO.[35] The CO derived from arterial pulse contour analysis is comparable to that obtained via PAC. Devices that use the pulse contour analysis for assessing CO include the PiCCO (Pulsion Medical Systems, Feldkirchen, Germany), FloTrac (Edwards Lifesciences, Irvine, CA), and LiDCO plus systems (LiDCO Cardiac Sensor Systems, Lake Villa, IL).[43] These devices provide data for hemodynamic assessment and involve less risk than the PAC. The systems, with the exception of the PiCCO system, are generally fast to set up. They provide SVV and PPV data and are better predictors of fluid responsiveness in mechanically ventilated patients than a static measurement of RAP or PAOP.[39] The pulse contour analysis provides an alternative to the PAC for measuring CO, even in patients who are hemodynamically unstable. Pulse contour analysis is inaccurate in patients with significant aortic insufficiency and those with peripheral vascular disease. The use of an intraaortic balloon counterpulsation also excludes the use of this technique. For illustration purposes (Fig. 9.25), the Vigileo system (Edwards Lifesciences, Irvine, CA) provides CCO, SV, SVV, and SVR data through an existing arterial line. The technology requires no manual calibration because the FloTrac algorithm automatically compensates for the continuously changing effects of vascular tone on hemodynamic parameters.[33]

The continuous measurement of SVV and PPV is only possible under full mechanical ventilation. Application of the pulse

TABLE 9.4 Interpretation Guidelines for Esophageal Doppler Monitoring

Waveform Alteration	Numerical Correlation	Interpretation
↓ Base width	↓ FTc	Hypovolemia
↑ Base width	↑ FTc	Euvolemia
↓ Waveform height	↓ PV or SV	Left ventricular failure
↑ Waveform height	↑ PV or SV	Hyperdynamic state (i.e., sepsis)
↓ Waveform height + ↓ base width	↓ FTc ↓ PV or SV	Elevated systemic vascular resistance

FTc, Corrected flow time; *PV,* peak velocity; *SV,* stroke volume.

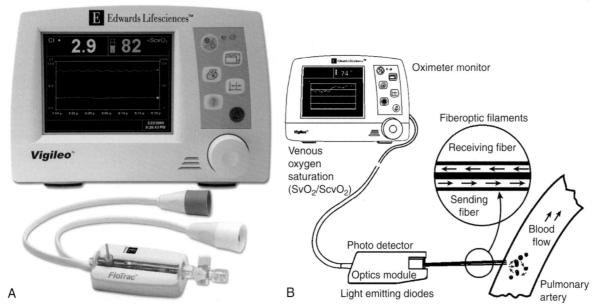

Fig. 9.25 A, Vigileo monitor. **B,** This monitor allows for the continuous monitoring of essential hemodynamic information, including stroke volume, providing rapid insight on a minimally invasive, easy-to-use platform. (Courtesy Edwards Lifesciences, Irvine, CA.)

contour analysis and the derived cardiac preload parameters are limited when cardiac dysrhythmias are present. Systemic vascular resistance and PPV are superior to the RAP and PAOP for predicting volume responsiveness.

CASE STUDY

Mr. J., a 44-year-old man with no previous medical history, presents to the emergency department with a chief complaint of severe abdominal pain, fever, and chills. He is subsequently admitted to the critical care unit after an open exploratory laparotomy during which it was found that he had a perforated appendix and diffuse peritonitis. Intraoperatively he had an estimated blood loss of 200 mL, and he received 1.5 L of crystalloid solution. He arrives at the critical care unit intubated and sedated with an arterial line, subclavian triple-lumen catheter, indwelling urinary catheter, and esophageal Doppler monitor in place. He is placed on mechanical ventilation with the following settings: assist/control mode at 12 breaths/min tidal volume, 700 mL; fraction of inspired oxygen, 1.0 (100%); and positive end-expiratory pressure, 5 cm H_2O. His initial vital signs and hemodynamic values are:

Heart rate	128 beats/min
Blood pressure	88/49 mm Hg
Mean arterial pressure	62 mm Hg
Respiratory rate	12 breaths/min
Right atrial pressure	3 mm Hg
Temperature	38.2°C (100.8°F)
Flow time corrected	250 ms
Peak velocity	120 cm/sec
Stroke volume	34 mL

The provider orders administration of a 250-mL infusion of 5% albumin. You administer the albumin and reassess his vital signs:

Heart rate	120 beats/min
Blood pressure	94/50 mm Hg
Mean arterial pressure	65 mm Hg
Right atrial pressure	5 mm Hg
Flow time corrected	280 ms
Peak velocity	120 cm/sec
Stroke volume	49 mL

The nurse reports the change in stroke volume and other parameters to the provider. The provider orders an additional 500-mL bolus of saline over 15 minutes. Mr. J.'s vitals are now:

Heart rate	110 beats/min
Blood pressure	94/50 mm Hg
Mean arterial pressure	65 mm Hg
Right atrial pressure	7 mm Hg
Flow time corrected	300 ms
Peak velocity	120 cm/sec
Stroke volume	50 mL

Questions

1. The 1.5 L of crystalloid solution the patient received during surgery should have provided adequate volume resuscitation. What was the rationale for the albumin bolus?
2. Discuss which hemodynamic parameters you would monitor to assess efficacy of the bolus of 250-mL 5% albumin and why.
3. The provider ordered an additional fluid bolus of 500 mL of normal saline. Evaluate the last set of vital signs to determine the patient's response.
4. Discuss how a passive leg raising test might have been used to determine fluid responsiveness with Mr. J. before giving the second fluid bolus.

SV optimization can be used clinically to determine preload responsiveness and treat patients with low SV or a low FTc.[22] A nurse-driven protocol to determine fluid needs and evaluate the patient for other alterations can be effective in maintaining the patient's overall hemodynamic stability.[23] After giving a fluid challenge of either crystalloids or colloids, assess SV response. If SV improves by at least 10%, continue giving fluid boluses until the SV response is less than 10%. If no response is noted after fluid administration, collaborate with the provider to determine if other therapies are needed to correct a high afterload state (vasodilators), low contractility state (inotropic agents), or low afterload state (vasopressors).

Passive Leg Raising to Assess Preload Responsiveness

Assessing a patient's response to passive leg raising (PLR) can be used to determine whether the patient is preload responsive, indicated by an increase in SV.[24] This allows the clinician to test for preload responsiveness before giving IV fluids. The PLR test consists of measuring the hemodynamic effects of leg elevation up to 45 degrees. The test is best performed starting from a semirecumbent position, as it allows for a larger increase in cardiac preload because it induces the shift of venous blood not only from the legs but also from the abdominal compartment.[27] The effects of PLR occur within the first minute of leg elevation, so it is important to assess the effects in real time. Pulse contour and Doppler technologies can all be used to determine preload responsiveness with a PLR test. The maneuver is effective in spontaneously breathing patients as well as those on mechanical ventilation. If the patient responds with an increase in SV of more than 10%, the patient is preload responsive and a fluid bolus is indicated.

REFERENCES

1. AACN Practice Alert. Pulmonary artery/central venous pressure monitoring in adults. *Crit Care Nurse.* 2016;36:e2–e18.
2. Ahrens T. Stroke volume optimization versus central pressure in fluid management. *Crit Care Nurs.* 2010;30(2):71–73.
3. Archer TL, Funk DJ, Moretti E, et al. Stroke volume calculation by esophageal Doppler integrates velocity over time and multiplies this "area under the curve" by the cross sectional area of the aorta. *Anesth Analg.* 2009;109(3):996.
4. Barone JE, Madlinger RV. Should an Allen test be performed before radial artery cannulation? *J Trauma.* 2006;61(2): 468–470.
5. Boev C, Xia Y. Nurse-physician collaboration and hospital-acquired infections in critical care. *Crit Care Nurs.* 2015;35(2):66–72.
6. Brashers V. Alterations of cardiovascular function. In: McCance KL, Huether SE, eds. *Pathophysiology: The Biological Basis for Disease in Adults and Children.* 8th ed. St. Louis, MO: Elsevier; 2019:1061–1067.
7. Bridges EJ. Pulmonary artery pressure monitoring: When, how, and what else to use. *AACN Advan Crit Care.* 2006;17(3): 286–303.

8. Chytra I, Pradl R, Bosman R, et al. Esophageal Doppler-guided fluid management decreases blood lactate levels in multiple-trauma patients: A randomized controlled trial. *Crit Care.* 2007;11(1):R24.

9. Compton FD, Zukunft B, Hoffmann C, et al. Performance of a minimally invasive uncalibrated cardiac output monitoring system (FloTrac/Vigileo) in haemodynamically unstable patients. *Br J Anaesth.* 2008;100(4):451–456.

10. Connors A, Speroff T, Dawson N, et al. The effectiveness of right heart catheterization in the initial care of critically ill patients: SUPPORT investigators. *JAMA.* 1996;276(11):889–897.

11. Crumlett H, Johnson A. Arterial catheter insertion (assist), care, and removal. In: Wiegand DLM, ed. *AACN Procedure Manual for Critical Care.* 7th ed. St. Louis, MO: Elsevier; 2017:501–522.

12. Dumont L, Harding AD. Development and implementation of a sepsis program. *J Emerg Nurs.* 2013;39(6):625–629.

13. Dunser MW, Takala J, Brunauer A. Re-thinking resuscitation: Leaving blood pressure cosmetics behind and moving forward to permissive hypotension and a tissue perfusion-based approach. *Crit Care.* 2013;17(326):1–8.

14. Goepfert MS, Richter HP, Eulenburg C, et al. Individually optimized hemodynamic therapy reduces complications and length of stay in the intensive care unit. *Anesthesiology.* 2013;119(4):824–836.

15. Gurgel ST, do Nascimento P Jr. Maintaining tissue perfusion in high-risk surgical patients: A systematic review of randomized clinical trials. *Anesth Analg.* 2010;112(6):1384–1391.

16. Hadian M, Angus DC. Protocolized resuscitation with esophageal Doppler monitoring may improve outcome in post-cardiac surgery patients. *Crit Care.* 2005;9(4):E7.

17. Hadian M, Kim HK, Severyn DA, et al. Cross-comparison of cardiac output trending accuracy of LiDCO, PiCCO, FloTrac and pulmonary artery catheters. *Crit Care.* 2006;14(6):R212.

18. Hall JE. *Guyton and Hall Textbook of Medical Physiology.* 13th ed. Philadelphia, PA: Saunders; 2015.

19. Harvey S, Young D, Brampton W, et al. Pulmonary artery catheters for adult patients in intensive care. *Cochrane Database Syst Rev.* 2006;3:CD003408.

20. Hollenberg SM. Hemodynamic monitoring. *Chest.* 2013;143(5):1480–1488.

21. Jansen TC, van Bommel J, Schoonderbeek FJ, et al. Early lactate-guided therapy in intensive care unit patients: A multicenter, open-label, randomized controlled trial. *Am J Respir Crit Care Med.* 2010;182(6):752–761.

22. Johnson A, Ahrens T. Stroke volume optimization: The new hemodynamic algorithm. *Crit Care Nurs.* 2015;35(1):11–27.

23. Joosten A, Hafiane R, Pustetto M, et al. Practical impact of decision support for goal-directed fluid therapy on protocol adherence: A clinical implementation study in patients undergoing major abdominal surgery. *J Clin Monit Comput.* 2019;33(1):15–24.

24. Lough ME. *Hemodynamic Monitoring: Evolving Technologies and Clinical Practice.* St. Louis, MO: Elsevier; 2016.

25. Marik PE, Baram M, Vahid B. Does central venous pressure predict fluid responsiveness? A systematic review of the literature and the tale of seven mares. *Chest.* 2008;134(1):172–178.

26. Marik PE, Cavallazzi R, Vasu T, et al. Dynamic changes in arterial waveform derived variables and fluid responsiveness in mechanically ventilated patients: A systematic review of the literature. *Crit Care Med.* 2009;37(9):2642–2647.

27. Marik PE, Monnet X, Teboul JL. Hemodynamic parameters to guide fluid therapy. *Ann Intensive Care.* 2011;1(1):1–9.

28. McCance KL, Cunningham S. Structure and function of the cardiovascular and lymphatic systems. In McCance KL, Huether SE, eds. *Pathophysiology: The Biological Basis for Disease in Adults and Children.* 8th ed. St. Louis, MO: Elsevier; 2019:1017–1048.

29. McVay R. Pulmonary artery catheter and pressure lines, troubleshooting. In: Wiegand DLM, ed. *AACN Procedure Manual for Critical Care.* 7th ed. St. Louis, MO: Elsevier; 2017:637–652.

30. McVay R. Pulmonary artery catheter insertion (assist) and pressure monitoring. In: Wiegand DLM, ed. *AACN Procedure Manual for Critical Care.* 7th ed. St. Louis, MO: Elsevier; 2017:609–629.

31. McVay R. Single-pressure and multiple-pressure transducer systems. In: Wiegand DLM, ed. *AACN Procedure Manual for Critical Care.* 7th ed. St. Louis, MO: Elsevier; 2017:653–663.

32. Napoli AM. Physiologic and clinical principles behind noninvasive resuscitation techniques and cardiac output monitoring. *Cardiol Res Pract.* 2012;531908.

33. Pagana KD, Pagana TJ. *Mosby's Manual of Diagnostic and Laboratory Tests.* 6th ed. St. Louis, MO: Elsevier; 2018.

34. Pasion E, Good L, Tizon J, et al. Evaluation of the monitor cursor-line method for measuring pulmonary artery and central venous pressures. *Am J Crit Care.* 2010;19(6):511–521.

35. Peyton PJ, Chong SW. Minimally invasive measurement of cardiac output during surgery and critical care: A meta-analysis of accuracy and precision. *Anesthesiology.* 2010;113(5):1220–1235.

36. Pike N, Peterson J. Alterations of cardiovascular function in children. In: McCance KL, Huether SE, eds. *Pathophysiology: The Biological Basis for Disease in Adults and Children.* 8th ed. St. Louis, MO: Elsevier; 2019.

37. ProCESS Investigators. A randomized trial of protocol-based care for early septic shock. *N Engl J Med.* 2014;370(18):1683–1693.

38. Rajaram SS, Desai NK, Kalra A, et al. Pulmonary artery catheters for adult patients in intensive care. *Cochrane Database Syst Rev.* 2013;(2): CD003408. doi:10.1002/14651858.CD003408.pub3.

39. Rhodes A, Evans LE, Alhazzani W, et al. Surviving Sepsis Campaign: International guidelines for the management of sepsis and septic shock: 2016. *Crit Care Med.* 2017;45:486–552.

40. Scott S. Cardiac output measurement techniques (invasive). In: Wiegand DLM, ed. *AACN Procedure Manual for Critical Care.* 7th ed. St. Louis, MO: Elsevier; 2017:553–568.

41. Shah MR, Hasselblad V, Stevenson LW, et al. Impact of the pulmonary artery catheter in critically ill patients: Meta-analysis of randomized clinical trials. *JAMA.* 2005;294(13):1664–1670.

42. Stover JF, Stocker R, Lenherr R, et al. Noninvasive cardiac output and blood pressure monitoring cannot replace an invasive monitoring system in critically ill patients. *BMC Anesthesiol.* 2009;9:6.

43. Swan HJ, Ganz W, Forrester J, et al. Catheterization of the heart in man with use of a flow-directed balloon-tipped catheter. *N Engl J Med.* 1970;283(9):447–451.

44. Taylor N. Pulmonary artery catheter insertion (perform). In: Wiegand DLM, ed. *AACN Procedure Manual for High Acuity,*

Progressive, and Critical Care. 7th ed. Philadelphia, PA: Saunders; 2017:601–608.

45. Thornburg K, Jaconson L, Giraud G, et al. Hemodynamic changes in pregnancy. *Semin Perinatol.* 2000;24(1):11–14.

46. U.S. Centers for Disease Control and Prevention. Central Line–Associated Bloodstream Infections: Resources for Patients and Healthcare Providers. http://www.cdc.gov/HAI/bsi/CLABSI-resources.html. Last reviewed February 7, 2011. Accessed February 13, 2019.

47. U.S. Centers for Disease Control and Prevention. Guidelines for the Prevention of Intravascular Catheter-Related Infections. http://www.cdc.gov/hicpac/pdf/guidelines/bsi-guidelines-2011.pdf. Published 2011. Accessed February 13, 2019.

Ventilatory Assistance

Lynelle N.B. Pierce, MS, RN, CCRN, CCNS, FAAN

Many additional resources, including self-assessment exercises, are located on the Evolve companion website at http://evolve.elsevier.com/Sole/.
- Animations
- Clinical Skills: Critical Care Collections
- Student Review Questions
- Video Clips

INTRODUCTION

The essential nursing interventions for all patients of maintaining an adequate airway and ensuring adequate breathing (ventilation) and oxygenation provide the framework for this chapter. Respiratory anatomy and physiology are reviewed to provide a basis for discussing ventilatory assistance. Assessment of the respiratory system includes physical examination, arterial blood gas (ABG) interpretation, and noninvasive methods for assessing gas exchange. Airway management, oxygen therapy, and mechanical ventilation, important therapies in the critical care unit, are also discussed.

REVIEW OF RESPIRATORY ANATOMY AND PHYSIOLOGY

The primary function of the respiratory system is gas exchange. Oxygen and carbon dioxide (CO_2) are exchanged via the respiratory system to provide adequate oxygen to the cells and to remove CO_2, the byproduct of metabolism, from the cells. The respiratory system is divided into (1) the upper airway, (2) the lower airway, and (3) the lungs. The upper airway conducts gas to and from the lower airway, and the lower airway provides gas exchange at the alveolar-capillary membrane. The anatomical structure of the respiratory system is shown in Fig. 10.1.

Upper Airway

The upper airway consists of the nasal cavity and the pharynx. The nasal cavity conducts air, filters large foreign particles, and warms and humidifies air. When an artificial airway is placed, these natural functions of the airway are bypassed. The nasal cavity also is responsible for voice resonance, smell, and the sneeze reflex. The throat, or pharynx, transports both air and food.

Lower Airway

The lower airway consists of the larynx, trachea, right and left mainstem bronchi, bronchioles, and alveoli. The larynx is the narrowest part of the conducting airways in adults and contains the vocal cords. The larynx is partly covered by the epiglottis, which prevents aspiration of food, liquid, or saliva into the lungs during swallowing. The passage through the vocal cords is the glottis (Fig. 10.2).

The trachea warms, humidifies, and filters air. Cilia in the trachea propel mucus and foreign material upward through the airway. At approximately the level of the fifth thoracic vertebra (sternal angle, or angle of Louis), the trachea branches into the right and left mainstem bronchi, which conduct air to the respective lungs. This bifurcation is referred to as the *carina*. The right mainstem bronchus is shorter, wider, and straighter than the left. The bronchi further branch into the bronchioles and finally the terminal bronchioles, which supply air to the alveoli. Mucosal cells in the bronchi secrete mucus that lubricates the airway and traps foreign materials, which are moved by the cilia upward to be expectorated or swallowed.

The alveoli are the distal airway structures and are responsible for gas exchange at the capillary level. The alveoli consist of a single layer of epithelial cells and fibers that permit expansion and contraction. The type II cells inside the alveolus secrete surfactant, which coats the inner surface and prevents it from collapsing. A network of pulmonary capillaries covers the alveoli. Gas exchange occurs between the alveoli and these capillaries.[49,69] The large combined surface area and single cell layer of the alveoli promote efficient diffusion of gases.

Lungs

The lungs consist of lobes; the left lung has two lobes, and the right lung has three lobes. Each lobe consists of lobules, or segments, that are supplied by one bronchiole. The top of each lung is the apex, and the lower part of the lung is the base.

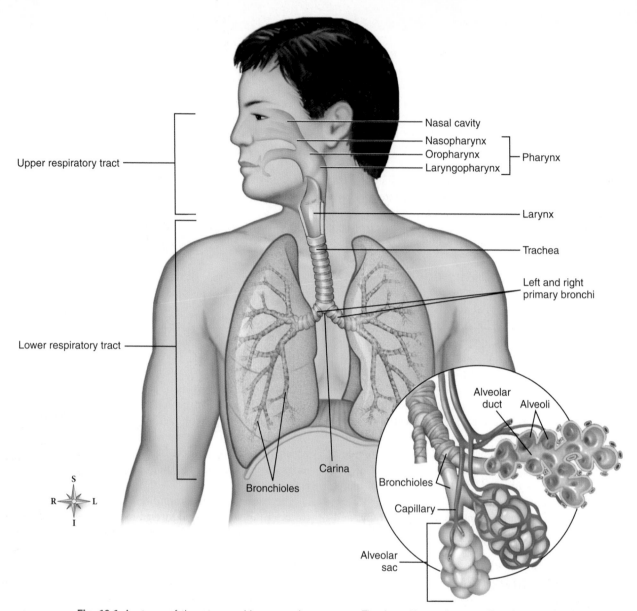

Fig. 10.1 Anatomy of the upper and lower respiratory tracts. The *inset* shows the grapelike clusters of alveoli and their rich blood supply, which supports the exchange of oxygen and carbon dioxide. (From Patton KT, Thibodeau GA. *Anatomy and Physiology.* 9th ed. St. Louis, MO: Elsevier; 2016.)

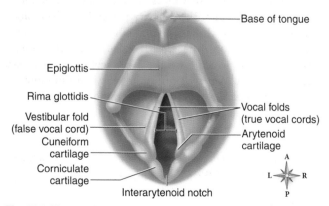

Fig. 10.2 The vocal cords and glottis. (From Patton KT, Thibodeau GA. *Anatomy and Physiology.* 9th ed. St. Louis, MO: Elsevier; 2016.)

The lungs are covered by pleura. The visceral pleura cover the lung surfaces, whereas the parietal pleura cover the internal surface of the thoracic cage. Between these two layers the pleural space is formed, which contains pleural fluid. This thin fluid lubricates the pleural layers so that they slide across each other during breathing and also holds the two pleurae together because it creates surface tension, an attractive force between liquid molecules. It is this surface tension between the two pleurae, opposing the tendency of the elastic lung to want to collapse, that leads to a pressure of -5 cm of water (H_2O) within the pleural space.[26] In disorders of the pleural space, such as pneumothorax, this negative pressure is disrupted, leading to collapse of the lung and the need for a chest tube.

PHYSIOLOGY OF BREATHING

The basic principle behind the movement of gas in and out of the lung is that gas travels from an area of higher to lower pressure. During inspiration, the diaphragm lowers and flattens and the intercostal muscles contract, lifting the chest up and outward to increase the size of the chest cavity. Subsequently, intrapleural pressure becomes even more negative than stated earlier, and intraalveolar pressure (the pressure in the lungs) becomes negative, causing air to flow into the lungs *(inspiration)*.[26] Expiration is a passive process in which the diaphragm and intercostal muscles relax and the lungs recoil. This recoil generates positive intraalveolar pressure relative to atmospheric pressure, and air flows out of the lungs *(expiration)*.[69]

Gas Exchange

The process of gas exchange (Fig. 10.3) consists of four steps: (1) ventilation, (2) diffusion at pulmonary capillaries, (3) perfusion (transport), and (4) diffusion to the cells.[12,26,69]

1. Ventilation is the movement of gases (oxygen and CO_2) in and out of the alveoli.
2. Diffusion of oxygen and CO_2 occurs at the alveolar-capillary membrane (Fig. 10.4). The driving force to move gas from

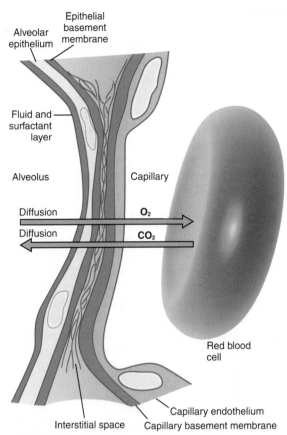

Fig. 10.4 Diffusion of oxygen and carbon dioxide at the alveolar-capillary membrane. (From Hall JE. *Guyton and Hall Textbook of Medical Physiology.* 13th ed. Philadelphia, PA: Saunders; 2016.)

the alveoli to the capillary and vice versa is the difference in gas pressure across the alveolar-capillary membrane. Gas molecules move from an area of higher to lower pressure via the process of diffusion. Oxygen pressure is higher in the alveoli than in the capillaries, thus promoting oxygen diffusion from the alveoli into the blood. Carbon dioxide pressure is higher in the capillaries, thus promoting diffusion of CO_2 into the alveoli for elimination during exhalation.
3. The oxygenated blood in the pulmonary capillary is transported via the pulmonary vein to the left side of the heart. The oxygenated blood is perfused, or transported to the tissues.
4. Diffusion of oxygen and CO_2 as a result of pressure gradients occurs at the cellular level, too. Oxygen diffuses from blood into the cells, and CO_2 leaves the cells and diffuses into the blood in a process called *internal respiration*. Carbon dioxide is transported via the vena cava to the right side of the heart and into the pulmonary capillaries, where it diffuses into the alveoli and is eliminated through exhalation.

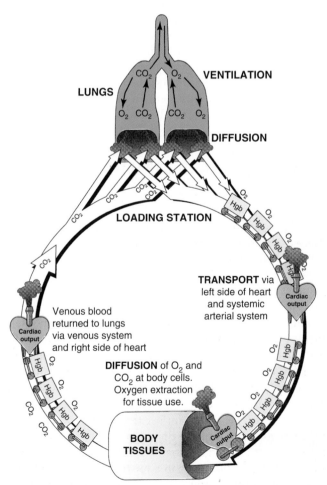

Fig. 10.3 Schematic view of the process of gas exchange. *Hgb,* Hemoglobin. (Modified from Alspach J. *AACN Instructor's Resource Manual for AACN Core Curriculum for Critical Care Nursing.* 4th ed. Philadelphia, PA: Saunders; 1992.)

? CRITICAL REASONING ACTIVITY

Based on your knowledge of clinical disorders, identify different clinical conditions that could cause problems with the following steps in gas exchange:
1. Ventilation
2. Diffusion
3. Perfusion (transportation)

Regulation of Breathing

The rate, depth, and rhythm of ventilation are controlled by respiratory centers in the medulla and pons. When the CO_2 level is high or the oxygen level is low, chemoreceptors in the respiratory center, carotid arteries, and aorta send messages to the medulla to regulate respiration. In persons with normal lung function, high levels of CO_2 stimulate respiration. However, patients with chronic obstructive pulmonary disease (COPD) maintain higher levels of CO_2 as a baseline, and their ventilatory drive in response to increased CO_2 levels is blunted. In these patients, the stimulus to breathe is hypoxemia, a low level of oxygen in the blood.[26]

Respiratory Mechanics

Work of Breathing. The work of breathing (WOB) is the amount of effort required for the maintenance of a given level of ventilation. When the lungs are not diseased, the respiratory muscles can manage the WOB and the respirations are unlabored. When lung disease is present, the respiratory pattern changes to manage the increased WOB, and the patient may use accessory muscles. As the WOB increases, more energy is expended to achieve adequate ventilation, which requires more oxygen and glucose to be consumed. If the WOB becomes too high, the muscles fatigue, respiratory failure ensues, and mechanical ventilatory support is warranted.[9,52]

Compliance. Compliance is a measure of the distensibility, or stretchability, of the lung and chest wall. The lungs are primarily made up of elastin and collagen fibers that in disease states become less elastic, leading to so-called stiff lungs. *Distensibility* refers to how easily the lung is stretched when the respiratory muscles work and expand the thoracic cavity. *Compliance*, a clinical measurement of the lung's distensibility, is defined as the change in lung volume per unit of pressure change.[52,69]

Various pathological conditions such as pulmonary fibrosis, acute respiratory distress syndrome (ARDS), and pulmonary edema lead to low pulmonary compliance. In these situations the patient must generate more work to breathe to create negative pressure to inflate the stiff lungs. Compliance is also decreased in obesity secondary to the increased mass of the chest wall.

In emphysema, destruction of lung tissue and enlarged air spaces cause the lungs to lose their elasticity, which increases compliance. The lungs are more distensible in this situation and require lower pressures for ventilation but may collapse during expiration, causing air to become trapped in the distal airways.

Monitoring changes in compliance provides an objective clinical indicator of changes in the patient's lung condition and ability to ventilate, especially the mechanically ventilated patient with decreased lung compliance. Compliance of the lung tissue is best measured under static conditions (no airflow) and is achieved by instituting a 2-second inspiratory hold maneuver with the mechanical ventilator.[9,52] Static compliance in patients with normal lungs usually ranges from 50 to 170 mL/cm H_2O.[69] This means that for every 1-cm H_2O change of pressure in the lungs, the volume of gas increases by 50 to 170 mL. A single measurement of compliance is not useful in monitoring patient progress; it is important to trend compliance over time.

Dynamic compliance is measured while gases are flowing during breathing; it measures not only lung compliance but also airway resistance to gas flow. The normal value for dynamic compliance is 50 to 80 mL/cm H_2O.[69] Dynamic compliance is easier to measure because it does not require breath holding or an inspiratory hold; however, it is not a pure measurement of lung compliance. A decrease in dynamic compliance may signify a decrease in compliance or an increase in resistance to gas flow.

The respiratory therapist (RT) or nurse measures compliance in the mechanically ventilated patient to identify trends in the patient's condition. Compliance can easily be obtained on most modern ventilators when the operator requests it using the menu options. Poor compliance requires higher ventilatory pressures to achieve adequate lung volume. Higher ventilatory pressures place the patient at increased risk for complications, such as volutrauma.

Resistance. *Resistance* refers to the opposition to the flow of gases in the airways. Factors that affect airway resistance are airway length, airway diameter, and the flow rate of gases. Airway resistance is increased when the airway is lengthened or narrowed, as with an artificial airway, or when the natural airway is narrowed by spasms (bronchoconstriction), the presence of mucus, or edema. Finally, resistance increases when gas flow is increased, as with increased breathing effort or when a patient requires mechanical ventilation. When resistance increases, more effort is required by the patient to maintain gas flow. If the patient is unable to generate the increased WOB, the amount of gas flow the patient produces decreases. Increasing airway resistance may result in reduced lung volume and inadequate ventilation.[9,26,69]

LUNG VOLUMES AND CAPACITIES

Air volume within the lung is measured with an instrument called a *spirometer*. Lung volumes and capacities (two or more lung volumes added together) are important for determining adequate pulmonary function and are shown graphically in Fig. 10.5.[26] Descriptions of the lung volumes and capacities are provided in Table 10.1. Measurements of lung volumes and capacities allow the practitioner to assess baseline pulmonary function and to monitor the improvement or progression of pulmonary diseases and patient response to therapy. For example, when the patient performs incentive spirometry, the nurse and RT assess the patient's inspiratory capacity and trend its improvement or decline over time and with interventions. Lung capacities decline gradually with aging.

RESPIRATORY ASSESSMENT

The ability to perform a physical assessment of the respiratory system is an essential skill for the critical care nurse. Assessment findings assist in identifying potential patient problems and in evaluating patient response to interventions. See the Lifespan Considerations box for information related to assessment of older patients and pregnant women.[44]

Older Adults

- ↓ Chest wall distensibility and expansion (costal cartilage calcifies)
- ↓ Alveolar surface area (enlarged alveoli)
- ↓ Alveolar elasticity
- ↓ Vital capacity and ventilatory reserves
- ↓ Diffusing capacity
- Lower PaO_2 levels on arterial blood gas
- ↓ Physiological compensatory mechanisms in response to hypercapnia or hypoxia
- ↓ Respiratory muscle strength and endurance
- Decreased cough and gag
- Increased risk for secretion retention and pneumonia, poor gas exchange, decrease in exercise tolerance, aspiration, respiratory depression caused by medications, respiratory distress and failure

Pregnant Women

- Edema and hyperemia of the upper airways
- ↓ FRC, decreased chest wall compliance
- Reduced tone of the esophagus
- ↑ Respiratory drive, larger V_T and minute ventilation due to increased progesterone.
- Respiratory alkalosis with a decreased bicarbonate
- Elevated diaphragm due to the enlarging uterus (up to 5 cm)
- ↑ O_2 consumption and CO_2 production
- Common causes of respiratory failure include pneumonia, pulmonary edema, asthma exacerbation, pulmonary embolism, amniotic fluid syndrome, pneumothorax
- Intubation failure is frequent in pregnant patients
- Apply mechanical ventilation as in nonpregnant women

FRC, Functional residual capacity; *PaO_2,* partial pressure of arterial oxygen; *V_T,* tidal volume.

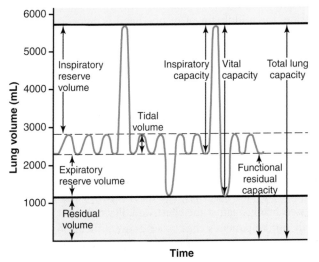

Fig. 10.5 Lung volumes and capacities. (From Hall JE. *Guyton and Hall Textbook of Medical Physiology.* 13th ed. Philadelphia, PA: Saunders; 2016.)

Health History

Ask several questions pertinent to the respiratory system when the health history is obtained:

1. Tobacco use: type, amount, and number of pack-years (number of packs of cigarettes per day × number of years smoking)
2. Occupational history such as coal mining, asbestos work, farming, and exposure to dust, fumes, smoke, toxic chemicals, paints, and insulation
3. History of symptoms such as shortness of breath, dyspnea, cough, anorexia, weight loss, chest pain, or sputum production; further assessment of sputum, including amount, color, consistency, time of day, and whether its appearance is chronic or acute
4. Use of oral and inhalant respiratory medications, such as bronchodilators and steroids
5. Use of over-the-counter or street inhalant drugs
6. Allergies: medication, food, or environmental
7. Dates of last chest radiograph and tuberculosis screening

Physical Examination

Inspection. Inspection provides an initial clue for potential acute and chronic respiratory problems. Inspect the head, neck, fingers, and chest for abnormalities.

Observe the chest for shape, breathing pattern, and chest excursion. During inspiration, chest wall excursion should be symmetrical. Asymmetrical excursion is usually associated with unilateral ventilation problems. The trachea is normally in a midline position; a tracheal shift may occur with a tension pneumothorax. Signs of acute respiratory distress include labored respirations, irregular breathing pattern, use of accessory muscles, asymmetrical chest movements, chest-abdominal asynchrony, open-mouthed breathing, or gasping breaths. Cyanosis is a late sign of hypoxemia and should not be relied on as an early warning of distress. Other indications of respiratory abnormalities include pallor or rubor, pursed-lip breathing, jugular venous distension, prolonged expiratory phase of breaths, poor capillary refill, clubbing of fingers, and a barrel-shaped chest.[69]

Count the respiratory rate (RR) for a full minute in critically ill patients. The normal RR is 12 to 20 breaths/min and expiration is usually twice as long as inspiration (inspiration-to-expiration ratio is 1:2). The normal breathing pattern is regular and even with an occasional sigh and is called *eupnea.* *Tachypnea,* a RR of greater than 20 breaths/min, may occur with anxiety, fever, pain, anemia, low partial pressure of oxygen (PaO_2), and elevated partial pressure of carbon dioxide ($PaCO_2$). *Bradypnea,* a RR of fewer than 10 breaths/min, may occur in central nervous system disorders, including administration or ingestion of central nervous system depressant medications or alcohol, severe metabolic alkalosis, and fatigue. The depth of respirations is as important as the rate and provides information about the adequacy of ventilation. Document and report alterations from normal rate and depth of respirations.

Several abnormal breathing patterns (Fig. 10.6) are possible and should be reported.[69] *Cheyne-Stokes respirations* are a cyclical respiratory pattern that occurs in central nervous system disorders and congestive heart failure. Deep, increasingly shallow respirations are followed by a period of apnea that lasts approximately 20 seconds, but the period may vary and progressively lengthen. Therefore the duration of the apneic period is timed for trending. The cycle repeats after each apneic period. *Biot's respirations,* or cluster breathing, are cycles of breaths that vary in depth and have varying periods of apnea. Biot's respirations are seen with brainstem injury. *Kussmaul respirations* are deep, regular, and rapid (usually

TABLE 10.1 Lung Volumes and Capacities

Name	Definition	Average	Formula
VOLUMES[a]			
Tidal volume (V_T)	Volume of a normal breath	500 mL	
Inspiratory reserve volume (IRV)	Maximum amount of gas that can be inspired at the end of a normal breath (over and above the V_T)	3000 mL	
Expiratory reserve volume (ERV)	Maximum amount of gas that can be forcefully expired at the end of a normal breath	1200 mL	
Residual volume (RV)	Amount of air remaining in the lungs after maximum expiration	1300 mL	
CAPACITIES			
Inspiratory capacity (IC)	Maximum volume of gas that can be inspired at normal resting expiration; the IC distends the lungs to their maximum amount	3500 mL	$IC = V_T + IRV$
Functional residual capacity (FRC)	Volume of gas remaining in the lungs at normal resting expiration	2500 mL	$FRC = ERV + RV$
Vital capacity (VC)	Maximum volume of gas that can be forcefully expired after maximum inspiration	4700 mL	$VC = V_T + IRV + ERV$
Total lung capacity (TLC)	Volume of gas in the lungs at end of maximum inspiration	6000 mL	$TLC = V_T + IRV + ERV + RV$

[a]Volumes are average in a 70-kg young adult. There is a range of normal values that varies by age, height, body size, and gender. Volumes are less in women than men when height and age are equal.

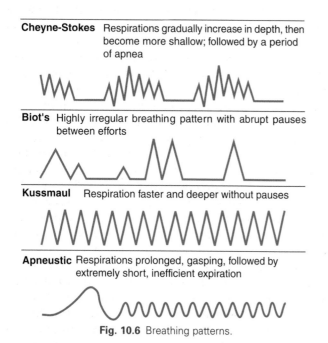

Cheyne-Stokes Respirations gradually increase in depth, then become more shallow; followed by a period of apnea

Biot's Highly irregular breathing pattern with abrupt pauses between efforts

Kussmaul Respiration faster and deeper without pauses

Apneustic Respirations prolonged, gasping, followed by extremely short, inefficient expiration

Fig. 10.6 Breathing patterns.

more than 20 breaths/min) and are commonly observed in diabetic ketoacidosis and other disorders that cause metabolic acidosis. *Apneustic respirations,* which are often associated with lesions to the pons, are gasping inspirations followed by short, ineffective expirations.

Palpation. Palpation is frequently performed simultaneously with inspection. Palpation is used to evaluate chest wall excursion, tracheal deviation, chest wall tenderness, subcutaneous crepitus, and tactile fremitus. The chest wall should not be tender to palpation; tenderness is usually associated with inflammation or trauma, including rib fractures. *Subcutaneous crepitus* or *subcutaneous emphysema* is the presence of air beneath the skin surface that has escaped from the airways or lungs. It is palpated with the fingertips and may feel like crunching rice cereal under the skin. Resist the temptation to palpate further because palpation promotes air dissection in the skin layers. Subcutaneous air indicates that air has escaped from the lungs or airways are no longer intact and may result from chest trauma, such as rib fractures, and from barotrauma.

Percussion. Percuss the chest to identify respiratory disorders such as hemothorax, pneumothorax, and consolidation. In percussion, the middle finger of one hand is tapped twice by the middle finger of the opposite hand placed against the patient's chest. The vibrations produced by tapping create different sounds, depending on the density of the underlying tissue being percussed. Five sounds may be audible on percussion: *resonance* (normal), *dullness* (tissue more dense than normal as in consolidation), *flatness* (absence of air as in lung collapse), *hyperresonance* (increased amount of air as in emphysema), and *tympany* (large amount of air as in pneumothorax).[36,69]

Auscultation. Assess lung sounds at least every 4 hours in critically ill patients using the diaphragm of the stethoscope pressed firmly against the chest wall. Place the stethoscope directly on the patient's chest; sounds are difficult to distinguish if they are auscultated through the patient's gown or clothing. The friction of chest hair on the stethoscope may mimic the sound of crackles; wetting the chest hair may reduce this sound. In addition, avoid resting the stethoscope tubing against skin or objects such as sheets, bed rails, or ventilator circuitry during auscultation.[36,52]

Use a systematic sequence during auscultation, comparing sounds from one side of the chest wall with those from the other (Fig. 10.7). If possible, perform auscultation with the patient sitting in an upright position and breathing deeply in and out through the mouth. If upright positioning is not feasible, auscultate the anterior and lateral chest wall. However,

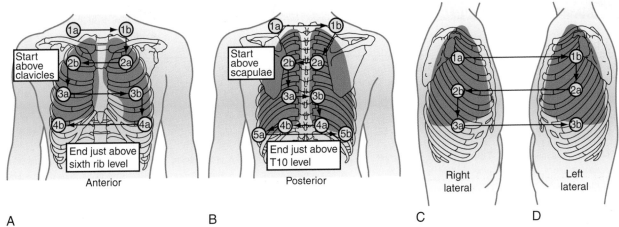

Fig. 10.7 Systematic method for palpation, percussion, and auscultation of the lungs in anterior (**A**), posterior (**B**), and lateral regions (**C** and **D**). Perform the techniques systematically to compare right and left lung fields.

take every opportunity to turn the patient and auscultate the chest posteriorly. When the patient has an artificial airway, auscultate the trachea for the presence of an air leak around the cuff of the artificial airway.[36]

Breath Sounds. Listen carefully for both normal and abnormal, or *adventitious,* breath sounds. Types of normal breath sounds include tracheal (larynx, trachea), bronchovesicular (large central airways), and vesicular (smaller airways). Be familiar with and report adventitious sounds including crackles, rhonchi, wheezes, pleural friction rub, and stridor (Table 10.2).[36] Breath sounds may be decreased because of the presence of fluid, air, or increased tissue density. Shallow respirations can also mimic decreased breath sounds; therefore encourage the patient to take deep breaths during auscultation. Document breath sounds and report abnormalities.

Arterial Blood Gas Interpretation

The ability to interpret ABG results rapidly is an essential critical care skill. Arterial blood gas results reflect oxygenation, adequacy of gas exchange, and acid-base status. Blood for ABG analysis is obtained from either a direct arterial puncture (radial, brachial, or femoral artery) or an arterial line. Arterial blood gases aid in patient assessment and are interpreted in conjunction with the patient's physical assessment findings, clinical history, and previous ABG values (Table 10.3). Noninvasive measures of gas exchange have reduced the frequency of ABG measurements.

Oxygenation. The ABG values that reflect oxygenation include the partial pressure of arterial oxygen (PaO_2) and the arterial oxygen saturation of hemoglobin (SaO_2). Approximately 3% of the available oxygen is dissolved in plasma. The remaining 97% of the oxygen attaches to hemoglobin in red blood cells, forming oxyhemoglobin.[26,69]

Partial pressure of arterial oxygen. The normal PaO_2 is 80 to 100 mm Hg at sea level. The PaO_2 decreases in older adults; the value for persons 60 to 80 years of age usually ranges from 60 to 80 mm Hg.

Arterial oxygen saturation of hemoglobin. The SaO_2 is the percentage of hemoglobin saturated with oxygen and is normally 92% to 99%. The SaO_2 is very important because it represents the primary way oxygen is transported to the tissues. The SaO_2 is measured directly from an arterial blood sample or continuously monitored indirectly with the use of a pulse oximeter (SpO_2).

Both the PaO_2 and the SaO_2 are used to assess oxygenation. Decreased oxygenation of arterial blood (PaO_2 <60 mm Hg) is referred to as *hypoxemia,* which may present with numerous symptoms, which are described in Box 10.1. A patient with a PaO_2 of less than 60 mm Hg requires immediate intervention with supplemental oxygen to treat the hypoxemia while further assessment is done to identify the cause. A PaO_2 of less than 40 mm Hg is life-threatening because oxygen is not available for metabolism. Without treatment, cellular death will occur.[9,26,69]

The relationship between the PaO_2 and the SaO_2 is shown in the S-shaped *oxyhemoglobin dissociation curve* (Fig. 10.8). The upper portion of the curve (PaO_2 >60 mm Hg) is flat. In this area of the curve, large changes in the PaO_2 result in only small changes in SaO_2. For example, the normal PaO_2 of 80 to 100 mm Hg is associated with an SaO_2 of 92% to 100%. If the PaO_2 decreases from 80 to 60 mm Hg, the SaO_2 decreases from 92% to 90%. Although this example reflects a drop in PaO_2, the patient is not immediately compromised because the hemoglobin responsible for carrying oxygen to all the tissues is still well saturated with oxygen.

The critical zone of the oxyhemoglobin dissociation curve occurs when the PaO_2 decreases to less than 60 mm Hg. At this point, the curve slopes sharply, and small changes in PaO_2 are reflected in large changes in the oxygen saturation (SpO_2). These changes in SaO_2 may cause a significant decrease in oxygen delivered to the tissues.[9,26]

As shown in Fig. 10.8, the oxyhemoglobin dissociation curve may shift under certain conditions. When the curve shifts to the right, a decreased hemoglobin affinity for oxygen exists; therefore oxygen is more readily released to the tissues. Conditions that cause a right shift include acidemia, increased temperature, and increased levels of the glucose metabolite 2,3-diphosphoglycerate (2,3-DPG), which occurs in anemia, chronic hypoxemia, and

TABLE 10.2 Adventitious Breath Sounds

Sound/Description	Cause	Clinical Significance	Additional Descriptors/Comments
Crackles—discontinuous, explosive, bubbling sounds of short duration	Air bubbling through fluid or mucus, or alveoli popping open on inspiration	Atelectasis, fluid retention in small airways (pulmonary edema), retention of mucus (bronchitis, pneumonia), interstitial fibrosis	Fine: soft, short duration Coarse: loud, longer duration Wet or dry May disappear after coughing, suctioning, or deep inspiration if alveoli remain inflated
Rhonchi—coarse, continuous, low-pitched, sonorous, or rattling sound	Air movement through excess mucus, fluid, or inflamed airways	Diseases resulting in airway inflammation and excess mucus (e.g., pneumonia, bronchitis, or excess fluid, as in pulmonary edema)	Inspiratory and/or expiratory; may clear or diminish with coughing if caused by airway secretions
Wheezes—high- or low-pitched whistling, musical sound heard during inspiration and/or expiration	Air movement through narrowed airway, which causes airway wall to oscillate or flutter	Bronchospasm, as in asthma, partial airway obstruction by tumor, foreign body or secretions, inflammation, or stenosis	High or low pitched; inspiratory and/or expiratory
Stridor—high-pitched, continuous sound heard over upper airway; a crowing sound	Air flowing through constricted larynx or trachea	Partial obstruction of upper airway, as in laryngeal edema, obstruction by foreign body, epiglottitis	Potentially life-threatening
Pleural friction rub—coarse, grating, squeaking, or scratching sound, as when two pieces of leather rub together	Inflamed pleura rubbing against each other	Pleural inflammation, as in pleuritis, pneumonia, tuberculosis, chest tube insertion, pulmonary infarction	Occurs during breathing cycle and is eliminated by breath holding Need to discern from pericardial friction rub, which continues despite breath holding

TABLE 10.3 Blood Gas Interpretation

Status	pH	PaCO$_2$	HCO$_3^-$	Base Excess
RESPIRATORY ACIDOSIS				
Uncompensated	↓ 7.35	↑ 45	Normal	Normal
Partially compensated	↓ 7.35	↑ 45	↑ 26	↑ +2
Compensated	7.35-7.45	↑ 45	↑ 26	↑ +2
RESPIRATORY ALKALOSIS				
Uncompensated	↑ 7.45	↓ 35	Normal	Normal
Partially compensated	↑ 7.45	↓ 35	↓ 22	↓ −2
Compensated	7.40-7.45	↓ 35	↓ 22	↓ −2
METABOLIC ACIDOSIS				
Uncompensated	↓ 7.35	Normal	↓ 22	↓ −2
Partially compensated	↓ 7.35	↓ 35	↓ 22	↓ −2
Compensated	7.35-7.45	↓ 35	↓ 22	↓ −2
METABOLIC ALKALOSIS				
Uncompensated	↑ 7.45	Normal	↑ 26	↑ +2
Partially compensated[a]	↑ 7.45	↑ 45	↑ 26	↑ +2
Compensated[a]	7.40-7.45	↑ 45	↑ 26	↑ +2
MIXED ACID-BASE DISORDERS				
Combined respiratory and metabolic acidosis	↓ 7.35	↑ 45	↓ 22	↓ −2
Combined respiratory and metabolic alkalosis	↑ 7.45	↓ 35	↑ 26	↑ +2

[a]Partially compensated or compensated metabolic alkalosis generally is rarely seen clinically because of the body's mechanism to prevent hypoventilation.

HCO$_3^-$, Bicarbonate; PaCO$_2$, partial pressure of carbon dioxide.

BOX 10.1 Signs and Symptoms of Hypoxemia

Integumentary System
- Pallor
- Cool, dry
- Cyanosis (late)
- Diaphoresis (late)

Respiratory System
- Dyspnea
- Tachypnea
- Use of accessory muscles

Cardiovascular System
- Tachycardia
- Dysrhythmias
- Chest pain
- Hypertension early, followed by hypotension
- Increased heart rate early, followed by decreased heart rate

Central Nervous System
- Anxiety
- Restlessness
- Confusion
- Fatigue
- Combativeness/agitation
- Coma

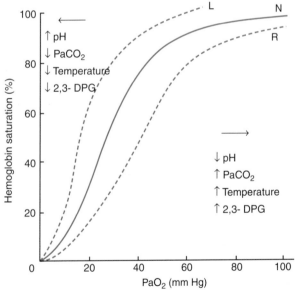

Fig. 10.8 Oxyhemoglobin dissociation curve. A partial pressure of oxygen (PaO_2) of 60 mm Hg correlates with an oxygen saturation of 90%. When the PaO_2 falls below 60 mm Hg, small changes in PaO_2 are reflected in large changes in oxygen saturation. Shifts in the oxyhemoglobin curve are shown. *L,* Left shift; *N,* normal; *R,* right shift. (From Weinberger SE, Cockrill BA, Mandel J. *Principles of Pulmonary Medicine.* 7th ed. Philadelphia, PA: Elsevier; 2019.)

low cardiac output states. When conditions exist where the curve has shifted to the right, the PaO_2 is higher than expected at the normal curve.[69]

When the curve shifts to the left, hemoglobin affinity for oxygen increases and hemoglobin clings to oxygen. Conditions that cause a left shift include alkalemia, decreased temperature, high altitude, carbon monoxide poisoning, and a decreased 2,3-DPG level. Common causes of decreased 2,3-DPG include administration of stored bank blood, sepsis, and hypophosphatemia.[26] With a left shift, the PaO_2 is lower than expected at the normal curve. Therefore if the patient's SpO_2 is 92%, obtain an ABG to assess for hypoxemia.

Ventilation and Acid-Base Status. Blood gas values that reflect ventilation and acid-base or metabolic status include the $PaCO_2$, pH, and bicarbonate (HCO_3^-).[26,69]

pH. The concentration of hydrogen ions (H^+) in the blood is referred to as the *pH.* The normal pH range is 7.35 to 7.45 (exact value, 7.40). If the H^+ level increases, the pH decreases (becomes <7.35) and the patient is said to have *acidemia.* Conversely, a decrease in H^+ level results in an increase in the pH (>7.45), and the patient is said to have *alkalemia.*

Partial pressure of arterial carbon dioxide. The partial pressure of carbon dioxide ($PaCO_2$) is CO_2 dissolved in arterial plasma. The $PaCO_2$ is regulated by the lungs and has a normal range of 35 to 45 mm Hg. A $PaCO_2$ of less than 35 mm Hg indicates respiratory alkalosis; a $PaCO_2$ greater than 45 mm Hg indicates respiratory acidosis. The respiratory system controls the $PaCO_2$ by regulating ventilation (the patient's rate and depth of breathing). If the patient hypoventilates, CO_2 is retained, leading to respiratory acidosis ($PaCO_2$ >45 mm Hg). Conversely, if a patient hyperventilates, excess CO_2 is excreted by the lungs, resulting in respiratory alkalosis ($PaCO_2$ <35 mm Hg).[69] Conditions that cause respiratory acidosis and alkalosis are noted in Box 10.2.

Sodium bicarbonate. Whereas H^+ ions are an acid in the body, HCO_3^- is a base, a substance that neutralizes or buffers acids. Bicarbonate is regulated by the kidneys. Its normal range is 22 to 26 mEq/L. An HCO_3^- level greater than 26 mEq/L indicates metabolic alkalosis, whereas an HCO_3^- level less than 22 mEq/L indicates metabolic acidosis. Conditions that cause metabolic acidosis and alkalosis are noted in Box 10.2.

Buffer systems. The body regulates acid-base balance through buffer systems, which are substances that minimize the changes in pH when either acids or bases are added. For example, acids are neutralized through combination with a base, and vice versa. The most important buffering system, the HCO_3^- buffer system, accounts for more than half of the total buffering and is activated as the H^+ concentration increases. Bicarbonate combines with H^+ to form carbonic acid (H_2CO_3), which breaks down into CO_2 (which is excreted through the lungs) and H_2O. The equation for this mechanism is as follows:

$$H^+ + HCO_3^- \rightarrow H_2CO_3 \rightarrow H_2O + CO_2$$

The HCO_3^- buffering system operates by using the lungs to regulate CO_2 and the kidneys to regulate HCO_3^-.[36,69]

Base excess or base deficit. The base excess or base deficit is reported on most ABG results. This laboratory value reflects the sum of all the buffer bases in the body, the total buffer base. The normal range for base deficit/base excess is −2 to +2 mEq/L. In metabolic acidosis, the body's buffers are used up in an attempt to neutralize the acids, and a base

BOX 10.2   Causes of Common Acid-Base Abnormalities

Respiratory Acidosis: Retention of CO_2
- Hypoventilation
- CNS depression (anesthesia, narcotics, sedatives, drug overdose)
- Respiratory neuromuscular disorders
- Trauma: spine, brain, chest wall
- Restrictive lung diseases
- Chronic obstructive pulmonary disease
- Acute airway obstruction (late phases)

Respiratory Alkalosis: Hyperventilation
- Hypoxemia
- Anxiety, fear
- Pain
- Fever
- Stimulants
- CNS irritation (e.g., central hyperventilation)
- Excessive ventilatory support (bag-valve-mask, mechanical ventilation)

Metabolic Acidosis
Increased Acids
- Diabetic ketoacidosis
- Renal failure
- Lactic acidosis
- Drug overdose (salicylates, methanol, ethylene glycol)

Loss of Base
- Diarrhea
- Pancreatic or small bowel fluid loss

Metabolic Alkalosis
Gain of Base
- Excess ingestion of antacids
- Excess administration of sodium bicarbonate
- Citrate in blood transfusions

Loss of Metabolic Acids
- Vomiting
- Nasogastric suctioning
- Low potassium and/or chloride
- Diuretics (loss of chloride and/or potassium)

CNS, Central nervous system; CO_2, carbon dioxide.

---

deficit occurs. In metabolic alkalosis, the total buffer base increases and the patient will have a base excess. All metabolic acid-base disturbances are accompanied by a change in the base excess/base deficit, making it a reliable indicator of metabolic acid-base disorders.[33] In pure respiratory acid-base disturbances, the base excess/base deficit is normal; however, once compensation occurs, the base excess/base deficit changes.

Compensation. Compensation involves mechanisms that normalize the pH when an acid-base imbalance occurs. The kidneys attempt to compensate for respiratory abnormalities, whereas the lungs attempt to compensate for metabolic problems. The lungs quickly respond to compensate for a primary metabolic acid-base abnormality. For example, in metabolic acidosis, the depth and rate of ventilation are increased in an effort to blow off more CO_2 (acid). Conversely, in metabolic alkalosis, the rate and depth of ventilation may be decreased in an effort to retain acid.[26]

The kidneys compensate for primary respiratory acid-base abnormalities by excreting excess H^+ and retaining HCO_3^-. The renal system activates more slowly, taking up to 2 days to regulate acid-base balance. The kidneys excrete HCO_3^- when respiratory alkalosis is present and retain HCO_3^- when respiratory acidosis is present.[26,34] The renal and respiratory systems exist in harmony to maintain acid-base balance (Fig. 10.9).

Steps in Arterial Blood Gas Interpretation. Systematic analysis of ABG values involves five steps.[52] Table 10.3 lists laboratory values associated with acid-base abnormalities. Critical ABG values are noted in the Laboratory Alert box.

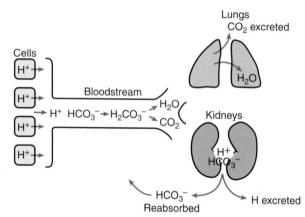

Fig. 10.9 The kidneys and lungs work together to compensate for acid-base imbalances in the respiratory or metabolic systems. HCO_3^-, Bicarbonate; H_2CO_3, carbonic acid. (Modified from Harvey MA. *Study Guide to the Core Curriculum for Critical Care Nursing*. 3rd ed. Philadelphia, PA: Saunders; 2000.)

! LABORATORY ALERT

Arterial Blood Gas Critical Values[a,b]

PaO_2 <60 mm Hg
$PaCO_2$ >50 mm Hg
pH <7.25 or >7.60

[a]Critical values vary by facility and laboratory.
[b]These are critical values only if they differ from baseline values (i.e., an acute change). Some patients with pulmonary disease tolerate highly "abnormal" arterial blood gas values.
PaCO2, Partial pressure of carbon dioxide; *PaO2*, partial pressure of arterial oxygen.

Step 1: Look at each number individually and label it. Decide whether the value is high, low, or normal, and label the finding. For example, a pH of 7.50 is high and labeled as *alkalemia.*

Step 2: Evaluate oxygenation. Oxygenation is analyzed by evaluating the PaO_2 and the SaO_2. Hypoxemia is present and considered a significant problem when the PaO_2 falls to less than 60 mm Hg or the SaO_2 falls to less than 90%. A complete assessment must consider the level of supplemental oxygen a patient is receiving when the ABG is drawn.

Step 3: Determine acid-base status. Assess the pH to determine the acid-base status. A pH of 7.4 is the absolute normal. If the pH is less than 7.4, the primary disorder is acidosis. If the pH is greater than 7.4, the primary disorder is alkalosis. Therefore even if the pH is within the normal range, noting whether it is on the acid or alkaline side of 7.40 is important.

Step 4: Determine whether primary acid-base disorder is respiratory or metabolic. Assess the $PaCO_2$, which reflects the respiratory system, and the HCO_3^- level, which reflects the metabolic system, to determine which one is altered in the same manner as the pH. The ABG results may reflect only one disorder (respiratory or metabolic). However, two primary acid-base disorders may occur simultaneously (mixed acid-base imbalance). For example, during cardiac arrest, both respiratory acidosis and metabolic acidosis commonly occur because of hypoventilation and lactic acidosis. Use the base excess to confirm your interpretation of the primary acid-base disturbance, especially if the disorder is mixed.

Step 5: Determine whether any form of compensatory response has taken place. *Compensation* refers to a return to a normal blood pH by means of respiratory or renal mechanisms. The system opposite the primary disorder attempts the compensation. For example, if a patient has respiratory acidosis, such as occurs in COPD (low pH, high $PaCO_2$), the kidneys respond by retaining more HCO_3^- and excreting H^+. Conversely, if a patient has metabolic acidosis, such as occurs in diabetic ketoacidosis (low pH, low HCO_3^-), the lungs respond by hyperventilation and excretion of CO_2 (respiratory alkalosis). If the $PaCO_2$ and the HCO_3^- are abnormal in the same direction, compensation is occurring.

Compensation may be absent, partial, or complete. Compensation is *absent* if the system opposite the primary disorder is within normal range. If compensation has occurred but the pH is still abnormal, compensation is referred to as *partial.* Compensation is *complete* if compensatory mechanisms are present and the pH is within normal range. The body does not overcompensate.[69] Examples of ABG compensation are shown in Box 10.3.

❓ CRITICAL REASONING ACTIVITY

Your patient has the following arterial blood gas results: pH, 7.28; PaO_2, 52 mm Hg; SaO_2, 84%; $PaCO_2$, 55 mm Hg; HCO_3^-, 24 mEq/L.

1. What is your interpretation of this arterial blood gas?
2. What clinical condition or conditions could cause the patient to have these arterial blood gas results?

BOX 10.3 Examples of Arterial Blood Gases and Compensation

Example 1

PaO_2	80 mm Hg (normal)
pH	7.30 (low; acidosis)
$PaCO_2$	50 mm Hg (high; respiratory acidosis)
HCO_3^-	22 mEq/L (normal)
SaO_2	95% (normal)

Interpretation: Normal oxygenation, respiratory acidosis; no compensation.

Example 2

PaO_2	80 mm Hg (normal)
pH	7.32 (low; acidosis)
$PaCO_2$	50 mm Hg (high; respiratory acidosis)
HCO_3^-	28 mEq/L (high; metabolic alkalosis)
SaO_2	95% (normal)

Interpretation: Normal oxygenation, partly compensated respiratory acidosis. The arterial blood gases are only partly compensated because the pH is not yet within normal limits.

Example 3

PaO_2	80 mm Hg (normal)
pH	7.36 (acid side of normal)
$PaCO_2$	50 mm Hg (high; respiratory acidosis)
HCO_3^-	29 mEq/L (high; metabolic alkalosis)
SaO_2	95% (normal)

Interpretation: Normal oxygenation, completely (fully) compensated respiratory acidosis. The pH is now within normal limits; therefore complete compensation has occurred.

HCO_3^-, Bicarbonate; $PaCO_2$, partial pressure of carbon dioxide; PaO_2, partial pressure of arterial oxygen; SaO_2, saturation of hemoglobin with oxygen in arterial blood.

Noninvasive Assessment of Gas Exchange

Intermittent ABG results have been the gold standard for the monitoring of gas exchange and acid-base status. Improvements in technology for noninvasive assessment of gas exchange by pulse oximetry and capnography have reduced the number of ABG samples obtained in critically ill patients.

Assessment of Oxygenation

Pulse oximetry. Pulse oximetry measures the saturation of oxygen in pulsatile blood (SpO_2), which reflects the SaO_2. The oxyhemoglobin dissociation curve (see Fig. 10.8) shows the relationship between SaO_2 and PaO_2 and provides the basis for pulse oximetry. The sensor that measures SpO_2 is placed on the patient's finger, toe, ear, or forehead where blood flow is not diminished. Light emitted from the sensor is absorbed by hemoglobin with oxygen or hemoglobin without oxygen, providing the necessary information for the device to calculate the percent hemoglobin saturated with oxygen in the pulsatile (arterial) blood. Pulse oximetry is measured continuously in critically ill patients, whereas SpO_2 values are sometimes "spot checked" in patients who are less acutely ill. Pulse oximetry measurements are trended to assess the effect of pathological conditions on the adequacy of oxygenation and to monitor a patient's response to treatment (e.g., ventilator changes, suctioning, inhalation therapy, body position changes). SpO₂ only measures oxygenation and cannot be used to assess adequacy of ventilation or CO_2 levels.[40]

To obtain accurate SpO₂ readings, place the sensor correctly on a warm, well-perfused area and ensure that an adequate pulsatile signal is detected. Several factors affect the accuracy of SpO₂ values. Artifact from patient motion or edema at the sensor site may prevent an accurate measurement. The SpO₂ measurements may be lower than the actual SaO₂ if the perfusion to the sensor site is reduced (e.g., limb ischemia or inflated blood pressure cuff) or in the presence of sunlight, fluorescent light, nail polish or artificial nails, and IV dyes. The SpO₂ measurements may be higher than the actual SaO₂ reported by ABG analysis if the patient has an abnormal hemoglobin, such as methemoglobin or carboxyhemoglobin.[26,33]

Assessment of Ventilation

End-tidal carbon dioxide monitoring. End-tidal carbon dioxide (ETCO₂) monitoring is the noninvasive measurement of alveolar CO_2 at the end of exhalation when CO_2 concentration is at its peak.[33,68] It reflects the alveolar CO_2 level, which in turn reflects the arterial CO_2 (PaCO₂), and is used to monitor and assess trends in ventilatory status. Expired gases are sampled from the patient's airway and are analyzed by a CO_2 sensor that uses infrared light to measure exhaled CO_2 at the end of inspiration. Both a numerical value and a waveform are provided for assessment of ventilation (Fig. 10.10).[33,41] The ETCO₂ sampling port and sensor are placed in the ventilator circuitry close to the patient's endotracheal tube (ETT) or the tracheostomy tube. A nasal cannula with a scoop is used in patients without an artificial airway.[41]

Normally, ETCO₂ values average 2 to 5 mm Hg less than the PaCO₂ in individuals with normal lung and cardiac function.[12] Each time an ABG is obtained, simultaneously note the ETCO₂ value. End-tidal carbon dioxide is subtracted from the PaCO₂, providing an index known as the *PaCO₂-ETCO₂ gradient.* The gradient is used to estimate the severity of pulmonary disease and to determine the baseline correlation between ETCO₂ and PaCO₂. For example, if a blood gas shows that the PaCO₂ is 40 mm Hg and simultaneously the ETCO₂ is noted to be 36 mm Hg, the PaCO₂-ETCO₂ gradient is +4, which is within the normal range. Conversely, if the PaCO₂ is 56 and the ETCO₂ is 32, the gradient is 24, indicating significant areas of the lung that are ventilated but not

perfused (dead space), affecting the exchange of CO_2 at the alveolar level. An example of a disease process that results in significant dead space is pulmonary embolism. Therapies targeted to improving matching of ventilation to perfusion in the lung can be implemented and their effects evaluated by determining if they reduce the ETCO₂ gradient. Knowing the gradient also allows for noninvasive assessment of the patient's ventilation by trend monitoring the ETCO₂ and inferring the PaCO₂ by use of the gradient.[41,52] Estimate the patient's PaCO₂ by adding the last calculated gradient to the ETCO₂.

Clinical applications of ETCO₂ monitoring include assessment of trends in alveolar ventilation; assessment of the patient's response to ventilator changes and respiratory treatments; confirmation and continuous monitoring of proper position of the endotracheal tube, including during transport; monitoring the integrity of the ventilator circuit, including detection of disconnection; trending CO_2 in patients with increased intracranial pressure to avoid inadvertent hyperventilation; and detection of blood flow during cardiac arrest (see Chapter 11).[41,59,68] The most common pitfall of ETCO₂ monitoring is believing that the value reflects only the patient's ventilatory status. Changes in exhaled CO_2 may occur because of changes not only in ventilation but also in CO_2 production (metabolism), transport of CO_2 to the lung (perfusion), and accuracy of the equipment. For example, a decreased ETCO₂ value could indicate decreased alveolar ventilation, a reduction in lung perfusion as in hypotension or pulmonary embolus, a reduction in metabolic production of CO_2 as in hypothermia or a return to normothermia after fever, or obstruction of the CO_2 sampling tube.[41,68]

Colorimetric carbon dioxide detector. Disposable colorimetric ETCO₂ detectors are routinely used after intubation to differentiate tracheal from esophageal intubation (Fig. 10.11). When CO_2 is detected, the color of the indicator changes, verifying correct tube placement.[8,33]

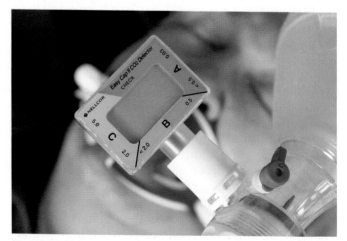

Fig. 10.11 Disposable colorimetric carbon dioxide (CO_2) detector for confirming endotracheal tube placement. Detection of CO_2 confirms tube placement in the lungs because the only source of CO_2 is the alveoli. (©2019 Medtronic. All rights reserved. Used with the permission of Medtronic.)

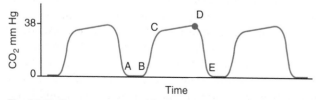

Fig. 10.10 Capnogram or graphic display of exhaled carbon dioxide *(CO₂)*. Rise in the waveform from *A* to *D* represents CO_2 leaving the lung. Point *D* is where end-tidal CO_2 is measured and represents the highest concentration of exhaled alveolar CO_2.

OXYGEN ADMINISTRATION

Oxygen is administered to treat or prevent hypoxemia. Oxygen may be supplied by various sources such as piped into wall devices, oxygen tanks, or oxygen concentrators. The amount of oxygen administered to the patient is described as the fraction of inspired oxygen (FiO_2) and is reported as a decimal (e.g., FiO_2 0.5). Oxygen concentrations are reported in percentages such as 50% oxygen. Devices can deliver low (<35%), moderate (35% to 60%), or high (>60%) oxygen concentrations.[29,33]

Oxygen delivery devices are classified into two general categories: low-flow systems (nasal cannula, simple face mask, partial-rebreather mask, and non-rebreather mask) and high-flow systems (air-entrainment or Venturi mask and high-flow nasal cannula).[8,29] Low-flow systems deliver oxygen at flow rates that are less than the patient's inspiratory demand for gas; total patient demand is not met. Low-flow system devices require the patient to entrain, or draw in, room air along with the delivered oxygen-enriched gas. The FiO_2 cannot be precisely controlled or predicted because it is determined not only by the amount of oxygen delivered but also by the patient's ventilatory pattern and thus the amount of air the patient entrains. For example, if the patient's ventilation increases, the delivered FiO_2 decreases because the patient entrains a larger percentage of room air. Conversely, if the patient's ventilation decreases, the oxygen delivered is less diluted and the FiO_2 rises. In high-flow systems, the flow of oxygen-enriched gas is sufficient for the patient's total inspiratory demand. The FiO_2 remains fairly constant. In general, for delivery of a consistent FiO_2 to a patient with a variable (deep, irregular, shallow) ventilatory pattern, use a high-flow system.

The successful administration of oxygen therapy is important in treating hypoxemia. When administering oxygen, consider not only the adequacy of the flow delivered by a device, but also fit and function. To ensure proper fit and function, inspect the patient's face to assess how well the oxygen delivery device is positioned and whether the airway is patent. The oxygen-connecting tubing is traced back to the gas source origin to ensure that it is connected. Finally, it is important to ensure that the gas source is oxygen, not air, and that it is turned on and set properly.

Humidification

Humidification of oxygen is recommended when oxygen flow is greater than 4 L/min to prevent the mucous membranes from drying. At lower flow rates, the patient's natural humidification system provides adequate humidity.[3,49,69] Monitor the quantity and consistency of the patient's secretions to determine the adequacy of humidification. If the secretions are thick despite adequate humidification of the delivered gases, the patient needs systemic hydration.

Humidification is also an important element of ventilator management. Maintain the inspired gas reaching the patient's airway at as close to 37°C and 100% relative humidity as possible.[29] Two approaches are used to provide humidification. One method functions by passing the dry gas through a water-based humidification system before it reaches the patient's airway. The second method is to attach a heat-moisture exchanger (HME) to the ventilator circuit. The HME functions as an artificial "nose" to warm and humidify the patient's inspired breath with his or her own expired moisture and body heat.

During mechanical ventilation, frequently inspect the humidification unit. If a water-based humidification is used, routine checks include maintaining the water reservoir level and removing condensate from loops in the ventilator circuit. During manipulation of the circuit tubing, it is important to prevent emptying the condensate into the patient's airway. This can lead to contamination of the patient's airway as well as breathing difficulty. If an HME is used, inspect it regularly for accumulation of patient secretions in the device, which could result in partial or complete obstruction, increased airway resistance, and increased WOB.[8,47]

Oxygen Delivery Devices

Nasal Cannula. The nasal cannula is relatively comfortable to wear and easy to secure on the patient. In adult patients, nasal cannulas provide oxygen concentrations between 24% and 44% oxygen at flow rates up to 6 L/min.[29,33] An increase in oxygen flow rate by 1 L/min generally increases oxygen delivery by 4% (e.g., 2 L/min nasal cannula delivers 28% of oxygen, whereas 3 L/min provides 32%). Flow rates higher than 6 L/min are not effective in increasing oxygenation because the capacity of the patient's anatomical reservoir in the nasopharynx is surpassed. An important nursing intervention for patients receiving oxygen via nasal cannula is to assess the nares and the skin above the ears for skin breakdown. It may be necessary to pad the tubing over the ear with gauze.

High-Flow Nasal Cannula. Oxygen delivered at rates ranging from 15 to 40 L/min is known as *high-flow therapy* and historically has been delivered with face masks. However, the delivery of high-flow therapy, which provides high concentrations of oxygen ranging from 60% to 90% and greater, is possible through a specifically designed high-flow nasal cannula (HFNC) and high-flow system that heats and humidifies the delivered gases. Compliance with therapy is usually better with the nasal cannula because the patient is more comfortable and can eat, drink, and talk. The high-flow system fills the patient's pharynx so that it becomes a reservoir of oxygen and generates low levels of positive pressure in the upper airway, thereby improving the oxygen delivered to the alveoli with each breath. The high flow rate also flushes expired CO_2 from the upper airway, which may explain why the patient's WOB may be decreased.[70] Collaborate with the RT to ensure that the water in the system remains sufficient to humidify the high flow of gas. A systematic review examined the effectiveness of HFNC relative to conventional oxygen therapy and noninvasive ventilation (NIV) in preventing the need for intubation. Compared with conventional therapy, HFNC was associated with a lower rate of endotracheal intubation, whereas no significant difference was found in the comparison with NIV. HFNC was better tolerated than NIV because it is more comfortable and there is a stable flow of warm, humidified gases with a reduced sense of dryness.[16,46]

Simple Face Mask. Placing a mask over the patient's face creates an additional oxygen reservoir beyond the patient's natural anatomical reservoir. Ensure that the mask has a tight fit and the flow rate is set to at least 5 L/min to prevent rebreathing CO_2. Oxygen is delivered at flow rates of 5 to 12 L/min, which provides concentrations of 30% to 60%.[35] Instruct the patient about the importance of wearing the mask as applied. Clean the inside of the mask as needed, and assess the skin for areas of pressure.[29]

Face Masks With Reservoirs. Both the partial-rebreather and the non-rebreather masks are similar to the design of a simple face mask, but with the addition of an oxygen reservoir bag. The reservoir increases the amount of oxygen available to the patient during inspiration and allows for the delivery of concentrations of 35% to 60% (partial-rebreather) or 60% to 80% (non-rebreather) depending on the flowmeter setting, the fit of the mask, and the patient's respiratory pattern. The main difference between these two devices is that the non-rebreather mask has one-way valves between the mask and reservoir bag and over one of the exhalation ports. These valves ensure that the patient breathes a high concentration of oxygen-enriched gas from the reservoir with each breath (Fig. 10.12). Set the flow rate on the meter to prevent the reservoir bag from deflating no more than one-half during inspiration for the partial rebreather and to prevent the bag from deflating for the non-rebreather.[29] Either mask may be used in the critically ill patient with severe hypoxemia in an effort to prevent the need for endotracheal intubation and mechanical ventilation.

Venturi or Air-Entrainment Mask. The Venturi or air-entrainment mask appears much like a simple face mask; however, it has a jet adapter placed between the mask and the tubing to the oxygen source. The jet adapters come in various sizes and are often color coded to the FiO_2 they deliver. The appropriate oxygen flow rate is often inscribed on the adapter (Fig. 10.13). The Venturi mask delivers a fixed FiO_2. Because the level of oxygen

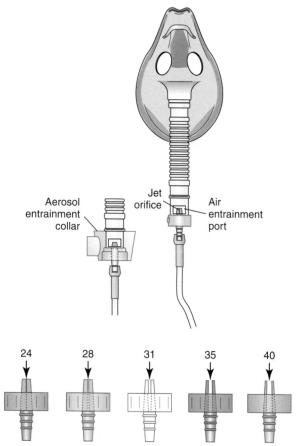

Fig. 10.13 Air-entrainment (Venturi) mask with various jet orifices. Each orifice provides a specific delivered fraction of inspired oxygen (FiO_2). (From Kacmarek RM, Dimas S, Mack CW. *The Essentials of Respiratory Care.* 4th ed. St. Louis, MO: Mosby; 2005.)

can be closely regulated, the Venturi mask is commonly used in the hypoxemic patient with chronic pulmonary disease for whom the delivery of excessive oxygen could depress the respiratory drive.[29,33]

Aerosol and Humidity Delivery Systems. The goal of adding humidity to the inspired gases is to prevent dehydration of the airways and secretions secondary to breathing dry medical gases. The high-humidity face mask or face tent is an option for patients who do not have artificial airways (Fig. 10.14). High-flow devices used for administering humidified oxygen to patients with an artificial airway are the T-piece and the tracheostomy mask/collar. Humidity is added through a nebulizer that delivers a fixed FiO_2. Set the initial flow rate at 10 L/min and adjust it so that a constant mist is seen coming from the exhalation port.[29,33,52]

Manual Resuscitation Bag (Variable Performance). A manual resuscitation bag, or bag-valve device, is used to ventilate and oxygenate a patient manually (see Chapter 11). The device is attached to a face mask or connected directly to an ETT or tracheostomy tube to ventilate the patient. When used on an emergency basis, ensure that the bag-valve device has a reservoir attached to increase the FiO_2. Set the oxygen flowmeter attached to the bag at 15 L/min.

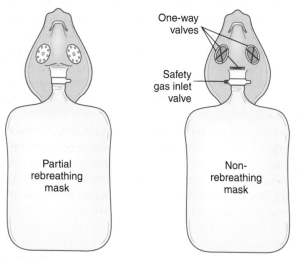

Fig. 10.12 Partial-rebreather and non-rebreather oxygen masks. (From Kacmarek RM, Dimas S, Mack CW. *The Essentials of Respiratory Care.* 4th ed. St. Louis, MO: Mosby; 2005.)

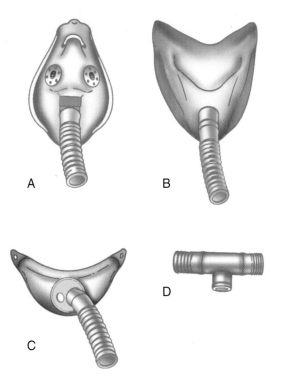

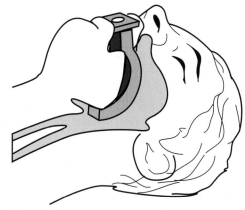

Fig. 10.15 Maintaining a patent airway with an oral airway. (Modified from Shilling A, Durbin CG. Airway management devices and advanced cardiac life support. In: Cairo JM, ed. *Mosby's Respiratory Care Equipment.* 10th ed. St. Louis, MO: Elsevier Health Sciences; 2018.)

Fig. 10.14 Devices used to apply high-flow, high-humidity oxygen therapy. **A,** Aerosol mask. **B,** Face tent. **C,** Tracheostomy collar. **D,** Briggs T-piece. (From Kacmarek RM, Stoller JK, Heuer AJ. *Egan's Fundamentals of Respiratory Care.* 11th ed. St. Louis, MO: Elsevier; 2017.)

BOX 10.4 Insertion of Oral Airway
1. Choose the proper size by measuring the airway on the patient. Airway should extend from the edge of the patient's mouth to the earlobe.
2. Suction mucus from the mouth using a tonsil (Yankauer) tip catheter.
3. Turn the airway upside down with its tip against the hard palate and slide airway into mouth until the soft palate is reached, then rotate the airway to match the curvature of the tongue into the proper position.
4. An alternative method to step 3 is to use a tongue blade to depress the patient's tongue while inserting the airway, matching its curvature to that of the tongue.
5. Advance tip to back of mouth. Ensure end of airway rests between the teeth but does not compress the lips against the teeth, which would cause injury.
6. Assess airway patency, breath sounds, and chest movement. Noises indicating upper airway obstruction should be absent.
7. Maintain proper head alignment after airway insertion.

AIRWAY MANAGEMENT

Positioning

A patent airway is essential to adequate ventilation and is a priority of nursing care. When the airway is partially or totally obstructed, the first method for reinstating a patent airway is proper head position with the head-tilt/chin-lift or jaw thrust. An airway adjunct such as the oral or nasopharyngeal airway may be needed to help maintain the airway.

Oral Airways

The oropharyngeal airway prevents the tongue from falling back and obstructing the pharynx (Fig. 10.15). It is indicated when the patient has a depressed level of consciousness. It may also be used to make ventilation with a manual resuscitation bag more effective or to prevent an unconscious patient from biting and occluding an ETT. It is contraindicated in a patient who is awake because it stimulates the gag reflex, resulting in discomfort, agitation, and possibly emesis. Choose the proper size oral airway: too short an airway forces the patient's tongue back into the pharynx and too long an airway stimulates the gag reflex.[37] The technique for inserting an oral airway is described in Box 10.4. When used, assess the lips and tongue for signs of pressure ulceration and suction the oropharynx of accumulated secretions as needed.

Nasopharyngeal Airways

The nasopharyngeal airway, also known as a *nasal airway* or *nasal trumpet*, is a soft rubber or latex tube placed in the nose that extends to the posterior portion of the pharynx (Fig. 10.16). It is indicated when an oropharyngeal airway is contraindicated or too difficult to place, such as when the patient's jaw is tight during a seizure, or if oral trauma is present. Nasopharyngeal airways are better tolerated than oral airways in the conscious patient, are more comfortable, and facilitate the passage of a suction catheter during nasotracheal suctioning.

The procedure for inserting a nasotracheal airway is described in Box 10.5. Complications of nasopharyngeal airways include insertion into the esophagus if the airway is too long, nosebleeds, and ulceration of the nares. Extended use of nasopharyngeal airways is not recommended because of an increased risk for sinusitis or otitis.[37]

Endotracheal Intubation

Intubation refers to the insertion of an ETT into the trachea through either the mouth or the nose. Advantages of oral versus nasal endotracheal intubation are listed in Box 10.6. The ETT

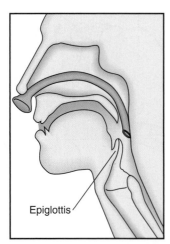

Fig. 10.16 The nasopharyngeal airway is used to relieve upper airway obstruction and to facilitate passage of a suction catheter.

BOX 10.5 Insertion of Nasal Airway

1. Choose the proper size by positioning the airway along the side of the face. The proper length airway extends from the nostril to the earlobe, or just past the angle of the jaw.
2. Generously lubricate the tip and sides of the nasal airway with a water-soluble lubricant.
3. If time allows, lubricate the nasal passage with a topical anesthetic.
4. Insert the airway medially and downward, not upward because the nasopharynx lies directly behind the nares. It may be necessary to rotate the airway slightly.
5. After insertion, assess airway patency, breath sounds, and chest movement.

(Fig. 10.17A) is made of a polyvinyl chloride or silicone material with a distal cuff (balloon) that is inflated via a one-way valve pilot balloon. The purpose of the cuff is to facilitate ventilation of the patient by sealing the trachea and allowing air to pass through, not around, the ETT. Standard ETT cuffs are the high-volume, low-pressure type, and most cuffs are inflated with air (some tubes have a foam-filled cuff). The pilot balloon and valve are used to monitor and adjust cuff pressure.[23]

ETTs capable of continuous suctioning of subglottic secretions have an extra suction port just above the cuff for removal of secretions that accumulate above the cuff (see Fig. 10.17B). Evidence shows a decrease in ventilator-associated pneumonia (VAP), but a meta-analysis found no differences in ventilator days, length of stay, ventilator-associated events, or mortality when these tubes are used (see Evidence-Based Practice box).[11] Despite strong evidence as to the outcomes associated with the subglottic secretion drainage endotracheal tube (SSD-ETT), the tubes have not been widely adopted. Primary reasons for nonuse are the higher costs associated with the devices and ensuring that patients who may benefit from the tube get intubated with the specialized devices. Nurses can assist in developing protocols for implementing the SSD-ETT in clinical practice, such as availability of the tube on crash carts and in the emergency department. Additional interventions are required when these tubes are in place. Continuous low-pressure suction not exceeding −20 mm Hg is applied to the suction lumen. Maintain patency of the suction lumen by administering a

---

BOX 10.6 Oral Versus Nasotracheal Intubation

Oral Intubation

Advantages
- Quickly performed, emergency airway
- Preferred method; less sinusitis and otitis media
- Larger tube facilitates secretion removal and bronchoscopy; creates less airway resistance
- Less kinking of tube

Disadvantages
- Discomfort
- Mouth care more difficult to perform
- Impairs ability to swallow
- May increase oral secretion production
- May cause irritation and ulceration of the mouth
- More difficult for patient to communicate by mouthing words
- Patient may bite on airway, reducing gas flow

Nasotracheal Intubation

Advantages
- Greater patient comfort and tolerance
- Better mouth care possible
- Fewer oral complications
- Facilitates swallowing of oral secretions
- Patient communication by mouthing words enhanced

Disadvantages
- More difficult to place
- Possible epistaxis during insertion
- Increases risk for sinusitis and otitis media
- Secretion removal may be more difficult to perform because of smaller tube diameter
- Increased work of breathing associated with smaller-diameter tube

---

bolus of air through the suction port as needed to relieve obstruction and maintain continuous suction.

Intubation is performed to establish an airway, assist in secretion removal, protect the airway from aspiration in patients with a depressed cough and gag, and provide mechanical ventilation. Personnel who are trained and skilled in intubation perform the procedure; these include anesthesiologists, nurse anesthetists, acute care nurse practitioners, emergency department physicians, intensivists, RTs, and some paramedics. Intubation may be performed emergently on a patient in cardiac or respiratory arrest, or electively in a patient with impending respiratory failure.[23]

It is important to be familiar with and be able to gather intubation equipment quickly. Know how to connect the laryngoscope blade to the handle, check to see that it illuminates properly, and change the bulb if indicated. Intubation equipment is frequently kept together in an emergency cart or special procedures box to facilitate emergency intubation (Fig. 10.18). If a patient requires intubation, notify the RT to obtain a ventilator, explain the procedure to the patient, remove dentures if present, gather all equipment, and ensure that suction equipment is in working order. During intubation, assist in positioning the patient, verify that the patient has a patent IV line for

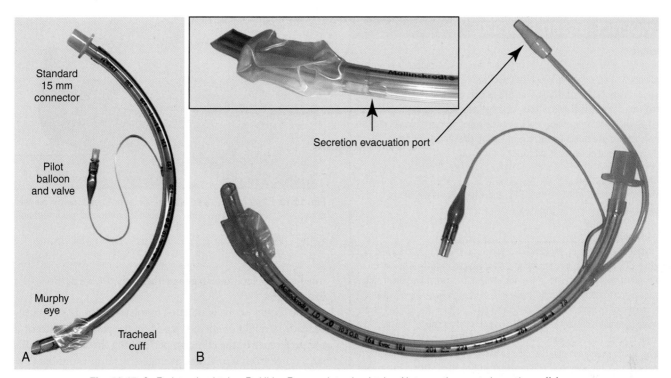

Fig. 10.17 A, Endotracheal tube. **B,** Hi-Lo Evac endotracheal tube. Note suction port above the cuff for removal of pooled secretions. (From Shilling A, Durbin CG. Airway management. In: Cairo JM, ed. *Mosby's Respiratory Care Equipment.* 10th ed. St. Louis, MO: Elsevier Health Sciences; 2018.)

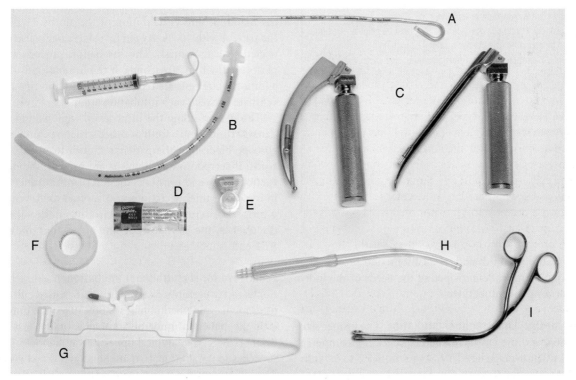

Fig. 10.18 Equipment used for endotracheal intubation: **A,** stylet (disposable); **B,** endotracheal tube with 10-mL syringe for cuff inflation; **C,** laryngoscope handle with attached curved blade *(left)* and straight blade *(right)*; **D,** water-soluble lubricant; **E,** colorimetric carbon dioxide detector to check tube placement; **F,** tape or **G,** commercial device to secure tube; **H,** Yankauer disposable pharyngeal suction device; **I,** Magill forceps (optional). Additional equipment, not shown, includes suction source and stethoscope.

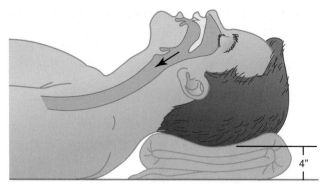

Fig. 10.19 Elevating the head with a blanket or folded towels places the patient in the "sniffing position" to facilitate endotracheal intubation.

lubricant to facilitate passage through the structures of the oropharynx.

The laryngoscope is attached to the appropriate size and type of blade (straight or curved) based on the patient's anatomy and the preference of the clinician performing the intubation. Blade sizes range from 0 to 4. The average-size adult is intubated with a size 3 blade.[2] Optional equipment includes a fiberoptic laryngoscope or equipment for video-assisted intubation.

Place the patient in a "sniffing" position to facilitate visualization of the glottis, or vocal cords. Place a folded towel or bath blanket under the head to achieve this position (Fig. 10.19). Time permitting, premedicate the patient with a sedative and possibly a paralytic agent to allow for easier manipulation of the mandible and visualization of the glottis. Hyperoxygenate the patient with 100% oxygen by using a bag-valve device connected to a face mask. The intubation procedure should be performed within 30 seconds. If the intubation is difficult and additional attempts are required to secure the airway, manually ventilate between each intubation attempt.

The person doing the intubation, while taking care not to damage the patient's teeth or other structures, inserts the laryngoscope blade into the patient's mouth to visualize the vocal cords. If secretions and vomitus are present, the oral cavity is suctioned. A rigid tonsil tip suction (e.g., Yankauer) is efficient in removing thick secretions and is often used. When the tube is properly inserted about 5 to 6 cm beyond the vocal cords into the trachea, the laryngoscope and stylet are removed and the ETT cuff is inflated.[2,23,37]

Procedure for Nasotracheal Intubation.
Nasotracheal intubation is rarely performed secondary to increased risk of sinusitis, otitis media, and pneumonia (see Box 10.6). The only indication is if the patient cannot be intubated orally because of oral trauma, surgery, or atypical upper airway anatomy. The two approaches to nasal intubation are blind and direct visualization.[2] The equipment for nasotracheal intubation is the same as for oral intubation with the addition of Magill forceps, which are used to guide the tube through the vocal cords in the direct visualization procedure. The naris selected for the ETT passage is prepared with a topical vasoconstricting agent to reduce bleeding from the highly vascular nares and an anesthetic agent such as water-soluble 2% lidocaine gel. The patient is positioned as

the administration of fluids and medications, and provide the necessary equipment while anticipating the needs of the individual performing the intubation.

Procedure for Oral Endotracheal Intubation.
The proper size ETT is chosen, and the cuff is inflated to check for symmetry and any leaks. The average-size ETT ranges from 7.5 to 8.0 mm for women and from 8.0 to 9.0 mm for men.[53] It is important that the ETT not be too small because a smaller-diameter ETT substantially increases airway resistance and the patient's WOB. A plastic-coated malleable stylet may be used to stiffen the ETT to facilitate insertion, but it should be placed carefully inside the ETT so that it does not protrude beyond the end of the ETT. The outside of the ETT is lubricated with a water-soluble

indicated by the preference of the person performing the intubation: semi-Fowler, high Fowler, or supine.

With nasal intubation, the correct placement level of the ETT at the naris is usually 28 cm for males and 26 cm for females.[37]

Verification of Endotracheal Tube Placement. Objective verification of correct placement of the ETT in the trachea (versus incorrect placement in the esophagus) is imperative and is performed through clinical assessment and confirmation devices. Clinical assessment includes auscultating the epigastrium and lung fields and observing for bilateral chest expansion. Failure to hear breath sounds while hearing air over the epigastrium represents esophageal rather than tracheal intubation. Breath sounds are equal bilaterally when the tube is placed correctly. Intubation of the right mainstem bronchus is common because the right mainstem is straighter than the left, and the ETT is occasionally placed deeper in the trachea than necessary. Right mainstem bronchus intubation is suspected when unilateral expansion of the right chest is observed during ventilation and the breath sounds are louder on the right than the left. Ensure that a portable chest radiograph is ordered to confirm tube placement.[23]

Devices to confirm ETT placement include either a handheld or disposable ETCO$_2$ detector or a bulb aspiration device (esophageal detector device). The disposable ETCO$_2$ detector is attached to the end of the ETT. This device changes color when CO$_2$ is detected and is a highly reliable method of confirming tracheal (versus esophageal) intubation; however, the detection of ETCO$_2$ is affected when cardiac output is profoundly depressed, as in cardiac arrest.[2,8,23,37] Another option is to attach an aspiration device that is similar to a bulb syringe. The device is compressed and deflated and is attached to the ETT. If the tube is in the trachea, the bulb inflates rapidly. If the tube is in the esophagus, filling is delayed. Pulse oximetry also assists in assessment of tube placement. Oxygen saturation will fall if the esophagus has been inadvertently intubated, and it may be decreased in right mainstem intubation.

The tip of the ETT should be approximately 3 to 4 cm above the carina. Once the placement is confirmed, record the centimeter depth marking at the teeth and gums or naris in the medical record. During each assessment, ensure that the tube remains in proper position as compared with the depth marking noted in the record after initial confirmation of placement. Collaborate with the RT to ensure that the ETT is properly secured with tape or a commercial device to prevent dislodging. Fig. 10.20 shows two methods for securing the ETT.

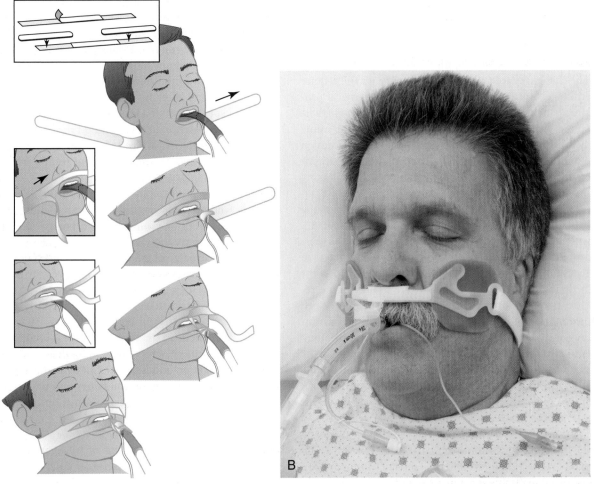

Fig. 10.20 Two methods for securing the endotracheal tube: tape (**A**) and harness device (**B**). Harness device shown is the SecureEasy Endotracheal Tube Holder. Nonelastic headgear reduces the risk of self-extubation. A soft bite block prevents tube occlusion. (**B,** Reprinted with permission, Cleveland Clinic Center for Medical Art & Photography © 2011–2019. All Rights Reserved.)

Tracheostomy

A tracheostomy tube provides an airway directly into the anterior portion of the neck. Tracheostomy tubes are indicated for long-term mechanical ventilation, long-term secretion management, protecting the airway from aspiration when the cough and gag reflexes are impaired, bypassing an upper airway obstruction that prevents placement of an ETT, and reducing the WOB associated with an ETT. The tracheostomy tube reduces the WOB because it is shorter than an ETT and airflow resistance is less.[20]

A tracheostomy is the preferred airway for the patient requiring a long-term airway. It is associated with greater comfort, decreased sedative and antipsychotic drug administration, less restraint use, and lower unplanned extubation. A patient may be permitted oral intake if swallowing studies demonstrate absence of aspiration. Oral hygiene is more easily performed, and some tube designs allow for talking and therefore facilitate patient communication. A speaking valve may be attached to most designs, which provides a mechanism for the patient to talk.

Optimal timing, early versus late, for when a tracheostomy should be performed is controversial. Recent prospective trials and evidenced-based guidelines have failed to demonstrate an effect of tracheostomy timing on outcomes, such as infectious complications, or critical care unit length of stay. Early tracheostomy, however, is associated with a reduced duration of mechanical ventilation and greater patient comfort.[53] If mechanical ventilation and an artificial airway are projected to be needed on a long-term basis, generally defined as more than 10 days, then a decision may be made to perform a tracheostomy. The challenges are predicting which patients will require long-term mechanical ventilation and avoiding a surgical procedure in a patient for whom it may not be indicated. Furthermore, studies that evaluate the effects of early versus late timing of tracheostomy placement vary considerably in study design and definition of *early* versus *late*. A collaborative, patient-centered approach should be used in decision making, taking into consideration the patient's and family's preferences.[28,53]

The tracheostomy has traditionally been a surgical technique performed in the operating room (OR). However, a percutaneous dilational tracheostomy (PDT) procedure may be performed safely at the bedside by a trained provider. Advantages of PDT are that the patient does not have to be transported to the OR, scheduling difficulties with the OR are avoided, time required for the procedure is shorter, cost is less than an open tracheostomy, and perioperative infection rates are less. Contraindications include inability to hyperextend the neck and patient inability to tolerate transient hypoxemia and hypercarbia. Other considerations include difficult anatomy such as morbid obesity and coagulopathy. The PDT is performed by making a small incision into the anterior neck down to the trachea. Once this location has been reached, the provider inserts a needle and sheath into the trachea. The needle is removed, and a guidewire is passed through the sheath. Progressively larger dilators are introduced over the guidewire until the patient's stoma is large enough to accommodate a tracheostomy tube.[45]

Collaboratively, the nurse and RT assist in the PDT procedure. Before the procedure, ensure that IV lines are accessible for administration of sedatives and analgesic medications. Position the patient for the procedure, and adjust the height of the bed relative to the individual performing the procedure. Gather all supplies and ensure that sterility is maintained throughout the procedure. Monitor physiological parameters continuously, and document values at least every 15 minutes throughout the PDT and for at least 1 hour after the procedure.[52]

The most significant postprocedure complication of PDT is accidental decannulation. When a patient undergoes a surgical tracheostomy, the trachea is surgically attached to the skin. This promotes prompt identification of the tract and reinsertion of the tracheal tube, should it become dislodged. With a PDT, the trachea is not secured in this way, and a mature tract takes approximately 2 weeks to form. Accidental decannulation and attempted reinsertion of the airway during this time may result in difficulty securing the airway, bleeding, tracheal injury, and death. Oral intubation may be required if the airway becomes dislodged or needs to be replaced.

Tracheostomy Tube Designs. Tracheostomy tubes come in a variety of sizes and styles and are primarily made of plastic. Design features are shown in Fig. 10.21. The flange lies against the patient's neck and has an opening on both ends for the placement of tracheostomy ties for securing the airway. Similar to the ETT, some tracheostomy tubes have a distal cuff and pilot balloon. An important part of the tracheostomy system is the obturator, which is inserted into the trachea tube during insertion. The rounded end of the obturator extends just beyond the end of the tracheostomy tube and creates a smooth tip, allowing for easy entry into the stoma. The obturator is removed after tube insertion to allow for air passage through the trachea. It must be kept in a visible location in the patient's room should emergency reinsertion of a misplaced tube be necessary. In this situation the obturator is inserted into the tracheostomy to create a rounded, smooth end promoting reentry into the stoma without tissue injury.[8]

Cuffed versus uncuffed tracheostomy tubes. Critically ill patients who need mechanical ventilation require cuffed tubes to ensure delivery of ventilation and prevent aspiration. The cuff may be a conventional low-pressure, high-volume type, or it may be constructed of foam. The foam-cuff tube may prevent trauma to the airway because of the low pressure exerted to the airway, and it is sometimes used for patients who have difficulty maintaining a good seal with conventional cuffed tracheostomy tubes. Many other types of tracheostomy tubes are available.[2,28,37] An uncuffed tracheostomy tube is used for long-term airway management in a patient who does not require mechanical ventilation and is at low risk of aspiration. For example, a patient with a neurological injury may require a tracheostomy for airway management and secretion removal.[53] Metal tracheostomy tubes are uncuffed.

Single- versus double-cannula tracheostomy tubes. Tracheostomy tubes may have one or two cannulas. A single-cannula tube does not have an inner cannula, whereas a double-cannula tube has both an inner and outer cannula. The inner cannula is removable to facilitate cleaning of the inner lumen and to prevent tube occlusion from accumulated secretions.

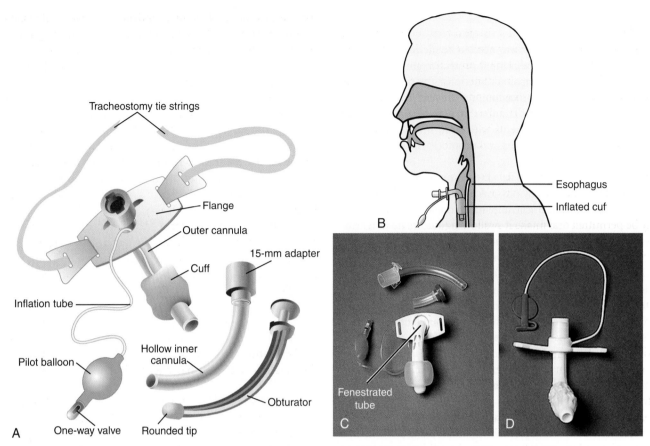

Fig. 10.21 A, General design features of the tracheostomy tube. **B,** Tracheostomy tube in place. **C,** Fenestrated tracheostomy tube (see text for description). **D,** Foam cuff tracheostomy tube. (From Lewis SL, Dirkson SR, Heitkemper MM, et al. *Medical-Surgical Nursing.* 9th ed. St. Louis, MO: Elsevier; 2014.)

Inner cannulas can be reusable or disposable. Cuffed tracheostomy tubes with disposable inner cannulas are commonplace in the critical care unit.

Fenestrated tracheostomy tube. The fenestrated tracheostomy tube has a hole in the outer cannula that allows air to flow above the larynx. The tube functions as a standard tracheostomy tube when the inner cannula is in place. When the inner cannula is removed, the fenestrated tracheostomy tube assists in weaning a patient from the tracheostomy by gradually allowing the patient to breathe through the natural upper airway. The fenestrated tube also allows the patient to emit vocal sounds, thereby facilitating communication. To use a cuffed fenestrated tracheostomy tube for speaking or to promote breathing through the natural airway, the inner cannula is carefully removed and the cuff is deflated. The inner cannula must be reinserted and the cuff reinflated for eating, suctioning, mechanical ventilation, or use of a bag-valve device.[2,28] It is difficult to get a proper fit for a fenestrated tracheostomy tube, which may result in increased airway resistance if the fenestrations are not properly positioned. Tubes with several fenestrations rather than a single fenestration are a lower risk. Furthermore, fenestrations may cause the formation of granulation tissue, resulting in airway compromise.[28] Regularly assess the amount of respiratory effort the patient exerts when breathing through the fenestration.

Speaking tracheostomy valves. One-way speaking valves are available to allow patients with a tracheostomy an opportunity to speak. Although these valves can be used in both ventilated and nonventilated patients, they can be used only in patients capable of initiating and maintaining spontaneous ventilation. Examples of these adjunctive devices include the Passy-Muir Valve (Passy-Muir, Inc., Irvine, CA) and the Shiley Phonate Speaking Valve (Covidien, Boulder, CO). For the speaking valve to work correctly, connect the valve to the tracheostomy tube, deflate the cuff on the tracheostomy tube, and allow the patient to breathe and exhale through the natural airway. The valve itself is a one-way device, allowing gas to enter through it into the tracheostomy tube and to the patient. Because this is a one-way valve, exhaled gas exits the trachea via the natural airway, past the deflated cuff of the tracheostomy tube, and through the vocal cords.[28,37]

If a speaking valve is used in conjunction with mechanical ventilation, it must be used with a tracheostomy tube, not an ETT. While the valve is in place, assess the patient's respiratory stability and tolerance. Monitor the patient's SpO_2, heart rate, RR, and blood pressure; observe the patient's anxiety level and perception of the experience; and assess the WOB.[28] The patient's ability to communicate provides an opportunity for the patient to describe feelings and participate in setting goals.

Endotracheal Suctioning

Patients with an artificial airway need to be suctioned to ensure airway patency because the normal protective ability to cough and expel secretions is impaired. Suctioning is performed according to a standard procedure to prevent complications such as hypoxemia, airway trauma, infection, and increased intracranial pressure in patients with head injury. Suctioning also stimulates the cough reflex and promotes the mobilization and removal of secretions.

Because suctioning is associated with complications, it is performed only as indicated by physical assessment and not according to a predetermined schedule. Indications for endotracheal suctioning include visible secretions in the tube, frequent coughing, sawtooth pattern on the flow-time waveform on the ventilator, presence of coarse crackles over the trachea, oxygen desaturation, a change in vital signs (e.g., increased or decreased heart rate or RR), dyspnea, restlessness, increased peak inspiratory pressure (PIP), high-pressure ventilator alarms in a volume mode of ventilation or decreased V_T in a pressure mode of ventilation, when the patency of the airway is questioned, when aspiration is suspected, or when a sputum specimen is indicated.[35,58,63]

It is common nursing practice to assess breath sounds after suctioning to determine effectiveness of the procedure. Suctioning removes secretions from the upper airways and trachea. Secretions in the lower airway that lead to adventitious sounds are rarely retrieved and therefore would not result in improved breath sounds over the lung fields. Auscultation over the trachea and reassessment of the ventilator flow-time waveform for resolution of a sawtooth pattern are recommended assessments.[63] The number of suction passes is usually one to three; however, suctioning should be continued until secretions are removed. Suction duration is limited to 10 to 15 seconds, and rest periods are provided between suction passes.[35,58]

Key points related to endotracheal suctioning are discussed in Box 10.7. Hyperoxygenate with 100% oxygen for 30 seconds before suctioning, during the procedure, and immediately after suctioning.[35,58] Most ventilators have a built-in suction mode that delivers 100% oxygen for a short period (e.g., 2 minutes).[9] Hyperoxygenation can also be administered with a bag-valve device. If the patient does not tolerate suctioning with hyperoxygenation alone, hyperinflation may be used. Hyperinflation involves the delivery of breaths 1 to 1.5 times the V_T and is performed by giving the patient three to five breaths before and between suctioning attempts using either the ventilator or the bag-valve device.[9]

The closed tracheal, or in-line, suction catheter is an alternative to the single-use suction catheter. The closed tracheal suction system consists of a suction catheter enclosed in a plastic sheath that is attached to the patient's ventilator circuit and airway (Fig. 10.22). Since the ventilator circuit remains closed during the suction procedure, the device assists in maintaining oxygenation, reduces symptoms associated with hypoxemia, maintains positive end-expiratory pressure (PEEP), and protects staff from the patient's secretions. Depending on the institution, closed suctioning may be used on all ventilated patients, or it may be used for specific indications such as for clinically

---

BOX 10.7 Key Points for Endotracheal Suctioning

- Suction only as indicated by patient, ventilator flow-time waveform, and airway pressure assessment.
- Choose the proper size device. The diameter of the suction catheter should be no more than half the diameter of the artificial airway.
- Assemble equipment: suction kit with two gloves or closed suction system (CSS), sterile saline for rinsing the catheter. The CSS is attached to the ventilator circuit, usually by a respiratory therapist.
- Set the suction regulator at 80 to 120 mm Hg.
- Use sterile technique for suctioning.
- Hyperoxygenate the patient via the ventilator circuit before, between, and after suctioning.
- Gently insert suction catheter. If resistance is met, pull back 1 cm before applying suction.
- Shallow suctioning prevents trauma to the mucosa. Deep suctioning has no benefit over shallow suctioning and results in more adverse events.[2]
- Suction the patient no longer than 10 to 15 seconds while applying intermittent or constant suction.
- Allow patient to recover between passes of the suction catheter.
- Repeat endotracheal suctioning until the airway is clear.
- Rinse the catheter with sterile saline after endotracheal suctioning is performed.
- Suction the mouth and oropharynx with a single-use suction catheter, suction swabs, or a tonsil suction device.
- Auscultate the lungs to assess effectiveness of suctioning, and document findings.
- Document the amount, color, and consistency of secretions.
- *Steps specific to closed suctioning* (in addition to those just noted):
  - Using the dominant hand, insert the suction catheter into the airway until resistance is met. Simultaneously, use the nondominant hand to stabilize the artificial airway.
  - Withdraw the suction catheter while depressing the suction valve; *be careful to not angle the wrist of the hand while withdrawing the catheter because kinking of the catheter and loss of suction may occur.*
  - Ensure that the CSS catheter is completely withdrawn from the airway. A marking is visible on the suction catheter when it is properly withdrawn.
  - Rinse the catheter after the procedure. Connect a small vial or syringe of normal saline for tracheal instillation (without preservatives) to the irrigation port, and simultaneously instill the saline into the port while depressing the suction control.
  - Keep the CSS suction catheter out of the patient's reach to avoid accidental self-extubation.

---

unstable patients receiving high levels of FiO_2 or PEEP, patients at risk for alveolar derecruitment, patients with contagious infections such as tuberculosis, or patients for whom frequent suctioning is required (e.g., six or more times per day).[34,58]

Do not routinely instill saline into the trachea during suctioning.[4] Saline instillation is associated with problems such as oxygen desaturation, washing organisms in the ETT into the lower airway, tachycardia, increased intracranial pressure and patient discomfort from excessive coughing, and bronchospasm. Purported benefits of liquefying secretions and increasing volume of secretions removed are not proven.[4,10] Adequate patient hydration and airway humidification, rather than saline instillation, facilitate secretion removal.

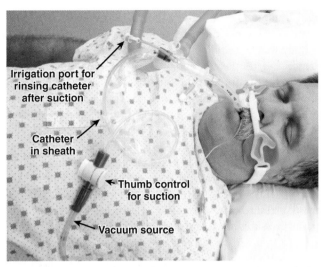

Fig. 10.22 Closed tracheal suction device. (Reprinted with permission, Cleveland Clinic Center for Medical Art & Photography © 2011-2019. All Rights Reserved.)

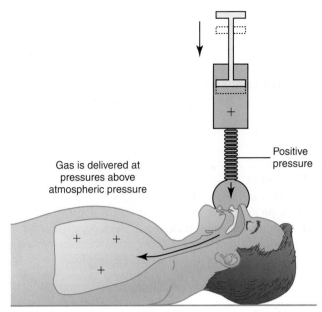

Fig. 10.23 Concept of positive-pressure ventilation.

MECHANICAL VENTILATION

The purpose of mechanical ventilation is to support the respiratory system until the underlying cause of respiratory failure can be corrected. Most ventilatory support requires an artificial airway; however, it may be applied without an artificial airway and is called *noninvasive ventilation.*

Indications

Mechanical ventilation is warranted for patients with acute respiratory failure who are unable to maintain adequate gas exchange as reflected in the ABGs. A clinical definition of respiratory failure is as follows:
- PaO_2 of 60 mm Hg or lower on an FiO_2 greater than 0.5 (oxygenation)
- $PaCO_2$ of 50 mm Hg or higher with a pH of 7.25 or less (ventilation)[26,34]

The patient may also demonstrate progressive physiological deterioration such as rapid, shallow breathing and an increase in the WOB as evidenced by increased use of the accessory muscles of ventilation, abnormal breathing patterns, and complaints of dyspnea. As life-saving therapy, mechanical ventilation supports the respiratory system while a treatment plan is instituted to correct the underlying abnormality.[9,34]

STUDY BREAK

1. Endotracheal tube (ETT) placement can be confirmed by all of the following except:
   A. ETCO$_2$ detector color change
   B. Auscultating breath sounds over the epigastrium and lung fields
   C. Fiberoptic bronchoscopy through the ETT to visualize the carina
   D. Chest x-ray

Positive-Pressure Ventilation

In the critical care setting, most patients are treated with positive-pressure ventilation. This method uses positive pressure to force air into the lungs via an artificial airway, as illustrated in Fig. 10.23. Movement of gases into the lungs using *positive pressure* is the opposite of the pressures created in the chest during spontaneous breathing. Spontaneous ventilation begins when energy is expended to contract the muscles of respiration. This enlarges the thoracic cavity, increases *negative pressure* within the chest and lungs, and results in the flow of air, at atmospheric pressure, into the lungs. If mechanical ventilators could mimic the intrathoracic pressures that occur during spontaneous ventilation, it would be ideal. Negative-pressure ventilators, which originated with the iron lung, perform in this manner; however, these ventilators are for management of chronic conditions. Many of the complications of mechanical ventilation are related to air being forced into the lungs under positive pressure.

Ventilator Settings

In most institutions in the United States and Canada, ventilators are set up and managed by RTs. However, the nurse must be familiar with selected values on the control panel or graphic interface unit to assess ventilator settings, patient response to ventilation, and alarms. Representative control panels and ventilator screens are shown in Fig. 10.24. Although the control panel of a microprocessor type of ventilator can appear overwhelming, it is important to learn to identify the common screen views that provide the settings and patient data that are integral to patient assessment. Know the basic ventilator settings: mode of ventilation, FiO_2, V_T in a volume mode of ventilation, inspiratory pressure setting in a pressure mode of ventilation, set RR rate, and PEEP. Additional settings of inspiratory-to-expiratory (I:E) ratio, sensitivity, and sigh are also discussed to provide a basis for the nurse to knowledgeably communicate with the RT and provider.[9,52]

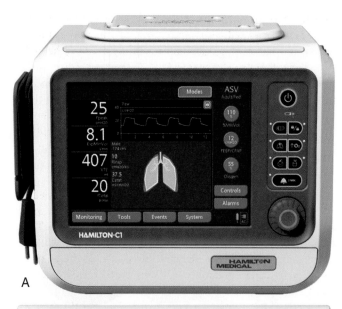

A

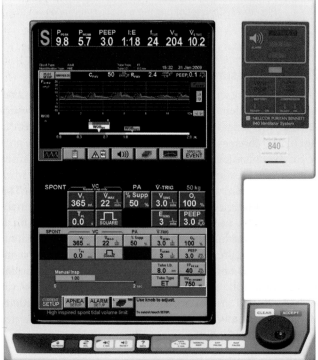

B

Fig. 10.24 Examples of mechanical ventilators and their control panels and graphic interface unit (GIU). **A,** Hamilton C1. **B,** Puritan Bennett 840 Ventilator GIU. (**A,** Copyright © by Hamilton Medical AG, 2018. All rights reserved. **B,** ©2019 Medtronic. All rights reserved. Used with the permission of Medtronic.)

Fraction of Inspired Oxygen. The FiO_2 is set from 0.21 (21% or room air) to 1.00 (100% oxygen). The initial FiO_2 setting is based on the patient's immediate physiological needs and is set to whatever value is necessary to maintain a PaO_2 between 60 and 100 mm Hg, or an SpO_2 of *at least* 90%. After the patient is stabilized, the setting is adjusted based on ABG or pulse oximetry values.

Tidal Volume. The amount of air delivered with each preset breath in a volume-controlled mode is the V_T. The V_T is dictated by body weight and by the patient's lung characteristics (compliance and resistance), and it is set to ensure that excessive stretch and pressure on the lung tissue is avoided. A starting point for the V_T setting is 4 to 8 mL/kg of ideal body weight with the lowest value recommended in patients with obstructive airway disease or ARDS.[6,9,33] The parameters monitored to avoid excessive pressure are the PIP and plateau airway pressure (Pplat). These pressures should remain below 40 cm H_2O and 30 cm H_2O, respectively, to prevent ventilator-induced lung injury (VILI).[6] The V_T setting can be reduced if the resulting airway pressures are nearing the maximum. Conversely, if the airway pressures are acceptable and a larger V_T is needed to remove CO_2, it can be increased. When choosing and adjusting the V_T setting, the goal is to achieve the lowest Pplat while maintaining gas exchange and patient comfort.

Inspiratory Pressure. The inspiratory pressure setting used with pressure modes of ventilation augments the flow of gas into the lungs. When the breath begins, the preselected amount of pressure is delivered and held constant throughout inspiration, thereby promoting the flow of gas into the lungs. No tidal volume is set. The tidal volume that the patient receives is determined by the compliance and resistance of the respiratory system (patient and ventilator). Lower inspiratory pressure settings are used when the patient's lungs are healthier, and high inspiratory pressures will be required when the lungs are more diseased.[9,52]

Respiratory Rate. The RR is the frequency of breaths (f) set to be delivered by the ventilator. The RR is set as near to physiological rates (14 to 20 breaths/min) as possible. Frequent changes in the RR are often required based on observation of the patient's WOB and comfort and assessment of the $PaCO_2$ and pH. During initiation of mechanical ventilation, many patients require full ventilatory support. The RR is selected based on the V_T, to achieve a minute ventilation (VE) that maintains an acceptable acid-base status (VE × RR × V_T). As the patient becomes capable of participating in the ventilatory work, the ventilator RR is decreased, or the mode of ventilation is changed, to encourage more spontaneous breathing.

Inspiratory-to-Expiratory Ratio. The I:E ratio is the duration of inspiration in comparison with expiration. In spontaneous ventilation, inspiration is shorter than expiration. When a patient undergoes mechanical ventilation, the I:E ratio is usually set at 1:2 to mimic the pattern of spontaneous ventilation; that is, 33% of the respiratory cycle is spent in inspiration and 66% in the expiratory phase. Longer expiratory times, an I:E ratio of 1:3 or 1:4, may be needed in patients with COPD to promote more complete exhalation and reduce air trapping.[33,47]

Inverse Inspiratory-to-Expiratory Ratio. Inspiratory-to-expiratory ratios such as 1:1, 2:1, and 3:1 are called *inverse I:E ratios.* An inverse I:E ratio is used to improve oxygenation in patients with noncompliant lungs, such as in ARDS. During

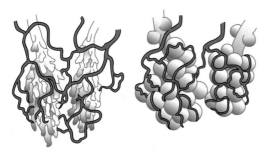

Fig. 10.25 Effect of application of positive end-expiratory pressure (PEEP) on the alveoli. (Modified from Pierce LNB. *Management of the Mechanically Ventilated Patient.* Philadelphia, PA: Saunders; 2007.)

the traditional I:E ratio of 1:2, alveoli in noncompliant lungs may not have sufficient time to reopen during the shorter inspiratory phase and may collapse during the longer expiratory phase. An inverse I:E ratio allows unstable alveoli time to fill and prevents them from collapsing because the next inspiration begins before the alveoli reach a volume where they can collapse.[33,47]

Positive End-Expiratory Pressure. Positive end-expiratory pressure (PEEP) is the addition of positive pressure into the airways during expiration. Positive end-expiratory pressure is measured in cm H_2O. Typical settings for PEEP are 5 to 20 cm H_2O, although higher levels may be used to treat refractory hypoxemia. Because positive pressure is applied at end-expiration, the airways and alveoli are held open, and oxygenation improves. Positive end-expiratory pressure increases oxygenation by preventing collapse of small airways and maximizing the number of alveoli available for gas exchange (Fig. 10.25). By recruiting more alveoli for gas exchange and by holding them open during expiration, the functional residual capacity improves, resulting in better oxygenation.[52]

Many mechanically ventilated patients routinely receive 3 to 5 cm H_2O of PEEP, a value often referred to as *physiological PEEP*. This small amount of PEEP is thought to mimic the normal "back pressure" created in the lungs by the epiglottis in the spontaneously breathing patient that is released by the displacement of the epiglottis by the artificial airway.

Positive end-expiratory pressure is often added to decrease a high FiO_2 that may be required to achieve adequate oxygenation. For example, a patient may require an FiO_2 of 0.80 to maintain a PaO_2 of 85 mm Hg. By adding PEEP, it may be possible to decrease the FiO_2 to a level where oxygen toxicity in the lung is not a concern (<0.5) while maintaining an adequate PaO_2.[9,52] Monitor the PEEP level by observing the pressure level displayed on the ventilator's analog and graphic displays. When no PEEP is set, the pressure reading on the graphic display should be zero at end-expiration. When PEEP is applied, the pressure reading does not return to zero at the end of the breath, and the display shows the amount of PEEP.

Although PEEP is often essential for treatment, it is associated with adverse effects associated with an increase in intrathoracic pressure. These problems include a decrease in cardiac output secondary to decreased venous return, volutrauma or barotrauma, and increased intracranial pressure resulting from

impedance of venous return from the head. Whenever the level of PEEP is increased, evaluate the patient's hemodynamic response through physical assessment and by available hemodynamic parameters. Management of decreased cardiac output secondary to PEEP includes ensuring that the patient has adequate intravascular volume (preload) and administering fluids as needed. If the cardiac output remains inadequate, an inotropic agent such as dobutamine should be considered. Optimal PEEP is defined as the amount of PEEP that affords the best oxygenation without resulting in adverse hemodynamic effects or pulmonary injury.[33,52]

Auto-PEEP. Auto-PEEP is the spontaneous development of PEEP caused by gas trapping in the lung resulting from insufficient expiratory time and incomplete exhalation. These trapped gases create positive pressure in the lung. Both set PEEP and auto-PEEP have the same physiological effects; therefore it is important to know when auto-PEEP is present so that it can be managed properly.[9,47,52]

Causes of auto-PEEP formation include rapid RR, high VE demand, airflow obstruction, and inverse I:E ratio ventilation. Auto-PEEP cannot be detected by the ventilator pressure manometer until a special maneuver is performed. This maneuver involves instituting a 2-second end-expiratory pause, which allows the ventilator to read the pressure deep in the lung. The airway pressure manometer reading therefore reflects total PEEP, which is the set PEEP and auto-PEEP added together. To determine auto-PEEP, the following calculation is performed:

$$\text{Auto-PEEP} = \text{Total PEEP} - \text{Set PEEP}$$

Sensitivity. Sensitivity determines the amount of patient effort needed to initiate gas flow through the circuitry on a patient-initiated breath. The sensitivity is set so that the ventilator is "sensitive" to the patient's effort to inspire. If the sensitivity is set too low, the patient must generate more work to trigger gas flow. If it is set too high, auto-cycling of the ventilator may occur, resulting in patient-ventilator dyssynchrony, because the ventilator cycles into the inspiratory phase when the patient is not ready for a breath.[9]

Patient Data

The nurse and RT ensure that the ventilator settings are consistent with the physician's orders. The ventilator control panel or graphic interface unit also provides valuable information regarding the patient's response to mechanical ventilation. These patient data include exhaled tidal volume (EV_T), PIP, and total RR.

Exhaled Tidal Volume. The EV_T is the amount of gas that comes out of the patient's lungs on exhalation. The EV_T is not a ventilator setting. It is data that indicate the patient's response to mechanical ventilation. This is the most accurate measure of the volume received by the patient and therefore is monitored at least every 4 hours and more often as indicated. Although the prescribed V_T is set on the ventilator control panel, it is not guaranteed to be delivered to the patient. Volume may be lost because of leaks in the ventilator circuit, around the cuff of the airway, or via a chest tube if there is a pleural air leak. The volume actually received by the patient, regardless of mode of ventilation, must be confirmed by monitoring the EV_T on the display panel of the ventilator. If the EV_T deviates from the set V_T by 50 mL or more, the nurse and RT must troubleshoot the system to identify the source of gas loss.

Peak Inspiratory Pressure. The PIP is the maximum pressure that occurs during inspiration. It is set in pressure modes of ventilation and is variable in volume modes of ventilation. The amount of pressure necessary to ventilate the patient increases with increased airway resistance (e.g., secretions in the airway, bronchospasm, biting the ETT) and decreased lung compliance (e.g., pulmonary edema, worsening infiltrate or ARDS, pleural space disease). The PIP should never be allowed to rise above 40 cm H_2O because higher pressures can result in ventilator-induced lung injury.[6,9,47]

Monitor and record the PIP at least every 4 hours and with any change in patient condition that could increase airway resistance or decrease compliance. Increasing PIP or values greater than 40 cm H_2O should be reported immediately so that interventions can be ordered to improve lung function, ventilator settings can be adjusted to reduce the inspiratory pressure, or both.

Total Respiratory Rate. The total RR equals the number of breaths delivered by the ventilator (set rate) plus the number of breaths initiated by the patient. Assessing the total RR provides data on the patient's contribution to the WOB or whether the ventilator is performing all of the work. The total RR is a very sensitive indicator of overall respiratory stability. For example, if the patient is on assist/control ventilation at a set RR of 10 breaths/min, and the total RR for 1 minute is 16, the patient is initiating 6 breaths above the set rate of 10. If the patient is on volume intermittent mandatory ventilation (VIMV) at a set RR of 8 breaths/min, and the total RR is 12 breaths/min with good spontaneous V_T for body weight, the patient is tolerating the mode of ventilation. If the patient's total RR increases to 26 breaths/min, this finding indicates that something has changed and the patient needs to be reassessed for causes of the increased rate, such as fatigue, pain, or anxiety. Treatment is based on the identified cause.

Modes of Mechanical Ventilation

Modes of mechanical ventilation describe how breaths are delivered to the patient. A mode is the method by which the patient and the ventilator interact to perform the respiratory cycle. They vary in degree of patient versus ventilator effort and may provide full to partial ventilatory support. A breath is *assisted* if the ventilator performs all or some of the work. A ventilator assists breathing using either pressure or volume as the control variable, the function that is controlled during inspiration. In volume-controlled modes of ventilation, a set V_T is delivered during inspiration. In pressure-controlled modes of ventilation, pressure is set and does not vary throughout inspiration.

In addition to understanding volume and pressure control as a classification scheme for modes of ventilation, other concepts helpful in understanding varying modes of ventilation include triggering, breath classification, and breath sequence.

- Triggering indicates what initiates inspiration. Breaths may be patient triggered or ventilator triggered.
- Breaths are classified as *spontaneous* or *mandatory*. A spontaneous breath is one where the patient controls both the start and the end of inspiration, whereas a mandatory breath is a breath delivered by the ventilator, independent of the patient.

A breath sequence is a particular pattern of spontaneous and/or mandatory breaths. The three possible breath sequences are continuous mandatory ventilation (CMV), intermittent mandatory ventilation (IMV), and continuous spontaneous ventilation (CSV). Continuous mandatory ventilation is commonly referred to as *assist/control*. In CMV every breath, whether triggered by the patient or the ventilator, is assisted by the ventilator, and there are no purely spontaneous breaths. IMV is a breath sequence in which spontaneous breaths are possible between mandatory breaths. In CSV every breath is initiated and ended by the patient. Knowledge of these terms will help the nurse understand the differences between the various modes of mechanical ventilation and how they work with the patient to perform the breath.[50]

Volume-Controlled Ventilation. In volume-controlled ventilation, V_T is constant for every breath delivered by the ventilator. The ventilator is set to allow airflow into the lungs until a preset volume has been reached. A major advantage of these modes is that the set V_T is delivered, regardless of changes in lung compliance or resistance. However, the PIP is variable and dependent on compliance and resistance, therefore the nurse should closely monitor for elevated PIP. Volume assist/control (V-A/C; Fig. 10.26A) and VIMV (see Fig. 10.26B) are volume-controlled modes of ventilation.

Volume assist/control. The volume assist/control (V-A/C) mode of ventilation delivers a preset number of breaths of a preset V_T. The patient may trigger additional breaths between the ventilator-initiated breaths by generating a negative inspiratory effort, and the ventilator will respond by delivering an assisted breath of the preset V_T. The V_T of the assisted breaths is constant for both ventilator-initiated and patient-triggered breaths. The V-A/C mode ensures that the patient receives adequate ventilation, regardless of patient effort. It is a full ventilatory support mode; therefore it is indicated when it is desirable for the ventilator to perform the bulk of the WOB. The only work the patient must perform is the negative inspiratory effort required to trigger the ventilator on the patient-initiated breaths. This mode is useful in patients who have a normal respiratory drive but whose respiratory muscles are too weak or unable to perform the WOB (e.g., patient emerging from general anesthesia or with pulmonary disease such as pneumonia). A disadvantage of V-A/C ventilation is that respiratory alkalosis may develop if the patient hyperventilates because of anxiety, pain, a neurological issue, or other factors. Respiratory alkalosis is treated or prevented by appropriately treating the underlying cause of tachypnea, or changing to VIMV. Another disadvantage is that the patient may rely on the ventilator and not

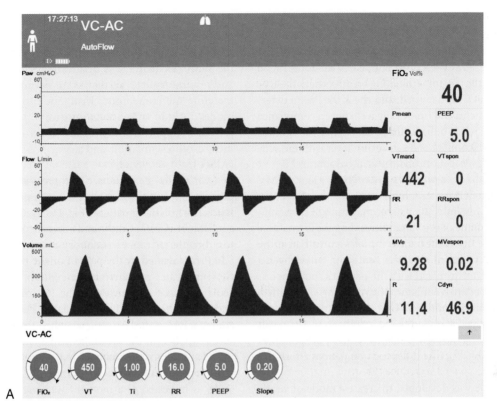

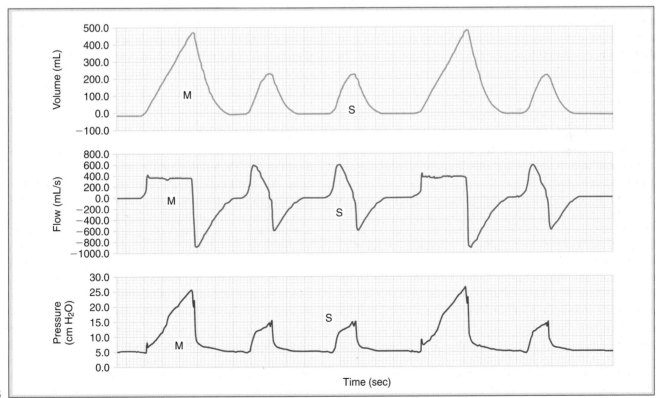

Fig. 10.26 Waveforms of volume-controlled ventilator modes. **A,** Volume assist/control (V-A/C) ventilation. The patient may trigger additional breaths above the set rate. The ventilator delivers the same volume for ventilator-triggered and patient-triggered (assisted) breaths. **B,** Volume intermittent mandatory ventilation (VIMV). Both spontaneous and mandatory breaths are graphed. Mandatory breaths receive the set tidal volume (V_T). V_T of spontaneous breaths depends on work the patient is capable of generating, lung compliance, and airway resistance. (**B,** From Cairo JM. *Mosby's Respiratory Care Equipment.* St. Louis, MO: Elsevier; 2018.)

attempt to initiate spontaneous breathing if all ventilatory demands are met.

During V-A/C ventilation, check the ventilator to ensure that the parameters are set as prescribed and assess the total RR to determine whether the patient is initiating breaths; check the EV_T to ensure that the set V_T is delivered; and check the PIP to determine whether it is increasing (indicating a change in compliance or resistance, which needs to be further evaluated). Also monitor the patient's sense of comfort and synchronization with the ventilator, oxygenation, ventilation, and the acid-base status.[47,52]

Volume intermittent mandatory ventilation. The VIMV mode of ventilation delivers a set number of breaths of a set V_T. Between mandatory breaths the patient may initiate spontaneous breaths. The volume of the spontaneous breaths is whatever the patient can generate. If the patient initiates a breath near the time a mandatory breath is due, the ventilator will deliver a mandatory breath synchronized with the patient's spontaneous effort to prevent patient-ventilator dyssynchrony. The difference between the VIMV and V-A/C is the volume of the patient-initiated breaths. Patient-initiated breaths in V-A/C result in the patient receiving the set V_T. In VIMV, the V_T of spontaneous breaths is variable because it depends on patient effort and lung characteristics.

The VIMV mode was developed to create a mode of ventilation where the patient can participate in the WOB and begin to recondition weak respiratory muscles. The VIMV mode is indicated when it is desirable to allow patients to contribute to the WOB and assist in maintaining a normal $PaCO_2$ or when hyperventilation has occurred in the V-A/C mode. The VIMV mode may be used for weaning patients from mechanical ventilation. As the VIMV rate is lowered, the patient initiates more spontaneous breaths, assuming a greater portion of the ventilatory work. As the patient demonstrates the ability to take on even more WOB, the mandatory breath rate is decreased accordingly. However, compared with other weaning modalities, VIMV is associated with the longest weaning and lowest success rate.[48,61]

During VIMV, monitor the total RR to determine whether the patient is initiating spontaneous breaths and the patient's ability to manage the WOB. If the total RR increases, assess the V_T of the spontaneous breaths for adequacy. An adequate spontaneous V_T is 5 mL/kg of ideal body weight. A rising total RR may indicate that the patient is beginning to fatigue, resulting in a more shallow and rapid respiratory pattern. This pattern may lead to atelectasis, a further increase in the WOB, and the need for greater ventilatory support. Monitor the EV_T of both the mandatory and the spontaneous breaths to ensure that the set V_T is being delivered with the mandatory breaths and that the spontaneous V_T is adequate. As in V-A/C ventilation, assess the PIP, the patient's sense of comfort, and synchronization with the ventilator, oxygenation, ventilation, and acid-base status.

Pressure Ventilation. In pressure ventilation the ventilator is set to allow air to flow into the lungs until a preset inspiratory pressure has been reached. The V_T the patient receives is variable and depends on lung compliance and airway and circuit resistance. Patients with normal lung compliance and low resistance will have better delivery of V_T for the amount of inspiratory pressure set. An advantage of pressure-controlled modes is that the PIP can be reliably controlled for each breath the ventilator delivers. A disadvantage is that hypoventilation and respiratory acidosis may occur because delivered V_T varies; therefore the nurse must closely monitor EV_T.[9,34,47,50] Pressure modes include continuous positive airway pressure (CPAP), pressure support (PS), pressure control, pressure-controlled inverse-ratio ventilation, and airway pressure release ventilation (APRV).

Continuous positive airway pressure. CPAP is positive pressure applied throughout the respiratory cycle to the spontaneously breathing patient (Fig. 10.27). The patient must have a reliable respiratory drive and adequate V_T because no mandatory breaths or other ventilatory assistance is given; therefore CPAP is classified as *CSV*. The patient performs all the WOB. CPAP provides pressure at end-expiration, which prevents alveolar collapse and improves the functional residual capacity and oxygenation. CPAP is identical to PEEP in its physiological effects. *CPAP* is the correct term when the end-expiratory pressure is applied in the spontaneously breathing patient. *PEEP* is the term used for the same setting when the patient is receiving any form of inspiratory assistance (e.g., V-A/C, VIMV, PS). CPAP is indicated as a mode of weaning when the patient has adequate ventilation but requires end-expiratory pressure to stabilize the alveoli and maintain oxygenation.[48] Because the ventilator is used to deliver CPAP during weaning, monitor the adequacy of the patient's EV_T, set alarms to detect low EV_T and apnea, and give back-up mechanical breaths in the event of apnea.

CPAP can also be administered via a nasal or face mask. Typically, a nasal CPAP system is used to keep the airway open in patients with obstructive sleep apnea in the home setting.

Pressure support. Pressure support is a mode of ventilation in which the patient's spontaneous respiratory activity is augmented by the delivery of a preset amount of inspiratory positive pressure. The patient must initiate every breath and determine when to end the inspiratory phase; therefore PS is classified as *CSV*. PS may be used as a stand-alone mode (Fig. 10.28) or in combination with other modes, such as IMV, to augment the V_T of the spontaneous breaths (Fig. 10.29). The positive pressure is applied throughout inspiration, thereby promoting the flow of gas into the lungs, augmenting the patient's spontaneous V_T, and decreasing the WOB associated with breathing through an artificial airway and the ventilatory circuit.[9,47,50,52] Typical levels of PS ordered for the patient are 6 to 12 cm H_2O. The V_T is variable, determined by patient effort, the amount of PS applied, and the compliance and resistance of the patient and ventilator system. Closely monitor exhaled V_T during PS; if it is inadequate, increase the level of PS. PS may increase patient comfort because the patient has greater control over the initiation and duration of each breath. PS promotes conditioning of the respiratory muscles because the patient works throughout the breath; this may facilitate weaning from the ventilator.

Pressure assist/control. Pressure assist/control (P-A/C) is a mode of ventilation in which there is a set RR, and every breath is augmented by a set amount of inspiratory pressure. If the

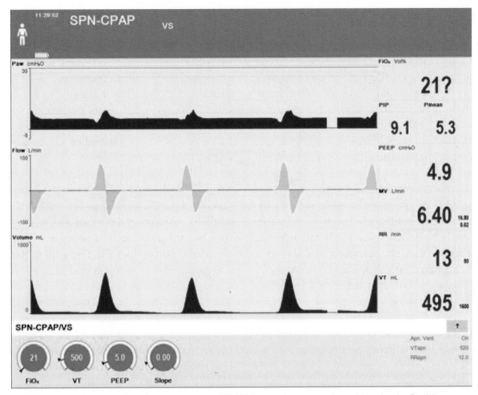

Fig. 10.27 Continuous positive airway pressure (CPAP) is a spontaneous breathing mode. Positive pressure at end-expiration splints alveoli and supports oxygenation. Note that the pressure does not fall to zero, indicating the level of CPAP.

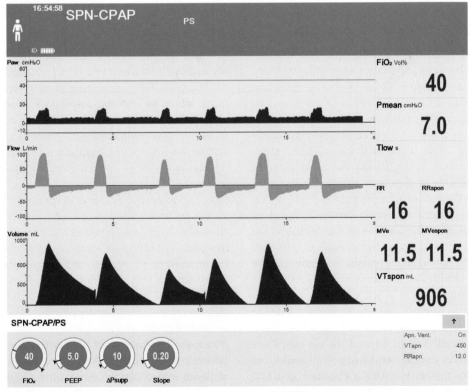

Fig. 10.28 Pressure support ventilation requires the patient to trigger each breath, which is then supported by pressure on inspiration. Patient may vary amount of time in inspiration, respiratory rate, and tidal volume (V_T).

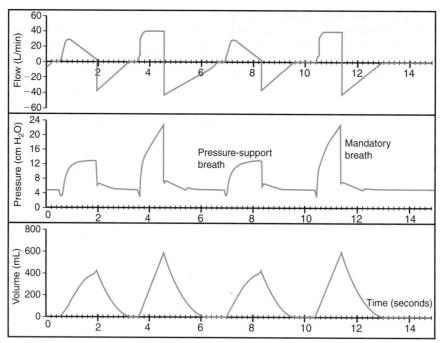

Fig. 10.29 Volume intermittent mandatory ventilation (VIMV) with pressure support (PS). VIMV breaths receive set tidal volume (V_T). Pressure support is applied to the spontaneous, patient-triggered breaths. (From Pierce LNB. *Management of the Mechanically Ventilated Patient.* Philadelphia, PA: Saunders; 2007.)

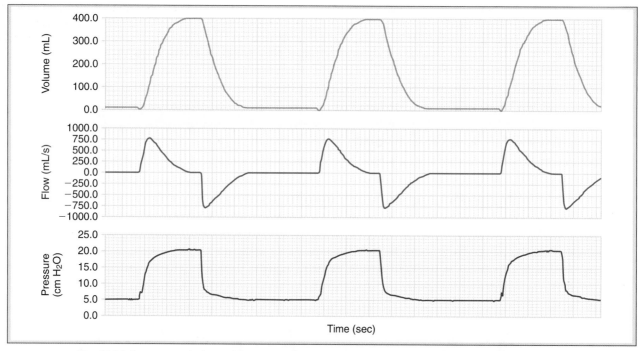

Fig. 10.30 Pressure assist/control ventilation. Patient can trigger additional breaths above the set rate. Patient- and ventilator-triggered breaths receive the same inspiratory pressure. (From Cairo JM. *Mosby's Respiratory Care Equipment.* St. Louis, MO: Elsevier; 2018.)

patient triggers additional breaths beyond the set rate, those breaths are augmented by the set amount of inspiratory pressure (Fig. 10.30); therefore P-A/C is classified as *CMV*. Just as with PS, there is no set V_T. The V_T the patient receives is variable and determined by the set inspiratory pressure, the patient's lung compliance, and circuit and airway resistance.

The typical pressure in P-A/C ranges from 15 to 25 cm H_2O, which is higher than a PS level because P-A/C is indicated for patients with ARDS or those with a high PIP during traditional volume ventilation. Because the lungs are noncompliant in these conditions, higher inspiratory pressure levels are needed to achieve an adequate V_T. Pressure assist/control reduces the risk of barotrauma while maintaining adequate oxygenation and ventilation. During P-A/C, be familiar with all ventilator settings: the level of pressure, the set RR, the FiO_2, and the level of PEEP. Monitor the total RR to evaluate whether the patient is initiating breaths and EV_T for adequacy of volume.

Pressure-controlled inverse-ratio ventilation. With pressure-controlled inverse-ratio ventilation (PC-IRV), the patient receives P-A/C ventilation as described, and the ventilator is set to provide longer inspiratory times. The I:E ratio is inversed to increase the mean airway pressure, open and stabilize the alveoli, and improve oxygenation. Pressure-controlled inverse-ratio ventilation is indicated for patients with noncompliant lungs such as in ARDS, when adequate oxygenation is not achieved despite high FiO_2, PEEP, or positioning. Because the reverse I:E ratio ventilation is uncomfortable, the patient must be sedated and possibly paralyzed to prevent ventilator dyssynchrony and oxygen desaturation.

Airway pressure–release ventilation. Airway pressure–release ventilation (APRV) is a mode of ventilation that provides two levels of CPAP, one during inspiration and the other during expiration, while allowing unrestricted spontaneous breathing at any point during the respiratory cycle (Fig. 10.31). APRV starts at an elevated pressure, the CPAP level or pressure high (P_{HIGH}), followed by a release pressure, pressure low (P_{LOW}). After the airway pressure release, the P_{HIGH} level is restored. The time spent at P_{HIGH} is known as *time high* and is generally prolonged, 4 to 6 seconds. The shorter release period (P_{LOW}) is known as *time low* and is generally 0.5 to 1.1 seconds. When observing the pressure waveform, APRV is similar to PC-IRV; however, unlike PC-IRV, the patient has unrestricted spontaneous breathing. The patient is more comfortable on APRV, and deep sedation or paralysis may not be needed. APRV assists in providing adequate oxygenation while lowering PIP. It is indicated as an alternative to V-A/C or P-A/C for patients with significantly decreased lung compliance, such as those with ARDS.[14,21,60]

Dual-controlled modes. Dual-controlled modes, also known as volume-assured modes, incorporate qualities of both volume- and pressure-controlled modes. Both the desired V_T and the pressure limit are set. The ventilator delivers gas to achieve the desired V_T while ensuring that the pressure remains below the set pressure limit. The ventilator monitors the EV_T and adjusts the inspiratory pressure on a breath-by-breath basis to ensure that the V_T is delivered using the lowest possible pressure. Pressure modes with a set volume are available on many ventilators; two of the more common ones are described here.[9,21,47,52,60]

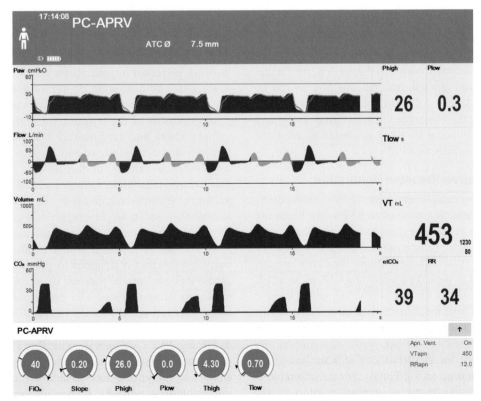

Fig. 10.31 Airway pressure release ventilation.

Pressure-regulated volume control. Pressure-regulated volume control (PRVC) is a control mode of ventilation in which the patient receives a preset number of breaths of a preset V_T that is given in the form of a pressure breath. The ventilator strives to achieve the target V_T using the lowest possible pressure. The ventilator determines the pressure needed to achieve the target breath by performing a calculation involving the pressure used for the previous breath, the target V_T, and the actual V_T of the previous breath. Inspiratory pressure is increased or decreased in a stepwise fashion to ensure the volume guarantee. If the measured V_T is too large, the pressure decreases. If it is too small, the pressure increases up to the upper pressure limit.[9]

Volume support. Volume support (VS) is a mode of ventilation that pressure supports every breath to a level that guarantees a preset V_T. The patient triggers every breath. The ventilator determines the pressure needed to achieve the target breath as described above for PRVC. The difference between these two modes is that VS is a spontaneous breathing mode and no RR is set, whereas PRVC is a controlled mode with a set number of breaths delivered each minute.

Mandatory minute ventilation. Mandatory minute ventilation (MMV) is an example of a closed-loop ventilation in which the level of support changes based on the patient's level of participation. With MMV the patient breathes spontaneously, yet a constant VE is guaranteed. The minimum ventilation is determined by the V_T and RR settings, which allows MMV to ensure that the patient always receives at least the set minimum VE ($VE = VT \times RR$). MMV works like volume-synchronized intermittent mandatory ventilation (V-SIMV); however, the mandatory breaths are provided only if spontaneous breathing is not sufficient and is below the prescribed minimum ventilation. When spontaneous breathing increases, fewer mandatory breaths are provided. Thus the patient can gradually take over more of the WOB. If the patient's spontaneous breathing is sufficient to achieve the set VE, no further mandatory breaths are applied. Spontaneous breaths can be supported with PS. At least 5 cm H_2O of PS is typically set to assist in overcoming the resistance of the artificial airway and ventilator circuit. Additional PS is set as needed to assist the patient in achieving an adequate V_T.[60]

Noninvasive Positive-Pressure Ventilation

Noninvasive positive-pressure ventilation (NPPV) is the delivery of mechanical ventilation without an ETT or tracheostomy tube. NPPV provides ventilation via (1) a face mask that covers the nose, mouth, or both; (2) a nasal mask or pillow; or (3) a full face mask (Fig. 10.32). Complications associated with an artificial airway, such as vocal cord injury and VAP, are reduced, and sedation needs are less. During NPPV, the patient can eat and speak and is free from the discomfort of an artificial airway. Treatment with NPPV may prevent the need for intubation in many patients.

NPPV is indicated for the treatment of acute exacerbations of COPD, cardiogenic pulmonary edema (along with other treatments), early hypoxemic respiratory failure in immunocompromised patients, and obstructive sleep apnea.

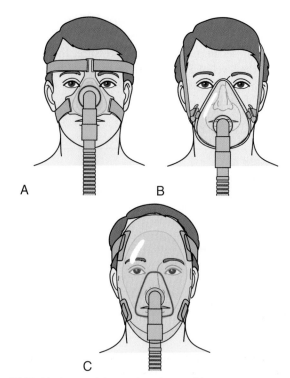

Fig. 10.32 Masks used for noninvasive positive-pressure ventilation. **A,** Nasal. **B,** Oronasal. **C,** Full face mask. (Redrawn from Mims BC, Toto KH, Luecke LE, et al. *Critical Care Skills.* 2nd ed. Philadelphia, PA: Saunders; 2003.)

NPPV has been used successfully in patients with asthma, pneumonia, postoperative respiratory failure, obesity hypoventilation syndrome, and other causes of acute respiratory failure. It may also be used to prevent reintubation in a patient who is experiencing respiratory distress following extubation and to provide ventilatory support while an acute problem is treated in patients for whom intubation is undesirable, such as those with "do not intubate" orders.[9,34,47,52] Its use is expanding beyond the critical care unit and even in settings outside of the hospital. Contraindications to NPPV include apnea and cardiovascular instability (hypotension, uncontrolled dysrhythmias, and myocardial ischemia). Relative contraindications, or factors that could contribute to noninvasive ventilation failure, include claustrophobia, impaired consciousness, high aspiration risk, viscous or copious secretions, inability to clear secretions, gastroesophageal surgery, recent craniofacial surgery trauma, and burns.[18]

NPPV can be delivered with critical care ventilators or a ventilator specifically designed to provide NPPV (Fig. 10.33). Modes delivered can be pressure or volume; however, pressure modes are better tolerated. The most common modes of ventilation delivered via NPPV are PS or pressure control with PEEP and CPAP.

During NPPV, collaborate with the RT to ensure that the right size and type of mask is chosen and that it fits snugly enough to prevent air leaks. Monitor the mask and the skin under the mask edges for signs of pressure injury. If signs of excess pressure are noted, reposition the mask, place a layer of

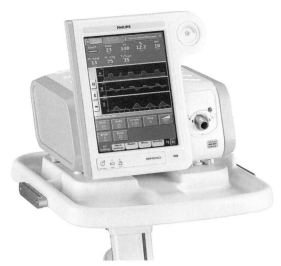

Fig. 10.33 The ventilator offers a range of conventional pressure modes, CPAP (continuous positive airway pressure), PCV (pressure-controlled ventilation), and S/T (spontaneous/timed). The volume-targeted AVAPS (average volume-assured pressure support) mode combines the attributes of pressure-controlled and volume-targeted ventilation. The optional PPV (pulse pressure variation) mode provides pressure ventilation in proportion to the patient's efforts. (Used with permission of Philips Respironics, Carlsbad, CA.)

wound care dressing on the skin as a protective shield, or select another mask type. If mouth breathing is a problem with the nasal mask, apply a chin strap or change the mask to an oronasal or full face mask.[18] Leakage of gases around the mask edges may lead to drying of the eyes and the need for eye drops. Monitor the mouth and airway passages for excessive drying, and add a humidification system as indicated. If the patient complains of nausea or vomits, gastric insufflation may be occurring, and gastric decompression may be indicated. Also monitor the total RR, the EV_T to ensure that it is adequate, and the PIP.

CRITICAL REASONING ACTIVITY

Your patient is being ventilated with noninvasive positive-pressure ventilation (NPPV) with a nasal mask. The patient is mouth breathing and the ventilator is alarming low exhaled tidal volume. What interventions should you take to ensure that the patient receives adequate ventilation?

High-Frequency Oscillatory Ventilation

High-frequency oscillatory ventilation (HFOV) delivers subphysiological tidal volumes at extremely fast rates (300 to 420 breaths/min). It is indicated in patients with noncompliant lungs and hypoxemia where conventional ventilation results in high airway pressures. This strategy stabilizes the alveoli and improves gas mixing, thereby improving oxygenation. The small tidal volumes limit peak pressure, preventing overdistension and protecting the lung from further injury. At the same time, collapse of the alveoli at end-expiration is limited through the use of higher end-expiratory pressure. HFOV is delivered

with a specialized ventilator that uses a diaphragm, much like a stereo speaker, driven by a piston creating a constant flow of gases into and out of the lung (Fig. 10.34). Ventilator settings control the amount, timing, and speed of piston movement. The nurse must learn new monitoring parameters when caring for a patient on HFOV.

Advanced Methods and Modes of Mechanical Ventilation

Microprocessor ventilators offer a wide range of options for mechanical ventilation. However, other forms of ventilatory support are available. These advanced techniques are usually ordered to treat patients with respiratory failure that is refractory to conventional treatment. These techniques include but are not limited to extracorporeal membrane oxygenation (ECMO), high-frequency jet ventilation, high-frequency percussive ventilation, and inhaled nitric oxide. Specialized equipment and training are essential for these advanced treatments. ECMO is increasingly being used to treat adults with refractory hypoxemia. Some hospitals have designated ECMO units to manage these complex, critically ill patients.

Respiratory Monitoring During Mechanical Ventilation

Nurses and RTs routinely monitor many parameters while a patient receives mechanical ventilation. Monitoring to assess the patient's response to treatment and to anticipate and plan for the ventilator weaning process includes physical assessment of the patient and assessment of the ventilator system: airway, circuitry, accuracy of ventilator settings, and patient data. Physical assessment includes vital signs and hemodynamic parameters, patient comfort and WOB, synchrony of patient's respiratory efforts with the ventilator, breath sounds, amount and quality of respiratory secretions, and assessment of the chest drain system if present. Evaluate ABG results, pulse oximetry, and $ETCO_2$ values to assess oxygenation and ventilation.[9,40,52] Patient data evaluated from the ventilator include EV_T (mandatory and spontaneous breaths), total RR, and PIP. Further assessment of the PIP may require direct measurements of airway resistance and static lung compliance. Check the ventilator system at least every 4 hours. The RT performs a more detailed assessment of the ventilator's functioning, including alarms and the appropriateness of alarm settings.[47]

Alarm Systems. Alarms are an integral part of a ventilator and warn of technical or patient events that require attention or action. Knowledge about troubleshooting alarms is essential. Follow two important rules to ensure patient safety:
1. Never shut off alarms. It is acceptable to silence alarms for a preset delay while working with a patient, such as during suctioning. However, alarms are never shut off.
2. Manually ventilate the patient with a bag-valve device if unable to troubleshoot alarms quickly or if equipment failure is suspected. Ensure that a bag-valve device is readily available at the bedside of every patient who is mechanically ventilated.

When an alarm sounds, the first thing to do is to look at the patient. If the patient is disconnected from the ventilator circuit, quickly reconnect the patient to the machine. If the

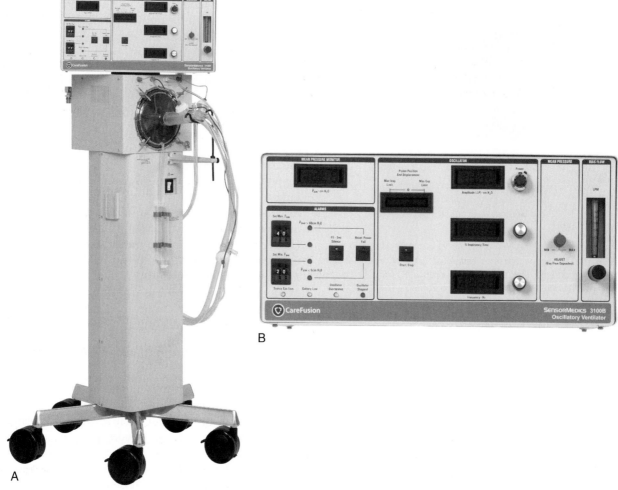

Fig. 10.34 A, Model 3100B High-Frequency Oscillatory Ventilator. **B,** Control panel of the 3100B. (©2020 Vyaire Medical, Inc., Mettawa, IL; Used with permission.)

circuit is connected to the airway, quickly assess whether the patient is in distress and whether he or she is adequately ventilated and oxygenated. Quickly assess the patient's level of consciousness, color, airway, RR, SpO_2 level, $ETCO_2$ value, heart rate, WOB, chest wall movement, and lung sounds. Observe the ventilator display to identify the status message related to the alarm, and silence the alarm while determining the cause of the alarm. Immediate action is required if the patient is in acute distress with labored respirations, an abnormal breathing pattern, pallor and diaphoresis, deterioration in breath sounds, or decreasing SpO_2. Quickly disconnect the patient from the ventilator and manually ventilate the patient with a bag-valve device while a second caregiver, often the RT, further assesses the problem. If the patient is not in respiratory distress, use the assessment data gathered to proceed with problem solving. Table 10.4 provides an overview of management of common ventilator alarms.

CRITICAL REASONING ACTIVITY

Your patient requires mechanical ventilation for treatment. The high peak pressure alarm has alarmed three times for a few seconds each time, even though you have just suctioned the patient. What nursing assessments and potential actions are warranted at this time?

Complications of Mechanical Ventilation

Numerous complications are associated with intubation and mechanical ventilation. Many complications can be prevented or treated rapidly through vigilant nursing care. Best practice includes implementation of the "ventilator bundle" for all mechanically ventilated patients to prevent complications and improve outcomes (see Clinical Alert box).

The absolute and relative value of each bundle component's impact on patient-centered outcomes is unclear. Recent evidence

! CLINICAL ALERT

Implementation of the Ventilator Bundle

The ventilator bundle of care should be implemented in all patients who receive mechanical ventilation.[31,39] This bundle is a group of evidence-based recommendations that has been demonstrated to improve outcomes. It is expected that all interventions in the bundle be implemented unless contraindicated. The interventions are as follows:

- Maintain head of bed elevation at 30 to 45 degrees.
- Interrupt sedation at least daily to assess readiness to wean from ventilator and extubate.
- Provide prophylaxis for deep vein thrombosis.
- Provide prophylaxis for peptic ulcer disease.
- Provide oral care with 0.12% chlorhexidine or other antiseptic solution.

TABLE 10.4 Management of Common Ventilator Alarms

Alarm	Description	Intervention
High peak pressure	Set 10 cm H_2O above average PIP Triggered when pressure increases anywhere in circuit Ventilator responds by terminating inspiratory phase to avoid pressure injury (barotrauma)	Assess for kinks in endotracheal tube or ventilator circuit and correct. Assess for anxiety and level of sedation or patient biting or gagging on tube; administer medications if warranted; use airway securing device with bite block. Observe for coughing; auscultate lung sounds for need for suctioning or bronchodilator. Use communication assistive devices for patient who is attempting to talk. Empty water from water traps if indicated. Assess for worsening pulmonary pathological conditions resulting in reduction in lung compliance (e.g., pulmonary edema) or increase in resistance (e.g., bronchospasm). Notify RT or physician if alarm persists.
Low pressure Low PEEP/CPAP	Set 10 cm H_2O below average PIP Set 3-5 cm H_2O below set PEEP/CPAP Triggered when pressure decreases in circuit	Assess for leaks in ventilator circuit or disconnection of ventilator circuit from airway; reconnect. If malfunction is noted, manually ventilate patient with bag-mask device. Notify RT to troubleshoot alarm.
Low exhaled V_T Low VE	Set 10% below the set V_T and the patient's average VE Ensures adequate alveolar ventilation	Assess for disconnection of ventilator circuit from airway; reconnect. Assess for disconnection in any part of the ventilator circuit; reconnect. Assess for leak in cuff of artificial airway by listening for audible sounds or bubbling of secretions around the airway and using device to measure cuff pressure; inflate as needed. Assess for new or increasing air leak in a chest drain system; connect if system related, notify provider if patient related. Assess for changes in lung compliance, increase in airway resistance, or patient fatigue on a pressure mode of ventilation.
High exhaled V_T High VE	Set 10% above the set V_T and the patient's average VE	Assess cause for increased RR or V_T such as anxiety, pain, hypoxemia, metabolic acidosis; treat. Assess for excess water in tubing; drain appropriately.
Apnea alarm	Set for <20 seconds Warns when no exhalation detected Ventilator will default to a backup controlled mode if alarm triggers	Assess for cause of lack of spontaneous respiratory effort (sedation, fatigue, respiratory arrest, neurological condition); physically stimulate patient; encourage patient to take a deep breath; reverse sedatives or narcotics. Manually ventilate patient and notify RT or provider to modify ventilator settings to provide more support such as a mode with mandatory breaths.

CPAP, Continuous positive airway pressure; *H₂O,* water; *PEEP,* positive end-expiratory pressure; *PIP,* peak inspiratory pressure; *RR,* respiratory rate; *RT,* respiratory therapist; *VE,* minute ventilation; *V_T,* tidal volume.

indicates that head-of-bed elevation, sedative infusion interruptions, spontaneous breathing trials, and thromboembolism prophylaxis appear beneficial, whereas daily oral care with chlorhexidine and stress ulcer prophylaxis may be harmful in some patients.[38] In the absence of updated practice guidelines, institutions should review the evidence in light of their patient populations and determine their approach to application of the latter two bundle components.

Airway Problems

Endotracheal tube out of position. If not properly secured, the ETT can become dislodged during procedures such as oral care, when changing the ETT securement device, during transport, or if the patient is anxious or agitated and attempts to pull out the tube. The ETT may be displaced upward, resulting in the cuff being positioned between or above the vocal cords. Conversely, the tube may advance too far into the airway and press on the carina or move into the right mainstem bronchus. Symptoms include absent or diminished breath sounds in the left lung and unequal chest excursion. Notify the provider of these findings so that the cuff can be let down, the tube gently retracted as needed, and the cuff properly reinflated.

Whenever the ETT is manipulated, assess for bilateral chest excursion, auscultate the chest for bilateral breath sounds after the procedure, and reassess tube position at the lip. A quick check of the centimeter markings can determine whether the tube has advanced or pulled out of position. When a serious airway problem cannot be resolved quickly, attempt to manually ventilate the patient. If the patient cannot be ventilated and the tube is not obviously displaced or the patient is not biting the airway, attempt to pass a suction catheter through the airway to determine whether it is obstructed. If the catheter cannot be passed and the patient has spontaneous respirations, deflate the cuff to allow air to pass around the tube. If the patient still cannot be adequately ventilated, remove the ETT and ventilate the patient with a bag-valve device with a mask while preparing for emergent reintubation.[1,9,13,33]

Unplanned extubation. The patient may intentionally or inadvertently remove the airway. The two most frequent methods by which self-extubation occurs are (1) by using the tongue and (2) by leaning forward or scooting downward so that the patient uses his or her hands to remove the tube.[1,13] Unplanned extubation (UE) can also occur as a result of patient care. For example, the tube can be dislodged if the ventilator circuit or closed suction catheter pulls on the ETT during procedures such as turning. Major risk factors for UE include agitation, especially when

BOX 10.8 Strategies for Unplanned or Self-Extubation

- Provide patient education regarding the purpose of the artificial airway and reassurance that it will be removed as soon as the patient can breathe independently.
- Provide adequate analgesia and sedation.
- Educate staff to assess for risk factors for self-extubation.
- Monitor all intubated patients vigilantly but especially those at high risk. Request that another staff member monitor the patient if the nurse needs to leave the area. Educate the family to assist in monitoring the patient.
- Apply protective devices only as needed after less restrictive methods have been exhausted (e.g., soft wrist restraints, arm immobilizers, mitts) according to hospital standards of practice.
- Adequately secure the endotracheal tube.
- Cut the end of the endotracheal tube to 2 inches beyond the fixation point.
- Provide support for the ventilator tubing and closed suction systems; keep these items out of the patient's reach.
- Use two staff members when applying or changing an ETT securement device.
- Identify one staff member to monitor the airway during patient movement and transport.
- Use professional communication techniques that ensure extubation in a timely manner when the patient meets established criteria.

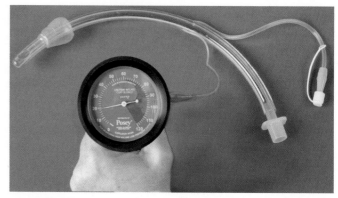

Fig. 10.35 Monitoring endotracheal tube cuff pressure. (Reprinted with permission, Cleveland Clinic Center for Medical Art & Photography © 2011–2019. All Rights Reserved.)

combined with inadequate sedation, inadequate surveillance, higher consciousness level, and presence of physical restraints.[1,13] Strategies for preventing UE are described in Box 10.8.

Laryngeal and tracheal injury. Damage to the larynx and trachea can occur because of tube movement and excess pressure exerted by the distal cuff. Prevent the patient from excessive head movement, especially flexion and extension, which result in the tube moving up and down in the airway, causing abrasive injury. An intervention for preventing tracheal damage from the cuff is routine cuff pressure monitoring (Fig. 10.35). Pressures should not exceed 25 to 30 cm H_2O (18 to 22 mm Hg).[2,34] Various commercial devices are available to measure cuff pressures quickly and easily.

Damage to the oral or nasal mucosa. Tape or commercial devices that secure the ETT and the tube itself can cause breakdown of the lip and oral mucosa (see Fig. 10.20). Nasal intubation may result in skin breakdown on the nares and also a higher risk of sinusitis. Ongoing assessment and skin care assist in preventing damage to the mouth and nose. Reposition the ETT frequently to prevent pressure necrosis.

STUDY BREAK

3. In which of the following situations would you try noninvasive ventilation?
   - A. A patient with COPD and right lower-lobe pneumonia with respiratory acidosis and increased WOB
   - B. A patient with a blood pressure of 65/35, heart rate of 150 beats/min, and respiratory rate of 39 breaths/min
   - C. A patient with pneumonia who has copious amounts of purulent, thick secretions
   - D. A 65-year-old man diagnosed with STEMI who has cardiogenic pulmonary edema

Pulmonary System

Trauma. *Barotrauma*, which means "pressure trauma," is the injury to the lungs associated with mechanical ventilation. In barotrauma, alveolar injury or rupture occurs as a result of excessive pressure, excessive peak inflating volume (volutrauma), or both.[6,17,50] Barotrauma may occur when the alveoli are overdistended, such as with positive-pressure ventilation, PEEP, and high V_T. Precipitating factors include diseases in which the lung has reduced compliance, such as ARDS and pneumonia associated with high PIP and mean airway pressures. The alveoli rupture or tear so that air escapes into various parts of the thoracic cavity, causing subcutaneous emphysema (air in the tissue space), pneumothorax or tension pneumothorax, pneumomediastinum, pneumopericardium, or pneumoperitoneum. Signs and symptoms of barotrauma include decreasing SpO_2, decreased breath sounds, tracheal shift, subcutaneous crepitus, new air leak or increase in air leak in a chest drainage system, and symptoms associated with hypoxemia.

A life-threatening complication is a *tension pneumothorax*. When tension pneumothorax occurs, pressurized air enters the pleural space. Air is unable to exit the pleural space and continues to accumulate. Air in the pleural space causes an increase in intrathoracic pressure, increasing amounts of lung collapse, shifting of the heart and great vessels to the opposite thorax (*mediastinal shift*), tachycardia, and hypotension. Treatment consists of immediate insertion of a chest tube or a needle thoracostomy. Whenever a pneumothorax is suspected in a patient receiving mechanical ventilation, remove the patient from the ventilator and ventilate with a bag-valve device until a needle thoracostomy or a chest tube insertion is performed.

Lung tissue injury induced by local or regional overdistending volume is called *volutrauma*. The damage that occurs to the lung is similar to the pathological findings of early ARDS and is the result of local stress and strain on the alveolar-capillary membrane. Volutrauma results in increased permeability of the alveolar-capillary membrane, pulmonary edema, accumulation of white blood cells and protein in the alveolar spaces, and reduced surfactant production. Because it is difficult to determine the exact distribution of volume in a patient's lung, pressure is used as a surrogate for volume. The PIP is kept below 40 cm

H_2O and/or the Pplat is kept at less than 30 cm H_2O as lung protective strategies to prevent both volutrauma and barotrauma.[6,9] Ventilator settings are adjusted to achieve these goals and may include reducing the V_T in a volume mode of ventilation or the inspiratory pressure in a pressure mode of ventilation.

Oxygen toxicity. The exposure of the pulmonary tissues to high levels of oxygen can lead to pathological changes. The degree of injury is related to the duration of exposure and to the FiO_2, not to the PaO_2. The first sign of oxygen toxicity, tracheobronchitis, is caused by irritant effects of oxygen. Prolonged exposure to high FiO_2 may lead to changes in the lung that mimic ARDS. Absorption atelectasis is another problem associated with high FiO_2. Nitrogen is needed to prevent collapse of the alveoli. When the FiO_2 is 1.0, alveolar collapse and atelectasis result from a lack of nitrogen in the distal air spaces. The goal is conservative oxygen therapy, targeting a PaO_2 of 70 to 100 mm Hg, or an SpO_2 of 90% to 92%, with an FiO_2 of 0.60 or less.[29,50] PEEP can also be adjusted to improve oxygenation in patients with collapsed alveoli.

Respiratory acidosis or alkalosis. Acid-base disturbances may occur secondary to V_T and RR settings on the ventilator. For example, if a patient is receiving V-A/C ventilation set at 10 breaths/min, but the patient's RR is 28 breaths/min because of pain or anxiety, respiratory alkalosis may occur. If the ventilator is set at a low RR (e.g., 2 to 6 breaths/min) and the patient does not have an adequate drive to initiate additional breaths, respiratory acidosis may occur. Ideally the V_T and RR are set to achieve a VE that ensures a normal $PaCO_2$ level.

Infection. Patients with artificial airways who are receiving mechanical ventilation are at an increased risk of VAP because normal upper airway defense mechanisms are bypassed. The principal mechanism for the development of VAP is aspiration of colonized gastric and oropharyngeal secretions. Factors that contribute to VAP include poor oral hygiene, aspiration, contaminated respiratory therapy equipment, poor hand washing by caregivers, breach of aseptic technique when suctioning, inadequate humidification or systemic hydration, and decreased ability to produce an effective cough because of the artificial airway. Specific strategies to reduce VAP include the following[31,39]:

- Avoid intubation and use noninvasive mechanical ventilation when possible.
- Implement the VAP bundle (see Clinical Alert: Implementation of the Ventilator Bundle box).
- Maintain and improve the patient's physical conditioning through early exercise and mobilization.
- Use an ETT with a lumen for aspirating subglottic secretions that pool above the airway cuff in patients likely to require intubation for longer than 48 to 72 hours.
- Ensure that secretions are aspirated from above the cuff before cuff deflation or tube removal.
- Maintain the ventilator circuit and change only if visibly soiled or malfunctioning.
- Prevent drainage of ventilator circuit condensate into the patient's airway. Always discard condensate and never drain it back into the humidifier.

- Practice proper hand hygiene and wear gloves when handling respiratory secretions.

Determination of VAP has low sensitivity and specificity. The Centers for Disease Control and Prevention, along with a team of experts, has recommended surveillance for ventilator-associated conditions, including infectious and noninfectious causes (see Clinical Alert: Ventilator-Associated Events box). See also Chapter 15.

> ### ! CLINICAL ALERT
> #### *Ventilator-Associated Events*
>
> The Centers for Disease Control and Prevention implemented surveillance for ventilator-associated events, including infectious and noninfectious types. Following a baseline period of stability or improvement for 2 or more days on mechanical ventilation, a ventilator-associated condition (VAC) is determined by indicators of worsening oxygenation: (1) need to increase the fraction of inspired oxygen by 0.20 or higher for 2 or more days or (2) need to increase positive end-expiratory pressure (PEEP) by 3 cm H_2O for 2 or more days. When VAC criteria are met, this alerts the caregiver that a clinically important pulmonary condition is developing such as atelectasis, pulmonary edema, pneumothorax, pneumonia, or acute respiratory distress syndrome. The health care team can then take action to diagnose the condition and initiate a plan of care. The presence of VAC predicts poor patient outcomes, including prolonged mechanical ventilation, increased length of stay in both the critical care unit and the hospital, and increased hospital mortality. They also may be preventable. The nurse plays an important role in monitoring for trends in worsening oxygenation and gathering assessment data to help determine the underlying cause.

From Centers for Disease Control and Prevention. Device Associated Module: Ventilator-Associated Event (VAE). http://www.cdc.gov/nhsn/PDFs/pscManual/10-VAE_FINAL.pdf. Published 2019. Accessed May 15, 2019.

Dysphagia and aspiration. Artificial airways increase the risk of upper airway injury, which in turn affects upper airway mechanics and protective reflexes, resulting in a swallowing disorder.[2,42] When the patient cannot effectively transfer food, liquids, and pills from the mouth to the stomach, quality of life and functional status are affected. Patients intubated 48 hours or longer are at risk for disordered swallowing, which can lead to aspiration, oxygen desaturation, pneumonia, and potentially reintubation. Reports of dysphagia following intubation vary widely, ranging from 3% to 62%, mostly because of varied assessment methods and instruments. Although oral feedings may be indicated after extubation or tracheostomy, dysphagia screening and/or a dysphagia (swallowing) evaluation is recommended prior to initiating oral intake.[32] Dysphagia screening is a pass/fail series of assessments to identify individuals who may either proceed to dietary intake or require a comprehensive referral to a speech-language pathologist prior to initiating oral intake.[32] In some institutions, a 3-ounce water swallow test followed by observation by a nurse, speech-language pathologist, or physician for clinical signs of aspiration has shown promise in identifying this potentially serious complication. This type of bedside screening for dysphagia is more common with stroke patients and is increasingly becoming the standard of care following extubation.[32] Diagnosis of a swallowing disorder is made by the speech-language pathologist using tests such as a bedside swallow evaluation or a fiberoptic endoscopic evaluation of swallow study. Review results of the swallowing evaluation and implement the treatment recommendations, such as specific food consistencies or body position when eating or drinking.[42]

Cardiovascular System. Hypotension and decreased cardiac output may occur with mechanical ventilation and PEEP, secondary to increased intrathoracic pressure, which can result in decreased venous return. The hemodynamic effects of mechanical ventilation are more pronounced in patients with hypovolemia or poor cardiac reserve. Patients with a high PIP who receive PEEP of greater than 8 cm H_2O may need hemodynamic monitoring to assess volume status and cardiac output.[50] Management of hypotension and decreased cardiac output involves the administration of volume to ensure an adequate preload, followed by administration of inotropic agents as necessary.

Gastrointestinal System. Stress ulcers and gastrointestinal bleeding may occur in patients who undergo mechanical ventilation. Stress ulcer prophylaxis is recommended. Initiate enteral feeding as soon as possible and monitor the patient for gross blood in the gastric aspirate and stools. Other interventions include identification and reduction of stressors, communication and reassurance, and administration of anxiolytic or sedative agents, as necessary based on standardized assessment tools (see Chapter 6).

Nutritional support is required for all patients who require mechanical ventilation (see Chapter 7). Early nutritional support may reduce the severity of disease and decrease complications and length of stay.[65] The type of formula may need to be modified for ventilated patients. Excess CO_2 production may occur with high-carbohydrate feedings and place a burden on the respiratory system to excrete the CO_2, increasing the WOB. Formulas developed for the patient with pulmonary disorders may be indicated.[65] Keep the head of the bed elevated 30 to 45 degrees during enteral feeding to reduce the risk of aspiration.[31,39]

Psychosocial Complications. Several psychosocial hazards may occur because of mechanical ventilation. Patients may experience stress and anxiety because they require a machine for breathing. If the ventilator is not set properly or if the patient resists breaths, patient-ventilator dyssynchrony may occur. The noise of the ventilator and the need for frequent procedures, such as suctioning, may alter sleep-wake patterns. In addition, the patient can become psychologically dependent on the ventilator.[24,25]

NURSING CARE

Nursing care of the patient who requires mechanical ventilation is complex. Use a holistic approach in patient care management. A detailed plan of care is described in the box titled Plan of Care for the Mechanically Ventilated Patient.

◎ PLAN OF CARE

For the Mechanically Ventilated Patient[64]

Patient Problem
Decreased Gas Exchange. Risk factors include respiratory muscle fatigue, acute respiratory failure, and metabolic factors.

Desired Outcomes
- Spontaneous ventilation with normal ABGs.
- Free of dyspnea or restlessness.
- No complications associated with mechanical ventilation.

*[handwritten: ambu bag if nurse accidently pulls it out
- pt. self extubated = greater chance to sustain airway so oxygen]*

Nursing Assessments/Interventions	Rationales
• Have bag-valve device and suctioning equipment readily available.	• Be prepared in the event of airway incompetency; maintain airway patency.
• Maintain artificial airway.	• Ensure maintenance of an adequate airway to facilitate mechanical ventilation.
• Secure ETT or tracheostomy with tape or commercial devices.	• Prevent unintended removal of artificial airway.
• Prevent unplanned extubation (see Box 10.8).	• Maintain an adequate airway by ensuring that artificial airway is in the proper position.
• Assess position of artificial airway:	
• Auscultate for bilateral breath sounds.	
• Evaluate placement on chest radiograph.	
• Once proper position is confirmed, note position of the tube at the lip line in the medical record.	
• Assess depth of tube (cm markings) during routine monitoring.	
• Monitor oxygenation and ventilation and respond to changes in:	• Ensure adequate oxygenation, ventilation, and acid-base balance.
• Vital signs	• Identify when ventilator setting changes are indicated.
• Total respiratory rate	
• Exhaled tidal volume of ventilator-assisted and patient-initiated breaths	
• Oxygen saturation	
• End-tidal CO_2	
• Mental status and level of consciousness	
• Signs and symptoms of hypoxemia (see Box 10.1)	
• ABGs	

PLAN OF CARE—cont'd

For the Mechanically Ventilated Patient

Nursing Assessments/Interventions	Rationales
• Assess respiratory status at least every 4 hours, including initiation of assisted or spontaneous breaths in the mechanically ventilated patient.	• Ensure that patient is breathing comfortably and is not expending excessive energy on the work of breathing.
• Change position of the ETT minimally every 24 hours.	• Prevent skin breakdown from the tube, tape, or airway securing device.
• Assess and document skin condition.	• Prevent aspiration of oral secretions and ventilator-associated pneumonia.
• Note placement of tube at lip line.	• Ensure that the tube remains in the proper position after manipulation.
• Use two staff members for procedure.	
• Suction secretions above the ETT cuff before repositioning tube.	
• After the procedure, assess position of tube at lip and auscultate for bilateral breath sounds.	
• Monitor cuff pressure of ETT or tracheostomy and maintain within therapeutic range.	• Prevent complications associated with overinflation or underinflation of ETT cuff.
• Maintain integrity of mechanical ventilator circuit.	• Ensure safe administration of mechanical ventilation.
• Monitor ventilator settings and respond to ventilator alarms.	• Ensure adequate oxygenation and ventilation.
• Keep tubing free of moisture by draining away from the patient or using water traps to collect condensate.	• Prevent aspiration of contaminated condensate.
• Assess prescribed ventilator settings every 2 hours (mode, set rate, V_T, FiO_2, PEEP).	• Ensure that patient is receiving therapy as ordered; promote patient safety.
• Ensure that alarms are on and respond to all ventilator alarms.	• Provide immediate intervention in response to specific alarm; promote patient safety.
• Assess PIP at least every 4 hours. Collaborate with RT to adjust ventilator settings to ensure that PIP does not exceed 40 cm H_2O.	• Identify elevations in PIP, which may indicate worsening lung function.
• Implement indicated therapies to improve pulmonary compliance (secretion removal, diuresis, mobilization) and reduce resistance (bronchodilators, keep tubing drained of condensate).	• Promote adequate oxygenation and ventilation.
• Assess tolerance to ventilatory assistance and monitor for patient-ventilator asynchrony. Notify RT and provider of potential need to adjust ventilator settings:	• Provide cues of condition improving or worsening; may indicate need for suctioning or need to adjust ventilator settings that are insufficient to meet patient's ventilatory needs.
• Patient's respiratory cycle out of phase with ventilator	
• High pressure and/or low EV_T alarms	
• Subjective report of breathlessness	
• Labored respirations, especially increased effort on inspiration	
• Tachypnea	
• Anxiety, agitation	
• Monitor serial chest radiographs.	• Assess for correct position of ETT and improvement or worsening of pulmonary conditions.
• Implement a multiprofessional plan of care to address underlying pulmonary condition:	• Mechanical ventilation only supports the respiratory system until the underlying condition is treated or resolved; well-coordinated team effort is essential to avoid fragmentation of care.
• Evaluate response to lung expansion, bronchial hygiene, and pulmonary medication therapies.	
• Mobilize patient as much as possible (i.e., turning, progressive upright mobility, lateral rotation therapy).	
• Consider pronation therapy to treat refractive hypoxemia in ARDS.	
• Ensure adequate hydration, nutrition, and electrolyte balance.	

Patient Problem
Potential for Insufficient Airway Clearance. Risk factors include ETT, inability to cough, thick secretions, fatigue.

Desired Outcomes
• Airway free of excessive secretions.
• Clear lung sounds.

Continued

◎ PLAN OF CARE—cont'd

For the Mechanically Ventilated Patient

Nursing Assessments/Interventions	Rationales
• Assess need for suctioning.	• Indicate possibility of airway obstruction with secretions and need for suctioning.
• Suction as needed according to standard of practice and assess for effectiveness (see Box 10.7).	• Remove secretions; maintain patent airway; improve gas exchange.
• If tracheal secretions are thick, assess hydration of patient and humidification of ventilator; avoid instillation of normal saline.	• Assist in thinning secretions for easier removal; saline has not shown to be effective and is associated with hypoxemia and increased risk of infection.
• Reposition the patient frequently and progress to upright as possible. Use lateral rotation and pronation therapy as indicated.	• Mobilize secretions; improve oxygenation.
• Collaborate with RT in the application and monitoring of secretion removal techniques, such as postural drainage and vibration or intrapulmonary vibration.	• Interventions from other team members may be needed to facilitate secretion removal.

Patient Problem

Fatigue With Decreased Exercise Tolerance. Risk factors include ineffective airway clearance, sleep-pattern disturbances, inadequate nutrition, pain, anemia, abdominal distension, debilitated condition, and psychological factors.

Desired Outcomes

- Liberation from mechanical ventilation.
- Adequate ABG values.
- Respiratory pattern and rate WNL.
- Effective secretion clearance.

Nursing Assessments/Interventions	Rationales
• Assess patient's readiness to wean (see Box 10.10).	• Identify readiness to begin the weaning process using validated parameters.
• Provide weaning method based on protocols and research evidence (see Box 10.9).	• Protocol-driven weaning is an effective strategy for systematic ventilator liberation that reduces ventilator days and critical care unit and hospital lengths of stay.
• Collaborate with the healthcare team to provide mechanical ventilation modes, patient coaching, and progressive mobility that supports respiratory muscle training.	• Promote respiratory conditioning that facilitates patient's ability to resume the work of breathing.
• Promote rest and comfort throughout the weaning process, especially between weaning trials; identify strategies that result in relaxation and comfort; ensure that environment is safe and comfortable.	• Facilitate weaning from mechanical ventilation.
• Support patient in setting goals for weaning.	• Promote rehabilitation and give patients some control in the process.
• Collaborate with the healthcare team to determine the most effective strategies for weaning those with severe dysfunctional breathing patterns.	• Various strategies may be needed to wean the patient; ongoing assessment is essential to determine the most effective strategy.
• Implement strategies that maximize tolerance of weaning:	• Maximize efforts to facilitate successful weaning.
• Titrate sedation and analgesia to a level at which patient is calm and cooperative with absence of respiratory depression.	
• Interrupt sedation at least once daily to determine if it is still indicated and reduce the overall amount of sedation accumulating. Restart at half the dose and titrate as needed.	
• Schedule weaning when patient is rested.	
• Avoid other procedures during weaning.	
• Position patient upright to allow for full expansion with abdominal compression on diaphragm.	
• Monitor phosphate levels because low phosphate affects respiratory muscle function.	
• Promote normal sleep-wake cycle.	
• Limit visitors to supportive persons.	
• Coach through periods of anxiety.	
• Terminate weaning if patient is unable to tolerate the process (see Box 10.11).	• Maintain adequate ventilation and gas exchange; prevent fatigue of respiratory muscles.
• Consider referring patients with prolonged ventilator dependence to an alternative setting, such as a long-term acute care hospital.	• Alternative settings specialize in weaning patients who are "difficult to wean."

ABG, Arterial blood gas; *ARDS,* acute respiratory distress syndrome; *cm H₂O,* centimeters of water; *CO₂,* carbon dioxide; *ETT,* endotracheal tube; *EV_T,* exhaled tidal volume; *FiO₂,* fraction of inspired oxygen; *PEEP,* positive end-expiratory pressure; *PIP,* peak inspiratory pressure; *RT,* respiratory therapist; *V_T,* tidal volume; *WNL,* within normal limits.

Adapted from Swearingen PL, Wright J. *All-in-One Nursing Care Planning Resource.* 5th ed. St. Louis, MO: Elsevier; 2019.

Communication

Communication difficulties are common because of the artificial airway. Patients identify lack of effective communication as a major stressor that elicits feelings of fear, frustration, isolation, anger, helplessness, anxiety, and sleeplessness.[25,66] Patients express a need to make themselves understood. They need constant re-orientation, reassuring words emphasizing a caregiver's presence, and point-of-care information that painful procedures done to them are indeed necessary and helpful. Increased frequency and repetition of explanations may help the patient cope with the experience of mechanical ventilation. In addition, touch, eye contact, and positive facial expressions are beneficial in relieving anxiety. Caregivers who attempt to individualize communication with intubated patients by using a variety of methods provide patients with a greater sense of control, encourage participation in their own care, and minimize cognitive disturbances.

Head nods, mouthing words, gestures, and writing are identi-fied as the most frequently used methods of nonverbal commu-nication among intubated patients, but they are often inhibited by wrist restraints. Communication with gestures and lip read-ing can convey some basic needs; however, augmentative devices may facilitate even better communication. Although writing is sometimes used, critically ill patients are often too weak or poorly positioned to write, or they lack the concentration to spell. Greater use of communication aids such as charts, com-munication boards, tablet computers with a communication app, and computer-generated voice devices could improve com-munication.[55] A picture board with icons representing basic needs and the alphabet that can be easily cleaned between pa-tients should be available in every unit. Family members can serve as a communication link between the patient and care providers. Reassure the patient that the loss of voice is tempo-rary and that speech will be possible after the tube is removed.[24]

Maintaining Comfort and Reducing Distress

Intubation, mechanical ventilation, advanced methods for ven-tilation (e.g., inverse-ratio ventilation), and suctioning contrib-ute to patient discomfort and distress. Patients often need both pharmacological and nonpharmacological methods to manage discomfort and to treat anxiety.[15,67] Strategies to promote patient comfort are discussed in depth in Chapter 6.

Medications

Commonly used medications include analgesics, sedatives, and neuromuscular blocking agents; many patients need a com-bination of these drugs. Medications are chosen based on the patient's hemodynamic stability, diagnosis, and the desired treatment goals. It is essential that the nurse, RT, and physician all use the same objective sedation and analgesia scoring systems to promote unambiguous assessment and communication. Nurse-driven decision trees or algorithms to guide initiation and titration of medications to targeted sedation and analgesia goals result in fewer days on sedation and mechanical ventila-tion. Sedation should be interrupted at least once daily to allow the patient to awaken and be reoriented and to determine if sedation is needed. A spontaneous breathing trial (SBT; weaning attempt) should be timed with sedation interruption.[15,51]

Analgesics, such as morphine and fentanyl, are administered to provide pain relief. Sedatives, such as dexmedetomidine, benzodiazepines, and propofol, are given to sedate the patient, reduce anxiety, and promote synchronous breathing with the ventilator. Benzodiazepines promote amnesia but are also as-sociated with an increase in delirium.[15] Patients who have acute lung injury or increased intracranial pressure or who require nontraditional modes of mechanical ventilation may require deep sedation or therapeutic paralysis with neuromuscular blocking agents (see Chapter 6).

When sedation is indicated, it must be titrated to a specific goal agreed upon by the multiprofessional team. Insufficient sedation may precipitate ventilator dyssynchrony and physio-logical alterations in thoracic pressures and gas exchange. Inad-equate sedation is also associated with unplanned extubation. Oversedation and prolonged sedation are associated with a longer duration of mechanical ventilation and lengths of stay in the critical care unit and hospital.[15] Prolonged duration of mechanical ventilation predisposes the patient to an increased risk of VAP, lung injury, and other complications. Depth of sedation also contributes to delayed weaning from mechanical ventilation. Because sedation, duration of mechanical ventila-tion, and ventilator weaning are interrelated, ensure that the patient is maintained on the lowest dose and lightest level of sedation possible. "Daily interruption," "sedation vacation," or a "spontaneous awakening trial" to evaluate the patient's cog-nitive status; to reduce the overall dose of sedation; and to determine what dose, if any, is needed to achieve a calm, coop-erative patient is an important nursing intervention.[15,51] Opti-mal sedation of the mechanically ventilated patient is present when patient-ventilator harmony exists and the patient re-mains capable of taking spontaneous breaths in readiness for weaning. Many patients achieve this state without sedative agents.

Nonpharmacological Interventions

Nonpharmacological, complementary, and alternative medi-cine strategies may reduce distress, promote patient-ventilator synchrony, and maintain a normal cognitive state.[67] Create a healing environment by involving the patient and family in the plan of care, reducing excess noise and light stimulation, pro-viding a reassuring presence, and minimizing unnecessary pa-tient stimulation to promote a normal sleep-wake cycle. Pro-vide adequate rest and frequent reorientation to prevent delirium. Implement a progressive mobility plan to reduce de-conditioning and promote endurance of the respiratory mus-cles to facilitate ventilator liberation. Daytime exercise may also promote a more restful nighttime sleep.

Meditation, guided imagery and relaxation, prayer, music therapy, massage, acupressure, therapeutic touch, herbal prod-ucts and dietary supplements, and family presence are non-pharmacological strategies to improve patient well-being. Ask the family and patient if they are already using complementary strategies and, if so, incorporate them as possible. The goal of incorporating these therapies into practice is to reduce patient distress, promote sleep, and create a healing environment con-ducive to reducing ventilator days.

CRITICAL REASONING ACTIVITY

You are caring for a patient who has been mechanically ventilated for 2 weeks. Physically, the patient meets all criteria to begin weaning from mechanical ventilation. What parameters should you monitor to assess tolerance of weaning?

WEANING PATIENTS FROM MECHANICAL VENTILATION

Mechanical ventilation is a therapy designed to support the respiratory system until the underlying disease or indication for mechanical ventilation is resolved. Weaning is the process of decreasing ventilator support and allowing the patient to assume a greater percentage of the work of ventilation. It may involve either an immediate shift from full ventilatory support to a period of breathing with minimal assistance (i.e., an SBT) or a gradual reduction in the amount of ventilator support. In general, patients who require short-term ventilatory support are liberated quickly.[22,48] Conversely, weaning patients who require long-term ventilatory support is often a slower process characterized by periods of success, as well as setbacks. Once the patient demonstrates the ability to breathe without the ventilator and both airway patency and airway protection is ensured, removal of the artificial airway is considered.[5]

Evidence-Based Approaches to Weaning

Weaning must be approached in a systematic fashion. Based on a comprehensive review of the research, evidence-based guidelines for ventilator weaning have been developed.[22,48]

Box 10.9 summarizes these guidelines. Weaning protocols usually are implemented by nurses and RTs, but computer-driven protocols reduce variability and result in a reduction of ventilator days and shorter stays in the critical care unit and hospital.[28,30] Regardless of strategy, the protocol should clearly define the method or screening tool to determine the patient's readiness to wean, the method and duration of the weaning trial, and criteria for extubation. Include methods to facilitate respiratory muscle work along with adequate rest in the weaning plan. See the QSEN Exemplar box for an example of teamwork and collaboration during the weaning process.[7]

Assessment for Readiness to Wean (Wean Screen)

Before initiating the weaning trial, screen the patient for readiness using parameters that have been associated with ventilator discontinuation success (Box 10.10). Screening assists in identifying patients who are ready to wean as well as those who are not ready, thereby protecting them against the risks associated with the stress of weaning.

Patients are usually able to wean when the underlying disease process is resolving and they are oxygenating with minimal support, are hemodynamically stable, and are able to initiate an inspiratory effort. Assessment of the neurological, cardiovascular, and respiratory systems provides a sufficient screen in most patients requiring a ventilator for only a short period. In many settings physiological respiratory parameters, referred to as weaning predictors, are also measured (see Box 10.10). The rapid shallow breathing index (RSBI) is easy to use and is the only measurement that has shown to be a true predictor of successful weaning.

BOX 10.9 Evidence-Based Guidelines for Weaning From Mechanical Ventilation

1. Identify causes for ventilator dependence if the patient requires ventilation for longer than 24 hours.
2. Conduct a formal assessment to determine a high potential for successful weaning:
   - Evidence of reversal of underlying cause of respiratory failure
   - Adequate oxygenation (PaO_2/FiO_2 >150-200; positive end-expiratory pressure <5-8 cm H_2O; FiO_2 <0.4-0.5) and pH greater than 7.25
   - Hemodynamic stability
   - Able to initiate an inspiratory effort
3. Conduct an SBT with inspiratory pressure augmentation (5-8 cm H_2O) rather than without (T-piece or CPAP). During the SBT, evaluate respiratory pattern, adequacy of gas exchange, hemodynamic stability, and comfort. A patient who tolerates an SBT for 30 to 120 minutes should be considered for permanent ventilator discontinuation.
4. If a patient fails an SBT, determine the cause of the failed trial. Provide a method of ventilatory support that is nonfatiguing and comfortable. Correct reversible causes, and attempt an SBT every 24 hours if the patient meets weaning criteria.
5. For patients who have been receiving mechanical ventilation for more than 24 hours, have passed an SBT, and are at high risk for extubation failure (i.e., hypercapnia, COPD, CHF, or other serious comorbidities), extubate to preventative NIV.[48]

6. For acutely hospitalized adults who have been mechanically ventilated for more than 24 hours, a physical conditioning plan using protocolized rehabilitation directed toward early mobilization should be used.[22]
7. Assess airway patency and the ability of the patient to protect the airway to determine whether to remove the artificial airway from a patient who has been successfully weaned. Perform a cuff leak test (CLT) in patients at high risk for postextubation stridor (i.e., traumatic intubation, intubation longer than 6 days, large ETT, female, or reintubation after unplanned extubation). For patients who fail a CLT, administer systemic steroids at least 4 hours before extubation.
8. Use protocols aimed at minimizing sedation.
9. Use either a personnel- or computer-driven ventilator liberation protocol.[22]
10. Consider a tracheostomy when it becomes apparent that the patient will require prolonged ventilator assistance.
11. Conduct slow-paced weaning in a patient who requires prolonged mechanical ventilation. Wean a patient to 50% of maximum ventilator support before daily SBT. Then initiate SBTs with gradual increase in duration of the SBT.
12. Unless evidence of irreversible disease exists (e.g., high cervical spine injury), do not consider a patient to be ventilator dependent until 3 months of weaning attempts have failed.
13. Transfer a patient who has failed weaning attempts but is medically stable to a facility that specializes in management of ventilator-dependent patients.

CHF, Congestive heart failure; *cm H₂O,* centimeters of water; *COPD,* chronic obstructive pulmonary disease; *CPAP,* continuous positive airway pressure; *FiO₂,* fraction of inspired oxygen; *NIV,* noninvasive ventilation; *PaO₂,* partial pressure of arterial oxygen; *SBT,* spontaneous breathing trial.

BOX 10.10 Assessment Parameters Indicating Readiness to Wean

Underlying Cause for Mechanical Ventilation Resolved
- Improved chest radiograph findings
- Minimal secretions
- Normal breath sounds

Adequate Oxygenation Without a High FiO₂ and/or a High PEEP
- PaO$_2$ greater than 60 mm Hg with FiO$_2$ of 0.4 or less
- PaO$_2$/FiO$_2$ greater than 150 to 200 (consider), ideally greater than 250
- PEEP less than 5 to 8 cm H$_2$O

Hemodynamic Stability
- Absence of hypotension
- Minimal vasopressor therapy

Adequate Respiratory Muscle Strength (Weaning Indices)
- Respiratory rate less than 25 to 30 breaths/min
- Rapid shallow breathing index less than 105
- Negative inspiratory force (maximum inspiratory pressure) −20 to −30 cm H$_2$O
- Spontaneous tidal volume 4 to 6 mL/kg IBW
- Vital capacity 10 to 15 mL/kg IBW
- Minute ventilation 5 to 10 L/min

Absence of Factors That Impair Weaning
- Infection
- Anemia
- Fever
- Sleep deprivation
- Pain
- Abdominal distension; bowel abnormalities (diarrhea or constipation)
- Mental readiness to wean: calm, minimal anxiety, motivated
- Minimal need for sedatives and other medications that may cause respiratory depression

cm H$_2$O, Centimeters of water; *FiO$_2$*, fraction of inspired oxygen; *IBW*, ideal body weight; *PaO$_2$*, partial pressure of arterial oxygen; *PEEP*, positive end-expiratory pressure.

⬧ QSEN EXEMPLAR

Teamwork and Collaboration

Successful weaning of patients from mechanical ventilation requires a team approach. Led by a clinical nurse specialist (CNS), a hospital-established multi-professional ventilator team was composed of a pulmonologist, critical care nurses, stepdown unit nurses, a respiratory therapist, a speech therapist, a physical therapist, a clinical pharmacist, a case manager, a social worker, a chaplain, and home care personnel. Every patient in the facility who was mechanically ventilated for more than 3 days received a comprehensive evaluation by the CNS. The CNS met with the patient, family, physician, and unit staff to identify potential issues that could affect the weaning process. Patients meeting criteria were then presented at the weekly "Vent Team" meeting. Individualized weaning plans were developed for each patient. Additional concerns related to mechanical ventilation, including nutrition, communication, mobility and function, pain and anxiety, infection risk, patient and family coping, end-of-life concerns, spirituality, and discharge preparation, were addressed, and plans of care were modified as required. Patient outcomes included improved transitions between nursing units, reduction in ventilator days, reduction in ventilator-acquired pneumonia, and reduced length of stay. Team members proactively worked with patients and families to address end-of-life issues and to plan terminal weaning as appropriate. A team approach was used to transition patients who required ongoing mechanical ventilation for conditions such as amyotrophic lateral sclerosis and spinal cord injury to the care of the family provider in the home setting.

Reference
Burns SM, Fisher C, Tribble SE, et al. The relationship of 26 clinical factors to weaning outcome. *Am J Crit Care*. 2012;21(1):52–58;quiz 59.

Patients who have complex critical illness or have been ventilated for more than 72 hours may have more physiological factors that affect successful weaning, such as inadequate nutrition and respiratory muscle deconditioning.[56] A tool that provides a more comprehensive or multidimensional assessment of weaning readiness, as well as a baseline score from which to measure patient progress once weaning begins, may guide the team through assessing a patient's strengths and factors that may interfere with successful weaning. The Burns Wean Assessment Program (BWAP) has been evaluated in patients weaning from mechanical ventilation.[7] The BWAP evaluates nonpulmonary factors that influence weaning success, such as hematocrit; fluids, electrolytes, and nutrition; anxiety, pain, and rest; bowel function; and physical conditioning and mobility. Pulmonary factors assessed with the BWAP include gas flow and WOB, airway clearance, respiratory muscle strength and endurance, and ABGs.

It is imperative that the nurse collaborate with an RT and the provider using data and weaning assessment tools to identify readiness for weaning and factors that may impede successful weaning. When a patient is successful at a weaning trial, these factors should be optimized to promote patient success in future weaning endeavors.

Weaning Process (Weaning Trial)

Table 10.5 describes weaning methods. Evidence-based practice guidelines recommend the use of an SBT for weaning. Pressure support, T-piece, and CPAP qualify as spontaneous breathing modes. The SBT with pressure augmentation (i.e., pressure support) has demonstrated a higher rate of extubation success and a trend toward lower critical care unit mortality than SBTs without pressure augmentation. An SBT for 30 to 120 minutes provides a direct assessment of spontaneous breathing capabilities and has been shown to be the most effective way to shorten the ventilator discontinuation process.[22,48]

Assess and monitor the patient throughout the weaning process. Organize patient care to ensure vigilant assessment throughout the trial. Explain the weaning procedure to the patient and family in a manner that promotes reassurance and minimizes anxiety. Ensure that the patient is adequately rested and positioned optimally for diaphragm function and lung expansion, such as sitting. Obtain baseline parameters: vital signs, heart

TABLE 10.5 Weaning Methods

	Description	Strategies
Spontaneous Breathing Trial (SBT) Trial of spontaneous breathing effort	Every breath is spontaneous, and patient performs all the WOB. Attempt daily if patient passes wean screen. Successful when patient remains stable for 30-120 min.	Daily or more often trial.
Reconditioning Trials Gradual exercising, or reconditioning of the respiratory muscles as patient can tolerate without inducing fatigue	Alternating periods of resting on full ventilator support with advancing periods of gradually reduced support. Gradual reconditioning indicated for deconditioned patients who are unsuccessful with SBT.	Ratio of rest periods to time on trial based on patient's response. Amount of time to liberate patient varies; may be days to weeks.

Mode	Spontaneous Breathing Trial (SBT) Strategy	Difficult or Prolonged Weaning
Pressure Support (PS) Provides inspiratory support to overcome resistance to gas flow through ventilator circuit and artificial airway	SBT = PS of 5 cm H_2O + 5 cm H_2O PEEP	Begin at level of PS that ensures nonlabored RR and V_T. Gradual reduction in PS in 2- to 5-cm H_2O increments. Gradually lengthen time interval on reduced levels of support. Discontinue when patient stable for 2 h or longer at 5 cm H_2O PS.
T-Piece Patient performs all the WOB No ventilator alarms for apnea, decreased V_T, etc. Requires high level of staff attention	Remove patient from ventilator and provide humidified oxygen via a T-piece adaptor attached to the ETT or tracheostomy tube.	May start with trial as short as 5 min. Increase time on T-piece as tolerated with adequate rest periods (6-8 h) on full ventilatory support. Discontinue when patient stable on T-piece for at least 2 h, often longer.
CPAP Useful when patient requires PEEP to maintain oxygenation Patient performs all the WOB Ventilator will provide alarms for apnea, high RR, or low EV_T	CPAP of 5 cm H_2O	CPAP of 5 cm H_2O. May start with trial as short as 5 min. Increase time on CPAP as tolerated with adequate rest periods (6-8 h) on full ventilatory support. Discontinue when patient on CPAP for at least 2 h, often longer.

cm H_2O, Centimeters of water; *CPAP,* continuous positive airway pressure; *ETT,* endotracheal tube; *EV_T,* exhaled tidal volume; *PEEP,* positive end-expiratory pressure; *RR,* respiratory rate; *V_T,* tidal volume; *WOB,* work of breathing.

rhythm, ABGs or pulse oximetry, ETCO$_2$ values, and neurological status. Monitor the patient during the weaning process for tolerance or intolerance to the procedure. Although the patient is required to increase participation in the WOB, ensure that the patient does not become fatigued by the weaning effort and become compromised. Indicators of tolerance include an unlabored respiratory pattern, adequate oxygenation and ventilation indices, hemodynamic stability, neurological stability, and patient comfort.[54] Box 10.11 defines the physiological parameters that constitute the integrated assessment to determine patient intolerance of the weaning process. If these signs of intolerance develop, stop the weaning trial and resume mechanical ventilation at ventilator settings that provide full ventilatory support.[9,19,43] However, thorough patient evaluation is necessary because reliance on a single parameter can delay ventilator liberation.

Many respiratory and nonrespiratory factors can influence weaning success. Increased oxygen demands occur with infection, fever, anemia, and pain, or asking the patient to perform another activity such as physical therapy during the trial can impair weaning. Other factors to assess for are decreased respiratory performance from malnutrition, overuse of sedatives or

BOX 10.11 Criteria for Discontinuing Weaning

Respiratory
- Respiratory rate greater than 35 breaths/min or less than 8 breaths/min
- Spontaneous V_T less than 5 mL/kg ideal body weight
- Labored respirations
- Use of accessory muscles
- Abnormal breathing pattern: chest/abdominal asynchrony
- Oxygen saturation less than 90%

Cardiovascular
- Heart rate changes more than 20% from baseline
- Dysrhythmias (e.g., premature ventricular contractions, bradycardia)
- Ischemia: ST-segment elevation
- Blood pressure changes more than 20% from baseline
- Diaphoresis

Neurological
- Agitation, anxiety
- Decreased level of consciousness

V_T, Tidal volume.

hypnotics, sleep deprivation, and abdominal distension. Factors involving equipment or technique, time of day, and method for weaning should also be examined. Psychological factors to evaluate include apprehension and fear, helplessness, and depression.[19] Systematically evaluate all potential factors to optimize successful weaning.

Extubation

If the patient demonstrates tolerance to the weaning procedure and can sustain spontaneous breathing for 90 to 120 minutes, the next step toward ventilator discontinuation is making the decision to extubate (remove the ETT). Prior to extubation, evaluate the need for airway secretion clearance; the patient must have a good cough and require suctioning no more than every 2 hours. If the patient has a tracheostomy, the patient may be liberated from the ventilator, but the tracheostomy is maintained to facilitate airway clearance. Also assess airway patency and the ability of the patient to protect the airway. Perform a cuff leak test (CLT) in patients at high risk for postextubation stridor. High risk includes traumatic intubation, intubation longer than 6 days, intubation with a large ETT, female, or reintubation after unplanned extubation. For patients who fail a CLT, administer systemic steroids at least 4 hours before extubation.[22] When the decision is made to extubate, suction the ETT thoroughly before removal. Also, suction the posterior oropharynx to remove secretions that may have pooled above the cuff, deflate the ETT cuff, and remove the ETT during inspiration. Once extubated, ask the patient to cough and speak and assess for stridor, hoarseness, changes in vital signs, or low SpO_2, which may indicate complications. Noninvasive ventilation may be used to avert reintubation in some patients.[27,46]

CASE STUDY

Mr. P., age 65 years, was transferred to the critical care unit from the emergency department after successful resuscitation from a cardiac arrest sustained out of the hospital. Initial diagnosis based on laboratory results and electrocardiography is acute anterior myocardial infarction. It is suspected that Mr. P. aspirated gastric contents during the cardiac arrest. He opens his eyes to painful stimuli. He is orally intubated with a size 7.5 mm endotracheal tube located at the 25-cm marking at the teeth. Placement was confirmed by auscultation, end-tidal carbon dioxide, and chest radiograph. He is receiving mechanical ventilation with volume assist-control ventilation, respiratory rate set at 12 breaths/min, fraction of inspired oxygen (FiO_2) of 0.40, positive end-expiratory pressure (PEEP) of 5 cm H_2O, and tidal volume of 700 mL. An arterial blood gas drawn on arrival to the critical care unit shows the following values: pH, 7.33; partial pressure of carbon dioxide ($PaCO_2$), 40 mm Hg; bicarbonate (HCO_3^-), 20 mEq/L; partial pressure of arterial oxygen (PaO_2), 88 mm Hg; and arterial oxygen saturation (SaO_2), 99%. A decision is made to maintain the current ventilator settings. The following day, Mr. P.'s chest radiograph shows progressive infiltrates. His oxygen saturation is dropping below 90%, and he is demonstrating signs of hypoxemia: increased heart rate and premature ventricular contractions. Arterial blood gas analysis now shows pH, 7.35; $PaCO_2$, 43 mm Hg; HCO_3^-, 26 mEq/L; PaO_2, 58 mm Hg; and SaO_2, 88%. The physician orders the FiO_2 increased to 0.50 and PEEP increased to 10 cm H_2O.

Questions

1. What were the results of Mr. P.'s first arterial blood gas analysis? What factors are contributing to these results?
2. What factor is contributing to Mr. P.'s worsening condition on the day after hospital admission?
3. Interpret the arterial blood gases done on the day after the cardiac arrest.
4. Why did the physician change the ventilator settings after the second set of arterial blood gases?
5. What must the nurse assess after the addition of the PEEP? Why is this especially important for Mr. P.?

REFERENCES

1. Ai ZP, Gao XL, Zhao XL. Factors associated with unplanned extubation in the intensive care unit for adult patients: A systematic review and meta-analysis. *Intensive Crit Care Nurs*. 2018;47: 62–68.
2. Altobelli NP. Airway management. In: Kacmarek RM, Stoller JK, Heuer AJ, eds. *Egan's Fundamentals of Respiratory Care*. 11th ed. St. Louis, MO: Elsevier; 2014:733–785.
3. Ari A, Fink J. Humidity and aerosol therapy. In: Cairo JM, ed. *Mosby's Respiratory Care Equipment*. 10th ed. St. Louis, MO: Elsevier; 2018:158–199.
4. Ayhan H, Tastan S, Iyigun E, et al. Normal saline instillation before endotracheal suctioning: "What does the evidence say? What do the nurses think?": Multimethod study. *J Crit Care*. 2015;30(4):762–767.
5. Baptistella AR, Sarmento FJ, da Silva KR, et al. Predictive factors of weaning from mechanical ventilation and extubation outcome: A systematic review. *J Crit Care*. 2018;48:56–62.
6. Brower RG, Matthay MA, Morris A, et al. Ventilation with lower tidal volumes as compared with traditional tidal volumes for acute lung injury and the acute respiratory distress syndrome. *N Engl J Med*. 2000;342(18):1301–1308.
7. Burns SM, Fisher C, Tribble SE, et al. The relationship of 26 clinical factors to weaning outcome. *Am J Crit Care*. 2012;21(1):52–58; quiz 59.
8. Cairo JM. *Mosby's Respiratory Care Equipment*. 10th ed. St. Louis, MO: Elsevier; 2018.
9. Cairo JM, Hinski ST. *Pilbeam's Mechanical Ventilation: Physiological and Clinical Applications*. 6th ed. St. Louis, MO: Elsevier; 2016.
10. Caparros AC. Mechanical ventilation and the role of saline instillation in suctioning adult intensive care unit patients: An evidence-based practice review. *Dimensions Crit Care Nurs*. 2014;33(4):246–253.
11. Caroff DA, Li L, Muscedere J, et al. Subglottic secretion drainage and objective outcomes: A systematic review and meta-analysis. *Crit Care Med*. 2016;44(4):830–840.
12. Cohen Z. Gas exchange and transport. In: Kacmarek RM, Stoller JK, Heuer AJ, eds. *Egan's Fundamentals of Respiratory Care*. 11th ed. St. Louis, MO: Elsevier; 2017:247–268.
13. Danielis M, Chiaruttini S, Palese A. Unplanned extubations in an intensive care unit: Findings from a critical incident technique. *Intensive Crit Care Nurs*. 2018;47:69–77.
14. Daoud EG. Airway pressure release ventilation: Translating clinical research to the bedside in acute respiratory distress syndrome. *Crit Care Shock*. 2015;18(1):7–15.

15. Devlin JW, Skrobik Y, Gelinas C, et al. Clinical practice guidelines for the prevention and management of pain, agitation/sedation, delirium, immobility, and sleep disruption in adult patients in the ICU. *Crit Care Med.* 2018;46(9):e825–e873.

16. Dries DJ. High-flow nasal cannula: Where does it fit? *Respir Care.* 2018;63(3):367–370.

17. Fan E, Del Sorbo L, Goligher EC, et al. An official American Thoracic Society/European Society of Intensive Care Medicine/Society of Critical Care Medicine clinical practice guideline: Mechanical ventilation in adult patients with acute respiratory distress syndrome. *Am J Respir Crit Care Med.* 2017;195(9):1253–1263.

18. Frazier SK. Noninvasive positive pressure ventilation: Continuous positive airway pressure (CPAP) and bilevel positive airway pressure (BiPAP). In: Wiegand DL, ed. *AACN Procedure Manual for High Acuity, Progressive, and Critical Care.* 7th ed. St. Louis, MO: Elsevier; 2017:249–260.

19. Frazier SK. Weaning mechanical ventilation. In: Wiegand DL, ed. *AACN Procedure Manual for High Acuity, Progressive, and Critical Care.* 7th ed. St. Louis, MO: Elsevier; 2017:277–285.

20. Freeman BD. Tracheostomy update: When and how. *Crit Care Clin.* 2017;33(2):311–322.

21. Gallagher JJ. Alternative modes of mechanical ventilation. *AACN Adv Crit Care.* 2018;29(4):396–404.

22. Girard TD, Alhazzani W, Kress JP, et al. An official American Thoracic Society/American College of Chest Physicians clinical practice guideline: Liberation from mechanical ventilation in critically ill adults. Rehabilitation protocols, ventilator liberation protocols, and cuff leak tests. *Am J Respir Crit Care Med.* 2017;195(1):120–133.

23. Goodrich CA. Endotracheal intubation (assist). In: Wiegand DL, ed. *AACN Procedure Manual for High Acuity, Progressive, and Critical Care.* 7th ed. St. Louis, MO: Elsevier; 2017:23–31.

24. Grossbach I, Stranberg S, Chlan L. Promoting effective communication for patients receiving mechanical ventilation. *Crit Care Nurse.* 2011;31(3):46–60.

25. Guttormson JL, Bremer KL, Jones RM. "Not being able to talk was horrid:" A descriptive, correlational study of communication during mechanical ventilation. *Intensive Crit Care Nurs.* 2015;31(3):179–186.

26. Hall JE. *Guyton and Hall Textbook of Medical Physiology.* 13th ed. Philadelphia, PA: Elsevier; 2016.

27. Hernandez G, Vaquero C, Colinas L, et al. Effect of postextubation high-flow nasal cannula vs noninvasive ventilation on reintubation and postextubation respiratory failure in high-risk patients: A randomized clinical trial. *JAMA.* 2016;316(15):1565–1574.

28. Hess DR, Altobelli NP. Tracheostomy tubes. *Respir Care.* 2014;59(6):956–971; discussion 971–973.

29. Heuer AJ. Medical gas therapy. In: Kacmarek RM, Stoller JK, Heuer AJ, eds. *Egan's Fundamentals of Respiratory Care.* 11th ed. St. Louis, MO: Elsevier; 2017:905–935.

30. Hirzallah FM, Alkaissi A, do Céu Barbieri-Figueiredo M. A systematic review of nurse-led weaning protocol for mechanically ventilated adult patients. *Nurs Crit Care.* 2019;24(2):89–96.

31. Institute for Healthcare Improvement. How-To Guide: Prevent Ventilator-Associated Pneumonia. http://www.ihi.org/resources/Pages/Tools/HowtoGuidePreventVAP.aspx. Published 2012.

32. Johnson KL, Speirs L, Mitchell A, et al. Validation of a postextubation dysphagia screening tool for patients after prolonged endotracheal intubation. *Am J Crit Care.* 2018;27(2):89–96.

33. Kacmarek RM, Dimas S, Mack CW. *Essentials of Respiratory Care.* St. Louis, MO: Elsevier; 2015.

34. Kacmarek RM, Stoller JK, Heuer AJ, et al. *Egan's Fundamentals of Respiratory Care.* 11th ed. St. Louis, MO: Elsevier; 2017.

35. Kaddoura MA. Effect of the essentials of critical care orientation (ECCO) program on the development of nurses' critical thinking skills. *J Contin Educ Nurs.* 2010;41(9):424–432.

36. Kallet RH. Bedside assessment of the patient. In: Kacmarek RM, Stoller JK, Heuer AJ, eds. *Egan's Fundamentals of Respiratory Care.* 11th ed. St. Louis, MO: Elsevier; 2017:320–344.

37. Kleiman AM, Shilling AM. Airway management devices and advanced cardiac life support. In: Cairo JM, ed. *Mosby's Respiratory Care Equipment.* 10th ed. St. Louis, MO: Elsevier; 2018:110–151.

38. Klompas M, Li L, Kleinman K, et al. Associations between ventilator bundle components and outcomes. *JAMA Intern Med.* 2016;176(9):1277–1283.

39. Klompas M, Branson R, Eichenwald EC, et al. Strategies to prevent ventilator-associated pneumonia in acute care hospitals: 2014 update. *Infect Control Hosp Epidemiol.* 2014;35(Suppl 2):S133–S154.

40. Lee DB. Oxygen saturation monitoring with pulse oximetry. In: Wiegand DL, ed. *AACN Procedure Manual for High Acuity, Progressive, and Critical Care.* 7th ed. St. Louis, MO: Elsevier; 2017:134–141.

41. Luehrs P. Continuous end-tidal carbon dioxide monitoring. In: Wiegand DL, ed. *AACN Procedure Manual for High Acuity, Progressive, and Critical Care.* 7th ed. St. Louis, MO: Elsevier; 2017:103–110.

42. Macht M, Wimbish T, Bodine C, et al. ICU-acquired swallowing disorders. *Crit Care Med.* 2013;41(10):2396–2405.

43. MacIntyre NR. The ventilator discontinuation process: An expanding evidence base. *Respir Care.* 2013;58(6):1074–1086.

44. McCance KL, Huether SE, Brashers VL, et al. *Pathophysiology: The Biologic Basis for Disease in Adults and Children.* 8th ed. St. Louis, MO: Elsevier; 2019.

45. Mehta C, Mehta Y. Percutaneous tracheostomy. *Ann Card Anaesth.* 2017;20(Suppl):S19–S25.

46. Ni YN, Luo J, Yu H, et al. Can high-flow nasal cannula reduce the rate of endotracheal intubation in adult patients with acute respiratory failure compared with conventional oxygen therapy and noninvasive positive pressure ventilation? A systematic review and meta-analysis. *Chest.* 2017;151(4):764–775.

47. Oakes DF, Shortall SP, Jones S. *Oakes' Ventilator Management: An Oakes Pocket Guide.* Coral Springs, FL: Respiratory Books; 2016.

48. Ouellette DR, Patel S, Girard TD, et al. Liberation from mechanical ventilation in critically ill adults: An official American College of Chest Physicians/American Thoracic Society clinical practice guideline: Inspiratory pressure augmentation during spontaneous breathing trials, protocols minimizing sedation, and noninvasive ventilation immediately after extubation. *Chest.* 2017;151(1):166–180.

49. Patton KT. *Anatomy & Physiology.* St. Louis, MO: Elsevier; 2016.

50. Pham T, Brochard LJ, Slutsky AS. Mechanical ventilation: State of the art. *Mayo Clin Proc.* 2017;92(9):1382–1400.

51. Pierce L, Berry S, Howard J, Udobi K, et al. Daily spontaneous awakening trial in the sedated mechanically ventilated patient in the surgical ICU. *Crit Care Med.* 2014;42(12):A1556–A1557.

52. Pierce LNB. *Management of the Mechanically Ventilated Patient.* Philadelphia, PA: Saunders; 2007.

53. Raimondi N, Vial MR, Calleja J, et al. Evidence-based guidelines for the use of tracheostomy in critically ill patients. *J Crit Care.* 2017;38:304–318.

54. Rose L. Strategies for weaning from mechanical ventilation: A state of the art review. *Intensive Crit Care Nurs.* 2015;31(4): 189–195.

55. Santiago C, Roza D, Porretta K, Smith O. The use of tablet and communication app for patients with endotracheal or tracheostomy tubes in the medical surgical intensive care unit: A pilot, feasibility study. *Can J Crit Care Nurs.* 2019;30(1):17–23.

56. Schreiber AF, Ceriana P, Ambrosino N, et al. Physiotherapy and weaning from prolonged mechanical ventilation. *Respir Care.* 2019;64(1):17–25.

57. Schwaiberger D, Karcz M, Menk M, et al. Respiratory failure and mechanical ventilation in the pregnant patient. *Crit Care Clin.* 2016;32(1):85–95.

58. Seckel M. Suctioning: Endotracheal or tracheostomy tube. In: Wiegand DL, ed. *AACN Procedure Manual for High Acuity, Progressive, and Critical Care.* 7th ed. St. Louis, MO: Elsevier; 2017:69–78.

59. Selby ST, Abramo T, Hobart-Porter N. An update on end-tidal CO_2 monitoring. *Pediatr Emerg Care.* 2018;34(12):888–892.

60. Singh PM, Borle A, Trikha A. Newer nonconventional modes of mechanical ventilation. *Emerg Trauma Shock.* 2014;7(3):222–227.

61. Sklar MC, Burns K, Rittayamai N, et al. Effort to breathe with various spontaneous breathing trial techniques: A physiologic meta-analysis. *Am J Respir Crit Care Med.* 2017;195(11): 1477–1485.

62. Slota M. *AACN Core Curriculum for Pediatric Critical Care Nursing.* 2nd ed. Philadelphia, PA: Saunders; 2006.

63. Sole ML, Bennett M, Ashworth S. Clinical indicators for endotracheal suctioning in adult patients receiving mechanical ventilation. *Am J Crit Care.* 2015;24(4):318–325.

64. Swearingen PL, Wright J. *All-in-One Nursing Care Planning Resource: Medical-Surgical,* Pediatric, Maternity, Psychiatric-Mental Health. St. Louis, MO: Mosby; 2018.

65. Taylor BE, McClave SA, Martindale RG, et al. Guidelines for the provision and assessment of nutrition support therapy in the adult critically ill patient: Society of Critical Care Medicine (SCCM) and American Society for Parenteral and Enteral Nutrition (A.S.P.E.N.). *Crit Care Med.* 2016;44(2):390–438.

66. Tembo AC, Higgins I, Parker V. The experience of communication difficulties in critically ill patients in and beyond intensive care: Findings from a larger phenomenological study. *Intensive Crit Care Nurs.* 2015;31(3):171–178.

67. Tracy MF, Chlan L. Nonpharmacological interventions to manage common symptoms in patients receiving mechanical ventilation. *Crit Care Nurse.* 2011;31(3):19–28.

68. Walsh BK, Crotwell DN, Restrepo RD. Capnography/capnometry during mechanical ventilation: 2011. *Respir Care.* 2011;56(4): 503–509.

69. West JB, Luks A. *West's Respiratory Physiology: The Essentials.* 10th ed. Philadelphia, PA: Wolters Kluwer; 2016.

70. Wittenstein J, Ball L, Pelosi P, et al. High-flow nasal cannula oxygen therapy in patients undergoing thoracic surgery: Current evidence and practice. *Curr Opin Anaesthesiol.* 2019;32(1):44–49.

11

Rapid Response Teams and Code Management

Deborah G. Klein, MSN, APRN, ACNS-BC, CCRN, FAHA, FAAN

Many additional resources, including self-assessment exercises, are located on the Evolve companion website at http://evolve.elsevier.com/Sole/.
- Animations
- Clinical Skills: Critical Care Collections
- Student Review Questions
- Video Clips

INTRODUCTION

Code, code blue, code 99, and *Dr. Heart* are terms frequently used in hospital settings to refer to emergency situations that require life-saving resuscitation and interventions. Codes are called when patients have a cardiac or respiratory arrest or a life-threatening cardiac dysrhythmia that causes a loss of consciousness. (The generic term *arrest* is used in this chapter to refer to these conditions.) Regardless of cause, patient survival and positive outcomes depend on prompt recognition of the situation and immediate institution of basic life support (BLS) and advanced cardiovascular life support (ACLS) measures. *Code management* refers to the initiation of a code and the life-saving interventions performed when a patient arrests.

Rapid response teams (RRTs) have been implemented to address changes in a patient's clinical condition *before* a cardiac or respiratory arrest occurs. The goal of RRTs is to prevent the cardiac or respiratory arrest from ever occurring. The Institute for Healthcare Improvement and The Joint Commission support efforts by hospitals to implement systems that enable healthcare workers to request additional assistance from specially trained individuals when the patient's condition appears to be worsening.[15]

This chapter discusses the role of RRTs in preventing cardiopulmonary arrest, the roles of the personnel involved in a code, and equipment that must be readily available to support interventions of the RRT or during a code. BLS and ACLS measures are presented, including medications commonly administered during a code. For the most up-to-date information, the reader should contact the American Heart Association (AHA) for current recommendations for BLS and ACLS or access materials on the AHA's website. Care of the patient after a code is discussed in this chapter, including the use of targeted temperature management (TTM).

In the absence of a written order from a physician to withhold resuscitative measures, cardiopulmonary resuscitation (CPR) and a code must be initiated when a patient has a cardiopulmonary arrest. Ideally, the physician, family, and patient (if possible) decide whether CPR is to be performed before resuscitative measures are needed. However, it is the physician who makes the decision to terminate resuscitation efforts in progress. Decisions about resuscitation status often create ethical dilemmas for the nurse, patient, and family (see Chapter 3).

All personnel involved in hospital patient care should have BLS training, including how to operate an automated external defibrillator (AED). This training is also recommended for the lay public and can be obtained through the Heartsaver courses offered by the AHA. ACLS provider training is available through the AHA and is strongly recommended for anyone working in critical care.

RAPID RESPONSE TEAMS

The RRT is designed to improve recognition of and response to clinical deterioration in patients and ensure that interventions are available quickly before an actual cardiopulmonary arrest. The goal is to improve patient outcomes and decrease hospital mortality.[22,23,35] Failure to recognize changes in a patient's condition until major complications, including death, have occurred is referred to as *failure to rescue*.[7] Conditions associated with failure to rescue or a delay in activation of RRT include acute respiratory failure, acute cardiac failure, acute changes in level of consciousness, hypotension, dysrhythmias, pulmonary edema, and sepsis.[29] Up to 80% of patients having an in-hospital cardiac arrest have signs of physiological instability as evidenced by changes in heart rate, blood pressure, and/or respiratory status in the 24 hours before cardiac arrest.[10,17] The RRT concept is based on three components: (1) identification of clinical deterioration that triggers early notification of a specific team of responders, (2) rapid intervention by the response team that includes both personnel and equipment that is brought to the patient, and (3) ongoing evaluation through data collection and analysis to improve prevention and response.[7,17]

The RRT is a resource team that can be called to the bedside 24 hours a day, 7 days a week, to assess patients outside the critical care unit and intervene as needed; the team also supports and educates the nursing staff.[38] The RRT is activated when a patient fulfills predefined criteria. These criteria include deterioration in heart rate, blood pressure, respirations, pulse oximetry saturation, mental status, urinary output, and laboratory values. Together, these are the components of an early warning score system that has been shown to predict cardiac arrest and death within 48 hours of measurement.[32] In addition, the RRT can be activated when a staff member is concerned about changes in a patient's condition. Some institutions empower family members to activate the RRT if they identify a change in the patient's condition.

Composition of the RRT varies based on institutional needs and resources. Some are composed of a critical care nurse, a respiratory therapist, and a physician. Other members may include an acute care nurse practitioner, a clinical nurse specialist, or a physician's assistant.[19] Once the RRT is activated, personnel and equipment are brought to the patient's bedside within minutes. The RRT carries equipment that ranges from a stethoscope to more complex monitoring equipment, including a portable electrocardiogram (ECG) monitor, pulse oximetry monitor, oxygen delivery system, IV supplies, and medications. Point-of-care testing equipment to perform a blood glucose measurement, arterial blood gas analysis, hemoglobin and hematocrit, and a basic metabolic panel may be available. ACLS algorithms, standing medical orders, and evidence-based protocols guide RRT interventions.

Data on RRT calls and patient outcomes are reviewed to develop strategies to prevent clinical deterioration and optimize outcomes. Research on the activation of RRTs demonstrated a reduction in cardiac arrests, length of stay, and incidence of acute illness such as respiratory failure, stroke, severe sepsis, and acute kidney injury.[41] Systematic literature reviews and meta-analyses evaluating outcomes have shown conflicting results, with one showing that RRTs are not associated with lower hospital mortality rates in hospitalized adults and others showing reduced rates of mortality and in-hospital cardiac arrest[5,6,22,35,39] (see Evidence-Based Practice: Outcomes of Rapid Response Teams). The use of RRTs to improve patient care by fostering end-of-life discussions between patients, their families, and healthcare providers has been introduced. Potential advantages include provision of palliative care, prevention of progression to cardiac arrest, and discussions about the likelihood of success with therapies in the critical care unit.[7,8,18,33,36]

Some institutions use the RRT to provide proactive rounding whereby a team member conducts rounds in the non–critical care units to identify high-risk patients and intervene preemptively. These activities have resulted in fewer cardiac arrests and code deaths, as well as increased RRT interventions and transfers to a higher level of care.[13]

STUDY BREAK

1. The goal of a rapid response team is to:
   A. Prevent cardiac and respiratory arrest
   B. Decrease critical care unit admissions
   C. Increase hospital length of stay
   D. Ensure that emergency equipment (code cart, defibrillator) are working properly

---

EVIDENCE-BASED PRACTICE
Outcomes of Rapid Response Teams

Problem

The goal of rapid response teams (RRTs) is to treat patients proactively to avoid cardiac arrest and reduce hospital mortality. Data are needed to evaluate outcomes.

Question

What are outcomes associated with RRTs?

Evidence

Solomon and colleagues reviewed the results of 30 studies related to outcomes of RRTs. Twenty-two studies were considered moderate- to good-quality studies. Meta-analysis found a reduction in both mortality and non–critical care unit inpatient cardiac arrests in both adult and pediatric inpatient populations. The presence of a physician on the team was not associated with improved outcomes.

Implications for Nursing

These data show positive outcomes associated with RRTs. Nurses are integral personnel on such teams. Trained, experienced personnel who practice under established protocols are essential to such teams to contribute to positive outcomes.

Level of Evidence

A—Meta-analysis

Reference

Solomon RS, Corwin GS, Barclay DC, et al. Effectiveness of rapid response teams on rates of in-hospital cardiopulmonary arrest and mortality: A systematic review and meta-analysis. *J Hosp Med.* 2016;11(6):438–444.

ROLES OF CAREGIVERS IN CODE MANAGEMENT

Prompt recognition of a patient's arrest and rapid initiation of BLS and ACLS measures are essential for improved patient outcomes. The first person to recognize that a patient has had an arrest should call for help, instruct someone to "call a code," call for a defibrillator or AED, and begin CPR. One-person CPR is continued until additional help arrives.

Code Team

Most hospitals have code teams that are designated to respond to codes (Table 11.1). Key personnel are notified via an overhead paging system or individual pagers to assist with code management. The code team usually consists of a physician, critical care or emergency department nurses, a nursing

TABLE 11.1 Roles and Responsibilities of Code Team Members

Team Member	Primary Role
Code leader (usually a physician)	Directs code Makes diagnoses and treatment decisions
Primary nurse	Provides information to code leader Measures vital signs Assists with procedures Administers medications
Second nurse	Coordinates use of the code cart Prepares medications Assembles equipment (intubation, suction)
Nursing supervisor	Controls the crowd Contacts the attending physician Assists with medications and procedures Ensures that a bed is available in critical care unit Assists with transfer of patient to critical care unit
Nurse or assistant	Records events on designated form
Anesthesiologist or nurse anesthetist	Intubates patient Manages airway and oxygenation
Respiratory therapist	Assists with ventilation and intubation Obtains blood sample for ABG analysis Sets up respiratory equipment/mechanical ventilator
Pharmacist or pharmacy technician	Assists with medication preparation Prepares IV infusions
ECG technician	Obtains 12-lead ECG
Chaplain	Supports family

ABG, Arterial blood gas; *ECG*, electrocardiogram.

supervisor, a nurse anesthetist or anesthesiologist, a respiratory therapist, a pharmacist or pharmacy technician, an ECG technician, and a chaplain. The code team responds to the code and works in conjunction with the patient's nurse and primary physician, if present. If a code team does not exist, any available trained personnel usually respond. Teamwork during a code is essential (see QSEN Exemplar box).

Code Leader. The person who directs, or runs, the code is responsible for making diagnoses and treatment decisions. The leader is usually a physician, preferably one who is experienced in code management, such as an intensivist or emergency medicine physician. However, the leader may be the patient's primary physician or another physician who is available and qualified for the task. If several physicians are present, one assumes responsibility for being the code leader and should be the only person giving orders for interventions, to avoid confusion and conflict. In some small hospitals, codes may be directed by a nurse trained in ACLS. In this situation, standing physician orders are needed to guide and support the nurse's decision making.

The code leader needs information about the patient to make treatment decisions, including the reason for the patient's hospitalization, current treatments and medications, the patient's code status, and the events that occurred immediately before the code. If possible, the code leader should not perform

✳ QSEN EXEMPLAR

Teamwork and Collaboration, Quality Improvement, and Evidence-Based Practice

Teamwork is essential for code teams. Advanced practice nurses on the hospital system code committee identified the need to improve multiprofessional team training for code responses. They identified that medical residents (who assume the role of code team leader) had significantly less clinical experience in codes and that perceptions of teamwork among code team members could be improved. They developed a 2-hour structured simulated team training program for nurses, respiratory therapists, and medical residents who participated in the code team on a regular basis. Perceptions of teamwork were significantly improved after the 2-hour simulated training exercise. Interactions with other disciplines, structured education related to teamwork, and facilitated debriefing assisted in enhancing teamwork among team members. Quality simulation is an effective way to improve teamwork and enhance code-response skills.

Reference

Mahramus T, Penoyer DA, Waterval EM, et al. Two hours of teamwork training improves teamwork in simulation cardiopulmonary events. *Clin Nurse Spec.* 2016; 30:284–291.

CPR or other tasks. The code leader should give full attention to assessment, diagnosis, and treatment decisions to direct resuscitative efforts.

Code Nurses

Primary nurse. The patient's primary nurse should be free to relate information to the person directing the code. The primary nurse may also start IV lines, measure vital signs, administer emergency medications, assist with procedures, or defibrillate the patient as directed by the code leader (if the primary nurse is qualified).

Second nurse. The major task of the second nurse is to coordinate the use of the code cart. This nurse must be thoroughly familiar with the layout of the cart and the location of items. This nurse locates, prepares, and labels medications and IV fluids and also assembles equipment for intubation, suctioning, and other procedures, such as central line insertion. An additional nurse or assistant records the code events on a designated form (code record).

Nursing supervisor. The nursing supervisor responds to the code to assist in whatever manner is needed. Frequently, more people respond to a code than are needed. One job of the supervisor is to limit the number of people involved in the code to only those necessary and those there for learning purposes. This approach decreases crowding and confusion. Other responsibilities may include contacting the patient's primary physician, relaying information to the staff and family, and ensuring that all necessary equipment is present and functioning. If the patient must be transferred to the critical care unit, the supervisor may also ensure that a critical care bed is available and coordinate the transfer.

Anesthesiologist or Nurse Anesthetist. The anesthesiologist or nurse anesthetist assumes control of the patient's ventilation and oxygenation. This team member intubates the patient to ensure an adequate airway and to facilitate ventilation. The primary or second nurse assists with the setup and checking of intubation equipment.

Respiratory Therapist. The respiratory therapist usually assists with manual ventilation of the patient before and after intubation. The therapist may also obtain a blood sample for arterial blood gas analysis, set up oxygen and ventilation equipment, and suction the patient. In some institutions, the respiratory therapist performs intubation.

Pharmacist or Pharmacy Technician. In some hospitals, a pharmacist or pharmacy technician responds to codes to prepare medications and mix IV infusions for administration. The pharmacist may also calculate appropriate medication doses based on the patient's weight. Frequently, pharmacy staff members are also responsible for bringing additional medications. At the termination of the code, pharmacy staff may replenish the code cart medications and ensure pharmacy charges to the patient's account.

Electrocardiogram Technician. In some hospitals, an ECG technician responds to codes. This person is available to obtain 12-lead ECGs that may be ordered to assist with diagnosis and treatment.

Chaplain. As a code team member, the hospital chaplain can be very helpful in comforting and waiting with the patient's family. The chaplain or other support person usually takes the family to a quiet, private area for waiting and remains with them during the code. This person may also be able to check on the patient periodically to provide the family with a progress report.

Other Personnel. Other personnel are available to run errands, such as taking blood samples to the laboratory or obtaining additional supplies. Only staff members necessary for the code remain in the room. Other team members care for the remaining patients on the unit.

> ### ❓ CRITICAL REASONING ACTIVITY
>
> You are the second nurse to respond to a code. The first nurse is administering cardiopulmonary resuscitation (CPR). Describe your first actions and their rationales.

EQUIPMENT USED IN CODES

After the first person to recognize a code calls for help and begins life-support measures, another team member immediately brings the code cart and defibrillator to the patient's bedside (Fig. 11.1). Code carts vary in organization and layout, but they all contain the same basic emergency equipment and medications. Many hospitals have standardized code carts so that anyone responding to a code is familiar with the location of the items on the cart. In other hospitals, the makeup and

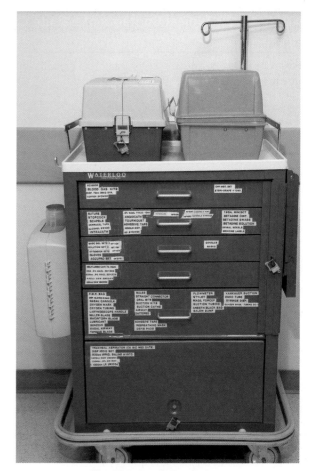

Fig. 11.1 A typical code cart.

organization of the code cart are unique to each unit. Whether carts are standardized or unique to an individual unit, nurses responding to codes must be familiar with them.

Most carts have equipment stored on top and in several drawers. Table 11.2 lists the equipment on a typical code cart. Equipment such as backboards and oxygen tanks may be attached to the cart. Larger equipment is stored on the top of the cart or in a large drawer; smaller items, such as medications and IV equipment, are in the smaller drawers.

A back or cardiac board is usually located on the back or side of the cart. Alternatively, some hospital bed headboards are removable for use as a cardiac board. Place the board under the patient as soon as possible to provide a hard, level surface to perform chest compressions. Either lift up or log roll the patient to one side to place the board. Care is taken to protect the patient's cervical spine if injury is suspected.

A monitor-defibrillator is located on top of the cart or on a separate cart. Monitor the patient's cardiac rhythm via the leads and electrodes or through adhesive electrode pads on this machine. A "quick look" at the patient's cardiac rhythm can also be obtained by placing the defibrillation paddles on the chest. In the hospital setting, continuous rhythm monitoring via the electrodes is preferable to intermittent use of the quick-look defibrillation paddles. The monitor must have a strip-chart recorder for documenting the patient's ECG rhythm for the code record. Monitor-defibrillator units also include capabilities for

TABLE 11.2 Typical Contents of a Code Cart

Main Items	Specific Supplies
Back	
Cardiac board	
Side	
Portable suction machine, bag-valve-mask device, and oxygen tubing	Oxygen tank Container for disposing of needles, syringes, and other sharp items
Top	
Monitor-defibrillator with recorder, clipboard with code record and medication calculation reference sheets	ECG leads, electrodes, conductive gel or adhesive electrode pads; possible transcutaneous pacemaker or combination unit
Airway equipment drawer or box	Oral and nasal airways, face masks, oxygen tubing, bag-valve-mask device, ETTs, stylet, laryngoscope handle with curved and straight blades, lubricating jelly, 10-mL syringes, tape, suction catheters or kits, portable suction device, oxygen flowmeter, end-tidal CO_2 detector
IV equipment drawer	IV catheters of various sizes, tape, syringes, tourniquet, needles and needleless adaptors, IV fluids (NS, Lactated Ringer's solution, and D_5W); IV tubing
Medication drawer or box	All IV push emergency medications in prefilled syringes if available, sterile water and NS for injection, and IV infusion emergency medications (see Table 11.4)
Miscellaneous supply drawer	Sterile and nonsterile gloves, nasogastric tubes, chest tubes, blood pressure cuff, blood collection tubes, sutures, pacemaker magnet, extra ECG recording paper, gauze pads, alcohol preps, face masks with shield, safety glasses, head cover, sterile gowns, scissors, sterile hemostat
Procedure kits	Arterial blood gas kit, peripheral IV start kit, tracheotomy tray, intraosseous insertion kit, central line insertion kit, chest tube insertion tray

CO_2, Carbon dioxide; *D_5W,* 5% dextrose in water; *ECG,* electrocardiogram; *ETTs,* endotracheal tubes; *NS,* normal saline.

transcutaneous pacing and an AED. Some patient care units use an AED for initial code management.

A bag with an attached face mask (bag-valve-mask device) and oxygen tubing is usually kept on the code cart. The tubing is connected to either a wall oxygen inlet or a portable oxygen tank on the code cart. Supplemental oxygen is always used with the bag-valve-mask device. Airway management supplies are located in one of the drawers. Some institutions have a separate box containing airway management supplies.

Another drawer contains IV supplies and solutions. Normal saline (NS) and Lactated Ringer's solution are the IV fluids most often used. A 5% dextrose in water solution (D_5W) in 250- and 500-mL bags is used to prepare vasoactive infusions.

Emergency medications fill another drawer or may be located in a separate box. These include IV push medications and medications that must be added to IV fluids for continuous infusions. Most IV push medications are available in prefilled syringes. Several medications that are given via a continuous infusion (e.g., lidocaine, dopamine) are also available as premixed bags. Medications are discussed in depth later (see Pharmacological Intervention During a Code later in the chapter).

Other important items on the cart include a suction device with a canister and tubing, suction catheters, nasogastric tubes, and a blood pressure cuff. Various kits used for tracheotomy, central line insertion, and intraosseous (IO) insertion may also be on the code cart.

The code cart and defibrillator are usually checked by nursing staff at designated time intervals (every shift or every 24 hours) to ensure that all equipment and medications are present and functional. Once the cart is fully stocked, keep it locked to prevent borrowing of supplies and equipment.

Ensure familiarity with the location of items on the cart by being responsible for checking it. Management of the code is more efficient when the nurse knows where items are located on the code cart and how to use them. Many institutions require nursing staff to participate in periodic mock codes to assist in maintaining skills. Multiprofessional team simulations also provide excellent opportunities for skill development.

RESUSCITATION EFFORTS

The flow of events during a code requires a concentrated team effort. BLS is provided until the code team arrives. Once help arrives, CPR is continued by the two-person technique. Priorities during cardiac arrest are high-quality CPR and early defibrillation. Other tasks, such as connecting the patient to an ECG monitor, starting IV lines, attaching an oxygen source to the bag-valve-mask device, and setting up suction, are performed by available personnel as soon as possible. The activities that occur during the code are summarized in Table 11.3. Often several activities are performed simultaneously.

The code team should be alerted to the patient's code status. Individuals may have advance directives documenting their wishes. The advance directive provides instructions to family

TABLE 11.3 Flow of Events During a Code

Priorities	Equipment From Cart	Intervention
Recognition of arrest		Assess code status, call for help, assess for absence of breathing or only gasping, initiate CPR
Arrival of code team, code cart, cardiac monitor-defibrillator, AED	Cardiac board Bag-valve-mask device with oxygen tubing Oxygen and regulator if not already at bedside	Place patient on cardiac board Ventilate with 100% oxygen and bag-valve-mask device Continue chest compressions
Identification of code leader		Assess patient Direct and supervise team members Solve problems Obtain patient history and determine events leading up to the code
Rhythm diagnosis	Cardiac monitor-defibrillator with ECG leads and adhesive electrode pads AED 12-lead ECG machine	Attach ECG leads or adhesive electrode pads, but do not interrupt CPR
Prompt defibrillation if indicated	Defibrillator/AED	Use correct algorithm
Intubation (if ventilation is inadequate and trained personnel are available)	Suction equipment Laryngoscope Endotracheal tube and other intubation equipment Stethoscope End-tidal CO_2 detector or waveform capnography	Connect suction equipment Intubate patient (interrupt CPR for no longer than 10 seconds) Confirm tube position with waveform capnography, an end-tidal CO_2 detector, or via clinical assessment by listening over bilateral lung fields; observe chest movement Secure endotracheal tube Oxygenate
Venous access	Peripheral or central IV equipment IO insertion kit IV tubing, infusion fluid (NS)	Insert peripheral IV into antecubital site(s) Insert IO needle Central venous catheter may be inserted by physician
Medication administration	Medications as ordered (and in anticipation, based on algorithms)	Use correct algorithm
Ongoing assessment of the patient's response to therapy during resuscitation		Assess frequently: 　Pulse generated with CPR 　Adequacy of artificial ventilation 　Arterial blood gases or other laboratory studies 　Spontaneous pulse after any intervention or rhythm change 　Spontaneous breathing with return of pulse 　Blood pressure, if pulse is present 　Decision to stop, if no response to therapy
Drawing arterial and venous blood specimens	Arterial puncture and venipuncture equipment	Draw specimens Treat as needed, based on results
Documentation	Code record	Accurately record events while resuscitation is in progress Record rhythm strips during the code
Controlling or limiting crowd		Dismiss those not required for bedside tasks
Family notification		Keep family informed of patient's condition Notify outcome with sensitivity Explore options for family presence during code
Transfer of patient to critical care unit		Ensure that a bed is assigned for the patient Transfer with adequate personnel and emergency equipment
Critique		Evaluate events of code and express feelings

AED, Automated external defibrillator; *CO_2*, carbon dioxide; *CPR*, cardiopulmonary resuscitation; *ECG*, electrocardiogram; *IO*, intraosseous; *NS*, normal saline.

members, physicians, and other healthcare providers (see Chapter 3).

Many states have implemented "no CPR" options. The patient, who usually has a terminal illness, signs a document requesting "no CPR" if there is a loss of pulse or if breathing stops. In some states, this document directs the patient to wear a "no CPR" identification bracelet. In the event of a code, the bracelet alerts the responders that CPR efforts are prohibited. The responders should respect the person's wishes.

Basic Life Support

The goal of BLS is to support or restore effective circulation, oxygenation, and ventilation with return of spontaneous circulation. Early CPR and rapid defibrillation with an AED are stressed.[2] CPR must be initiated immediately in the event of an arrest to improve the patient's chance of survival.

BLS providers must be trained in the use of an AED (see Electrical Therapy later in the chapter). Assessment is a part of each step, and the steps are performed in order (Box 11.1). The following summary is adapted from the 2015 AHA standards.[2,21]

Responsiveness. The first intervention is to assess responsiveness by tapping or shaking a patient and shouting, "Are you okay?" If the patient is unresponsive, call for help by shouting to fellow caregivers or by using the nurse-call system. Position the patient on his or her back, turning the head and body as a unit to prevent injury.

BOX 11.1   Steps in Basic Cardiac Life Support

Determine Responsiveness
- Tap and shout, "Are you all right?"
- Shout for help or activate the emergency response system and get the AED or defibrillator.
- Look at chest for absence of breathing or only gasping and simultaneously check carotid pulse for 5 to 10 seconds.

Assess and Support Circulation
- Verify if pulse is definitely felt within 10 seconds.
- If normal breathing with pulse, monitor until help arrives.
- If normal breathing absent with a pulse, open airway and start rescue breathing at 1 breath every 5 or 6 seconds (10 to 12 breaths/min). Check pulse every 2 minutes.
- If breathing absent with no pulse, begin cycles of CPR with chest compressions at rate of 100 to 120 compressions per minute (30 compressions to every 2 breaths).

Provide Rapid Defibrillation
- If no pulse, check for shockable rhythm with a monitor-defibrillator or AED.
- Provide shocks as indicated.
- Follow each shock immediately with CPR, beginning with compressions.

AED, Automated external defibrillator; *CPR,* cardiopulmonary resuscitation.
Modified from Kleinman ME, Brennan EE, Goldberger ZD, et al. Part 5: Adult basic life support and cardiopulmonary resuscitation quality: 2015 American Heart Association guidelines update for cardiopulmonary resuscitation and emergency cardiovascular care. *Circulation.* 2015;132(Suppl 2):S414–S435.

Circulation and Chest Compressions. The next step is to look for the absence of breathing or only gasping and simultaneously check for the presence or absence of the carotid pulse within 10 seconds to detect bradycardia. Assess the pulse even if the patient is attached to a cardiac monitor, because artifact or a loose lead may mimic a cardiac dysrhythmia. Check the carotid pulse on the side nearest the nurse.

If a pulse is present without normal breathing, initiate rescue breathing at a rate of 10 to 12 breaths/min, or 1 breath every 5 to 6 seconds. Assess the pulse every 2 minutes for no longer than 10 seconds. If the pulse is absent, begin chest compressions. Place the patient supine on a firm surface (e.g., cardiac board).

Proper hand position is essential for performing compressions. The location for compressions is the lower half of the sternum in the center of the chest between the nipples. Place the heel of one hand on the lower half of the sternum. Place the heel of the second hand on top of the first hand so that the hands are overlapped and parallel. Using both hands, begin compressions by depressing the sternum at least 2 inches for the average adult and then let the chest return (recoil) to its normal position after each compression. Perform compressions at a rate of at least 100 to 120 per minute ("hard and fast"). The compression-ventilation ratio is 30 compressions to 2 breaths.

Minimize interruptions in chest compressions to less than 10 seconds. Continue CPR until the monitor-defibrillator or AED arrives, adhesive electrode pads are placed, and the AED is ready to analyze the rhythm. Provide shocks as indicated. After each shock, immediately resume CPR, beginning with compressions for 2 minutes.

Airway. There are two methods for opening the airway to provide breaths: the head-tilt/chin-lift method (Fig. 11.2) and the jaw-thrust maneuver. The head-tilt/chin-lift method is performed if there is no evidence of head or neck trauma by placing one hand on the victim's forehead and tilting the head back. Place the fingers of the other hand under the bony part of the patient's lower jaw near the chin. Lift the jaw to bring the chin forward. Usually, two people are needed to perform the jaw thrust and provide breaths with a bag-valve-mask device. Use a jaw thrust if a head or neck injury is suspected.

The first person who arrives to help activates the code team. Some units and emergency departments have an emergency call

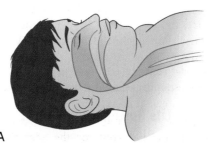
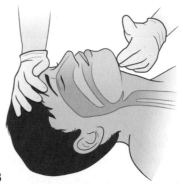

A   B

Fig. 11.2 Head-tilt/chin-lift technique for opening the airway, **A,** Obstruction by the tongue. **B,** Head-tilt/chin-lift maneuver lifts tongue, relieving airway obstruction.

system that can be activated from the patient's room by pressing a button. If alone and an emergency call system is not available, press the nurse-call system and begin CPR. When the call is answered, state, "Call a code!"

Breathing. Barrier devices must be available in the workplace for individuals who are expected to perform CPR. In the hospital setting, these include a pocket mask at every patient's bedside. Critical care units often have a bag-valve-mask device available for each patient. Personnel are trained to use the bag-valve-mask device effectively.

Ventilation of the patient with a bag-valve-mask device requires that an open airway be maintained. Frequently, an oral airway is used to keep the airway patent and to facilitate ventilation. Connect the bag-valve-mask device to an oxygen source set at 15 L/min. Position the face mask to seal over the patient's mouth and nose after the airway is opened. Manually ventilate the patient with the bag-valve-mask device (Fig. 11.3). During CPR, deliver two breaths during a pause in compressions. Each breath is delivered over approximately 1 second.

Advanced Cardiovascular Life Support

For cardiac or respiratory emergencies, many institutions follow the AHA standards for ACLS. The tools of management are the BLS survey followed by the ACLS survey.[21]

The BLS survey focuses on early CPR and rapid defibrillation. The ABCDs of ACLS are the same as for BLS: airway, breathing, and compressions or circulation. The "D" refers to differential diagnosis, or searching, finding, and treating reversible causes.

Airway. Airway management involves reassessment of the original techniques established in BLS. Endotracheal intubation provides definitive airway management and, if needed, is performed by properly trained personnel during the resuscitation effort.[21] The benefit of endotracheal intubation is weighed against the effects of interrupting chest compressions. If bag-valve-mask ventilation is adequate, endotracheal

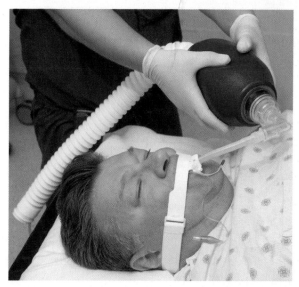

Fig. 11.4 Ventilation with a bag-valve device connected to an endotracheal tube. (Reprinted with permission, Cleveland Clinic Center for Medical Art & Photography © 2011–2019. All Rights Reserved.)

intubation may be deferred until the patient fails to respond to initial CPR and defibrillation or until spontaneous circulation returns.

Techniques of endotracheal intubation are discussed in Chapter 10. Once intubated, the patient is manually ventilated with a bag-valve device attached to the endotracheal tube (ETT; Fig. 11.4). The bag-valve device should have a reservoir and be connected to an oxygen source to deliver 100% oxygen. Chest compressions are not stopped for ventilations. Chest compressions are delivered continuously at a rate of 100 to 120 per minute. Ventilations are delivered at a rate of 1 breath every 6 seconds or approximately 10 breaths/min.

Breathing. Breathing assessment determines whether the ventilatory efforts are causing the chest to rise. If the patient is intubated, confirm ETT placement by continuous waveform capnography (discussed in more detail later in the chapter) or with the use of an end-tidal carbon dioxide ($ETCO_2$) detector (Fig. 11.5).[21] Listen for bilateral breath sounds and observe chest movement with ventilation as part of the assessment. If no chest expansion is present with bag-valve ventilation, the ETT has mistakenly been placed in the esophagus and must be removed immediately. Obtain a chest radiograph after the code to confirm placement.

Circulation. Circulation initially focuses on chest compressions, attachment of electrodes and leads to the monitor-defibrillator, rhythm identification, IV and/or IO access, and medication administration. If ventricular fibrillation (VF) or pulseless ventricular tachycardia (VT) is identified, deliver high-energy unsynchronized shocks, followed by 2 minutes of chest compressions with ventilation. Then establish IV access for medication administration. A patent IV catheter is necessary during an arrest for the administration of fluids and medications. IO cannulation is recommended by the AHA as the primary alternative to IV access.[21] IO cannulation provides

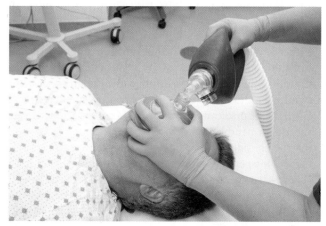

Fig. 11.3 Rescue breathing with bag-valve-mask device. (Reprinted with permission, Cleveland Clinic Center for Medical Art & Photography © 2011–2019. All Rights Reserved.)

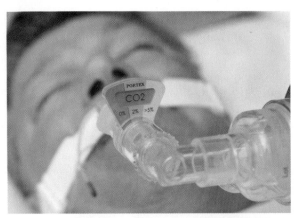

Fig. 11.5 End-tidal carbon dioxide detector connected to an endotracheal tube. Exhaled carbon dioxide reacts with the device to create a color change, indicating correct endotracheal tube placement. (Reprinted with permission, Cleveland Clinic Center for Medical Art & Photography © 2011–2019. All Rights Reserved.)

access to the bone marrow and is a rapid, safe, and reliable route for administering medications, blood, and IV fluids during resuscitation. Commercially available kits facilitate IO access in adults. Endotracheal administration of medications may be considered; however, tracheal absorption of medications is poor, and optimal dosing is not known. Medications that can be administered through the ETT until IV access is established include epinephrine, atropine, and lidocaine.[21]

Most critically ill patients have IV access. If the patient does not have IV access or needs additional IV access, insert a large-bore peripheral IV catheter. The antecubital vein is the first target for IV access. Other areas for IV insertion include the dorsum of the hands and the wrist. If a peripheral IV cannot be started, the physician inserts a central line for IV access. The IO route is an option if IV access is difficult.

NS is the preferred IV fluid because it expands intravascular volume better than dextrose. When any medication is administered by the peripheral IV route, it is best followed with a 20-mL bolus of IV fluid and elevation of the extremity for about 10 to 20 seconds to enhance delivery to the central circulation.

Differential Diagnosis. Differential diagnosis involves searching for, finding, and treating reversible causes of the cardiopulmonary arrest. Cardiac dysrhythmias that result in cardiac arrests have many possible causes (Box 11.2). The lethal dysrhythmias include VF or pulseless VT, asystole, and pulseless electrical activity (PEA). Other dysrhythmias that may lead to a cardiopulmonary arrest include symptomatic bradycardias and symptomatic tachycardias. Algorithms for treating these rhythm disorders have been established by the AHA.[21] Because these algorithms periodically change, they are not reproduced here; rather, critical actions in the management of these dysrhythmias are summarized in the following sections.

Recognition and Treatment of Dysrhythmias

Ventricular Fibrillation and Pulseless Ventricular Tachycardia. The most common initial rhythms in witnessed sudden cardiac arrest are VF or pulseless VT. When VF is present, the

BOX 11.2	**Reversible Causes of Cardiac Arrest**
H's	**T's**
Hypovolemia	**T**ension pneumothorax
Hypoxia	**T**amponade, cardiac
Hydrogen ion (acidosis)	**T**oxins (drug overdose)
Hypokalemia or hyperkalemia	**T**hrombosis, pulmonary
Hypothermia	**T**hrombosis, coronary (massive myocardial infarction)

Modified from Link MS, Berkow LC, Kudenchuk PJ, et al. Part 7: Adult advanced cardiovascular life support: 2015 American Heart Association guidelines update for cardiopulmonary resuscitation and emergency cardiovascular care. *Circulation.* 2015;132(18 Suppl 2):S444–S464.

heart quivers and does not pump blood. The treatments for VF and for pulseless VT are the same.

Critical actions.

- Initiate the BLS survey. Begin CPR until a defibrillator is available. Defibrillate as soon as possible because early CPR and rapid defibrillation increase the chance of survival and a good neurological outcome.
- Give one shock and resume CPR, beginning with chest compressions. If a biphasic defibrillator is available, use the dose at which that defibrillator has been shown to be effective for terminating VF (typically 120 to 200 joules [J]). If the dose is not known, use the maximum dose available. If a monophasic defibrillator is available, use an initial shock of 360 J and use 360 J for subsequent shocks. Resume CPR immediately, beginning with chest compressions for 2 minutes. After 2 minutes of CPR, check rhythm. Monophasic versus biphasic defibrillation is discussed later in the chapter (see Electrical Therapy).
- If VF or VT persists, continue CPR, charge the defibrillator, and obtain IV or IO access. Give one shock (with a biphasic defibrillator, use same or higher joules as for the first shock; with a monophasic defibrillator, use 360 J). Resume CPR immediately, beginning with chest compressions for 2 minutes.
- After IV or IO access is available, administer epinephrine, 1 mg IV or IO every 3 to 5 minutes, if VF persists. Check rhythm after 2 minutes of CPR. If VF or VT persists, resume CPR immediately, beginning with chest compressions for 2 minutes, and charge the defibrillator.
- Give one shock (with a biphasic defibrillator, use same or higher joules as for the first shock; with a monophasic defibrillator, use 360 J). Resume CPR immediately for 2 minutes.
- Consider giving an antidysrhythmic medication either before or after the shock; however, there is no evidence that an antidysrhythmic medication given during a cardiac arrest increases survival or neurological outcome.[21] Amiodarone or lidocaine may be considered for VF or VT unresponsive to defibrillation.[28] Dosages and administration are discussed later in the chapter (see Pharmacological Intervention During a Code).
- Reassess the patient frequently. Search for and treat the underlying cause of the cardiac arrest. Check for return of pulse, spontaneous respirations, and blood pressure. Resume CPR if appropriate.

Pulseless Electrical Activity and Asystole. The goal in treating any rhythm without a pulse is to determine and treat the probable underlying cause. PEA, an organized rhythm without a pulse, is often associated with clinical conditions that can be reversed if they are identified early and treated appropriately.[21] Asystole, the absence of electrical activity on the ECG, has a poor prognosis. It is essential to search for and treat reversible causes of asystole for resuscitation efforts to be successful.

Critical actions.

- Initiate the BLS survey. Initiate CPR for 2 minutes. Obtain IV or IO access. Endotracheal intubation is performed only if ventilations with a bag-valve-mask device are ineffective.
- Consider possible causes and treat (see Box 11.2).
- Confirm asystole by ensuring that lead and cable connections are correct, ensuring that the power is on, and verifying asystole in another lead. An additional lead confirms or rules out the possibility of a fine VF.
- Check rhythm for no longer than 10 seconds. If no rhythm is present (e.g., asystole), resume CPR for 2 minutes. If organized electrical activity is present, palpate a pulse for at least 5 seconds but no longer than 10 seconds. If no pulse is present (e.g., PEA), resume CPR starting with chest compressions for 2 minutes.
- After IV or IO access is available, administer epinephrine, 1 mg IV or IO every 3 to 5 minutes. CPR is not stopped for drug administration. Consider endotracheal intubation.
- Resume CPR for 2 minutes and then check the rhythm and pulse.
- Continue the ACLS survey while identifying underlying causes and initiating related interventions.
- Consider termination of resuscitative efforts if a reversible cause is not rapidly identified and treated and the patient fails to respond to the BLS and ACLS surveys. The decision to terminate resuscitative efforts in the hospital is the responsibility of the treating physician and is based on consideration of many factors, including time from collapse to CPR, time from collapse to first defibrillation attempt (if a shockable rhythm is present), comorbid disease, pre-arrest state, initial rhythm at time of arrest, and response to resuscitative measures. In intubated patients, failure to achieve an $ETCO_2$ of greater than 10 mm Hg by continuous waveform capnography after 20 minutes of CPR may also be considered in deciding when to end resuscitative efforts.[21]

Symptomatic Bradycardia. The category of symptomatic bradycardia encompasses two types: bradycardia, a heart rate less than 60 beats/min (e.g., third-degree heart block), and symptomatic bradycardia, any heart rhythm that is slow enough to cause hemodynamic compromise (Box 11.3). If bradycardia is the cause of the symptoms, the heart rate is typically less than 50 beats/min. The cause of the bradycardia must be considered. For example, hypotension associated with bradycardia may be caused by dysfunction of the myocardium or hypovolemia, rather than by a conduction system or autonomic nervous system disturbance.

BOX 11.3 Signs and Symptoms of Poor Perfusion Associated With Bradycardia

Signs
- Hypotension
- Orthostatic hypotension
- Diaphoresis
- Pulmonary congestion
- Pulmonary edema

Symptoms
- Chest pain
- Shortness of breath
- Decreased level of consciousness
- Weakness
- Fatigue
- Dizziness
- Syncope

Critical actions.

- Perform ACLS survey. Maintain a patent airway and assist breathing as necessary. Provide oxygen if patient is hypoxic as determined by pulse oximetry. Monitor blood pressure, heart rate, and pulse oximetry. Obtain a 12-lead ECG. Establish IV access. Search for and treat possible contributing factors.
- Determine whether signs and symptoms of poor perfusion are present and whether they are related to the bradycardia (see Box 11.3). If adequate perfusion is present, observe and monitor.
- If poor perfusion is present, administer atropine, 0.5 mg IV every 3 to 5 minutes to a total dose of 3 mg. Atropine is not indicated in second-degree atrioventricular (AV) block type II or in third-degree AV block.
- If atropine is ineffective, prepare for transcutaneous pacing. Analgesics or sedatives may be needed because patients often find the pacing stimulus that is delivered with this therapy uncomfortable.
- Consider epinephrine or dopamine infusion if pacing is not effective. Either may be used with symptomatic bradycardia if low blood pressure is associated with the bradycardia.

STUDY BREAK

2. Signs and symptoms of poor perfusion associated with bradycardia include:
   A. Hypertension, diaphoresis, dizziness
   B. Decreased level of consciousness, hypotension, cough
   C. Chest pain, hypotension, shortness of breath
   D. Fatigue, abdominal pain, fever

Unstable Tachycardia. Tachycardia is defined as a heart rate greater than 100 beats/min. *Unstable tachycardia* occurs when the heart beats too fast for the patient's clinical condition. The treatment of this group of dysrhythmias involves the rapid recognition that the patient is symptomatic and that the signs and symptoms are caused by the tachycardia. If the heart rate is less than 150 beats/min, it is unlikely that the symptoms of instability are caused by the tachycardia. Synchronized cardioversion and antidysrhythmic therapy may be needed.[21]

Critical actions.

- Perform the BLS and ACLS surveys. Assess the patient and recognize the signs of cardiovascular instability, including increased work of breathing (tachypnea, intercostal retractions, paradoxical abdominal breathing) and hypoxia as determined by pulse oximetry. Provide supplemental oxygen, assess blood pressure, and establish IV access. Determine cardiac rhythm.

- Assess the degree of instability. If the patient has hypotension, acutely altered mental status, signs of shock, chest discomfort, or acute heart failure, prepare for synchronized cardioversion. If the ECG complex is regular and narrow, consider administration of adenosine.
- If cardioversion is indicated, premedicate with sedation if the patient is conscious. Cardioversion is an uncomfortable procedure.
- Perform synchronized cardioversion at the appropriate energy level. Supraventricular tachycardia and atrial flutter often respond to an energy dose of 50 to 100 J. If the initial attempt with 50 J fails, the energy dose is increased stepwise for subsequent attempts. In cases of unstable atrial fibrillation, start at 200 J (monophasic) or 120 to 200 J (biphasic) and increase the energy dose stepwise for subsequent cardioversion attempts. Cardioversion for monomorphic ventricular tachycardia with a pulse should be initiated at 100 J (monophasic or biphasic) and increased stepwise for subsequent attempts.[21]
- Reassess the patient and rhythm, and consider further monitoring and antidysrhythmic therapy including adenosine, procainamide, or amiodarone.

Electrical Therapy

The therapeutic use of electrical current has expanded with the addition and increased use of the AED. This section addresses the use of electricity in code management for the purposes of defibrillation, cardioversion, and transcutaneous (external) pacing.

Defibrillation. The only effective treatment for VF and pulseless VT is defibrillation. VF deteriorates into asystole if not treated. VF may occur as a result of coronary artery disease, myocardial infarction, electrical shock, drug overdose, near drowning, or acid-base imbalance.

Definition. *Defibrillation* is the delivery of an electrical current to the heart through the use of a defibrillator (Fig. 11.6). The current can be delivered through the chest wall via external paddles or adhesive electrode pads ("hands-off" defibrillation) connected to cables. Smaller internal paddles may be used to deliver current directly to the heart during cardiac surgery when the chest is open and the heart is visualized. Defibrillation works by completely depolarizing the heart and disrupting the impulses that are causing the dysrhythmia. This allows the sinoatrial node or other pacemaker to resume control of the heart's rhythm.

Defibrillation delivers energy or current in waveforms. *Monophasic* waveforms deliver current in one direction; *biphasic* waveforms deliver current that flows in a positive direction for a specified duration and then reverses and flows in a negative direction. Biphasic defibrillation uses fewer joules than monophasic defibrillation. Biphasic defibrillation is at least as

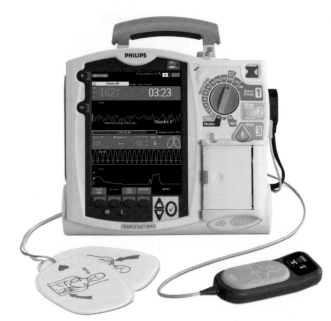

Fig. 11.6 Defibrillator. (Courtesy Philips Healthcare, Andover, MA.)

effective as monophasic defibrillation and in some reports is more effective in converting VF with fewer shocks.[21]

Procedure. Use of conductive materials during defibrillation reduces transthoracic impedance and enhances the flow of electrical current through the chest structures. Conductive materials include paddles with electrode paste, gel pads, and adhesive electrode pads.

Two methods exist for paddle or adhesive electrode pad placement for external defibrillation. In the *anterior method,* one paddle or adhesive electrode pad is placed at the second intercostal space to the right of the sternum, and the other paddle or adhesive electrode pad is placed at the fifth intercostal space, midaxillary line, to the left of the sternum (Fig. 11.7). An alternative method is *anterior-posterior placement.* Adhesive electrode pads are used to facilitate correct positioning. The anterior electrode pad is placed at the left anterior precordial area, and the posterior electrode pad is placed at the left posterior-infrascapular area or at the posterior-infrascapular area (Fig. 11.8).

The amount of energy delivered is measured in joules, or watt-seconds. For monophasic defibrillation, 360 J is used for all shocks. For biphasic defibrillation, refer to the manufacturer's instructions for the amount of joules to be delivered to the patient. If the recommended dose is unknown, use the maximum dose available.[21]

For the shock to be effective, some type of conductive medium must be placed between the paddles and the skin. If paddles are used, completely cover them with gel to conduct the electricity. Commercially prepared defibrillator gel pads are available that facilitate defibrillation and prevent burns on the patient's skin that may occur when paddles are used. Adhesive electrode pads used in hands-off defibrillation also have conductive gel and are recommended instead of paddles to enhance the delivery of the electrical current.[21,23] Adhesive electrode pads reduce the risk of current arcing, facilitate monitoring of

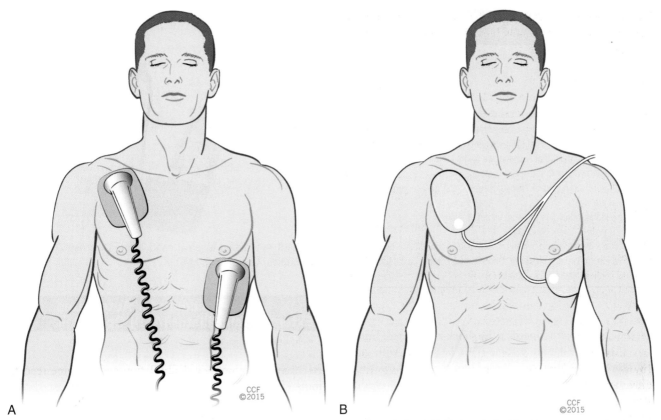

Fig. 11.7 Standard placement of paddles or adhesive electrode pads for defibrillation. **A,** Paddle placement. **B,** Anterior placement of adhesive electrode pads for defibrillation or transcutaneous pacing.

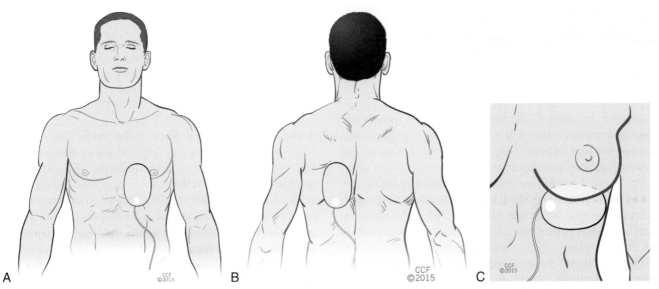

Fig. 11.8 Adhesive electrode pad placement for defibrillation or transcutaneous pacing. **A,** Anterior. **B,** Posterior. **C,** Anterior in females.

the patient's underlying rhythm, and allow the rapid delivery of a shock when needed.

Charge the defibrillator to the desired setting. Place the paddles firmly on the patient's chest to facilitate skin contact and reduce the impedance to the flow of current. Implement safety measures to prevent injury to the patient and to personnel

assisting with the procedure. Ensure that all personnel are standing clear of the bed and visually check to see that no one is in contact with the patient or bed. It is important that this step not be omitted when hands-off defibrillation is used. The announcement "Clear. I am going to shock on three" provides an audible check that no one is touching the patient. "One, two,

BOX 11.4 Procedure for External Defibrillation

- Apply adhesive electrode pads or gel pads to the patient's chest (or apply conductive gel to paddles).
- Turn on the defibrillator.
- Select the energy level.
- If using paddles, position the paddles on the patient's chest.
- If using adhesive electrode pads, connect the electrode cable to the defibrillator.
- Ensure that all personnel (including yourself) are clear of the patient, the bed, and any equipment that is connected to the patient.
- Charge the defibrillator to the desired setting.
- Shout, "Clear. I am going to shock on three," and look to verify that all personnel are clear.
- If using paddles, apply firm pressure on both paddles.
- Shout, "One, two, three. Shocking."
- Deliver shock by depressing buttons on each paddle simultaneously. If using adhesive electrode pads, press the "Shock" button on the defibrillator.
- Resume cardiopulmonary resuscitation.

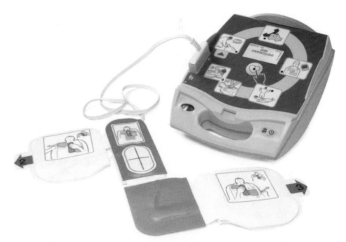

Fig. 11.9 Automated external defibrillator. (Courtesy ZOLL Medical Corporation, Chelmsford, MA.)

BOX 11.5 Procedure for Automated External Defibrillator (AED) Operation

- Turn the power on.
- Attach the AED connecting cable to the AED "box."
- Attach the adhesive electrode pads to the patient:
  - Place one electrode pad on the upper right sternal border directly below the clavicle.
  - Place the other electrode pad lateral to the left nipple, with the top margin of the pad a few inches below the axilla.
  - The correct position of the electrode pads is often displayed on the electrode pads.
- Attach the AED connecting cable to the adhesive electrode pads (if not already connected).
- Clear personnel from the patient (no one should be touching the patient) and press the "Analyze" button to start rhythm analysis.
- Listen or read the message: "Shock indicated" or "No shock indicated."
- Clear personnel from the patient and press the "Shock" button if shock is indicated.

three, shocking" is announced as the shock is delivered. Immediately after defibrillation, resume CPR, beginning with chest compressions for 2 minutes, followed by a check of the patient's rhythm and pulse. Record rhythm strips during the procedure to document response. The procedure for defibrillation is summarized in Box 11.4.

Complications of defibrillation include burns on the skin and damage to the heart muscle. Arcing of electricity or a spark can occur if the paddles are not firmly placed on the skin, excessive conductive gel is used, or the skin is wet. Arcing has also been observed when patients have medication patches with aluminized backing (e.g., nitroglycerin, nicotine, pain medication); remove such patches and clean the area before defibrillation. Remove body jewelry, such as nipple rings, before defibrillation to reduce the risk for arcing during the procedure.

Automated External Defibrillation. The AED extends the range of personnel trained in the use of a defibrillator and shortens the time between code onset and defibrillation. The AED is considered an integral part of emergency cardiac care.

Definition. The AED is an external defibrillator with rhythm analysis capabilities (Fig. 11.9). It is used to achieve early defibrillation. Because of the ease of use, AEDs may be placed on medical-surgical patient units, in emergency response vehicles, and in public places.

The AED should be used only if the patient is in cardiac arrest (unresponsive, absent or abnormal breathing, and no pulse). Confirmation that the patient is in cardiac arrest must be obtained before the AED is attached.[21]

Procedure. Attach the AED to the patient by two adhesive pads and connecting cable. Each adhesive electrode pad depicts an image of correct placement on the chest. These pads serve a dual purpose: recording the rhythm and delivering the shock. AEDs eliminate the need for training in rhythm recognition because these microprocessor-based devices analyze the surface ECG signal. The AED "looks" at the patient's rhythm numerous times to confirm the presence of a rhythm for which

defibrillation is indicated. The semiautomatic "shock advisory" AED charges the device and "advises" the operator to press a button to defibrillate. The fully automated AED requires only that the operator attach the defibrillation pads and turn on the device (Box 11.5). Both models deliver AHA-recommended energy levels for the treatment of VF or pulseless VT. They are not designed to deliver synchronous shocks and will shock VT if the rate exceeds preset values.

Cardioversion

Definition. Cardioversion is the delivery of a shock that is synchronized with the patient's cardiac rhythm. The purpose of cardioversion is to disrupt an ectopic pacemaker that is causing a dysrhythmia and to allow the sinoatrial node to take control of the rhythm. During an emergency situation, cardioversion is used to treat patients with VT, atrial flutter, atrial fibrillation, or supraventricular tachycardia who have a pulse but are developing symptoms related to poor perfusion, such as hypotension and a decreased level of consciousness. Elective cardioversion is used to treat stable atrial flutter and atrial fibrillation.

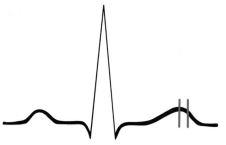

Fig. 11.10 Approximate location of the vulnerable period. (From Conover MB. *Understanding electrocardiography*. 4th ed. St. Louis, MO: Mosby; 2003.)

Cardioversion is similar to defibrillation except that the delivery of energy is synchronized to occur during ventricular depolarization (peak of the QRS complex). Delivering the shock during the QRS complex prevents the shock from being delivered during repolarization (T wave), which is often called the vulnerable period. If a shock is delivered during this vulnerable period (Fig. 11.10), VF may occur. Because the purpose of cardioversion is to disrupt the rhythm rather than completely depolarize the heart, less energy is usually required. Cardioversion can be performed with energy levels as low as 50 J. The amount of energy is gradually increased until the rhythm is converted.

? CRITICAL REASONING ACTIVITY

A surgical patient on a general nursing unit has just been successfully defibrillated with the use of an AED by the nursing staff. He is being manually ventilated with a bag-valve-mask device. Identify the current nursing priorities and their rationales.

Procedure. The procedure for cardioversion (Box 11.6) is similar to that for defibrillation. However, set the defibrillator in the "synchronous" mode for the cardioversion. The R waves are sensed by the machine and are indicated by "spikes" or other markings on the monitor of the defibrillator (Fig. 11.11). Verify that all R waves are properly sensed. When it is time to deliver the shock, depress the buttons on the paddles until the shock has been delivered because energy is discharged only during the QRS complex. If a patient is undergoing cardioversion on a nonemergency basis, sedate the patient before the procedure. Record rhythm strips during cardioversion to document response.

Special Situations. Patients at risk for sudden cardiac death may have an implantable cardioverter-defibrillator (ICD) and/ or permanent pacemaker that delivers shocks directly to the heart muscle if a life-threatening dysrhythmia is detected. These devices are easily identified because they create a hard lump beneath the skin of the upper chest or abdomen. If a patient with a permanent pacemaker or ICD requires defibrillation, avoid placing the paddle near the generator during the procedure. Although damage to the device rarely occurs, the device can absorb much of the current of defibrillation from the

BOX 11.6 Procedure for Synchronized Cardioversion

- Ensure that emergency equipment is readily available.
- Explain the procedure to the patient.
- Attach monitor leads to the patient. Ensure that the monitor displays the patient's rhythm clearly without artifact.
- Apply the adhesive electrode pads (recommended) or defibrillator gel pads to the patient's chest (or apply conductive gel to the paddles).
- Turn on the defibrillator to "synchronous" mode.
- Observe the rhythm on the monitor to determine that the R wave is properly sensed and marked (usually with a spike) (see Fig. 11.11).
- Sedate the conscious patient unless unstable or rapidly deteriorating.
- Select the appropriate energy level.
- If using paddles, position the paddles on the patient's chest and apply firm pressure.
- Announce, "Charging defibrillator. Stand clear." Ensure that all personnel (including yourself) are clear of the patient, the bed, and any equipment that is connected to the patient.
- Press the "Charge" button on the defibrillator.
- Shout, "Clear. I am going to shock on three," and look to verify that all personnel are clear.
- Shout, "One, two, three. Shocking."
- Deliver synchronized shock by depressing the buttons on each paddle simultaneously or press the shock button on the defibrillator if using adhesive electrode pads. Keep the buttons depressed until the shock has been delivered.
- After the cardioversion, observe the patient's heart rhythm and palpate pulse to determine effectiveness.

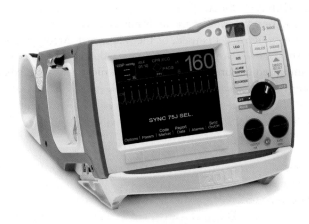

Fig. 11.11 ZOLL R Series monitor-defibrillator with marked R waves for cardioversion. (Courtesy ZOLL Medical Corporation, Chelmsford, MA.)

adhesive electrode pads or paddles, block the shock delivery, and reduce the chance of success. Place the adhesive electrode pad or paddle on either side and not directly on top of the implanted device.[21]

A patient may have an ICD with dual-chamber pacing capabilities. Be familiar, whenever possible, with the type of therapy the patient's device has been programmed to deliver. By the time VF or VT is recognized on the monitor, the ICD should recognize the rhythm. If a successful shock by the ICD has not occurred by the time the rhythm is noted on the monitor, initiate standard code management protocols. If external defibrillation is unsuccessful, change the location of the adhesive electrode pads or paddles on the chest. Anterior-posterior placement may be more effective than anterior-apex placement.

External defibrillation of a patient while the ICD is firing does not harm the patient or the ICD. ICDs and permanent pacemakers are insulated from damage caused by conventional external defibrillation. There is no danger to personnel if the ICD discharges while staff members are touching the patient. However, the shock may be felt and has been compared to the sensation of contact with an electrical outlet. Assess the pacing and sensing thresholds of the pacemaker or ICD after external defibrillation.

Transcutaneous Cardiac Pacing

Definition. Transcutaneous (external noninvasive) cardiac pacing is used during emergency situations to treat symptomatic bradycardia (hypotension, acutely altered mental status, ischemic chest pain, signs of shock, heart failure) that has not responded to atropine. Transcutaneous pacing is not recommended for asystole. In this method of pacing, the heart is stimulated with externally applied, adhesive electrode pads that deliver the electrical impulse. Impulse conduction occurs across the chest wall to stimulate the cardiac contraction.

The transcutaneous pacemaker may be a freestanding unit with a monitor and a pacemaker. Most models incorporate a monitor, a defibrillator, and an external pacemaker into one system (Fig. 11.12). The advantages of transcutaneous pacemakers include easy operation in an emergent situation, minimal training, and none of the risks associated with invasive pacemakers.

Procedure. The procedure for transcutaneous pacing (Box 11.7) involves the placement of adhesive electrode pads anteriorly and posteriorly on the patient (see Fig. 11.8). Connect the electrodes to the external pacemaker, allowing for hands-off pacing. Set the pacemaker in either asynchronous or demand mode. Some devices permit only demand pacing. In

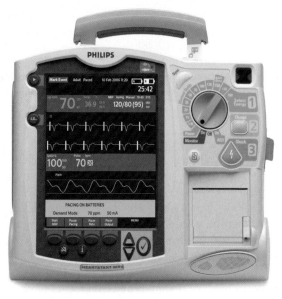

Fig. 11.12 Transcutaneous pacemaker-defibrillator. (Courtesy Philips Healthcare, Andover, MA.)

BOX 11.7   Procedure for Transcutaneous Pacing

- If the patient is alert, explain the procedure.
- Clip excess hair from the patient's chest. Do not shave hair.
- Apply the posterior adhesive electrode pad on the patient's back to the left of the thoracic spine.
- Apply the anterior adhesive electrode pad to the chest. The electrode is centered at the fourth intercostal space to the left of the sternum.
- Connect the electrode cable to the pacemaker generator.
- Turn the unit on. Choose pacing mode (asynchronous or demand).
- Set the pacemaker parameters for heart rate (60 beats/min) and output (2 mA above the dose at which consistent capture is observed) according to the manufacturer's instructions.
- Adjust the heart rate based on the patient's clinical response.
- Assess the adequacy of pacing:
  - Pacemaker spike and QRS complex (capture)
  - Palpable pulse
  - Heart rate and rhythm
  - Blood pressure
  - Level of consciousness
- Observe for patient discomfort. The patient may need sedation and/or analgesia.
- Anticipate follow-up treatment (e.g., insertion of a temporary transvenous pacemaker).

the asynchronous mode, the pacemaker generates a rhythm without regard to the patient's own rhythm. In the demand mode, the pacemaker fires only if the patient's heart rate falls below a preset limit determined by the operator (e.g., 60 beats/min). Adjust the output, in milliamperes (mA), to stimulate a paced beat, usually 2 mA higher than the dose at which consistent capture is observed.

Assess the electrical and mechanical effectiveness of pacing. The electrical activity is verified by a pacemaker "spike." The spike is followed by a broad QRS complex (Fig. 11.13). Mechanical activity is verified by palpation of a pulse during electrical activity. In addition, the patient has signs of improved cardiac output, including increased blood pressure and improved skin color and skin temperature. If the external pacemaker is effective, the patient may need to have a temporary transvenous pacemaker inserted, depending on the cause of the bradycardia.

The alert patient who requires transcutaneous pacing may experience some discomfort. Because the skeletal muscles are stimulated, as well as the heart muscle, the patient may experience a tingling, twitching, or thumping feeling that ranges from mildly uncomfortable to intolerable. Sedation, analgesia, or both may be indicated.

PHARMACOLOGICAL INTERVENTION DURING A CODE

Medications that are administered during a code depend on several factors: the cause of the arrest, the patient's cardiac rhythm, the physician's preference, and the patient's response. The goals of treatment are to reestablish and maintain optimal cardiac function, to correct hypoxemia and acidosis, and to

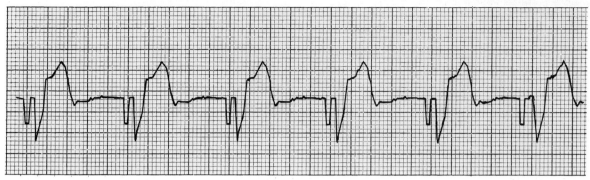

Fig. 11.13 Electrical capture of transcutaneous pacemaker. Notice the pacemaker spikes followed by a wide QRS complex and a tall T wave.

suppress dangerous cardiac ectopic activity. In addition, medications are used to achieve a balance between myocardial oxygen supply and demand, to maintain adequate blood pressure, and to relieve heart failure. Because of the rapid and profound effects these medications can have on cardiac activity and hemodynamic function, continuous ECG monitoring is essential, and hemodynamic monitoring may be instituted as soon as possible after the code. IV push medications given peripherally are followed by flushing with at least 20 mL of IV fluid to ensure central circulation. In addition, because of the precise dosages and careful administration required with these medications,

use infusion pumps to deliver continuous infusions. Titrate IV dosages slowly, while monitoring clinical effectiveness.

The following medications are included in ACLS guidelines and represent those medications most frequently used in code management.[21] Actions, uses, and dosages for each medication, as well as side effects and nursing implications, are discussed in this section and are summarized in Table 11.4.

Oxygen

Oxygen is essential to resuscitation and has several pharmacological considerations. Oxygen is used to treat hypoxemia,

TABLE 11.4 PHARMACOLOGY

Medications Frequently Used in Code Management

Medication	Action/Uses	Dose/Route	Side Effects	Nursing Implications
Adenosine (Adenocard)	Slows conduction in AV node and interrupts AV nodal reentry circuits *Use:* Initial drug of choice for supraventricular dysrhythmias	6 mg rapid IV push over 1-2 sec, followed by 20 mL rapid NS flush; if no response in 1-2 min, give 12 mg repeat dose and flush; may repeat 12 mg dose if necessary	Lightheadedness, headache, dizziness, facial flushing, dyspnea, bronchospasm, and chest pain; may cause asystole up to 15 sec	Half-life 10 sec; higher dose needed with theophylline, lower dose with dipyridamole or after cardiac transplantation Inform patient about potential effects of the medication
Amiodarone (Cordarone)	↓ Membrane excitability, prolongs action potential to terminate VT or VF *Use:* Treatment and prophylaxis of recurrent VF and hemodynamically unstable VT; rapid atrial dysrhythmias	*Cardiac arrest:* 300 mg IV/IO push followed by 150 mg IV/IO in 3-5 min if needed *Recurrent VF/VT:* 150 mg IV over 10 min (15 mg/min); may repeat 150 mg IV q10 min as needed; followed by 360 mg infusion for 6 h (1 mg/min), then 540 mg for next 18 h (0.5 mg/min), for a maximum dose of 2.2 g over 24 h	Bradycardia, headache, hypotension; use with caution on preexisting conduction system abnormalities	Monitor for symptomatic sinus bradycardia, PR, QRS, and QT prolongation. Central venous catheter infusion site preferred with in-line filter
Atropine	↑ SA node automaticity and AV node conduction activity *Use:* Symptomatic bradycardia	*Bradycardia:* 0.5 mg IV q3-5 min to maximum dose of 3 mg 1-2 mg in 10 mL NS or sterile water may be given via ETT	Tachycardia, headache, increased myocardial oxygen consumption and ischemia	Consider transcutaneous pacing, dopamine infusion, or epinephrine infusion if atropine is ineffective
Dopamine (Intropin)	*Moderate doses:* stimulates beta receptors to ↑ cardiac contractility *High doses:* stimulates alpha receptors *Use:* Hypotension not related to hypovolemia	*Moderate doses* (2-10 mcg/kg/min): ↑ contractility and cardiac output *High doses* (10-20 mcg/kg/min): vasoconstriction and ↑ systemic vascular resistance *IV infusion:* 400-800 mg in 250 mL D₅W = 1600-3200 mcg/mL; infuse at 2-5 mcg/kg/min and titrate as needed to maximum 50 mcg/kg/min	Tachycardia, increased dysrhythmias	Extravasation may cause necrosis and sloughing Administer through a central line if possible

Continued

☉ TABLE 11.4　PHARMACOLOGY—cont'd

Medications Frequently Used in Code Management

Medication	Action/Uses	Dose/Route	Side Effects	Nursing Implications
Epinephrine (Adrenalin)	↑ Cardiac contractility, ↑ heart rate, peripheral vasoconstriction, and ↑ arterial blood pressure; improves coronary and cerebral perfusion *Use:* VF, pulseless VT, PEA, asystole; consider after atropine as an alternative infusion to dopamine in symptomatic bradycardia	1 mg IV/IO, or 2-2.5 mg in 10 mL sterile water or NS via ETT; may repeat q3-5 min *IV infusion:* 1 mg in 250 mL D$_5$W or NS; infuse at 2-10 mcg/min and titrate as needed	Tachycardia, hypertension	In a cardiac arrest, may be used as a continuous infusion for hypotension
Lidocaine (Xylocaine)	Suppresses ventricular dysrhythmias, raises fibrillation threshold *Use:* Alternative to amiodarone in cardiac arrest from VF and VT	*VF/VT:* 1-1.5 mg/kg IV/IO, followed by 0.5-0.75 mg/kg q5-10 min to maximum of three doses or 3 mg/kg; may be given by ETT at dose of 2-4 mg/kg in 10 mL sterile water or NS; follow with continuous IV infusion at 1-4 mg/min *IV infusion:* 1 g in 250 mL or 2 g in 500 mL D$_5$W = 4 mg/mL	Neurological toxicity (lethargy, confusion, tinnitus, muscle twitching, paresthesia, seizures), bradycardia if serum lidocaine level is excessive	Lower dose if impaired hepatic blood flow
Magnesium	Essential for enzyme reactions and sodium-potassium pump, ↓ postinfarction dysrhythmias *Use:* Torsades de pointes, hypomagnesemia	*Cardiac arrest:* 1-2 g in 10 mL of D$_5$W IV/IO over 5-20 min *Nonarrest:* 1-2 g in 50-100 mL of D$_5$W IV over 5-60 min	Flushing, bradycardia, hypotension, respiratory depression	Monitor serum magnesium levels
Norepinephrine (Levophed)	Stimulates alpha receptors to cause arterial and venous vasoconstriction Stimulates beta receptors to increase contractility *Use:* Hypotension uncorrected by other medications	Continuous IV infusion at 0.1-0.5 mcg/kg/min (0.5-1 mcg/min), titrated upward as needed to a maximum of 30 mcg/min *IV infusion:* 4 mg in 250 mL D$_5$W	Myocardial ischemia	Extravasation may cause necrosis and sloughing Administer through a central line if possible
Oxygen	↑ Arterial oxygen content and tissue oxygenation *Use:* Cardiopulmonary arrest, chest pain, hypoxemia	100% in a code via bag-valve device with mask		Monitor pulse oximetry values
Sodium bicarbonate	Counteracts metabolic acidosis by binding with hydrogen ions to produce water and carbon dioxide *Use:* Preexisting metabolic acidosis, hyperkalemia, or tricyclic antidepressant overdose	1 mEq/kg IV push initially; subsequent doses based on bicarbonate levels		Ensure adequate CPR, oxygenation, and ventilation Guide administration according to laboratory values

AV, Atrioventricular; *CPR,* cardiopulmonary resuscitation; *D$_5$W,* 5% dextrose in water solution; *ETT,* endotracheal tube; *IO,* intraosseous; *NS,* normal saline; *PEA,* pulseless electrical activity; *q,* every; *SA,* sinoatrial; *VF,* ventricular fibrillation; *VT,* ventricular tachycardia.
Based on data from Link MS, Berkow LC, Kudenchuk PJ, et al. Part 7: Adult advanced cardiovascular life support: 2015 American Heart Association guidelines update for cardiopulmonary resuscitation and emergency cardiovascular care. *Circulation.* 2015;132(18 Suppl 2):S444–S464; Gahart BL, Nazareno AR, Ortega MQ. *2019 Intravenous Medications.* St. Louis, MO: Elsevier; 2019.

which exists in any arrest situation as a result of lack of adequate gas exchange, inadequate cardiac output, or both. Artificial ventilation without supplemental oxygen does not correct hypoxemia. In addition, the success of other medications and interventions, such as defibrillation, depends on adequate oxygenation and normal acid-base status.

Oxygen can be delivered by a bag-valve-mask device, a bag-valve device attached to an ETT, or other airway adjuncts. During an arrest, 100% oxygen is administered.

Epinephrine (Adrenalin)

Epinephrine is a potent vasoconstrictor. Because of its alpha-adrenergic and beta-adrenergic effects (Box 11.8), epinephrine increases systemic vascular resistance and arterial blood pressure, as well as heart rate, contractility, and automaticity of cardiac pacemaker cells. Because of peripheral vasoconstriction, blood is shunted to the heart and brain. Epinephrine also increases myocardial oxygen requirements.

BOX 11.8 Effects of Adrenergic Receptor Stimulation

Alpha
- Vasoconstriction
- Increased contractility

Beta$_1$
- Increased heart rate
- Increased contractility

Beta$_2$
- Vasodilation
- Relaxation of bronchial, uterine, and gastrointestinal smooth muscle

? CRITICAL REASONING ACTIVITY

Your patient has an implantable cardioverter-defibrillator (ICD) or permanent pacemaker. How would care and treatment of this patient differ in a code situation?

Epinephrine is indicated for the restoration of cardiac electrical activity in an arrest. In addition, epinephrine increases automaticity and the force of contraction, an effect that makes the heart more susceptible to successful defibrillation. Epinephrine is used to treat VF or pulseless VT that is unresponsive to initial defibrillation, asystole, and PEA.

During a code, epinephrine may be given by the IV or IO route or through an ETT. The IV dosage is 1 mg and is repeated every 3 to 5 minutes as needed. When given through the ETT, 2 to 2.5 mg is diluted in 10 mL of NS or sterile water.

Epinephrine may be administered by continuous infusion to increase the heart rate or blood pressure. Dilution is 1 mg in 250 or 500 mL of D$_5$W or NS. Start the infusion at 1 mcg/min and titrate within a range of 2 to 10 mcg/min according to the patient's response. In a situation other than cardiac arrest, because epinephrine increases myocardial oxygen requirements, monitor the patient closely for signs of myocardial ischemia.

STUDY BREAK
3. The first medication given to a patient in ventricular fibrillation unresponsive to initial defibrillation is:
   A. Atropine
   B. Epinephrine
   C. Amiodarone
   D. Lidocaine

Atropine

Atropine is used to increase heart rate by decreasing vagal tone. It is indicated for patients with symptomatic bradycardia. Routine use of atropine during PEA or asystole is no longer recommended because it is unlikely to be of benefit.[21] For symptomatic bradycardia, administer atropine 0.5 mg IV and repeat every 3 to 5 minutes as needed (for a total of 3 mg) to maintain a heart rate greater than 60 beats/min or until adequate tissue perfusion is achieved as indicated by blood pressure and level of consciousness. If atropine is ineffective in maintaining the heart rate and adequate tissue perfusion, consider transcutaneous pacing, dopamine infusion (2 to 10 mcg/kg/min), or an epinephrine infusion (2 to 10 mcg/min). If necessary, atropine may

be given via an ETT. The dose for ETT administration is 1 to 2 mg diluted in 10 mL of NS or sterile water. Use atropine cautiously in patients with acute coronary ischemia or myocardial infarction because the increased heart rate may worsen ischemia or increase infarction size.[21]

Amiodarone (Cordarone)

Amiodarone is a unique antidysrhythmic possessing some characteristics of all groups of antidysrhythmic medications. It reduces membrane excitability, and by prolonging the action potential and retarding the refractory period, it facilitates the termination of VT and VF. It also has alpha-adrenergic and beta-adrenergic blocking properties. Many antidysrhythmic agents, despite their effectiveness in suppression of dysrhythmias, also have a propensity to exacerbate dysrhythmias. This property is known as *proarrhythmia* or *prodysrhythmia*. Administration of amiodarone is rarely associated with prodysrhythmia. Amiodarone has the added benefit of dilating coronary arteries and increasing coronary blood supply. It also decreases systemic vascular resistance, and in patients with impaired left ventricular function it can improve cardiac function.

IV amiodarone is indicated for treatment and prophylaxis of recurring VF and unstable VT refractory to other treatment. In cardiac arrest, amiodarone or lidocaine may be considered for VF and pulseless VT that are not responsive to defibrillation.[28] Amiodarone is also given in supraventricular tachycardia for rate control or conversion of atrial fibrillation or flutter, especially in patients with heart failure. During cardiac arrest, administer a loading dose of 300 mg IV or IO. If VF or pulseless VT persists, give a second loading dose of 150 mg IV or IO in 3 to 5 minutes. For recurrent VF or pulseless VT, administer a bolus dose of 150 mg IV over 10 minutes (15 mg/min) and repeat every 10 minutes as needed. This may be followed by an infusion of 360 mg over the next 6 hours (1 mg/min) and then a maintenance infusion of 540 mg over the next 18 hours (0.5 mg/min) for a maximum cumulative dose of 2.2 g over 24 hours. Adverse reactions include hypotension and bradycardia, which can be prevented by slowing the infusion rate or treating the patient with fluids, vasopressors, chronotropic medications, or temporary pacing.

Lidocaine (Xylocaine)

Lidocaine is an antidysrhythmic drug that suppresses ventricular ectopic activity. It depresses the ventricular conduction system and reduces automaticity. In cardiac arrest, amiodarone or lidocaine may be considered for VF and pulseless VT that is unresponsive to defibrillation.[28] Lidocaine is also used in the suppression of ventricular ectopy (premature ventricular contractions).

During a code, administer a bolus dose of 1 to 1.5 mg/kg of lidocaine by IV or IO push. Give additional boluses of 0.5 to 0.75 mg/kg every 5 to 10 minutes, as needed, until a maximum of three doses or a total of 3 mg/kg has been given. If IV or IO access is not available, 2 to 4 mg/kg of lidocaine diluted in 10 mL of NS or sterile water may be given through the ETT.

If lidocaine is successful in treating the cardiac dysrhythmia, a continuous infusion may be started at 1 to 4 mg/min. There is

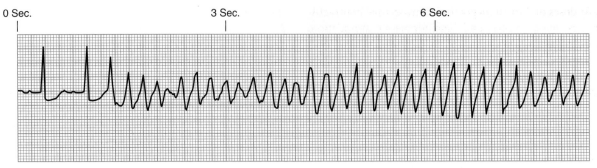

Fig. 11.14 Torsades de pointes. The QRS complex seems to spiral around the isoelectric line. (From Urden LD, Stacy KM, Lough ME. *Critical Care Nursing: Diagnosis and Management.* 8th ed. St. Louis, MO: Mosby; 2018.)

inadequate evidence to support the routine use of lidocaine after cardiac arrest.[21] Dilution is 1 g mixed in 250 mL of D_5W, or 2 g can be mixed in 500 mL of D_5W. Both solutions deliver 4 mg/mL, the standard dilution.

Decrease dosages of lidocaine in patients with impaired hepatic blood flow (as occurs in heart failure or left ventricular dysfunction) and in elderly patients. Monitor serum drug levels, and assess the patient for central nervous system disturbances that may indicate lidocaine toxicity. Common side effects of lidocaine include lethargy, confusion, tinnitus, muscle twitching, seizures, bradycardia, and paresthesias.

Adenosine (Adenocard)

Adenosine is the initial drug of choice for the diagnosis and treatment of supraventricular dysrhythmias. Adenosine slows conduction through the AV node and interrupts AV node reentrant electrical conduction, which is the cause of most supraventricular dysrhythmias. It is effective in restoring normal sinus rhythm in patients with paroxysmal supraventricular tachycardia, including that caused by Wolff-Parkinson-White syndrome. Adenosine does not convert supraventricular rhythms that do not involve the sinoatrial or AV node, such as atrial fibrillation, atrial flutter, atrial tachycardia, and VT. However, adenosine may produce a brief AV node block, thereby assisting with the diagnosis of these rhythms.

Adenosine has an onset of action of 10 to 40 seconds and a duration of 1 to 2 minutes; therefore it is administered rapidly. The initial dose is a 6 mg IV push over 1 to 2 seconds, followed by a 20 mL rapid saline flush. A period of asystole lasting as long as 15 seconds may occur after adenosine administration due to suppression of AV node conduction. A second and third dose of 12 mg may be given 1 to 2 minutes later if the first dose is ineffective in converting the rhythm. Common side effects include transient facial flushing (from mild dilation of blood vessels in the skin), dyspnea, coughing (from mild bronchoconstriction), and chest pain.

Magnesium

Magnesium is essential for many enzyme reactions and for the function of the sodium-potassium pump. It also acts as a calcium channel blocker tand slows neuromuscular transmission. Hypomagnesemia is associated with a high frequency of cardiac dysrhythmias, including refractory VF. Magnesium administered via the IV route may terminate or prevent recurrent torsades de pointes in patients who have a prolonged QT interval. *Torsades de pointes* is a form of VT characterized by QRS complexes that change amplitude and appearance (polymorphic) and appear to twist around the isoelectric line (Fig. 11.14). The QRS complexes may deflect downward for a few beats and then upward for a few beats. When VF or pulseless VT cardiac arrest is associated with torsades de pointes, 1 to 2 g of magnesium sulfate diluted in 10 mL of D_5W is given IV or IO over 5 to 20 minutes.[28] In nonarrest situations, a loading dose of 1 to 2 g mixed in 50 to 100 mL of D_5W is given over 5 to 60 minutes. Slower rates are recommended in a stable patient. The side effects of rapid magnesium administration include hypotension, bradycardia, flushing, and respiratory depression. Serum magnesium levels are monitored to avoid hypermagnesemia.

Sodium Bicarbonate

A patient who has experienced an arrest quickly becomes acidotic. The acidosis results from two sources: no blood flow during the arrest and low blood flow during CPR. Effective ventilation with supplemental oxygen and rapid restoration of tissue perfusion by CPR and spontaneous circulation are the best mechanisms to correct these causes of acidosis.

Limited data support the administration of sodium bicarbonate during cardiac arrest.[23] Sodium bicarbonate buffers the increased numbers of hydrogen ions present in metabolic acidosis. It is beneficial in treating preexisting metabolic acidosis, hyperkalemia, and tricyclic antidepressant overdose.

The initial dosage of sodium bicarbonate is 1 mEq/kg by IV push. When possible, guide bicarbonate therapy by the bicarbonate concentration or calculated base deficit from arterial blood gas analysis or laboratory measurement. Do not mix or infuse sodium bicarbonate with any other medication because it may precipitate or cause deactivation of other medications.

Dopamine (Intropin)

The indication for dopamine is symptomatic hypotension in the absence of hypovolemia. It is the second-line medication for symptomatic bradycardia (after atropine). Its effects are dose related. At doses of 2 to 10 mcg/kg/min, myocardial contractility increases due to alpha- and beta-adrenergic stimulation, causing enhanced cardiac contractility, increased cardiac output, increased heart rate, and increased blood pressure. At doses greater than 10 mcg/kg/min, systemic vascular resistance markedly increases as a result of generalized vasoconstriction produced from alpha-adrenergic stimulation. At doses greater than 20 mcg/kg/min, marked vasoconstriction occurs. Myocardial workload is increased without an increase in coronary blood supply, a situation that may cause myocardial ischemia.

Administer dopamine by continuous IV infusion starting at 2 to 5 mcg/kg/min, and titrate the dose according to patient response. A dilution of 400 to 800 mg of dopamine in 250 to 500 mL of D5W delivers 1600 to 3200 mcg/mL. Administer the lowest dose necessary for blood pressure control to minimize side effects and to ensure adequate perfusion of vital organs.

In addition to causing myocardial ischemia, dopamine may cause cardiac dysrhythmias such as tachycardia and premature ventricular contractions. Necrosis and sloughing of tissue may occur if the drug infiltrates; therefore it should be infused into a central line if possible. Phentolamine, 5 to 10 mg in 10 to 15 mL of NS, can be injected into the infiltrated area to prevent necrosis.

Cardiac arrest after cardiac surgery presents different challenges that are not addressed by ACLS algorithms. Most cardiac arrests occur within the first 24 hours after surgery from VF, cardiac tamponade, and major bleeding. Defibrillation is performed for VF. Emergency resternotomy (opening the chest) is performed to relieve tamponade and control bleeding. In 2017 the Society of Thoracic Surgeons published an expert consensus document for the resuscitation of patients who arrest after cardiac surgery. The protocol includes specific recommendations (Box 11.9).[34]

ⓘ LIFESPAN CONSIDERATIONS

Older Adults

- Older adults have an increased incidence of complications from chest compressions, including rib fractures, sternal fractures, pneumothorax, and hemothorax.
- Cardiopulmonary resuscitation (CPR) is less likely to be effective in patients older than 70 years of age who have comorbidities, unwitnessed arrest, terminal dysrhythmias (asystole, pulseless electrical activity), CPR duration greater than 15 minutes, metastatic cancer, sepsis, pneumonia, renal failure, trauma, or acute or sustained hypotension.[31]
- Declines in hepatic and renal functioning may result in higher-than-desired serum drug concentrations and adverse drug reactions with standard therapeutic dosing regimens.
- The beta-adrenergic receptors on the myocardium are less responsive to changes in heart rate and cardiac contractility. Heart rate responses to beta-blockers (propranolol, metoprolol) and parasympathetic medications (atropine) are less. Moreover, a decline in heart rate and slowing of conduction through the atrioventricular (AV) node result in a narrow therapeutic range for cardiovascular medications.

Pregnant Women[16]

- The pregnant woman is placed supine for chest compressions on a firm backboard.
- Manual left uterine displacement (LUD) is used to relieve aortocaval compression during resuscitation or chest compressions.
- Chest compression rate and depth and medication selection and doses are the same in pregnant patients as in nonpregnant patients.
- Hypoxemia is always considered as a cause of cardiac arrest. Oxygen reserves are lower and metabolic demands higher during pregnancy, and early ventilator support may be necessary.
- After successful resuscitation, place the pregnant woman in the full lateral decubitus position. If this is not possible due to patient monitoring, airway control, and/or IV access, maintain continuous manual LUD.

BOX 11.9 Recommendations for the Resuscitation of Patients Who Arrest After Cardiac Surgery

- Management is a multiprofessional activity with defined roles, including designated members preparing for resternotomy (instruments, sterile field)
- Ventricular fibrillation is managed with three sequential attempts at defibrillation; if not successful, start cardiopulmonary resuscitation (CPR) and give 300 mg amiodarone bolus through a central venous catheter; continue CPR with one shock or defibrillation until emergency resternotomy is performed within 5 minutes
- Asystole or extreme bradycardia is managed with pacing if pacing wires available; if not successful, start CPR; transcutaneous pacing is considered, followed by emergency resternotomy within 5 minutes
- Pulseless electrical activity (PEA) is managed by CPR while simultaneously excluding reversible causes (tension pneumothorax, tamponade, or hemorrhage) followed by emergency resternotomy within 5 minutes
- Epinephrine is not routinely given due to the danger of extreme hypertension with the potential of graft failure and hemorrhage

Data from Society of Thoracic Surgeons Task Force on Resuscitation After Cardiac Surgery. The Society of Thoracic Surgeons expert consensus for the resuscitation of patients who arrest after cardiac surgery. *Ann Thor Surg.* 2017;103(3):1005–1020.

DOCUMENTATION OF CODE EVENTS

Maintain a detailed chronological record of all interventions during a code. One of the first actions of the nurse team leader is to ensure that someone is assigned to record information throughout the code. Documentation includes the time the code is called, the time CPR is started, any actions that are taken, and the patient's response (e.g., presence or absence of a pulse, heart rate, blood pressure, cardiac rhythm). Document intubation and defibrillation (including the energy levels used), along with the patient's response. Accurately record the time and sites of IV initiations, types and amounts of fluids administered, and medications and dosages given. Record rhythm strips to document events and response to treatment. Many hospitals have standardized code records (Fig. 11.15) that list actions and medications and include spaces for entering the time of each intervention and any comments. If possible, record information directly on the code record during the code to ensure that all information is obtained. The code record is signed by the code team and becomes part of the patient's permanent record. Documentation of code events using a tablet computer is being investigated.[27]

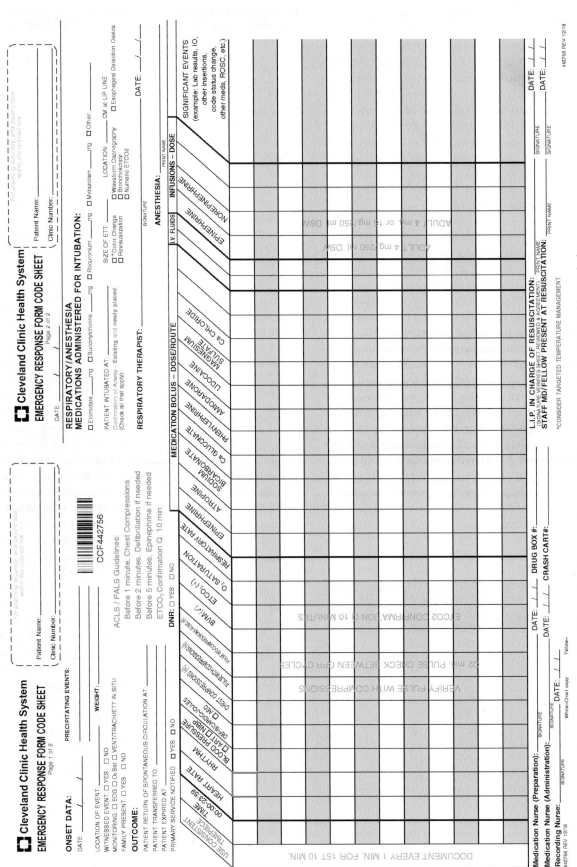

Fig. 11.15 Sample of a code record used for documenting activities during a code. (Reprinted with permission, Cleveland Clinic Center for Art & Photography © 2019. All rights reserved.)

CARE OF THE PATIENT AFTER RESUSCITATION

Systematic post–cardiac arrest care after return of spontaneous circulation (ROSC) can improve patient survival with good quality of life.[5] Postresuscitation goals include optimizing cardiopulmonary function and tissue perfusion, transporting the patient to an appropriate critical care unit capable of providing post–cardiac arrest care, and identifying and treating the precipitating causes of the arrest to help prevent another arrest. This is achieved by advanced airway placement, maintenance of blood pressure and oxygenation, control of dysrhythmias, advanced neurological monitoring, and the use of TTM.

After ROSC, an adequate airway and support of breathing must be initiated. The unconscious patient will require an advanced airway or endotracheal intubation. When securing the ETT, avoid ties that pass circumferentially around the patient's neck to prevent obstruction of venous return to the brain. Elevate the head of the bed to 30 degrees, if tolerated, to reduce the incidence of cerebral edema, aspiration, and pulmonary infection.

Waveform capnography is recommended to confirm and continuously monitor the position of the ETT, especially during patient transport.[5] Waveform capnography measures the partial pressure of CO_2 at the end of expiration (ETCO$_2$). It can be continuously measured as a numerical value with a graphic display of the exhaled waveform over time (Fig. 11.16). A heated sensor is placed in the airway circuit between the ETT and the ventilator tubing. The exhaled gas flows directly over the sensor, providing a measurement of ETCO$_2$. When the ETT is correctly placed, a normal waveform is seen with ETCO$_2$ rising on expiration, sustaining a plateau, and returning to baseline on inspiration (see Fig. 11.16). A sudden loss of ETCO$_2$ with a waveform at baseline indicates incorrect ETT placement or cardiac arrest. The patient's airway should be assessed immediately. The normal range of ETCO$_2$ is 35 to 40 mm Hg. Waveform capnography should be used in addition to breath sound auscultation and direct visualization of the larynx. If it is not available, an ETCO$_2$ detector placed on the ETT (see Fig. 11.5) or an esophageal detector device may be used.

Although 100% oxygen may have been used during the initial resuscitation, the lowest inspired oxygen concentration that is adequate to maintain oxygen saturation (SpO$_2$) at 94% or greater (as measured by pulse oximetry) and the partial pressure of oxygen (PaO$_2$) at approximately 100 mm Hg (as determined by arterial blood gas measurement) are used. Excessive ventilation (too fast or too much) is avoided because it may increase intrathoracic pressure and decrease cardiac output. The decrease in the partial pressure of carbon dioxide (PaCO$_2$) seen with hyperventilation can also decrease cerebral blood flow. Manual ventilations with a bag-valve device are performed at 10 to 12 breaths/min and titrated to achieve an ETCO$_2$ of 35 to 40 mm Hg or a PaCO$_2$ of 35 to 45 mm Hg.

The major determinant of CO_2 delivery to the lungs is cardiac output. If ventilation is relatively constant, ETCO$_2$ will correlate with cardiac output during CPR. Therefore waveform capnography could be used to evaluate the effectiveness of CPR compressions.[21] Obtain a chest radiograph soon after arrival in the critical care unit to verify ETT placement.

Continuous ECG monitoring continues after ROSC, during transport to the critical care unit, and throughout the critical care stay until no longer deemed necessary. Obtain IV access if not already established, and verify the position and function of all IV catheters. Replace an IO catheter emergently placed during the code with IV access. If the patient is hypotensive (systolic blood pressure <90 mm Hg), consider administration of fluid boluses of 1 to 2 L Lactated Ringer's solution or NS. Cold fluid may be used if TTM will be initiated but is no longer recommended in the prehospital setting.[5] Vasoactive medications, including dopamine (2 to 10 mcg/kg/min), norepinephrine (0.1 to 0.5 mcg/kg/min), or epinephrine (2 to 10 mcg/min), may be initiated and titrated to achieve a systolic blood pressure of 90 mm Hg or a mean arterial blood pressure of 65 mm Hg.[4] Metabolic acidosis may be seen after cardiac arrest and is often corrected as adequate perfusion is restored. Record blood pressure and heart rate at least every 30 minutes during continuous infusions of vasoactive medications. If antidysrhythmic medications were used successfully during the code, additional doses may be repeated to achieve adequate blood levels, or continuous infusions may be administered. Other medications may be given to improve cardiac output and myocardial oxygen supply.

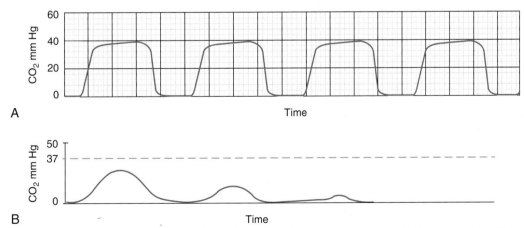

Fig. 11.16 Waveform capnography. **A,** Normal waveform indicating adequate ventilation pattern (end-tidal carbon dioxide [ETCO$_2$] 35 to 40 mm Hg). **B,** Abnormal waveform indicating airway obstruction or obstruction in breathing circuit (ETCO$_2$ decreasing).

One of the most common causes of cardiac arrest is cardiovascular disease and coronary ischemia.[21] Therefore obtain a 12-lead ECG as soon as possible to determine the presence of ST-segment elevation or a new bundle branch block. If there is a high suspicion of acute myocardial infarction, implement protocols for treatment and coronary reperfusion. Additional tubes and lines may be inserted after the code: an arterial line and pulmonary artery catheter for hemodynamic assessment; an indwelling urinary catheter to monitor urinary output hourly; and a nasogastric tube for gastric decompression.

Neurological prognosis is difficult to determine during the first 72 hours after a cardiac arrest. This time frame is usually extended in patients who are being cooled.[5] Therefore perform serial neurological assessments, including response to verbal commands or physical stimulation, pupillary response to light, presence of corneal reflex, spontaneous eye movement, gag, cough, and spontaneous breaths. Patients with post–cardiac arrest cognitive dysfunction may display agitation. In addition, the presence of an ETT may result in pain, discomfort, and anxiety. Intermittent or continuous IV sedation, analgesia, or both can be used to achieve specific goals (see Chapter 6). Seizure activity is common after cardiac arrest. Serial head computed tomography scans are performed if the patient is comatose. Electroencephalography (EEG) monitoring is performed for the diagnosis of seizures and then monitored continuously in comatose patients.[5] Management of patient care continues to focus on the differential diagnosis to identify reversible causes of the arrest and the underlying pathophysiology, including electrolyte abnormalities. Hyperglycemia may occur after cardiac arrest. The optimal blood glucose concentration and strategies are not known[5] (see Laboratory Alert box, which summarizes critical electrolyte values).

Emotional support is an important aspect of care after an arrest. Fear of death or of a recurrence of arrest is common. Survivors often feel the need to discuss their experience in depth, and nurses should listen objectively and provide psychological support. In addition to the patient, many other people are affected when a code occurs. Family members, roommates and other patients, and staff members are all affected by the emergency.

Research supports the benefits of family presence during a code. Families who have been present during a code describe the benefits as knowing that everything possible was being done for their loved one, feeling supportive and helpful to the patient and staff, sustaining patient-family relationships, providing a sense of closure on a life shared together, and facilitating the grief process.[9,25,26,40] Family members should be given the option of being present at the bedside (see Chapter 2).[1]

Targeted Temperature Management After Cardiac Arrest

The higher the body temperature is after a cardiac arrest, the poorer is the neurological recovery. Lower body temperature after cardiac arrest is associated with better neurological recovery.[3,12] Fever resulting from brain injury or ischemia exacerbates the degree of permanent neurological damage after cardiac arrest and contributes to an increased length of stay.[11] For patients who are comatose in whom the initial cardiac rhythm was either VF or pulseless VT after out-of-hospital cardiac arrest, TTM (32°C to 36°C for 24 hours) is likely to be effective in improving neurological function and survival compared to no TTM.[3,4,14]

! LABORATORY ALERT

Electrolyte Values

Laboratory Test	Normal Range	Critical Value[a]	Significance
Sodium (Na+)	136-145 mEq/L	<120 or >160 mEq/L	Implications for polarization of heart muscle via K+/Na+ pump
Potassium (K+)	3.5-5 mEq/L	<2.5 or >6.5 mEq/L	Affects cardiac conduction and contraction
			Maintains cardiac cell homeostasis
			ECG:
			Hypokalemia: depressed ST segment, flat or inverted T wave, presence of U wave
			Hyperkalemia: tall, peaked T wave, prolonged PR interval, flattened P wave, widening of QRS; can progress to asystole
Calcium (Ca++) (total)	9-10.5 mg/dL	<6 or >13 mg/dL	Affects cardiac cell action potential and contraction
			ECG:
			Hypocalcemia: prolonged QT interval
			Hypercalcemia: shortened QT interval
Magnesium (Mg++)	1.3-2.1 mEq/L	<0.5 or >3 mEq/L	Affects contraction of cardiac muscle and promotes vasodilation that may reduce preload, alter cardiac output, and reduce systemic blood pressure
			ECG:
			Hypomagnesemia: ↑ cardiac irritability with cardiac dysrhythmias (torsades de pointes), tachycardia, flat or inverted T waves, ST segment depression
			Hypermagnesemia: slowing of cardiac conduction, bradycardia, prolonged PR and QT intervals

[a]Critical values vary by facility and laboratory.
ECG, Electrocardiogram.

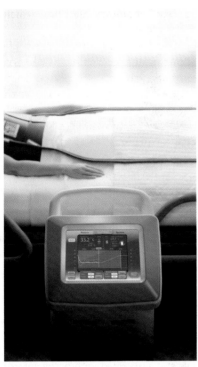

Fig. 11.17 Arctic Sun 5000 Temperature management system. (© 2019 C.R. Bard, Inc., Covington, GA. Used with permission.)

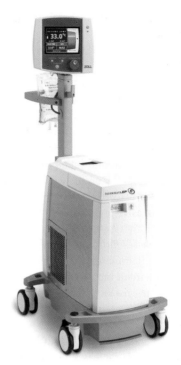

Fig. 11.18 Thermagard XP Temperature Management System. (Courtesy ZOLL Medical Corporation, Chelmsford, MA.)

Hypothermia decreases the metabolic rate by 6% to 7% for every decrease of 1°C in temperature. Because the cerebral metabolic rate for oxygen is the main determinant of cerebral blood flow, inducing hypothermia may improve oxygen supply and reduce oxygen consumption in the ischemic brain. The AHA recommends that comatose adult patients (i.e., those who lack meaningful response to verbal commands) with ROSC after cardiac arrest be cooled to 32°C to 36°C (a temperature selected) and maintained for 24 hours.[5]

Although data support cooling to 32°C to 36°C, the optimal temperature has not been determined. There may be a subgroup of patients after cardiac arrest who may benefit from lower (32°C to 34°C) or higher (36°C) temperature.[5] In addition, the optimal method, time of onset and duration, and rewarming rate are not known. However, there is evidence that attainment of a temperature below 34°C within 3.5 hours of ROSC may be beneficial.[30] Multiple methods for inducing hypothermia include ice packs, cooling blankets, specialized cooling pads that adhere to the skin, ice-cold isotonic IV fluids, and an endovascular device using a central catheter with an external heat exchange system. Several cooling systems are commercially available to initiate and maintain hypothermia. In one system, iced solution is circulated through specialized external pads that adhere to the skin (Fig. 11.17). Another system uses an endovascular catheter that circulates iced solution through a closed system of balloons (Fig. 11.18). Both systems have closed feedback, allowing continuous adjustment in the temperature of the iced solution to maintain a core preset temperature.

There are three phases of TTM: rapid induction to the selected core body temperature, maintenance of this temperature

for 24 hours, and slow rewarming to normothermia (37°C). Hypothermia should be initiated as soon as possible after resuscitation. The patient's core body temperature is continuously monitored with the use of an esophageal thermometer, a bladder catheter with temperature probe, or a pulmonary artery catheter if one is placed. Axillary, oral, and tympanic temperature probes do not measure core body temperature changes and are not used during TTM. A secondary source of temperature measurement is considered, especially if a closed feedback cooling system is used for temperature management.

Anticipate shivering during cooling and rewarming as part of the normal physiological response to a change in body temperature. Shivering increases oxygen consumption especially during the induction of hypothermia, when it actually generates heat, making it more difficult to cool the body. Control shivering with IV sedatives, analgesics, and neuromuscular blockade medications; however, these medications can also mask seizure activity. Therefore EEG monitoring is recommended to identify any seizure activity that occurs during TTM.[5]

Physiological changes during TTM significantly alter medication pharmacokinetics (absorption, distribution, metabolism, and excretion) and pharmacodynamics (physiological effects, mechanism of action, and relationship of medication concentration and effect). Medication selection, dosing, and monitoring of potential medication-therapy interactions is essential to avoid potential complications (see Evidence-Based Practice: Medication Distribution and Metabolism During Targeted Temperature Management [TTM]).[37]

❓ CRITICAL REASONING ACTIVITY

Some hospitals are now considering allowing family members to be present during a code. How could the presence of family members affect the management of the code? What factors should you consider before permitting family members to be present?

Adverse effects associated with hypothermia include bradycardia, bleeding, infection, and metabolic and electrolyte disturbances.[20,24] Coagulopathy occurs with hypothermia, and any bleeding is controlled before hypothermia is induced. Bleeding may be seen after invasive procedures (e.g., coronary angiography with antiplatelet therapy or anticoagulation) but is not associated with increased mortality.[20] Hypothermia suppresses ischemia-induced inflammatory reactions that occur after cardiac arrest, resulting in an increased risk of infection. Pneumonia is common in unconscious patients and may not be related to hypothermia. Bloodstream infections have occurred more frequently with the use of endovascular catheters compared with noninvasive cooling methods, but these infections have not been associated with increased mortality.[20] Ensure that infection prevention strategies are followed, including correct central line maintenance, prevention of ventilator-associated events, and good hand-washing technique.

Hyperglycemia occurs with hypothermia because of increased stress and the release of endogenous and exogenous catecholamines. Manage hyperglycemia with an IV insulin infusion to achieve appropriate glycemic control. During cooling, potassium, magnesium, phosphate, and calcium levels may decrease and are corrected as needed. During the rewarming process, these electrolyte levels may rise. Some hypothermia protocols require that potassium replacement stop 8 hours before initiation of slow, controlled rewarming to prevent increased potassium levels.

After 24 hours of cooling, rewarming proceeds slowly (0.25°C/h to 0.5°C/h) to prevent sudden vasodilation, hypotension, and shock. After normothermia is achieved, implement strategies to prevent fever, which is easily achieved by leaving the devices used to cool in place.[5,11]

STUDY BREAK

4. The three phases of targeted temperature management (TTM) are:
   A. Slow induction to targeted temperature, maintenance of this temperature for 12 hours, rapid rewarming to 37°C
   B. Rapid induction to 30°C, maintenance of this temperature for 12 hours, slow rewarming to 37°C
   C. Slow induction to 33°C, maintenance of this temperature for 48 hours, rapid rewarming to 35°C
   D. Rapid induction to targeted temperature, maintenance of this temperature for 24 hours, slow rewarming to 37°C

EVIDENCE-BASED PRACTICE

Medication Distribution and Metabolism During Targeted Temperature Management (TTM)

Problem

During the three phases of TTM (rapid induction, maintenance of goal temperature for 24 hours, and slow rewarming to normothermia), there are changes in medication pharmacokinetics (absorption, distribution, metabolism, and excretion) and pharmacodynamics (physiological effects, mechanism of action, and relationship of medication concentration and effect). These changes can result in toxic or subtherapeutic medication serum concentrations, leading to adverse effects, suboptimal effects, or heightened drug interactions. Knowledge of these changes permits appropriate dosing and safe medication use during each phase of TTM.

Question

What are the effects of TTM after cardiac arrest on medication pharmacokinetics and pharmacodynamics?

Evidence

Sunjic and colleagues completed a systematic search of the literature for relevant studies and clinical and observational trials of physiological changes and medication pharmacokinetic and pharmacodynamic alterations during TTM. Changes in medication absorption, distribution, metabolism, and excretion during TTM alter medication selection and dosing in the management of shivering, sedation and analgesia, electrolyte disturbances, coagulopathy, seizures, and cardiovascular support. All will affect neurological evaluation, time to recovery of consciousness, and evaluation of seizures.

Implications for Nursing

Organ dysfunction after cardiac arrest and physiological changes associated with TTM can have a profound effect on medication pharmacokinetics and pharmacodynamics. Knowledge of these changes and anticipation of potential interactions is important to maintain therapeutic effects and prevent adverse effects. Careful selection and dosing of medications is essential so as to not adversely affect neurological recovery. TTM protocols, including preferred medication options, are valuable tools for clinicians.

Level of Evidence

A—Meta-analysis

Reference

Sunjic KM, Webb AC, Sunjic I, et al. Pharmacokinetic and other considerations for drug therapy during targeted temperature management. *Crit Care Med.* 2015;43(10):2228–2238.

REFERENCES

1. American Association of Critical-Care Nurses. AACN Practice Alert: Family Presence During Resuscitation and Invasive Procedures. https://www.aacn.org/~/media/aacn-website/clincial-resources/practice-alerts/famvisitpafeb2016ccnpages.pdf. Published February 2016. Accessed February 19, 2019.
2. American Heart Association. *Highlights of the 2015 American Heart Association Guidelines for CPR and ECC.* Dallas, TX: American Heart Association; 2015.
3. Arrich J, Holzer M, Havel C, et al. Hypothermia for neuroprotection in adults after cardiopulmonary resuscitation (review). *Cochrane Database Syst Rev.* 2016;2:1–52.

4. Bernard SA, Gray TW, Buist MD, et al. Treatment of comatose survivors of out-of-hospital cardiac arrest with induced hypothermia. *N Engl J Med.* 2002;346(8):557–563.

5. Callaway CW, Donnino MW, Fink EL. Part 8: Post-cardiac arrest care: 2015 American Heart Association guidelines update for cardiopulmonary resuscitation and emergency cardiovascular care. *Circulation.* 2015;132(Suppl 1):S465–S482.

6. Chan PS, Jain R, Nallmothu BK. Rapid response teams: A systematic review and meta-analysis. *Arch Intern Med.* 2010;170(1):18–26.

7. DeVita MA, Bellomo R, Hillman K, et al. Findings of the first consensus conference on medical emergency teams. *Crit Care Med.* 2006;34(12):2463–2478.

8. Downar J, Rodin D, Barua R, et al. Rapid response teams, do not resuscitate orders, and potential opportunities to improve end-of-life care: A multicenter retrospective study. *J Crit Care.* 2013;28(4):498–503.

9. Flanders SA, Strasen JH. Review of evidence about family presence during resuscitation. *Crit Care Nurs Clin North Am.* 2014;26(4):533–550.

10. Galhotra S, DeVita MA, Simmons RL, et al. Mature rapid response system and potentially avoidable cardiopulmonary arrests in hospital. *Qual Saf Health Care.* 2007;16:260–265.

11. Gebhardt K, Guyette FX, Doshi AA, et al. Prevalence and effect of fever on outcome following resuscitation after cardiac arrest. *Resuscitation.* 2013;84:1062–1067.

12. Geocadin RG, Wijdicks E, Armstrong MJ, et al. Practice guideline summary: Reducing brain injury following cardiopulmonary resuscitation. *Am Acad Neurol.* 2017;88:2141–2149.

13. Guirgis F, Gerdik C, Wears RL, et al. Proactive rounding by the rapid response team reduces inpatient cardiac arrests. 2013;84(12):1668–1673.

14. Hypothermia after Cardiac Arrest Study Group. Mild therapeutic hypothermia to improve the neurologic outcome after cardiac arrest. *N Engl J Med.* 2002;346(8):549–556.

15. Institute for Healthcare Improvement. Rapid Response Teams. http://www.ihi.org/topics/RapidResponseTeams/Pages/default.aspx. Published 2018. Accessed December 14, 2018.

16. Jeejeebhoy FM, Zelop CM, Lipman S, et al. Cardiac arrest in pregnancy: A scientific statement from the American Heart Association. *Circulation.* 2015;132:1747–1773.

17. Jones DA, DeVita MA, Bellomo R. Rapid response teams. *N Engl J Med.* 2011;365(2):139–146.

18. Jones D, Moran J, Winters B, et al. The rapid response team and end-of-life care. *Crit Care.* 2013;19(6):616–623.

19. Kapu AN, Wheeler AP, Lee B. Addition of acute care nurse practitioners to medical and surgical rapid response teams: A pilot project. *Crit Care Nurse.* 2014;34(1):51–59.

20. Karcioglu O, Topacoglu H, Dikme O, et al. A systematic review of safety and adverse effects in the practice of therapeutic hypothermia. *Am J Emerg Med.* 2018;36:1886–1894.

21. Link MS, Berkow LC, Kudenchuk PJ, et al. Part 7: Adult advanced cardiovascular life support: 2015 American Heart Association guidelines update for cardiopulmonary resuscitation and emergency cardiovascular care. *Circulation.* 2015;132(18 Suppl 2):S444–S464.

22. Muharaj R, Raffaele I, Wendon J. Rapid response systems: A systematic review and meta-analysis. *Crit Care.* 2015;19:254.

23. Neumar RW, Otto CW, Link MS, et al. Part 8: Adult advanced cardiovascular life support: 2010 American Heart Association guidelines for cardiopulmonary resuscitation and emergency cardiovascular care. *Circulation.* 2010;122(18 Suppl 3):S729–S767.

24. Nielsen N, Sunde K, Hovdenes J, et al. Adverse events and their relation to mortality in out-of-hospital cardiac arrest patients treated with therapeutic hypothermia. *Crit Care Med.* 2011;39(1):57–64.

25. Oczkowski SJ, Mazzetti I, Cupido C, et al. The offering of family presence during resuscitation: A systematic review and meta analysis. *J Intensive Care.* 2015;3(41).

26. Oczkowski SJ, Mazzetti I, Cupido C, et al. Family presence during resuscitation: A Canadian Critical Care Society position paper. *Can Respir J.* 2015;22(4):201–205.

27. Pearce JM, Yuen TC, Borah MH, et al. Tablet-based cardiac arrest documentation: A pilot study. *Resuscitation.* 2014;85(12):266–269.

28. Panchal AR, Berg KM, Kudenchuk PJ, et al. 2018 American Heart Association focused update on advanced cardiovascular life support use of antiarrhythmic drugs during and immediately after cardiac arrest. *Circulation.* 2018;138:e1–e10.

29. Reardon PM, Fernando SM, Murphy K, et al. Factors associated with delayed rapid response team activation. *J Crit Care.* 2018;46:73–78.

30. Schock RB, Janata A, Peacock F, et al. Time to cooling is associated with resuscitation outcomes. *Ther Hypothermia Temp Man.* 2016;6(4):208–217.

31. Seder DB, Patel N, McPherson J, et al. Geriatric experience following cardiac arrest at six interventional cardiology centers in the United States 2006–2011: Interplay of age, do-not-resuscitate order, and outcomes. *Crit Care Med.* 2014;42(2):289–295.

32. Smith ME, Chiovaro JC, O'Neil M, et al. Early warning system scores for clinical deterioration in hospitalized patients: A systematic review. *Ann Am Thorac Soc.* 2014;11(9):1454–1465.

33. Smith RL, Hayashi VN, Young IM, et al. The medical emergency team call: A sentinel event that triggers goals of care discussion. *Crit Care Med.* 2014;42(2):322–327.

34. Society of Thoracic Surgeons Task Force on Resuscitation After Cardiac Surgery. The Society of Thoracic Surgeons expert consensus for the resuscitation of patients who arrest after cardiac surgery. *Ann Thor Surg.* 2017;103(3):1005–1020.

35. Solomon RS, Corwin GS, Barclay DC, et al. Effectiveness of rapid response teams on rates of in-hospital cardiopulmonary arrest and mortality: A systematic review and meta-analysis. *Hosp Med.* 2016;11(6):438–445.

36. Sulistio M, Franco M, Vo A, et al. Hospital rapid response team and patients with life-limiting illness: A multicenter retrospective cohort study. *Pall Med.* 2015;29(4):302–309.

37. Sunjic KM, Webb AC, Sunjic I, et al. Pharmacokinetic and other considerations for drug therapy during targeted temperature management. *Crit Care Med.* 2015;43(10):2228–2238.

38. Thomas K, Force MV, Rasmussen D, et al. Rapid response teams: Challenges, solutions, and benefits. *Crit Care Nurse.* 2007;27(1):20–27.

39. Tirkkonen J, Tamminen T, Skrifvars MB. Outcome of adult patients attended by rapid response teams: A systematic review of the literature. *Resuscitation.* 2017;112:43–52.

40. Toronto CE, LaRocco SA. Family perception of and experience with family presence during cardiopulmonary resuscitation: An integrative review. *Clin Nurs.* 2018;28:32–46.

41. Winters BD, Weaver SJ, Pfoh ER, et al. Rapid-response systems as a patient safety strategy: A systematic review. *Ann Int Med.* 2013;158(5 Part 2):417–425.

PART III

Nursing Care During Critical Illness

Shock, Sepsis, and Multiple Organ Dysfunction Syndrome

Christina Marie Canfield, MSN, RN, ACNS-BC, CCRN-E

Many additional resources, including self-assessment exercises, are located on the Evolve companion website at http://evolve.elsevier.com/Sole/.
- Animations
- Clinical Skills: Critical Care Collections
- Student Review Questions
- Video Clips

INTRODUCTION

Shock is a clinical syndrome characterized by inadequate tissue perfusion that results in cellular, metabolic, and hemodynamic derangements. Impaired tissue perfusion occurs when there is an imbalance between cellular oxygen supply and cellular oxygen demand. Shock can result from ineffective cardiac function, inadequate blood volume, or inadequate vascular tone.

Shock is associated with many causes and a variety of clinical manifestations. The effects are not isolated to one organ system; instead, all body systems can be affected. Shock can progress to multiple organ dysfunction syndrome (MODS) unless compensatory mechanisms reverse the process or clinical interventions are successfully implemented.[33] Patient responses to shock and treatment strategies vary, producing challenges in assessment and management for the multiprofessional healthcare team.

This chapter discusses the various clinical conditions that create the shock state, including hypovolemic shock, cardiogenic shock, distributive shock (anaphylactic, neurogenic, and septic shock), and obstructive shock. The progression of shock to MODS is also explained. The pathophysiology, clinical presentation, and definitive and supportive management of each type of shock state are described.

REVIEW OF ANATOMY AND PHYSIOLOGY

The cardiovascular system is a closed, interdependent system composed of the heart, blood, and vascular bed. Arteries, arterioles, capillaries, venules, and veins make up the vascular bed. The microcirculation, the portion of the vascular bed between the arterioles and the venules, is the most significant portion of the circulatory system for cell survival. It delivers oxygen and nutrients to cells, removes the waste products of cellular metabolism, and regulates blood volume. Vessels of the microcirculation constrict or dilate selectively to regulate blood flow to cells in need of oxygen and nutrients.

The structure of the microcirculation is tailored to the function of the tissues and organs it supplies, but all vascular beds have common structural characteristics (Fig. 12.1). As oxygenated blood leaves the left side of the heart and enters the aorta, it flows through progressively smaller arteries until it flows into an arteriole. Arterioles are lined with smooth muscle, which allows the small vessels to change diameter to direct and adjust blood flow to the capillaries. From the arteriole, blood enters a metarteriole, a smaller vessel that branches from the arteriole at right angles. Metarterioles are partially lined with smooth muscle, which allows them to adjust their diameter and regulate blood flow into capillaries.

Blood next enters the capillary network by passing through a muscular precapillary sphincter. Capillaries are narrow, thin-walled vascular networks that branch off the metarterioles. This network configuration increases the surface area, which allows greater fluid and nutrient exchange. It also decreases the velocity of the blood flow to prolong transport time through the capillaries. Capillaries have no contractile ability and are not responsive to vasoactive chemicals, electrical or mechanical stimulation, or pressure across their walls. The precapillary sphincter is the only means of regulating blood flow into a capillary. When the precapillary sphincter constricts, blood flow is diverted away from a capillary bed and directed to one that supplies tissues in need of oxygen and nutrients. The capillary bed lies close to the cells of the body, a position that facilitates the delivery of oxygen and nutrients to the cells.

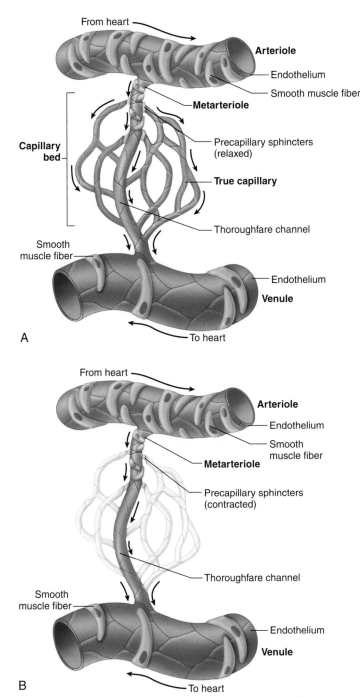

Fig. 12.1 Microcirculation. Control of blood flow through the capillary network is regulated by altering the tone of the precapillary sphincters surrounding arterioles and metarterioles. **A,** Sphincters are relaxed, permitting blood flow to enter the capillary bed. **B,** With sphincters contracted, blood flows into the thoroughfare channel, bypassing the capillary bed. (From Patton K, Thibodeau G. *Anatomy & Physiology.* 10th ed. St. Louis, MO: Elsevier; 2019.)

After nutrients are exchanged for cellular waste products in the capillaries, blood enters a venule. These small, muscular vessels are able to dilate and constrict, offering postcapillary resistance for the regulation of blood flow through capillaries. Blood then flows from the venule and enters the larger veins of the venous system. Another component of the microcirculation consists of the arteriovenous anastomoses that connect arterioles directly to venules. These muscular vessels can shunt blood away from the capillary circulation and send it directly to tissues in need of oxygen and nutrients.

Blood pressure is determined by cardiac output and systemic vascular resistance (SVR). Blood pressure is decreased by a reduction in cardiac output (hypovolemic, cardiogenic, or obstructive shock) or SVR (neurogenic, anaphylactic, or septic shock). Changing pressures within the vessels as blood moves from an area of high pressure in the arteries to lower pressures in the veins facilitates the flow of blood. The force of resistance opposes blood flow, and as resistance increases, blood flow decreases. Resistance is determined by three factors: vessel length, blood viscosity, and vessel diameter. Increased resistance occurs with increased vessel length, increased blood viscosity, and decreased vessel diameter. Vessel diameter is the most important determinant of resistance.

As the pressure of blood within the vessel decreases, the diameter of the vessel decreases, resulting in decreased blood flow. The critical closing pressure and the resultant cessation of blood flow occur when blood pressure decreases to a point at which it is no longer able to keep the vessel open.

Delivery of oxygen (DO_2) to tissues and cells is required for the production of cellular energy (i.e., adenosine triphosphate [ATP]). Oxygen delivery requires an adequate hemoglobin level to carry oxygen, adequate lung function to oxygenate the blood and saturate the hemoglobin (SaO_2), and adequate cardiac function (i.e., cardiac output [CO]) to transport the oxygenated blood to the cells. Impairment of DO_2 or increased consumption of oxygen by the tissues (VO_2) decreases the oxygen reserve (indicated by the mixed venous oxygen saturation [SvO_2]), which may result in tissue hypoxia, depletion of the supply of ATP, lactic acidosis, organ dysfunction, and death.

Pathophysiology

Diverse events can initiate the shock syndrome. Shock begins when the cardiovascular system fails to function properly because of an alteration in at least one of the four essential circulatory components: blood volume, myocardial contractility, blood flow, or vascular resistance. In healthy circumstances, these components function together to maintain circulatory homeostasis. When one of the components fails, the others compensate. However, as compensatory mechanisms fail, or if more than one of the circulatory components is affected, a state of shock ensues. Shock states are classified according to which component is adversely affected (Table 12.1).

Shock is not a single clinical entity but a life-threatening response to alterations in circulation resulting in impaired tissue

TABLE 12.1	**Classification of Shock**
Type of Shock	**Physiological Alteration**
Cardiogenic	Inadequate myocardial contractility
Distributive (anaphylactic, neurogenic, septic)	Inadequate vascular tone
Hypovolemic	Inadequate intravascular volume
Obstructive	Obstruction of blood flow

perfusion. As the delivery of adequate oxygen and nutrients decreases, impaired cellular metabolism occurs. Cells convert from aerobic to anaerobic metabolism. Less energy in the form of ATP is produced. Lactic acid, a byproduct of anaerobic metabolism, causes tissue acidosis. Cells in all organ systems require energy to function, and this resultant tissue acidosis impairs cellular metabolism. Shock is not selective in its effects; all cells, tissues, and organ systems suffer as a result of the physiological response to the stress of shock and decreased tissue perfusion. The end result is organ dysfunction because of decreased blood flow through the capillaries that supply the cells with oxygen and nutrients (Fig. 12.2).

STUDY BREAK

1. Alteration in which of the following components does not contribute to development of shock?
   A. Myocardial contractility
   B. Capillary refill
   C. Vascular resistance
   D. Blood volume

Stages of Shock

The response to shock is highly individualized, and a pattern of stages progresses at unpredictable rates. If each stage of

shock is not recognized and treated promptly, progression to the next stage occurs. The pathophysiological events and associated clinical findings for each stage are summarized in Table 12.2.

Stage I: Initiation. The process of shock is initiated by subclinical hypoperfusion that is caused by inadequate DO_2, inadequate extraction of oxygen, or both. No obvious clinical indications of hypoperfusion are seen in this stage, although hemodynamic alterations, such as a decrease in cardiac output, can occur.

Stage II: Compensatory Stage. The sustained reduction in tissue perfusion initiates a set of neural, endocrine, and chemical compensatory mechanisms in an attempt to maintain blood flow to vital organs and to restore homeostasis. During this stage, symptoms become apparent, but shock is potentially reversible with minimal morbidity if appropriate interventions are initiated.

Neural compensation. Baroreceptors (which are sensitive to pressure changes) and chemoreceptors (which are sensitive to chemical changes) located in the carotid sinus and aortic arch detect the reduction in arterial blood pressure. Impulses are relayed to the vasomotor center in the medulla oblongata,

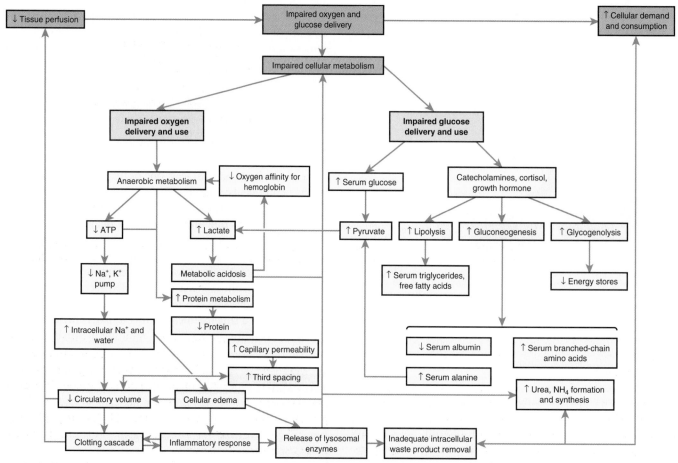

Fig. 12.2 Impairment of cellular metabolism by shock. *ATP,* Adenosine triphosphate; *K^+,* potassium; *Na^+,* sodium; *NH_4,* ammonia. (From McCance K, Huether S. *Pathophysiology: The Biologic Basis for Disease in Adults and Children.* 8th ed. St. Louis, MO: Elsevier; 2019.)

TABLE 12.2 Stages of Shock

Stage of Shock	Physiological Events	Clinical Presentation
I. Initiation	**Decreased tissue oxygenation caused by:** ↓ Intravascular volume (hypovolemic shock) ↓ Myocardial contractility (cardiogenic shock) Obstruction of blood flow (obstructive shock) ↓ Vascular tone (distributive shock) 　Mediator release (septic shock) 　Histamine release (anaphylactic shock) 　Suppression of SNS (neurogenic shock)	No observable clinical indications ↓ CO may be assessed with invasive hemodynamic monitoring
II. Compensatory	**Neural compensation by SNS** ↑ Heart rate and contractility Vasoconstriction Redistribution of blood flow to essential organs Bronchodilation **Endocrine compensation** (RAAS, ADH, glucocorticoid release) Renal reabsorption of sodium, chloride, and water Vasoconstriction Glycogenolysis and gluconeogenesis **Chemical compensation**	↑ Heart rate (except in neurogenic shock) Narrowed pulse pressure Thirst Cool, moist skin Oliguria Diminished bowel sounds Restlessness progressing to confusion Hyperglycemia ↑ Urine specific gravity and ↓ creatinine clearance Rapid, deep respirations causing respiratory alkalosis
III. Progressive	Progressive tissue hypoperfusion Anaerobic metabolism with lactic acidosis Failure of sodium-potassium pump Cellular edema	Dysrhythmias ↓ BP with narrowed pulse pressure Tachypnea Cold, clammy skin Decreased capillary refill Mottling Anuria Absent bowel sounds Lethargy progressing to coma Hyperglycemia resistant to insulin ↑ BUN, creatinine, and potassium Respiratory and metabolic acidosis
IV. Refractory	Severe tissue hypoxia with ischemia and necrosis Worsening acidosis SIRS MODS	Life-threatening dysrhythmias Severe hypotension despite vasopressors Respiratory and metabolic acidosis Acute respiratory failure ARDS DIC Hepatic dysfunction or failure Acute kidney injury Myocardial ischemia, infarction, or failure Cerebral ischemia or infarction

ADH, Antidiuretic hormone; *ARDS*, acute respiratory distress syndrome; *BP*, blood pressure; *BUN*, blood urea nitrogen; *CO*, cardiac output; *DIC*, disseminated intravascular coagulation; *MODS*, multiple organ dysfunction syndrome; *RAAS*, renin-angiotensin-aldosterone system; *SIRS*, systemic inflammatory response syndrome; *SNS*, sympathetic nervous system.

stimulating the sympathetic branch of the autonomic nervous system to release epinephrine and norepinephrine from the adrenal medulla.

In response to the catecholamine release, heart rate and myocardial contractility increase to improve cardiac output. Dilation of the coronary arteries increases perfusion to the myocardium to meet the increased demands for oxygen. Systemic vasoconstriction and redistribution of blood occur. Arterial vasoconstriction improves blood pressure, whereas venous vasoconstriction augments venous return to the heart, increasing preload and cardiac output. Blood is shunted from the kidneys, gastrointestinal tract, and skin to the heart and brain. Bronchial smooth muscles relax, and respiratory rate and depth are increased, improving gas exchange and oxygenation. Additional catecholamine effects include increased blood glucose levels as the liver is stimulated to convert glycogen to glucose for energy production; dilation of pupils; peripheral vasoconstriction; and increased sweat gland activity resulting in cool, moist skin.

Endocrine compensation. In response to the reduction in blood pressure, messages are relayed to the hypothalamus, which stimulates the anterior and posterior pituitary glands.

The anterior pituitary gland releases adrenocorticotropic hormone (ACTH), which acts on the adrenal cortex to release glucocorticoids and mineralocorticoids (e.g., aldosterone). Glucocorticoids increase the blood glucose level by increasing the conversion of glycogen to glucose (glycogenolysis) and causing the conversion of fat and protein to glucose (gluconeogenesis).

Mineralocorticoids act on the renal tubules, causing the reabsorption of sodium and water, resulting in increased intravascular volume and blood pressure. The renin-angiotensin-aldosterone system (Fig. 12.3) is stimulated by a reduction of pressure in the renal arterioles and by a decrease in sodium levels as sensed by the juxtaglomerular apparatus of the kidney. In response to decreased renal perfusion, the juxtaglomerular apparatus releases renin. Renin circulates in the blood and reacts with angiotensinogen to produce angiotensin I. Angiotensin I circulates through the lungs, where it forms angiotensin II, a potent arterial and venous vasoconstrictor that increases blood pressure and improves venous return to the heart. Angiotensin II also activates the adrenal cortex to release aldosterone.

Antidiuretic hormone (ADH) is released by the posterior pituitary gland in response to the increased osmolality of the blood that occurs in shock. The overall effects of endocrine compensation result in an attempt to combat shock by providing the body with glucose for energy and by increasing the intravascular blood volume.

STUDY BREAK

2. Which of the following describes the endocrine response during the compensatory stage of shock?
   A. Increased reabsorption of sodium and water
   B. Suppression of renin release
   C. Inhibition of angiotensin II
   D. Inhibition of antidiuretic hormone

Chemical compensation. As pulmonary blood flow is reduced, ventilation-perfusion imbalances occur. Initially, alveolar ventilation is adequate, but the perfusion of blood

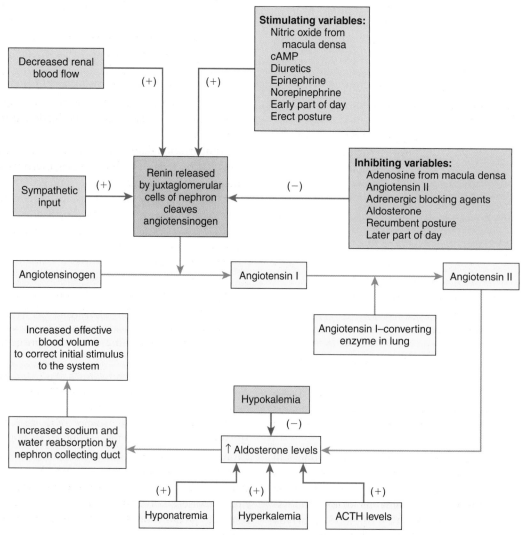

Fig. 12.3 Feedback mechanisms regulating aldosterone secretion. *ACTH,* Adrenocorticotropic hormone; *cAMP,* cyclic adenosine monophosphate. (From McCance K, Huether S. *Pathophysiology: The Biologic Basis for Disease in Adults and Children.* 8th ed. St. Louis, MO: Elsevier; 2019.)

through the alveolar capillary bed is decreased. Chemoreceptors located in the aorta and carotid arteries are stimulated in response to the low oxygen tension in the blood. Consequently, the rate and depth of respirations increase. As the patient hyperventilates, carbon dioxide is excreted, and respiratory alkalosis occurs. A reduction in carbon dioxide levels and the alkalotic state cause vasoconstriction of cerebral blood vessels. Coupled with the reduced oxygen tension, vasoconstriction may lead to cerebral hypoxia and ischemia. The overall effects of chemical compensation result in an attempt to combat shock by increasing oxygen supply; however, cerebral perfusion may decrease.

Stage III: Progressive Stage. If the cause of hypoperfusion is not corrected or the compensatory mechanisms continue without reversing the shock, profound hypoperfusion and further deterioration result. Vasoconstriction continues in the systemic circulation. Although this effect shunts blood to vital organs, the decreased blood flow leads to ischemia in the extremities, weak or absent pulses, and altered body defenses. Prolonged vasoconstriction results in decreased capillary blood flow and cellular hypoxia. The cells convert to anaerobic metabolism, producing lactic acid, which leads to metabolic acidosis. Anaerobic metabolism produces less ATP than aerobic metabolism, which reduces the energy available for cellular metabolism. The lack of ATP causes failure of the sodium-potassium pump. Sodium and water accumulate within the cell, resulting in cellular swelling and a further reduction in cellular function.

The microcirculation exerts the opposite effect and dilates to increase the blood supply to meet local tissue needs. Whereas the arterioles remain constricted in an attempt to keep vital organs perfused, the precapillary sphincters relax, allowing blood to flow into the capillary bed. Meanwhile, postcapillary sphincters remain constricted. As a result, blood flows freely into the capillary bed but accumulates in the capillaries as blood flow exiting the capillary bed is impeded. Capillary hydrostatic pressure increases, and fluid is pushed from the capillaries into the interstitial space, causing interstitial edema.

The intravascular-to-interstitial fluid shift is further aggravated by the release of histamine and other inflammatory mediators that increase capillary permeability, along with the loss of proteins through enlarged capillary pores, which decreases capillary oncotic pressure. As intravascular blood volume decreases, the blood becomes more viscous, and blood flow slows. This situation causes capillary sludging as red blood cells, platelets, and proteins clump together. The loss of intravascular volume and capillary pooling further reduce venous return to the heart and cardiac output.

Coronary artery perfusion pressure is decreased. The ischemic pancreas releases myocardial depressant factor (MDF), decreasing myocardial contractility. Cardiac output, blood pressure, and tissue perfusion continue to decrease, contributing to worsening cellular hypoxia. At this point, the patient shows classic signs and symptoms of shock. This phase of shock responds poorly to fluid replacement alone, and reversal requires aggressive interventions.

Stage IV: Refractory Stage. Prolonged inadequate tissue perfusion that is unresponsive to therapy ultimately contributes to MODS and death. A large volume of the blood remains pooled in the capillary bed, and the arterial blood pressure is too low to support perfusion of the vital organs.

Dysrhythmias occur because of the failure of the sodium-potassium pump, which results from decreased ATP, hypoxemia, ischemia, and acidosis. Cardiac failure may occur because of ischemia, acidosis, and the effects of MDF.

Endothelial damage in the capillary bed and precapillary arterioles, along with damage to the type II pneumocytes, which make surfactant, leads to acute respiratory distress syndrome (ARDS). Hypoxemia causes vasoconstriction of the pulmonary circulation and pulmonary hypertension. Ventilation-perfusion mismatch occurs because of disturbances in ventilation and perfusion. Pulmonary edema may result from disruption of the alveolar-capillary membrane, ARDS, heart failure, or overly aggressive fluid resuscitation.

When cerebral perfusion pressure is significantly impaired, loss of autoregulation occurs, resulting in brain ischemia. Cerebral infarction may occur. Sympathetic nervous system dysfunction results in massive vasodilation, depression of cardiac and respiratory centers (resulting in bradycardia and bradypnea), and loss of normal thermoregulation.

Renal vasoconstriction and hypoperfusion of the kidney decrease the glomerular filtration rate. Prolonged ischemia causes acute kidney injury with acute tubular necrosis. Metabolic acids accumulate in the blood, worsening the metabolic acidosis caused by lactic acid production during anaerobic metabolism.

Hypoperfusion damages the reticuloendothelial cells, which recirculate bacteria and cellular debris, thereby predisposing the patient to bacteremia and sepsis. Damaged hepatocytes impair the liver's ability to detoxify drugs, toxins, and hormones; conjugate bilirubin; or synthesize clotting factors. Hepatic dysfunction decreases its ability to mobilize carbohydrate, protein, and fat stores, resulting in hypoglycemia.

Pancreatic ischemia causes the release of MDF, which impairs cardiac contractility. Hyperglycemia may occur because of endogenous corticosteroids, exogenous corticosteroids, or insulin resistance. Hyperglycemia results in dehydration and electrolyte imbalances related to osmotic diuresis, impairment of leukocyte function causing decreased phagocytosis and increased risk of infection, depression of the immune response, impairment in gastric motility, shifts in substrate availability from glucose to free fatty acids or lactate, negative nitrogen balance, and decreased wound healing.

Ischemia and increased gastric acid production caused by glucocorticoids increase the risk of stress ulcer development. Prolonged vasoconstriction and ischemia lead to the inability of the intestinal walls to act as intact barriers to prevent the migration of bacteria out of the gastrointestinal tract. This may result in the translocation of bacteria from the gastrointestinal tract into the lymphatic and vascular beds, increasing the risk of sepsis.

Hypoxia and the release of inflammatory cytokines impair blood flow and result in microvascular thrombosis. Sluggish blood flow, massive tissue trauma, and consumption of clotting factors may cause disseminated intravascular coagulation (DIC). The bone marrow releases white blood cells, causing leukocytosis early in shock and then leukopenia as depletion of white blood cells in blood and in bone marrow occurs. Tissue injury caused by widespread ischemia stimulates the development of systemic inflammatory response syndrome (SIRS) with a massive release of mediators of the inflammatory process.

Poor renal function, respiratory failure, and impaired cellular function aggravate the existing state of acidosis, which contributes to further fluid shifts, loss of vasomotor tone, and relative hypovolemia. Alterations in the cardiovascular system and continued acidosis reduce the heart rate, impair myocardial contractility, and further decrease cardiac output and tissue perfusion. Cerebral ischemia occurs because of the reduction in cerebral blood flow. Consequently, the sympathetic nervous system is stimulated, an effect that aggravates the existing vasoconstriction, increasing afterload and decreasing cardiac output. Prolonged cerebral ischemia eventually causes the loss of sympathetic nervous system response, and vasodilation and bradycardia result. The patient's decreasing blood pressure and heart rate cause a lethal decrease in tissue perfusion, MODS that is unresponsive to therapy, brain death, and cardiopulmonary arrest.

Systemic Inflammatory Response Syndrome

SIRS is widespread inflammation that can occur in patients with diverse disorders such as ARDS, infection, trauma, shock, pancreatitis, or ischemia.[33] It may result from or lead to MODS.

The inflammatory cascade maintains homeostasis through a balance between proinflammatory and antiinflammatory processes. Although inflammation is normally a localized process, SIRS is a systemic response associated with the release of mediators. The mediators increase the permeability of the endothelial wall, shifting fluid from the intravascular space into extravascular spaces, including the interstitial space. Intravascular volume is reduced, resulting in relative hypovolemia. Other mediators cause microvascular clotting, impaired fibrinolysis, and widespread vasodilation.

ASSESSMENT

An understanding of the pathophysiology of shock and identification of patients at risk are essential for the prevention of and timely response to shock. Assessment focuses on three areas: history, clinical presentation, and laboratory studies. Review the patient's history first and then assess the systems most sensitive to a lack of oxygen and nutrients. The patient's history may include an identifiable predisposing factor or cause of the shock state.

Clinical Presentation

Multiple body systems are affected by the shock syndrome. The clinical presentation specific to each classification of shock is discussed later.

> **! CLINICAL ALERT**
>
> *Shock*
>
> Assessment findings in the initial stages of shock include increased heart rate and respiratory rate; decreased urine output; cool, moist skin; and restlessness or confusion. These signs and symptoms are related to the body's attempt to compensate and restore homeostasis. Later signs of shock include hypotension, dysrhythmia(s), respiratory distress, decreased responsiveness, anuria, and skin mottling. These symptoms are the result of decreased organ and tissue perfusion.

Central Nervous System. The central nervous system is the most sensitive to changes in the supply of oxygen and nutrients. It is the first system affected by changes in cellular perfusion. Initial responses of the central nervous system to shock include restlessness, agitation, and anxiety. As the shock state progresses, the patient becomes confused and lethargic because of the decreased perfusion to the brain. As shock progresses, the patient becomes unresponsive.

Cardiovascular System. A major focus of assessment is blood pressure, and it is important to know the patient's baseline blood pressure. During the compensatory stage, innervation of the sympathetic nervous system increases myocardial contractility and vasoconstriction, which results in a normal or slightly elevated systolic pressure, an increased diastolic pressure, and a narrowed pulse pressure. As the shock state progresses, systolic blood pressure decreases, but diastolic pressure remains normal or increased, resulting in a narrowed pulse pressure. The narrowed pulse pressure may precede changes in heart rate or be accompanied by tachycardia.[13]

Definitions vary, but a systolic blood pressure of less than 90 mm Hg is considered hypotension. If the patient has hypertension, a decrease in systolic pressure of 40 mm Hg from the usual systolic pressure is considered severely hypotensive. Noninvasive automated blood pressure in shock is often inaccurate because of peripheral vasoconstriction. Arterial pressure monitoring may be indicated to obtain accurate readings and guide therapy.

Evaluate the rate, quality, and character of major pulses (i.e., carotid, radial, femoral, posterior tibial, and dorsalis pedis). In shock states, the pulse is often weak and thready. The pulse rate is increased, usually greater than 100 beats/min, through stimulation of the sympathetic nervous system as a compensatory response to the decreased cardiac output and increased demand of the cells for oxygen.

Normal compensatory responses to shock are often altered if the patient is taking certain medications. Negative inotropic agents, such as beta-blocking agents (e.g., propranolol, metoprolol), are widely used in the treatment of angina, hypertension, and dysrhythmias. These agents work primarily by blocking the effects of the beta branch of the sympathetic nervous system, resulting in decreased heart rate and cardiac output. A patient who is taking these medications has an altered ability to respond to the stress of shock and may not exhibit the typical signs and symptoms, such as tachycardia.

Assessment of the jugular veins provides information on the volume and pressure in the right side of the heart. It is an indirect method of evaluating the central venous pressure. Jugular venous distension is noted in patients with obstructive or cardiogenic shock. Neck veins are flat in those with hypovolemic shock.

Capillary refill assesses the ability of the cardiovascular system to maintain perfusion to the periphery. The normal response to pressure on the nail beds is blanching, and the color returns to a normal pink hue in 1 to 2 seconds after the pressure is released. A delay in the return of color indicates peripheral vasoconstriction. Capillary refill provides a quick assessment of overall cardiovascular status, but this assessment is not reliable in a patient who is hypothermic or has peripheral circulatory problems.

Assessment of fluid responsiveness is an important consideration for the management of shock. Only about 50% of patients respond adequately to fluid administration and demonstrate clinically significant increases in stroke volume as defined by an increase of 10% to 15% or greater.[45] Central venous pressure monitoring has traditionally been used to assess fluid responsiveness; however, it has been found to be a poor discriminator for predicting fluid responsiveness.[5,22,45]

The *passive leg raise* is a dynamic and predictive indicator of fluid responsiveness. Blood volume from the lower body is mobilized to the heart and temporarily mimics a fluid bolus during the passive leg raise. The resultant increase in preload causes an increase in cardiac output. Perform the passive leg raise by placing the patient in a semirecumbent position with the head of bed at 45 degrees. Record baseline measurements and then lower the head of bed and elevate the legs at 45 degrees. Measure stroke volume, cardiac output or cardiac index, or systolic blood pressure within 30 to 90 seconds after raising the legs.[45]

A pulmonary artery (PA) catheter may be a useful tool for diagnosing and treating the patient in shock. The risks associated with catheter insertion and central line–associated bloodstream infection must be weighed against the clinical information obtained from this invasive diagnostic device.[60] The PA catheter provides information on cardiac dynamics, fluid balance, and effects of vasoactive medications. Preload, which is measured by right atrial pressure (RAP) for the right ventricle and by the pulmonary artery occlusion pressure (PAOP) for the left ventricle, is used to assess fluid balance. Cardiac output and index, afterload, and stroke work indices can also be assessed with a PA catheter (see Chapter 9). Table 12.3 describes hemodynamic values and alterations in each classification of shock.

Use of PA catheters in the management of shock is decreasing as newer, less invasive technology has been introduced. Devices that use pulse contour methods for hemodynamic assessment (see Chapter 9) provide stroke volume variation (SVV), pulse pressure variation (PPV), continuous cardiac output, and other hemodynamic parameters that better predict fluid responsiveness. Outcomes of using these newer devices continue to be evaluated (see Evidence-Based Practice box).

EVIDENCE-BASED PRACTICE

Dynamic Assessment of Fluid Responsiveness in Goal-Directed Therapy

Problem

Over the past decade, the use of central venous pressure (CVP) to guide goal-directed therapy has been called into question, as the evidence has found CVP to be a poor predictor of fluid responsiveness. The use of dynamic indices such as stroke volume variation, changes in stroke volume, and pulse pressure variation may be better methods of evaluating fluid responsiveness and directing therapy. Dynamic measures accurately predict fluid responsiveness; however, their impact on clinically relevant outcomes has not yet been established.

Clinical Question

What is the impact on clinical outcomes of goal-directed therapy incorporating dynamic assessment of fluid responsiveness (FT-DYN) when compared to the standard of care?

Evidence

A meta-analysis of 13 randomized control trials was conducted analyzing the outcomes of 1652 patients who underwent acute volume resuscitation with either standard care or FT-DYN. Standard care included fluid administration based on weight, clinical examination, or static indicators. FT-DYN encompasses stroke volume variation greater than 10% to 15%, pulse pressure variation greater than 10%, and an increase in stroke volume of 10%. A variety of patients were represented in the study, including abdominal surgery, septic shock, and cardiac surgery patients. FT-DYN was associated with decreased mortality, critical care unit length of stay, and duration of mechanical ventilation compared to standard care. The study did not find a difference in hospital length of stay nor in the incidence of renal impairment between FT-DYN and standard care.

Conclusions

The use of dynamic assessments for fluid resuscitation in goal-directed therapy may be more advantageous than static measures. The analysis finds that patients who were treated using dynamic measures had overall better outcomes; however, further research is needed.

Implications for Nursing

Understanding new technology regarding dynamic measures and developing knowledge and skill in interpretation of assessment findings better guide resuscitation and reduce adverse events (i.e., prolonged ventilation, extended critical care unit length of stay). Depending on the type of shock, advocate for the use of dynamic measures that are less invasive and do not require a central line unless warranted (e.g., patients in cardiogenic shock likely will need more invasive monitoring).

Level of Evidence

A—Meta-analysis

Reference

Bednarczyk JM, Fridfinnson JA, Kumar A, et al. Incorporating dynamic assessment of fluid responsiveness into goal-directed therapy: A systematic review and meta-analysis. *Crit Care Med.* 2017;45(9):1538–1545.

TABLE 12.3 **Hemodynamic Alterations in Shock States**

Hemodynamic Parameter (Normal Value)	Hypovolemic Shock	Cardiogenic Shock	Obstructive Shock	DISTRIBUTIVE SHOCK		
				Septic Shock	Anaphylactic Shock	Neurogenic Shock
Heart rate (60-100 beats/min)	High	High	High	High	High	Normal to low
Blood pressure	Normal to low	Normal to low	Normal to low	Normal to low	Normal to low	Normal to low
Cardiac output (4-8 L/min)	Low	Low	Low	High then low	Normal to low	Normal to low
Cardiac index (2.5-4.0 L/min/m²)	Low	Low	Low	High then low	Normal to low	Normal to low
RAP (2-6 mm Hg)	Low	High	High	Low to variable	Low	Low
PAOP (8-12 mm Hg) or PADP (8-15 mm Hg)	Low	High	High if impaired diastolic filling or high LV afterload Low if high RV afterload	Low to variable	Low	Low
SVR (770-1500 dynes/sec/cm⁻⁵)	High	High	SVR high PVR high	Low to variable	Low	Low
SvO₂ (60%-75%)	Low	Low	Low	High then low	Low	Low

LV, Left ventricular; *PADP*, pulmonary artery diastolic pressure; *PAOP*, pulmonary artery occlusion pressure; *PVR*, pulmonary vascular resistance; *RAP*, right atrial pressure; *RV*, right ventricular; *SvO₂*, mixed venous oxygen saturation; *SVR*, systemic vascular resistance.

🛈 LIFESPAN CONSIDERATIONS

Older Adults

- Changes in immunological function with age are referred to as immunosenescence. These changes result in impaired immune responses and inflammatory dysregulation, which may affect the aging body's ability to respond to infection.[4]
- As the body ages, the left ventricular wall thickens, ventricular compliance decreases, and calcification and fibrosis of the heart valves occur. Stroke volume and cardiac output are reduced. The sensitivity of the baroreceptors is decreased, and the heart rate is less responsive to sympathetic nervous system stimulation in the early stage of shock. Arterial walls lose elasticity, increasing systemic vascular resistance, which increases the myocardial oxygen demand and decreases the responsiveness of the arterial system to the effects of catecholamines.
- Aging decreases lung elasticity, alveolar perfusion, and alveolar surface area and causes thickening of the alveolar-capillary membrane. These changes limit the body's ability to increase oxygen levels and improve tissue perfusion during shock states.[37]
- The ability of the kidney to concentrate urine decreases with age, which limits the body's ability to conserve water when required.[16]
- Skin turgor decreases, making fluid status assessment more difficult. Dehydration is common and may increase the risk for hypovolemia.[18]

Pregnant Women

- Factors affecting maternal oxygenation also affect fetal oxygenation. Priority is given to resuscitation of the mother and administration of oxygen. Include an obstetrician and neonatologist (if indicated) on the multiprofessional team.
- Consider left lateral positioning to prevent compression of the vena cava.
- Assess fetal heart tones; consult obstetrical nurses for assistance.
- Assess pregnant women for signs and symptoms of uterine hemorrhage.[12]

Breastfeeding Women

- Establish a plan for continued breastfeeding, expressing milk, or suppressing milk supply, if indicated.
- The multiprofessional team must be aware of the breastfeeding plan so that medications and nutrition are prescribed accordingly.[12]

Critical care management involves optimizing cardiac output and minimizing myocardial oxygen consumption. If an oximetric PA catheter is inserted, SvO₂ is measured (see Chapter 9). The SvO₂ reflects the amount of oxygen bound to hemoglobin in the venous circulation and reflects the balance between DO₂ and VO₂. If the SvO₂ is less than 60%, the DO₂ is inadequate or the VO₂ is excessive. The SvO₂ is decreased in all forms of shock except in early septic shock, in which poor oxygen extraction causes the SvO₂ value to be high. SvO₂ is useful in identifying the type of shock and in evaluating the effectiveness of treatment.

Respiratory System. In the early stage of shock, respirations are rapid and deep. The respiratory center responds to shock and metabolic acidosis with an increase in respiratory rate to eliminate carbon dioxide. Direct stimulation of the medulla by chemoreceptors alters the respiratory pattern. As the shock state progresses, metabolic wastes accumulate and cause generalized muscle weakness, resulting in shallow breathing with poor gas exchange. Increased capillary permeability leads to interstitial edema and changes in breath sounds (e.g., crackles).[33]

Interpret pulse oximetry values (SpO₂) cautiously because decreased peripheral circulation may result in inaccurate readings. Arterial blood gas analysis provides a more accurate assessment of oxygenation and ventilation.

Renal System.

Renal hypoperfusion and decreased glomerular filtration rate cause oliguria (urine output <0.5 mL/kg/h). The renin-angiotensin-aldosterone system is activated, which promotes the retention of sodium and reabsorption of water in the kidneys, further decreasing urinary output. This prerenal cause of acute kidney injury is manifested by concentrated urine and an increased blood urea nitrogen level, but the serum creatinine level remains normal. If the decreased perfusion is prolonged, acute tubular necrosis, a form of intrarenal failure, occurs, and creatinine levels increase.

Gastrointestinal System.

Hypoperfusion of the gastrointestinal system slows intestinal activity, which results in decreased bowel sounds, increased gastric residual, distension, nausea, and constipation.[36] Paralytic ileus and ulceration with bleeding may occur with prolonged hypoperfusion. Hyperpermeability leads to the translocation of organisms into systemic circulation.

Hypoperfusion of the liver leads to decreased function and alterations in liver enzyme levels such as lactate dehydrogenase (LDH) and aspartate aminotransferase (AST). If decreased perfusion persists, the liver is not able to produce coagulation factors, detoxify drugs, or neutralize invading microorganisms. Clotting disorders, drug toxicity concerns, and increased susceptibility to infection occur. Signs and symptoms of decreased liver function include increased ammonia and bilirubin levels, irritability, ascites, and jaundice. The patient's urine may appear dark, and stools may become light or clay colored.[33]

Hematologic System.

The interaction between inflammation and coagulation enhances clotting and inhibits fibrinolysis, leading to clotting in the microcirculatory system and bleeding. Increased consumption of platelets and clotting factors occurs, causing a consumptive coagulopathy. The inability of the liver to manufacture clotting factors also contributes to the coagulopathy. A decreased platelet count, decreased clotting factors, and prolonged clotting times are seen with coagulopathy. Petechiae and ecchymosis may occur, along with blood in the urine, stool, gastric aspirate, and tracheal secretions. Clotting in the microcirculation causes peripheral ischemia manifested by symmetrical cyanosis of the hands, feet, or face and necrosis of digits and extremities. Leukocytosis frequently occurs, especially in early septic shock. Leukopenia occurs later because of consumption of white blood cells.

Integumentary System.

Evaluate skin color, temperature, texture, turgor, and moisture level. Cyanosis may occur, but it is a late and unreliable sign. The patient may exhibit central cyanosis observed in the mucous membranes of the mouth and nose or peripheral cyanosis that is evident in the nails and earlobes. Note that assessment of skin turgor is often an unreliable indicator of hydration in older adults, as they have decreased skin elasticity.[18]

Skin mottling is a common sign of hypoperfusion. Mottling is an irregular, patchy skin discoloration that usually appears around the knees. As hypoperfusion progresses, the mottling extends the length of the leg from the knee toward the groin and toes. It may also be observed in other areas of peripheral circulation such as the fingers and ears.[1,24] The skin mottling score is a noninvasive bedside tool used to evaluate the severity of mottling and overall tissue perfusion; scores range from 0 (no mottling) to 5 (extreme mottling of the leg extending into the groin region). Higher scores are associated with increased mortality.[23]

Laboratory Studies

Laboratory studies assist in the differential diagnosis of the patient in shock (see Laboratory Alert box). However, by the time many of the laboratory values are abnormal, the patient is in the later stages of shock. The clinical picture is often more useful for early diagnosis and immediate treatment.

The serum lactate level is a measure of the overall state of shock, regardless of the cause. The lactate level is an indicator of decreased oxygen delivery to the cells and the adequacy of treatment. Elevated lactate levels produce an acidic environment and decreased arterial pH. The serum lactate level correlates with the degree of hypoperfusion, meaning the higher the lactate level, the more significant the hypoperfusion.

MANAGEMENT

Management of the patient in shock consists of identifying and treating the cause of the shock as rapidly as possible. Direct care toward correcting or reversing the altered circulatory component (e.g., blood volume, myocardial contractility, obstruction, vascular resistance) and reversing tissue hypoxia. Implement fluid, pharmacological, and mechanical therapies to maintain tissue perfusion and improve oxygen delivery. Interventions include increasing the cardiac output and cardiac index, increasing the hemoglobin level, increasing the arterial oxygen saturation, and minimizing oxygen consumption. Specific management for each classification of shock is discussed later in the chapter.

In addition to treatment specific to the shock state, it is important to implement basic nursing interventions to prevent complications associated with decreased perfusion, hemodynamic alterations, and immobility. For example, these conditions increase the patient's risk for developing a pressure injury, and therapeutic interventions are warranted.[25,41,42] See the Plan of Care for the Patient in Shock and the Collaborative Plan of Care for the Critically Ill Patient in Chapter 1.

Maintain Circulating Blood Volume and Adequate Hemoglobin Level

Regardless of the cause, shock produces profound alterations in fluid balance. Patients with absolute hypovolemia (hypovolemic shock) or relative hypovolemia (distributive shock) require the administration of IV fluids to restore intravascular volume, maintain oxygen-carrying capacity, and establish the

! LABORATORY ALERT

Shock

Laboratory Test	Normal Range	Critical Value[a]	Significance
Chemistry Studies			
Glucose	74-106 mg/dL	<50 or >450 mg/dL	↑ Impairs immune response ↑ Diuresis ↓ Level of consciousness
Blood urea nitrogen	10-20 mg/dL	>100 mg/dL	↑ Hypoperfusion (prerenal failure) ↑ Gastrointestinal bleeding and catabolism
Creatinine	*Female:* Up to age 60, 0.5-1.1 mg/dL >61, 0.5-1.2 mg/dL *Male:* Up to age 60, 0.6-1.3 mg/dL >61, 0.7-1.3 mg/dL	>4 mg/dL	↑ Acute kidney injury
Sodium	136-145 mEq/L	<120 or >160 mEq/L	↓ Hemodilution from replacement with excessive hypotonic fluid ↑ Hemoconcentration from fluid loss
Chloride	98-106 mEq/L	<80 or >115 mEq/L	↑ Excess infusion of normal saline; may cause hyperchloremic acidosis
Potassium	3.5-5.0 mEq/L	<3 or >6.1 mEq/L	↓ Excessive loss of potassium ↑ Impaired elimination from acute kidney injury Observe for cardiac dysrhythmias
Lactic acid (lactate)	0.6-2.2 mmol/L (5-20 mg/dL)	>4 mmol/L	↑ Hypoxia leading to anaerobic metabolism and production of lactic acid
AST	0-35 units/L	>1600 units/L	↑ Hepatic impairment
LDH	100-190 units/L	N/A	↑ Hepatic impairment, renal impairment, intestinal ischemia, or myocardial infarction
Hematology Studies			
WBCs	5000-10,000/mm³	<2000 or >40,000/mm³	↑ Stress response; significant increase indicates infection ↓ Late shock due to consumption of WBCs
Hemoglobin	Male 14-18 g/dL Female 12-16 g/dL	<7 g/dL	↓ Blood loss
Hematocrit	Male 42%-52% Female 37%-47%	<21% or >65%	↓ Blood loss ↑ Dehydration and hemoconcentration
Arterial Blood Gases			
pH	7.35-7.45	<7.25 or >7.65	↑ Early shock: respiratory alkalosis due to hyperventilation ↓ Late shock: metabolic acidosis due to lactic acidosis and respiratory failure
$PaCO_2$	35-45 mm Hg	<20 or >60 mm Hg	↓ Early shock: respiratory alkalosis due to hyperventilation
PaO_2	80-100 mm Hg	<40 mm Hg	↓ Hypoxemia; may indicate pulmonary edema or ARDS
HCO_3^-	21-28 mEq/L	<10 or >40 mEq/L	↓ Late shock: metabolic acidosis caused by hypoxia, anaerobic metabolism, and lactic acidosis
Base deficit/excess	−2 to +2 mEq/L	<−3 mEq/L or >+3 mEq/L	Represents the number of buffering anions in the blood. A negative value (base deficit) indicates metabolic acidosis (e.g., lactic acidosis). A positive value (base excess) indicates metabolic alkalosis or a compensatory response to respiratory acidosis.

[a]Critical values vary by facility and laboratory.
ARDS, Acute respiratory distress syndrome; *AST*, aspartate aminotransferase; HCO_3^-, bicarbonate; *LDH*, lactate dehydrogenase; $PaCO_2$, partial pressure of arterial carbon dioxide; PaO_2, partial pressure of arterial oxygen; *WBCs*, white blood cells.

hemodynamic stability necessary for optimal tissue perfusion. The choice of fluid and the volume and rate of infusion depend on the type of fluid lost, the patient's hemodynamic status, and coexisting conditions.

Benefits of IV fluid administration include increased intravascular volume, increased venous return to the right side of the heart, optimal stretching of the ventricle, improved myocardial contractility, and increased cardiac output. Do not withhold initial fluid resuscitation because of preexisting heart failure.[7,49]

Goal-directed therapy with assessment of fluid volume responsiveness should follow initial resuscitation.[5,8,49] Fluid administration is adjusted based on changes in blood pressure, urine output, hemodynamic values, diagnostic test results, and the clinical picture of the patient's response to treatment. Values obtained from hemodynamic monitoring also assist in monitoring the effects of treatment. Volume replacement usually continues until an adequate mean arterial pressure (MAP) of 65 to 70 mm Hg is achieved and evidence of end-organ tissue perfusion is reestablished, as evidenced by improvement in the level of consciousness, urinary output, and peripheral perfusion.

IV Access. Patients in severe shock may require immediate, rapid volume replacement as well as IV medication administration. The patient in shock requires a minimum of two IV catheters: one in a peripheral vein and ideally one in a central vein. Peripheral access through a large catheter (i.e., 16-gauge) in a large vein in the antecubital fossa provides a route for rapid administration of fluids and medications. Establishing IV routes in a patient in shock is challenging because peripheral vasoconstriction and venous collapse make access difficult. Ultrasound may be used to guide peripheral IV insertion but requires additional training.

Intraosseous (IO) access is used during emergent situations if peripheral access is not readily obtainable.[44] Intraosseous access should be established quickly, and both fluids and medications can be given through the device. An IO needle is most commonly inserted into the proximal tibia but may also be inserted in the distal tibia and proximal humerus.[44]

A central venous catheter is often inserted for large-volume replacement and can be used to trend hemodynamic parameters. Central venous catheters are commonly inserted into the subclavian, internal jugular, or femoral veins. An upper body insertion site is preferred over the femoral vein.[60]

Multilumen catheters, which provide multiple access ports, allow the concurrent administration of fluid, medication, and blood products. A PA catheter may be inserted to monitor hemodynamic pressures and guide fluid replacement. However, a PA catheter is not routinely recommended unless patient management decisions depend on information provided by PA measurements.[49]

Fluids often need to be infused at a rapid rate. Several strategies can be used for rapid administration of fluids, including a pressure bag, large-bore infusion tubing, or a rapid-infusion device. Infusion pumps are recommended to rapidly and accurately administer large volumes of fluids. Administration of large volumes of room-temperature fluids can rapidly drop core body temperature and cause hypothermia. Because fluid-related hypothermia can adversely affect cardiac contractility and coagulopathies, large volumes of fluids are infused through warming devices (Fig. 12.4).

Fluid Challenge. A fluid challenge is often performed to assess the patient's hemodynamic response to fluid administration. Typically, a rapid infusion of 250 mL (up to 2 L) of a crystalloid solution is initiated. Resultant increases in preload and cardiac output are expected. The patient's response depends on the type of shock. Patients experiencing cardiogenic shock with ventricular dysfunction may demonstrate signs of fluid overload after administration of very small volumes of fluid, whereas patients with distributive shock will continue to demonstrate vasodilation-associated hypotension. Nursing responsibilities include obtaining baseline hemodynamic measurements (e.g., blood pressure, MAP, urine output, respiratory rate, SVV, CVP, passive leg raise), administering the fluid challenge, and assessing the patient's response.[5]

Types of Fluids. The choice of fluids depends on the cause of the volume deficit and the patient's clinical status. Although the nurse is not responsible for selecting the infusion or transfusion, it is important to understand the rationale for the prescribed fluid and the expected effects of therapy.

Crystalloids, colloids, blood, and blood products are given alone or in combination to restore intravascular volume. Crystalloid infusions are a first line to resuscitative therapy in shock.[28,29]

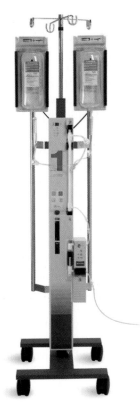

Fig. 12.4 Level 1 rapid infuser. (Courtesy Smiths Medical, Rockland, MA.)

Crystalloids are classified by tonicity. Isotonic solutions have approximately the same tonicity as plasma (osmolality of 250 to 350 mOsm/L). Lactated Ringer's solution and normal saline are isotonic solutions that are commonly infused. These solutions move freely from the intravascular space into the tissues. Lactated Ringer's solution closely resembles plasma, and there is evidence to support that administration of Lactated Ringer's solution may be a more appropriate first choice for fluid resuscitation than 0.9% normal saline.[46,51] Although normal saline is an isotonic solution, its side effects include hypernatremia, hypokalemia, and hyperchloremic metabolic acidosis.[14,46,51]

Solutions of 5% dextrose in water and 0.45% normal saline are hypotonic and are not used for fluid resuscitation. Hypotonic solutions rapidly leave the intravascular space, causing interstitial and intracellular edema.

When large volumes of crystalloids are infused, the patient is at risk for hemodilution of red blood cells and plasma proteins. Hemodilution of red blood cells impairs oxygen delivery if the hematocrit value is decreased, and the cardiac output cannot increase enough to compensate. Hemodilution of plasma proteins decreases colloid osmotic pressure and places the patient at risk for pulmonary edema.[11,33] Elderly patients are at increased risk for pulmonary edema and cardiac dysfunction and may require invasive hemodynamic monitoring to guide fluid resuscitation.

Blood loss should be treated with blood products and hemorrhage control. If blood products are not readily available and the patient is unstable, crystalloids may be administered to maintain hemodynamic stability at a 1:1 ratio of crystalloids to blood loss.[19]

Colloids contain proteins that increase osmotic pressure. Osmotic pressure holds and attracts fluid into blood vessels, thereby expanding plasma volume. Because colloids remain in the intravascular space longer than crystalloids, smaller volumes of colloids may be given in shock states. Albumin and plasma protein fraction (Plasmanate) are naturally occurring colloid solutions that are infused when the decreased volume is caused by a loss of plasma rather than blood, such as in peritonitis and bowel obstruction. Colloids are avoided when there is an increase in capillary permeability, as in sepsis, septic shock, anaphylactic shock, and early burn injury. Administration of colloids has not been shown to reduce mortality (compared to crystalloids) and is more costly.[28,49,51] In addition, colloid administration during initial fluid resuscitation has been associated with a statistically significant increase in 2-year mortality rates in patients with severe traumatic brain injury.[50]

Typing and crossmatching of albumin and plasma protein fraction are not required, but a consent for administration may be necessary, as they are derivatives of blood. Refer to hospital policy for guidance. Pulmonary edema is a potential complication of colloid administration. It results from increased pulmonary capillary permeability or increased capillary hydrostatic pressure in the pulmonary vasculature created by rapid plasma expansion.

Hetastarch (Hespan) is a semisynthetic starch colloid solution that acts as a plasma expander but carries less risk of pulmonary edema. Side effects include altered prothrombin time (PT) and activated partial thromboplastin time (aPTT) and the potential for circulatory overload. Resuscitation with starch solutions may increase the use of renal replacement therapy in critically ill patients.[29]

Blood products, packed red blood cells, fresh frozen plasma (FFP), and platelets are administered to treat major blood loss. Typing and crossmatching of these products are performed to identify the patient's blood type (A, B, AB, or O) and Rhesus (Rh) factor to ensure compatibility with the donor blood and prevent transfusion reactions. In extreme emergencies, patients are transfused with type-specific or uncrossmatched O-negative blood, which is considered the universal donor blood type. Rh factor negative, uncrossmatched type O blood should be administered to women of childbearing age in emergency situations to avoid fetal health problems in the event of pregnancy.

Transfusions require an IV access with at least a 20-gauge, preferably an 18-gauge or larger, catheter. A 22- or 23-gauge needle or catheter may be used in adults with small veins. Administer only normal saline solutions with blood; other solutions cause red blood cells to aggregate, swell, and burst. Never infuse IV medications in the same port with blood. Follow hospital policy to ensure patient and blood identification before starting a transfusion.

Administer transfusions with a blood filter to trap debris and clots. Assess the patient's vital signs frequently during a blood transfusion to monitor for adverse reactions. Signs and symptoms of a transfusion reaction include fever, chills, rash, petechiae, respiratory distress, and hypotension.[15] In the event of a reaction, stop the transfusion, disconnect the transfusion tubing from the IV access site, and keep the vein open with an IV infusion of normal saline solution. Continue to assess the patient, and notify the provider and laboratory. Send all transfusion equipment (bag, tubing, and remaining solutions) and any blood or urine specimens obtained to the laboratory according to hospital policy. Document the events of the reaction, interventions performed, and patient's response to treatment.

Transfusion administration time varies with the type of blood product used and the patient's condition. During transfusion, document the blood product administered, baseline vital signs, start and completion time of the transfusion, volume of blood and fluid administered, assessment of the patient during the transfusion, and any nursing actions taken.

Packed red blood cells increase the blood volume and provide more oxygen-carrying capability. One unit of packed red blood cells increases the hematocrit value by about 3% and the hemoglobin value by 1 g/dL. Typing and crossmatching of packed red blood cells are required. Red blood cells tend to aggregate because of the fibrinogen coating; therefore washed red blood cells may be given. Administration of 10 or more units of packed red cells is associated with decreased 2,3-diphosphoglycerate (2,3-DPG) levels, causing a shift of the oxyhemoglobin dissociation curve to the left, which impairs the delivery of oxygen to the tissues. Stored blood is anticoagulated with citrate, which leads to the chelating of calcium.[30] Therefore monitor ionized calcium levels when transfusing large volumes of packed red blood cells.

Fresh frozen plasma is administered to replace all clotting factors except platelets. One unit of FFP is usually given for every 1 to 2 units of packed red blood cells transfused.[34,58] Typing and crossmatching of FFP are required.

Platelets are given rapidly to help control bleeding caused by low platelet counts (usually <50,000/mm³). Do not administer platelets under pressure, as this can negatively affect their function. Typing of platelets, but not crossmatching, is required.

Although control of hemorrhage is a treatment priority, transfusions are often needed. If massive transfusion is needed, defined as requiring 5 units or more of blood within a 3-hour period (varying definitions exist), protocols recommend giving a ratio of 1:1:1 (packed red blood cells, FFP, and platelets).[59] Some centers administer fresh whole blood, if available, rather than component therapy.

Maintain Arterial Oxygen Saturation and Ventilation

Airway maintenance is a priority (see Chapter 10). Administer oxygen to increase arterial oxygen tension, thereby improving tissue oxygenation. Oxygen administration methods range from nasal cannula to mechanical ventilation, depending on the patient's condition.

Mechanical ventilation also assists in maintaining adequate ventilation as reflected by a normal partial pressure of arterial carbon dioxide ($PaCO_2$) level. Another benefit of mechanical ventilation in a patient with shock is to reduce the work of breathing and the associated increase in oxygen consumption. Strategies to prevent ventilator-induced lung injury, such as low tidal volume ventilation, are implemented if mechanical ventilation is needed.[63] Additional treatment with analgesia, sedation, with or without neuromuscular blockade may be required to reduce oxygen demand (see Chapters 6 and 10).

Pharmacological Support

Pharmacological management of shock is based on manipulation of the determinants of cardiac output: heart rate, preload, afterload, and contractility. Fig. 12.5 shows therapies used to

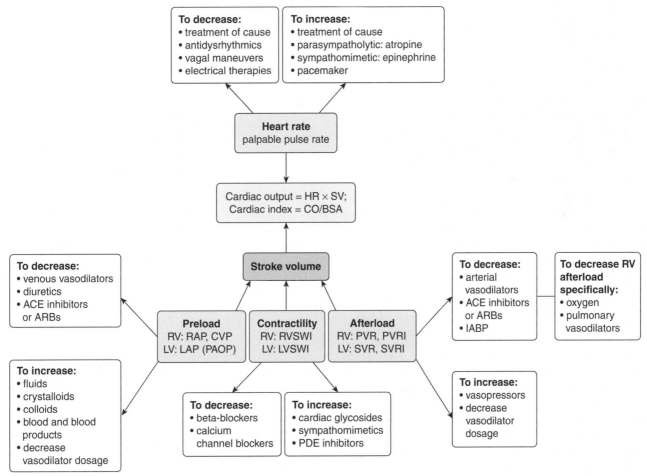

Fig. 12.5 Therapeutic manipulations to optimize cardiac output and/or minimize myocardial oxygen consumption. *ACE,* Angiotensin-converting enzyme; *ARB,* angiotensin receptor blocker; *BSA,* body surface area; *CO,* cardiac output; *CVP,* central venous pressure; *HR,* heart rate; *IABP,* intraaortic balloon pump; *LAP,* left atrial pressure; *LV,* left ventricle; *LVSWI,* left ventricular stroke work index; *PAOP,* pulmonary artery occlusion pressure; *PDE,* phosphodiesterase; *PVR,* pulmonary vascular resistance; *PVRI,* pulmonary vascular resistance index; *RAP,* right atrial pressure; *RV,* right ventricle; *RVSWI,* right ventricular stroke work index; *SV,* stroke volume; *SVR,* systemic vascular resistance; *SVRI,* systemic vascular resistance index. (Modified from Dennison RD. *Pass CCRN!* 5th ed. St. Louis, MO: Mosby; 2019.)

manipulate these parameters. Many medications are vesicants and are preferably administered through a central venous catheter. Assess effectiveness of medications through noninvasive and invasive hemodynamic monitoring (see Chapter 9). Older adults are particularly sensitive to the physiological effect of medications and the deleterious effects of polypharmacy, which requires closer monitoring. Medications commonly administered in shock are listed in Table 12.4.

Cardiac Output. Low or high heart rates and dysrhythmias decrease cardiac output. Chronotropic and antidysrhythmic medications are administered as indicated.

TABLE 12.4 PHARMACOLOGY

Medications Commonly Used for Treating Shock

Medication	Action and Use	Dose and Route[a]	Side Effects	Nursing Implications
Dobutamine (Dobutrex)	Stimulates primarily beta$_1$ receptors to ↑ contractility (cardiogenic and distributive shock) and ↑ HR and causes vasodilation in low-CO states	*Continuous infusion:* Initial, 0.5-1 mcg/kg/min IV Maintenance, 2-20 mcg/kg/min IV Titrate based on response Central venous catheter preferred	Headache Anxiety Tachycardia Dysrhythmias Hypotension Palpitations Chest pain Dyspnea Nausea, vomiting Paresthesia	Monitor BP, HR, ECG, PAP, PAOP, SVR, CO, and CI. Use cautiously in patients with hypertension, myocardial ischemia, or ventricular dysrhythmias. Titrate so HR does not increase by more than 10% of baseline. Replace volume before initiation of infusion. Do not administer with alkaline solutions.
Dopamine (Intropin)	Used in low-CO states or vasodilatory states (distributive shock) to restore vascular tone Dose-dependent effect At 2-10 mcg/kg/min stimulates beta$_1$ receptors, which ↑ contractility and HR At 10-20 mcg/kg/min, stimulates alpha receptors, which causes vasoconstriction and ↑ SVR	*Continuous infusion:* Initial, 2-10 mcg/kg/min IV Maintenance, 2-20 mcg/kg/min IV Titrate by 5-10 mcg/kg/min q 10 to 30 minutes until targets achieved to a maximum of 50 mcg/kg/min Central venous catheter preferred	Headache Tachycardia Dysrhythmias Palpitations Chest pain in patients with coronary artery disease Dyspnea Nausea, vomiting	Monitor HR, BP, ECG, PAP, PAOP, SVR, CO, CI, and urine output. Treat cause of ↓ BP before initiating (e.g., hypovolemia treated with fluid resuscitation). Consider norepinephrine if 20 mcg/kg/min is ineffective. Dosing greater than 20 mcg/kg/min decreases perfusion to the kidneys. Wean slowly. Tissue necrosis if extravasation; treat extravasation with phentolamine (Regitine). Do not administer with alkaline solutions.
Epinephrine	Used in hypotensive states to produce constriction of vascular smooth muscle Promotes bronchodilation in anaphylactic shock	**Septic shock and hypotension** *Continuous infusion:* Initial, 0.05-2.0 mcg/kg/min IV Maintenance, titrate in increments of 0.05-0.2 mcg/kg/min q 10-15 min to target MAP. **Anaphylactic shock** *Intramuscular/subcutaneous:* 0.3 mg, IM into anterior thigh preferred; can be given through clothing *Intravenous:* Bolus: 0.1 mg of a 0.1 mg/mL solution administered over 5 to 10 minutes Continuous infusion: Initial, 2-15 mcg/min with crystalloid Central venous catheter preferred	Anxiety Chest pain Hypertension Tachycardia Pulmonary edema Dyspnea	Monitor HR, BP, ECG, and chest pain. Assess and correct volume depletion before and during administration. Tissue necrosis if extravasation; treat extravasation with phentolamine (Regitine).
Norepinephrine (Levophed)	Stimulates alpha receptors, which causes vasoconstriction Used in vasodilatory states (distributive shock) to restore vascular tone Stimulation of beta receptors, which ↑ contractility and HR	*Continuous infusion:* Initial, 0.5-1 mcg/min IV Maintenance, 2-4 mcg/min; titrate to maintain desired BP range; maximum dose, 30 mcg/min Central venous catheter preferred	Anxiety Headache Tremor Dizziness Tachycardia Ventricular dysrhythmias Hypertension Chest pain Metabolic (lactic) acidosis	Monitor BP, HR, ECG, urine output, and neurological status. Tissue necrosis if extravasation; treat extravasation with phentolamine (Regitine). Do not administer with alkaline solutions.

✦ **TABLE 12.4 PHARMACOLOGY—cont'd**

Medications Commonly Used for Treating Shock

Medication	Action and Use	Dose and Route[a]	Side Effects	Nursing Implications
Phenylephrine (Neo-Synephrine)	Stimulates alpha receptors, which causes vasoconstriction Used in vasodilatory states (distributive shock) to restore vascular tone	*Bolus:* 40-100 mcg IV, repeat q 1-2 minutes, not to exceed 200 mcg *Continuous infusion:* Initial, 10-35 mcg/min Maintenance, titrate to maintain desired BP range; maximum dose, 200 mcg/min Central venous catheter preferred	Anxiety Restlessness Headache Tremor Reflex bradycardia Ventricular dysrhythmias Hypertension Palpitations Chest pain Nausea, vomiting Paresthesia	Monitor HR, BP, and ECG. Treat reflex bradycardia with atropine.
Vasopressin	Vasoconstriction through smooth muscle contraction of all parts of capillaries, arterioles, and venules Used in vasodilatory states (distributive shock) to restore vascular tone	*Continuous infusion:* Initial, 0.01-0.03 unit/min IV Maintenance, titrate by 0.005 units/min q 10-15 minutes to desired BP; maximum dose, 0.07 units/min Central venous catheter preferred	Fever Tremor Headache Seizures Coma Bradycardia Chest pain and myocardial ischemia Hypertension Hyponatremia Abdominal cramps	Monitor HR, BP, ECG, and urine output. Tissue necrosis if extravasation; treat extravasation with phentolamine (Regitine).
Nitroglycerin	Vasodilation by direct smooth muscle relaxation, predominantly venous Used in preload and/or afterload reduction (cardiogenic shock) Dose-dependent effect Arterial dilation only if infusion >1 mcg/kg/min	*Continuous infusion:* Initial, 5 mcg/min IV infusion Maintenance, increase by 5 mcg/min q 3-5 min until desired results are achieved. If no response is seen at 20 mcg/min, increase by 10-20 mcg/min until desired results achieved (control of chest pain and decreased preload) Peripheral venous catheter acceptable	Headache Apprehension Dizziness Flushing Syncope Tachycardia Hypotension Palpitations Weakness	Monitor HR, BP, and urine output. Monitor RAP, PAP, PAOP, SVR, CO, and CI if pulmonary artery catheter in place. Use cautiously in cases of hypotension. Administer in glass bottle with non–polyvinyl chloride tubing.
Nitroprusside (Nipride)	Vasodilation by direct smooth muscle relaxation, predominantly arterial Used in preload and/or afterload reduction (cardiogenic shock)	*Continuous infusion:* Initial, 0.3 mcg/kg/min IV infusion Maintenance, titrate by 0.5 mcg/kg/min to achieve desired BP; maximum dose, 10 mcg/kg/min Peripheral venous catheter acceptable	Headache Tinnitus Dizziness Diaphoresis Apprehension Hypotension Tachycardia Palpitations Hypoxemia (from nitroprusside-induced intrapulmonary thiocyanate toxicity) Nausea, vomiting Abdominal pain	Monitor HR, BP, urine output, and neurological status. Monitor for patient thiocyanate toxicity (metabolic acidosis, confusion, hyperreflexia, and seizures). Serum thiocyanate levels drawn daily if drug is used longer than 72 h. Treatment includes amyl nitrate, sodium nitrate, and/or sodium thiosulfate. Protect from light by wrapping with opaque material such as aluminum foil.

[a] All medications are administered by volumetric infusion pump.
BP, Blood pressure; *CI,* cardiac index; *CO,* cardiac output; *ECG,* electrocardiogram; *HR,* heart rate; *MAP,* mean arterial pressure; *PAOP,* pulmonary artery occlusion pressure; *PAP,* pulmonary artery pressure; *q,* every; *RAP,* right atrial pressure; *SVR,* systemic vascular resistance.
From Gahart B, Nazareno A. *Gahart's 2019 Intravenous Medications.* 35th ed. St. Louis, MO: Elsevier; 2019.

Preload. In hypovolemic and distributive shock, fluid administration is the primary treatment to increase preload. In cardiogenic shock, the myofibrils are overstretched, and strategies to reduce the preload are implemented. Medications that reduce preload include venous vasodilators and diuretics.

Afterload. Afterload is low in distributive shock. In this situation, medications that cause vasoconstriction are administered to increase vascular tone and tissue perfusion pressure. Examples of vasoconstrictive medications include phenylephrine, norepinephrine, epinephrine, and vasopressin. These medications increase blood pressure and SVR. A negative effect of medications that increase afterload is an increase in myocardial oxygen demand. Accurate measurement and calculation of SVR and pulmonary vascular resistance (PVR) using a PA catheter assists in assessment.

Do not administer vasopressor medications to treat hypovolemic shock until hypovolemia is corrected with volume replacement. Administration of vasopressors in hypovolemia causes vasoconstriction and further diminishes tissue perfusion.

In cardiogenic shock, afterload must be reduced. The use of arterial vasodilators to reduce afterload may be limited by the patient's blood pressure. When hypotension prevents the use of arterial vasodilators, an intraaortic balloon pump (IABP) is used to decrease afterload as discussed later in the chapter and in Chapter 13.

Contractility. Medications that increase contractility, inotropic agents such as dobutamine and digoxin, may be administered in cardiogenic shock.

Other Medications. Other medications used to manage shock include sedatives, analgesics, insulin, corticosteroids, and antibiotics. Although respiratory acidosis is treated by improving ventilation, metabolic acidosis caused by lactic acidosis is best treated by improving oxygen delivery, SaO_2, hemoglobin level, and cardiac output. Monitor arterial blood gas analysis and serum lactate levels to guide treatment.

Insulin therapy should be initiated when two consecutive blood glucose levels are greater than 180 mg/dL. The goal is to maintain a blood glucose level of 180 mg/dL or less.[49] Low-molecular-weight heparin is often prescribed for deep vein thrombosis prophylaxis. Peptic ulcer prophylaxis is often initiated with an H_2-receptor antagonist or proton pump inhibitor.

Body Temperature

Monitor the patient's temperature and implement care to maintain a normal body temperature. Fever is defined as a core temperature above 38.2°C.[64] Increased body temperature increases oxygen demand and can negatively affect the already stressed cardiovascular system.[10]

Hypothermia is defined as a drop in core body temperature below 35°C.[40] Hypothermia causes dysrhythmias, depresses cardiac contractility, and reduces cardiac output, ultimately decreasing oxygen delivery. The coagulation pathway is altered, and platelet function is impaired in hypothermia, which can result in significant coagulopathies. Anticipate hypothermia when fluids are infused rapidly, and proactively use warming methods (e.g., fluid warmer, heated forced air blankets, blankets around the patient's head). Keep the patient warm and comfortable, avoiding hyperthermia.

Nutritional Support

Nutritional support is essential for patient survival. The goals of nutritional support are to initiate enteral intake as soon as possible and to maintain sufficient caloric intake to assist the healing process. Early administration of enteral nutrition may assist with maintenance of gut integrity and reduction of insulin resistance.[21,48,49] Nutritional requirements of the patient in shock depend on the degree of hemodynamic stability; the cause of shock; and the patient's age, gender, and preexisting diseases. Overfeeding patients in the early phases of shock is associated with adverse outcomes.[47,49]

Enteral feeding is the preferred method; however, administration of enteral nutrition may be limited by paralytic ileus, gastric dilation, or both, which are common in shock. Total parenteral nutrition is given if patients are unable to tolerate enteral feeding (see Chapter 7).

Psychological Support

Nursing interventions focus on identifying the effect of the illness on the patient and the family. Provide information that is essential for the psychological well-being of the patient and family and that may help give them a sense of understanding and control of the situation. Since shock has a high mortality, initiate a discussion regarding the patient's goals of care and life-sustaining therapies (see Chapters 2, 3, and 4).

◎ PLAN OF CARE

For the Patient in Shock

Patient Problem

Decreased Multisystem Tissue Perfusion. Risk factors include decreased blood volume (i.e., hypovolemic shock), decreased myocardial contractility (i.e., cardiogenic shock), impaired circulatory blood flow (i.e., obstructive shock), and widespread vasodilation (i.e., septic, anaphylactic, or neurogenic shock).

Desired Outcomes

- Vital signs and hemodynamic parameters within normal limits (see Table 12.3).
- Oxygen saturation 90% or greater.
- Balanced intake and output.
- Urine output at least 0.5 mL/kg/h.
- Normal serum and urine laboratory values and ABG results.
- Absence of complications (ARDS, DIC, acute kidney injury, hepatic failure, MODS).
- Normal mentation.

Nursing Assessments/Interventions	Rationales
• Monitor for early symptoms of shock (see Table 12.2).	• Initiate early support to improve outcomes and reduce risk of complications, organ dysfunction, and death.

◎ PLAN OF CARE—cont'd

For the Patient in Shock

Nursing Assessments/Interventions	Rationales
• Establish IV access; use large-bore catheters (16 gauge); and obtain central venous access, if possible.	• Provide rapid medication and fluid administration.
• Control bleeding through the application of pressure or surgical intervention.	• Reduce risk of infiltration and irritation of peripheral site.
• Administer fluids as ordered (e.g., crystalloids, colloids, blood products).	• Prevent blood loss.
• Consider warming fluids before and during infusing.	• Maintain tissue perfusion.
• Replace blood components as indicated; obtain laboratory specimen for type and crossmatch.	• Reduce hypothermia
• Evaluate patient's response to fluid challenges and blood product administration such as improved vital signs, level of consciousness, urinary output, hemodynamic values, and serum and urine laboratory values.	• Replace volume loss associated with blood loss; prevent transfusion reaction. • Monitor response to treatment.
• Monitor for clinical indications of fluid overload (↑ HR, ↑ RR, dyspnea, crackles) when fluids are administered rapidly.	• Assess for signs of volume overload in response to treatment.

• Monitor cardiopulmonary status:
  • HR   • Capillary refill
  • RR   • Mottling
  • BP   • Hemodynamic values
  • MAP   • Cardiac rhythm
  • Skin color • Neck veins
  • Temperature • Lung sounds
  • Moisture
	• Monitor response to treatment.

• Monitor level of consciousness.	• Assess perfusion of the central nervous system.

• Monitor gastrointestinal status:
  • Abdominal distension
  • Bowel sounds
  • Gastric pH
  • Vomiting
  • Large enteral feeding residual
	• Assess perfusion of the gastrointestinal system.

• Monitor fluid balance:
  • I&O
  • Daily weights
  • Amount and type of drainage (chest tube, nasogastric, wounds)
	• Evaluate need for continued fluid volume support.
	• Alterations in fluid balance may indicate end organ damage (i.e., acute kidney injury).

• Monitor serial serum values:
  • Hct   • Platelets
  • Hgb   • ABGs
  • WBC   • Chemistry profile
  • PT   • Lactate
  • aPTT   • Cultures
  • D-dimer
	• Evaluate physiological status and response to treatment.

• Administer medications as prescribed and based on the classification of shock (see Table 12.4).	• Improve outcomes and reduce complications.
• Evaluate patient response to interventions and adjust treatments accordingly; monitor for complications.	• Monitor patient response to determine need for modification of treatment and/or nursing care.

ABG, Arterial blood gas; *aPTT,* activated partial thromboplastin time; *ARDS,* acute respiratory distress syndrome; *BP,* blood pressure; *DIC,* disseminated intravascular coagulation; *Hct,* hematocrit; *Hgb,* hemoglobin; *HR,* heart rate; *I&O,* intake and output; *MAP,* mean arterial pressure; *MODS,* multiple organ dysfunction syndrome; *PT,* prothrombin time; *RR,* respiratory rate; *WBC,* white blood cell.
Adapted from Swearingen PLW, Wright JD. *All-in-One Nursing Care Planning Resource.* 5th ed. St. Louis, MO: Elsevier; 2019.

CLASSIFICATIONS OF SHOCK

Table 12.5 summarizes the classifications of shock.

Hypovolemic Shock

Hypovolemic shock occurs when the circulating blood volume is inadequate to fill the vascular network. Intravascular volume deficits may be caused by external or internal losses of blood or fluid. In these situations, the intravascular blood volume is depleted and unavailable to transport oxygen and nutrients to tissues. The severity of hypovolemic shock depends on the degree of volume loss, the type of fluid lost, and the age and preinjury health status of the patient.

External volume deficits include loss of blood, plasma, or body fluids. The most common cause of hypovolemic shock is hemorrhage. External loss of blood may occur after traumatic

TABLE 12.5	Summary of Classifications of Shock		
Classification	**Possible Causes**	**Clinical Presentation**	**Management**
Hypovolemic shock	*External loss of blood:* • GI hemorrhage • Surgery • Trauma *External loss of fluid:* • Diarrhea • Diuresis • Burns *Internal sequestration of blood/fluid:* • Hemoperitoneum • Retroperitoneal hemorrhage • Hemothorax • Hemomediastinum • Dissecting aortic aneurysm • Femur or pelvic fracture • Ascites • Pleural effusion	↑ HR ↓ BP Tachypnea Oliguria Cool, pale skin Decreased mentation Flat neck veins ↓ CO, CI, RAP, PAP, PAOP ↑ SVR ↓ SvO$_2$ ↑ Hematocrit if from dehydration ↓ Hematocrit if from blood loss	Eliminate and treat the cause Replace lost volume with appropriate fluid
Cardiogenic shock	Myocardial infarction Myocardial contusion Cardiomyopathy Myocarditis Severe heart failure Dysrhythmias Valvular dysfunction Ventricular septal rupture	↑ HR Dysrhythmias ↓ BP Chest pain Tachypnea Oliguria Cool, pale skin ↓ Mentation Left ventricular failure Right ventricular failure ↓ CO, CI ↑ RAP, PAP, PAOP, SVR ↓ SvO$_2$	Improve contractility with inotropic medications Mechanical circulatory support Emergency revascularization Optimize preload Reduce afterload Prevent or treat dysrhythmias
Obstructive shock	*Impaired diastolic filling:* • Cardiac tamponade • Tension pneumothorax • Constrictive pericarditis • Compression of great vein *Increased right ventricular afterload:* • Pulmonary embolism • Severe pulmonary hypertension • Increased intrathoracic pressure *Increased left ventricular afterload:* • Aortic dissection • Systemic embolization • Aortic stenosis • Abdominal hypertension	↑ HR Dysrhythmias ↓ BP Chest pain Dyspnea Oliguria Cool, pale skin Decreased mental status Jugular venous distension Cardiac tamponade: muffled heart sounds, pulsus paradoxus Tension pneumothorax: diminished breath sounds on affected side, tracheal shift away from affected side Pulmonary embolism: right ventricular failure Aortic dissection: ripping chest pain, pulse differences between left and right side, widened mediastinum ↓ CO, CI ↑ or Normal RAP, PAP, PAOP ↑ PVR, SVR ↓ SvO$_2$	Eliminate source of obstruction or compression Pericardiocentesis for cardiac tamponade Fibrinolytics, anticoagulants for PE Emergency decompression for tension pneumothorax

TABLE 12.5	Summary of Classifications of Shock—cont'd		
Classification	**Possible Causes**	**Clinical Presentation**	**Management**
Anaphylactic shock	*Foods:* fish, shellfish, eggs, milk, wheat, strawberries, peanuts, tree nuts (pecans, walnuts), food additives *Medications:* antibiotics, ACE inhibitors, aspirin, local anesthetics, narcotics, barbiturates, contrast media, blood and blood products, allergic extracts *Bites or stings:* venomous snakes, wasps, hornets, spiders, jellyfish, stingrays, deer flies, fire ants *Chemicals:* latex, lotions, soap, perfumes, iodine-containing solutions	↑ HR; dysrhythmias ↓ BP Chest pain Tachypnea Flushed, warm to hot skin Oliguria Restlessness, change in LOC, seizures Nausea, vomiting, abdominal cramping, diarrhea Dyspnea, cough, stridor, wheezing, dysphagia Urticaria, angioedema, hives ↓ CO, CI ↓ RAP, PAP, PAOP, SVR ↓ SvO$_2$ ↑ IgE	Remove offending agent or slow absorption: remove stinger; apply ice to sting or bite; discontinue drug, dye, blood; lavage stomach if antigen ingested; flush skin with water Maintain airway, oxygenation, and ventilation; intubation may be necessary Modify or block the effects of mediators: epinephrine, antihistamines, steroids Maintain MAP
Neurogenic shock	General or spinal anesthesia Epidural block Spinal cord injury at or above the level of T6 *Medications:* barbiturates, phenothiazines, sympathetic blocking agents	↓ HR ↓ BP Hypothermia Warm, dry, flushed skin Oliguria Neurological deficit ↓ CO, CI ↓ RAP, PAP, PAOP, SVR ↓ SvO$_2$	Eliminate and treat the cause Maintain MAP Maintain adequate heart rate VTE prophylaxis
Septic shock	*Immunosuppression:* • Extremes of age • Malnutrition • Alcoholism or drug abuse • Malignancy • History of splenectomy • Chronic health problems • Immunosuppressive therapies *Significant bacteremia:* • Invasive procedures and devices • Traumatic wounds or burns • GI infection or untreated disease • Peritonitis • Food poisoning • Prolonged hospitalization	↑ HR ↑ RR ↓ BP Temperature >38.3°C or <36°C WBC >12/mm^3 or <4/mm^3 Lactate >4 mmol/L or >2 mmol/L after fluid resuscitation Confusion Widened pulse pressure Skin warm, flushed Poor capillary refill Mottling Oliguria ↑ CO, CI ↓ RAP, PAP, PAOP, SVR ↑ SvO$_2$, then ↓	Obtain blood cultures Administer antibiotics within 1 h of diagnosis Obtain lactate level Administer fluid bolus of at least 30 mL/kg in the first 3 h; additional fluid resuscitation guided by hemodynamic status Administer vasopressors if systolic BP <90 mm Hg or MAP <65 mm Hg after fluid bolus Good hand-washing techniques Avoid invasive procedures Identify source of infection Meticulous oral and airway care Meticulous catheter and wound care Avoid NPO status: initiate and maintain enteral nutrition Antibiotics as indicated by culture results Maintain MAP >65 mm Hg

ACE, Angiotensin-converting enzyme; *BP,* blood pressure; *CI,* cardiac index; *CO,* cardiac output; *GI,* gastrointestinal; *HR,* heart rate; *IgE,* immunoglobulin E; *LOC,* level of consciousness; *MAP,* mean arterial pressure; *NPO,* nothing by mouth; *PAOP,* pulmonary artery occlusion pressure; *PAP,* pulmonary artery pressure; *PE,* pulmonary embolism; *PVR,* pulmonary vascular resistance; *RAP,* right atrial pressure; *SvO$_2$,* mixed venous oxygen saturation; *SVR,* systemic vascular resistance; *VTE,* venous thromboembolism; *WBC,* white blood cell.

injury, surgery, or obstetric delivery or with coagulation alterations (hemophilia, thrombocytopenia, DIC, and anticoagulant medications). External plasma losses may be seen in patients with burn injuries who have significant fluid shifts from the intravascular space to the interstitial space (see Chapter 21). Excessive external loss of fluid may occur through the gastrointestinal tract because of suctioning, upper gastrointestinal bleeding, vomiting, diarrhea, reduction in oral fluid intake, or fistulas; through the genitourinary tract as a result of excessive diuresis, diabetes mellitus with polyuria, diabetes insipidus, or Addison disease; or through the skin due to diaphoresis without fluid and electrolyte replacement.

Blood or body fluids may be sequestered within the body outside the vascular bed. For example, blood may sequester secondary to a ruptured spleen or liver, hemothorax, hemorrhagic pancreatitis, fractures of the femur or pelvis, and dissecting aneurysm. Other forms of internal sequestration of body fluids include ascites, peritonitis, and intestinal obstruction (whereby fluid leaks from the intestinal capillaries into the lumen of the intestine).

Assess for both obvious and subtle fluid losses. Weigh dressings; measure drainage from chest or nasogastric tubes; monitor potential sites for bleeding, such as surgical wounds, or IV or intraarterial catheter sites after removal; and consider insensible losses, such as perspiration. Measure abdominal girth periodically in patients in whom occult bleeding may be suspected or in those with ascites. Obtain daily weights by using the same scale with the patient wearing the same clothing at approximately the same time each day. If a bed scale is used, ensure that the equipment and tubing do not touch the bed. Evaluate the hematocrit to help determine whether blood or fluid was lost. In a patient with blood loss, the hematocrit is decreased, whereas in a patient with fluid loss, the hematocrit is increased.

Hypovolemic shock results in a reduction of intravascular volume and a decrease in venous return to the right side of the heart. Ventricular filling pressures (preload) are reduced, resulting in decreased stroke volume and cardiac output. As the cardiac output decreases, blood pressure and tissue perfusion also

decrease. Fig. 12.6 summarizes the pathophysiology of hypovolemic shock.

Patients with hypovolemic shock present with signs and symptoms as a result of poor organ perfusion, including altered mentation ranging from lethargy to unresponsiveness; rapid, deep respirations; cool, clammy skin with weak, thready pulses; tachycardia; and oliguria. Hypovolemic shock resulting from hemorrhage is classified according to the volume of blood lost and the resultant effects on the level of consciousness, vital signs, and urine output (Table 12.6).

An increase in abdominal girth may indicate abdominal bleeding or fluid loss into the abdomen. Consider monitoring intraabdominal pressures to assess for abdominal compartment syndrome (ACS). ACS can compound hypovolemic shock via obstructive shock, leading to rapid patient deterioration if not emergently decompressed. Ultrasonography is performed to detect abdominal bleeding or fluid loss. Particularly in trauma patients, a focused assessment with sonography for trauma (FAST) exam is used to evaluate the torso for free fluid, which may be indicative of noncompressible torso hemorrhage (see Chapter 20). If fluid is found, computed tomography (CT) may be obtained to pinpoint sources of bleeding in the hemodynamically stable patient or to locate possible abscesses in the potentially septic patient. In the hemodynamically unstable

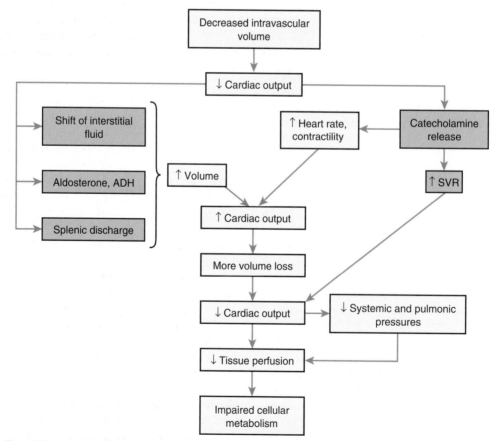

Fig. 12.6 Hypovolemic shock. Hypovolemic shock becomes life-threatening when compensatory mechanisms *(orange boxes)* are overwhelmed by continuous loss of intravascular volume. *ADH,* Antidiuretic hormone; *SVR,* systemic vascular resistance. (From McCance K, Huether S. *Pathophysiology: The Biologic Basis for Disease in Adults and Children.* 8th ed. St. Louis, MO: Elsevier; 2019.)

TABLE 12.6 Severity of Hemorrhagic Shock

Indicators	CLASS			
	I Compensated	II Mild	III Moderate	IV Severe
Blood loss (% blood volume)	<15%	15%-30%	30%-40%	>40%
Blood loss (mL)	750-1000	1000-1500	1500-2000	>2000
Heart rate (beats/min)	<100	100-120	120-140	>140
Blood pressure	Normal	Orthostatic changes	Decreased	Greatly decreased
Respiratory rate (breaths/min)	Normal	Normal to mildly increased	Moderate tachypnea	Marked tachypnea
Urine output (mL/h)	Normal	Normal	Decreased	Significantly decreased
Glasgow Coma Scale score	Normal	Normal	Decreased	Decreased
Need for blood products	Monitor for need	Possible need	Yes	Massive transfusion protocol

Modified from American College of Surgeons' Committee on Trauma. *Advanced Trauma Life Support (ATLS) Program for Doctors: Student Manual.* 10th ed. Chicago, IL: American College of Surgeons; 2018.

bleeding patient, either interventional radiology or surgical intervention is warranted.

Management of hypovolemic shock focuses on identifying, treating, and eliminating the cause of hypovolemia and replacing lost fluid. Consider the type of fluid lost when determining fluid replacement. Treatment can include surgery, antidiarrheal medication for diarrhea, reversal of anticoagulation, and insulin for hyperglycemia. The type of fluid lost is considered when determining fluid replacement.

Isotonic crystalloids such as Lactated Ringer's solution are typically used first, although blood and blood products may be administered if the patient is bleeding.[51] Limit fluid resuscitation with crystalloids to no more than 3 liters within the first 6 hours of hypovolemic shock resuscitation.[9] Over-resuscitation with crystalloids dilutes the blood and impairs oxygen-carrying capacity and clotting factors, which can lead to decreased tissue perfusion and increased bleeding.[9] Monitor the patient's response to therapy by assessing oxygenation, blood pressure, pulse, level of consciousness, capillary refill, and urine output.[9,39,58]

Cardiogenic Shock

Cardiogenic shock can occur when the heart fails to act as an effective pump. A decrease in myocardial contractility results in decreased cardiac output and impaired tissue perfusion. Cardiogenic shock is one of the most difficult types of shock to treat and carries a hospital mortality rate as high as 51%.[61]

The most common cause of cardiogenic shock is extensive left ventricular myocardial infarction. The degree of myocardial damage correlates with the likelihood of cardiogenic shock. If 40% or more of the left ventricle is damaged, the likelihood of cardiogenic shock increases.[6] Other causes of cardiogenic shock include dysrhythmias, congenital abnormalities, cardiomyopathy, myocarditis, valvular dysfunction, severe heart failure, and structural disorders.[61]

The pathophysiology of cardiogenic shock can be understood by reviewing the dynamics of cardiac output and stroke volume. When damage to the myocardium occurs, contractile force is reduced, and stroke volume decreases. Ventricular filling pressures increase because blood remains in the cardiac chambers. Cardiac output and ejection fraction decrease, causing hypotension. Increased left ventricular end-diastolic pressure creates pulmonary congestion with resultant hypoxia. A progressive decrease in cardiac output leads to further impairment of coronary artery perfusion and tissue perfusion. Neurohormonal mechanisms trigger peripheral vasoconstriction with retention of sodium and water, which in turn increases preload.[6] Fig. 12.7 illustrates the pathophysiology of cardiogenic shock.

Increased demand is placed on the myocardium as it attempts to increase perfusion to the cells. The heart rate increases as a compensatory mechanism, increasing the oxygen demand of an overworked myocardium. Compensatory mechanisms may increase myocardial oxygen requirements, which may further increase infarction size.

The clinical presentation of cardiogenic shock includes manifestations of left ventricular failure (S3 heart sound, crackles, dyspnea, hypoxemia, hypotension) and right ventricular failure (jugular venous distension, peripheral edema, hepatomegaly). Hemodynamic monitoring via PA catheter or less invasive technologies may be useful for assessment and monitoring response to treatment.[6,61] In cardiogenic shock, cardiac output and cardiac index decrease; however, RAP, pulmonary artery pressure (PAP), and PAOP increase as pressure and volume back up into the pulmonary circulation and the right side of the heart. Chest radiograph, 12-lead electrocardiogram, and transthoracic or transesophageal echocardiogram may assist in diagnosis of cardiogenic shock.[61]

Treatment of cardiogenic shock focuses on promoting myocardial contractility, decreasing the myocardial oxygen demand, and increasing the oxygen supply to the damaged tissue. Administer oxygen to increase oxygen delivery to the ischemic muscle and preserve myocardial tissue.[61]

Aggressive management after a myocardial infarction includes percutaneous coronary interventions, with or without intracoronary stent placement; fibrinolytic agents when primary percutaneous coronary intervention is not available; glycoprotein IIb/IIIa inhibitors; and beta-blockers to limit the size of the infarction. Pain relief and rest reduce the workload of the heart and the infarct size.

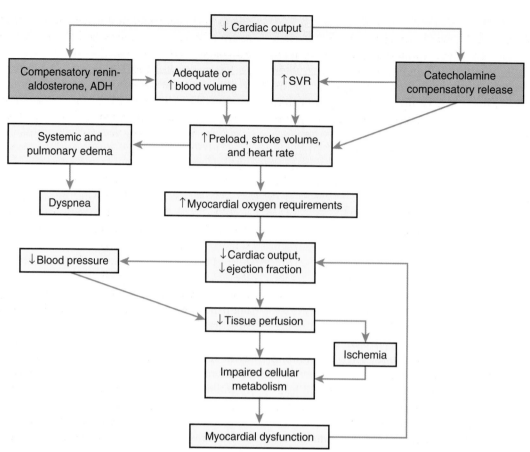

Fig. 12.7 Cardiogenic shock. Cardiogenic shock becomes life-threatening when compensatory mechanisms *(orange boxes)* increase myocardial oxygen requirements. *ADH,* Antidiuretic hormone; *SVR,* systemic vascular resistance. (From From McCance K, Huether S. *Pathophysiology: The Biologic Basis for Disease in Adults and Children.* 8th ed. St. Louis, MO: Elsevier; 2019.)

Medications are administered to decrease preload (RAP and PAOP), decrease afterload (SVR), increase stroke volume, increase cardiac index, and increase contractility (see Table 12.4). Diuretics (e.g., furosemide) and venous vasodilators (e.g., morphine, nitroglycerin, nitroprusside) reduce preload and venous return to the heart. Nitroglycerin at low doses (<1 mcg/kg/min) causes venous vasodilation to decrease preload. At higher doses (>1 mcg/kg/min), arterial vasodilation decreases afterload. Administer medications cautiously because they may cause hypotension, further contributing to cellular hypoperfusion.

Positive inotropic medications (e.g., dobutamine) are given to increase the contractile force of the heart. As contractility increases, ventricular emptying improves, filling pressures decrease (RAP and PAOP), and stroke volume improves. The improved stroke volume increases cardiac output and improves tissue perfusion. However, positive inotropic medications also increase myocardial oxygen demand and must be used cautiously in patients with myocardial ischemia.

Afterload reduction may be achieved by the cautious administration of arterial vasodilators (e.g., nitroprusside) to decrease SVR, increase stroke volume, and increase cardiac index. Closely monitor blood pressure to keep the MAP above 65 mm Hg to ensure organ perfusion. Significant hypotension may limit the use of arterial vasodilators because coronary artery perfusion pressure may be reduced and worsen myocardial ischemia. In this situation, afterload reduction is achieved through the insertion of an IABP.

The IABP is a mechanical circulatory support device that provides *counterpulsation therapy* concurrently with pharmacological support. The IABP improves coronary artery perfusion, reduces afterload, and improves perfusion to vital organs. Desired outcomes for a patient in cardiogenic shock with an IABP include decreased SVR, diminished symptoms of myocardial ischemia (i.e., chest pain, ST-segment elevation), and increased stroke volume and cardiac output.

Other mechanical circulatory devices may be required to temporarily support a failing ventricle that has not responded to IABP therapy and pharmacological therapy.[20] The devices are used to treat cardiogenic shock by allowing the ventricle to recover or to support the patient awaiting cardiac transplantation. Examples include the Impella (Abiomed, Danvers, MA), TandemHeart (LivaNova, Houston, TX), or extracorporeal membrane oxygenation (ECMO). These devices can support the left ventricle, the right ventricle, or both ventricles.[3] Additional information about the IABP and other mechanical assist devices is provided in Chapter 13.

Distributive Shock

Distributive shock, also known as vasogenic shock, describes several types of shock that manifest with widespread vasodilation and decreased SVR, including neurogenic, anaphylactic, and septic shock. Vasodilation increases the vascular capacity, but the blood volume is unchanged, resulting in relative hypovolemia. This causes a decrease in venous return to the right side of the heart and a reduction in ventricular filling pressures. Anaphylactic shock and septic shock are also complicated by an increase in capillary permeability, which decreases intravascular volume, further compromising venous return. In all forms of distributive shock, stroke volume, cardiac output, and blood pressure eventually decrease, resulting in decreased tissue perfusion and tissue hypoxia leading to impaired cellular metabolism.

Neurogenic Shock. Neurogenic shock occurs when a disturbance in the nervous system affects the vasomotor center in the medulla. In healthy persons, the vasomotor center initiates sympathetic stimulation of nerve fibers that travel down the spinal cord and out to the periphery, where they innervate the smooth muscles of the blood vessels and cause vasoconstriction. In neurogenic shock, there is an interruption of impulse transmission or a blockage of sympathetic outflow that results in vasodilation, inhibition of baroreceptor response, and impaired thermoregulation. These reactions produce vasodilation with decreased SVR, venous return, preload, and cardiac output and a relative hypovolemia. Fig. 12.8 summarizes the pathophysiology of neurogenic shock.

Causes of neurogenic shock include direct and indirect insults to the nervous system. Spinal cord injuries are the most common cause of neurogenic shock, specifically those above the level of T4, but can occur in patients with injuries as low as T6.[56]

Neurogenic shock may also result from surgical intervention, cerebral ischemia, and injury to the medulla or be triggered by extreme stress or severe pain.[52,55,56]

The most profound features of neurogenic shock are bradycardia with hypotension from the decreased sympathetic activity. The skin is frequently warm, dry, and flushed. Hypothermia develops from uncontrolled heat loss. Venous pooling in the lower extremities promotes the formation of deep vein thrombosis, which increases the risk of a pulmonary embolism.

Management focuses on treating the cause, including reversal of contributing medications or glucose administration for hypoglycemia. Immobilization of spinal injuries with traction devices (halo brace to maintain alignment) or surgical intervention to stabilize the injury assists in preventing severe neurogenic shock.[56] For patients receiving spinal anesthesia, elevate the head of the bed to prevent the progression of the spinal blockade up the cord. Infuse IV fluids to treat hypotension, but administer fluids cautiously to prevent fluid overload and cerebral or spinal cord edema.

Vasopressors are frequently required to restore vascular tone and maintain perfusion. Alpha- and beta-adrenergic medications, such as dopamine and norepinephrine, are preferred. Pure alpha-adrenergic agents, such as phenylephrine, are associated with persistent bradycardia and are avoided.[56] The target MAP for patients with a spinal injury may be as high as 85 to 90 mm Hg in the first 7 days to improve spinal cord perfusion.[56] Hypothermia is common; however, initiate rewarming slowly because rapid rewarming may cause vasodilation and worsen the patient's hemodynamic status. Atropine is administered for symptomatic bradycardia, but a temporary or permanent pacemaker may be required.

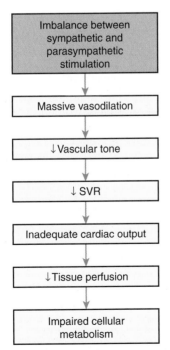

Fig. 12.8 Neurogenic shock. *SVR,* Systemic vascular resistance. (From McCance K, Huether S. *Pathophysiology: The Biologic Basis for Disease in Adults and Children.* 8th ed. St. Louis, MO: Elsevier; 2019.)

STUDY BREAK

3. In neurogenic shock, decreased sympathetic activity results in:
   A. Hypertension and tachycardia
   B. Cool diaphoretic skin and fine tremors
   C. Hypotension and bradycardia
   D. Hyperthermia and low respirations

Anaphylactic Shock. A severe allergic reaction can precipitate a second form of distributive shock known as anaphylactic shock. Antigens, which are foreign substances to which someone is sensitive, initiate an antigen-antibody response. Table 12.5 lists some common antigens (foods, medications, animal bites or stings, chemicals) that cause anaphylaxis.

After an antigen enters the body, the antibodies (i.e., immunoglobulin E [IgE]) produced attach to mast cells and basophils. The greatest concentrations of mast cells are found in the lungs, around blood vessels, in connective tissue, and in the uterus. Mast cells are also found to a lesser extent in the kidneys, heart, skin, liver, and spleen and in the omentum of the gastrointestinal tract. Basophils circulate in the blood. Mast cells and basophils contain histamine and histamine-like substances, which are potent vasodilators.

The initial exposure (primary immune response) to the antigen does not usually cause harmful effects, but subsequent exposures to the antigen may cause an anaphylactic reaction (secondary immune response). The antigen-antibody reaction causes cellular breakdown and the release of powerful vasoactive mediators from the mast cells and basophils. The mediators cause bronchoconstriction, excessive mucus secretion, vasodilation, increased capillary permeability, inflammation, gastrointestinal cramps, and cutaneous reactions that stimulate nerve endings, causing itching and pain. Fig. 12.9 summarizes the pathophysiology of anaphylactic shock. The combined effects result in decreased blood pressure, relative hypovolemia caused by vasodilation and fluid shifts, and symptoms of anaphylaxis that primarily affect the dermal, respiratory, and gastrointestinal systems.

Obtain a thorough history of allergies and medication reactions, especially reactions to medications with similar structures. If patients are allergic to penicillin, they are likely to have a reaction to other beta-lactam antibiotics.[2] Monitor the response to IV administration of medications, particularly antibiotics. Collaborate with the clinical pharmacist if a medication must be administered to a patient in whom a known or suspected allergy exists. In this situation, a small amount of medication may be given as a test dose or prior to administration of the full dose.[53]

Transfusion of blood or blood products can also result in allergic reactions. Observe the patient receiving any of these products closely for any signs of an allergic reaction (e.g., sudden shortness of breath, hives, tachycardia, hypotension, anxiety).

The clinical presentation of anaphylactic shock includes flushing, pruritus, urticaria, and angioedema (swelling of eyes, lips, tongue, hands, feet, and genitalia). Cough, runny nose, nasal congestion, hoarseness, dysphonia, and dyspnea are common because of upper airway obstruction from edema of the larynx, epiglottis, or vocal cords. Stridor may occur as a result of laryngeal edema. Lower airway obstruction may result from diffuse bronchoconstriction and cause wheezing and chest tightness. Tachycardia and hypotension occur, and the patient

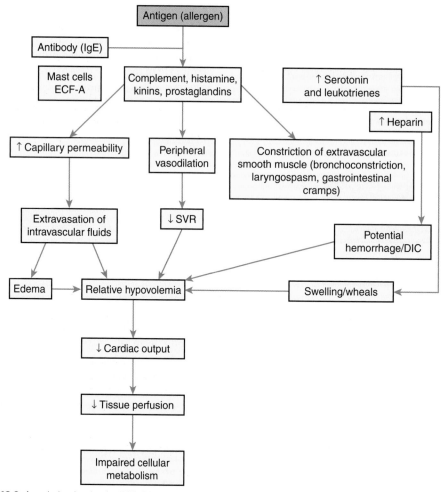

Fig. 12.9 Anaphylactic shock. *DIC,* Disseminated intravascular coagulation; *ECF-A,* eosinophil chemotactic factor of anaphylaxis; *IgE,* immunoglobulin E; *SVR,* systemic vascular resistance. (From McCance K, Huether S. *Pathophysiology: The Biologic Basis for Disease in Adults and Children.* 8th ed. St. Louis, MO: Elsevier; 2019.)

may show signs of pulmonary edema. Gastrointestinal symptoms of nausea, vomiting, cramping, abdominal pain, and diarrhea may also occur. Neurological symptoms include lethargy and decreased consciousness. Elevated levels of IgE are seen on laboratory analysis.

Goals of therapy are to remove the antigen, reverse the effects of the mediators, and promote adequate tissue perfusion. If the anaphylactic reaction results from medications, contrast dye, or blood or blood products, immediately stop the infusion and support airway, ventilation, and circulation. Laryngeal edema may be severe enough to require intubation or cricothyrotomy if swelling is so severe that an endotracheal tube cannot be placed. Administer oxygen to keep the SpO_2 greater than 90%. Remove the offending agent; for example, remove a stinger, administer antivenom, stop the medication, or flush the skin to remove a tropical allergen.

Epinephrine is the medication of choice for treating anaphylactic shock.[26] Epinephrine is an adrenergic agent that promotes bronchodilation and vasoconstriction. Anaphylaxis is often treated with epinephrine autoinjectors (EpiPens), as many allergic individuals carry this life-saving medication. The epinephrine dosage for those who weigh at least 66 pounds (30 kg) is 0.3 mg (intramuscular or subcutaneous), which can be repeated every 10 to 15 minutes. To block histamine release, diphenhydramine (Benadryl), an H1-receptor blocker, or ranitidine, an H_2-receptor blocker, may decrease some of the cutaneous symptoms of anaphylaxis, but both are considered second-line treatment.[26] Corticosteroids such as methylprednisolone (Solu-Medrol) are used to reduce inflammation. IV epinephrine, fluid replacement, positive inotropic medications, and vasopressors may be required.

❓ CRITICAL REASONING ACTIVITY

Identify the type of shock associated with the following hemodynamic changes:
1. Bradycardia, decreased SVR, decreased SvO_2
2. Tachycardia, decreased SVR, increased SvO_2
3. Decreased RAP, PAP, and PAOP; increased SVR; decreased SvO_2

PAOP, Pulmonary artery occlusion pressure; *PAP*, pulmonary artery pressure; *RAP*, right atrial pressure; *SvO₂*, mixed venous oxygen saturation; *SVR*, systemic vascular resistance.

Septic Shock. Sepsis is a clinical emergency.[49] Septic shock is a subset of the diagnosis of sepsis. *Sepsis* is defined as life-threatening organ dysfunction caused by a dysregulated host response to infection.[49] *Septic shock* is a life-threatening complication of sepsis in which the underlying circulatory and cellular or metabolic abnormalities are profound enough to substantially increase mortality. The definitions and diagnostic criteria are presented in Table 12.7. The criteria provide a tool for recognizing and diagnosing sepsis quickly, prompting the search for an infectious source, and initiating the appropriate therapy.

Invasion of the host by a microorganism or an infection begins the process that may progress to sepsis, followed by septic shock, which progresses to MODS. After a microorganism has invaded the host, an inflammatory response is initiated to restore homeostasis. For reasons not completely understood, the inflammatory response may progress to septic shock and MODS (Fig. 12.10).

Cytokines are proinflammatory or antiinflammatory. Proinflammatory cytokines include tumor necrosis factor, interleukin-1α, and interleukin-1β. They produce pyrogenic responses and initiate the hepatic response to infection. Antiinflammatory

TABLE 12.7 Sepsis Continuum: Definitions, Diagnostic Criteria, and Management

Clinical Condition and Definition	Diagnostic Criteria	Management

Sepsis: Life-threatening organ dysfunction caused by a dysregulated host response to infection	Suspected or known source of infection
	AND two or more indicators of systemic inflammation:
	    Temperature >38.3°C or <36°C
	    HR >90 beats/min
	    RR >20 breaths/min
	    WBC >12 mm³ or <4 mm³ or 10% bands
		Obtain blood cultures
		Administer antibiotics
		Obtain lactate; repeat lactate within 6 h of identification
		Monitor for hypotension
		Maintain adequate ventilation and oxygenation
		Remove source of infection

Septic shock: Sepsis that results in circulatory and cellular or metabolic dysfunction	Sepsis
	AND end-organ dysfunction as evidenced by two or more of the following:
	    SBP <90 mm Hg or MAP <65 mm Hg
	    Urine output <0.05 mL/kg/h × 2 h or creatinine >2.0 mg/dL
	    Creatinine >0.5 mg/dL above baseline if history of chronic kidney disease
	    Platelets <100,000 mm³
	    INR >1.5 or aPTT >60 seconds
	    Serum lactate >4 mmol/L or serum lactate >2 mmol/L after fluid resuscitation
	    New need for noninvasive or invasive ventilation
		Administer antibiotics within 1 h of diagnosis
		Remove source of infection
		Maintain adequate ventilation and oxygenation
		Maximize oxygen delivery; minimize oxygen demand
		Administer at least 30 mL/kg of IV crystalloid fluid within the first 3 h
		Administer vasopressors to maintain a target MAP >65 mm Hg
		Administer vasoactive medications
		Correct acid-base abnormalities
		Monitor and support organ function

aPTT, Activated partial thromboplastin time; *HR,* heart rate; *INR,* international normalized ratio; *MAP,* mean arterial pressure; *RR,* respiratory rate; *SBP,* systolic blood pressure; *WBC,* white blood cell.

Modified from Levy M, Evans L, Rhodes A. The Surviving Sepsis Campaign bundle. *Crit Care Med.* 2018;46(6):997–1000; Rhodes A, Evans L, Alhazzani W, et al. Surviving Sepsis Campaign. *Crit Care Med.* 2017;45(3):486–552.

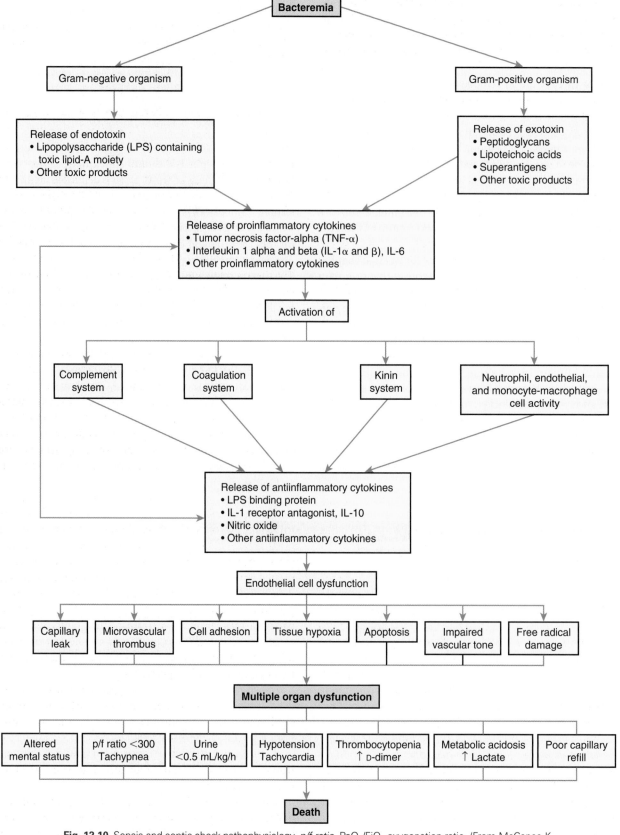

Fig. 12.10 Sepsis and septic shock pathophysiology. *p/f ratio,* PaO$_2$/FiO$_2$ oxygenation ratio. (From McCance K, Huether S. *Pathophysiology: The Biologic Basis for Disease in Adults and Children*. 8th ed. St. Louis, MO: Elsevier; 2019.)

cytokines, including nitric oxide, lipopolysaccharide, and interleukin-1 receptor antagonist, are compensatory, ensuring that the effect of the proinflammatory mediators does not become destructive. In sepsis, continued activation of proinflammatory cytokines overwhelms the antiinflammatory cytokines, and excessive systemic inflammation results.

A state of enhanced coagulation occurs through stimulation of the coagulation cascade, with a reduction in the levels of activated protein C and antithrombin III. This results in the generation of thrombin and the formation of microemboli that impair blood flow and organ perfusion. Fibrinolysis is activated in response to the activation of the coagulation cascade to promote clot breakdown. However, activation is followed by inhibition, further promoting coagulopathy. This imbalance among inflammation, coagulation, and fibrinolysis results in systemic inflammation, widespread coagulopathy, and microvascular thrombi that impair tissue perfusion, leading to MODS.

Inflammatory mediators also damage the endothelial cells that line blood vessels, producing profound vasodilation and increased capillary permeability. Initially, this results in tachycardia, hypotension, and low SVR. Although norepinephrine and the renin-angiotensin-aldosterone system are activated in response to this clinical state, the molecules are unable to enter the cells, and hypotension and vasodilation persist. In contrast, the plasma levels of the ADH are low despite the presence of hypotension. The exact mechanism that creates this low concentration is unknown; however, continuous administration of vasopressin is a second-line intervention when combined with norepinephrine for blood pressure support in septic shock.[49]

Once sepsis is present, it can progress to septic shock. Septic shock is identified in patients with persistent hypotension requiring vasopressor medication to maintain a MAP greater than 65 mm Hg and a serum lactate level greater than 2 mmol/L despite adequate volume resuscitation.[49]

Factors that increase the risk of developing sepsis include immunosuppression or situations that cause significant bacteremia (see Table 12.5). Tools are available to identify patients with suspected infection who are at risk for sepsis. The Sequential Organ Failure Assessment (SOFA) evaluates coagulation; respiration; and hepatic, cardiovascular, central nervous system, and renal function.[17,32,62] The patient's risk of morbidity and mortality increases with the score. The quick Sequential Organ Failure Assessment (qSOFA) tool uses just three criteria—respiratory rate greater than 22 breaths/min, Glasgow Coma Scale greater than 15, and a systolic blood pressure of 100 mm Hg or lower—to identify patients who are likely to have poorer outcomes.[17,32] The SOFA better predicts risk of death for patients with an infection while in the critical care unit. The qSOFA better identifies patients at high risk of death in the hospital.[17] Sepsis can advance to septic shock with signs of end-organ perfusion, including hypotension, chills, decreased urine output, decreased skin perfusion, poor capillary refill, skin mottling, decreased platelets, petechiae, hyperglycemia, and unexplained changes in mental status.[49]

❓ CRITICAL REASONING ACTIVITY

Consider factors in the critically ill patient that increase susceptibility to the development of sepsis and septic shock. Describe nursing interventions to reduce the risk of infection.

Infection prevention efforts include proper hand washing, use of aseptic technique, and awareness of at-risk patients. Most critically ill patients are debilitated and have many potential portals of entry for bacterial invasion. Meticulous technique is required during procedures such as suctioning, dressing changes, and wound care and when handling catheters or tubes. Maintain an awareness of patient-specific baseline assessment criteria such as mental status and vital signs. Frequently assess for signs and symptoms of infection, including elevated or decreased temperature, increased heart rate, increased respiratory rate, hypotension, and changes in mentation. Evaluate wounds and IV and device insertion sites for signs and symptoms of infection. Review laboratory results, including white blood cell count, differential counts, and cultures for the identification of infection.[57]

Infections caused by gram-negative organisms are associated with a high financial burden due to antimicrobial resistance and high morbidity and mortality.[31] Common sites of infection include the pulmonary system, urinary tract, gastrointestinal system, and wounds. Urinary tract infection is an often overlooked cause of secondary bloodstream infections, especially in older adults. Minimize the use of indwelling urinary catheters by daily assessing their need and promptly removing unnecessary catheters.[35]

Gram-positive bacteria such as *Staphylococcus aureus* can lead to sepsis and septic shock. These bacteria release a potent toxin that exerts its effects within hours. Gram-positive infection has been associated with the use of tampons in menstruating women (toxic shock syndrome), but it is also seen after vaginal and cesarean delivery and in patients with surgical wounds, abscesses, infected burns, abrasions, insect bites, herpes zoster, cellulitis, septic abortion, and osteomyelitis. The bacteria may be transmitted from mother to newborn. Management includes antimicrobial therapy, removal of the source of infection if possible, fluid resuscitation, and vasoactive medication to improve cardiac performance.

Pneumonia is a common trigger for sepsis.[43] Infection-related, ventilator-associated conditions such as pneumonia are significant risk factors for sepsis. Implement nursing interventions to ventilated patients to reduce the risk of ventilator-associated conditions (see Chapter 10). For example, provide regular oral care, monitor sedation, and assess readiness to wean and extubate.[54]

Timely identification of the causative organism and the initiation of appropriate antibiotics improve survival of patients with sepsis or septic shock.[27,49] Remove invasive devices if they are suspected to be a source of infection. Surgery may be required to locate the source of infection, drain an abscess, or debride necrotic tissue.

BOX 12.1 Surviving Sepsis Campaign Bundles

Within 1 hour of sepsis recognition:

- Measure lactate level. Re-measure if initial lactate is >2 mmol/L
- Obtain blood cultures prior to administration of antibiotics
- Administer broad-spectrum antibiotics
- Rapidly administer 30 ml/kg crystalloid for hypotension or lactate ≥4 mmol/L
- Apply vasopressors if patient is hypotensive during or after fluid resuscitation to maintain MAP ≥65 mm Hg

MAP, Mean arterial pressure.
From Levy MM, Evans LE, Rhodes A. The Surviving Sepsis Campaign bundle: 2018 update. *Crit Care Med.* 2018;46(6):997–1000.

Obtain culture and sensitivity tests of blood and other suspicious sources before initiation of antibiotics. The Surviving Sepsis Campaign international guidelines recommend obtaining these cultures first unless doing so will delay the initial administration of antibiotics by more than 45 minutes.[49] Choice of the initial antibiotic is directed toward the most likely organism. Empirical and broad-spectrum antibiotics are frequently initiated within 1 hour of identification of sepsis.[27,49] The antibiotic regimen is modified, if indicated, after culture and sensitivity results are available.

Early goal-directed therapy decreases the mortality rate among patients with sepsis and septic shock, and it should be initiated within the first hour of sepsis recognition (Box 12.1).[28,49] Early goal-directed therapy includes IV fluid resuscitation to maintain a MAP greater than 65 mm Hg.[8,27,28,49]

Isotonic crystalloid solutions are infused for fluid resuscitation. Avoid colloids, as they are likely to leak out of the vascular bed into the interstitium because of increased capillary permeability. Administer vasopressors to increase SVR and MAP if hypoperfusion persists despite aggressive fluid resuscitation. Norepinephrine is the first choice for vasopressor support.[49] A low dose of vasopressin (0.03 unit/min) or epinephrine may be added if norepinephrine administration alone does not adequately increase MAP to greater than 65 mm Hg. Vasopressin causes vasoconstriction without the adverse effects of tachycardia and ventricular ectopy seen with catecholamines, such as dopamine or norepinephrine. Phenylephrine is not recommended because it is a pure vasoconstrictor that results in decreased stroke volume.[49] Dopamine may be administered in bradycardic patients who have a low risk of tachyarrhythmia.[49] Dobutamine may be added to increase the myocardial contractility and improve the cardiac index and oxygen delivery in patients who have persistent hypoperfusion despite adequate fluid resuscitation and use of vasopressors.[49] Transfusion of packed red blood cells is recommended when hemoglobin is less than 7 g/dL; platelets may be transfused if the platelet count is less than 10,000 mm[3].[49] IV hydrocortisone is not routinely administered but may be given if hemodynamic instability persists despite adequate fluid resuscitation and vasopressor therapy.[49]

Hyperglycemia and insulin resistance are common in the patient with sepsis. Although aggressive management of blood glucose is no longer advocated, institute a blood glucose management protocol when two consecutive blood glucose levels are greater than 180 mg/dL.[49]

Pyrogens (polypeptides that produce fever) aid in activation of the immune response. Treatment of fever has no clear effect on mortality but may be considered.[10] Treatment of fever includes administration of antipyretics (acetaminophen, ibuprofen, or aspirin). Avoid overcooling because hypothermia adversely affects oxygen delivery and may result in shivering, which increases oxygen consumption.

✹ QSEN EXEMPLAR
Quality Improvement

The nurse in the critical care unit identified lack of consistent documentation of "time zero" (the time at which sepsis or septic shock is identified) for patients transferred from the emergency department with sepsis. The nurse noted that time zero was inconsistently communicated during verbal handoff and documentation was not always located in the same place in the electronic medical record. Lack of a standardized way to communicate time zero often led to confusion and missed opportunities to adhere to the sepsis bundle guidelines. The nurse collaborated with nursing leadership, nursing quality, and nursing informatics to create a standardized area for time zero documentation in the electronic medical record. Standardized documentation of time zero led to improved adherence with sepsis bundle guidelines and provided a framework for development of a sepsis tracking tool within the electronic medical record.

Obstructive Shock

Obstructive shock (extracardiac obstructive shock) occurs when a blockage or compression impairs circulatory blood flow. Causes of obstructive shock include impaired diastolic filling (cardiac tamponade, tension pneumothorax, constrictive pericarditis, compression of the great veins), increased right ventricular afterload (pulmonary embolism, severe pulmonary hypertension, increased intrathoracic pressures), and increased left ventricular afterload (aortic dissection, systemic embolization, aortic stenosis). Obstruction of the heart or great vessels impedes venous return to the right side of the heart or prevents effective pumping action of the heart. This results in decreased cardiac output, hypotension, decreased tissue perfusion, and impaired cellular metabolism (Fig. 12.11).

Common clinical findings in obstructive shock include chest pain, dyspnea, jugular venous distension, and hypoxia. Other findings depend on the cause. Cardiac tamponade manifests with muffled heart sounds, hypotension, and pulsus paradoxus. *Pulsus paradoxus* is a decrease in systolic blood pressure of more than 10 mm Hg during inspiration. Tension pneumothorax is characterized by diminished breath sounds on the affected side and tracheal shift away from the affected side. Massive pulmonary embolism manifests with clinical indications of right ventricular failure (jugular venous distension, peripheral edema, hepatomegaly). Aortic dissection is characterized by complaints of ripping chest pain that radiates to the back; pulse differences between the left and right side; and a widened mediastinum on the chest radiograph, echocardiogram, or CT scan.

Obstructive shock may be prevented or treated by aggressive interventions to relieve the source of the compression or

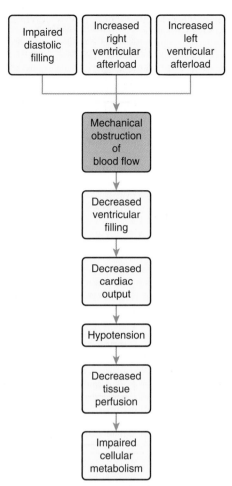

Fig. 12.11 Obstructive shock.

obstruction. Cardiac tamponade is treated by a *pericardiocentesis*, or the removal of fluid from the pericardial sac. A tension pneumothorax from blunt or penetrating chest injuries is relieved by a needle *thoracentesis* to remove the accumulated intrathoracic pressure. The risk of pulmonary embolism is reduced by early surgical reduction of long bone fractures, devices to enhance circulation in immobile patients (e.g., intermittent pneumatic compression devices), range-of-motion exercises, and prophylactic anticoagulant therapy.

MULTIPLE ORGAN DYSFUNCTION SYNDROME

MODS is the progressive dysfunction of two or more organ systems as a result of an uncontrolled inflammatory response to severe illness or injury.[33] Organ dysfunction can progress to organ failure and death. The most common causes of MODS are sepsis and septic shock; however, MODS can occur after any severe injury or disease process that activates a massive systemic inflammatory response, which includes any classification of shock. The immune system and the body's response to stress can cause maldistribution of circulating volume, global tissue hypoxia, and metabolic alterations that damage organs. MODS frequently leads to a persistent, prolonged state known as *chronically critically ill.*[38] The risk of death associated with MODS is 54% when two organ systems fail and increases to 100% when five organ systems fail.[33]

Damage to organs may be primary or secondary. In *primary MODS,* there is direct injury to an organ from shock, trauma, burn injury, or infection with impaired perfusion that results in dysfunction. Decreased perfusion may be localized or systemic. The stress response and inflammatory response are activated, with the release of catecholamines and activation of mediators that affect cellular activity (Fig. 12.12).

Secondary MODS is a consequence of widespread systemic inflammation that results in dysfunction of organs not involved with the initial insult. It occurs in response to altered regulation of the acute immune and inflammatory responses. Failure to control the inflammatory response leads to excessive production of inflammatory cells and biochemical mediators that cause widespread damage to vascular endothelium and organ damage. The interaction of injured organs then leads to self-perpetuating inflammation with maldistribution of blood flow and hypermetabolism.

Maldistribution of blood flow refers to the uneven distribution of flow to various organs and between the large vessels and capillary beds. It is caused by vasodilation, increased capillary permeability, selective vasoconstriction, and impaired microvascular circulation. This impaired blood flow leads to impaired tissue perfusion and decreased oxygen supply to the cells. The organs most severely affected are the lungs, splanchnic bed, liver, and kidneys.

Hypermetabolism with altered carbohydrate, fat, and lipid metabolism is initially compensatory to meet the body's increased demands for energy. Eventually, hypermetabolism becomes detrimental, placing tremendous demands on the heart as cardiac output increases up to twice the normal value. Hyperglycemia occurs as gluconeogenesis by the liver increases and glucose use by the cells decreases.

Decreased oxygen delivery to the cells from maldistribution of blood flow and increased oxygen needs of the cells from hypermetabolism create an imbalance in oxygen supply and demand. In MODS, the amount of oxygen consumed depends on the amount of oxygen that can be delivered to the cells. Hypoxemia, cellular acidosis, and impaired cellular function result, leading to multiple organ failure.

The clinical picture of MODS is caused by inflammatory mediator damage, tissue hypoxia, and hypermetabolism. Damage to the organs is usually sequential rather than simultaneous. The first system frequently affected is the pulmonary system, with ARDS developing within 12 to 24 hours after the initial insult. Coagulopathy frequently develops, followed by renal, hepatic, and intestinal impairment.[33] Failure of the cardiovascular system or neurological system is frequently fatal. MODS progresses from minor dysfunction of one or more organs to multiple organs requiring support.

Criteria used in the diagnoses of organ dysfunction are described in Table 12.8. Pulmonary dysfunction manifests with tachypnea, hypoxemia despite high levels of supplemental oxygen, and chest radiographic changes. Hematological dysfunction manifests with petechiae, bleeding, thrombocytopenia, prolonged PT and aPTT, increased fibrin split products, and a positive D-dimer. The earliest sign of hepatic dysfunction is hypoglycemia, which is followed by jaundice, increased levels of liver enzymes and bilirubin, prolonged PT, and decreased

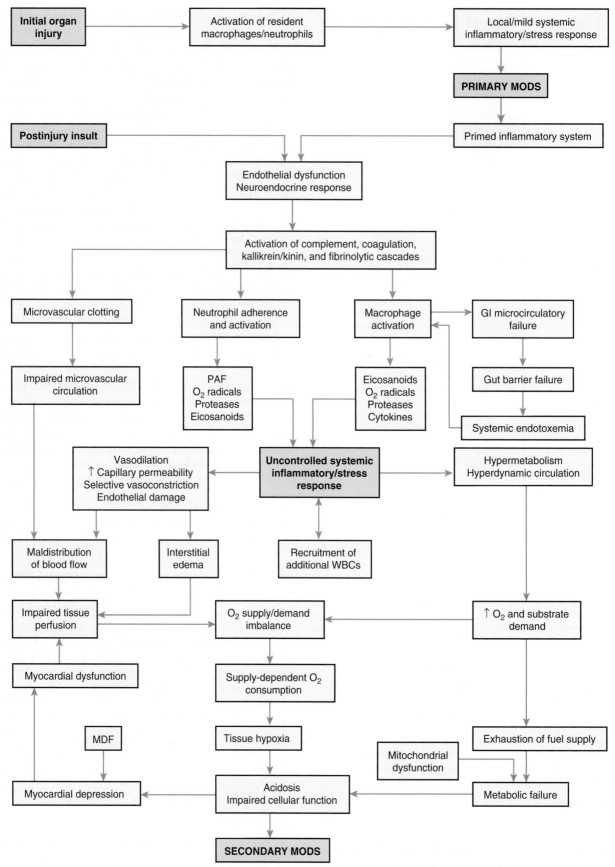

Fig. 12.12 Pathogenesis of multiple organ dysfunction syndrome (MODS). *GI,* Gastrointestinal; *MDF,* myocardial depressant factor; *PAF,* platelet-activating factor; *WBCs,* white blood cells. (Modified from McCance K, Huether S. *Pathophysiology: The Biologic Basis for Disease in Adults and Children.* 8th ed. St. Louis, MO: Elsevier; 2019.)

TABLE 12.8 Multiple Organ Dysfunction Syndrome

System	Dysfunction	Clinical Presentation
Pulmonary	Acute respiratory distress syndrome	Predisposing factor such as shock or sepsis
		Unexplained hypoxemia ($\downarrow$ PaO_2, $\downarrow$ SaO_2)
		Dyspnea
		Tachypnea
		PaO_2/FiO_2 ratio <300 for acute lung injury and <200 for ARDS
		Bilateral pulmonary infiltrates on chest radiograph
		PAOP <18 mm Hg
Cardiovascular	Hyperdynamic	Increased oxygen consumption
		Increased cardiac output
		Tachycardia
	Hypodynamic	Myocardial depression
		Decreased oxygen consumption
		Decreased cardiac output
Hematologic	Disseminated intravascular coagulation	Fibrin split products >1:40 or D-dimer >2 mg/L
		Thrombocytopenia
		Prolonged PT and aPTT
		INR >1.5
		Bleeding
		Petechiae
Renal	Acute tubular necrosis	Oliguria
		$\uparrow$ Serum creatinine, $\uparrow$ BUN
		Urinary sodium >20 mEq/L
Liver	Hepatic dysfunction/ failure	$\uparrow$ Serum bilirubin
		$\uparrow$ AST, ALT, LDH
		Jaundice
		Hepatomegaly
		$\uparrow$ Serum ammonia
		$\downarrow$ Serum albumin
CNS	Cerebral ischemia or infarction	Lethargy
		Altered level of consciousness progressing to unresponsiveness
		Hyperthermia
		Hypothermia
Metabolic	Lactic acidosis	$\uparrow$ Serum lactate level

ALT, Alanine transaminase; *aPTT*, activated partial thromboplastin time; *AST*, aspartate transaminase; *BUN*, blood urea nitrogen; *CNS*, central nervous system; *FiO₂*, fraction of inspired oxygen; *INR*, International Normalized Ratio; *LDH*, lactic dehydrogenase; *PaO₂*, partial pressure of arterial oxygen; *PAOP*, pulmonary artery occlusion pressure; *PT*, prothrombin time; *SaO₂*, arterial oxygen saturation.

albumin. The first indication of intestinal dysfunction is frequently intolerance of enteral feedings with abdominal distension and increased retention volumes. Renal dysfunction progresses from oliguria to anuria, increased levels of blood urea nitrogen and creatinine, and fluid and electrolyte imbalance.

Tachycardia (frequently with dysrhythmias), hypotension, and hemodynamic alterations indicate cardiovascular dysfunction. Cerebral dysfunction manifests with confusion, a change in the level of consciousness, and focal neurological signs such as hemiparesis. The final response to MODS is hypotension unresponsive to fluids and vasopressors, followed by cardiac arrest.

Management of MODS focuses on prevention and support. Eliminate or control the initial source of inflammation, and avoid a secondary insult. Remove potential sites of infection. Medical interventions include debriding necrotic tissue, draining abscesses, reducing the number of invasive procedures performed, and removing hematomas. Goals are to control infection, provide adequate tissue oxygenation, restore intravascular volume, and support organ function. Administer antibiotics and implement treatment to maintain SpO₂ at 88% to 92% and SvO₂ at greater than 70%. Initiate aggressive fluid therapy with isotonic crystalloid solutions early during systemic vasodilation to promote oxygen delivery to the tissues.

Support must be provided for each organ. Respiratory failure is managed with mechanical ventilation with low tidal volumes, high oxygen concentrations, and positive end-expiratory pressure (PEEP) (see Chapters 10 and 15).[63] Adequate nutrition and metabolic support are provided with enteral feedings (see Chapter 7). Acute kidney injury is managed with continuous renal replacement therapies or hemodialysis (see Chapter 16). Inotropic medications (low-dose dopamine or dobutamine) or vasopressor medications (norepinephrine or vasopressin) may be needed to maximize cardiac contractility and maintain cardiac output.

CASE STUDY

Ms. C., a 43-year-old woman, had complaints of shortness of breath and tachycardia when she was evaluated in the emergency department. Her medical history was significant for pulmonary sarcoidosis (an autoimmune disease) treated with oral prednisone daily. She reported a history of a dog bite to the right arm 7 days earlier. She did not receive treatment after the bite.

Initial assessment in the emergency department revealed the following: weight, 75 kg; temperature, 37.9°C (100.2°F); blood pressure, 85/54 mm Hg; heart rate, 138 beats/min; respiratory rate, 28 breaths/min; and oxygen saturation, 91% on room air. Blood cultures were obtained. Initial laboratory results included the following: white blood cell count, 31,300/mm³; hemoglobin, 12.8 g/dL: hematocrit, 38.5%; platelet count, 50,000/mm³; blood urea nitrogen, 13 mg/dL; creatinine, 2.12 mmol/L; and lactate, 5 mmol/L. Three liters of Lactated Ringer's solution and a broad-spectrum antibiotic were administered.

The patient was admitted to the critical care unit for further treatment. An arterial catheter was placed in her left radial artery, and a central venous catheter was placed in her right jugular vein. An infusion of norepinephrine was initiated after fluid resuscitation. She required endotracheal intubation due to increased work of breathing. Blood cultures were positive for *Pasteurella multocida*, a common pathogen transmitted by dog bites. Antibiotic coverage was adjusted to reflect the blood culture results. She was extubated on hospital day 5 and transitioned out of the critical care unit on hospital day 7.

Questions
1. What type of shock did Ms. C. demonstrate on arrival to the emergency department?
2. What components of her history and assessment support this diagnosis?
3. Ms. C. weighs 75 kg. Given weight-based recommendations, how much crystalloid infusion was indicated for *initial* resuscitation in this case of shock?

REFERENCES

1. Ait-Oufella H, Bakker J. Understanding clinical signs of poor tissue perfusion during septic shock. *Intens Care Med.* 2016;42(12):2070–2072.
2. Alharbi H. Antibiotic skin testing in the Intensive Care Unit: A systematic review. *Crit Care Nurse.* 2019;39(6):e1–e9.
3. Asber SR, Shanahan KP, Lussier L, et al. Nursing management of patients requiring acute mechanical circulatory support devices. *Crit Care Nurse.* 2020;40(1):e1–e11.
4. Bandaranayake T, Shaw AC. Host resistance and immune aging. *Clin Geriatr Med.* 2016;32(3):415–432.
5. Bednarczyk JM, Fridfinnson JA, Kumar A, et al. Incorporating dynamic assessment of fluid responsiveness into goal-directed therapy: A systematic review and meta-analysis. *Crit Care Med.* 2017;45(9):1538–1545.
6. Braile-Sternieri MCVB, Mustafa EM, Ferreira VRR, et al. Main considerations of cardiogenic shock and its predictors: Systematic review. *Cardiol Res.* 2018;9(2):75–82.
7. Bridges E, McNeill MM, Munro N. Research in review: Advancing critical care practice. *Am J Crit Care.* 2017;26(1):77–88.
8. Brotfain E, Koyfman L, Toledano R, et al. Positive fluid balance as a major predictor of clinical outcome of patients with sepsis/septic shock after ICU discharge. *Am J Emerg Med.* 2016;34(11):2122–2126.
9. Cannon JW. Hemorrhagic shock. *N Eng J Med.* 2018;378(4):370–379.
10. Chiumello D, Gotti M, Vergani G. Paracetamol in fever in critically ill patients—An update. *J Crit Care.* 2017;38:245–252.
11. Claure-Del Granado R, Mehta RL. Fluid overload in the ICU: Evaluation and management. *BMC Nephrol.* 2016;17(1):109.
12. Crozier T. General care of the pregnant patient in the intensive care unit. *Semin Respirat Crit Care Med.* 2017;38(02):208–217.
13. De Backer D. Detailing the cardiovascular profile in shock patients. *Crit Care.* 2017;21(Suppl 3):311.
14. de-Madaria E, Herrera-Marante I, González-Camacho V, et al. Fluid resuscitation with lactated Ringer's solution vs normal saline in acute pancreatitis: A triple-blind, randomized, controlled trial. *United Eur Gastroenterol J.* 2018;6(1):63–72.
15. Delaney M, Wendel S, Bercovitz RS, et al. Transfusion reactions: Prevention, diagnosis, and treatment. *Lancet.* 2016;388(10061):2825–2836.
16. Denic A, Glassock RJ, Rule AD. Structural and functional changes with the aging kidney. *Adv Chronic Kidney Dis.* 2016;23(1):19–28.
17. Donnelly JP, Safford MM, Shapiro NI, et al. Application of the Third International Consensus Definitions for Sepsis (Sepsis-3) Classification: A retrospective population-based cohort study. *Lancet Infect Dis.* 2017;17(6):661–670.
18. El-Sharkawy AM, Watson P, Neal KR, et al. Hydration and outcome in older patients admitted to hospital (the HOOP prospective cohort study). *Age Ageing.* 2015;44(6):943–947.
19. Fodor GH, Habre W, Balogh AL, et al. Optimal crystalloid volume ratio for blood replacement for maintaining hemodynamic stability and lung function: An experimental randomized controlled study. *BMC Anesthesiol.* 2019;19(1):21.
20. Hajjar LA, Teboul J-L. Mechanical circulatory support devices for cardiogenic shock: State of the art. *Crit Care.* 2019;23(1):76.
21. Harvey SE, Parrott F, Harrison DA, et al. A multicentre, randomised controlled trial comparing the clinical effectiveness and cost-effectiveness of early nutritional support via the parenteral versus the enteral route in critically ill patients (CALORIES). *Health Technol Asses.* 2016;20(28):1–144.

22. Jalil BA, Cavallazzi R. Predicting fluid responsiveness: A review of literature and a guide for the clinician. *Am J Emerg Med.* 2018;36(11):2093–2102.
23. Jouffroy R, Saade A, Tourtier JP, et al. Skin mottling score and capillary refill time to assess mortality of septic shock since pre-hospital setting. *Am J Emerg Med.* 2019;37(4):664–671.
24. Kakihana Y, Ito T, Nakahara M, Yamaguchi K, Yasuda T. Sepsis-induced myocardial dysfunction: Pathophysiology and management. *J Intens Care.* 2016;4(1):22.
25. Kayser SA, VanGilder CA, Ayello EA, Lachenbruch C. Prevalence and analysis of medical device-related pressure injuries: Results from the International Pressure Ulcer Prevalence Survey. *Adv Skin Wound Care.* 2018;31(6):276–285.
26. Lee SE. Management of anaphylaxis. *Otolaryngol Clin N Am.* 2017;50(6):1175–1184.
27. Lester D, Hartjes T, Bennett A. CE: A review of the revised sepsis care bundles. *Am J Nurs.* 2018;118(8):40–49.
28. Levy MM, Evans LE, Rhodes A. The Surviving Sepsis Campaign bundle: 2018 update. *Crit Care Med.* 2018;46(6):997–1000.
29. Lewis SR, Pritchard MW, Evans DJ, et al. Colloids versus crystalloids for fluid resuscitation in critically ill people. *Cochrane Database Sys Rev.* 2018;8:CD000567.
30. Li K, Xu Y. Citrate metabolism in blood transfusions and its relationship due to metabolic alkalosis and respiratory acidosis. *Int J Clin Exp Med.* 2015;8(4):6578–6584.
31. MacVane SH. Antimicrobial resistance in the intensive care unit: A focus on gram-negative bacterial infections. *J Intens Care Med.* 2017;32(1):25–37.
32. Makic MBF, Bridges E. CE: Managing sepsis and septic shock. *Am J Nurs.* 2018;118(2):34–39.
33. Martin LL, Cheek DJ, Morrise SE. Shock, multiple organ dysfunction syndrome and burns in adults. In: McCance KL, Huether SE, eds. *Pathophysiology: The Biologic Basis for Disease in Adults and Children.* 8th ed. St. Louis, MO: Elsevier; 2019:1543–1571.
34. McQuilten ZK, Crighton G, Brunskill S, et al. Optimal dose, timing and ratio of blood products in massive transfusion: Results from a systematic review. *Trans Med Rev.* 2018;32(1):6–15.
35. Melzer M, Welch C. Does the presence of a urinary catheter predict severe sepsis in a bacteraemic cohort? *J Hosp Infect.* 2017;95(4):376–382.
36. Meng M, Klingensmith NJ, Coopersmith CM. New insights into the gut as the driver of critical illness and organ failure. *Curr Opin Crit Care.* 2017;23(2):143–148.
37. Meschiari CA, Ero OK, Pan H, Finkel T, Lindsey ML. The impact of aging on cardiac extracellular matrix. *GeroSci.* 2017;39(1):7–18.
38. Mira JC, Gentile LF, Mathias BJ, et al. Sepsis pathophysiology, chronic critical illness, and persistent inflammation-immuno suppression and catabolism syndrome. *Crit Care Med.* 2017;45(2):253–262.
39. Moore K. The physiological response to hemorrhagic shock. *J Emerg Nurs.* 2014;40(6):629–631.
40. Morrison G. Management of acute hypothermia. *Medicine.* 2017;45(3):135–138.
41. Muntlin Athlin Å, Engström M, Gunningberg L, Bååth C. Heel pressure ulcer, prevention and predictors during the care delivery chain—When and where to take action? A descriptive and explorative study. *Scand J Trauma Resuscit Emerg Med.* 2016;24(1):134.
42. National Pressure Ulcer Advisory Panel. Pressure Ulcer Prevention Points. https://www.npuap.org/resources/educational-and-clinical-resources/pressure-injury-prevention-points/. Published April 2019.

43. Novosad SA, Sapiano MRP, Grigg C, et al. Vital signs: Epidemiology of sepsis: Prevalence of health care factors and opportunities for prevention. *MMWR Morbid Mortal Weekly Rep.* 2016;65(33):864–869.

44. Petitpas F, Guenezan J, Vendeuvre T, et al. Use of intra-osseous access in adults: A systematic review. *Crit Care.* 2016;20(1):102.

45. Pickett JD, Bridges E, Kritek PA, Whitney JD. Passive leg-raising and prediction of fluid responsiveness: Systematic review. *Crit Care Nurs.* 2017;37(2):32–47.

46. Reddy S, Weinberg L, Young P. Crystalloid fluid therapy. *Crit Care.* 2016;20:59.

47. Reignier J, Boisramé-Helms J, Brisard L, et al. Enteral versus parenteral early nutrition in ventilated adults with shock: A randomised, controlled, multicentre, open-label, parallel-group study (NUTRIREA-2). *Lancet.* 2018;391(10116):133–143.

48. Reignier J, Van Zanten ARH, Arabi YM. Optimal timing, dose and route of early nutrition therapy in critical illness and shock: The quest for the Holy Grail. *Intens Care Med.* 2018;44(9):1558–1560.

49. Rhodes A, Evans LE, Alhazzani W, et al. Surviving Sepsis Campaign: International guidelines for management of sepsis and septic shock. *Crit Care Med.* 2017;45(3):486–552.

50. Rossi S, Picetti E, Zoerle T, et al. Fluid management in acute brain injury. *Curr Neurol Neurosci Rep.* 2018;18(11):74.

51. Semler MW, Rice TW. Saline is not the first choice for crystalloid resuscitation fluids. *Crit Care Med.* 2016;44(8):1541–1544.

52. Singhal V, Aggarwal R. Spinal shock. In: Prabhakar H, ed. *Complications in Neuroanesthesia.* London, England: Academic Press; 2016:89–94.

53. Solensky R, Khan D, et al. Drug allergy: An updated practice parameter. *Ann Allergy Asthma Immunol.* 2010;105(4):259–273.

54. Speck K, Rawat N, Weiner NC, et al. A systematic approach for developing a ventilator-associated pneumonia prevention bundle. *Am J Infect Control.* 2016;44(6):652–656.

55. Standl T, Annecke T, Cascorbi I, et al. The nomenclature, definition and distinction of type. *Dtsch Arztebl Int.* 2018;115(45):757–768.

56. Stein DM, Knight WA. Emergency neurological life support: Traumatic spine injury. *Neurocrit Care.* 2017;27(Suppl 1):170–180.

57. Swearingen PL. *All-in-One Nursing Care Planning Resource: Medical-Surgical, Pediatric, Maternity, and Psychiatric-Mental Health.* 5th ed. St. Louis, MO: Elsevier; 2018.

58. Thibeault S. Massive transfusion for hemorrhagic shock. *Crit Care Nurs Clin N Am.* 2015;27(1):47–53.

59. Thomasson RR, Yazer MH, Gorham JD, et al. International assessment of massive transfusion protocol contents and indications for activation. *Transfusion.* 2019;59(5):1637–1643.

60. Timsit J-F, Rupp M, Bouza E, et al. A state of the art review on optimal practices to prevent, recognize, and manage complications associated with intravascular devices in the critically ill. *Intens Care Med.* 2018;44(6):742–759.

61. van Diepen S, Katz JN, Albert NM, et al. Contemporary management of cardiogenic shock: A scientific statement from the American Heart Association. *Circulation.* 2017;136(16):e232–e268.

62. Vincent J-L, de Mendonca A, Cantraine F, et al. Use of the SOFA score to assess the incidence of organ dysfunction/failure in intensive care units: Results of a multicenter, prospective study. *Crit Care Med.* 1998;26(11):1793–1800.

63. Walkey AJ, Goligher EC, Del Sorbo L, et al. Low tidal volume versus non–volume-limited strategies for patients with acute respiratory distress syndrome: A systematic review and meta-analysis. *Ann Am Thorac Soc.* 2017;14(Suppl_4):S271–S279.

64. Walter EJ, Hanna-Jumma S, Carraretto M, Forni L. The pathophysiological basis and consequences of fever. *Crit Care.* 2016;20(1):200.

Cardiovascular Alterations

Colleen Walsh-Irwin, DNP, RN, ANP-BC, AACC, FAANP

Many additional resources, including self-assessment exercises, are located on the Evolve companion website at http://evolve.elsevier.com/Sole/.
- Animations
- Clinical Skills: Critical Care Collections
- Student Review Questions
- Video Clips

INTRODUCTION

Care of the patient with decreased cardiac function presents unique challenges because of potential serious hemodynamic changes that can affect the prognosis of the critically ill patient. The critical care nurse needs both theoretic knowledge and practice-related understanding of the common cardiac diseases to have the sound clinical judgment necessary for making rapid and accurate decisions and responding with optimal interventions. The purpose of this chapter is to identify and explore common cardiac alterations that are likely to be encountered by the critical care nurse caring for adult patients with compromised cardiac status and to describe the nursing care to optimize patient outcomes.

NORMAL STRUCTURE AND FUNCTION OF THE HEART

The heart muscle is approximately the size of a person's closed fist and lies within the mediastinal space of the thoracic cavity—between the lungs, directly under the lower half of the sternum, and above the diaphragm (Fig. 13.1). It is covered by the *pericardium*, which has an inner visceral layer and an outer parietal layer. Certain diseases can cause this covering to become inflamed and can subsequently diminish the effectiveness of the heart as a pump. Several cubic milliliters of lubricating fluid are present between these layers. Some pathological conditions can increase the amount and the consistency of this fluid, affecting the pumping ability of the heart. The heart muscle itself is composed of three layers. The outer layer, or *epicardium,* covers the surface of the heart and extends to the great vessels; the middle muscular layer, or *myocardium,* is responsible for the heart's pumping action; and the inner endothelial layer, or *endocardium,* covers the heart valves and the small muscles associated with the opening and closing of those valves. These

layers are damaged or destroyed when a patient has a myocardial infarction (MI).

Functionally, the heart is divided into right-sided and left-sided pumps that are separated by a septum. The right side is considered a low-pressure system, whereas the left side is a high-pressure system. Each side has an atrium that receives the blood and a ventricle that pumps the blood out. Blood travels from the atria to the ventricles by means of a pressure gradient between the chambers. The right atrium receives deoxygenated blood from the body through the superior vena cava and the inferior vena cava. The right ventricle pumps the deoxygenated blood to the lungs through the pulmonary artery for oxygen and carbon dioxide exchange. The left atrium receives the newly oxygenated blood by way of the pulmonary veins from the lungs, and the left ventricle pumps the oxygenated blood through the aorta to the systemic circulation (Fig. 13.2).

The four cardiac valves maintain the unidirectional blood flow through the chambers of the heart. The valves also assist in producing the pressure gradient needed between the chambers for the blood to flow through the heart. There are two types of valves: the atrioventricular (AV) valves, which separate the atria from the ventricles, and the semilunar (SL) valves, which separate the pulmonary artery from the right ventricle and the aorta from the left ventricle (Fig. 13.3). The AV valves are the tricuspid valve, which lies between the right atrium and the right ventricle, and the mitral valve, located between the left atrium and the left ventricle. Each AV valve is anchored by chordae tendineae to the papillary muscles on its ventricular floor. The SL valves are the pulmonic valve, which lies between the right ventricle and the pulmonary artery, and the aortic valve, located between the left ventricle and the aorta. These SL valves are not anchored by chordae tendineae. Instead, their closing is passive and is caused by differences in pressure between the chamber and the respective great vessel.

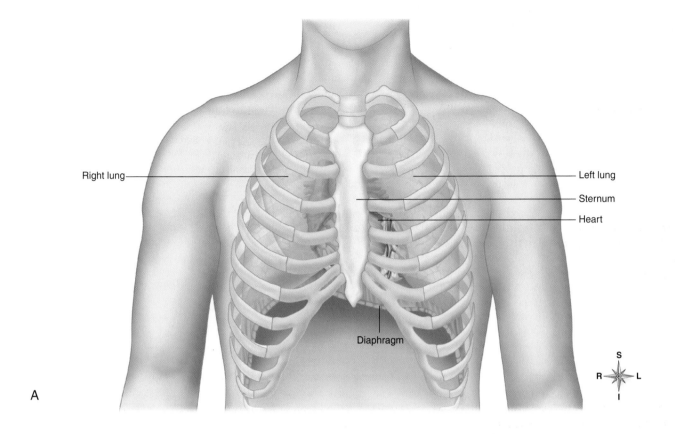

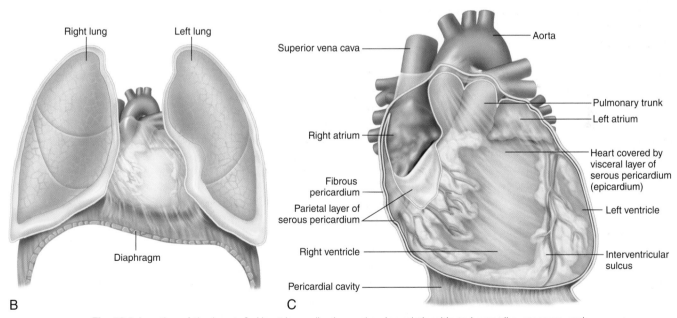

Fig. 13.1 Location of the heart. **A,** Heart in mediastinum showing relationship to lungs, ribs, sternum, and other thoracic structures. **B,** Anterior view of isolated heart and lungs. Portions of the parietal pleura and pericardium have been removed. **C,** Detail of heart resting on diaphragm with pericardial sac opened.

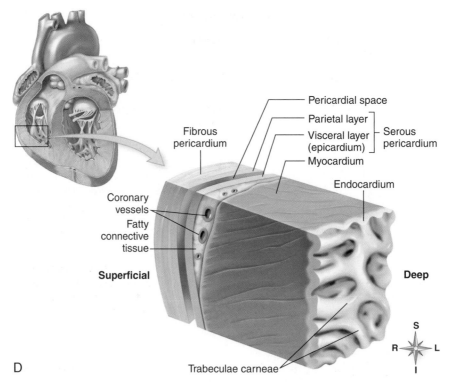

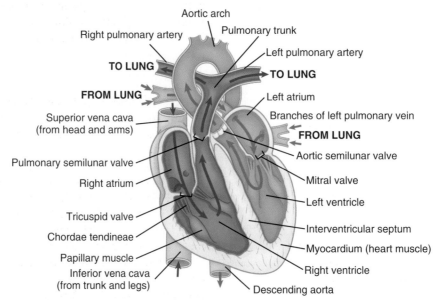

Fig. 13.1 cont'd, D, Transverse section of cadaver specimen and color drawing of thoracic structures at the level of the sixth thoracic (T6) vertebra (inferior aspect). (From Patton KT, Thibodeau GA. *Anatomy and Physiology.* 10th ed. St. Louis, MO: Elsevier; 2019.)

Fig. 13.2 Structures that direct blood flow through the heart. *Arrows* indicate path of blood flow through chambers, valves, and major vessels. (From Huether S, McCance K. *Understanding Pathophysiology.* 6th ed. St. Louis, MO: Elsevier; 2017.)

Autonomic Control

The autonomic nervous system (sympathetic and parasympathetic) exerts control over the cardiovascular system. The sympathetic nervous system releases norepinephrine, which has alpha- and beta-adrenergic effects. Alpha-adrenergic effects cause arterial vasoconstriction. Beta-adrenergic effects increase sinus node discharge (positive chronotropic effect), increase the force of contraction (positive inotropic effect), and accelerate the AV conduction time (positive dromotropic effect). The parasympathetic nervous system releases acetylcholine through stimulation of the vagus nerve. It causes a decrease in sinus node discharge and slows conduction through the AV node.

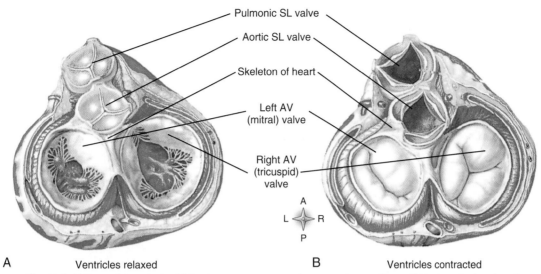

Fig. 13.3 **A,** The atrioventricular *(AV)* valves in the open position and the semilunar *(SL)* valves in the closed position. **B,** The AV valves in the closed position and the SL valves in the open position. (From Patton KT, Thibodeau GA. *Anatomy and Physiology.* 10th ed. St. Louis, MO: Elsevier; 2019.)

In addition to this innervation, receptors help control cardiovascular function. The first group of receptors is the *chemoreceptors,* which are sensitive to changes in partial pressure of arterial oxygen (PaO_2), partial pressure of arterial carbon dioxide ($PaCO_2$), and pH blood levels. Chemoreceptors stimulate the vasomotor center in the medulla; this center controls vasoconstriction and vasodilation. The second group of receptors is the *baroreceptors,* which are sensitive to stretch and pressure. If blood pressure (BP) increases, the baroreceptors cause the heart rate to decrease. If BP decreases, the baroreceptors stimulate an increase in heart rate (Fig. 13.4).

STUDY BREAK

1. The left atrium receives oxygenated blood from which vessel?
   A. Pulmonary artery
   B. Pulmonary vein
   C. Right ventricle
   D. Superior vena cava

Coronary Circulation

Many cardiac problems result from a complete or partial occlusion of a coronary artery. The blood supply to the myocardium is derived from the coronary arteries that branch off the aorta immediately above the aortic valve (Fig. 13.5). Two major branches exist: the left coronary artery, which splits into the left anterior descending and left circumflex branches, and the right coronary artery. Knowledge of the portion of the heart that receives its blood supply from a particular coronary artery allows the critical care nurse to anticipate problems related to occlusion of that vessel (Box 13.1). Variations in branching and in the exact placement of the coronary arteries are common.

Blood flow to the coronary arteries occurs during ventricular diastole, when the aortic valve is closed, and the sinuses of Valsalva are filled with blood. Myocardial fibers are relaxed at this time, promoting blood flow through the coronary vessels. The coronary veins return blood from the coronary circulation back into the heart through the coronary sinuses to the right and left atria.

Other Cardiac Functions

Knowledge of the properties of cardiac muscle and the normal conduction system of the heart is essential because many patients have cardiac dysrhythmias (see Chapter 8). Hemodynamic concepts of the cardiovascular system are also important in understanding pathological disorders such as heart failure (HF) (see Chapter 9).

Heart Sounds

The vibrations produced by vascular walls, flowing blood, heart muscle, and heart valves create sound waves known as heart sounds. Auscultation of these sounds with a stethoscope over the heart provides valuable information about valve and cardiac function (Fig. 13.6). Ventricular systole occurs when the pulmonic and aortic valves open to allow blood to be pumped to the lungs (right ventricle, pulmonic valve) and to the systemic circulation (left ventricle, aortic valve). Ventricular diastole occurs when the tricuspid and mitral valves open to allow the ventricles to fill with blood.

The first heart sound is known as S_1. This sound has been described as "lub." It is caused by closure of the tricuspid and mitral valves. It is best heard at the apex of the heart (fifth intercostal space, left midclavicular line) and represents the beginning of ventricular systole (see Fig. 13.6, mitral valve site).

The second heart sound, or S_2, has been described as "dub." It is caused by closure of the pulmonic and aortic valves. It is best heard at the second intercostal space at the left or right sternal border and represents the beginning of ventricular diastole. The first and second heart sounds are best heard with the diaphragm of the stethoscope.

A third heart sound, known as S_3 or ventricular gallop, is a normal variant in young adults but usually represents a pathological

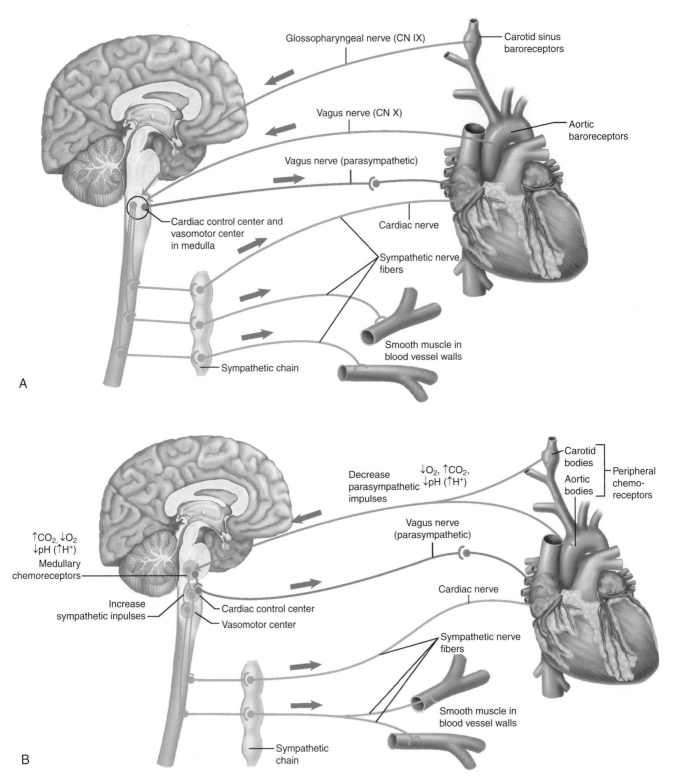

Fig. 13.4 A, Vasomotor pressoreflexes. **B,** Vasomotor chemoreflexes. (From Patton KT, Thibodeau GA. *Anatomy and Physiology*. 10th ed. St. Louis, MO: Elsevier; 2019.)

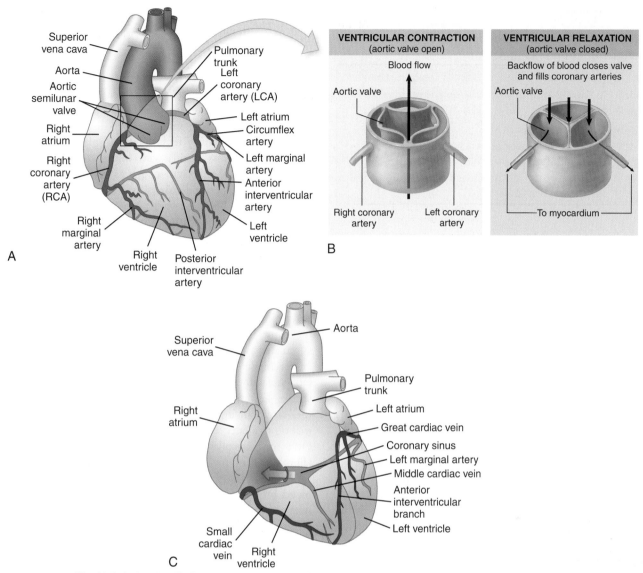

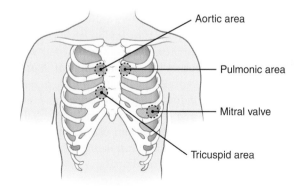

Fig. 13.5 A, Arteries. B, Coronary artery openings from the aorta. Placement of the coronary artery opening behind the leaflets of the aortic valve allows the coronary arteries to fill during ventricular relaxation. C, Veins. Both A and C are anterior views of the heart. Vessels near the anterior surface are more darkly colored than vessels of the posterior surface seen through the heart. (From Patton KT, Thibodeau GA. *The Human Body in Health & Disease*. 8th ed. St. Louis, MO: Elsevier; 2018.)

BOX 13.1 Coronary Artery Distribution

Right Coronary Artery
- Right atrium
- Right ventricle
- Sinoatrial node
- Atrioventricular bundle
- Posterior portion of the left ventricle

Left Anterior Descending Artery
- Anterior two-thirds of the intraventricular septum
- Anterior left ventricle

Circumflex Artery
- Left atrium

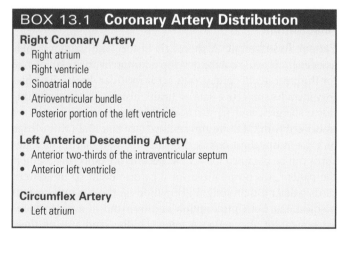

Fig. 13.6 Chest areas from which each valve sound is best heard. (Modified from Hall JE, Guyton AC. *Guyton and Hall Textbook of Medical Physiology*. 13th ed. Philadelphia, PA: Saunders; 2016.)

TABLE 13.1   Grading of Heart Murmurs

Intensity of Murmur Graded from I to VI Based on Increasing Loudness

Grade I	Lowest intensity, usually not audible by inexperienced providers
Grade II	Low intensity, usually audible by inexperienced providers
Grade III	Medium intensity without a thrill
Grade IV	Medium intensity with a thrill
Grade V	Loudest murmur, audible when stethoscope is placed on the chest; associated with a thrill
Grade VI	Loudest intensity, audible when stethoscope is removed from chest; associated with a thrill

process in an older adult. The sound is caused by rapid left ventricular filling and may be produced when the heart is already overfilled or poorly compliant. The S_3 sound is low pitched and can best be heard with the bell of the stethoscope at the fifth intercostal space, at the left midclavicular line. It occurs immediately after S_2. Together with S_1 and S_2, S_3 produces a "lub-dubba" or "ken-**tuk′**e" sound. S_3 is often heard in patients with HF or fluid overload.

A fourth heart sound, known as S_4 or atrial gallop, is produced from atrial contraction that is more forceful than normal. Together with S_1 and S_2, S_4 produces a "te-lubb-dubb" or "**ten′**-ne-see" sound. S_4 can be normal in elderly patients, but it is often heard after an acute myocardial infarction (AMI), when the atria contract more forcefully against ventricles distended with blood.

In the severely failing heart, all four sounds may be heard, producing a "gallop" rhythm, so named because it sounds like the hoofbeats of a galloping horse. It can best be heard with the bell of the stethoscope at the fifth intercostal space, at the left midclavicular line. It is often documented as S_4, S_1, S_2, S_3 because of the order in which the sounds are heard. A summation gallop occurs when the third and fourth heart sounds are superimposed; it is usually an indication of heart disease.

Heart Murmur

A heart murmur is a sound caused by turbulence of blood flow through the valves of the heart. A murmur is usually a rumbling, blowing, harsh, or musical sound. It is important to determine the sound, anatomical location, loudness, and intensity of a murmur and whether extra heart sounds are heard. Table 13.1 presents a grading of heart murmurs. Murmurs are audible when a septal defect is present, when a valve (usually aortic or mitral) is stenosed, or when the valve leaflets fail to approximate (valve insufficiency). The presence of a new murmur warrants special attention, particularly in a patient with AMI. A papillary muscle may have ruptured, causing the mitral valve to not close correctly, which can be indicative of severe damage and impending complications (HF and pulmonary edema). Auscultation of heart sounds is a skill developed from practice in listening to many different patients' hearts and correlating the sounds heard with the patients' pathological conditions.

CORONARY ARTERY DISEASE

Coronary artery disease (CAD) is a broad term used to refer to the narrowing or occlusion of the coronary arteries. Other terms used to describe CAD include coronary heart disease and atherosclerotic cardiovascular disease (ASCVD).

Pathophysiology

CAD is the progressive narrowing of one or more coronary arteries by atherosclerosis. CAD results in ischemia when the internal diameter of the coronary vessel is reduced by 50% or more (Fig. 13.7).[7]

Atherosclerosis is an inflammatory disease that progresses from endothelial injury to fatty streak, plaque, and complex lesion. The process begins with injury to the endothelium caused by cardiac risk factors such as smoking, hypertension, diabetes, and hyperlipidemia (Box 13.2). Once injury occurs, endothelial cells become inflamed, causing release of cytokines. Macrophages adhere to the injured endothelium and release enzymes and toxic oxygen radicals that create oxidative stress, oxidize low-density lipoproteins (LDLs), and further injure the vessel. Inflammation with additional oxidative stress and activation of macrophages occurs. Oxidized LDLs penetrate the arterial wall and are engulfed by macrophages, creating foam cells that release cytokines, tissue factor, reactive oxygen species, metalloproteinases, and growth factor. Cytokines and LDLs stimulate vascular smooth cell proliferation, which leads to vascular remodeling (Fig. 13.8). Accumulation of foam cells leads to fatty streak formation.[8] With age, most individuals develop fatty streaks, accumulations of serum lipoproteins in the intima of the vessel wall, in their coronary arteries. The dysfunctional formation of a fatty streak leads to the presence of fibrotic plaque. Over time, a collagen cap is formed from connective tissue (fibroblasts and macrophages) and LDL[7] (see Fig. 13.7C).

Plaques may rupture, causing the contents to interact with blood, producing a thrombus. The thrombus can occlude a coronary artery, with resulting injury and infarction. Rupture of the plaque starts the coagulation cascade, leading to the initiation of thrombin production, conversion of fibrinogen to fibrin, and platelet aggregation at the site. After injury to the endothelium, platelets are exposed to proteins that bind to receptors, causing adhesion of platelets at the site of injury. Next, the platelets are activated and change shape. They release thromboxane A_2, which in turn binds to thromboxane receptors that enhance platelet activation, vasoconstriction, and plaque progression. At the same time, the platelets aggregate with one another. This process of adhesion, activation, and aggregation causes a rapidly growing thrombus that compromises coronary blood flow.[7]

Assessment

Patient Assessment. A thorough history and cardiovascular assessment provide data to develop a comprehensive plan of care for the critically ill patient with cardiovascular disease. The history includes subjective data on health history, prior hospitalizations, allergies, and family health history. Several risk factors associated with CAD are also assessed (see Box 13.2). Knowledge of prior hospitalizations is also important so that medical records can be obtained for review. Records are especially useful if the patient was hospitalized for a cardiac event or underwent cardiac diagnostic testing. Information on the patient's current medications, both prescription and over-the-counter, includes assessment of the patient's understanding and use of these medications. For example, when considering nitroglycerin

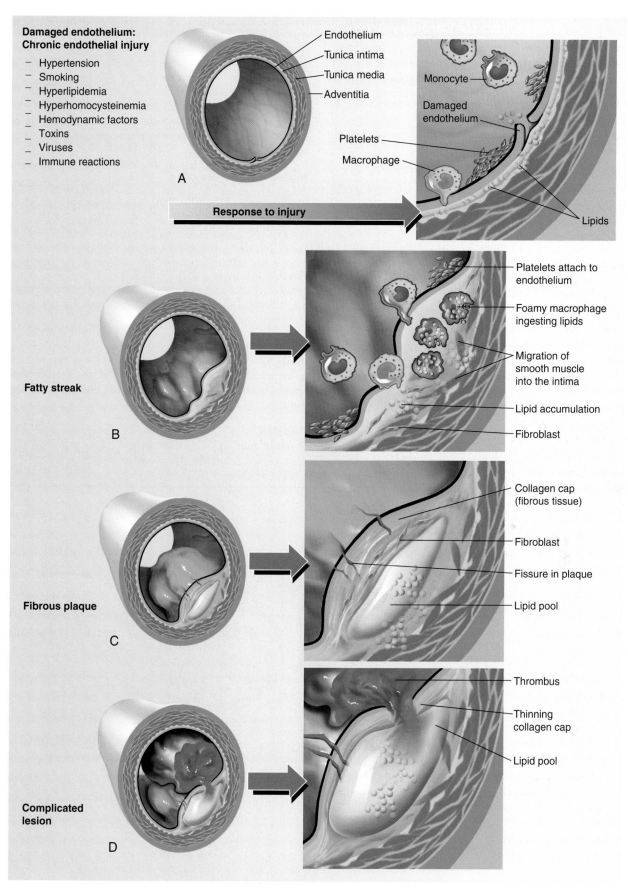

Fig. 13.7 Progression of atherosclerosis. **A,** Damaged endothelium. **B,** Fatty streak and lipid core formation. **C,** Fibrous plaque (raised plaques are visible: some are yellow; others are white). **D,** Complicated lesion (thrombus is red; collagen is blue). (From Huether S, McCance K. *Understanding Pathophysiology.* 6th ed. St. Louis, MO: Elsevier; 2017.)

BOX 13.2 Risk Factors for Coronary Artery Disease

Several risk factors predispose an individual to coronary artery disease (CAD). Some risk factors cannot be changed (e.g., gender, heredity, age). Other risk factors are modifiable, including smoking, high blood cholesterol, high blood pressure (BP), physical inactivity, overweight or obesity, and diabetes.

Gender
Men have a greater risk of heart attacks than women, and they have heart attacks earlier in life.

Heredity
A family history of early heart disease is an unmodifiable risk for CAD. A positive history is defined as having a first-degree relative (i.e., parent, sister, brother, or child) with CAD diagnosed before age 55 years in male relatives or before age 65 years in female relatives.

Age
Men in their mid-40s or older, and women once they reach menopause, are considered to be at higher risk for CAD.

Smoking
Smokers have a higher risk of CAD. Smoking increases low-density lipoprotein (LDL) levels and damages the endothelium of coronary vessels. These are predisposing factors for the development of atherosclerosis. Smoking also causes vasoconstriction of coronary vessels, thus decreasing blood flow to the heart muscle itself.

High Blood Cholesterol
Serum cholesterol or lipid levels play a key role in the development of atherosclerosis. An elevated total cholesterol value (>200 mg/dL) is considered a risk factor for CAD. Cholesterol is insoluble in plasma and must be transported by lipoproteins that are soluble. High-density lipoproteins (HDLs) are considered the "good" cholesterol. HDLs assist in transporting cholesterol to the liver for

removal. A high HDL level (>40 mg/dL for men and >50 mg/dL for women) may reduce the incidence of CAD, whereas a low HDL level (<40 mg/dL) may be considered a risk factor for developing CAD.

LDLs are considered the "bad" cholesterol. LDLs transport and deposit cholesterol in the arterial vessels, thus facilitating the process of atherosclerosis. Other non-HDL lipoproteins also contribute to the development of CAD. Very-low–density lipoproteins are largely composed of triglycerides and contribute to an increased risk of CAD.

High Blood Pressure
Though there are many hypertension guidelines, most agree that a BP greater than 140/90 mm Hg or taking antihypertensive medication is a risk factor for CAD. Hypertension causes direct injury to the vasculature, leading to the development of CAD. Oxygen demands are also increased. The heart muscle enlarges and weakens over time, thereby increasing the workload of the heart.

Physical Inactivity
Lack of physical activity is a risk factor for CAD. Regular aerobic exercise reduces the incidence of CAD. Exercise also helps control other risk factors such as high BP, diabetes, and obesity.

Overweight and Obesity
Obesity increases the atherogenic process and predisposes persons to CAD. In addition, obesity is related to hypertension and diabetes, two other major risk factors. The waist-to-hip ratio and body mass index (BMI) are important assessments.

Diabetes
Diabetes is associated with increased levels of LDL and triglycerides. Glycation associated with diabetes decreases the uptake of LDL by the liver and increases the hepatic synthesis of LDL.

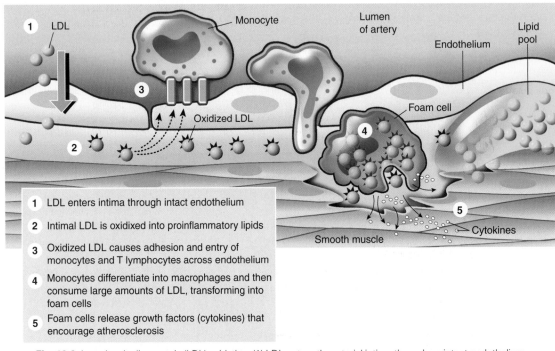

1 LDL enters intima through intact endothelium

2 Intimal LDL is oxidixed into proinflammatory lipids

3 Oxidized LDL causes adhesion and entry of monocytes and T lymphocytes across endothelium

4 Monocytes differentiate into macrophages and then consume large amounts of LDL, transforming into foam cells

5 Foam cells release growth factors (cytokines) that encourage atherosclerosis

Fig. 13.8 Low-density lipoprotein (LDL) oxidation. (1) LDL enters the arterial intima through an intact endothelium. (2) and (3) Inflammation and oxidized LDL cause endothelial cells to express adhesion molecules that bind monocytes and other inflammatory and immune cells. Monocytes penetrate the vessel wall, becoming macrophages. (4) Lipid-laden macrophages are called "foam cells." (5) Foam cells accumulate and form the fatty streak, and many inflammatory cytokines and enzymes are released that injure the vessel wall. (From McCance KL, Huether SE, eds. *Pathophysiology: The Biologic Basis for Disease in Adults and Children.* 8th ed. St. Louis, MO: Elsevier; 2019.)

BOX 13.3   Assessment of Daily Activities

- What, if any, is the critically ill patient's exercise routine, including the type, amount, and regularity of the activity?
- What is the critically ill patient's daily food pattern and intake?
- What is the critically ill patient's sleep pattern?
- What are the critically ill patient's habitual social patterns in using tobacco, alcohol, medications, coffee, tea, and caffeinated sodas?

⚠ CLINICAL ALERT
PQRST Assessment of the Patient With Chest Pain

- P = Provocation
- Q = Quality
- R = Region/Radiation
- S = Severity
- T = Timing (when began) and Treatment

(NTG) administration, it is necessary to know the history of the patient's use of phosphodiesterase type 5 inhibitors taken for erectile dysfunction, such as sildenafil (Viagra), tadalafil (Cialis), or vardenafil (Levitra). These medications potentiate the hypotensive effects of nitrates such as NTG; therefore their concurrent use is contraindicated. It is also important to determine whether the patient has any food or medication allergies.

A psychosocial or personal history is important for the planning of the critically ill patient's care. This history includes information related to daily activities such as sleep, diet, and exercise (Box 13.3).

Before beginning the physical examination, determine recent and recurrent symptoms that may be related to the patient's current problems. Such symptoms include the presence or absence of fatigue, fluid retention, dyspnea, irregular heartbeat (palpitations), and chest pain (see Clinical Alert box). The physical examination itself encompasses all body systems and is not limited to the cardiovascular system. Because all body systems are interrelated and interdependent, it is imperative that a total evaluation be completed regarding the physical status of the patient. Patients whose primary problems are cardiovascular most commonly exhibit alterations in circulation and oxygenation. Therefore all systems are examined from this perspective.

The examination is performed in an orderly, organized manner and involves the techniques of inspection, palpation, percussion, and auscultation. A baseline assessment summary is provided in Table 13.2.

STUDY BREAK

2. When assessing chest pain using the PQRST mnemonic, the P refers to which of the following?
   A. Place
   B. Pressure
   C. Prevention
   D. Provocation

Diagnostic Studies. Many diagnostic studies are fundamental for the care and treatment of critically ill patients with CAD. The following paragraphs describe common diagnostic studies the cardiac patient may encounter.

12-Lead electrocardiography (ECG). This noninvasive test, also commonly referred to as ECG or EKG, is usually preliminary to most other tests performed. It is useful for identification of rhythm disturbances; pericarditis; pulmonary diseases; left ventricular hypertrophy; and myocardial ischemia, injury, and infarction. The importance of this basic test should not be underestimated.

TABLE 13.2   Major Systems Assessment for Cardiovascular Disease

System	Assessment
Neurological	Level of consciousness and orientation to person, place, time, events; presence of hallucinations, depression, withdrawal, restlessness, apprehensiveness, irritability, cooperativeness, response to tactile stimuli; type and location of pain; how pain is relieved; trembling; pupils (size, equality, response); paresthesias; eye movements; hand grips (strength and equality); leg movement
Skin	Color (mottling, cyanosis, pallor), temperature, dryness, turgor, presence of rashes, broken areas, pressure areas, urticaria, incision site, wounds
Cardiovascular	BP (bilaterally); apical heart rate and radial pulses; pulse deficit; monitor leads on patient in correct anatomical placement; regularity of rhythm, presence of ectopy; PR, QRS, and QT intervals; heart sounds; presence of abnormalities (rubs, gallops, clicks); neck vein distension with head of bed at what angle; edema (sacral and dependent); calf pain; varicosities; presence of pulses: bilateral carotid, radial, femoral, posterior tibial, dorsalis pedis; capillary refill in extremities; hemodynamic measurements; temporary pacemaker settings; medications to maintain BP or rhythm
Respiratory	Rate, depth, and quality of respirations; oxygen needs; accessory muscle use; cough, sputum: type, color, suctioning frequency; symmetry of chest expansion and breath sounds, breath sounds (crackles, wheezing); interpretation of ABGs; chest tube with description of drainage, fluctuation in water seal, bubbling, suction applied; tracheostomy or endotracheal tube; ventilator used; ventilator settings; ventilator rate versus patient's own breaths
Gastrointestinal	Abdominal size and softness, bowel sounds, nausea and vomiting, bowel movement, dressing and/or drainage, NG tube with description of drainage, feeding tube: type and frequency of feedings, drains
Genitourinary	Voiding or indwelling urinary catheter, urine color, quality, and quantity; vaginal or urethral drainage
IV	Volume of fluid, type of solution, rate; IV site condition
Wounds	Dry or drainage: type, color, amount, odor; hematoma, inflamed, drains, Hemovac, dressing changes, cultures

ABG, Arterial blood gas; *BP,* blood pressure; *NG,* nasogastric.

Chest radiography. This study is usually performed in the anteroposterior view. Chest radiography is used to detect cardiomegaly, cardiac positioning, degree of fluid infiltrating the pulmonary space or pericardial space, and other structural changes that may affect the physical ability of the heart to function in a normal manner.

Holter or event monitors. The Holter or event devices are used to detect suspected dysrhythmias. The Holter monitor is a small portable recorder (about the size of a large cellular phone) connected to the patient by three to five electrodes. The recorder is worn for 24 to 48 hours. Event monitors come in different models; some models are leadless and can be worn for longer periods. The patient engages in normal daily activities and keeps a log of all activities and symptoms during the monitoring period. The recording is analyzed for abnormalities and correlated with the documented activities and symptoms.

Exercise tolerance test (ETT). In this noninvasive test, also known as a stress test, the patient is connected to an ECG machine while exercising. Physical stress causes an increase in myocardial oxygen consumption. If oxygen demand exceeds supply, ischemia may result. The stress test is used to document exercise-induced ischemia and can identify those individuals who are prone to cardiac ischemia during activity, even though their resting ECGs are normal. The exercise usually involves pedaling a stationary bike or, more commonly, walking on a treadmill. The patient is constantly monitored, BP is checked at intervals, and the ECG printout is analyzed at the end of the testing period. Changes in the ST segments of the ECG can indicate ischemia. Beta-blockers are often withheld on the morning of an ETT so that an adequate heart rate can be attained during the test. Patients return to their room or go home after the heart rate returns to baseline.

Pharmacological stress testing. If a patient is physically unable to perform the exercise required by an ETT, a pharmacological stress test can be done. This test is done in conjunction with radionuclide scintigraphy or echocardiography. Medications such as regadenoson, dipyridamole, or adenosine are used to cause vasodilation of normal coronary arteries. If an area of a blood vessel is stenosed, it does not dilate and shows up as hypoperfusion on radionuclide scanning or as hypokinesis on echocardiography. Alternatively, dobutamine can be used to increase heart rate and contractility. Areas that are not perfused well because of blockages are evident when scanned.

Nuclear stress testing. This test can be done with exercise to increase the sensitivity of the test. It is used for patients who have an ECG that precludes accurate interpretation of ST-segment changes, and it is also used in conjunction with medications for patients who cannot walk on a treadmill. Technetium-99m and thallium-201 are radionuclides given intravenously to image the heart at rest and under stress (induced by either exercise or use of a pharmacological agent). The stress images are compared with the resting images. Perfusion defects seen on rest and stress images are evidence of infarct, whereas defects observed on stress images that are normal during the rest study indicate ischemia.

Echocardiography. This is a noninvasive imaging procedure that uses ultrasound to visualize the cardiac structures and the motion and function of cardiac valves and chambers. A transducer placed on the chest wall sends ultrasound waves at short intervals. The reflected sound waves, termed *echoes,* are displayed on a graph for interpretation. Echocardiography is used to assess valvular function, evaluate congenital defects, measure the size of cardiac chambers, evaluate cardiac disease progression, evaluate ventricular function, diagnose myocardial tumors and effusions, and, to a lesser degree, measure cardiac output. Ventricular function is evaluated by measuring the left ventricular ejection fraction (LVEF). The LVEF is the percentage of blood ejected from the left ventricle during systole, normally 55% to 60%.

Transesophageal echocardiography (TEE). This test provides ultrasonic imaging of the heart as viewed from behind the heart. In TEE, an ultrasound probe is fitted on the end of a flexible gastroscope, which is inserted into the posterior pharynx and advanced into the esophagus. This technique provides a clear picture of the heart because the esophagus lies against the back of the heart and parallel to the aorta. TEE is indicated to visualize prosthetic heart valves, mitral valve function, aortic dissection, vegetative endocarditis, congenital heart defects in adults, cardiac masses and tumors, and embolic phenomena. It is also used intraoperatively to assess left ventricular function. Patients should fast (except for medications) for 6 to 8 hours before the examination. During the procedure, vital signs, cardiac rhythm, and oxygen saturation are monitored. After the procedure, the patient is unable to eat until the gag reflex returns. A rare complication of TEE is esophageal perforation. The signs of perforation are sore throat, dysphagia, stiff neck, and epigastric or substernal pain that worsens with breathing and movement or pain in the back, abdomen, or shoulder.

Multigated blood acquisition study (MUGA). The MUGA scan is used to assess left ventricular function. An isotope is injected, and images of the heart are taken during systole and diastole to assess the LVEF of the heart. An LVEF of 55% to 60% and symmetrical contraction of the left ventricle are considered normal test results. This test will not be as accurate in patients with irregular heart rhythms.

Cardiac magnetic resonance imaging (MRI). An MRI is a noninvasive test used to evaluate tissues, structures, and blood flow. The technique uses magnetic resonance to create images of hydrogen ions as they are emitted, picked up, and fed into a computer. The computer reconstructs the image, which can be used to differentiate between healthy and ischemic tissue. MRI is used to diagnose or evaluate CAD, aortic aneurysm, congenital heart disease, left ventricular function, cardiac tumors, thrombus, valvular disease, and pericardial disorders. One of the advantages of MRI is that it does not involve exposure to ionizing radiation. A contrast agent can be used with MRI to enhance results.

MRI cannot be performed on patients with cochlear implants or some types of brain clips (used to treat cerebral aneurysms). It generally cannot be performed on patients with pacemakers or defibrillators, although some of these devices are MRI compatible. The test can be very stressful for patients who are claustrophobic, and in such situations open MRI may be indicated. Cardiac monitors that are designed for use in MRI suites have been developed to ensure adequate monitoring of critically ill patients during the procedure.

Cardiac computed tomography (CT). The cardiac CT scan is a noninvasive way to image the heart three-dimensionally. It is used to evaluate for CAD, valvular disease, pericardial disease, and aneurysms and to map the pulmonary veins before ablation. When used with contrast, it is called CT angiography.

Positron emission tomography (PET). A PET scan is a noninvasive way to study cardiac tissue perfusion. Radioactive isotopes are injected intravenously to enable the imaging.

Cardiac catheterization and angiography. A cardiac catheterization is an invasive procedure that can be divided into two stages (right-sided and left-sided catheterization). It is used to measure pressures in the chambers of the heart, cardiac output, and blood gas content; to confirm and evaluate the severity of lesions within the coronary arteries; and to assess left ventricular function.

Right-sided catheterization is performed by placing a pulmonary artery catheter in the femoral or brachial vein and then carefully advancing it into the right atrium, right ventricle, and pulmonary artery. The healthcare provider measures pressures in the right atrium, right ventricle, and pulmonary artery, as well as the pulmonary artery occlusion pressure. Oxygen saturations can be measured if indicated to detect disease (i.e., valve disease or septal defect).

Left-sided catheterization is performed to visualize coronary arteries, to determine the area and extent of lesions within native vessel walls and bypass grafts, to evaluate angina-related spasms, to locate areas of infarct, and to perform interventions such as percutaneous angioplasty or stent placement.

Left-sided catheterization is performed by cannulation of a femoral, brachial, or radial artery. The procedure entails positioning a catheter into the aorta at the proximal end of the coronary arteries. Dye is injected into the arteries, and a radiographic picture is recorded as the dye progresses or fails to progress through the coronary circulation. In addition, dye is injected into the left ventricle, and the amount of dye ejected with the next systole is measured to determine the LVEF.

After the procedure, the catheters are removed. There are numerous vascular closure devices (VCDs) to prevent bleeding from the arterial site: a sealing device made of collagen (e.g., Angio-Seal), a clip-mediated device (e.g., StarClose), a suture device (e.g., Perclose), and a hemostatic bandage (e.g., QuikClot). For the radial artery, a compression device (e.g., TR Band) can be used (Fig. 13.9). If a VCD is not used, apply firm pressure to the site for 15 to 30 minutes. Commercial devices are available to assist in applying pressure to the site. Depending on the diagnostic study results and the patient's status, patients are usually discharged within 4 to 8 hours after completion of the test.

Nursing care for a patient undergoing cardiac catheterization involves preprocedure education (the procedure will be performed using local anesthesia, and the patient may feel a warm or hot flush sensation or flutter of the catheter as it moves about) and postprocedure instruction. The postprocedure routine is described in Box 13.4.

Electrophysiology. An electrophysiology study is an invasive procedure that involves the introduction of an electrode catheter percutaneously from a peripheral vein or artery into the cardiac chamber or sinuses and the performance of programmed electrical stimulations of the heart. Electrophysiology studies aid in recording intracardiac ECGs, diagnosing cardiac conduction defects, evaluating the effectiveness of antiarrhythmic medications, determining the proper choice of pacemaker programming, and mapping the cardiac conduction system before ablation.

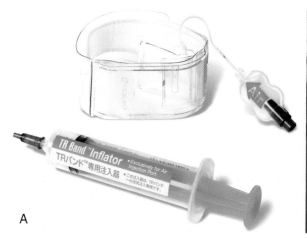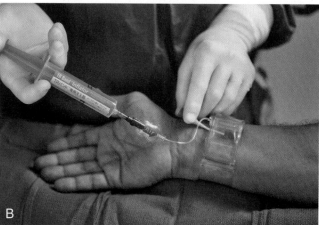

Fig. 13.9 TR Band Radial Compression Device. (©2020 Terumo Medical Corporation. All rights reserved.)

BOX 13.4 Nursing Care After Cardiac Catheterization and Angiography

- Maintain the patient on bed rest (time varies depending on the size of the catheter used, the access site, and the method for preventing arterial bleeding).
- Keep the extremity used for catheter insertion immobile.
- Observe the insertion site for bleeding or hematoma, especially if the patient is receiving postprocedure anticoagulant therapy.
- Mark the hematoma with a marker around its outer perimeter to aid in assessing for an increase in bleeding.
- Assess for bruits.
- Maintain head-of-bed elevation no higher than 30 degrees (if femoral access).
- Monitor peripheral pulses, color, and sensation of the extremity distal to insertion site (every 15 minutes × 4; every 30 minutes × 4; every 1 hour × 2). In addition, monitor the opposite extremity pulse to assess for presence of equal pulses, and for color and sensation bilaterally.
- Observe cardiac rhythm.
- Encourage fluid intake if not contraindicated.
- Monitor intake and output.
- Observe for an adverse reaction to dye (angiography).
- Assess for chest pain, back pain, and shortness of breath and notify health-care provider.

Laboratory Diagnostics. Other diagnostic measures include the evaluation of serum electrolytes and cardiac enzymes. Because many books are available regarding reading and interpretation of the laboratory values, this section presents a brief overview of the more important blood studies that should or may have to be assessed in the patient with a cardiovascular alteration.

Serum electrolytes. Electrolytes are important in maintaining the function of the cardiac conduction system. Imbalances in sodium, potassium, calcium, and magnesium can result in cardiac dysrhythmias. Therefore analysis of serum electrolytes is a routine part of the assessment and treatment of the cardiac patient. Table 13.3 reviews ECG changes that may alert the nurse to possible electrolyte abnormalities.

Cardiac enzymes—troponin I and troponin T. Serum troponin levels aid in the early diagnosis of AMI. Levels are normally undetectable in healthy people but become elevated as early as 1 hour after myocardial cell injury. Testing for troponin can be done quickly in the field or in the emergency department. The normal value of troponin I is less than 0.03 ng/L, and that of troponin T is less than 0.1 ng/L.[26]

LIFESPAN CONSIDERATIONS

Several lifespan factors must be considered for the patient with cardiovascular disease. Cardiovascular issues can occur as a result of pregnancy. Women are delaying pregnancy, which increases risks during pregnancy. In addition, women with a history of heart defects and cardiovascular disease are choosing to become pregnant. Older adults also need special consideration.

Older Adults

- Exercise caution when administering medications. Older adults have greater sensitivity to medications and may require lower dosages for some medications. Conversely, dosages may have to be increased for medications taken for long periods of time.
- Monitor closely for signs of medication effectiveness, adverse reactions, and possible interactions with other medications.
- Provide information in an easy-to-understand form and reinforce teaching. Consider having a family member or other caregiver present when providing teaching. Use teach-back to ensure understanding.
- Careful monitoring and continuous assessment are warranted postprocedure and in the postoperative period. Circulation decreases with aging. In addition, anesthesia and a major surgical procedure contribute to changes in level of consciousness and circulation.
- Always involve family members or close friends in care of older adults. These individuals can assist the patient as they adjust to changes in treatment, activity, diet, and medications.
- Older adults may need assistance to maintain activities of daily living.
- Rehabilitation may be an important treatment after interventions, AMI, or surgery. Facilitate rehabilitation and encourage older adults to adhere to the set regimen to progress to maximum cardiac and vascular function.

Pregnant Women

- Several cardiovascular conditions can occur during pregnancy. Some are more severe than others.
  - Peripartum cardiomyopathy may occur if heart failure occurs late in pregnancy or in the postpartum period.
  - Pregnancy-induced hypertension occurs in about 6% to 8% of women.
  - Acute myocardial infarction (AMI) is rare but can occur in women with a history of coronary artery disease (CAD) or from a spontaneous clot since pregnancy increases the risks of blood clots.
  - A heart murmur may be noted secondary to increased blood volume in pregnancy. If noted, a cardiac workup is indicated.
  - Increased heart rate is a physiological response to pregnancy and increased blood volume. Although dysrhythmias may occur, most do not require treatment.
- Women with a history of cardiovascular disease can have a successful pregnancy with close observation during pregnancy, labor, and delivery. It is important to discuss pregnancy plans with the obstetrician and cardiologist prior to pregnancy.
  - If the pregnant woman requires antidysrhythmic medications, the effects of the medication on the fetus must be considered.
  - Women with valvular disorders or artificial heart valves need to be monitored closely during pregnancy. The risk for endocarditis is higher. Those with artificial heart valves may need to change anticoagulants during pregnancy.
  - Heart failure can develop or worsen in pregnancy secondary to increased blood volume.
  - Babies of women with a history of a congenital heart defect may have a greater risk of developing a heart defect as well. Prenatal evaluation for defects is indicated.
  - Planning and careful monitoring during delivery and in the immediate postpartum period are essential to reduce stress on the body associated with delivery. Vaginal delivery is often possible.

TABLE 13.3 ECG Changes Associated With Electrolyte Imbalances

Electrolyte Abnormality	ECG Abnormality
Increased calcium	Prolonged PR interval Shortened QT interval
Decreased calcium	Prolonged QT interval
Increased potassium	Narrowed, elevated T waves AV conduction changes Widened QRS complex
Decreased potassium	Prolonged U wave Prolonged QT interval

AV, Atrioventricular; *ECG,* electrocardiography.
From Pagana KP, Pagana TJ. *Mosby's Manual of Diagnostic and Laboratory Tests.* Vol 6. 6th ed. St. Louis, MO: Elsevier; 2018.

STUDY BREAK
3. Which of the following is considered a normal left ventricular ejection fraction (LVEF)?
   A. 30%
   B. 40%
   C. 50%
   D. 60%

Patient Problems

Because CAD is a broad diagnostic area, patients may present with several problems. With the complications of CAD, such as angina, MI, and HF, the problems are more specific. Patient problems for those with CAD include the following[31]:

- Acute Pain (Angina) due to decreased oxygen supply to the myocardium
- Fatigue with Decreased Exercise Tolerance due to generalized weakness and imbalance between oxygen supply and demand occurring with tissue ischemia secondary to MI
- Need for Health Teaching due to unfamiliarity with the disease process and lifestyle implications of CAD

Interventions

Nursing Interventions. Nursing interventions encompass health assessment and patient education. Assessment of the patient's psychosocial status and family support, as well as the history and physical examination findings, are used to guide interventions. Instruct the patient about risk factor modification and signs and symptoms of progression of CAD that warrant medical treatment.

Medical Management. The goal of medical management is to reduce the risk factors for progression of CAD. Strategies for risk factor modification include a low-fat, low-cholesterol diet; exercise; weight loss; smoking cessation; and control of other risks such as diabetes and hypertension. The American Heart Association and the American College of Cardiology revised the cholesterol guidelines in 2018. Rather than recommending therapy to reach a specific LDL level, statin therapy is now recommended based on a patient history of clinical ASCVD, diabetes mellitus, LDL level, and CAD risk. Clinical ASCVD includes history of AMI, acute coronary syndrome (ACS), stable or unstable angina, coronary or other arterial revascularization, stroke, transient ischemic attack (TIA), or peripheral arterial disease presumed to be of atherosclerotic origin. The new guidelines match a patient's risk with the intensity of dose of a statin (Fig. 13.10 and Box 13.5).

Medications to reduce serum lipid levels. Lipid-lowering medications include statins, bile acid resins, ezetimibe, nicotinic acid, and a newer class of medications called proprotein convertase subtilisin/kexin type 9 (PCSK9) inhibitors (Table 13.4). The statins are officially classified as 3-hydroxy-3-methylglutaryl-coenzyme A (HMG-CoA) reductase inhibitors.

The statins lower LDL by slowing the production of cholesterol and increasing the liver's ability to remove LDL from the body and are well tolerated by most individuals. Some commonly prescribed medications include lovastatin, atorvastatin, pravastatin, simvastatin, and rosuvastatin. It is recommended that some statins be given as a single dose in the evening because the body makes more cholesterol at night.[30] Rosuvastatin can be taken at any time due to its long half-life. A disadvantage of statins is that they can cause liver damage; therefore ensure that the patient has liver enzymes measured periodically. Rarely, the medications cause myopathies; instruct patients to contact their healthcare provider if they develop any muscle aches. Statins are considered to be the best treatment for cholesterol management. Other medications may be prescribed for patients who are intolerant of statins.[30]

The bile acid resins combine with cholesterol-containing bile acids in the intestines to form an insoluble complex that is eliminated through feces. Bile acid resins include cholestyramine and colestipol. These medications lower LDL levels by 10% to 20%. The medications are mixed in liquid and are taken twice daily. Side effects include nausea and flatulence; therefore the medications are contraindicated in biliary obstruction. The medications interfere with absorption of many medications; therefore it is recommended that other medications be given 1 hour before, or 2 to 4 hours after, administration of the resins to promote absorption.[12]

Ezetimibe (Zetia) works in the digestive tract by blocking the absorption of cholesterol from food. It is often used in conjunction with other cholesterol-reducing medications. Ezetimibe can cause liver disease; therefore liver function tests must be monitored, and the medication is contraindicated in patients with severe hepatic disease. When added to a statin, ezetimibe reduces cardiovascular events.[10]

Nicotinic acid, or niacin, reduces total cholesterol, LDL, and triglyceride levels, and it increases HDL. The medication is available over the counter; however, its use in lowering cholesterol must be done under the supervision of a healthcare provider. A long-acting, once-daily dose is available by prescription, but it has a higher incidence of liver toxicity. The medication dosage is gradually increased to the maximum effective daily dose. Common side effects include a metallic taste in the mouth, flushing, and increased feelings of warmth. Major side effects include hepatic dysfunction, gout, and hyperglycemia. Because nicotinic acid affects the absorption of other medications, it must be given separately from other

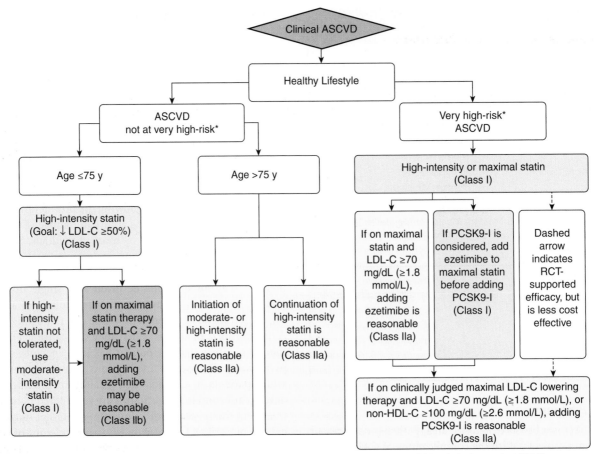

Fig. 13.10 Secondary prevention statin recommendations for the treatment of blood cholesterol. *ASCVD,* Atherosclerotic cardiovascular disease; *HDL-C,* high-density lipoprotein cholesterol; *LDL-C,* low-density lipoprotein cholesterol; *PCSK9-I,* proprotein convertase subtilisin/kexin type 9 inhibitor; *RCT,* randomized controlled trial. (From Grundy SM, Stone NJ, Bailey AL, et al. 2018 AHA/ACC/AACVPR/AAPA/ABC/ACPM/ADA/ AGS/APhA/ASPC/NLA/PCNA guideline on the management of blood cholesterol. *J Am Coll Cardiol.* 2019;73[24]:3234–3237.)

BOX 13.5	Intensity of Statin Therapy	
High-Intensity Statin Therapy	**Moderate-Intensity Statin Therapy**	**Low-Intensity Statin Therapy**
Daily dose lowers LDL-C, on average, by approximately ≥50%	*Daily dose lowers LDL-C, on average, by approximately 30% to 50%*	*Daily dose lowers LDL-C, on average, by <30%*
Atorvastatin 40-80 mg	Atorvastatin 10-20 mg	Simvastatin 10 mg
Rosuvastatin 20-40 mg	Rosuvastatin 5-10 mg	Pravastatin 10-20 mg
	Simvastatin 20-40 mg	Lovastatin 20 mg
	Pravastatin 40-80 mg	Fluvastatin 20-40 mg
	Lovastatin 40 mg	
	Fluvastatin XL 80 mg	
	Fluvastatin 40 mg bid	
	Pitavastatin 1-4 mg	

bid, Twice daily; *LDL-C,* low-density lipoprotein cholesterol.
Modified from Grundy SM, Stone NJ, Bailey AL, et al. 2018 AHA/ACC/AACVPR/AAPA/ABC/ACPM/ADA/AGS/APhA/ASPC/NLA/ PCNA guideline on the management of blood cholesterol. *J Am Coll Cardiol.* 2019;73(24):3234–3237.

medications. Administering niacin at night with food or taking 325 mg of nonenteric-coated aspirin 30 minutes before the niacin dose can reduce some of the side effects.

If triglyceride levels are elevated, patients may be prescribed agents that specifically lower triglyceride levels. One such agent is gemfibrozil, a fibric acid derivative that lowers triglycerides and increases HDL levels. This medication is associated with many gastrointestinal side effects.

If a patient does not respond adequately to single-medication therapy, combined-medication therapy is considered to lower LDL levels further. For example, statins may be combined with bile acid resins, ezetimibe, or PCSK9 inhibitors. PCSK9 inhibitors are approved by the US Food and Drug Administration (FDA) for treatment of heterozygous familial hypercholesteremia and for those patients with ASCVD who require additional LDL lowering.[28] Carefully monitor patients when two or more lipid-lowering agents are given simultaneously.

Medications to prevent platelet adhesion and aggregation. Medications are often prescribed for the patient with CAD to reduce platelet adhesion and aggregation. A single dose (81 to 325 mg) of an enteric-coated aspirin per day is commonly prescribed. To prevent platelet aggregation, other agents may be prescribed with aspirin, such as clopidogrel (Plavix), prasugrel (Effient), or ticagrelor (Brilinta).

TABLE 13.4 PHARMACOLOGY

Medications for Lowering Cholesterol and Triglycerides

Medication	Action/Use	Dose/Route	Side Effects	Nursing Implications
Antilipemic Agents (HMG-CoA Reductase Inhibitors)				
Lovastatin (Altocor, Mevacor)	Competitively inhibits HMG-CoA reductase, which affects cholesterol biosynthesis; lowers total and LDL-C levels; increases HDL-C; used to lower total cholesterol and LDL-C and to help reduce the risk of AMI and stroke	10-60 mg PO once daily (in the evening) or in two divided doses	Headache, dizziness, constipation, hepatic dysfunction, and increased creatine phosphokinase (CPK) levels, myopathy, rhabdomyolysis	Administer with evening meal. Report severe muscle pain or weakness, which can be a sign of rhabdomyolysis, a serious side effect. Obtain baseline liver function and lipid profile tests before starting therapy, 6 weeks later, and periodically or when dose is increased. Do not give in pregnancy. Instruct patient about a low-cholesterol diet.
Atorvastatin (Lipitor)	Same	10-80 mg PO daily	Same	Same
Fluvastatin (Lescol)	Same	20-80 mg daily PO at bedtime	Same	Same
Pravastatin (Pravachol)	Same	10-80 mg daily PO at bedtime	Same	Same
Rosuvastatin (Crestor)	Same	5-40 mg daily PO at bedtime	Same	Same
Simvastatin (Apo-Simvastatin, Zocor)	Same	5-80 mg daily PO at bedtime	Same	The FDA has mandated no more new prescriptions of 80 mg. (Patients who have been stable for >1 yr may continue to take 80 mg/day.) Maximum dose of 20 mg for patients taking amiodarone, amlodipine, or ranolazine, and 10 mg for patients taking verapamil or diltiazem. Contraindicated in patients taking gemfibrozil; antifungal medications; antibiotics such as erythromycin, clarithromycin; and HIV protease inhibitors
Antilipemic Agents (Bile Acid Sequestrants)				
Cholestyramine (Prevalite, Questran, Questran Light)	Forms a nonabsorbable complex with bile acids in the intestine, inhibiting enterohepatic reuptake of intestinal bile salts, which increases the fecal loss of bile salt–bound LDL-C; used to manage hypercholesterolemia	*Powder:* 4-24 g 1-2 times a day *Tablet:* 4-16 g 1-2 times a day	Constipation, heartburn, nausea, flatulence, vomiting, abdominal pain, headache	Mix powder with fluid or applesauce. Do not take dry; avoid inhaling product. Take other medications at least 1 h before taking this medication. Report any stomach cramping, pain, blood in stool, or unresolved nausea or vomiting. Monitor cholesterol and triglyceride levels before and during therapy. Use during pregnancy must be cautious, weighing risks versus benefits.
Colesevelam (Welchol)	Same	625 mg, 3 tablets bid with meals	Same	Same
Ezetimibe (Zetia)	Inhibits absorption of cholesterol in the small intestine	*Tablet:* 10 mg daily PO with or without food	Headache, dizziness, diarrhea, sore throat, runny nose, sneezing, joint pain	Monitor for signs of liver failure. Follow low-cholesterol, low-fat diet. Keep a written list of all prescription and nonprescription medicines, as well as vitamins, minerals, or other dietary supplements.
Antilipemic Agent (Niacin)				
Niacinamide (Niacin)	Inhibits VLDL synthesis Used for adjunctive treatment of hyperlipidemia	*Immediate release:* 1-2 g PO 2-3 times daily; max 6 g/day *Extended release:* 500 mg PO once daily at bedtime; titrate in 500-mg intervals (up to 2 g) q 4 wk based on tolerability and efficacy; maintenance, 1 to 2 g PO once daily; max 2 g/day	Headache, flushing, hepatic toxicity, bloating, flatulence, nausea	Take as directed and not to exceed recommended dosage. Should be taken after meals. Report persistent GI disturbances or changes in color of urine or stool. Take with aspirin to reduce flushing.

Continued

TABLE 13.4   PHARMACOLOGY—cont'd

Medications for Lowering Cholesterol and Triglycerides

Medication	Action/Use	Dose/Route	Side Effects	Nursing Implications
Antilipemic Agent (Fibric Acid)				
Gemfibrozil (Lopid)	Inhibits biosynthesis of VLDL, increases HDL-C, and decreases triglycerides; treatment of hypertriglyceridemia in patients who have not responded to dietary intervention	600 mg bid PO	Dyspepsia, abdominal pain, fatigue, headache, diarrhea, nausea	Administer before breakfast and dinner. May take with milk or meals if GI upset occurs. Report severe abdominal pain, nausea, or vomiting. Use during pregnancy must be weighed against the possible risks.
Fenofibrate (Tricor)	Same	48-145 mg PO once daily	Nausea, abdominal pain, increased liver enzymes, rash, headaches	Same
Adenosine Triphosphate-citrate Lyase (ACL) Inhibitor				
Bempedoic acid (Nexletol)	Lowers LDL-C by inhibiting cholesterol synthesis in the liver. Used to treat heterozygous familial hypercholesterolemia or patients who require additional lowering of LDL-C	One tablet (180 mg) PO once daily	Flu-like symptoms, abdominal or back pain, elevated liver enzymes, muscle spasms, anemia, bronchitis, gout, tendon rupture	May take with or without food. Observe for serious complications of gout and tendon rupture. Monitor closely if also on statin therapy.

AMI, Acute myocardial infarction; *bid,* twice daily; *FDA,* US Food and Drug Administration; *GI,* gastrointestinal; *HDL-C,* high-density lipoprotein cholesterol; *HMG-CoA,* 3-hydroxy-3-methylglutaryl-coenzyme A; *LDL-C,* low-density lipoprotein cholesterol; *max,* maximum; *PO,* orally; *q,* every; *VLDL,* very-low–density lipoprotein.
From Skidmore-Roth L. *Mosby's 2019 Nursing Drug Reference.* 32nd ed. St. Louis, MO: Elsevier; 2019.

Patient Outcomes

Several outcomes are expected after treatment. These include relief of pain; less anxiety related to the disease; adherence to health behavior modification to reduce cardiovascular risks; and the ability to describe the disease process, causes, factors contributing to the symptoms, and the procedures for disease or symptom control.

ANGINA

Angina is chest pain or discomfort caused by myocardial ischemia that is attributed to an imbalance between myocardial oxygen supply and demand. CAD and coronary artery spasms are common causes of angina.

Pathophysiology

Angina (from the Latin word meaning "squeezing") is the chest pain associated with myocardial ischemia. It is transient and does not cause cell death, but it may be a precursor to cell death from MI. The neural pain receptors are stimulated by accelerated metabolism, chemical changes and imbalances, and/or local mechanical stress resulting from abnormal myocardial contractions. The level of oxygen circulating via the vascular system to the myocardial cells decreases, causing ischemia to the tissue resulting in pain.

Angina occurs when oxygen demand is higher than oxygen supply. Box 13.6 shows factors influencing oxygen supply and demand that may result in angina.

Types of Angina

Different types of angina exist: stable angina, unstable angina, and variant (Prinzmetal's) angina. *Stable angina* occurs with exertion and is relieved by rest. It is sometimes called chronic

---

BOX 13.6   Factors That Influence Oxygen Demand and Supply

Increased Oxygen Demand
- *Increased heart rate:* exercise, tachydysrhythmias, fever, anxiety, pain, thyrotoxicosis, medications, ingestion of heavy meals, adapting to extremes in temperature
- *Increased preload:* volume overload
- *Increased afterload:* hypertension, aortic stenosis, vasopressors
- *Increased contractility:* exercise, medications, anxiety

Reduced Oxygen Supply
- Coronary artery disease
- Coronary artery spasms
- Anemia
- Hypoxemia

exertional angina. *Unstable angina* pain is often more severe, may occur at rest, and requires more frequent nitrate therapy. It is sometimes described as crescendo (increasing) in nature. During an unstable episode, the ECG may show ST-segment depression, T-wave inversion, or no changes at all. The patient has an increased risk of MI within 18 months after onset of unstable angina; therefore medical or surgical interventions, or both, are warranted. Patients are often hospitalized for diagnostic workup and treatment. The treatment of unstable angina is discussed more completely later in the chapter (see Acute Coronary Syndrome).

Variant, or *Prinzmetal's,* angina is caused by coronary artery spasms. It often occurs at rest and without other precipitating factors. The ECG shows a marked ST elevation (usually seen only in AMI) during the episode. The ST segment returns to normal after the spasm subsides. AMI can occur with prolonged coronary artery spasm, even in the absence of CAD.

Assessment

Assessment of the patient with actual or suspected angina involves continual observation of the patient and monitoring of signs, symptoms, and diagnostic findings. The patient must be monitored for the type and degree of pain (see Clinical Alert box).

! CLINICAL ALERT

Symptoms of Angina

- Pain is frequently retrosternal, left pectoral, or epigastric. It may radiate to the jaw, left shoulder, or left arm.
- Pain may be associated with dyspnea, lightheadedness, or diaphoresis.
- Pain can be described as chest pressure, burning, squeezing, heavy, or smothering.
- Pain usually lasts 1 to 5 minutes.
- Classic placing of clenched fist against the chest (sternum) may be seen or may be absent if the sensation is confused with indigestion.
- Pain usually begins with exertion and subsides with rest.

STUDY BREAK
4. Which of following types of angina is associated with ST-segment elevation?
   A. Exercise-induced
   B. Prinzmetal's
   C. Smoking-induced
   D. Stable

The precipitating factors for anginal pain include physical or emotional stress, exposure to temperature extremes, and ingestion of a heavy meal. It is important to know what factors alleviate the anginal pain, including stopping activity or exercise and taking NTG sublingual tablets or spray.

Diagnostic Studies. Diagnostic studies for angina include the following: history and physical examination, including assessment of pain and precipitating factors; laboratory data, including cardiac enzymes (cardiac troponin I, cardiac troponin T levels), complete blood count to assess for anemia (hemoglobin and hematocrit values), and cholesterol and triglyceride levels; ECGs during resting periods; stress testing; and coronary angiography. Complications of untreated angina or unstable angina include AMI, HF, dysrhythmias, psychological depression, and sudden death.

Patient Problems

Patients with angina have many problems amenable to nursing interventions. These include the following[31]:
- Acute Pain (angina) due to decreased oxygen supply to the myocardium
- Anxiety due to actual or perceived threat of death, change in health status, threat to self-concept or role, unfamiliar people and environment, medications, preexisting anxiety disorder, uncertainty
- Need for Health Teaching due to unfamiliarity with current health status and prescribed therapies

Interventions

Nursing Interventions. Nursing interventions for the patient with angina are aimed at assessing the patient's description of pain, noting exacerbating factors and measures used to relieve the pain; evaluating whether this is a chronic problem (stable angina) or a new presentation; assessing for indications for obtaining an ECG to evaluate ST-segment and T-wave changes; monitoring vital signs during chest pain and after nitrate administration; and monitoring the effectiveness of interventions. Instruct the patient to relax and rest at the first sign of pain or discomfort and to notify the nurse at the onset of any type of chest pain so that nitrates and oxygen can be administered. Offer assurance and emotional support by explaining all treatments and procedures and encouraging questions. Assess the patient's knowledge level regarding the causes of angina, diagnostic procedures, the treatment plan, and risk factors for CAD. For those patients who smoke, assess readiness to quit and encourage participation in a smoking cessation program. Refer patients who wish to stop smoking to the American Heart Association, American Lung Association, American Cancer Society, or other organizations for support groups and interventions.

Medical Interventions. Unstable angina is treated by conservative management, early intervention with percutaneous intervention, or surgical revascularization. Conservative intervention includes the administration of nitrates, beta-adrenergic blocking agents, calcium channel blocking agents, and ranolazine (Table 13.5). Angioplasty, stenting, and bypass surgery are interventional approaches to revascularization.

Nitrates are the most common medications for angina. They are direct-acting smooth muscle relaxants that cause vasodilation of the peripheral or systemic vascular bed. Nitrate therapy is beneficial because it decreases myocardial oxygen demand.

TABLE 13.5 PHARMACOLOGY

Common Medications Used to Treat Common Cardiovascular Problems

Medication	Action/Use	Dose/Route	Side Effects	Nursing Implications
Nitrates				
Nitroglycerin Nitro-Dur, Nitrostat)	Directly relaxes smooth muscle, causing vasodilation of the systemic vascular bed; decreases myocardial oxygen demands; secondary effect is vasodilation of responsive coronary arteries	*SL:* 0.4 mg q 5 min for up to 3 doses *Topical:* 0.5-2 inches q 6 h *Transdermal:* one patch each day *IV:* continuous infusion started at 5 mcg/min and titrated up to a max of 200 mcg/min	Headache, flushing, tachycardia, dizziness, orthostatic hypotension	Instruct patient to call 911 if chest pain does not subside after the third SL dose. For topical dosing, patient should have a nitrate-free interval (10-12 h/day) to avoid development of tolerance. Do not take nitrate with medications used to treat erectile dysfunction (e.g., vardenafil, tadalafil, sildenafil).
Isosorbide dinitrate (Isordil)	Same	*PO:* 5-40 mg bid-tid		Same
Beta-Blockers				
Metoprolol (Lopressor, Toprol XL)	Blocks beta-adrenergic receptors, resulting in decreased SNS response such as decreased heart rate, blood pressure, and cardiac contractility; used to treat angina, acute myocardial infarction, dysrhythmias and heart failure, hypertension	*PO:* 50-100 mg bid *PO Toprol XL:* 12.5-200 mg daily *IV:* 5 mg	Bradycardia, hypotension, AV blocks, asthma attacks, fatigue, impotence; may mask hypoglycemic episodes	Teach patient to take pulse and blood pressure on a regular basis. Black box warning: do not stop abruptly. Monitor for worsening signs of heart failure.
Labetalol (Trandate)	Same	*PO:* 200-400 mg bid *IV:* 2 mg over 2 min at 10-min intervals; slow IVP	Same	Acts on alpha, beta$_1$, and beta$_2$ receptors. During IV administration, monitor blood pressure continuously; max effect occurs within 5 min.
Carvedilol (Coreg)	Same	*PO:* 3.125-50 mg bid		Same; take with meals. Dose is doubled q 2 wk until desired effect is obtained.
Calcium Channel Blockers				
Verapamil	Inhibits the flow of calcium ions across cellular membranes, with resulting increased coronary blood flow and myocardial perfusion and decreased myocardial oxygen requirements; used to treat hypertension, tachydysrhythmias, vasospasms, and angina	*PO:* 80-120 mg tid; max daily dose is 480 mg	Dizziness, flushing, headaches, bradycardia, atrioventricular blocks, hypotension	Teach patient to monitor pulse and blood pressure, especially if taking nitrates or beta-blockers. Tablets cannot be crushed or chewed. Instruct patient to make position changes slowly.
Diltiazem (Cardizem, Cardizem CD)	Same	*PO:* 30 mg qid *PO sustained release:* 120-360 mg daily, max 480-540 mg	Same	Same
Antiplatelet Agents				
Aspirin	Inhibits clotting mechanisms within the clotting cascade or prevents platelet aggregation; used for unstable angina, acute myocardial infarction, and coronary interventions	*PO:* 81-325 mg daily	Bleeding, epigastric discomfort, bruising, gastric ulceration	Instruct patient to take medication with food. Do not crush or chew the enteric-coated forms.

TABLE 13.5 PHARMACOLOGY—cont'd

Common Medications Used to Treat Common Cardiovascular Problems

Medication	Action/Use	Dose/Route	Side Effects	Nursing Implications
Clopidogrel (Plavix)	Same	*PO:* 300-mg loading dose, then 75 mg/day (in combination with aspirin)	Same	Same
Prasugrel (Effient)	Same	*PO:* 60-mg loading dose, then 10 mg/day	Same	Anemia, edema, headaches, dizziness. Not recommended for patients >75 years of age, weighing <60 kg, or with history of TIA.
Ticagrelor (Brilinta)	Same	*PO:* 180-mg (two 90-mg tablets) loading dose (in combination with 325 mg aspirin), then 90 mg/day (with 81 mg aspirin)	Same	Contraindicated in patients with history of intracranial hemorrhage, active pathological bleeding, or severe hepatic impairment. The risk of bleeding is higher with ticagrelor.
Glycoprotein IIb/IIIa Inhibitors				
Tirofiban (Aggrastat)	Antiplatelet agent and Gp IIb/IIIa inhibitor; acts by binding to the Gp IIb/IIIa receptor site on the surface of the platelet; used in patients with acute coronary syndromes and coronary intervention	*IV:* 0.4 mcg/kg/min for 30 min, then continue at 0.1 mcg/kg/min for 12-24 h. Reduce loading and maintenance infusion by 50% in patients with impaired renal function (creatinine clearance <30 mL/min).	Bleeding, bruising, hemorrhage, thrombocytopenia, and hypotension	Observe and teach patient bleeding precautions and activities to avoid that may cause injury. Assess infusion insertion site for bleeding or hematoma formation. Assess puncture site used for coronary intervention frequently. Tirofiban stops working when the infusion is discontinued. Platelet function is restored 4 h after stopping the infusion.
Eptifibatide (Integrilin)	Same	*IV:* 180 mcg/kg loading dose over 2 min, max 22.6 mg, followed by continuous infusion of 2 mcg/kg/min for 18-24 h or until hospital discharge. Reduce maintenance dose by 50% (to 1 mcg/kg/min) in patients with creatinine clearance <50 mL/min; contraindicated if creatinine clearance is <10 mL/min.	Same	Eptifibatide stops working when the infusion is discontinued. Platelet function is restored 4 h after stopping the infusion.
Antithrombin Agents				
Heparin	Enhances inhibitory effects of antithrombin III, preventing conversion of fibrinogen to fibrin and prothrombin to thrombin; used to prevent or delay thrombus formation	*IV:* 80 units/kg bolus, followed by infusion of 18 units/kg/h, titrated to aPTT.	Bleeding, bruising, thrombocytopenia	Monitor aPTT. Monitor for signs of bleeding and hematoma formation. The aPTT should be monitored aggressively, and the patient should be evaluated closely for signs and symptoms of bleeding.
Enoxaparin (Lovenox)	Same	*Subcutaneous:* 1 mg/kg q 12 h, in conjunction with aspirin. For patients with creatinine clearances <30 mL/min, dosage is 1 mg/kg q 24 h for treatment and 30 mg daily for prophylaxis.	Bleeding, bruising, local site hematomas, hemorrhage	Instruct patient to report persistent chest pain and unusual bleeding or bruising. Do not rub the site after giving the injection.
Analgesic				
Morphine	Binds to opioid receptors in the CNS and causes inhibition of ascending pain pathways, altering perception and response to pain; used for pain relief and anxiety reduction during acute MI	*IV:* 2-4 mg IVP q 5-10 min.	Hypotension, respiratory depression, apnea, bradycardia, nausea, restlessness	Titrated for chest pain. Monitor level of consciousness, blood pressure, respiratory rate, and oxygen saturation during therapy. Effects are reversed with naloxone (Narcan).

Continued

| TABLE 13.5 | PHARMACOLOGY—cont'd | | | |

Common Medications Used to Treat Common Cardiovascular Problems

Medication	Action/Use	Dose/Route	Side Effects	Nursing Implications
Angiotensin-Converting Enzyme Inhibitors				
Enalapril (Vasotec)	Prevents the conversion of AI to AII, resulting in lower levels of AII, which causes an increase in plasma renin activity and a reduction of aldosterone secretion; also inhibits the remodeling process after myocardial injury; used to treat hypertension and heart failure and after MI	*PO:* 2.5-40 mg bid.	Hypotension, bradycardia, renal impairment, cough, orthostatic hypotension	Monitor urine output. Monitor potassium levels. Avoid use of NSAIDs. Instruct patient to avoid rapid change in position (e.g., from lying to standing). Contraindicated in pregnancy.

AI, Angiotensin I; *AII,* angiotensin II; *aPTT,* activated partial thromboplastin time; *AV,* atrioventricular; *bid,* twice daily; *CNS,* central nervous system; *Gp,* glycoprotein; *IVP,* intravenous push; *max,* maximum; *MI,* myocardial infarction; *NSAIDs,* nonsteroidal antiinflammatory drugs; *PO,* orally; *q,* every; *qid,* four times daily; *SL,* sublingual; *SNS,* sympathetic nervous system; *TIA,* transient ischemic attack; *tid,* three times daily.
From Skidmore-Roth L. *Mosby's 2019 Nursing Drug Reference.* 32nd ed. St. Louis, MO: Elsevier; 2019.

The vasodilating effect relieves pain and lowers BP. Nitroglycerin (NTG) is available in quick-acting forms such as sublingual tablets or spray, or as an IV infusion. Long-acting nitrates are delivered orally or by ointments and skin patches (transdermal). Oral isosorbide is another vasodilator. Side effects of these vasodilators include headache, flushing, tachycardia, dizziness, and orthostatic hypotension.[30] Avoid nitrates if a right ventricular infarct is suspected.[5] Instructions for NTG therapy are detailed in Box 13.7.

Beta-adrenergic blocking agents may also be used to treat angina. These agents block adrenergic receptors, thereby decreasing heart rate, BP, and cardiac contractility.[30] The side effects of these medications include bradycardia, AV block, asthma attacks, depression, erectile dysfunction, hypotension, memory loss, and masking of hypoglycemic episodes (except for sweating). Instruct the patient to take these medications as prescribed, to not stop them abruptly, and to monitor heart rate and BP at regular intervals. Instruct patients with diabetes to monitor blood glucose levels since hypoglycemic symptoms may be masked.

Calcium channel blockers inhibit the flow of calcium ions across cellular membranes, an effect that causes direct increases in coronary blood flow and myocardial perfusion.[30] In addition to angina, these medications are used to treat tachydysrhythmias, vasospasms, and hypertension. Calcium channel blockers are divided into two categories: dihydropyridines and nondihydropyridines. Dihydropyridines are primarily used to treat hypertension. These medications typically end in the suffix "-pine" (e.g., amlodipine). Nondihydropyridines such as verapamil and diltiazem are more effective for treatment of angina and dysrhythmias. The side effects of calcium channel blockers include dizziness, flushing, headaches, decreased heart rate, and hypotension. Ankle edema is a major side effect with the dihydropyridine-type calcium channel blocker. Instruct the patient to monitor BP for hypotension and heart rate for bradycardia,

BOX 13.7   Instructions Regarding Nitroglycerin

If the client is discharged on sublingual or buccal nitroglycerin, instruct client to do the following:

- Have tablets readily available.
- Take a tablet before strenuous activity and in stressful situations.
- Take one tablet when chest pain occurs and another every 5 minutes up to a total of three times if necessary; obtain emergency medical assistance if pain persists.
- Place the tablet under the tongue or in the buccal pouch and allow it to dissolve thoroughly.
- Store tablets in a tightly capped, original container away from heat and moisture.
- Replace tablets every 6 months or sooner if they do not relieve discomfort.
- Avoid rising to a standing position quickly after taking nitroglycerin.
- Recognize that dizziness, flushing, and mild headache are common side effects.
- Report fainting, persistent or severe headache, blurred vision, or dry mouth.
- Avoid drinking alcoholic beverages.
- Caution against use of medications for erectile dysfunction (e.g., Viagra, Levitra, Cialis) when taking nitrates because hypotensive effects are exaggerated.

If nitroglycerin skin patches are prescribed:

- Provide instructions about correct application, skin care, the need to rotate sites and to remove the old patch, and frequency of change.
- The patch should be worn no more than 12–14 h/day to prevent development of nitrate tolerance.

From Skidmore-Roth L. *Mosby's 2014 Nursing Drug Reference.* St. Louis, MO: Mosby; 2014.

especially if the agents are taken in combination with nitrates and beta-blockers.

Outcomes

The outcomes for patients with angina are that they will verbalize relief of chest discomfort, appear relaxed and comfortable, verbalize an understanding of angina pectoris and its management, describe their own cardiac risk factors and strategies to reduce them, and perform activities within limits of their ischemic disease, as evidenced by absence of chest pain or discomfort and no ECG changes reflecting ischemia.

ACUTE CORONARY SYNDROME

ACS includes the diagnoses of stable angina, unstable angina, and AMI. AMI is defined as myocardial necrosis caused by ischemia.[29] Prompt recognition and treatment result in improved outcomes for all ACSs.

Pathophysiology

ACS is caused by an imbalance between myocardial oxygen supply and demand. This imbalance is the result of decreased coronary artery perfusion. Most cases of ACS are secondary to atherosclerosis. Other causes include coronary artery spasm, coronary embolism, and blunt trauma. Reduced blood flow to an area of the myocardium causes significant and sustained oxygen deprivation to myocardial cells. Normal functioning is disrupted as ischemia and injury lead to eventual cellular death. Myocardial dysfunction occurs as more cells become involved.

Prolonged ischemia from cessation of blood flow to the cardiac muscle results in infarction and evolves over time. Cardiac cells can withstand ischemic conditions for 20 minutes; after that period, irreversible myocardial cell damage and cellular death begin. The amount of cell death increases, extending from the endocardium to the epicardium as the duration of the occlusion increases. The extent of cell death determines the size of the infarct. Contractility in the infarcted area becomes impaired. A nonfunctional zone and a zone of mild ischemia with potentially viable tissue surround the infarct. The ultimate size of the infarct depends on the fate of this ischemic zone. Early interventions, such as administration of thrombolytics, can restore perfusion to the ischemic zone and can reduce the area of myocardial damage.

Classification of an MI has been changed recently to reflect the anatomical causes of the infarction rather than the ECG changes. Type I is a spontaneous MI and occurs because of plaque rupture, leading to occlusion of the artery. Type II is an MI secondary to ischemic imbalance, in which injury is due to an imbalance between myocardial oxygen supply and/or demand. Type II may be caused by coronary endothelial dysfunction, coronary vasospasm, embolism, arrhythmias, anemia, respiratory failure, hypotension, and shock.[11] Most infarcts occur in the left ventricle; however, right ventricular infarction occurs in approximately one-third of patients with inferior wall infarction.[5] The treatment for a right ventricular infarct is usually fluid therapy. Patients with right ventricular infarctions require cardiac pacing more frequently than those with left ventricular infarcts secondary to conduction defects, which are common.

The severity of the MI is determined by the success or failure of the treatment and by the degree of collateral circulation present at that particular part of the heart muscle. The collateral circulation consists of the alternative routes, or channels, that develop in the myocardium in response to chronic ischemia or regional hypoperfusion. Through this small network of extra vessels, blood flow to the threatened myocardium can be improved.

Assessment

Patient Assessment. Patient assessment includes close observation to identify the classic signs and symptoms of ACS. For men, chest pain is the paramount symptom. It may be severe, crushing, tight, squeezing, or simply a feeling of pressure. It can be precordial, substernal, or in the back, and it can radiate to the arms, neck, or jaw. The skin may be cool, clammy, pale, and diaphoretic; the patient's color may be dusky or ashen; and slight hyperthermia may be present. The patient may be dyspneic and tachypneic and may feel faint or have intermittent loss of sensorium. Nausea and vomiting commonly occur. Hypotension may be present and is often associated with dysrhythmias, particularly ventricular ectopy, bradycardia, tachycardia, or heart block. The type of dysrhythmia present depends on the area of the MI. The patient may be anxious or restless or may exhibit certain behavioral responses, including denial, depression, and a sense of impending doom. For women, chest pain may not be the most obvious symptom.[13] See Box 13.8 and Clinical Alert box.

BOX 13.8 Cardiovascular Disease in Women

Cardiovascular disease is the leading cause of death in women, and more women than men die of heart disease.

Risk Factors

- *Age:* Women are at higher risk at age 55, whereas men are at higher risk at age 45.
- *Family history:* Heart disease in a first-degree relative is considered premature if it occurred before age 65 for women or before age 55 for men. Heart disease in a first-degree female relative is a more potent risk factor than heart disease in a male relative.
- *Hypertension:* The risk of heart failure due to hypertension is greater in women.
- *Diabetes:* Diabetes is a greater risk factor for heart disease in women than in men. Risk for fatal heart disease in diabetic women is 3.5 times higher than in nondiabetic women.
- *Dyslipidemia:* More than half of US women have dyslipidemia, which becomes worse as women age and become menopausal.

- *Smoking:* Women smokers die earlier than men smokers in relation to their nonsmoker counterparts. In addition, the use of oral contraceptives in women smokers increases their risk of acute myocardial infarction.
- *Physical activity:* Women tend to be more sedentary than men.

Symptoms of Ischemia

Women are less likely than men to have chest pain during acute coronary syndrome. Women tend to have less severe symptoms and less specific symptoms, such as dyspnea, nausea, vomiting, diaphoresis, syncope, fatigue, and palpitations.

Treatment of Coronary Artery Disease in Women

Although treatment is the same for men and women, women often receive less optimal medical therapy and lifestyle counseling. Women have higher postoperative morbidity and mortality rates, a poorer quality of life postoperatively, and a higher incidence of depression.

Data from Gulati MM, Merz CNB. Cardiovascular disease in women. In: Zipes DP, Libby P, Bonow RO, et al, eds. *Braundwald's Heart Disease: A Textbook of Cardiovascular Medicine.* 11th ed. Philadelphia, PA: Elsevier; 2019:1767-1779.

Acute Coronary Syndrome in Women

Women are less likely than men to have chest pain in acute coronary syndrome (ACS), and they are more likely to have atypical signs and symptoms such as fatigue, diaphoresis, indigestion, arm or shoulder pain, nausea, and vomiting.

Some individuals have ischemic episodes without knowing it; this is known as a *silent* infarction. Silent infarctions occur with no presenting signs or symptoms and are more common in patients with diabetes secondary to neuropathy. Assessment of a patient experiencing ACS takes all the foregoing signs and symptoms into account during the history and physical examination. Risk factors for ACS are also considered.

Diagnosis

Diagnosis of ACS is based on symptoms, analysis of a 12-lead ECG, and cardiac enzyme values. Typical angina, atypical angina, and noncardiac chest pain are described in Table 13.6.

TABLE 13.6 Chest Pain Differences in Angina

Type of Angina	Characteristic of Chest Pain
Typical angina	Pain or discomfort that is (1) retrosternal, (2) provoked by exercise and/or emotion, and (3) relieved by rest and/or nitroglycerin
Atypical angina	Sharp or knifelike, brought on by respiratory movements or coughing; abdominal pain
Nonanginal (or noncardiac) chest pain	Pain that is reproducible with movement or palpation of the chest wall or arms, constant pain that persists for many hours or brief episodes that last a few seconds or less

From Bonaca MP, Sabatine MS. Approach to the patient with chest pain. In: Zipes DP, Libby P, Bonow RO, et al, eds. *Braunwald's Heart Disease: A Textbook of Cardiovascular Medicine*. Philadelphia, PA: Elsevier; 2019:1059-1068.

Inspect the ECG for ST-segment elevation (>1 mm) in two or more contiguous leads. ST-segment depression ($\geq$0.5 mm) and new-onset left bundle branch block also suggest an AMI. The type of AMI is determined by the particular coronary artery involved and the blood supply to that area (Table 13.7).

Elevated serum cardiac enzyme levels (troponin I and troponin T) are used to confirm the diagnosis of AMI. These tests are ordered immediately when a diagnosis of ACS is suspected and periodically (usually every 6 to 8 hours) during the first 24 hours to assess for increasing levels. Emergency cardiac catheterization may be performed in institutions with interventional cardiology services.

Patient Problems. Problems for the patient with ACS are described in the Plan of Care for the Patient With Acute Coronary Syndrome. In addition, many problems and interventions apply from the Collaborative Plan of Care for the Critically Ill Patient (Chapter 1).

Complications

Complications of AMI include cardiac dysrhythmias, HF, thromboembolism, rupture of a portion of the heart (ventricular wall, interventricular septum, or papillary muscle), pericarditis, infarct extension or recurrence, and cardiogenic shock (Chapter 12). Dysrhythmias, HF, and pericarditis are discussed later in this chapter.

Medical Interventions

Treatment goals for AMI are to establish reperfusion, reduce infarct size, prevent and treat complications, and provide emotional support and education. Medical treatment of AMI is aimed at relieving pain, providing adequate oxygenation to the myocardium, preventing platelet aggregation, and restoring blood flow to the myocardium through thrombolytic therapy or acute interventional therapy (e.g., angioplasty). Hemodynamic monitoring is also used to assess cardiac function and to monitor fluid balance in some patients.

TABLE 13.7 Myocardial Infarction by Site, Electrocardiographic Changes, and Complications

Location of MI	Primary Site of Occlusion	Primary ECG Changes	Complications
Inferior MI	RCA (80%-90%) LCX (10%-20%)	II, III, aV_F	First- and second-degree heart block, right ventricular infarction
Inferolateral MI	LCX	II, III, aV_F, V_5, V_6	Third-degree heart block, left HF, cardiomyopathy, left ventricular rupture
Posterior MI	RCA or LCX	No lead truly looks at the posterior surface. Look for reciprocal changes in V_1 and V_2—tall, broad R waves; ST depression; and tall T waves. Posterior leads V_7, V_8, and V_9 may be recorded and evaluated.	First-, second-, and third-degree heart blocks; HF; bradydysrhythmias
Anterior MI	LAD	V_2-V_4	Third-degree heart block, HF, left bundle branch block
Anterior-septal MI	LAD	V_1-V_3	Second- and third-degree heart block
Lateral MI	LAD or LCX	V_5, V_6, I, aVL	HF
Right ventricular	RCA	V_4R. Right precordial leads V_1R-V_6R may be recorded and evaluated.	Increased RAP, decreased cardiac output, bradydysrhythmias, heart blocks, hypotension, cardiogenic shock

ECG, Electrocardiographic; *HF*, heart failure; *LAD*, left anterior descending coronary artery; *LCX*, left circumflex artery; *MI*, myocardial infarction; *RAP*, right atrial pressure; *RCA*, right coronary artery.

◎ PLAN OF CARE

For the Patient With Acute Coronary Syndrome

Patient Problem

Acute Pain. Risk factors include decreased oxygen supply to the myocardium and reduced circulation.

Desired Outcomes

- Within 30 minutes from the onset of pain, the patient's perception of pain decreases, as documented by a pain scale.
- Objective indicators, such as grimacing and diaphoresis, are absent or decreased.

Assessments/Interventions	Rationales
• Assess location, character, and severity of the pain. Record severity on a subjective 0 (no pain) to 10 (worst pain) scale.	• Establish baseline and monitor trends in pain and response to treatment.
• Assess HR and BP during episodes of chest pain. Be alert to and report significant findings: increased HR and changes in SBP >20 mm Hg from baseline.	• Assess changes that indicate increased myocardial O_2 demands and need for prompt medical intervention.
• Administer humidified O_2 as prescribed.	• Hypoxia is common because of decreased perfusion and creates additional stress to the compromised myocardium.
	• Humidity prevents drying of the oral and nasal mucosa.
• Notify the provider if pain is unrelieved.	• Alternative treatments, or additional dosages of medications, may be needed.
	• Unrelieved pain may indicate the need for additional workup.
• If prescribed or per protocol, increase IV NTG infusion in increments of 10 mcg if pain persists, and monitor SBP. Notify the provider if SBP <90 mm Hg, HR <60 beats/min, or RR <10 breaths/min. Monitor for headache.	• NTG lowers BP.
	• An SBP ≥90 mm Hg prevents worsening ischemia secondary to hypotension.
	• Headache is associated with dilation of cerebral blood vessels.
• As prescribed, add IV morphine sulfate in small increments (2 mg). Monitor HR, RR, and BP.	• Relieve pain.
	• Decrease heart rate, BP, RR, and anxiety.
• Obtain ECG per protocol and monitor cardiac rhythm.	• ECG patterns may reveal ischemia: ST- or T-wave changes, new Q waves, or left bundle branch block.
• Stay with the patient and provide reassurance during periods of pain.	• Reduce anxiety and lessen the angina.
• Maintain the patient in a recumbent position with the HOB elevated no higher than 30 degrees during angina and NTG administration.	• Minimize the potential for headache or hypotension by enabling better blood return to the heart and head.
• Emphasize to the patient the importance of immediately reporting chest pain.	• Facilitate prompt treatment to decrease morbidity and mortality.
• Instruct the patient to avoid activities and factors known to cause stress.	• Stress may precipitate angina.
• Implement complementary and alternative strategies:	• Reduction in stress and anxiety may reduce pain.
• Relaxation techniques	
• Soothing music	
• Biofeedback, meditation	
• Yoga	
• Administer beta-blockers as prescribed. Use with caution in asthmatics because medication antagonizes pulmonary vasodilation.	• Reduce workload of the heart and myocardial O_2 demand, improving myocardial oxygenation.
• Instruct patient to rise slowly from a recumbent or seated position.	• Avoid orthostatic hypotension.
• Administer long-acting nitrates (isosorbide preparations) and/or topical nitrates as prescribed.	• Prevent future angina attacks, lower BP, and decrease O_2 demand.
• Administer ACE inhibitor as prescribed.	• Downregulate the RAAS and reduce BP.
	• Improve long-term survival.
• Administer calcium channel blockers as prescribed.	• Decrease coronary artery vasospasm, dilate coronary arteries, and increase blood flow to the myocardium.
• Administer thrombolytic agents, including aspirin as prescribed.	• Reduce platelet aggregation
• Observe bleeding precautions and review with patient.	• Medications increase the risk for bleeding.
• Administer antihyperlipidemic agents and triglyceride-lowering agents as prescribed.	• Reduce total cholesterol, LDH, and triglyceride levels.
• Administer stool softeners as prescribed.	• Straining at stool or constipation can increase myocardial demand.

ACE, Angiotensin-converting enzyme; *BP,* blood pressure; *ECG,* electrocardiogram; *HOB,* head of bed; *HR,* heart rate; *LDH,* lactate dehydrogenase; *NTG,* nitroglycerin; *O_2,* oxygen; *RAAS,* renin-angiotensin-aldosterone system; *SBP,* systolic blood pressure.
Adapted from Swearingen PL, Wright JD. *All-in-One Nursing Care Planning Resource.* 5th ed. St. Louis, MO: Elsevier; 2019.

Pain Relief. The initial pain of AMI is treated with morphine sulfate administered by the IV route. The dose is 2 to 4 mg IV push over 5 minutes. Observe the patient for hypotension and respiratory depression (see Table 13.5).

Nitrates. NTG may be given to reduce the ischemic pain of AMI. NTG is a vasodilator and increases coronary perfusion. It is usually started at doses of 5 to 10 mcg/min IV and titrated to a total dose of 50 to 200 mcg/min until chest pain is absent, pulmonary artery occlusion pressure decreases, and/or systolic BP decreases. Do not give nitrates to patients who have used phosphodiesterase inhibitors within the last 24 to 48 hours,[3] and administer cautiously to patients with inferior or right ventricular infarctions to avoid profound hypotension.

Oxygen. Oxygen has been traditionally administered via nasal cannula at 4 to 6 L/min to treat and prevent hypoxemia in AMI and maintain oxygen saturation at greater than 90%. However, recent guidelines suggest that routine use of supplemental oxygen may not be necessary in patients with uncomplicated ACS without signs of HF or hypoxemia.[5]

Antidysrhythmics. Dysrhythmias are common after AMI. Antidysrhythmic medications are administered when the heart's natural pacemaker develops an abnormal rate or rhythm (see Chapter 8).

Prevention of Platelet Aggregation. Alterations in platelet function contribute to occlusion of the coronary arteries. Aspirin (325 mg) is given immediately to all patients with suspected ACS. Aspirin blocks synthesis of thromboxane A_2, thus inhibiting aggregation of platelets. In addition, a thienopyridine, such as clopidogrel (Plavix), prasugrel (Effient), or ticagrelor (Brilinta), or a glycoprotein (Gp) IIb/IIIa inhibitor may be added.[3] Heparin is used with other antiplatelet agents.

Percutaneous Coronary Intervention. Primary percutaneous coronary intervention (PCI) at a PCI-capable hospital should be performed as part of the management of AMI with ST-segment elevation (STEMI) within 12 hours after the initiation of ischemic symptoms. PCI should be performed within 120 minutes after first medical contact with either emergency medical service personnel or emergency department staff. Primary PCI is more effective than thrombolysis in opening acutely occluded arteries when it can be rapidly performed by experienced interventional cardiologists. Placement of bare metal stents or drug-eluting stents is common during PCI. If patients come to a facility without PCI capabilities, they should be transferred to a PCI-capable facility to receive a PCI within 120 minutes after first medical contact or triaged to receive fibrinolytic therapy at the receiving facility.[5]

Fibrinolytic Therapy. The goals of fibrinolytic therapy are to dissolve the clot that is occluding the coronary artery and to increase blood flow to the myocardium. For treatment to be considered, the patient must have been symptomatic for less than 12 hours. However, the best outcomes occur in patients who are treated within 1 to 2 hours of the onset of symptoms.[5] Table 13.8 lists common thrombolytic agents. Important considerations in the use of thrombolytics include the following:
- Fibrinolysis reduces mortality and salvages myocardium in STEMI or bundle-branch involvement in AMI.
- Fibrinolysis is not effective in the treatment of unstable angina or AMI without ST-segment elevation (NSTEMI).
- Thrombolysis should be instituted within 30 to 60 minutes of arrival. The sooner the treatment is initiated, the better the outcome.
- The worst possible complication of fibrinolysis is intracranial hemorrhage.
- Bleeding from puncture sites commonly occurs.

Nursing care of the patient includes rapid identification of whether the patient is a suitable candidate for IV thrombolytics, screening for contraindications, and prompt administration of thrombolytics. Next, secure three vascular access lines and obtain necessary laboratory data. Initiate cardiac monitoring and

---

TABLE 13.8 PHARMACOLOGY

Thrombolytics

Medication	Dose/Route	Half-Life
Alteplase (tissue plasminogen activator [t-PA])	*3-h infusion:* For adults weighing ≥65 kg, 100-mg dose; administer 60 mg over the first hour (6-10 mg as IV bolus over 1-2 min, followed by infusion of remaining dose), 20 mg over second hour, and 20 over third hour For adults weighing <65 kg, 1.25 mg/kg dose; administer 60% first hour (0.075 mg/kg as an IV bolus, followed by infusion of remaining dose), 20% over second hour, and 20% over third hour *Accelerated 90-min infusion:* For adults weighing >67 kg, 100-mg dose; administer 15-mg bolus IV over 1-2 min, followed by infusion of 50 mg over the first 30 min and 35 mg over next 60 min For adults weighing ≤67 kg, 15-mg bolus IV over 1-2 min, followed by infusion of 0.75 mg/kg over the first 30 min (not to exceed 50 mg) and 0.50 mg/kg over next 60 min (not to exceed 35 mg)	4-5 min
Reteplase (r-PA)	10 units IV bolus; repeat 10-unit dose in 30 min; administer over 2 min. Give through a dedicated IV line. Do not give repeat bolus if serious bleeding occurs after first IV bolus	13-16 min
Tenecteplase (TNK)	Total dose 30-50 mg, based on weight (see package insert) given IV over 5 secs	20-24 min
Streptokinase (SK)	1.5 million units IV infusion over 60 min	23 min

Data from Skidmore-Roth L. *Mosby's 2019 Nursing Drug Reference.* 32nd ed. St. Louis, MO: Elsevier; 2019; Urden LD, Stacy KM, Lough ME. *Critical Care Nursing Diagnosis and Management.* 8th ed. St. Louis, MO: Elsevier; 2018.

document rhythm before starting the infusion, at routine intervals throughout the infusion, and at the end of the infusion. Finally, monitor the patient for complications, including reperfusion dysrhythmias (premature ventricular contractions, sinus bradycardia, accelerated idioventricular rhythm, or ventricular tachycardia [VT]), oozing at venipuncture sites, gingival bleeding, reocclusion or reinfarction, and symptoms of hemorrhagic stroke.

Medications. Several medications may be ordered for the patient with ACS. Patients whose chest pain symptoms are suggestive of serious illness need immediate assessment in a monitored unit and early therapy, including an IV line, oxygen, aspirin, NTG, and morphine. Early therapy consists of aspirin, heparin or low-molecular-weight heparin, nitrates, beta-blockers, clopidogrel, bivalirudin, and fondaparinux.

Nitrates. Nitrates are vasodilators that reduce pain, increase venous capacitance, and reduce platelet adhesion and aggregation. Sublingual NTG is often given in the emergency department. IV NTG is effective for relieving ischemia (see Table 13.5).

Beta-blockers. Beta-blockers are used to decrease heart rate, BP, and myocardial oxygen consumption. Morbidity and mortality after AMI have been reduced by the use of beta-blockers. Beta-blockers should be started within 24 hours after ACS begins unless otherwise contraindicated. Carefully assess the patient for hypotension and bradycardia.

Angiotensin-converting enzyme inhibitors. ACS can cause the area of ventricular damage to change shape or *remodel*. The ventricle becomes thinner and balloons out, thus reducing contractility. Cardiac tissue surrounding the area of infarction undergoes changes that can be categorized as (1) myocardial stunning (a temporary loss of contractile function that persists for hours to days after perfusion has been restored); (2) hibernating myocardium (tissue that is persistently ischemic and undergoes metabolic adaptation to prolong myocyte survival until perfusion can be restored); and (3) myocardial remodeling (a process mediated by angiotensin II, aldosterone, catecholamines, adenosine, and inflammatory cytokines that causes myocyte hypertrophy and loss of contractile function in areas of the heart distant from the site of infarction). Angiotensin-converting enzyme inhibitors (ACEIs) should be started within 24 hours to reduce the incidence of ventricular remodeling. The medications may be discontinued if the patient exhibits no signs of ventricular dysfunction (see Table 13.5). ACEIs should be prescribed for patients with unstable angina; NSTEMI; STEMI with an LVEF of 40% or less; or a history of hypertension, diabetes, or chronic kidney disease, unless contraindicated. The most common side effect with ACEIs is cough, which is chronic and nonproductive. If side effects occur with an ACEI, angiotensin II receptor blockers (ARBs) should be initiated.[3]

Novel Stem Cell Treatment. Autologous bone marrow stem cell therapy is being used to prevent ventricular remodeling and improve cardiac function. The stem cells are implanted into mapped areas of dysfunctional and viable myocardium. Research has shown improvement in LVEF in some trials, but more research is needed.[24]

❓ CRITICAL REASONING ACTIVITY

You are taking care of a 58-year-old male patient who was readmitted to the unit after a myocardial infarction (MI) because of recurrent chest pain, shortness of breath, and the need for IV nitroglycerin. Prioritize your actions at this time. What assessment findings regarding MI would concern you? What pertinent information from the patient's history would you want to obtain? What diagnostic tests do you anticipate?

Patient Outcomes

Patient outcomes are generalized to encompass the wide spectrum of patients who have experienced an AMI, uncomplicated or complicated, and have required medical or surgical intervention. Outcomes include adequate cardiac output, ability to tolerate progressive activity, verbalization of relief of pain and fear, and demonstration of positive coping mechanisms.

INTERVENTIONAL CARDIOLOGY

Several interventions are used to treat ACS. Primary PCI is recommended for treatment of acute STEMI. The goal is reperfusion of the affected area to reduce ischemia and to prevent further damage to the myocardium. PCI includes percutaneous transluminal coronary angioplasty (PTCA), rotational atherectomy, laser atherectomy, thrombectomy, and intracoronary stenting. An early, invasive PCI procedure is indicated for patients with unstable angina or NSTEMI who are hemodynamically unstable, continue to have angina, or have an elevated risk for clinical events. For the purpose of this book, only PTCA and stenting are discussed. The postprocedure care for all patients who undergo PCI consists of the same interventions.

Percutaneous Transluminal Coronary Angioplasty

The purpose of PTCA is to compress intracoronary plaque in order to increase blood flow to the myocardium. It is usually the treatment of choice for patients with uncompromised collateral flow, noncalcified lesions, and lesions not present at bifurcations of vessels. PTCA is performed in the cardiac catheterization laboratory. A balloon catheter is inserted into the femoral, brachial, or radial artery, threaded into the occluded coronary artery, and advanced with the use of a guidewire across the lesion. The balloon is inflated under pressure one or several times to compress the lesion (Fig. 13.11). The optimal goal after PTCA is open coronary arteries (Fig. 13.12). PTCA is rarely done without stenting, but it is usually done to dilate the artery before placement of a bare metal or drug-eluting stent or in the instance of very small vessels.[22]

Complications. Complications of PTCA are commonly due to the angiography and include hematoma at the catheter insertion site, MI, stroke or TIA, pseudoaneurysm, dysrhythmias, infection, acute kidney injury, and coronary artery dissection. Mortality rates are less than 1% for PTCA.[22]

Coronary Stent

Coronary stents are tubes that are implanted at the site of stenosis to widen the arterial lumen by squeezing atherosclerotic

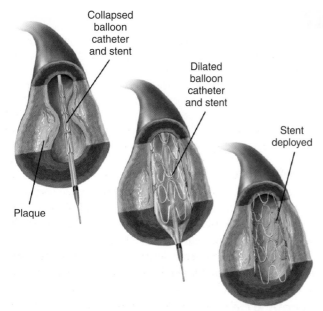

Fig. 13.11 Cardiac stent. (From Good VS, Kirkwood PL. *Advanced Critical Care Nursing.* 2nd ed. St. Louis, MO: Elsevier; 2018.)

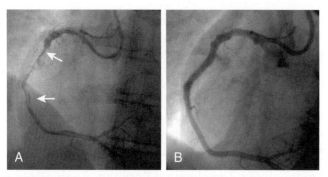

Fig. 13.12 A, Thrombotic occlusion of the right coronary artery *(arrows).* **B,** Right coronary artery is opened and blood flow is restored after angioplasty and placement of a 4-mm stent. (From Lewis SL, Dirkson L, Heitkemper M, Bucher L. *Medical-Surgical Nursing: Assessment and Management of Clinical Problems.* 9th ed. St. Louis, MO: Mosby; 2014.)

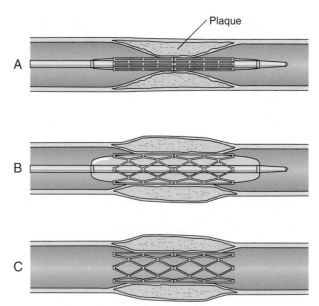

Fig. 13.13 Placement of a coronary artery stent. **A,** The stent is positioned at the site of the lesion. **B,** The balloon is inflated, expanding the stent. The balloon is then deflated and removed. **C,** The implanted stent is left in place. (From Lewis SL, Dirkson L, Heitkemper M, Bucher L. *Medical-Surgical Nursing: Assessment and Management of Clinical Problems.* 9th ed. St. Louis, MO: Mosby; 2014.)

plaque against the artery's walls (as does PTCA). The stent also keeps the lumen open by providing structural support. Approximately 90% of PCI procedures involve stent placement.[22] Stent designs differ, but most designs have springs, slots, or mesh tubes; some resemble the spiral bindings used in notebooks. Stents are tightly wrapped around a balloon catheter, which is inflated to implant the stent.

The procedure for placing a stent is similar to the procedure in PTCA. The patient first undergoes cardiac angiography for identification of occlusions in coronary arteries. Next, the balloon catheter bearing the stent is inserted into the coronary artery, and the stent is positioned at the desired site. The balloon is inflated, thereby expanding the stent, which squeezes the atherosclerotic plaque and intimal flaps against the vessel wall. After the balloon is deflated and removed, the stent remains, holding the plaque and other matter in place and providing structural support to keep the artery from collapsing (Fig. 13.13).

Aggressive anticoagulation therapy before, during, and after the stent procedure is necessary to prevent coagulation. Before sheath removal, monitor peripheral perfusion because the sheath may occlude the femoral artery. Monitor peripheral pulses, skin color, and temperature, and inspect the insertion site for any oozing or bleeding. After sheath removal, maintain hemostasis with manual pressure, a femoral compression device, or an arterial puncture sealing device.

Pain management and proper hydration aid in recovery. Retroperitoneal bleeding or impaired perfusion may occur after sheath removal. Restenosis can occur as a result of neointimal (new intimal cell) growth resulting from the body's natural defense when the inner intimal lining is injured, even slightly, as happens with stent placement. Gp IIb/IIIa inhibitors are used after stent placement to prevent acute reocclusion through prevention of platelet aggregation. With the use of second-generation stents and dual antiplatelet therapy, restenosis rates have declined to approximately 1% in the first year after stenting.[22]

After a stent procedure, a patient must take antiplatelet agents such as aspirin and clopidogrel, prasugrel, or ticagrelor. Aspirin, 81 mg, is used indefinitely. Oral clopidogrel, 75 mg/day, is commonly added to aspirin for 3 to 12 months; it may be used for as little as 30 days or given indefinitely depending on the type and location of the stent.

Therapies in intracoronary stenting have advanced, including drug-eluting stents that are completely bioabsorbable. Drug-eluting stents have the benefit of being coated with an antiproliferative medication that reduces in-stent thrombosis. The medication is released slowly over time to reduce the risk of neointimal growth.[22]

❓ CRITICAL REASONING ACTIVITY

You are caring for a 63-year-old woman who has just returned to the cardiac care unit after placement of a drug-eluting stent to the right coronary artery. Her proximal right coronary artery had a 90% occlusive lesion. She has an occlusive device (TR Band) in place to the right radial artery. She is receiving IV nitroglycerin and eptifibatide (Integrilin).

1. What type of dysrhythmia would you anticipate if her right coronary artery were to reocclude?
2. Prioritize your actions on her arrival.
3. What type of assessment would you perform regarding the right radial TR Band?

Surgical Revascularization

Surgical approaches used for revascularization include coronary revascularization by coronary artery bypass grafting (CABG), minimally invasive CABG, and transmyocardial revascularization (TMR).

❓ CRITICAL REASONING ACTIVITY

Many patients now come into the hospital on the same day that cardiac surgery is performed. Discuss methods for teaching patients effectively given this situation.

Coronary Artery Bypass Grafting. CABG is a surgical procedure in which the ischemic areas of the myocardium are revascularized by implantation of a graft from the internal mammary artery (IMA) or the coronary occlusion is bypassed with a graft from the saphenous vein or the radial artery. The indications for CABG are chronic stable angina that is refractory to other therapies, significant left main coronary artery occlusion (>50%), triple-vessel CAD, unstable angina pectoris, left ventricular failure, lesions not amenable to PCI, and PCI failure.

CABG is performed in the operating room while the patient receives general anesthesia and is intubated. One approach is to make a midsternal, longitudinal incision into the chest cavity. Surgery is done either with cardiopulmonary bypass or without it (i.e., *off-pump*). During cardiopulmonary bypass, blood is pumped through an oxygenator, or heart-lung machine, to receive oxygen. Cardioplegia solution is used to stop the heart so that the surgery can be performed.

The coronary arteries are visualized, and a segment of the saphenous vein is grafted or anastomosed to the distal end of the affected vessel, with the proximal end of the graft vessel anastomosed to the aorta (Fig. 13.14). The IMA is often used

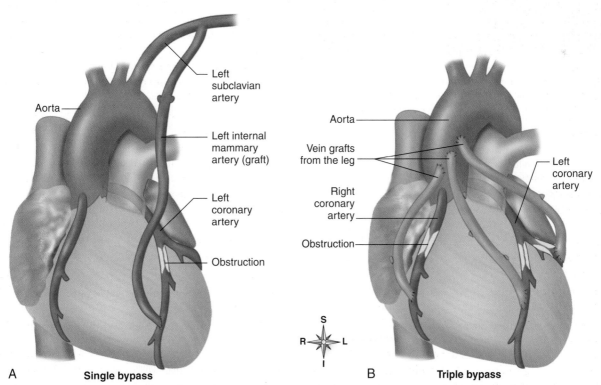

Fig. 13.14 Options for coronary artery bypass surgery. **A,** Internal mammary artery is "rerouted" to bypass the obstruction. **B,** Vessels are "harvested" from other parts of the body and used to construct detours around blocked coronary arteries. Artificial vessels can also be used. (From Patton KT, Thibodeau GA. *Human Body in Health and Disease.* 6th ed. St. Louis, MO: Elsevier; 2018.)

to create an artery-to-artery graft. IMA revascularization has better long-term patency than saphenous vein grafts. It is the preferred graft for lesions of the left anterior descending coronary artery.

Once grafting is done, the cardiopulmonary bypass (if used) is progressively discontinued, chest and mediastinal tubes are inserted, and the chest is closed. Box 13.9 provides information related to chest and mediastinal tubes.

Minimally Invasive Coronary Artery Surgery. Minimally invasive cardiac surgery–coronary artery bypass grafting (MICS CABG) has been evaluated as an alternative to the standard methods for CABG. This alternative allows for a thoracotomy approach instead of a sternotomy, resulting in shorter hospital stay and earlier recovery postoperatively. It is done without cardiopulmonary bypass. However, no clinical trials have shown improvement in quality of life with MICS CABG. The Minimally Invasive Coronary Surgery Compared to Sternotomy Coronary Artery Bypass Grafting Randomized Controlled (MIST) trial is underway to evaluate the quality of life and postoperative recovery in patients with MICS CABG compared to those with traditional CABG with sternotomy.[14]

Off-pump coronary artery bypass (OPCAB) is not as widely used as it has been in the past due to several studies that showed no mortality benefit, though there were decreases shown in bleeding and the need for transfusions. It is also associated with less renal and respiratory failure; however, there is a lower incidence of complete revascularization and a lower graft patency rate. Patients with severe ventricular dysfunction, left main disease, ongoing ischemia, and pulmonary hypertension are at higher risk for poor outcomes and more likely to have to be converted to on-pump. Therefore candidates for OPCAB have to be chosen carefully, and there is a higher learning curve for surgeons training to perform OPCAB.[27]

Robotically assisted cardiac surgery is another type of minimally invasive surgery. The cardiac surgeons use a computer console to control surgical instruments on thin robotic arms. Robotic coronary artery bypass grafting can be done on-pump or off-pump for single-vessel or multivessel disease.[6]

Management After Cardiac Surgery. Patients are usually admitted directly to the critical care unit after cardiac surgery. The patient often has a pulmonary artery catheter, arterial

---

BOX 13.9   Key Points for Maintaining Pleural Chest and Mediastinal Tubes

Definitions

- *Pleural chest tube:* The tube is inserted into the pleural space to maintain the normal negative pressure and to facilitate respiration. It is inserted after cardiac surgery if the pleural space has been opened. It is also inserted as treatment for pneumothorax or hemothorax.
- *Mediastinal tube:* The tube is inserted into the mediastinal space to provide drainage after cardiac surgery.
- *Drainage system:* A water-seal system assists in maintaining negative pressures (chest tube). Some devices are designed to function without water (dry). Suction (up to 20 cm H_2O) is often applied to facilitate drainage.
- *Autotransfusion:* This is defined as reinfusion of autologous drainage from the system back to the patient.

Baseline Assessment

- Ensure that all connections are tight: insertion site to the chest drainage system and suction control chamber to the suction unit.
- Confirm that the dressing over the insertion site is dry and intact.
- Palpate for subcutaneous crepitus around the insertion site and chest wall.
- Auscultate breath sounds bilaterally.
- Observe the color and consistency of fluid in the collecting tubing (a more accurate assessment than fluid in the drainage system); mark the fluid level on the drainage system.
- Assess the drainage system for proper functioning (read instructions for the device being used).
- Check the water in the water-seal chamber; the water level should fluctuate with respirations in chest tubes (not in mediastinal tubes).
- Check suction control and be sure that suction is on, if ordered.
- Check for intermittent bubbling in the water-seal chamber; it indicates an air leak from the pleural space (pleural tube).

Maintaining the Chest Drainage System

- Keep the tubing coiled on the bed near the patient.
- Record drainage in the medical record according to protocol; notify the provider of excessive drainage. (The volume to report is determined by unit parameters or written order; it varies depending on the purpose of the tube and the time since insertion.)
- Change the dressing according to unit protocol.
- Splint the insertion site to facilitate coughing and deep breathing.
- Ensure that drainage flows into the drainage system by facilitating gravity drainage; milking or stripping of tubes is not recommended because these procedures generate high negative pressures in the system.
- If the patient is transported (or ambulated), disconnect the drainage system from suction and keep it upright below the level of the chest. Do not clamp the tube.
- Obtain chest radiographic studies immediately after insertion and usually daily thereafter.

Assisting With Removal

- Chest and mediastinal tubes are usually removed by the provider.
- Ensure adequate pain medication before removal.
- Apply an occlusive dressing to the site after removal.
- A chest radiographic study is usually done after removal.

Autotransfusion

- An autotransfusion collection system is attached to the chest drainage device.
- Anticoagulants may be ordered to be added to the autotransfusion system (citrate-phosphate-dextrose, acid-phosphate-dextrose, or heparin); these are not usually necessary with mediastinal drainage.
- Reinfuse drainage within the time frame specified by unit policy. It is recommended that reinfusion begin within 6 hours after initiation of the collection and reinfused to the patient within a 4-hour period.
- Evacuate air from the autotransfusion bag; air embolism may occur unless all air is removed.
- Attach a microaggregate filter and infuse via gravity or a pressure bag.

BOX 13.10 Nursing Interventions After Cardiac Surgery

- Monitor for hypotension; administer fluids and vasopressors as ordered or based on protocol.
- Assess for hypovolemia; monitor and trend output from the pleural chest and mediastinal tubes and urine output.
- Monitor hemodynamic pressures, SvO$_2$, stroke index, cardiac index, PAOP, and RAP; treat the patient per protocol.
- Rewarm the patient gradually (if applicable).
- Monitor and treat fluid volume status and electrolytes, hemoglobin, hematocrit, renal function, and coagulation studies.
- Provide pain relief.
- Monitor for complications: intraoperative AMI, dysrhythmias, heart failure, cardiac tamponade, thromboembolism, impaired renal function, pneumonia, pneumothorax, pleural effusion, cerebral ischemia, and stroke.
- Wean from mechanical ventilation per protocol; extubate; promote pulmonary hygiene every 1 to 2 hours while the patient is awake.
- Assess wounds and provide incisional care per hospital protocol.
- Gradually increase the patient's activity.
- Provide emotional support to the patient and family.

AMI, Acute myocardial infarction; *PAOP*, pulmonary artery occlusion pressure; *RAP*, right atrial pressure; *SvO$_2$*, mixed venous oxygen saturation.

catheter, peripheral IV lines, temporary pacemaker wires, pleural chest tubes, mediastinal tubes, and an indwelling urinary catheter. The patient is usually mechanically ventilated in the immediate postoperative period. Assess the patient often and provide rapid intervention to help the patient recover from anesthesia and to prevent complications. The nurse-to-patient ratio is often 1:1 during the first few hours after surgery or until the patient is extubated. Nursing care for these patients is summarized in Box 13.10.

Complications of Cardiac Surgery. Closely monitor patients postoperatively for complications such as dysrhythmias (atrial fibrillation, atrial flutter, VT, ventricular fibrillation), AMI, shock, pericarditis, pericardial effusion, and cardiac tamponade. The critical care nurse caring for a patient who has just undergone CABG must have quick critical thinking skills and the ability to assess the whole picture while prioritizing interventions that must be performed.

MECHANICAL THERAPIES

Transmyocardial Laser Revascularization

In transmyocardial laser revascularization (TMLR), a high-energy laser creates channels from the epicardial surface into the ischemic myocardium of the left ventricular. The purpose of TMLR is to increase perfusion directly to the heart muscle. It is performed on patients in conjunction with CABG or for those who are poor candidates for CABG or PCI and whose symptoms are refractory to medical treatment. To do this procedure, a surgeon makes an incision on the left side of the chest and inserts a laser device into the chest cavity. With the laser, the surgeon makes 1-mm channels through the heart's left ventricle in between heartbeats. TMLR does not replace CABG or

angioplasty as a common method of treating CAD. TMLR may be used for patients who are high-risk candidates for a second bypass or angioplasty, such as patients whose blockages are too diffuse to be treated with bypass alone.[19]

Enhanced External Counterpulsation

Enhanced external counterpulsation (EECP) is a treatment for angina that may be used when the patient is not a candidate for bypass surgery or PCI. Cuffs are wrapped around the patient's legs to increase arterial BP and retrograde aortic blood flow during diastole. Sequential pressure, using compressed air, is applied from the lower legs to the upper thighs. These treatments take place over the course of a few hours per day for several weeks. There are no definitive data showing that EECP reduces ischemia; however, treatment reduces angina and improves quality of life.[23]

CARDIAC DYSRHYTHMIAS

Cardiac dysrhythmias (Chapter 8) have many causes, such as CAD, AMI, electrolyte imbalances, and HF. Emergency treatment of dysrhythmias includes medications, transcutaneous pacemakers, and cardioversion and defibrillation (Chapter 11). Other medication given to manage dysrhythmias are shown in Table 13.9. Additional surgical and electrical treatments are discussed in the following sections.

Radiofrequency Catheter Ablation

Radiofrequency catheter ablation is a method that is used to treat dysrhythmias when medications, cardioversion, or both are not effective or not indicated. The objective of catheter ablation is to permanently interrupt electrical conduction or activity in a region of arrhythmogenic cardiac tissue. Indications for radiofrequency catheter ablation include the presence of dysrhythmias such as VT, atrial fibrillation, atrial flutter, and AV nodal reentry tachycardia. The most predominant group are those patients with symptomatic paroxysmal atrial fibrillation.

Radiofrequency ablation is performed percutaneously. The procedure begins with a diagnostic electrophysiology study to map the areas to be ablated. A catheter with an electrode is positioned at the accessory (abnormal) pathway, and mild, painless radiofrequency energy (similar to microwave heat) is transmitted to the pathway, causing coagulation and necrosis in the conduction fibers without destroying the surrounding tissue. This stops the area from conducting the extra impulses that cause the tachycardia. After each ablation attempt, the patient is retested until there is no recurrence of the tachycardic rhythm.

Current guidelines report that for patients with atrial fibrillation (AF) and heart failure with reduced ejection fraction (HFrEF), catheter ablation may be superior to pharmacological management in quality of life, functional status, and improved ejection fraction (EF). However, another randomized control trial showed that ablation was not superior to medication therapy in outcomes such as death, stroke, bleeding, or cardiac arrest.[16]

TABLE 13.9 PHARMACOLOGY

Medications Used to Treat Dysrhythmias

Medication	Actions/Use	Dose/Route	Side Effects	Nursing Implications
Diltiazem (Cardizem)	Inhibits calcium ion influx into vascular smooth muscle and myocardium; used in atrial fibrillation/flutter, SVT	*IV:* 0.25 mg/kg actual body weight over 2 min; may repeat in 15 min at dose of 0.35 mg/kg actual body weight *Infusion:* 5-15 mg/h × 24 h	Hypotension, edema, dizziness, bradycardia	Often used in conjunction with digoxin for rate control. Not used in heart failure. Observe for dysrhythmias.
Amiodarone (Cordarone)	Prolongs action potential phase 3; used for atrial fibrillation/flutter, SVT, ventricular dysrhythmias	*IV:* 150 mg IV over 10 min (15 mg/min). Follow with infusion of 360 mg over next 6 h at 1 mg/min; maintenance infusion of 540 mg over remaining 18 h (0.5 mg/min) *PO:* For life-threatening dysrhythmias, administer loading dose of 800-1600 mg/day for 1-3 wk; decrease dose to 600-800 mg/day for 1 mo, then decrease to lowest therapeutic dose, usually 400 mg/day	Bradycardia, complete atrioventricular block, hypotension Multiple side effects (thyroid, pulmonary, hepatic, neurological, dermatological)	Has a long half-life. Monitor cardiac rhythm. Obtain baseline pulmonary and liver function tests.
Flecainide (Tambocor)	Decreases conduction in all parts of the heart; stabilizes cardiac membrane; used for ventricular dysrhythmias	*PO:* 50-100 mg q 12 h; increase as needed, not to exceed 400 mg/day	Hypotension, bradycardia, heart block, blurred vision, respiratory depression	Interacts with many other medications; check medication guide. Monitor cardiac rhythm. Monitor intake and output. Assess electrolytes. Assess for CNS symptoms.
Sotalol (Betapace)	Nonselective beta-blocker; used for ventricular dysrhythmias	*PO:* 80 mg bid; increase to 240-320 mg/day	Hematologic disorders, bronchospasm	Monitor BP and heart rate. Check baseline liver and renal function. Monitor hydration. Watch for QT prolongation; requires continuous cardiac monitoring at the initiation of therapy. Teach patient not to decrease medication abruptly.
Ibutilide (Corvert)	Prolongs duration of action potential and refractory period; used for atrial fibrillation/flutter	*IV:* 1 mg IV push over 10 min; may repeat after 10 min	Hypotension, bradycardia, sinus arrest, QT prolongation, torsades de pointes, ventricular tachycardia	Monitor cardiac rhythm. Assess for CNS symptoms. Use is usually restricted to electrophysiology personnel.
Propafenone (Rythmol)	Stabilizes cardiac membranes; slows conduction velocity; used for ventricular dysrhythmias	*PO:* 150 mg q 8 h; 450-900 mg/day	Ventricular dysrhythmias, heart failure, dizziness, nausea/vomiting, altered taste	Monitor cardiac rhythm. Use in patients without structural heart disease.

bid, Twice daily; *BP,* blood pressure; *CNS,* central nervous system; *PO,* orally; *q,* every; *SVT,* supraventricular tachycardia.
From Skidmore-Roth L. *Mosby's 2019 Nursing Drug Reference.* 32nd ed. St. Louis, MO: Elsevier; 2019.

Pacemakers

Temporary pacemakers are used to treat patients urgently who are waiting for a permanent pacemaker placement or to treat transient bradydysrhythmias. Temporary pacemakers include external (transcutaneous) and transvenous types. External pacing requires the attachment of large electrodes to the chest (see Chapter 11). This type of pacing is quite uncomfortable for the patient because of the current of electricity that is required to pace the heart; therefore it is used only on an emergency basis. In transvenous pacing, a wire is passed through the venous system into the heart and connected to an external pulse generator. This type is more comfortable but is associated with multiple complications, including ventricular dysrhythmias, cardiac tamponade, infection, and venous thrombosis.[20]

Permanent pacemakers are used to treat conduction disturbances of the heart. Guidelines for the treatment of patients with bradycardia and conduction delays were most recently updated in 2018. The indications include sinus node dysfunction, AV block, neurocardiogenic syncope, and some

TABLE 13.10 The NASPE/BPEG Generic (NBG) Pacemaker Code

Position:	I	II	III	IV	V
Category:	Chamber(s) Paced	Chamber(s) Sensed	Response to Sensing	Rate Modulation	Multisite Pacing
	O = None	**O** = None	**O** = None	**O** = None	**O** = None
	A = Atrium	**A** = Atrium	**T** = Triggered	**R** = Rate modulation	**A** = Atrium
	V = Ventricle	**V** = Ventricle	**I** = Inhibited		**V** = Ventricle
	D = Dual (A + V)	**D** = Dual (A + V)	**D** = Dual (T + I)		**D** = Dual (A + V)
Manufacturer's Designation:	**S** = Single (A or V)	**S** = Single (A or V)			

BPEG, British Pacing and Electrophysiology Group (currently known as the Heart Rhythm Society); *NASPE,* North American Society of Pacing and Electrophysiology.
From Bernstein AD, Daubert J-C, Fletcher RD, et al. The revised NASPE/BPEG generic code for antibradycardia, adaptive-rate, and multisite pacing. *J Pacing Clin Electrophysiol.* 2002;25:260–264.

tachycardias (i.e., tachycardia-bradycardia syndrome).[20] Biventricular pacemakers are used to treat HF and are discussed later, along with implantable cardioverter-defibrillators. Pacemakers are inserted in the operating room, cardiac catheterization laboratory, or electrophysiology laboratory, depending on the facility. The patient may require atrial and/or ventricular pacing. Leads are inserted through the venous system and into the right atrium and/or right ventricle. A pulse generator is attached to the leads and implanted under the skin, usually on the left side of the chest. Pacemakers are powered by lithium batteries that last approximately 7 to 10 years, at which point a new pulse generator is implanted and attached to the existing functioning leads.

Pacemakers are referred to by a lettered code used to describe their basic function. This code has been modified by the North American Society of Pacing and Electrophysiology and the British Pacing and Electrophysiology Group, currently known as the Heart Rhythm Society. The code uses three or five letters to define the chamber paced, chamber sensed, response to pacing, rate responsiveness (if rate response is being used), and multisite pacing (Table 13.10).

Cardiac resynchronization therapy (CRT) is permanent pacing with an additional lead placed in the left ventricle. It is indicated for patients with HF who have a widened QRS complex and an LVEF of 35% or less and have remained symptomatic despite maximum medical therapy.[21] CRT involves biventricular pacing to synchronize contractions of both ventricles. This improves symptoms of HF, decreases mortality, and decreases hospital readmissions. It can be implanted as a pacemaker device or, as is more common, in combination with a defibrillator.

Defibrillators

Implantable cardioverter-defibrillators (ICDs) are placed in patients for primary or secondary prevention of potentially lethal dysrhythmias. In primary prevention, they are indicated for patients who are at risk for sudden cardiac death, such as patients with HF, patients who have genetic mutations that put them at risk for ventricular dysrhythmias, and those who have certain congenital and structural heart diseases. In secondary prevention, ICDs are implanted in patients who have survived cardiac arrest or sustained VT. Current indications for ICD

therapy are listed in Box 13.11. ICDs detect tachydysrhythmias and, when necessary, deliver a shock to the heart to stop the abnormal heart rhythm.

ICDs are implanted in the same manner as pacemakers by electrophysiologists (cardiologists who specialize in cardiac rhythms). All ICDs are developed to include pacemaker capabilities in the rare instance when the patient needs backup pacing after receiving an ICD shock.

Pacemaker and ICD functions are periodically checked in the office and at home using telemonitoring. These checks help to ensure proper functioning of the device and to determine when the battery needs to be replaced. Instruct the patient to carry a wallet identification card at all times. Box 13.12 lists patient and family teaching points. Although newer devices are MRI compatible, patients who have older devices are restricted from undergoing an MRI.

BOX 13.11 Class I Indications for an Implantable Cardioverter-Defibrillator

- Cardiac arrest resulting from VT or VF not produced by a transient or reversible cause or in the event of acute MI when revascularization cannot be done
- Spontaneous sustained VT in association with structural heart disease
- Syncope of undetermined origin with clinically relevant, hemodynamically significant sustained VT or VF induced during electrophysiological study
- Nonsustained VT in patients with coronary artery disease, prior MI, left ventricular dysfunction, and sustained VT or inducible VF during electrophysiological study
- Patients with LVEF of 30% or less at least 40 days after MI and who are in NYHA Class I 3 months after coronary revascularization
- ICD therapy is indicated in patients with nonischemic dilated cardiomyopathy who have an LVEF of 35% or less and who are in NYHA functional class II or III
- ICD therapy is indicated in patients with nonsustained VT due to prior MI, LVEF of 40% or less, and inducible VF or sustained VT at electrophysiological study

ICD, Implantable cardioverter-defibrillator; *LVEF,* left ventricular ejection fraction; *MI,* myocardial infarction; *NYHA,* New York Health Association; *VF,* ventricular fibrillation; *VT,* ventricular tachycardia.
Modified from Swerdlow CD, Wang PJ, Zipes DP. Pacemakers and implantable cardioverter-defibrillators. In: Zipes DP, Libby P, Bonow RO, et al, eds. *Braunwald's Heart Disease: A Textbook of Cardiovascular Medicine.* 11th ed. Philadelphia, PA: Elsevier; 2019:780-806.

BOX 13.12 Patient and Family Teaching for an Implantable Cardioverter-Defibrillator

Preprocedural Teaching
- Device and how it works
- Lead and generator placement
- Implantation procedure
- Educational materials from the manufacturer

Postprocedural Teaching
- Site care and symptoms of complications
- Hematoma at the site, most common when the patient takes anticoagulant or antiplatelet medications
- Restricting activity of the arm on the side of the implant
- Identification (MedicAlert jewelry and ICD card)
- Diary of an event if the device fires
- Response if the device fires (varies, ranging from falling, tingling, or discomfort to no awareness of the shock); family members need to help in assessment
- Safety measures:
  - Avoid strong magnetic fields (no magnetic resonance imaging).
  - Avoid sources of high-power electricity.
  - Keep cellular phones at least 6 inches from the ICD.
  - Inform airline security personnel about the device; avoid the metal detector; the security wand may be used but should not be left over the device.
  - The defibrillator therapy must be turned off for surgical procedures using electrocautery.
- Everyday activities:
  - Hair dryers, microwaves, and razors are safe.
  - Sexual activity can be resumed; tachycardia associated with sexual activity may cause the device to fire; rate adjustments may be needed; if shock occurs during sexual activity, it will not harm the partner.
  - Avoid driving for 6 months if there is a history of sudden cardiac arrest.
- Replacement of the device
- Instruction of family members in cardiopulmonary resuscitation and in how to contact emergency personnel
- Support groups in the local community

ICD, Implantable cardioverter-defibrillator.

HEART FAILURE

HF is a complex clinical syndrome that results from the heart's inability to pump blood sufficiently to meet the metabolic demands of the body. HF can result from any structural or functional cardiac disorder that impairs the ability of the ventricle to fill or eject blood. CAD is the primary underlying cause of HF; however, several nonischemic causes have been identified, including hypertension, valvular disease, exposure to myocardial toxins, myocarditis, untreated tachycardia, alcohol abuse, and in 20% to 30% of cases unidentifiable causes (which result in idiopathic dilated cardiomyopathy).[21]

The cardinal manifestations of HF are dyspnea, fatigue, exercise intolerance, and fluid retention, which may lead to pulmonary and peripheral edema. Signs and symptoms of HF consist of progressive exertional dyspnea, paroxysmal nocturnal dyspnea, orthopnea, fatigue, loss of appetite, abdominal bloating, nausea or vomiting, and eventual organ system dysfunction, particularly the renal system as the HF advances.

The American Heart Association and American College of Cardiology developed a classification system for HF. A patient is classified by stage (A through D) based on the result of a physical examination, diagnostic tests, and clinical symptoms. This terminology helps in understanding that HF is often a progressive condition that worsens over time. HF can be asymptomatic (stages A and B, pre-HF) or symptomatic (stages C and D). HF also has a classification system based on symptoms. The New York Heart Association (NYHA) Heart Failure Symptom Classification System is used to determine functional limitations, and it is an indicator of prognosis. The categories range from class I, which refers to no symptoms with activity, to class IV, which indicates dyspnea with little or no exertion. The two classification systems can be used with each other (Table 13.11).[21]

Pathophysiology

HF is defined as impaired cardiac function of one or both ventricles. Patients can either have preserved ejection fraction (HFpEF) or have a reduced ejection fraction (HFrEF). Patients with HFpEF have an LVEF of 50% or greater, and those with HFrEF have an LVEF of less than 40%. Those with LVEF values between 40% and 50% are considered borderline.[17]

In left-sided HF, the left ventricle cannot pump efficiently. The ineffective pumping action causes a decrease in cardiac output, leading to poor perfusion. The volume of blood remaining in the left ventricle increases after each beat. As this

TABLE 13.11 ACC/AHA 2001 Staging Compared With NYHA Functional Classification

ACC/AHA		NYHA	
Category	**Definition**	**Category**	**Definition**
A	At high risk of developing HF but without structural heart disease or symptoms of HF	None	
B	Structural heart disease or symptoms of HF	I	Asymptomatic
C	Structural heart disease with prior or current symptoms of HF	II	Symptomatic with moderate exertion
		III	Symptomatic with minimal exertion
		IV	Symptomatic with rest
D	Refractory HF requiring specialized interventions	IV	Symptomatic with rest

ACC, American College of Cardiology; *AHA,* American Heart Association; *HF,* heart failure; *NYHA,* New York Heart Association.
Modified from Januzzi JL, Mann, D.L. Approach to the patient with heart failure. In: Zipes DP, Libby P, Bonow RO, et al, eds. *Braunwald's Heart Disease: A Textbook of Cardiovascular Medicine.* 11th ed. Philadelphia, PA: Elsevier; 2019:403-417.

BOX 13.13 Causes of Heart Failure

- Myocardial infarction
- Coronary artery disease
- Familial cardiomyopathy
- Hypertension
- Valvular heart disease
- Tachydysrhythmias and bradydysrhythmias
- Toxins: cocaine, ethanol, chemotherapy agents
- Viral or infectious agents
- High-output states
- Infiltrative disease: amyloid sarcoid
- Cor pulmonale
- Metabolic disorders
- Nutritional disorders
- Anemia

volume increases, it backs up into the left atrium and pulmonary veins and into the lungs, causing congestion. Eventually, fluid accumulates in the lungs and pleural spaces, causing increased pressure in the lungs. Gas exchange (oxygen and carbon dioxide) in the pulmonary system is impaired. The backflow can continue into the right ventricle and right atrium and into the systemic circulation (right-sided HF). Right-sided dysfunction is usually a consequence of left-sided HF; however, it can be a primary cause of HF after a right ventricular MI, or it may occur secondary to pulmonary pathology.[18] Selected causes of HF are noted in Box 13.13.

When gas exchange is impaired and carbon dioxide levels increase, the respiratory rate increases to help eliminate the excess carbon dioxide. This phenomenon causes the heart rate to increase, pumping more blood to the lungs for gas exchange. The increased heart rate results in the pumping of more blood from the systemic circulation into the cardiopulmonary circulation, which is already dangerously overloaded, and thus a vicious cycle ensues.

As the heart begins to fail to meet the body's metabolic demands, several compensatory mechanisms are activated to improve cardiac output and tissue perfusion. The most noteworthy of these neurohormonal systems are the renin-angiotensin-aldosterone system and the adrenergic nervous system. These interrelated systems act in concert to redistribute blood to critical organs in the body by increasing peripheral vascular tone, heart rate, and contractility. The activation of these diverse systems may account for many of the symptoms of HF and may contribute to the progression of the syndrome. Although these responses are initially viewed as compensatory, many of them are or become counterregulatory and lead to adverse effects.[15]

The *renin-angiotensin-aldosterone system* plays a major role in the pathogenesis and progression of HF. Angiotensin II is a potent vasoconstrictor and promotes salt and water retention by stimulation of aldosterone release. Sodium reabsorption increases, and this, in turn, increases blood volume. In patients with impaired function, the heart is unable to handle the extra volume effectively, resulting in edema (peripheral, visceral, and hepatic) (Fig. 13.15).

The *adrenergic nervous system* is activated in HF. Although this is initially beneficial in preserving cardiac output and systemic BP, chronic activation is deleterious. Activation (1) produces tachycardia, thereby decreasing preload and contributing to a decrease in stroke index; (2) causes vasoconstriction, which increases afterload, further decreasing stroke index; and (3) increases contractility, which increases myocardial oxygen demand, thereby decreasing contractility and possibly decreasing stroke index.[15] These changes are progressive. In time, the ventricle dilates, hypertrophies, and becomes more spherical. This process of cardiac remodeling generally precedes symptoms by months or even years.

Assessment

Patient assessment includes identification of the cause of both right-sided and left-sided HF, the signs and symptoms, and precipitating factors as well as results of diagnostic studies. Signs and symptoms of HF are presented in Box 13.14.

Diagnosis

In diagnosing HF, it is important to identify the etiology or precipitating factors and to determine whether ventricular dysfunction is present; therapies are different for different causes. Ischemia is responsible for most cases of HF, and identifying ischemia as a cause of HF is important because most of these patients can benefit from revascularization.

Diagnosis of the patient with suspected HF includes the following:

- A complete *history,* including precipitating factors
- *Physical examination,* including assessment of the following:
  - Intravascular volume, with examination of neck veins and presence of hepatojugular reflux
  - Presence or absence of edema
  - Perfusion status, which includes BP, quality of peripheral pulses, capillary refill, and temperature of extremities
  - Lung sounds, which may not be helpful. In many cases the lung fields are clear when the patient is obviously congested, a reflection of chronicity of the disease and adaptation.
- *Chest radiographic study* to view heart size and configuration and to check the lung fields to determine whether they are clear or opaque (i.e., fluid filled).
- *Hemodynamic monitoring.* Invasive monitoring may be done to assess mixed venous oxygen saturation, stroke index, cardiac index, and pulmonary artery pressures, especially in those who do not respond to conventional therapy. Noninvasive methods of determining hemodynamic parameters may also be used (see Chapter 9).

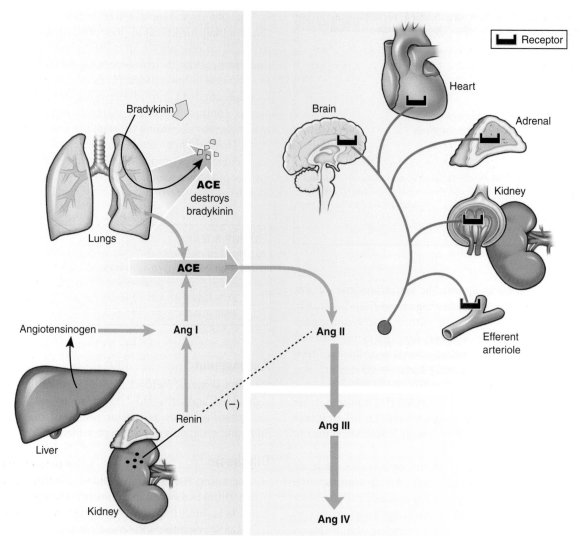

Fig. 13.15 Angiotensins and the organs affected. The *shaded blue area* is the classical pathway of biosynthesis that generates the renin and angiotensin I *(Ang I)*. Angiotensinogen is synthesized in the liver and released into the blood, where it is cleaved to form angiotensin I by renin secreted by cells in the kidneys. Angiotensin-converting enzyme *(ACE)* in the lung catalyzes the formation of angiotensin II *(Ang II)* from angiotensin I and destroys the potent vaso-dilator, bradykinin. Further cleavage generates the angiotensins III and IV *(Ang III and Ang IV)*. The *reddish shading* shows the organs affected by angiotensin II, including the brain, heart, adrenals, kidney, and the kidney's efferent arterioles. The *dashed line* shows the inhibition of renin by angiotensin II. (From McCance KL, Huether SE, eds. *Pathophysiology: The Biologic Basis for Disease in Adults and Children.* 8th ed. St. Louis, MO: Elsevier; 2019.)

BOX 13.14 Signs and Symptoms of Heart Failure

Left-Sided Heart Failure: Poor Pump
- Dyspnea or orthopnea
- Cheyne-Stokes respiration
- Paroxysmal nocturnal dyspnea
- Cough (orthopnea equivalent)
- Fatigue or activity intolerance
- Pulmonary crackles
- Weight gain
- Somnolence
- Elevated pulmonary artery occlusion pressure
- S_3 and S_4 gallop
- Tachycardia
- Tachypnea

Right-Sided Heart Failure: Excess Volume
- Jugular venous distention
- Edema
- Loss of appetite, nausea, vomiting
- Increased abdominal girth

- *Noninvasive imaging of cardiac structures.* The single most useful test in evaluating patients with HF is the echocardiogram, which can evaluate ventricular enlargement, wall motion abnormalities, and valvular structures. It can also be used to determine the LVEF.
- *Measurement of arterial blood gases* to assess oxygenation and acid-base status.
- *Serum electrolytes.* Many electrolyte imbalances are seen in patients with HF. A low serum sodium level is a sign of advanced or end-stage disease; a low potassium level is associated with diuresis; a high potassium level is seen in renal impairment; blood urea nitrogen and creatinine levels are elevated in low perfusion states, in renal impairment, or with overdiuresis.
- *Complete blood count* to assess for anemia.
- *B-type (brain) natriuretic peptide* (BNP). BNP is a cardiac hormone that is secreted by ventricular myocytes in

response to wall stretch. Assays of BNP and its prohormone, proBNP, are useful in the diagnosis of patients with dyspnea of unknown etiology. BNP is a good marker for differentiating between pulmonary and cardiac causes of dyspnea.[26] Plasma concentrations of BNP reflect the severity of HF. In decompensated HF, the BNP concentration increases as a response to wall stress or stretch. As the HF is treated, BNP is used to assess the response to therapies. The normal BNP concentration is less than 100 pg/mL. A BNP level greater than 500 pg/mL is highly specific and indicates increased mortality risk in the short term. Patients are at increased risk for readmission and death if the BNP concentration remains persistently elevated at the time of discharge. BNP is not a good indicator of HF for patients with chronic renal insufficiency.

- *Liver function studies.* The liver often becomes enlarged with tenderness because of hepatic congestion. Serum transaminase and bilirubin levels are elevated with diminished liver function. Function usually returns once the patient is treated and euvolemic.

- *ECG.* Intraventricular conduction delays are common. Left bundle branch blocks are often associated with structural abnormalities. Patients frequently have premature ventricular contractions, premature atrial contractions, and atrial dysrhythmias. Sinus tachycardia at rest implies substantive cardiac decompensation, and detection of this occurrence is essential.

TABLE 13.12 Medication Subsets for Heart Failure

Medication	Management of Heart Failure
ACEIs	Slow disease progression, improve exercise capacity, and decrease hospitalization and mortality
Angiotensin II receptor antagonists	Reduce afterload and improve cardiac output; can be used for patients with ACEI cough
Hydralazine/isosorbide dinitrate	Vasodilator effect; useful in patients intolerant to ACEIs
Diuretics	Manage fluid overload
Aldosterone antagonists	Manage HF associated with LV systolic dysfunction (<35%) while receiving standard therapy, including diuretics
Digoxin	Improve symptoms, exercise tolerance, and quality of life; no effect on mortality
Beta-blockers	Manage HF associated with LV systolic dysfunction (<40%); well tolerated in most patients, including those with comorbidities such as diabetes mellitus, chronic obstructive lung disease, and peripheral vascular disease

ACEI, Angiotensin-converting enzyme inhibitor; *HF,* heart failure; *LV,* left ventricular.

? CRITICAL REASONING ACTIVITY

A patient has been hospitalized three times in the past 2 months for chronic heart failure. What teaching and other interventions can you implement to prevent rehospitalization after discharge?

Interventions

Medical and nursing interventions for the patient with HF consist of a threefold approach: (1) treatment of the existing symptoms, (2) prevention of complications, and (3) treatment of the underlying cause. For example, some patients with HF can be treated by controlling hypertension or by repairing or replacing abnormal heart valves.

Treatment of existing symptoms includes the following:
1. *Improve pump function, fluid removal, and enhanced tissue perfusion* (Tables 13.12 and 13.13).
   a. First-line medications include ACEIs, ARBs, and diuretics. Once symptoms and volume status are stable, a beta-blocker is added. Use of an ACEI plus a beta-blocker is the cornerstone of treatment for HF. ARBs are indicated for those patients who are intolerant of ACEIs.[21]
   b. Additional medication therapies include digoxin, spironolactone, eplerenone, hydralazine, and nitrates.
   c. Inotropes—dobutamine, dopamine, and milrinone—have failed to demonstrate improved mortality in the treatment of severe decompensated HF, although they may improve symptoms at end-of-life.

   d. Nesiritide is administered IV to patients with acutely decompensated HF who have dyspnea at rest or with minimal activity. The best candidates for therapy are those who have clinical evidence of fluid overload, increased central venous pressure, or both. BP should be monitored closely because hypotension can occur.
2. *Reduce cardiac workload and oxygen consumption*
   a. Ultrafiltration is sometimes used for hospitalized patients with HF to remove sodium and reduce water retention. Access is needed, and the risks may not outweigh the benefits. Results from clinical trials have been mixed.[9]
   b. Mechanical circulatory support devices (MCSDs) are capable of partial to complete circulatory support for short- to long-term use. They assist the failing heart and maintain adequate circulatory pressure. MCSDs attach to the patient's own heart, leaving the patient's heart intact, and they have the potential for removal (Box 13.15 and Table 13.14).
   c. Biventricular pacing may be used for cardiac resynchronization therapy in patients with chronic HF who exhibit dyssynchronous contraction of the left ventricle resulting from abnormal electrical conduction pathways. Biventricular pacing involves placement of a ventricular lead in the right ventricle and another lead down the coronary sinus to the left ventricle. Both ventricles are stimulated simultaneously, resulting in a synchronized contraction that improves cardiac performance and exercise tolerance and decreases hospitalizations and mortality.

TABLE 13.13 **PHARMACOLOGY**

Specific Medications for Heart Failure

Medication	Action/Use	Dose/Route	Side Effects	Nursing Implications
Angiotensin-Converting Enzyme Inhibitors (ACEIs)				
Enalapril (Vasotec)	Prevents the conversion of AI to AII, causing an increase in plasma renin activity and a reduction of aldosterone secretion; also inhibits the remodeling process after myocardial injury; used to treat hypertension, heart failure, and patients after myocardial infarction	*PO:* 2.5-20 mg bid	Hypotension, bradycardia, renal impairment, cough, orthostatic hypotension	Do not give IV enalapril to patients with unstable heart failure or AMI. Monitor urine output and potassium levels. Avoid use of NSAIDs. Avoid rapid change in position, such as from lying to standing. Contraindicated in pregnancy.
Fosinopril (Monopril)	Same	*PO:* 10-40 mg daily	Same	Same
Captopril (Capoten)	Same	*PO:* 6.25-150 mg tid	Same	Same
Lisinopril (Prinivil, Zestril)	Same	*PO:* 5-40 mg daily	Same	Same
Diuretics				
Furosemide (Lasix)	Inhibits reabsorption of sodium and chloride in the ascending loop of Henle; used for the management of edema or fluid volume overload	*PO/IV:* 20-600 mg daily	Orthostatic hypotension, vertigo, gout, hypokalemia, cramping, diarrhea or constipation, hearing impairment, tinnitus (rapid IV administration)	Monitor laboratory results, especially potassium levels. Monitor cardiovascular and hydration status regularly. In decompensated patients, use IV route until euvolemic status is reached. Administer first dose early in the day and second dose late in afternoon to prevent sleep disturbance.
Bumetanide (Bumex)	Same	*PO/IV/IM:* 0.5-10 mg daily	Same	Same
Torsemide (Demadex)	Same	*PO/IV:* 10-200 mg daily (max 200 mg daily)	Same	Same
Metolazone (Zaroxolyn)	Same	*PO:* 5-20 mg daily	Same	Increased diuretic effect occurs when given with loop diuretics. Administer 30 min before IV loop diuretic.
Ethacrynic acid (Edecrin)	Same	*PO:* 25-200 mg daily or q 12 h	Same	Same. Used when patient has a sulfa allergy.
Beta-Blockers				
Metoprolol tartrate (Lopressor)	Blocks beta-adrenergic receptors with resulting decreased sympathetic nervous system responses such as decreases in HR, BP, and cardiac contractility in heart failure; may improve systolic function over time; used to treat angina, acute myocardial infarction, and heart failure	*PO:* 50-450 mg daily *IV:* 5 mg IVP	Bradycardia, hypotension, atrioventricular blocks, asthma attacks, fatigue, impotence; may mask hypoglycemic episodes	Teach patient to take pulse and blood pressure on regular basis. Patient should not abruptly stop taking these medications. Start on the lowest dose and titrate to the max dose possible depending on BP and HR.
Metoprolol succinate (Toprol XL)	Same	*PO:* 25-200 mg daily	Same	Same
Carvedilol (Coreg)	Same	*PO:* 12.5-50 mg daily	Same	Same. Better tolerated on a full stomach.
Bisoprolol (Concor)	Same	*PO:* 2.5-20 mg daily	Same	Same

TABLE 13.13 PHARMACOLOGY—cont'd

Specific Medications for Heart Failure

Medication	Action/Use	Dose/Route	Side Effects	Nursing Implications
Aldosterone Receptor Antagonists				
Spironolactone (Aldactone)	Competes with aldosterone for receptor sites in distal renal tubules, increasing sodium chloride and water excretion while conserving potassium and hydrogen ions; may block the effect of aldosterone on arterial smooth muscle; used to manage edema associated with excessive aldosterone secretion	*PO:* 25-200 mg daily	Hyperkalemia, gynecomastia	Monitor serum potassium and renal function; medication is potassium sparing.
Eplerenone (Inspra)	Same	*PO:* 50 mg daily; increase to 50 mg bid if inadequate response after 4 wk	Hyperkalemia	Monitor BP closely, especially at 2 wk. Monitor potassium and sodium levels.
Inotropes				
Digoxin (Lanoxin)	Augments cardiac output by increasing contractility and enhancing tissue perfusion; used to treat cardiac decompensation from heart failure, shock, or renal failure	*PO/IV:* 0.125-0.5 mg daily	Heart block, asystole, visual disturbances (blurred or yellowed vision), confusion/mental disturbances, nausea, vomiting, diarrhea	Monitor serum concentrations; toxicity can be life-threatening. Monitor potassium levels; hypokalemia increases risk of digoxin toxicity. Monitor HR and notify provider if rate is <50 beats/min. Treatment of digoxin toxicity is digoxin immune fab (DigiFab).
Dobutamine (Dobutrex)	Same	*IV infusion:* 2-40 mcg/kg/min titrated to desired response	Increased HR, ventricular ectopy, hypotension, angina, headache, nausea, local inflammatory changes	Administer into large vein via infusion device. May be used in outpatient settings in patients with end-stage heart failure. Monitor heart rate and rhythm and BP closely.
Dopamine (Intropin)	Same	*IV infusion:* 1-50 mcg/kg/min titrated to desired response	Frequent ventricular ectopy, tachycardia, angina, vasoconstriction, headache, nausea, or vomiting. Extravasation can cause tissue necrosis and sloughing.	Administer into large vein via infusion device. Monitor heart rate and rhythm and BP closely. Dopamine is frequently used to treat hypotension and is often used with dobutamine, which increases cardiac output. Monitor the IV site frequently.
Milrinone (Primacor)	Same	*IV:* Loading dose of 50 mcg/kg over 10 min, followed by continuous infusion at 0.375-0.75 mcg/kg/min	Same	Same as dobutamine.
Inamrinone (Inocor)	Same	*IV:* Loading dose of 0.75 mg/kg over 2-3 min, followed by continuous infusion of 5-10 mcg/kg/min. May give additional bolus of 0.75 mcg/kg/min 30 min after starting therapy. Do not exceed total daily dose of 10 mg/kg.	Same	Same as dobutamine. Do not administer furosemide and inamrinone through the same IV line because precipitation occurs.

Continued

TABLE 13.13 PHARMACOLOGY—cont'd

Specific Medications for Heart Failure

Medication	Action/Use	Dose/Route	Side Effects	Nursing Implications
Brain Natriuretic Peptide (BNP)				
Nesiritide (Natrecor)	Vasodilates both veins and arteries; has a positive neurohormonal effect by decreasing aldosterone and positive renal effects by increasing diuresis and natriuresis; used for decompensated congestive heart failure	*IV:* Loading dose of 2 mcg/kg followed by infusion of 0.01 mcg/kg/min	Hypotension, enhanced diuresis, electrolyte imbalances (hypokalemia)	Patients usually respond quickly to therapy. Infusions typically run for 24 h but can continue for days in the severely decompensated patient.
Nitrates				
Nitroglycerin (Tridil)	Directly relaxes smooth muscle, which causes vasodilation of the peripheral vascular bed; decreases myocardial oxygen demands; used to reduce afterload, elevated systemic vascular resistance	*IV infusion:* 5 mcg/min, titrated to a max of 200 mcg/min	Headache, dizziness, flushing, orthostatic hypotension	Monitor BP closely. Titrate to effect.
Angiotensin Receptor Blockers (ARBs)				
Valsartan (Diovan)	Selective and competitive AII receptor antagonist; blocks the vasoconstrictor and aldosterone-secreting effects of AII; used to treat hypertension, heart failure; used in patients who cannot tolerate ACEIs	*PO:* 40 mg daily bid up to 320 mg total daily dose	Hypotension, diarrhea, dyspepsia, upper respiratory tract infection	Avoid use of NSAIDs, such as indomethacin or naproxen, which can cause renal impairment.
Candesartan (Atacand)	Same	*PO:* 4-32 mg daily	Same	Same

AI, Angiotensin I; *AII,* angiotensin 2; *AMI,* acute myocardial infarction; *bid,* twice daily; *BP,* blood pressure; *HR,* heart rate; *IM,* intramuscular; *IVP,* intravenous push; *max,* maximum; *NSAIDs,* nonsteroidal antiinflammatory drugs; *PO,* orally; *q,* every; *tid,* three times daily.

d. Nursing measures that reduce cardiac workload and oxygen consumption include scheduling of rest periods and encouraging patients to modify their activities of daily living. Activity is advanced as tolerated. Patients with HF derive tremendous benefit from formal cardiac rehabilitation to improve activity tolerance and endurance.

3. *Optimize gas exchange through supplemental oxygen and diuresis.*

a. Evaluate the airway, the degree of respiratory distress, and the need for supplemental oxygenation by pulse oximetry, arterial blood gas measurement, or both. Patients are more comfortable in semi-Fowler's position. Adjust oxygen delivery. Consider noninvasive ventilatory support such as continuous positive airway pressure (CPAP) or intermittent noninvasive positive-pressure ventilation (NPPV). CPAP and NPPV have demonstrated effectiveness in the management of HF and often reduce the need for intubation.[9]

b. Diurese aggressively. Administer IV diuretics; furosemide, torsemide, and bumetanide are the preferred agents.

BOX 13.15 Mechanical Circulatory Support

Patients with advanced heart failure or cardiogenic shock may require mechanical circulatory support (MCS) to augment or replace ventricular function. MCS therapy is being used to treat not only patients in the hospital, but also long-term outpatients.[3] With the increase in the incidence of heart failure as well as a shortage of organ donors, the demands for MCS have escalated.

Various MCS devices (MCSDs) exist that support the left ventricle, right ventricle, or both. MCSDs are indicated as a bridge to recovery, a bridge to cardiac transplantation, or destination (i.e., permanent) therapy.[1]

Bridge to recovery (BTR) MCSDs are used for patients with acute heart failure or cardiogenic shock who have an expectation for recovery but who have failed optimal medical therapy. These devices include the intraaortic balloon pump (IABP; Fig. 13.16), ventricular assist device (VAD; Fig. 13.17), and systems such as extracorporeal life support (ECLS), previously known as extracorporeal membrane oxygenation (ECMO).[1] Short-term therapy can last from hours to several days, allowing time for organ recovery or placement of a long-term MCSD.

Bridge to transplantation (BTT) is used for patients who are unlikely to recover from their cardiogenic shock or decompensated heart failure and who are candidates for heart transplantation. These patients have significant symptoms at rest, often require inotropes, are hemodynamically stable, and do not have significant end-organ damage. They are candidates for a left ventricular assist devices (LVAD), which may require surgery with cardiopulmonary bypass for implantation.[1]

Destination therapy (DT) is used for those patients who require long-term support for chronic heart failure that is refractory to medical therapy and who are not candidates for heart transplantation. DT requires major surgery that requires the patient to be hemodynamically stable with no significant end-organ damage. DT improves quality of life and decreases mortality despite the significant risk involved (stroke, infection, bleeding, and device malfunction).[1]

Patients requiring MCSDs need specialized nursing care.[2] During the early postoperative period, nursing management is focused on avoiding potential

BOX 13.15 Mechanical Circulatory Support—cont'd

complications such as low pump flow, bleeding, infection, organ dysfunction, and cardiac dysrhythmias. Monitor for adequate systemic perfusion (i.e., urine output, mentation, capillary refill) and laboratory values (i.e., electrolytes, mixed venous oxygenation saturation [SvO_2], serum lactate level, white blood cell count, metabolic panel, and coagulation studies). During the late postoperative period, nursing management shifts toward patient and family education and preparation for discharge. Educate patients about infection prevention measures, medication management, nutrition, mobility, and signs and symptoms of complications. Before discharge, patients must demonstrate proper management of their devices, including troubleshooting, battery changes, and emergency responses. The goals of therapy are to optimize functional capacity, improve quality of life, and facilitate integration back into the community.

References

1. Aaronson KD, Pagana FD. Mechanical circulatory support. In: Zipes DP, Libby P, Bonow RO, Mann DL, Tomaselli GF, eds. *Braunwald's Heart Disease: A Textbook of Cardiovascular Medicine.* 11th ed. Philadelphia, PA: Elsevier; 2019:568-579.
2. Casida JM, Abshire M, Widmar B, Combs P, Freeman R, Baas L. Nurses' competence caring for hospitalized patients with ventricular assist devices. *Dimens Crit Care Nurs.* 2019;38(1):38–49.
3. Peberdy MA, Gluck JA, Ornato JP, et al. Cardiopulmonary resuscitation in adults and children with mechanical circulatory support: A scientific statement from the American Heart Association. *Circulation.* 2017;135(24):e1115–e1134.

TABLE 13.14 Temporary and Long-Term Mechanical Circulatory Support

Type	Indications	Description
Temporary		
CentriMag	Short-term univentricular or biventricular support	Continuous-flow pump that produces blood flow from 0-10 L/min. Blood flow is produced by rotation of a magnetically suspended impeller, eliminating contact between components. Placed either through an open chest or by percutaneous methods.
Impella LP 2.5 and Impella LP 5.0	Short-term left ventricular support	Continuous-flow pump that has a percutaneously inserted catheter, allowing flows of 2.5 L/min or 5 L/min for the version that requires a surgical cutdown for implantation. The catheter is placed retrograde across the aortic valve to pull blood from the left ventricle, which is returned to ascending aorta.
TandemHeart	Short-term left or right ventricular support	Percutaneously inserted device that provides continuous flow up to 5 L/min. LVAD: Inflow is obtained from a catheter positioned in the left atrium (by a transseptal approach), and outflow is through the femoral artery. RVAD: Inflow is obtained from a catheter positioned in the right atrium, and outflow is through the pulmonary artery. Device allows for transport to a center for long-term therapy.
Long-Term HeartWare	Long-term left ventricular support as bridge to transplantation or destination therapy	A continuous flow rotary pump with centrifugal design that produces nonpulsatile flow. FDA approved for bridge to transplant. Its small size allows for placement above the diaphragm in the pericardial space. The pump has no points of mechanical contact, which reduces damage to red blood cells.
HeartMate II	Long-term left ventricular support	An electrically driven rotary pump that produces nonpulsatile flow. FDA approved for bridge to transplantation and destination therapy. Smaller size allows for implantation in patients with body surface area <1.5 m². Anticoagulation and antiplatelet therapy are required.

FDA, US Food and Drug Administration; *LVAD,* left ventricular assist device; *RVAD,* right ventricular assist device.
From Urden LD, Stacy KM, Lough ME. *Critical Care Nursing Diagnosis and Management.* 8th ed. Maryland Heights, MO: Elsevier; 2018.

Ethacrynic acid is useful if the patient has a serious sulfa allergy. These agents are characterized by quick onset; diuresis is expected 15 to 30 minutes after administration. IV loop diuretic administration is preferred over IV thiazide diuretic administration. The goal is to achieve euvolemia, which may take days. After the patient is euvolemic, oral medications are restarted.

c. Control of sodium and fluid retention sometimes involves fluid restriction of 2 L/day and sodium restriction of 2 g/day. Sodium restriction alone may provide substantial benefits for patients with HF. Discuss management of fluid balance and the importance of avoiding excess intake of sodium, water, or both. Initiate a consult with a dietitian for dietary management and additional teaching.

d. Daily weights are a priority in these patients.

Nurses make a tremendous impact by teaching and enforcing these concepts throughout the hospital stay. Patients may find it easier to continue these habits at discharge if their importance is stressed throughout hospitalization (see QSEN Exemplar box).

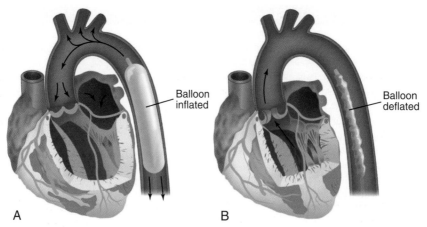

Fig. 13.16 Mechanisms of action of intraaortic balloon pump. **A,** Diastolic balloon inflation augments coronary blood flow. **B,** Systolic balloon deflation decreases afterload. (From Urden LD, Stacy KM, Lough ME. *Critical Care Nursing: Diagnosis and Management.* 8th ed. Maryland Heights, MO: Elsevier; 2019.)

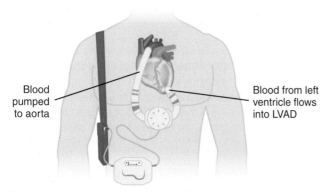

Fig. 13.17 Left ventricular assist device *(LVAD)* system. (From Urden LD, Stacy KM, Lough ME. *Critical Care Nursing: Diagnosis and Management.* 8th ed. Maryland Heights, MO: Elsevier; 2019.)

Pulmonary artery (PA) pressure management (CardioMEMS HF System, Abbott, Abbott Park, IL) is a relatively new way of managing patients with HF from home. A PA sensor is implanted into the distal branch of the descending pulmonary artery and the patient's PA pressures are monitored remotely. The CHAMPION trial showed a 33% reduction in hospitalization for patients with CardioMEMS.[1]

Cardiac transplantation is a therapeutic option for patients with end-stage HF (see Transplant Considerations box). Patients who have severe cardiac disability refractory to expert management and who have a poor prognosis for 6-month survival are optimal candidates. For many patients with symptomatic HF and ominous objective findings (LVEF <20%, stroke volume <40 mL, severe ventricular dysrhythmias), timing of the surgery is difficult. Another consideration is quality of life, which is a judgment made between the patient and provider.

Once the crisis stage has passed and the patient is stabilized, the precipitating factors for the complications must be addressed and treated. Treatment consists of surgical or catheter-based interventions as addressed earlier for a patient with an MI, such as CABG, PTCA or stent, and pharmacological therapy (ACEIs, beta-blockers); valve replacement or repair for valvular heart disease; restoration of sinus rhythm if atrial fibrillation or flutter and tachydysrhythmias are present; and management of risk factors such as hypertension, hyperlipidemia, diabetes, and obesity. Compliance with medications and sodium restriction is continually and vigilantly readdressed.

Complications

Complications of HF can be devastating. Interventions must be provided to avoid extending the existing conditions or allowing the development of new, life-threatening complications. Two specific complications for which patients are monitored are pulmonary edema and cardiogenic shock.

Pulmonary Edema. The failing heart is sensitive to increases in afterload. Pulmonary edema develops in some patients with HF when they become hypertensive. The pulmonary vascular system becomes full and engorged. The results are increasing volume and pressure of blood in pulmonary vessels, increasing

TRANSPLANT CONSIDERATIONS

Heart Transplantation

Criteria for Transplant Recipients

Indications for heart transplant are those individuals who are younger than 70 years of age with end-stage heart disease that is not treatable by other medical or surgical therapies. The Adult Heart Allocation Criteria for Medical Urgency Status is used to classify patients. Scores range from Status 1 (patient has a nondischargeable, surgically implanted, nonendovascular biventricular support device) to Status 6.[1] Transplantation is not indicated for those with major systemic disease, including cancer, active smoker or substance abuse, HIV, severe infection, and severe neurological deficits.

Patient Management

After transplantation, management focuses on optimizing preload, afterload, and contractility. Vasoactive medications and mechanical circulatory support (intraaortic balloon pump, left or right ventricular support) may be indicated.[4]

Immunosuppressive therapy targets different processes in the rejection process: induction, maintenance, and rejection. Induction therapy (antithymocyte agents and interleukin-2 receptor blockers) is initiated in the immediate posttransplant period when the risk for rejection is greatest. Maintenance therapy consists of medications that inhibit T-cell proliferation and differentiation, deplete lymphocytes, and inhibit macrophages. These medications include a calcineurin inhibitor (cyclosporine [Neoral] or tacrolimus [Prograf]), a steroid (methylprednisolone), and an antiproliferative agent (mycophenolate mofetil [CellCept], azathioprine [Imuran], or sirolimus). Complications associated with immunosuppressive therapy include nephrotoxicity, hypertension, diabetes, hyperlipidemia, bone loss, and infection.[3,4]

Complications

Infection is the leading cause of death in the first year after transplantation. In the early postoperative period nosocomial infections predominate, including pneumonia, wound and urinary tract infections, and sepsis.[2] Opportunistic infections predominate 1 to 6 months after heart transplantation. Causative organisms include cytomegalovirus (CMV), herpes simplex virus, varicella zoster (shingles), *Pneumocystis carinii*, *Aspergillus*, and *Candida*.

CMV has been a significant cause of morbidity and mortality after heart transplantation. After 6 months, most infections are community acquired and patients are instructed to avoid contact with anyone who is ill, avoid environments high in dust or mold, and use good hand-washing practices. A high index of suspicion must be maintained, as fever can be masked by the effects of the immunosuppressive medications.[2]

Preventing Rejection

Compliance with immunosuppressive medication is essential to reduce the risk of rejection. *Hyperacute rejection* occurs within minutes or hours of transplantation, is caused by preformed antibodies against the donor, and rarely occurs. *Primary graft dysfunction* occurs within 24 hours of transplantation. It presents as left and/or right ventricular failure. Aggressive management includes vasoactive medications, mechanical circulatory support, or retransplantation. *Acute cellular rejection* occurs 3 to 6 months after transplantation and involves the activation and proliferation of T lymphocytes with destruction of cardiac tissue. *Humoral* or *antibody-mediated rejection* involves B-cell mediated production of immunoglobulin G antibody against the transplanted organ. Significant hemodynamic compromise and shock can occur, resulting in death.

Rejection is diagnosed by endomyocardial biopsy initially performed weekly for 4 to 6 weeks and then at increasingly longer periods based on clinical presentation and cardiac function. Symptoms of rejection may be subtle and include weight gain, shortness of breath, fatigue, abdominal bloating, or fever. Management may include high-dose methylprednisolone; augmenting current maintenance immunosuppression with tacrolimus (Prograf), mycophenolate mofetil (CellCept), rapamycin, or orthoclone; and/or plasmapheresis.

Cardiac allograft vasculopathy (CAV), also known in the past as *chronic rejection*, is an accelerated form of diffuse arteriosclerosis that remains one of the principal limiting factors to long-term survival in cardiac transplant recipients. It can result in myocardial ischemia, infarction, heart failure, ventricular dysrhythmias, and death.

References

1. Organ Procurement and Transplantation Network. Adult Heart Allocation Criteria for Medical Urgency Status. https://optn.transplant.hrsa.gov/learn/professional-education/adult-heart-allocation/. Published 2018. Accessed April 10, 2019.
2. Fishman J. Infection in organ transplantation. *Am J Transplant*. 2017;17(4):856–879.
3. Koomalsingh K, Kobashigawa JA. The future of cardiac transplantation. *Ann Cardiothorac Surg*. 2018;7(1):135–142.
4. Vega E, Schroder J, Nicoara A. Postoperative management of the heart transplantation patients. *Best Pract Res Clin Anaesthesiol*. 2017;31(2):201–213.

pressure in pulmonary capillaries, and leaking of fluid into the interstitial spaces of lung tissue.

Pulmonary edema greatly reduces the amount of lung tissue space available for gas exchange and results in clinical symptoms of extreme dyspnea, cyanosis, severe anxiety, diaphoresis, pallor, and blood-tinged, frothy sputum. Arterial blood gas results indicate severe respiratory acidosis and hypoxemia.

Patients with persistent volume overload may be candidates for continuous IV diuretics, ultrafiltration, or hemodialysis. Loop diuretics given as an IV bolus are considered along with an IV infusion. Furosemide is the most commonly used loop diuretic, with the dose adjusted upward if the patient is currently receiving oral doses. The diuretic effect occurs in 30 minutes and peaks in 1 to 2 hours.[30] IV torsemide or bumetanide are alternative loop diuretics.

Continuous infusion of loop diuretics is considered if the patient does not respond to intermittent dosing. In addition, combinations of diuretics with different mechanisms of action are considered. Thiazide diuretics such as metolazone are often added. Monitor the urinary output hourly to assess the effectiveness of the diuretic therapy.

Although diuretic therapy is important, it is also critical to lower the BP and cardiac filling pressures. IV NTG is administered and titrated until the BP is controlled, resulting in a reduction in both preload and afterload. Patients who do not demonstrate improvement in symptoms require more aggressive treatment. An NTG infusion is initiated at 10 to 20 mcg/min, and the initial titration is in increments of 10 mcg/min at intervals of 3 to 5 minutes, guided by patient response. The maximum dose is 200 mcg/min. Other care requirements for the administration of NTG include the use of non–polyvinyl chloride tubing.

Cardiogenic Shock. Cardiogenic shock is the most acute and ominous form of pump failure. Cardiogenic shock can be seen after a severe MI and with dysrhythmias, decompensated HF, pulmonary embolus, cardiac tamponade, and ruptured abdominal aortic aneurysm (AAA). Often the outcome of cardiogenic shock is death. Cardiogenic shock and its treatment are discussed in depth in Chapter 12. Outcomes for the patient with HF are included in Plan of Care for the Patient With Heart Failure.

◎ PLAN OF CARE

For the Patient With Heart Failure[a]

Patient Problem

Fluid Overload. Risk factors include compromised regulatory mechanisms occurring with decreased cardiac output.

Desired Outcomes
- Less shortness of breath.
- Increased urinary output.
- Peripheral edema is decreased.
- Weight loss occurs and becomes stable within 2 to 3 days.

Assessments/Interventions	Rationales
• Assess I&O, including insensible losses from diaphoresis and respirations.	• Decreased cardiac output reduces renal blood flow, which may result in decreased urine output.
• Assess daily morning weight; record and report steady losses or gains.	• Identify fluid retention and fluid loss; guide titration of diuretics.
• Assess for dependent edema (legs, ankles, feet, and sacrum).	• Identify fluid retention; guide early treatment, decreasing the potential for rehospitalization.
• Assess lung sounds for signs of fluid retention (i.e., crackles or wheezing).	• Indicate fluid retention.
• Monitor for jugular vein distension and ascites.	• Indicators of fluid overload.
• Monitor for abnormal laboratory results:	• Indicators of fluid imbalance or side effects of medications.
• Increased urine specific gravity	
• Decreased Hct	
• Increased urine osmolality	
• Hyponatremia	
• Hypokalemia	
• Hypochloremia	
• Monitor IV flow rate; use an infusion pump for IV fluid administration.	• Prevent volume overload during IV infusion.
• Limit fluid intake per provider orders.	
• Prevent volume overload.	
• Unless contraindicated, provide ice chips or ice pops.	• Provide comfort and reduce thirst while providing minimal amounts of fluid.
• Provide frequent mouth care to reduce dry mucous membranes.	• Small amounts of room-temperature water also relieve thirst.
• Administer diuretics as prescribed and record the patient's response. Use loop diuretics with caution in renal failure or hypokalemia.	• Promote normovolemia by reducing fluid accumulation and blood volume.
• Administer morphine sulfate if prescribed.	• Hypokalemia is a common side effect of loop diuretics.
	• Induce vasodilation and decrease venous return to the heart; relieve acute anxiety and decrease RR.
• A reduced-sodium diet (1-2 g/day) is recommended.	• Hypernatremia can increase fluid retention.
• Teach patients and families about the importance of adhering to a low-sodium diet.	

Patient Problem

Anxiety. Risk factors include an actual or potential life-threatening situation, change in health status, unfamiliar medication, and uncertainty.

Desired Outcomes
- Communicates anxieties and concerns.
- Expresses ways to increase physical and psychological comfort.

Assessments/Interventions	Rationales
• Assess for and acknowledge the patient's anxieties and concerns.	• Reduce anxiety.
• Provide opportunities for the patient and significant other to express their feelings.	• Demonstrate support and caring.
• Be reassuring and supportive.	
• Assist the patient in being as comfortable as possible, ensuring prompt pain relief and supportive positioning.	• Promote an overall sense of well-being and positive outcomes.
• Create and maintain a calm and quiet environment.	• Prevent or reduce sensory overload that may cause increased anxiety.
• Explain all treatment modalities, especially those that may be uncomfortable (e.g., O₂ face mask, IV therapy, invasive testing).	• Reduce anxiety and enable a sense of control.

[a]Also refer to Collaborative Plan of Care for the Critically Ill Patient in Chapter 1.

Hct, Hematocrit; *HF,* heart failure; *I&O,* intake and output; *O₂,* oxygen; *RR,* respiratory rate.

Adapted from Swearingen PL, Wright JD. *All-in-One Nursing Care Planning Resource.* 5th ed. St. Louis, MO: Elsevier; 2019.

PERICARDITIS

Pericarditis is acute or chronic inflammation of the pericardium. It may occur as a consequence of AMI or secondary to trauma, infection, radiation therapy, connective tissue diseases, or cancer.[7] The pericardium has an inner and an outer layer with a small amount of lubricating fluid between the layers. When the pericardium becomes inflamed, the amount of fluid between the two layers increases (pericardial effusion). This squeezes the heart, restricts its action, and may result in cardiac tamponade. Chronic inflammation can result in constrictive pericarditis, which leads to scarring. The epicardium may thicken and calcify (see Fig. 13.1).

The patient with pericarditis usually has precordial pain; this pain may radiate to the shoulder, neck, back, and arm and often mimics the pain associated with an AMI. Other signs and symptoms may include a pericardial friction rub, dyspnea, weakness, fatigue, a persistent temperature elevation, increased white blood cell count, increased sedimentation rate, and increased anxiety level.[7] *Pulsus paradoxus* may be noted during auscultation of the BP. Pain due to pericarditis is usually positional and pleuritic (worse with inspiration and cough).

Detection of a *pericardial friction rub* is the most common method of diagnosing pericarditis. The friction rub is usually heard best on inspiration with the diaphragm of the stethoscope placed over the second, third, or fourth intercostal space at the sternal border. It is best heard when the patient is leaning forward. Friction rubs have been described as grating, scraping, squeaking, or scratching sounds. This rubbing sound results from an increase in fibrous exudate between the two irritated pericardial layers.

The ECG is abnormal in 90% of patients with acute pericarditis. On the ECG, diffuse concave ST-segment elevation and PR-segment deviations opposite to P-wave polarity are often seen. T waves progressively flatten and invert, with generalized T-wave inversions present in most or all leads.[7] An echocardiogram is also useful in diagnosis to visualize the effusion. A diagnosis of pericarditis requires at least two of the following four criteria: chest pain characteristic of pericarditis, a pericardial rub, ECG changes characteristic of pericarditis, and new or worsening pericardial effusion.[7]

The treatment of patients with pericarditis involves relief of pain (analgesic agents or antiinflammatory agents such as colchicine or ibuprofen) and treatment of other systemic symptoms.

Approximately 15 to 50 mL of fluid is present in the pericardial space. Excess fluid compresses the heart chambers, limits the filling capacity of the heart, and may result in tamponade. Treatment of cardiac tamponade includes inserting a needle into the pericardial space to remove the fluid (pericardiocentesis). In extreme cases, surgery may be required to remove part of the pericardium (pericardial window).

VALVULAR HEART DISEASE

Valvular heart disease (VHD) affects approximately 2.5% of the population, with the largest percentage of patients older than 65 years of age. The most common type of VHD is aortic stenosis, followed by mitral regurgitation, aortic regurgitation, and mitral stenosis. Causes include degenerative changes, congenital defects, rheumatic heart disease, ischemic heart disease, and endocarditis. VHD can be initially identified on physical examination by the presence of a murmur on auscultation. Research has revealed that physical examination is not reliable in diagnosing the severity of VHD.[25] An echocardiogram is done to confirm the diagnosis and denote its severity. Treatment of VHD consists of surgery to repair or replace the valve.

ENDOCARDITIS

Infective endocarditis (IE) occurs when microorganisms circulating in the bloodstream attach to an endocardial surface. It is caused by various microbes and frequently involves the heart valves. Endocarditis is increasing in incidence and affects approximately 15 in 100,000 people in the United States. Certain preexisting heart conditions increase the risk for endocarditis, including implantation of an artificial (prosthetic) heart valve, a history of previous endocarditis, and heart valves damaged by conditions such as rheumatic fever, congenital heart defects, or valve defects. Increasing use of cardiac implantable devices and prevalence of drug use have resulted in increased prevalence of IE. *Staphylococcus aureus* accounts for 40% of cases of IE.[32]

Infectious lesions, referred to as *vegetations,* form on the heart valves. These lesions have irregular edges, creating a cauliflower-like appearance. The mitral valve is the most commonly affected valve. The vegetative processes can grow to involve the chordae tendineae, papillary muscles, and conduction system. Therefore the patient may have dysrhythmias or acute HF.

The clinical presentation of patients with acute infectious endocarditis includes high fever and shaking chills. Other manifestations include night sweats, cough, weight loss, general malaise, weakness, fatigue, headache, musculoskeletal complaints, new murmurs, and symptoms of HF. Abnormal physical findings associated with septic emboli may also be seen, including Janeway lesions (lesions on the palms and soles that are often hemorrhagic), Osler nodes (red-purple lesions on fingers or toes), splinter hemorrhages, and Roth spots (retinal hemorrhages). Skin lesions are referred to as the peripheral stigmata of endocarditis.[4]

Treatment of endocarditis involves diagnosing the infective agent and treating with the appropriate IV antibiotics for 2 to 6 weeks. Valve replacement surgery may be indicated in severe cases.[4] Prevention is important, and antibiotic prophylaxis is recommended for high-risk patients before procedures are undertaken.

VASCULAR ALTERATIONS

The aorta is the largest blood vessel in the body in both length and diameter. Shaped like a walking cane, the aorta is an artery that carries blood from the heart. It extends from the aortic valve to the abdomen. Its many branches supply blood to all other areas of the body. The aorta is divided into the thoracic aorta and the abdominal aorta[6] (Fig. 13.18).

EVIDENCE-BASED PRACTICE

Transcatheter Aortic Valve Replacement for the Treatment of Aortic Stenosis

Problem

Traditionally, surgical repair of the aortic valve was the only treatment for severe aortic stenosis in symptomatic patients. Transcatheter aortic valve replacement (TAVR) is an option for patients considered at high risk for surgical aortic valve replacement (SAVR). Novel treatment options are needed to treat those patients who need repair of their aortic valve and are at intermediate risk for SAVR.

Clinical Question

Is TAVR a safe alternative for those patients at intermediate risk for SAVR?

Evidence

Lazkani and colleagues conducted a meta-analysis of randomized and nonrandomized trials comparing SAVR and TAVR. Eleven studies met the criteria for inclusion: four randomized control trials (RCTs) and seven observational studies. The PRISMA checklist for RCTs and the MOOSE criteria for observational studies were used. This was the largest meta-analysis to date and included 5647 intermediate-risk patients. The incidence of 30-day, 1-year, and greater than 2-year all-cause mortality and cardiac mortality was similar between SAVR and TAVR. TAVR had a lower incidence of acute kidney injury and atrial fibrillation, whereas SAVR had a lower incidence of permanent pacemaker implantation and aortic insufficiency. They concluded that TAVR, which is a minimally invasive therapy, is as effective as SAVR for intermediate-risk patients.

Implications for Nursing

Patients with severe aortic stenosis who are symptomatic have a poor prognosis. TAVR offers an option for those patients who are deemed to be at intermediate risk for SAVR. It is important for nurses to be aware of novel therapies that might benefit their patients. Care of the patient who has undergone TAVR is similar to that of any postoperative surgical patient and involves evaluation of the patient for any hemodynamic changes and complications. Common postoperative complications in TAVR include stroke, bleeding, acute kidney failure, and dysrhythmias.

Level of Evidence

A—Meta-analysis

Reference

Lazkani M, Singh N, Howe C, et al. An updated meta-analysis of TAVR in patients at intermediate risk for SAVR. *Cardiovasc Revasc Med.* 2019;20(1):57–69.

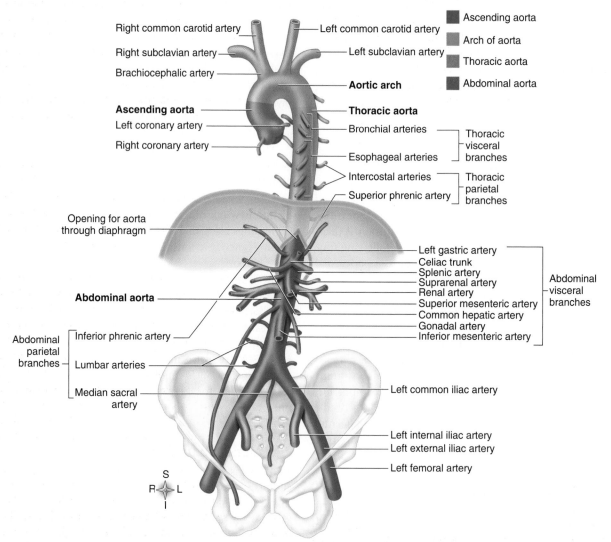

Fig. 13.18 Anatomy of the aorta and its major branches. (From Patton KT, Thibodeau GA. *Anatomy and Physiology.* 10th ed. St. Louis, MO: Elsevier; 2019.)

The thoracic aorta is divided into the ascending aorta, the aortic arch, and the descending aorta. The thoracic aorta begins at the aortic root, which supports the bases of the three aortic valve leaflets.[8] The rounded segment (cane handle) includes the ascending aorta and the aortic arch. Branches of the ascending aorta include the right and left coronary arteries, which feed the myocardium. The arch vessels include the innominate artery, which branches into the right subclavian artery and the right common carotid artery, and the left common carotid and left subclavian arteries. These branches send blood to the head and upper extremities. The descending thoracic aorta (the long segment of the cane) lies to the left of midline in the chest. Branches of the descending aorta are the intercostal arteries, which provide the major blood supply to the distal spinal cord.

The abdominal aorta begins at the level of the diaphragm. At the umbilicus it bifurcates into the two iliac arteries. Abdominal branches include the celiac artery, the superior and inferior mesenteric arteries, and the renal arteries.[8]

Aortic Aneurysms

The word *aneurysm* comes from the Greek *aneurysma*, which means "widening." An aneurysm is a diseased area of an artery causing dilation and thinning of the wall. An aneurysm may be classified as a false (pseudoaneurysm) or a true aneurysm (Fig. 13.19). A false aneurysm results from a complete tear in the arterial wall (see Fig. 13.19C). Blood leaks from the artery to form a clot. Connective tissue is then laid down around this cavity. One example of a false aneurysm is an arterial wall tear resulting from an arterial puncture in the groin area. Anastomotic

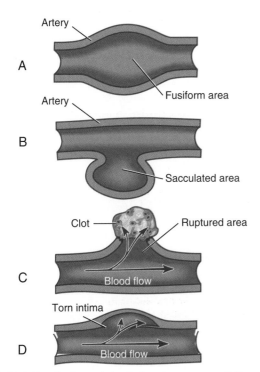

Fig. 13.19 A, True fusiform abdominal aortic aneurysm. **B,** True saccular aortic aneurysm. **C,** False aneurysm, or pseudoaneurysm. **D,** Aortic dissection. (From Lewis SL, Dirkson L, Heitkemper M, Bucher L. *Medical-Surgical Nursing: Assessment and Management of Clinical Problems.* 9th ed. St. Louis, MO: Mosby; 2014.)

aneurysms are false aneurysms found at any graft-host artery anastomosis. True aneurysms include fusiform (see Fig. 13.19A), saccular (see Fig. 13.19B), and dissecting (see Fig. 13.19D) aneurysms. Fusiform or spindle-shaped aneurysms are usually found in the abdominal aorta and are the most common type. A saccular aneurysm is a bulbous pouching of the artery and is usually found in the thoracic aorta. Aortic aneurysms are divided into thoracic aortic, thoracoabdominal aortic, and abdominal aortic types.[8]

Atherosclerosis and degeneration of elastin and collagen are the underlying causes in most cases. Aneurysms are also associated with certain connective tissue disorders such as Marfan syndrome (see Genetics box) or Ehlers-Danlos syndrome. Aneurysms are frequently hereditary, with predominance in males. Risk factors for atherosclerosis, such as age, smoking, hyperlipidemia, hypertension, and diabetes, are also risk factors for aortic aneurysms.[8]

Most aneurysms are asymptomatic and are found on routine physical examination or during testing for another disease entity. Back or abdominal pain may be seen with AAAs. The goal of treatment is avoidance of rupture, which is dramatic and often fatal. Risk of rupture is related to the size of the aneurysm, with aneurysms larger than 6 cm carrying the greatest risk. Patients should be monitored closely for changes in size of the aneurysm.

Treatment of an aneurysm is based on the patient's symptoms and the size of the aneurysm. Thoracic aortic or thoracoabdominal aortic aneurysms larger than 5.5 to 6.0 cm, and AAAs 5.0 cm or larger, are usually surgically repaired. Patients with smaller aneurysms are followed up diagnostically for any change in size. For patients with small AAAs, smoking cessation is emphasized because smokers have a fivefold increase in risk compared with nonsmokers.[8]

Aortic Dissection. Aortic dissection is a life-threatening emergency that requires immediate medical attention. Dissection is a tear in the intimal layer of the vessel that creates a "false lumen," causing blood flow diversion into the false lumen. Sudden, severe chest pain is the most common presenting symptom of aortic dissection. Dissections are classified by the Stanford and the DeBakey categories.

Stanford categories include type A (proximal) and type B (distal). Type A involves the ascending aorta; it is the more concerning type because dissection can extend into the coronary and arch vessels. It usually manifests as severe anterior chest pain. Type B is confined to the descending thoracic and abdominal aorta and is often associated with pain between the scapulae.

DeBakey categories include types I, II, and III. Type I dissections begin in the ascending aorta and may extend all the way to the iliac arteries. Type II dissections involve only the ascending aorta. Type III dissections start in the descending aorta and continue downward to just above (type IIIA) or just below (type IIIB) the diaphragm.[8]

Ascending dissections are more common in younger patients, especially those with Marfan syndrome. Immediate treatment is directed at controlling systolic BP to 100 to 120 mm Hg and decreasing the force of contraction of the heart. Therefore beta-blockers are the initial pharmacological treatment of choice. Emergency surgery is warranted to prevent death. Once rupture occurs, the overall mortality rate is high.[8]

Nursing Assessment

Knowledge of anatomy is the key factor in the treatment and care of patients with aortic aneurysms. Presentation of symptoms, intraoperative risk, and postoperative care are often location dependent. Blood flow to the aortic branches may be hindered by the aneurysm itself, or embolization of thrombus may cause signs and symptoms such as chest pain, TIAs, arm paresthesia with arch location, transient paralysis with descending aorta involvement, or abdominal or flank pain with AAA. In addition, systolic BP may be different in each arm if the dissection occludes one of the subclavian arteries. A murmur may be auscultated if the dissection results in aortic regurgitation.[8]

Diagnostic Studies

1. *Physical examination.* Disparity in BP measurements may be observed between the right and left arms or between the arms and legs, or a diminished pulse may be found in one of the limbs. Palpation reveals decreased or absent peripheral pulses. The patient may have a history of paresthesia, TIAs, lower extremity or buttock claudication, and/or back or abdominal pain.

2. *Imaging studies.* Abdominal ultrasound, computed tomography, angiography, TEE, and MRI are accurate diagnostic tools for AAA.

Treatment

Open surgical or endovascular repair is the treatment for large aortic aneurysms, especially acute type A aortic dissections. The open or conventional repair of an aortic aneurysm is the endo aneurysmal repair (Fig. 13.20). This surgery generally requires a median sternotomy approach.[8]

Uncomplicated type B aortic dissections are often treated medically because of the high mortality rates associated with surgical repair. Acute type B aortic dissections that are complicated are more likely to be treated with endovascular aneurysm repair.[8] This method is less invasive than open repair; it involves percutaneous stent placement in the descending thoracic or thoracoabdominal aorta. Through a small opening in the exposed femoral artery, an intraluminal sheathed stent is introduced, placed, and deployed with fluoroscopic guidance. Care of the vascular surgery patient is detailed in Box 13.16.

⚕ GENETICS

Marfan Syndrome

Marfan syndrome (MFS) is an autosomal dominant inherited disorder that causes pathology in connective tissue. Mutations within the *FBN1* gene cause this disorder.[3] The *FBN1* gene codes for the synthesis of fibrillin-1. Fibrillin migrates out of the cell to provide a matrix that binds proteins, ultimately resulting in thread-like filaments called microfibrils. Microfibrils, in turn, form elastic fibers that allow skin, ligaments, and blood vessels to stretch. Microfibrils also support rigid tissues such as heart valves, bones, and the lens of the eyes.

MFS has a wide range in age at onset of symptoms and severity of disease. It is an example of a genetic disorder that has both high (but not complete) clinical penetrance and variable expression.[1] *Penetrance* refers to the proportion of individuals with a specific gene who exhibit signs and symptoms of the disorder.[3] *Variable expression* refers to the range of signs and symptoms that occur in individuals with the same gene variation.[4] Researchers have identified more than 1300 *FBN1* polymorphisms, but not all mutations are associated with phenotypic MFS.[2]

Genetic studies have progressed from gene identification in MFS to building an understanding of how fibrillin-1 variations contribute to tissue fragility. This aspect of gene-related investigation, called *proteomics,* involves the study of protein structure and function. One example of proteomics is the interaction between fibrillin-1 and a growth factor pathway.[5] The reduced amount and quality of extracellular fibrillin-1 activates growth factors in an attempt to repair the tissue. Overgrowth occurs, contributing to signs and symptoms such as tall and slender build, heart murmurs, an abnormally curved spine, or extreme nearsightedness.

The diagnosis of MFS is based on the presence of a positive family history and the number of organ systems with Marfan-related defects. More than 90% of patients with MFS have mutations of the *FBN1* gene.[3] Although genetic testing is sensitive to MFS, it is not specific because *FBN1* variations are also associated with other hereditary connective tissue disorders such as bicuspid aortic valve and Ehlers-Danlos syndrome. About 1 in 4 individuals with MFS have a de novo or new mutation in the *FBN1* gene.[3]

MFS results in tissue fragility. The clinical manifestations most commonly associated with MFS are aortic aneurysm (especially thoracic); dilation of the root of the aorta where it connects to the left ventricle; tall stature with especially long arms, legs, fingers, and toes; a protruding or indented sternum; enlargement

of the dural membrane surrounding the lower spine or brainstem (i.e., dural ectasia); and dislocation of the lens of the eye.[5] Individuals can also have blebs or emphysema-like changes in the lung with possible spontaneous pneumothorax, inguinal or incisional hernias, skin stretch marks (i.e., striae), joint hypermobility, and visual disorders such as myopia or early cataracts.[3]

Clinicians tailor management of MFS to each individual's manifestation of the disease. For those who have aortic manifestations of MFS, management includes prescribing beta-blockers and angiotensin-converting enzyme inhibitors or selective angiotensin-2 receptor blockers to control blood pressure and slow the progression of widening in the aorta.[6] Clinicians also advise patients to restrict contact sports and weight lifting. Definitive treatment consists of surgical intervention to prevent aortic dissection. Patients with MFS and their family members may be referred by clinicians for genetic testing and genetic counseling, including psychosocial support.

Genetic terms: *autosomal dominant, de novo mutation, polymorphism, single nucleotide polymorphism (SNP), phenotype, penetrance, variable expression, proteomics.*

References

1. Jorde LB. Genes and genetic disease. In: McCance S, Huether K, eds. *Pathophysiology.* 8th ed. Philadelphia, PA: Elsevier; 2019.
2. Muino-Mosquera L, Steijns F, Audenaert T, et al. Tailoring the American College of Medical Genetics and Genomics and the Association for Molecular Pathology guidelines for the interpretation of sequenced variants in the *FBN1* gene for Marfan syndrome: Proposal for a disease- and gene-specific guideline. *Circ Genom Precis Med.* 2018;11(6):e002039.
3. National Institutes of Health. Marfan Syndrome. https://ghr.nlm.nih.gov/condition/marfan-syndrome. Published May 2018. Accessed February 18, 2019.
4. National Institutes of Health. What Are Reduced Penetrance and Variable Expressivity? https://ghr.nlm.nih.gov/primer/inheritance/penetranceexpressivity. Published March 3, 2020. Accessed March 14, 2020.
5. Prockop DJ, Bateman JF. Heritable Disorders of Connective Tissue. In: Jameson J, Fauci AS, Kasper DL, et al., eds. *Harrison's Principles of Internal Medicine,* 20e New York, NY: McGraw-Hill. http://accessmedicine.mhmedical.com/content.aspx?bookid=2129&sectionid=192530885. Accessed March 14, 2020.
6. Seo GH, Kim YM, Kang E, et al. The phenotypic heterogeneity of patients with Marfan-related disorders and their variant spectrums. *Medicine (Baltimore).* 2018;97(20):e10767.

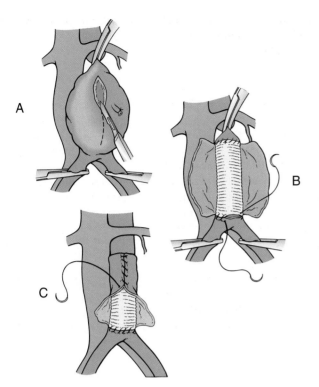

Fig. 13.20 Surgical repair of an abdominal aortic aneurysm. **A,** The aneurysmal sac is incised. **B,** The synthetic graft is inserted. **C,** The native aortic wall is sutured over the synthetic graft. (From Lewis SL, Dirksen RD, Heitkemper MM, et al. *Medical-Surgical Nursing: Assessment and Management of Clinical Problems.* 9th ed. St. Louis, MO: Mosby; 2014.)

BOX 13.16 Nursing Interventions After Aortic Surgery

- Monitor vital signs every 1 hour (postrecovery stage); assess for tachycardia and irregular rhythms.
- Blood pressure: Keep the patient normotensive. Hypertension causes bleeding; give vasodilators per protocol. Hypotension causes organ ischemia; give fluids and vasoconstrictors.
- Monitor hemodynamic pressures: SvO_2, stroke index, cardiac index, PAOP, and RAP; treat per protocols.
- Assess for hypovolemia: Monitor output from chest tubes, drains, and urine output every 1 hour.
- Assess for hypothermia; rewarm the patient per protocol.
- Monitor fluid and electrolytes, hemoglobin, hematocrit, renal function, and coagulation studies.
- Monitor the radial, dorsalis pedis, and posterior tibial pulses every 1 hour; use Doppler studies as needed. Assess the ankle-brachial index every 2 hours or as ordered.
- Monitor for complications: Intraoperative AMI, dysrhythmias, heart failure, cardiac tamponade, thromboembolism, impaired renal function, pneumonia, pneumothorax, pleural effusion, cerebral ischemia, stroke.
- Implement ventilator bundle of care (Chapter 10); wean from mechanical ventilation and extubate as soon as possible; promote pulmonary hygiene.
- Assess wounds and provide incisional care per protocol.
- Organize nursing care; control environmental stimuli.
- Gradually increase the patient's activity.
- Provide emotional support to the patient and family; assess the family's level of understanding; discuss the postoperative course.
- For abdominal aneurysm, assess for ischemic colitis.

AMI, Acute myocardial infarction; *PAOP,* pulmonary artery occlusion pressure; *RAP,* right atrial pressure; *SvO2,* mixed venous oxygen saturation.

CASE STUDY

Mr. P. was admitted to the emergency department with the complaint of sudden onset of substernal chest pain while he was mowing his lawn. He took aspirin and three sublingual nitroglycerin tablets every 5 minutes en route. Mr. P. states that his pain has gone from a 7 to a 3, on a scale from 0 to 10.

The cardiac monitor shows he is in a sinus rhythm. His blood pressure is 150/88 mm Hg, his pulse is 96 beats/min, and his respiratory rate is 24 breaths/min and nonlabored. The nurse starts two IV lines, gives Mr. P. another nitroglycerin tablet, and proceeds to obtain a brief history.

Mr. P. is a 68-year-old white male who weighs 220 lb and has a history of hypertension and diabetes. He smokes 1½ packs of cigarettes per day. He is allergic to penicillin.

The monitor alarms, and the nurse identifies the rhythm as ventricular fibrillation. The nurse calls a code and begins cardiopulmonary resuscitation. Mr. P. is defibrillated with 200 J using the biphasic defibrillator. After defibrillation, his rhythm is regular sinus with frequent premature ventricular contractions. His blood pressure is 92/56 mm Hg. His pupils are 4 mm, equal and reactive. His respiratory rate is 16 breaths/min, and his oxygen saturation is 92%. He is not fully awake at this time, but he is moving all of his extremities. A 150-mg IV bolus of amiodarone is given over 10 minutes, and an infusion is started at 1 mg/min. Laboratory tests and arterial blood gas measurements are ordered, along with a 12-lead electrocardiogram (ECG). Consultation by the cardiologist is requested.

Mr. P.'s cardiac enzyme results return as follows:

Troponin I	0.5 ng/mL
Troponin T	0.4 ng/mL

His electrolyte values are as follows:

Sodium	143 mEq/L
Potassium	3.4 mEq/L
Chloride	109 mEq/L
Carbon dioxide	34 mEq/L
Glucose	354 mg/dL
Magnesium	1.5 mEq/L

Arterial blood gas values are as follows:

pH	7.32
$PaCO_2$	49 mm Hg
PaO_2	77 mm Hg
Bicarbonate	24 mEq/L
SaO_2	92%

A 12-lead ECG shows ST elevation in leads V_2, V_3, and V_4. Mr. P. is diagnosed with an acute anterior myocardial infarction. His oxygen is increased to 6 L/min by nasal cannula. Based on these assessment and study results, tissue plasminogen activator (t-PA) is administered.

Questions

1. What do Mr. P.'s cardiac enzyme values indicate about the time and extent of his myocardial infarction?
2. What complications may be anticipated for Mr. P. related to the infusion of t-PA? What parameters would the nurse need to monitor?
3. What assessments would indicate that the t-PA was effective?
4. What risk factors for coronary artery disease should be addressed before Mr. P.'s discharge to reduce his risk of another myocardial infarction?

REFERENCES

1. Abraham WT, Stevenson LW, Bourge RC, et al. Sustained efficacy of pulmonary artery pressure to guide adjustment of chronic heart failure therapy: Complete follow-up results from the CHAMPION randomised trial. *Lancet*. 2016;387(10017):453–461.

2. Al-Mallah MH, Farah I, Al-Madani W, et al. The impact of nurse-led clinics on the mortality and morbidity of patients with cardiovascular diseases: A systematic review and meta-analysis. *J Cardiovasc Nurs*. 2016;31(1):89–95.

3. Amsterdam EA, Wenger NK. The 2014 American College of Cardiology ACC/American Heart Association guideline for the management of patients with non-ST-elevation acute coronary syndromes: Ten contemporary recommendations to aid clinicians in optimizing patient outcomes. *Clin Cardiol*. 2015;38(2): 121–123.

4. Baddour LMF, W.K, Suri RM, et al. Cardiovascular infections. In: Zipes DP, Libby P, Bonow RO, Mann DL, Tomaselli GF, eds. *Braunwald's Heart Disease: A Textbook of Cardiovascular Medicine*. 11th ed. Philadelphia, PA: Elsevier; 2019:442–461 .

5. Bohula EAM, David A. ST-elevation myocardial infarction: Management. In: Zipes DP, Libby P, Bonow RO, Mann DL, Tomaselli GF, eds. *Braunwald's Heart Disease: A Textbook of Cardiovascular Medicine*. 11th ed. Philadelphia, PA: Elsevier; 2019:1483–1509.

6. Bonatti JH, F, Prud'Homme D, Mick S. Robotic coronary artery bypass grafting. In: Selke F, Ruel M, eds. *Atlas of Cardiac Surgical Techniques*. 2nd ed. Philadephia, PA: Elsevier; 2019:103–113.

7. Brashers VL. Alterations in cardiovascular function. In: McCance KL, Huether SE, eds. *The Biologic Basis for Disease in Adults and Children*. 8th ed. St. Louis, MO: Mosby; 2019:1059–1114.

8. Braverman ACS, M. Diseases of the aorta. In: Zipes DP, Libby P, Bonow RO, Mann DL, Tomaselli GF, eds. *Braunwald's Heart Disease: Textbook of Cardiovascular Medicine*. 11th ed. Philadelphia, PA: Elsevier; 2019:1295–1327.

9. Felker GMT, JR. Diagnosis and management of acute heart failure. In: Zipes DP, Libby P, Bonow RO, Mann DL, Tomaselli GF, eds. *Braunwald's Heart Disease: A Textbook of Cardiovascular Medicine*. 11th ed. Philadelphia, PA: 2019:462–489.

10. Giugliano RP, Cannon CP, Blazing MA, et al. Benefit of adding ezetimibe to statin therapy on cardiovascular outcomes and safety in patients with versus without diabetes mellitus: Results from IMPROVE-IT (Improved Reduction of Outcomes: Vytorin Efficacy International Trial). *Circulation*. 2018;137(15):1571–1582.

11. Goyal A, Gluckman TJ, Levy A, et al. Translating the fourth universal definition of myocardial infarction into clinical documentation: Ten pearls for frontline clinicians. *Cardiol Mag*. 2018;47(11):34–36.

12. Grundy SM, Stone NJ, Bailey AL, et al. 2018 AHA/ACC/AACVPR/AAPA/ABC/ACPM/ADA/AGS/APhA/ASPC/NLA/PCNA guideline on the management of blood cholesterol. *J Am Coll Cardiol*. 2019;73(24):3168–3209.

13. Gulati MM, C.N.B. Cardiovascular disease in women. In: Zipes DP, Libby P, Bonow RO, Mann DL, Tomaselli GF, eds. *Braundwald's Heart Disease: A Textbook of Cardiovascular Medicine*. 11th ed. Philadelphia, PA: Elsevier; 2019:1767–1779.

14. Guo MH, Wells GA, Glineur D, et al. Minimally Invasive coronary surgery compared to STernotomy coronary artery bypass grafting: The MIST trial. *Contemp Clin Trials*. 2019;78:140–145.

15. Hasenfuss GM, D.L. Pathophysiology of heart failure. In: Zipes DP, Libby P, Bonow RO, Mann DL, Tomaselli GF, eds. *Braundwald's Heart Disease: A Textbook of Cardiovascular Medicine*. 11th ed. Philadelphia, PA: Elsevier; 2019:442–461.

16. January CT, Wann LS, Calkins H, et al. 2019 AHA/ACC/HRS focused update of the 2014 AHA/ACC/HRS guideline for the management of patients with atrial fibrillation: A report of the American College of Cardiology/American Heart Association Task Force on Clinical Practice Guidelines and the Heart Rhythm Society. *Heart Rhythm*. 2019.

17. Januzzi JLM, D.L. Approach to the patient with heart failure. In: Zipes DPL, P, Bonow RO, Mann DL, Tomasello GF, Braunwald, E, ed. *Braunwald's Heart Disease: a textbook of cardiovascular medicine*. 11 ed. Philadelphia, PA: Elsevier; 2019;16(8):e66–e93.

18. Konstam MA, Kiernan MS, Bernstein D, et al. Evaluation and management of right-sided heart failure: A scientific statement from the American Heart Association. *Circulation*. 2018;137(20):e578–e622.

19. Konstanty-Kalandyk J, Piatek J, Kedziora A, et al. Ten-year follow-up after combined coronary artery bypass grafting and trans-myocardial laser revascularization in patients with disseminated coronary atherosclerosis. *Lasers Med Sci*. 2018;33(7):1527–1535.

20. Kusumoto FM, Schoenfeld MH, Barrett C, et al. 2018 ACC/AHA/HRS guideline on the evaluation and management of patients with bradycardia and cardiac conduction delay: Executive summary: A report of the American College of Cardiology/American Heart Association Task Force on Clinical Practice Guidelines, and the Heart Rhythm Society. *J Am Coll Cardiol*. 2019;74(7):932–987.

21. Mann D. Management of heart failure patients with reduced ejection fraction. In: Zipes DP, Libby P, Bonow RO, Mann DL, Tomaselli GF, eds. *Braunwald's Heart Disease: A Textbook of Cardiovascular Medicine*. 11th ed. Philadelphia, PA: Elsevier; 2019:490–522.

22. Mauri LB, Deepak L. Percutaneous coronary intervention. In: Zipes DP, Libby P, Bonow RO, Mann DL, Tomaselli GF, eds. *Braunwald's Heart Disease: A Textbook of Cardiovascular Medicine*. 11th ed. Philadelphia, PA: Elsevier; 2019:49–69.

23. Morrow DAdL, J.A. Stable ischemic heart disease. In: Zipes DP, Libby P, Bonow RO, Mann DL, Tomaselli GF, eds. *Braunwald's Heart Disease: A Textbook of Cardiovascular Medicine*. 11th ed. Philadelphia, PA: Elsevier; 2019:1209–1270.

24. Nguyen PK, Rhee JW, Wu JC. Adult stem cell therapy and heart failure, 2000 to 2016: A systematic review. *JAMA Cardiol*. 2016;1(7):831–841.

25. Otto CMB, R.O. Approach to the patient with valvular heart disease. In: Zipes DP, Libby P, Bonow RO, Mann DL, Tomaselli GF, eds. *Braunwald's Heart Disease: A Textbook of Cardiovascular Medicine*. 11th ed. Philadelphia, PA: Elsevier; 2019:1383–1388.

26. Pagana K, Pagana TJ. *Mosby's Manual of Diagnostic and Laboratory Tests*. Vol 6. 6th ed. St. Louis, MO: Elsevier; 2018.

27. Riberio IBG, J.B, Fortier JH, et al. Off pump coronary artery bypass grafting. In: Selke F, Ruel M, eds. *Atlas of Cardiac Surgical Techniques*. 2nd ed. Philadelphia, PA: Elsevier; 2019:49–69.

28. Rosenson RS, Hegele RA, Fazio S, et al. The evolving future of PCSK9 inhibitors. *J Am Coll Cardiol*. 2018;72(3):314–329.

29. Scirica BML, P, Morrow DA. ST-elevation myocardial infarction: Pathophysiology and clinical evolution. In: Zipes DP, Libby P, Bonow RO, Mann DL, Tomaselli GF, eds. *Braunwald's Heart Disease: A Textbook of Cardiovascular Medicine*. 11th ed. Philadelphia, PA: Elsevier; 2019:1095–1122.

30. Skidmore-Roth L. *Mosby's 2019 Nursing Drug Reference*. 32nd ed. St. Louis, MO: Elsevier; 2019.

31. Swearingen PL, Wright JD. *All-in-One Nursing Care Planning Resource*. 5th ed. St. Louis, MO: Elsevier; 2019.

32. Wang A, Gaca JG, Chu VH. Management considerations in infective endocarditis: A review. *JAMA*. 2018;320(1):72–83.

Nervous System Alterations

Christina Amidei, RN, PhD, CNRN, FAAN

Many additional resources, including self-assessment exercises, are located on the Evolve companion website at http://evolve.elsevier.com/Sole/.
- Animations
- Clinical Skills: Critical Care Collections
- Student Review Questions
- Video Clips

INTRODUCTION

The central and peripheral nervous systems are responsible for producing consciousness and higher mental functions, movement, sensation, and reflex activity. When these structures are damaged, a person's ability to provide self-care and interact with the environment may be greatly altered. This chapter discusses the pathophysiology, assessment, and nursing and medical management related to common neurological problems such as increased intracranial pressure (ICP), head and traumatic brain injury (TBI), meningitis, status epilepticus (SE), cerebrovascular diseases, and spinal cord injury (SCI).

ANATOMY AND PHYSIOLOGY OF THE NERVOUS SYSTEM

Cells of the Nervous System

The nervous system is composed of two types of cells: neurons and neuroglia. The *neuron,* or nerve cell, is the basic functional unit of the nervous system and serves as the transmitter of nerve impulses (Fig. 14.1). Each neuron is unique in character, and its features are determined by its specific function. During nerve transmission, *dendrites* receive an electrical impulse from other neurons. The electrical impulse is transmitted along the *axon* of the neuron to the *synaptic knobs,* which release neurotransmitters into the synapse. Once in the synapse, the neurotransmitters bind to available receptor sites, usually on a nerve or muscle cell.

Neurotransmitter binding propagates receptor membrane depolarization and continuation of impulse transmission. Postsynaptic responses may be excitation or inhibition, depending on the type of neurotransmitter released. Acetylcholine, norepinephrine, dopamine, serotonin, glutamate, gamma-aminobutyric acid (GABA), substance P, and endorphins are common neurotransmitters released. It is generally believed that each neuron releases only one type of neurotransmitter at its nerve terminals.[2]

Degeneration of neurons or failure of neurons to release or take up neurotransmitters can be associated with nervous system dysfunction.

Some axons are surrounded by a white protein-lipid complex *(myelin)* that is formed by Schwann cells in the peripheral nervous system (PNS) and by oligodendrocytes in the central nervous system (CNS). Periodic constrictions along the axon lack myelin; these areas, known as nodes of Ranvier, facilitate fast and efficient impulse conduction (see Fig. 14.1). The speed of impulse conduction depends on both the thickness of the myelin and the distance between nodes. Loss of myelin (i.e., demyelination) slows or alters neuronal function and is characteristic of diseases such as multiple sclerosis.

Neuroglial cells (glia) constitute the supportive tissue of the CNS. These cells are approximately 5 to 10 times as numerous as neurons. Most primary CNS tumors originate from glial cells and are thus termed gliomas. Four types of glial cells exist, each with specific functions. *Microglia* act as phagocytic scavenger cells when nervous tissue is damaged. *Astrocytes* are star-shaped cells that play a critical role in transport of nutrients, gases, and waste products among neurons, the vascular system, and cerebrospinal fluid (CSF); in the formation of scar tissue in the brain; and in the function of the blood-brain barrier. *Oligodendrocytes* are responsible for myelin formation. *Ependymal* cells produce specialized glial tissue that forms the lining of the ventricles of the brain and the central canal of the spinal cord; they also play a role in production of CSF.

Cerebral Circulation

The cerebral circulation must provide sufficient blood to supply oxygen, glucose, and nutrients to the cerebral tissues. The brain does not have any energy stores and is dependent on aerobic metabolism. Therefore even a brief interruption in blood supply may result in significant ischemic tissue damage. The brain receives approximately 750 mL of blood per minute, or 15% to 20% of the total resting cardiac output.[14]

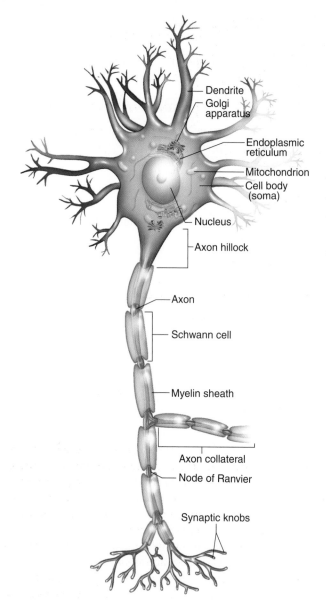

Fig. 14.1 Structure of a typical neuron. (From Patton KT, Thibodeau GA, Douglas MM. *Essentials of Anatomy and Physiology.* St. Louis, MO: Mosby; 2012.)

The blood supply of the brain arises from two major sets of arteries, the carotid arteries (anterior circulation) and the vertebral arteries (posterior circulation). Specifically, the left common carotid artery originates from the aortic arch, and the right common carotid artery originates from the innominate artery. The common carotid arteries then branch to form the external and internal carotid arteries. The external carotid artery supplies the face, scalp, and other extracranial structures. Each internal carotid artery terminates by dividing into anterior cerebral and middle cerebral arteries (MCA). The anterior cerebral artery and its branches supply the medial aspects of the motor cortex and the frontal lobes. The MCA comprises the principal blood supply of the frontal, temporal, and parietal lobes. Most strokes involve the MCA.

The paired vertebral arteries originate from the subclavian arteries and enter the skull through the foramen magnum. The

vertebral arteries and their branches supply the upper spinal cord, medulla, and cerebellum before joining at the pons to form the basilar artery. The basilar artery sends branches to the cerebellum, medulla, pons, and internal ear. Then the basilar artery bifurcates and terminates as the posterior cerebral arteries, which serve the medial portions of the occipital and inferior temporal lobes.

These two arterial systems interconnect at the base of the brain via communicating arteries. The posterior communicating artery connects the internal carotid artery to the posterior cerebral artery, and the anterior communicating artery connects the two anterior cerebral arteries. This interconnection is known as the cerebral arterial circle (of Willis) at the base of the brain (Fig. 14.2).

Cerebral veins, which do not have a muscle layer or valves, empty blood into venous sinuses located throughout the cranium. Because the venous sinuses play a role in absorption of CSF, they parallel the ventricular system, rather than the arterial system as in most other organs. The venous blood is emptied into the internal jugular vein and, ultimately, into the superior vena cava, which returns the blood to the heart.

Cerebral Metabolism

Glucose is the brain's sole source of energy for cellular function. Because the brain is unable to store glucose, it requires a continuous supply of glucose to maintain normal brain metabolism. If the cerebral glucose level drops below 70 mg/dL, confusion may develop. Seizures and decreased responsiveness may occur if the glucose level continues to decrease. Cellular damage develops when the brain glucose level drops to less than 20 mg/dL.[1,2]

Aerobic metabolism is used to meet cerebral energy demands because anaerobic metabolism produces only a minimal amount of adenosine triphosphate (ATP). If the brain is deprived of oxygen, even for a few minutes, metabolism changes from aerobic to the less efficient anaerobic cellular metabolism, resulting in energy failure and neurological deficits.

Maintaining a constant *cerebral blood flow (CBF)* is essential to sustain normal cerebral metabolism. In the absence of adequate blood flow, cell membrane integrity is lost, allowing extracellular fluid to flow into the cell, causing edema within the cell. The extracellular environment becomes acidotic as a result of lactic acid production from anaerobic metabolism, and cellular damage ensues. Neurological manifestations occur owing to slowing of electrical activity. If an anoxic state lasts for 5 minutes or longer at normal body temperature, cerebral neurons are destroyed and cannot regenerate.[1]

A process called autoregulation ensures continuous CBF regardless of the mean arterial pressure (MAP). *Autoregulation* is defined as the ability of cerebral blood vessels to adjust their diameter to arterial pressure changes within the brain.[1] If a rapid increase in MAP occurs, the cerebral vessels constrict to prevent excessive distension of the cerebral arteries. Conversely, if the MAP drops, the cerebral blood vessels dilate to maintain normal CBF and to prevent cerebral ischemia.

The cerebral vessels are also sensitive to the chemical regulators that maintain CBF, such as the partial pressure of arterial carbon dioxide ($PaCO_2$) or oxygen (PaO_2) and the hydrogen

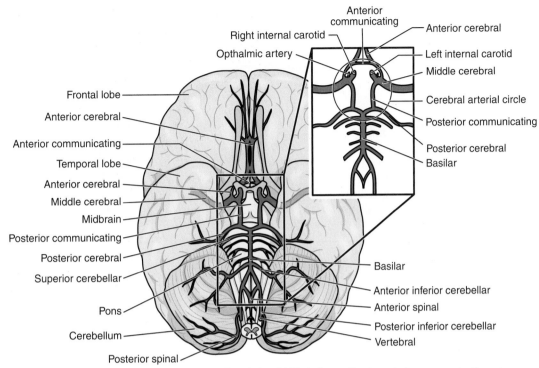

Fig. 14.2 Arterial blood supply of the brain. The circle of Willis is formed by the anterior communicating artery, which joins together the two anterior cerebral arteries, and the posterior communicating arteries, which arise from the internal carotid arteries and connect to the posterior cerebral arteries.

ion concentration. Carbon dioxide is the most potent agent influencing CBF. When $PaCO_2$ is greater than 45 mm Hg, cerebral blood vessels vasodilate, increasing CBF. A low $PaCO_2$ causes the cerebral arteries to constrict, leading to decreased CBF and decreased tissue perfusion. Cerebral arteries are less sensitive to changes in PaO_2. When PaO_2 is less than 50 mm Hg, cerebral vessels dilate to increase CBF and oxygen delivery. If the PaO_2 is not raised, anaerobic metabolism begins, resulting in lactic acid accumulation. An increased hydrogen ion concentration further increases vasodilation to facilitate the removal of acidic end products from cerebral tissue.[1]

Blood-Brain Barrier System

The *blood-brain barrier system* protects the brain from toxic elements and disease-causing organisms that may circulate in the blood. The blood-brain barrier operates on the concept of tight junctions between adjacent cells and selective permeability that prevents the free movement of materials from the vascular bed into the brain. Typically, large molecules do not cross the blood-brain barrier, whereas small molecules cross easily. Water, carbon dioxide, oxygen, and glucose freely cross the cerebral capillaries. The movement of other substances into the brain is dependent on their chemical dissociation, lipid solubility, and protein-binding potential. Infections, tumors, and certain other disease states may also alter the blood-brain barrier.

Ventricular System and Cerebrospinal Fluid

The four *ventricles* of the adult brain are hollow spaces lined by ependymal cells. Specialized epithelium in the ventricular wall, called the *choroid plexus*, produces CSF. A smaller amount of

CSF is secreted from the ependymal cells that line the ventricles. CSF is continually secreted from these surfaces at a rate of about 500 mL/day, or about 20 mL/h.[1] On average, 150 mL of CSF is contained in the ventricles and subarachnoid space. The CSF plays a role in metabolic function of the brain and provides a cushioning effect during head movement.

CSF flows from the two lateral ventricles into the third ventricle through the foramen of Monro. From the third ventricle, CSF flows through the aqueduct of Sylvius into the fourth ventricle. From there, the CSF flow is directed through the foramina of Luschka and Magendie into the cisterna and the subarachnoid space (Fig. 14.3). After circulating around the brain and spinal cord, CSF is reabsorbed into the venous sinuses of the brain through the arachnoid villi, which are dural projections from the arachnoid space. If flow out of the ventricular system is blocked, obstructive hydrocephalus occurs. Scarring or inflammation of the arachnoid villi prevents CSF resorption, causing communicating hydrocephalus.

FUNCTIONAL AND STRUCTURAL DIVISIONS OF THE CENTRAL NERVOUS SYSTEM

Meninges

Meninges cover the brain and spinal cord and consist of three layers: dura mater, arachnoid mater, and pia mater (see Fig. 14.3). The *dura mater* is the outermost covering and has two layers. The outer surface adheres to the skull, and the inner layer produces prominent folds (falx cerebri, tentorium cerebelli, falx cerebelli) that subdivide the interior cranial cavity to

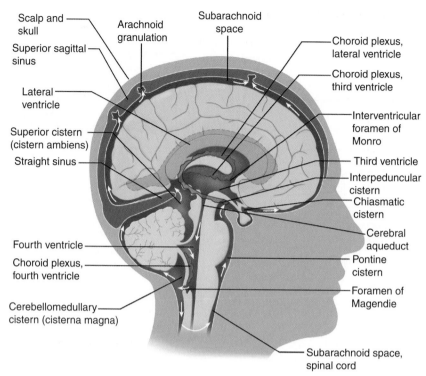

Fig. 14.3 Flow pattern of cerebrospinal fluid within the ventricles of the brain and the surrounding subarachnoid space. (From Schapira A. *Neurology and Clinical Neuroscience.* St. Louis, MO: Mosby; 2017.)

support and protect the brain. The inner dura mater also covers the spinal cord. The *arachnoid mater* is located inside the dura mater. It is a delicate, avascular layer that loosely encloses the brain and spinal cord. The *pia mater* closely adheres to the brain's outer surface and contains a network of blood vessels. The pia mater surrounding the spinal cord is less vascular.

Actual or potential spaces exist between the meningeal layers. The epidural space is a potential space between the skull and the outer dura mater. The subdural space lies between the dura mater and the arachnoid mater and is filled with a small amount of lubricating fluid. The subarachnoid space, a considerable area between the arachnoid mater and the pia mater, contains circulating CSF. In addition, the subarachnoid space has a vast network of arteries traveling through it.

Brain (Encephalon)

The brain is approximately 2% of body weight. Brain weight and size decrease with aging, primarily because of neuronal loss. The brain is divided into three major areas: the cerebrum, the brainstem, and the cerebellum.

Cerebrum

The *cerebrum* is composed of the right and left cerebral hemispheres, basal ganglia, and diencephalon. The cerebral hemispheres are separated by a deep longitudinal fissure. The *corpus callosum* consists of fibers that travel from one hemisphere to the other, providing intricate connections between the two hemispheres.

Each person has a dominant hemisphere. The left hemisphere specializes in language for most individuals and dominates

skilled and gesturing hand movements. The right hemisphere specializes in the perception of certain nonverbal auditory stimuli, such as music. Processing visual information and determining spatial relationships are also functions of the right hemisphere. The two sides of the brain communicate with each other to facilitate coordinated interactions.

The surface of each hemisphere appears wrinkled because of the numerous raised areas called *gyri* (Fig. 14.4). Each gyrus folds into another, causing the convoluted appearance and substantially increasing the surface area of the brain. The surface of the cerebral hemisphere is approximately six cells deep and is called the *cerebral cortex,* or gray matter. Beneath the cortex is a layer of white matter, consisting of mostly myelinated axons, which serve as association and projection pathways.

A *fissure,* or *sulcus,* is a separation in the cerebral hemisphere. The fissures serve as important divisions or landmarks (see Fig. 14.4). The longitudinal fissure separates the cerebral hemispheres into left and right sections. The lateral, or Sylvian, fissure divides the frontal and temporal lobes of the cerebrum. The central, or Rolandic, fissure separates the frontal and parietal lobes. The parieto-occipital fissure separates the occipital lobe from the parietal and temporal lobes.

Each lobe of the cerebrum has a specific function. Knowledge of the functions for each lobe (Table 14.1) guides assessment and facilitates localization of the patient's problem.

The *diencephalon,* located on the inferior surface (see Fig. 14.4), connects the brainstem to the cerebrum and the midbrain. It is divided into four paired regions: thalamus, hypothalamus, subthalamus, and epithalamus. The *thalamus* is the largest structure within the diencephalon; it integrates all

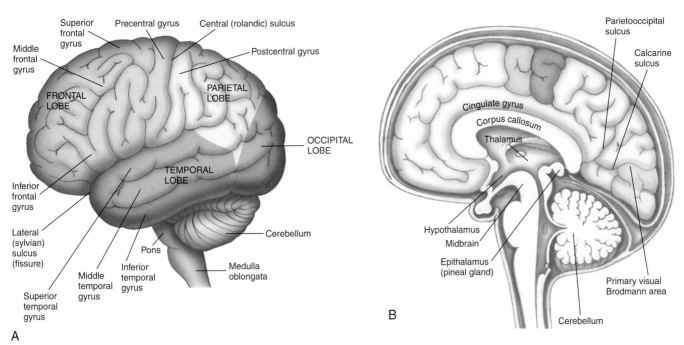

Fig. 14.4 Cerebral hemispheres and structures of the brain. **A,** Lateral external view. **B,** Midsagittal view. (From Patton KT, Thibodeau GA. *Anthony's Textbook of Anatomy and Physiology.* 20th ed. St. Louis, MO: Mosby, 2013.)

TABLE 14.1	**Functions of the Cerebral Hemispheres**
Structure	**Function**
Frontal lobes	Conscious thought, abstract thinking, judgment, voluntary movement on opposite side of the body; prefrontal areas are responsible for affect, memory, and concentration; motor expression of language in Broca's area on the left side in most individuals
Parietal lobes	Processing, association, and interpretation of sensory information from opposite side of the body
Temporal lobes	Processing, association, and interpretation of auditory information; comprehension of language in Wernicke's area on the left side in most individuals; medial portion is responsible for memory and social behavior
Occipital lobes	Visual processing and interpretation
Basal ganglia	Motor control of fine body movements

bodily sensations except smell. The thalamus assists in recognizing pain, touch, and temperature and relays sensory information to the cerebrum. It also plays a role in emotions, arousal and alertness, and complex reflexes. The *hypothalamus* acts as a regulatory center for the autonomic nervous system (ANS). The general functions of the hypothalamus include temperature control, water balance, control of appetite and thirst, cardiovascular regulation, sleep-wake cycle, circadian rhythms, and sexual activity. The hypothalamus also controls the release of hormones from the pituitary gland.

Brainstem. The *brainstem* is at the central core of the brain and controls vital functions. The major divisions of the brainstem are the midbrain, pons, and medulla (see Fig. 14.4). The *midbrain,* also known as the mesencephalon, is a short segment of brainstem lying between the diencephalon and the pons. It contains nuclei of cranial nerves III (oculomotor) and IV (trochlear). The midbrain relays impulses to and from the cerebrum and lower brainstem. It also serves as the center for auditory and visual reflexes. The *pons* is seated between the

midbrain and the medulla. It contains nuclei of cranial nerves V (trigeminal), VI (abducens), VII (facial), and VIII (vestibulocochlear), and it connects the cerebellum to the brainstem. In conjunction with the medulla, the pons controls the rate and duration of respirations. The *medulla oblongata* is situated between the pons and the spinal cord. It contains nuclei of cranial nerves IX (glossopharyngeal), X (vagus), XI (accessory), and XII (hypoglossal). The medulla regulates the basic rhythm of respiration, rate and strength of the pulse, and vasomotor activity. In addition, neurons within the medulla regulate certain reflexes, including sneezing, swallowing, coughing, and vomiting.

Cerebellum. The *cerebellum* is located posterior to the brainstem (see Fig. 14.4). It is connected to the brainstem at the pons by three paired cerebellar peduncles. The peduncles receive input from the spinal cord and brainstem and send it to the cerebellar cortex. The functions of equilibrium, fine movement, muscle tone, balance, and coordination are mediated by the cerebellum.

Specialized Systems Within the Central Nervous System.
The *limbic system* provides primitive control of emotional responses and arousal. Structures of the limbic system include the amygdala (reward and fear stimuli), hippocampus (long-term memory), cingulate gyrus (attention and cognition), and connections to the hypothalamus and thalamus. The *reticular activating system* (RAS) consists of diffuse fibers that begin in the lower brainstem and connect to various locations in the cerebral cortex. The RAS controls arousal, the sleep-wake cycle, selective attention, and perceptual awareness. If the RAS is intact, a person is aware and attentive. When the RAS is impaired, the person experiences inattention, alterations in the sleep-wake cycle, or decreased arousal, which is manifested as coma.

Spinal Cord

The *spinal cord* is surrounded by the vertebral column and meninges. It begins as an extension from the medulla and ends at the first lumbar vertebra. The dura and arachnoid layers of the meninges surround the spinal cord and contain CSF.

The *spinal cord* has 31 segments: 8 cervical, 12 thoracic, 5 lumbar, 5 sacral, and 1 coccygeal (Fig. 14.5). The spinal nerves, originating at each segment of the spinal cord, are part of the PNS. They transmit information to and from the periphery and the spinal cord. These nerves innervate the skin and musculature of most of the body. Each spinal nerve consists of a *dorsal root* (posterior) and *ventral root* (anterior). The dorsal roots convey afferent impulses (sensory input) into the spinal cord from skin segments that represent specific areas of the body known as *dermatomes*. The ventral roots carry efferent impulses (muscle signals) from the spinal cord to specific areas of the body known as *myotomes*. A dermatome and myotome chart traces the spinal nerves to their point of skin or muscle innervation and provides anatomical clues about level of injury or dysfunction (Fig. 14.6).

The spinal nerves interconnect in three areas: the cervical, brachial, and lumbosacral plexuses. The *cervical plexus* includes spinal nerves C1 to C4 and innervates the muscles of the neck and shoulders. The phrenic nerve originates in this plexus and supplies the diaphragm. The *brachial plexus* comprises spinal nerves C5 to C8 and T1 and innervates the arms via the radial and ulnar nerves. The *lumbosacral plexus* is formed by spinal nerves L1 to L5 and S1 to S3. The femoral nerve arises from the lumbar plexus and the sciatic nerve from the sacral plexus; both nerves innervate the legs (see Fig. 14.5).

The cross-sectional size of the spinal cord varies by level, but structures remain the same at all levels. The H-shaped gray matter comprises the center of the cord. The anterior gray matter contains *sensory fibers* that convey sensory impulses from organs and muscles to the spinal cord. The posterior gray matter relays motor impulses from the spinal cord to skeletal muscles. The white matter of the cord consists of fibers that connect with gray matter; together, they comprise the ascending (sensory) and descending (motor) pathways.

Peripheral Nervous System

The PNS comprises the 12 paired cranial nerves, 31 paired spinal nerves, and the ANS. The 12 pairs of *cranial nerves* originate in the brain and brainstem and exit from the cranial cavity. Cranial nerves have sensory or motor functions, or both. These nerves are primarily responsible for the innervation of structures in the head and neck. A summary of the functions of the cranial nerves and their assessment in the critically ill patient is provided in Table 14.2.

The ANS comprises motor nerves that innervate visceral effectors: cardiac muscle; smooth muscle; adrenal medulla; and various glands, including salivary, gastric, and sweat glands. The ANS controls visceral activities at an unconscious level. The ANS consists of the *sympathetic nervous system* and the *parasympathetic nervous system*. These parallel systems act to regulate visceral organs in opposing ways—one system stimulates effectors and the other inhibits—to maintain homeostasis.

The *sympathetic nervous system* is known as the thoracolumbar system because the nerve fibers originate in the thoracic and lumbar regions of the spinal cord. This system contains a chain of ganglia located on each side of the vertebrae. The sympathetic nervous system is sometimes called the *fight-or-flight* system because it is activated and dominates during stressful periods. Most sympathetic neurons release the neurotransmitter norepinephrine at the visceral effector. Sympathetic impulses cause vasoconstriction in the skin and viscera, vasodilation in the skeletal muscles, an increase in the heart rate and force of contraction, an increase in blood pressure

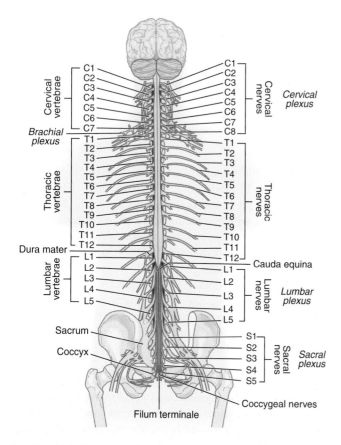

Fig. 14.5 Spinal nerves and nerve plexuses as they relate to vertebral level. The names of the vertebrae are listed on the left, and the corresponding spinal nerves and plexuses are listed on the right.

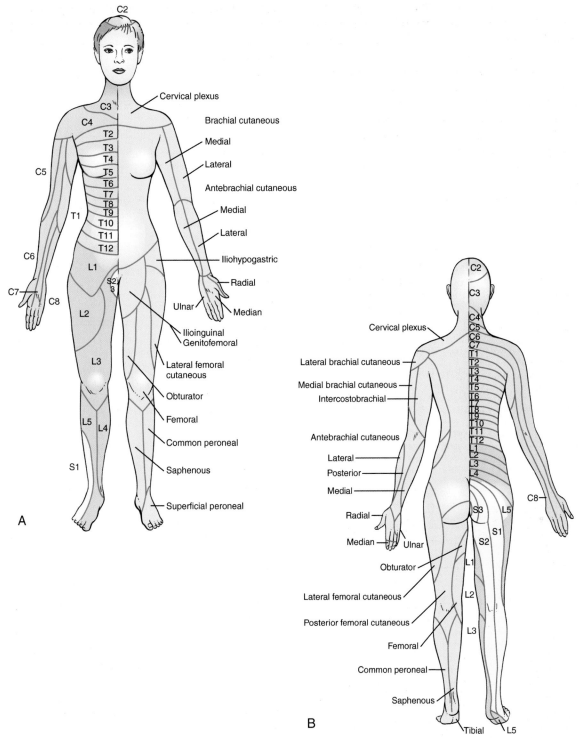

Fig. 14.6 Segmental distribution of the spinal nerves. **A,** Distribution in the front. **B,** Distribution in the back. (Sartz MH. *Textbook of Physical Diagnosis.* 7th ed. St. Louis, MO: Mosby; 2014.)

(BP), dilation of the bronchioles, an increase in sweat gland activity, dilation of the pupils, a decrease in peristalsis, and contraction of the pilomotor muscles (gooseflesh).

The *parasympathetic nervous system* is known as the craniosacral system because the preganglionic fibers originate at certain cranial nerves and in the sacral spinal cord. The axons are long, and ganglia are situated adjacent to or within specific organs. The parasympathetic system is dominant in nonstressful situations. It stimulates visceral activities associated with maintenance of normal functions. The effects of parasympathetic nervous system stimulation induce the return of systems to a normal state of functioning. All neurons within the parasympathetic nervous system release the neurotransmitter acetylcholine at the visceral effector.

TABLE 14.2 The Cranial Nerves and Their Assessment in the Critically Ill Patient

Nerve	Major Functions	Assessment
I—Olfactory (S)	Smell	Evaluate ability to identify familiar smells. Important to assess with basilar skull fracture or surgery on the skull base.
II—Optic (S)	Visual acuity	Assess gross ability to see and field of peripheral vision.
III—Oculomotor (M)	Movement of eyes; pupillary constriction and accommodation	Evaluate pupil size (mm), shape, and equality with bright penlight or pupillometer in dimly lit room. Assess for direct and consensual reaction to light; rate as brisk, sluggish, or nonreactive.
IV—Trochlear (M)	Movement of eyes	Evaluate voluntary movement of eyes together—up, down, laterally, and diagonally (tests CNs III, IV, and VI). In unconscious patients with stable cervical spine, assess *oculocephalic reflex* (doll's eye): turn the patient's head quickly from side to side while holding the eyes open. Note movement of eyes. The doll's eye reflex is present and cranial nerve intact if the eyes move bilaterally in the opposite direction of the head movement. Do not check if neck is unstable. Assess for nystagmus.
V—Trigeminal (S/M)	Chewing; sensation of scalp, face, teeth	Assess corneal reflex; observe for bilateral blink.
VI—Abducens (M)	Movement of eyes	See CN IV.
VII—Facial (M)	Facial expression; lacrimation, salivation; taste anterior tongue	Assess facial muscles for symmetry; if possible, ask patient to open eyes, arch eyebrows, smile, frown, and puff cheeks.
VIII—Auditory (S)	Hearing (cochlear)	Assess response to verbalization (gross hearing ability).
	Equilibrium (vestibular)	In the unconscious patient, the caloric irrigation test is done to assess the *oculovestibular reflex* (may be more sensitive than the doll's eye): elevate the head of bed to 30 degrees to assess for intact tympanic membrane; irrigate the ear canal with cold water. Bilateral eye movement toward the irrigated ear indicates an intact reflex.
IX—Glossopharyngeal (S/M)	Swallowing; taste posterior tongue; general sensation pharynx	CNs IX and X are evaluated together. Evaluate cough and gag reflex in response to suctioning the endotracheal tube and pharynx. Assess ability to manage oral secretions by swallowing.
X—Vagus (S/M)	Swallowing and laryngeal control; parasympathetic function	See CN IX.
XI—Spinal accessory (M)	Movement of head and shoulders	Assess ability to move and shrug shoulders and turn head.
XII—Hypoglossal (M)	Movement of tongue	If patient able to follow commands, assess ability to protrude and/or move tongue from side to side.

CN, Cranial nerve; *M,* motor; *S,* sensory; *S/M,* sensory and motor.

STUDY BREAK
1. All of the following are true about the brainstem functions except:
   A. The brainstem is responsible for temperature control.
   B. Mechanisms that regulate respiratory rhythm are located in the brainstem.
   C. The brainstem connects the cerebellum to the rest of the brain.
   D. Nuclei for most cranial nerves are located in the brainstem.

Assessment

A thorough history provides information about the patient's condition. Ideally, the patient is the primary source of the historical data. If the patient is unable to give a history, obtain information from family or friends about symptoms, onset, progression, and chronology of the event. Comorbidities and contributing factors must also be considered. If pain is a presenting symptom, obtain information about the location, onset, type, duration, presence of other symptoms, and what makes the pain better or worse. Some changes occur with aging (see Lifespan Considerations box).

An initial baseline neurological assessment, along with ongoing assessments, assists in monitoring the patient's condition and the response to treatments and nursing interventions. When performing a neurological assessment, focus on mental status; level of consciousness (LOC); and cranial nerve, motor, and sensory function. Because many neurological changes represent life-threatening conditions that require emergent treatment, immediately report adverse assessment findings to the physician.

👤 LIFESPAN CONSIDERATIONS

Effects of Age on the Nervous System

Older Adults

- In older adults, the effects of certain medications used to decrease intracranial pressure (e.g., osmotic and loop diuretics, barbiturates) are closely monitored because of decreased ability to absorb, metabolize, and/or excrete these medications.
- Assess for preexisting renal insufficiency and diuretic use because diuretics may place older adults at risk for hypokalemia or hyponatremia when used to reduce intracranial pressure.
- In the older adult, elevating the head of the bed to decrease intracranial pressure may compromise an already diminished cerebral blood flow. Continuous assessment of neurological function and/or cerebral perfusion pressure is necessary to prevent decreasing blood flow to the brain.
- Central cord syndrome is more common in older adults and may result from hyperextension of an osteoarthritic spine.
- Subdural hematomas are more common in older adults because as the brain atrophies with aging, it shrinks away from the dura and stretches bridging veins, which may easily tear. A large amount of blood can accumulate in the subdural space before the patient demonstrates overt signs and symptoms. Subtle mental status changes are often the first finding and are easily misinterpreted as signs of normal aging.

❗ CLINICAL ALERT

Neurological Assessment

Perform the neurological assessment with the nurse who just cared for the patient as part of hand-off report. This ensures complete understanding of the prior documented assessment by the receiving nurse and quick recognition of neurological changes.

Mental Status. When assessing a patient's mental status, assess consciousness (awareness of self and the environment), cognition (the ability to produce a response, including expressive and receptive language), and memory.

The Glasgow Coma Scale (GCS; Fig. 14.7) is a commonly used standardized tool that assesses consciousness and cognition. Evaluate the patient's ability to speak, open the eyes, and produce a motor response to verbal command or noxious stimuli. A noxious stimulus may include firm pressure applied to the nail bed, a trapezium squeeze, supraorbital pressure, or sternal pressure. Apply noxious stimuli only if the patient fails to respond to verbal stimuli. Care is taken to avoid injury when applying noxious stimuli.

The best response in each of the three categories of eye opening, verbal response, and motor response is scored, and the three scores are summed. GCS scores range from 3 (deep coma) to 15 (normal functioning). A GCS of 8 or less is consistent with coma. Several conditions limit application of the GCS, including medications, such as sedatives and neuromuscular blockade, and concurrent injuries, such as SCI. GCS is a measure of consciousness and cognition; it does not replace neurological assessment of specific brain function.

Additional scales used to monitor overall status in critical care settings have been gaining acceptance. The full outline of unresponsiveness (FOUR) score, which evaluates eye

Glasgow Coma Scale				
Eyes	Open		Spontaneously	4
			To verbal command	3
			To pain	2
			No response	1
Best motor response	To verbal command		Obeys	6
	To painful stimulus		Localizes pain	5
			Flexion-withdrawal	4
			Flexion-abnormal (Decorticate rigidity)	3
			Extension (Decerebrate rigidity)	2
			No response	1
Best verbal response			Oriented and converses	5
			Disoriented and converses	4
			Inappropriate words	3
			Incomprehensible sounds	2
			No response	1
Total				3-15

Fig. 14.7 The Glasgow Coma Scale is a measure of consciousness based on eye opening, movement, and verbal responses. Each response is given a number, and the three scores are summed. Scores range from 3 to 15.

response, motor response, breathing pattern, and brainstem reflexes, is one scale in use.[17,27] Scores on this scale range from 0 to 16, with lower scores indicating lower level of responsiveness. This scale may be more reliable than the GCS in lower levels of responsiveness and is predictive of poor outcomes but has not been systematically studied.[27] Although additional scales, such as the AVPU (alert, responds to voice and pain, unresponsive) scale and the Reaction Level Scale, are used in some settings, they have not been widely adopted.[27]

❓ CRITICAL REASONING ACTIVITY

What interventions can you teach families to assist in the care and rehabilitation of patients with prolonged unconsciousness after a head injury or cranial surgery?

Language. Assess fluency and spontaneity of speech, word-finding ability, and comprehension. If the patient is intubated and responsive, ask the patient to perform simple verbal commands such as pointing to the clock, blinking the eyes, or raising the right arm. Language skills may also be evaluated by asking the patient to write responses.

Language deficits are common in neurological disorders. *Expressive dysphasia* is a deficit in language output or speech production caused by a dysfunction in the dominant frontal lobe. It varies from mild word-finding difficulty to complete loss of both verbal and written communication skills. The inability to comprehend language and follow commands is called *receptive dysphasia*. Receptive dysphasia indicates dysfunction in the dominant temporal lobe. A nonintubated patient with receptive problems can speak spontaneously, but the verbal response does not follow the context of the conversation. An intubated patient with receptive aphasia may appear to be responsive but is unable to follow simple verbal commands.

Memory. Evaluate both short- and long-term memory. To assess *short-term memory,* ask the patient to recall the names of three common words or objects (e.g., chair, clock, blue) after a 3-minute interval. Test *long-term memory* by asking the patient questions about the distant past (e.g., birth place, year of birth, year of graduation from school, year of marriage). If intubated and responsive, the patient can write the answers.

Cranial Nerve Function. On initial baseline neurological assessment, assess all cranial nerves. Focused cranial nerve assessments may be conducted depending on the anatomy involved. Table 14.2 presents assessments that can be done in patients who are critically ill, who often have a decreased LOC.

Pupil examination is the most critical component of cranial nerve assessment. Assess pupils for size, shape, equality, and direct and consensual response to light. Normal pupil diameter ranges from 1.5 to 6 mm. Measurement with a millimeter scale is the most reliable method of determining size and equality. A pupillometer may provide a more objective measure than manual testing.[21] Unequal pupils *(anisocoria)* occur normally in approximately 10% of the general population. Otherwise, inequality of pupils is a sign of a pathological process. A change in pupil reaction to light in one or both eyes is an important sign that may indicate increasing ICP or neurological deterioration. Hypoxia and medications may also influence pupillary size and reactivity to light.

Motor Function. Assess all extremity movement, muscle strength, muscle tone and posture, and coordination. Assess muscle groups for symmetry, and complete a more comprehensive assessment if the patient is able to follow commands. If the patient does not follow commands, assess motor response to noxious stimuli. Ask the patient to move the extremities on command, or observe the patient's ability to move around in bed. Grade muscle strength of the extremities on a five-point scale (Table 14.3). The grading is based on the ability to move muscle groups, hold a position against gravity, and maintain that position against resistance.

It is important to assess each limb because differences between the right and left sides and between upper and lower extremities can occur. In persons with SCI, individual muscle function by myotome (Table 14.4) is assessed to identify the level of injury. *Hemiplegia* exists when one side of the patient's body is affected. *Paraplegia* exists when two of the same extremities are paralyzed. *Quadriplegia* or *tetraplegia* exists when all four extremities are paralyzed.

In a conscious patient, check for *arm drift* to detect subtle weakness. Ask the patient to close the eyes and stretch out the arms with palms up for 20 to 30 seconds. A downward drift of the arm or pronation of the palm indicates subtle weakness in the involved extremity.

TABLE 14.3 Grading Scale for Motor Responses

Numerical Rating	Motor Response
0	Unable to lift the arm or leg to command or in response to painful stimuli
1	Flicker of movement is felt or seen in the muscle(s) of the limb
2	Moves the limb but unable to raise the extremity off the bed
3	Able to lift the extremity off the bed briefly but does not have the strength to maintain the lift
4	Able to lift the extremity off the bed but has difficulty resisting the examiner ("I am going to push your right arm/leg down, so try to prevent me from doing that.")
5	Able to lift the extremity off the bed and maintain the position against resistance

TABLE 14.4 Spinal Nerve Innervation (Myotomes) of Major Muscle Groups

Spinal Nerve	Muscle Group Movement	Assessment Technique
C4-C5	Shoulder abduction	Shoulders shrugged against downward pressure of examiner's hands
C5	Elbow flexion (biceps)	Arm pulled up from resting position against resistance
C7	Elbow extension (triceps)	From the flexed position, arm straightened out against resistance
	Thumb–index finger pinch	Index finger held firmly to thumb against resistance to pull apart
C8	Hand grasp	Hand grasp strength evaluated
L2	Hip flexion	Leg lifted from bed against resistance
L3	Knee extension	From flexed position, knee extended against resistance
L4	Foot dorsiflexion	Foot pulled up toward nose against resistance
S1	Foot plantar flexion	Foot pushed down (stepping on the gas) against resistance

Assess muscle tone by taking each extremity through passive range of motion. Normal muscle tone shows slight resistance to range of motion. Flaccid muscles have diminished muscle tone, with no resistance to movement. Increased muscle tone is manifested as spasticity or rigidity.

Coordination of movement is under cerebellar control. Ask the patient to perform rapid alternating movements, such as touching the finger to the nose or running the heel down the shin bilaterally. These tests require the patient to be able to follow verbal commands. Incoordination or exaggerated movements may indicate cerebellar injury.

Abnormal posturing may be observed in unconscious patients with brain damage. These include flexor (decorticate)

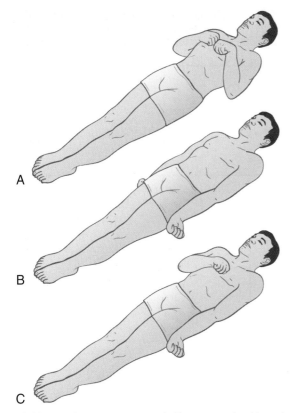

Fig. 14.8 Abnormal motor responses. **A,** Flexor posturing (decorticate). **B,** Extensor posturing (decerebrate). **C,** Flexor posturing on right side and extensor posturing on left side.

or extensor (decerebrate) posturing (Fig. 14.8). *Flexor posturing* involves rigid flexion and adduction of the arms, wrist flexion with clenched fists, and extension and internal rotation of the legs. It usually occurs secondary to damage of the corticospinal tract. *Extensor posturing* is the result of a midbrain or pons lesion. In this posture, the arms and legs are rigidly extended, and the feet are in plantar extension. The forearms may be pronated and abducted, and the wrists and fingers are flexed. Abnormal posturing can occur in response to noxious stimuli, such as suctioning or pain, or it may be spontaneous. Different posturing may be noted on each side of the body.

Reflexes. There are three types of reflexes: deep tendon, superficial, and pathological. *Deep tendon reflexes* (DTRs) are obtained by a brisk tap of a reflex hammer on the tendons of a muscle group to elicit a motor response. The biceps reflex assesses spinal nerve roots C5-C6; brachioradialis, C5-C6; triceps, C7-C8; patellar, L2-L4; and Achilles tendon, S1-S2. DTRs are graded according to the response elicited: 0, no reflex; 1+, hypoactive; 2+, normal; 3+, increased but normal; 4+, very brisk, hyperreflexive, clonus. Alterations in DTRs may indicate damage of the spinal cord or brain. In spinal shock, DTRs are absent below the level of injury initially; return of DTRs signals resolution of spinal shock. Aging and metabolic factors, such as thyroid dysfunction or electrolyte abnormalities, may diminish DTRs.

Superficial reflexes are elicited by touching or stroking a specific area and observing the motor response. The corneal reflex is a superficial reflex, as are the palpebral, gag, abdominal, cremasteric, and anal reflexes.

Pathological reflexes are typically present at birth, disappear with maturing of the nervous system, then reappear as a consequence of impaired neurological function. The most common pathological reflex is the Babinski reflex. When the sole of the patient's foot is lightly stroked, the normal response is plantar flexion of the toes. A Babinski reflex is present when dorsiflexion of the great toe with fanning of the other toes is observed with stimulation. In an adult, the presence of a Babinski reflex is a sign of an upper motor neuron lesion and damage to the corticospinal tract. Other pathological reflexes include the suck (sucking motions in response to touching the lips), snout (lip pursing in response to touching the lips), palmar (grasp in response to stroking the palm), and palmomental (contraction of the facial muscle in response to stimulation of the thenar eminence near the thumb) reflexes in adults.

Sensory Function. Sensory assessment evaluates the patient's ability to discriminate a sharp stimulus (such as a pinprick), position sense, and temperature. Sensory function in the skin is supplied by a single spinal nerve or sensory dermatome (see Fig. 14.6). For example, the ability to sense a superficial pinprick on the lateral forearm, thumb, and index finger tests innervation of the C6 dermatome. To assess position sense, instruct the patient to close the eyes. Move the patient's thumb or big toe up or down, or leave it in a neutral position, and ask the patient to identify the pattern of movement. To discriminate temperature, ask the patient to identify the sensation when a hot or cold container is touched to the skin. Sensation cannot be assessed in coma but is implied if the patient responds to painful stimulation.

Respiratory Assessment. Assess the respiratory pattern and rate as part of the neurological assessment. Changes in the respiratory pattern can indicate neurological deterioration. Table 14.5 describes abnormal respiratory patterns seen in neurological disorders. These patterns may be obscured in mechanically ventilated patients.

TABLE 14.5 Anatomical Correlates of Abnormal Respiratory Patterns in Neurological Disorders

Abnormal Pattern	Anatomical Correlate
Cheyne-Stokes respiration	Bilateral deep cerebral lesion or some cerebellar lesions
Central neurogenic hyperventilation	Lesions of the midbrain and upper pons
Apneustic	Lesions of the middle to lower pons
Cluster breathing	Lesions of the lower pons or upper medulla
Ataxic respirations	Lesions of the medulla

TABLE 14.6   Components of the Hourly Neurological Assessment for Patients With Increased Intracranial Pressure, Head Injury, or Acute Stroke

Mental Status	Focal Motor	Pupils	Brainstem/Cranial Nerves
Glasgow Coma Scale • Assesses level of consciousness, expressive language, ability to follow commands	Move all extremities Strength of all extremities (compare right and left sides) Motor response	Size Shape Reaction to light (direct and consensual) Extraocular movements	Corneal reflex • Present: immediate blinking bilaterally • Diminished: blinking asymmetrically • Absent: no blinking Cough, gag, swallow reflex • Observe for excessive drooling • Observe for cough/swallow reflex

Hourly Assessment. Neurological parameters are assessed based on the ordered frequency (often hourly) and the severity of the patient's condition. Reassessment is also done if changes are noted. Table 14.6 contains the components of an hourly neurological assessment for patients with increased ICP, head injury, or acute stroke. Focused assessments are performed based on the patient's specific condition. Document all findings per unit protocol and report abnormal findings to the physician immediately.

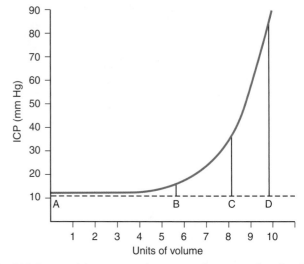

Fig. 14.9 Intracranial pressure–volume curve. Between points *A* and *B*, intracranial compliance is present. Intracranial pressure *(ICP)* is normal, and increases in intracranial volume are tolerated without large increases in ICP. As compliance is lost, small increases in volume result in large and dangerous increases in ICP (points *C* and *D*).

INCREASED INTRACRANIAL PRESSURE

A commonly encountered problem in the critical care setting is increased ICP. Many neurological problems are associated with increased ICP, such as brain injury and stroke. Sustained increases in ICP compound the extent of brain injury and can be life-threatening. Therefore it is important to assess and maintain ICP within normal limits.

Pathophysiology

The rigid cranial vault contains three types of noncompressible contents: brain tissue, blood, and CSF. The pressure exerted by the combined volumes of these three components is ICP. If the volume of any one of these components increases, the volume of one or both of the other compartments must decrease proportionally or an increase in ICP occurs (Monro-Kellie doctrine). This compensation is called *compliance* (Fig. 14.9). With adequate compliance, an increase in intracranial volume is compensated by displacement of CSF into the spinal subarachnoid space, displacement of blood into the venous sinuses, or both. The ICP remains normal despite increases in volume (flat part of curve). As compensatory mechanisms are exhausted, a small increase in volume leads to a large increase in ICP (steep part of curve).

As compliance decreases, ICP increases and CBF decreases. When CBF decreases, the brain becomes hypoxic, carbon dioxide levels increase, and acidosis occurs. In response to these changes, the cerebral blood vessels dilate to increase CBF. This compensatory response further increases intracranial volume, creating a vicious cycle that can be life-threatening (Fig. 14.10).

Normal ICP ranges from 0 to 15 mm Hg. Increased ICP is defined as a pressure of 20 mm Hg or greater persisting for 5 minutes or longer; it is a life-threatening event. Sustained increases in ICP can lead to *herniation*, which is caused by shifting of brain tissue from an area of high pressure to one of lower pressure. Herniation syndromes are classified as supratentorial (cingulate, central, and uncal herniation) or infratentorial (cerebellar tonsil herniation). These herniation syndromes are described in Table 14.7 and shown in Fig. 14.11.

Along with MAP, the ICP determines cerebral perfusion pressure (CPP), which is the pressure required to perfuse the brain. CPP is calculated as the difference between MAP and ICP (CPP = MAP − ICP). The normal CPP in an adult is between 60 and 100 mm Hg; it must be maintained at 70 mm Hg or greater in those with brain pathology. Any factor that decreases MAP and/or increases ICP decreases the CPP. CPP determines CBF; therefore ischemia or infarction can occur if the CPP is inadequate. Measures to promote adequate CPP include lowering of increased ICP

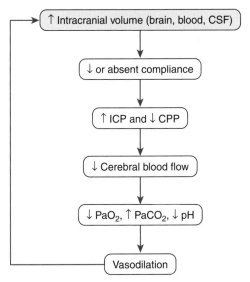

Fig. 14.10 Pathophysiology flow diagram for increased intracranial pressure. *CPP,* Cerebral perfusion pressure; *CSF,* cerebrospinal fluid; *ICP,* intracranial pressure; *PaCO₂,* partial pressure of arterial carbon dioxide; *PaO₂,* partial pressure of arterial oxygen.

or, if this is not possible, increasing MAP to offset the effects of ICP on CPP. Often MAP will rise in the presence of increased ICP; lowering MAP in this circumstance actually may decrease CPP and should be prevented.[1,5]

Causes of Increased Intracranial Pressure

Factors that increase ICP are associated with increased brain volume, increased cerebral blood volume (CBV), and increased CSF.

Increased Brain Volume. A common cause of increased brain volume is cerebral edema, which is an increase in the water content of the brain tissue. Cytotoxic edema and vasogenic edema are two categories of cerebral edema; they may occur independently or together. *Cytotoxic cerebral edema* is characterized by intracellular swelling of neurons, most often as a result of hypoxia and hypo-osmolality. Hypoxia causes decreased ATP production, leading to the failure of the sodium-potassium pump in the cellular membrane. This allows sodium, chloride, and water to enter the cell while potassium exits. Cytotoxic edema is associated with brain ischemia or hypoxic events such as stroke or cardiac arrest. It is also seen with hypo-osmolar

TABLE 14.7	**Herniation Syndromes**	
Syndrome	**Definition**	**Symptoms**
Cingulate	Shift of brain tissue from one cerebral hemisphere under the falx cerebri to the other hemisphere	No specific symptoms; may have focal motor deficit; herniation may compromise cerebral blood flow
Central	Downward shift of cerebral hemispheres, basal ganglia, and diencephalon through the tentorial notch that compresses the brainstem	Early • Decrease in LOC • Motor weakness • Cheyne-Stokes respiration • Small, reactive pupils Late • Coma • Pupils dilated and fixed • Abnormal flexor posturing, progressing to abnormal extensor posturing • Unstable vital signs progressing to cardiopulmonary arrest
Uncal	Unilateral lesion forces uncus of temporal lobe to displace through the tentorial notch, compressing the midbrain Symptoms can progress rapidly	Early • Decreased LOC • Increased muscle tone • Positive Babinski reflex • Cheyne-Stokes respiration, progressing to central neurogenic hyperventilation • Ipsilateral dilated pupil • Weakness Late • Pupils dilated and fixed • Paralyzed eye movements • Contralateral hemiplegia • Abnormal flexor posturing, progressing to abnormal extensor posturing • Unstable vital signs progressing to cardiopulmonary arrest
Cerebellar tonsil	Displacement of cerebellar tonsils through foramen magnum, compressing the pons and medulla	Alterations in respiratory and cardiopulmonary function, rapidly progressing to cardiopulmonary arrest

LOC, Level of consciousness.

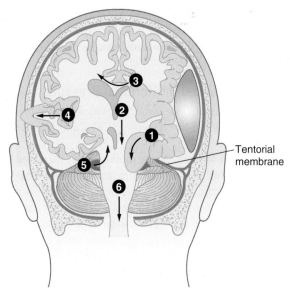

Fig. 14.11 Types of brain herniation. Herniation can occur above and below the tentorial membrane. Supratentorial: *1*, uncal (transtentorial); *2*, central; *3*, cingulate; *4*, transcalvarial (external herniation through an opening in the skull). Infratentorial: *5*, upward herniation of cerebellum; *6*, cerebellar tonsillar moves down through the foramen magnum. (From Huether SE, McCance KL. *Understanding Pathophysiology.* 6th ed. St. Louis, MO: Mosby, 2017.)

conditions, including water intoxication and hyponatremia. *Vasogenic cerebral edema* occurs as a result of increased capillary permeability. With increased permeability, osmotically active substances (proteins) leak into the brain interstitium and draw water from the vascular system, leading to an increase in fluid in the extracellular space and consequently an increase in ICP. Brain injuries, brain tumors, meningitis, and abscesses are common causes of vasogenic cerebral edema. It is important to distinguish between the two types of edema where possible, as treatment may differ.

Increased Cerebral Blood Volume. Several mechanisms increase CBV. These include loss of autoregulation, physiological responses to decreased cerebral oxygenation, increased metabolic demand, and obstruction of venous outflow.

Within normal limits, the cerebral vasculature exhibits pressure and chemical autoregulation. Autoregulation provides a constant CBV and CPP over a wide range of MAPs. Pathological states such as head injury or hypertension often lead to a loss of autoregulation. Without autoregulation, hyperemia may occur, leading to increased ICP.[1,2]

Decreased cerebral oxygenation leads to cerebral vasodilation in an attempt to improve oxygen delivery. Hypercapnia also causes vasodilation in the brain. Any factor that results in hypoxemia or hypercapnia, such as ineffective ventilation, airway obstruction, or endotracheal suctioning, can contribute to an increase in ICP.

CBF may increase to augment oxygen supply in response to increased metabolic demands. Several factors increase oxygen demands, including fever, physical activity, pain, shivering, and seizures.[1,5] Grouping nursing activities together (e.g., bathing, suctioning, turning) may also increase metabolic demands. Although sleep and rest are important, oxygen demands are

higher during rapid eye movement (REM) sleep. Increases in ICP may be noted during any of these situations.

Obstruction of venous outflow results in increased CBV and increases ICP. Hyperflexion, hyperextension, or rotation of the neck or tightly applied tracheostomy or endotracheal tube ties may compress the jugular vein, inhibit venous return, and cause central venous engorgement. A tumor or abscess can compress the venous structures, causing an outflow obstruction. Mechanisms that increase intrathoracic or intraabdominal pressure also impair venous return (e.g., coughing, vomiting, posturing, isometric exercise, Valsalva maneuver, positive end-expiratory pressure, hip flexion).

Increased Cerebrospinal Fluid. Hydrocephalus, an increase in CSF, can increase ICP. Hydrocephalus may occur in any circumstance in which CSF flow is obstructed, such as with a tumor of the third ventricle, or absorption is blocked, due to subarachnoid hemorrhage (SAH) or infection (meningitis, encephalitis), or when excess CSF is produced.

Assessment

Assess vital signs and perform a thorough neurological examination with emphasis on LOC and motor and cranial nerve function. Pupillary changes often correlate with ICP changes and are the most critical cranial nerve assessment. Hypertension is common early with increased ICP and represents a compensatory mechanism to augment CPP. Cushing's triad is a late sign of increased ICP and consists of systolic hypertension with a widening pulse pressure, bradycardia, and irregular respirations. It often signifies irreversible damage.

Monitoring Techniques. Invasive monitoring of ICP, cerebral oxygenation, and other physiological parameters may be used to augment the clinical assessment.

Intracranial pressure monitoring. ICP monitoring is used to correlate objective data with the clinical picture and to determine cerebral perfusion. Monitoring is indicated for patients who have a GCS score between 3 and 8 due to a severe brain insult.[12,14] It is used to assess response to therapy (e.g., after administration of osmolar diuretic) or to augment the neurological assessment.

ICP monitoring systems are classified by location of device or type of transducer system. Devices can be placed in one of the ventricles; in the parenchyma; or in the subarachnoid, epidural, or subdural spaces (Fig. 14.12). Each site has advantages and disadvantages (Table 14.8). Ventricular devices are most commonly used for monitoring because they also allow therapeutic interventions. A ventricular catheter system, also known as a *ventriculostomy,* may be connected to a drainage bag to drain CSF in a controlled manner to relieve increased ICP or to remove blood products after SAH. The ventricular catheter system allows continuous monitoring only, continuous CSF drainage only, or both monitoring and CSF drainage, depending on patient need and system used.

The transducer system may be a microchip sensor device, a fiberoptic catheter, or a fluid-filled system.[1] The fluid-filled system is most often used for ICP monitoring. This system is similar to that used for hemodynamic monitoring with a few exceptions. Flush the pressure tubing with sterile normal saline

TABLE 14.8 Intracranial Pressure Monitoring Devices

Device	Location	Advantages	Disadvantages
Intraventricular catheter (ventriculostomy) or fiberoptic transducer	Lateral ventricle of non-dominant hemisphere; may be tunneled or bolted	Therapeutic or diagnostic removal of CSF to control ICP Good ICP waveform quality Accurate and reliable	Highest risk for infection (2%-5%) Risk for hemorrhage Longer insertion time Rapid CSF drainage may result in collapsed ventricle CSF leakage around insertion site
Subarachnoid bolt or screw	Subarachnoid space	Inserted quickly Does not penetrate brain	Bolt can become occluded with clots or tissue, causing a dampened waveform CSF leakage may occur CSF drainage not possible
Epidural sensor or transducer	Between the skull and the dura	Least invasive Low risk of infection Low risk of hemorrhage Recommended in patients at risk for meningitis or other CNS infections	Indirect measure of ICP Less accurate and reliable CSF drainage not possible
Parenchymal fiberoptic catheter	1 cm into brain tissue	Inserted quickly Accurate and reliable Good ICP waveform quality	CSF drainage not possible Catheter relatively fragile Expensive

CNS, Central nervous system; CSF, cerebrospinal fluid; ICP, intracranial pressure.
Data from Bader MK, Littlejohns L, Olson D. *AANN Core Curriculum for Neuroscience Nursing.* 6th ed. Chicago, IL: American Association of Neuroscience Nurses; 2016.

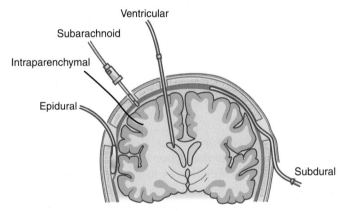

Fig. 14.12 Intracranial pressure monitoring sites. (From Lewis SL, Dirksen SR, Heitkemper MM, et al. *Medical Surgical Nursing: Assessment and Management of Clinical Problems.* 9th ed. St. Louis, MO: Mosby; 2017.)

without preservatives (because preservatives may damage brain tissue), and *do not use* pressurized fluid or flush the system. Zero reference the air-fluid interface at the level of the foramen of Munro. Observe the ICP waveform on a channel on the bedside monitor, and record the mean ICP pressure.

Catheters with internal microchip sensors and fiberoptic catheters have the transducer built into the tip of the catheter. These devices only need to be zero referenced before insertion. They are connected via a cable to a stand-alone monitor provided by the manufacturer. Some devices can be connected to the bedside monitor for an additional display of ICP and waveforms.[1]

ICP monitoring systems allow nurses to observe an ICP waveform pattern.[5] The normal intracranial pulse waveform has three defined peaks of decreasing height that correlate with the arterial pulse waveform and are identified as P_1, P_2, and P_3 (Fig. 14.13). P_1 (percussion wave) is fairly consistent in shape and amplitude; it represents the blood being ejected from the heart and correlates with cardiac systole. Extreme hypotension

or hypertension produces changes in P_1. P_2 (tidal wave) represents intracranial brain bulk. It is variable in shape and is related to the state of compliance. Decreased compliance exists when P_2 is equal to or higher than P_1. It also is helpful in predicting the risk for increases in ICP. P_3 (dicrotic wave) follows the dicrotic notch and represents closure of the aortic valve, correlating with cardiac diastole. Smaller peaks that follow the three main peaks vary among individual patients.[6]

✳ QSEN EXEMPLAR

Safety; Teamwork and Collaboration

A nurse notices that stopcock covers on the external ventricular drainage (EVD) system are the same red color as those used on the arterial pressure and IV lines, making it difficult to distinguish lines and contributing to potential for inadvertent injection of medications into the EVD system. The nurse recognizes that inadvertent injection of medications into the EVD system could contribute to severe neurotoxicities. The nurse brings the issue to a staff meeting for discussion and learns that several staff members have experienced a near-miss event related to challenges with line identification. The nurse works with the unit manager to develop a task force to identify options that would facilitate a more clear system for line identification. One task force member identified additional stopcock color options, while another investigated options for different EVD systems. A third nurse surveyed other institutions in the area for additional solutions. Staff nurses were encouraged to provide suggestions. Options were reviewed with the supply management team to determine availability and cost. Two potential solutions were identified: line labels specifying line type, and stopcock covers of different colors for different types of lines. The two options were presented by the task force to the entire critical care team, and staff nurses voted on the choice they believed to be most appropriate. Different-colored stopcock covers were ultimately used for each line type. Signs were made and posted above each patient bed providing a legend for stopcock cover colors. The nurse worked with the staff educator to inform nurses about the change in stopcock cover color. The nurse worked with the clinical nurse specialist to conduct episodic audits of appropriate stopcock cover use and any additional near-miss events.

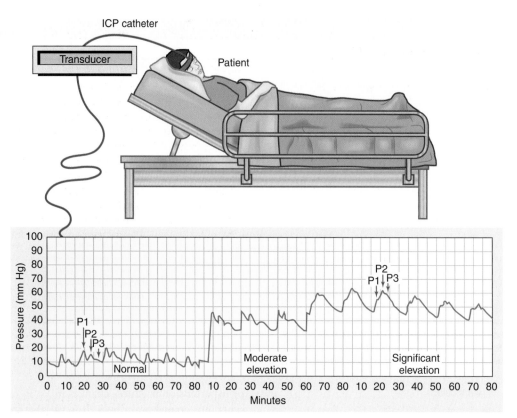

Fig. 14.13 Intracranial pressure *(ICP)* monitoring can be used to continuously measure ICP. The ICP tracing shows normal, elevated, and plateau waves. At high ICP, the P_2 peak is higher than the P_1 peak, and the peaks become less distinct and plateau. (From Lewis SL, Dirksen SR, Heitkemper MM, et al. *Medical Surgical Nursing: Assessment and Management of Clinical Problems.* 9th ed. St. Louis, MO: Mosby; 2017.)

Cerebral oxygenation monitoring. CBF and brain oxygen use may be monitored by *jugular vein oxygen saturation* (S_jO_2). The technology is similar to that for measurement of mixed venous oxygen saturation (SvO_2) in the pulmonary artery. S_jO_2 is monitored via a fiberoptic catheter inserted retrogradely through the internal jugular vein into the jugular venous bulb. Placement of the catheter is verified by a neck radiograph. Oxygen saturation of venous blood is measured as it leaves the brain and provides a global measure of cerebral oxygenation. The normal value is 60% to 70%. Values less than 50% suggest cerebral ischemia. However, because the jugular vein drains only a portion of the brain, normal values do not ensure adequate perfusion to all brain areas.[1,27,28]

The *partial pressure of oxygen within brain tissue* ($PbtO_2$) can be measured by placing a monitoring probe directly into the brain white matter and attaching it to a stand-alone monitor. The probe may be inserted into the damaged portion of the brain to measure regional oxygenation, or it may be inserted into an undamaged portion of the brain to measure global oxygenation. In a patient with TBI, the goal of therapy is to maintain an adequate $PbtO_2$. Current studies recommend a $PbtO_2$ greater than 20 mm Hg. However, the science of brain tissue oxygenation is evolving, and target values may change. Values may also be device specific; therefore it is important to review the manufacturer's literature. Management of low $PbtO_2$ is directed at treating the underlying cause.[1,27,28]

Other physiological monitoring. Hemodynamic monitoring may be used to monitor fluid status and to assist in maintaining adequate cerebral perfusion (see Chapter 9). Continuous monitoring of arterial oxygen saturation via pulse oximetry (SpO_2) and of end-tidal carbon dioxide levels is useful to ensure adequate gas exchange in the neurological patient. Periodic arterial blood gas samples may also be obtained.

Continuous bedside electroencephalographic (EEG) monitoring provides recording of electrical activity in the brain and correlation with ICP monitoring. In some cases, continuous EEG monitoring is used to assess the effects of sedation and neuromuscular blockade medications. Bispectral index monitoring provides a numerical indicator of brain electrical activity (see Chapter 6). Microdialysis is an evolving technology used to measure metabolic markers in the brain.[28] A catheter with a semipermeable membrane is inserted into brain tissue, and a dialysate solution is continuously perfused at an ultralow rate (0.1 to 0.5 μL/min), causing solutes to diffuse across the membrane for sampling. The dialysate is analyzed for biochemical changes. Data obtained from microdialysis can be used to adjust therapies and predict outcomes.

Diagnostic Testing

The initial baseline and ongoing *laboratory tests* obtained in a patient with increased ICP include the following:

- Arterial blood gases, SpO_2, end-tidal carbon dioxide
- Complete blood count, with an emphasis on hematocrit, hemoglobin, and platelets

EVIDENCE-BASED PRACTICE

Positioning for Neurodynamic Stability

Problem

Increased intracranial pressure (ICP), decreased cerebral perfusion pressure (CPP), and decreased brain tissue oxygenation have been associated with poor outcomes after traumatic brain injury (TBI). Commonly used nursing interventions, such as head elevation and repositioning, may adversely affect these neurodynamic parameters.

Clinical Question

What is the optimal position for patients with TBI that promotes neurodynamic stability?

Evidence

Several researchers have investigated the effect of body position on neurodynamics. Head elevation and repositioning are interventions nurses use to maximize systemic and cerebral oxygenation and protect skin while preventing other complications. However, head elevation to 30 degrees and 45 degrees and lateral positioning produced variable neurodynamic responses in severely brain-injured adults.[1,2,5] Multiple neurodynamic measures were used to clarify understanding of these responses. Head elevation to at least 30 degrees significantly decreased ICP but also decreased CPP because of a decrease in mean arterial pressure. Lateral positioning, particularly to the left, with 15-degree head elevation was associated with an increase in ICP, a decrease in CPP, and a decrease in cerebral oxygenation, but not in all patients.[1,2,5] Prone positioning has been reported to increase systemic oxygenation but is also associated with increased ICP and decreased CPP in some patients.[4] Recent guidelines direct arterial pressure measurement be obtained at the same level as ICP monitoring. Subsequent research indicated that placement of the arterial blood pressure transducer can influence CPP values obtained.[3] Collectively, study findings suggest that responses to head elevation and repositioning are highly individualized and depend, in part, on cerebral autoregulatory integrity but also on placement of the arterial pressure monitoring device.

Implications for Nursing

No one position or degree of head elevation is optimal for patients with TBI. Carefully monitor patient response to head elevation and position change, and when adverse changes are noted, consider alternative positions. The left lateral position, with or without head elevation, warrants the greatest attention. If prone positioning is indicated for treatment of respiratory failure, use with caution and closely observe the neurological status during use.[4] No single measure of neurodynamics is beneficial in monitoring response to position change, so multimodality monitoring of response to head elevation and repositioning should be used. Nurses should be aware that arterial pressure transducer placement may also influence interpretation of CPP values that guide assessment of response to head of bed elevation and position change.

Level of Evidence

B—Well-designed controlled studies

References

1. Kim MN, Edlow BL, Durduran T, et al. Continuous optical monitoring of cerebral hemodynamics during head-of-bed manipulation in brain-injured adults. *Neurocrit Care.* 2014;20(3):443–453.
2. Ledwith MB, Bloom S, Maloney-Wilensky E, et al. Effect of body position on cerebral oxygenation and physiologic parameters in patients with acute neurological conditions. *J Neurosci Nurs.* 2010;42(5):280–287.
3. McNett M, Libvesay S, Yeager S, et al. The impact of head-of-bed positioning and transducer location on cerebral perfusion pressure measurement. *J Neurosci Nurs.* 2018;50(6):322–326.
4. Roth C, Ferbert A, Deinsberger W, et al. Does prone positioning increase intracranial pressure? A retrospective analysis of patients with acute brain injury and acute respiratory failure. *Neurocrit Care.* 2014;21(2):186–191.
5. Ugras GA, Yuksel A, Temiz Z, et al. Effect of different head-of-bed elevations and body positions on intracranial pressure and cerebral perfusion pressure in neurosurgical patients. *J Neurosci Nurs.* 2018;50(4):247–251.

- Coagulation profile, including prothrombin time, international normalized ratio (INR), and activated partial thromboplastin time (aPTT) because brain injury may induce a coagulopathy
- Electrolytes, blood urea nitrogen, creatinine, liver function, and serum osmolality

Radiological studies and other diagnostic tests that may be performed on a patient with increased ICP include the following:[23,29,34]

- Computed tomography (CT) scan (usually without contrast) to assess the potential for a worsening intracranial mass effect.
- Magnetic resonance imaging (MRI) to provide anatomical detail of pathology contributing to increased ICP.
- CBF monitoring, in which a transcutaneous Doppler device (a noninvasive technology) measures the velocity of arterial flow and allows for indirect monitoring of CBF at the bedside. Transcutaneous Doppler measurements are correlated with ICP values to assess the patient's response to treatment and nursing interventions. Monitoring is particularly useful to detect vasospasm in patients with a cerebral aneurysm. Vasospasm is manifested by an increase in velocity.
- Evoked potential monitoring, a noninvasive procedure in which sensory stimuli are applied and the electrical potentials created are recorded. Each potential is recorded and stored in a computer, and an average curve is calculated. Brainstem auditory evoked potentials evaluate brainstem function and can be conducted on a conscious or unconscious patient or even during surgery. Somatosensory evoked potentials measure peripheral nerve responses and are helpful in evaluating spinal cord function.
- An EEG may be obtained to identify seizure activity or lack of electrical activity, which may be consistent with brain death. It can also be used to monitor brain activity in patients who are in an induced coma.

Patient Problems

Refer to the Plan of Care for the Patient With Traumatic Brain Injury, Increased Intracranial Pressure, or Acute Stroke for a detailed description of patient problems, specific nursing interventions, and selected rationales. Other interventions are discussed in the Collaborative Plan of Care for the Critically Ill Patient in Chapter 1.

Management

Medical and Nursing Interventions (Nonsurgical). The goal of management is to maintain an ICP of less than 20 mm Hg while maintaining the CPP at greater than 70 mm Hg.[1] The first task is to prevent an increase in ICP. If the ICP is elevated, therapy is

◎ PLAN OF CARE

For the Patient With Traumatic Brain Injury, Increased Intracranial Pressure, or Acute Stroke

Patient Problem

Potential for Increased Intracranial Pressure. Risk factors include underlying brain injury, volume overload, fever pain, seizures, positional factors, or increased intrathoracic or intraabdominal pressure.

Desired Outcomes

- Prevention of increased intracranial pressure (ICP <20 mm Hg).
- Neurological status stable or improved from baseline.
- Stable vital signs.
- Optimal fluid balance.
- Absence of seizures.

Nursing Assessments/Interventions	Rationales
• Assess neurological status hourly, including level of consciousness, pupillary function (other cranial nerve functions as indicated), strength and equality in bilateral extremity movements, superficial and deep tendon reflex activity, and sensory function where appropriate.	• Detect changes indicative of increased ICP.
• Monitor ICP and CPP; notify provider if ICP >20 mm Hg sustained for more than 5 min or if CPP <70 mm Hg.	• Ensure adequate cerebral perfusion (CPP >70 mm Hg).
• Maintain airway; monitor SpO_2 and $ETCO_2$, or ABGs, for evidence of hypoxemia/hypercapnia; hyperoxygenate the patient before and after suctioning.	• Ensure adequate cerebral perfusion; prevent cerebral vasodilation.
• Monitor VS; be alert to changes in respiratory pattern, fluctuations in BP, bradycardia, widening pulse pressure.	• Detect responses to increased ICP; however, these signs occur very late.
• Maintain patient's head in a neutral position; maintain HOB elevation that keeps ICP and CPP within normal ranges.	• Facilitate cerebral venous drainage and prevent increased ICP.
• Monitor fluid volume status by measuring I&O, skin turgor, daily weight, breath sounds, CVP if available; ensure precise delivery of IV fluids; administer osmotic diuretics as ordered.	• Prevent fluid volume excess or deficit, both of which can affect ICP.
• Evaluate patient's response to nursing interventions; space activities to avoid increases in ICP.	• Prevent sustained elevations in ICP; ICP should return to normal values within 5 min after completion of activities.
• Prevent increases in intrathoracic and intraabdominal pressure through proper positioning, avoiding coughing and Valsalva maneuver.	• Facilitate cerebral venous drainage and prevent increased ICP.
• If patient is hyperthermic, administer treatments to reduce temperature to normal. Mild hypothermia may be ordered.	• Reduce cerebral metabolic demands.
• Administer antiepileptic medications as ordered to prevent seizures; if seizures occur, treat promptly.	• Seizures increase CBF and can increase ICP.
• Administer medications as needed for pain.	• Pain may contribute to increased ICP.
• Weigh daily.	• Monitor fluid volume status (all interventions).
• Monitor I&O hourly.	
• Monitor laboratory results (electrolytes, serum, and urine osmolality).	
• Assess skin and mucous membranes.	

Patient Problem

Potential for Decreased Cerebral Tissue Perfusion. Risk factors include increased ICP and decreased cerebral blood flow.

Desired Outcomes

- Vital signs within normal limits.
- Improved cerebral perfusion.
- Neurological status within normal limits.

Nursing Assessments/Interventions	Rationales
• Assess neurological status hourly using GCS, FOUR score, or NIHSS; monitor VS.	• Assess for alterations in ICP.
• Assess for restlessness, anxiety, or mental status changes as early indicators of altered cerebral tissue perfusion. Institute safety precautions as needed.	• Mental status changes are often the earliest indicators of altered tissue perfusion. • Mental status changes may predispose the patient to injury.
• Perform interventions to prevent and treat increased ICP.	• Ensure adequate cerebral tissue perfusion.
• Maintain head in a midline position.	
• Elevate HOB >30 degrees.	
• Assess and treat pain.	
• Maintain BP within desired range with prescribed medications; maintain IV fluid therapy.	• Decreases in BP and hypovolemia may decrease CPP.

◎ PLAN OF CARE—cont'd

For the Patient With Traumatic Brain Injury, Increased Intracranial Pressure, or Acute Stroke

Patient Problem

Delirium. Risk factors include impaired cerebral functioning, decreased physiological reserve, or decreased brain oxygenation.

Desired Outcomes
- Optimal thought processes.
- Improved attention, memory, and judgment.
- Appropriate response with an improved level of orientation.

Nursing Assessments/Interventions	Rationales
• Assess the patient for signs and symptoms of delirium using a standardized delirium assessment tool.	• Delirium is multifactorial and may be reversible if assessed and treated early.
• Assess for treatable causes of delirium.	• Use of a standardized delirium assessment tool assists in accurate detection of the syndrome.
• Reorient frequently; place a clock or calendar within patient's view.	• Provide reorientation to place and time.
• Explain activities clearly and simply in a calm manner; allow adequate time for response.	• Provide information; prevents anxiety.
• Instruct the family in methods to deal with patient's altered thought processes.	• Provide ongoing reorientation.
• Maintain a consistent and fairly structured routine.	• Facilitate reorientation.
• Allow for frequent rest periods for the patient.	• Promote energy conservation and recovery.
• Create a safe environment for the patient; avoid use of restraints.	• Delirium may predispose the patient to injury.
	• Restraints may increase delirium.

ABG, Arterial blood gas; *BP*, blood pressure; *CBF*, cerebral blood flow; *CPP*, cerebral perfusion pressure; *CVP*, central venous pressure; *ETCO₂*, end-tidal carbon dioxide; *FOUR*, full outline of unresponsiveness; *GCS*, Glasgow Coma Scale; *HOB*, head of bed; *ICP*, intracranial pressure; *I&O*, intake & output; *NIHSS*, National Institutes of Health Stroke Scale; *SpO₂*, arterial oxygen saturation via pulse oximetry; *VS*, vital signs.
Adapted from Swearingen PL, Wright JD. *All-in-One Nursing Care Planning Resource.* 5th ed. St. Louis, MO: Elsevier; 2019.

---

instituted to decrease ICP and then identify the cause of increased ICP. Once the cause is discovered, management is centered on permanently decreasing the high ICP, maintaining CPP, maintaining the airway, providing ventilation and oxygenation, and decreasing the metabolic demands placed on the injured brain.

Nursing actions to manage intracranial pressure. Position the patient to minimize ICP and maximize CPP. Elevate the head of the bed to 30 degrees and keep the head in a neutral midline position to facilitate venous drainage and decrease the risk of venous obstruction. It is important to evaluate BP response to head elevation.[19] Raising the head of the bed may decrease MAP, thereby decreasing CPP. Hemodynamically unstable patients may need to be cared for in a flat position. Patients with increased ICP can be turned from side to side. During any position change or change in elevation of the head of the bed, it is imperative to monitor and document the patient's individualized cerebral and hemodynamic response. If the CPP does not return to the baseline value within 5 minutes after the position change, reposition the patient to the position that maximized CPP.[28]

Because endotracheal suctioning is associated with hypoxemia, suction the patient only when necessary. Preoxygenate the patient with 100% oxygen before and between suction attempts and for 1 minute after the procedure. Limit each suction pass to less than 10 seconds, with no more than two suction passes. Maintain the head in a neutral position during the suctioning procedure.

Several nursing activities are associated with increases in ICP. These include turning, repositioning, and hygiene measures. Elevated ICP resulting from nursing care is usually temporary, and the ICP should return to the resting baseline value within a few minutes. Sustained increases in ICP lasting longer than 5 minutes should be prevented. Spacing nursing care activities allows for rest between activities. If ICP pressure monitoring is available, monitor the ICP in response to care and other interventions.

Family presence has been shown to decrease ICP. However, caution family members to avoid excess stimulation of the patient or unpleasant conversations that may emotionally stimulate the patient (e.g., discussing prognosis, condition, deficits, restraints) because this can cause an elevation in ICP.[1] Assess the patient's physiological response to visitors.

❓ CRITICAL REASONING ACTIVITY

You are caring for Mr. S., who has sustained a traumatic brain injury from a motor vehicle crash, presenting with a Glasgow Coma Scale score of 6. He has an intraventricular catheter for continuous measurement of intracranial pressure (ICP). His ICP has been stable at 13 mm Hg for the past 4 hours. The alarm on the monitor sounds because his ICP is now 20 mm Hg. What are your priority assessments and interventions at this time?

Medical management. Medical management of increased ICP includes the following: adequate oxygenation and ventilation; cautious, limited use of hyperventilation; osmotic and loop diuretics; euvolemic fluid administration; maintenance of BP; and reduction of metabolic demands. Corticosteroids are useful for reducing cerebral edema associated with brain tumors and meningitis, but studies do not support administration of corticosteroids to reduce ICP associated with other intracranial conditions.[12,29] Table 14.9 identifies medications commonly used for patients with increased ICP.

TABLE 14.9 **PHARMACOLOGY**

Frequently Used Medications in Nervous System Alterations

Medication	Actions/Use	Dose/Route	Side Effects	Nursing Implications
Mannitol	Osmotic diuretic Pulls water from brain interstitium into plasma Used to treat ↑ ICP	0.5-1 g/kg IV over 5-10 min, then 0.25-2.0 g/kg IVP q 4-12 h as needed depending on ICP, CPP, serum osmolality	Hypotension, dehydration, electrolyte disturbances, tachycardia Rebound cerebral edema when used for more than one dose	Neurological assessment every hour Monitor ICP, CPP, serum osmolality, electrolytes, ABGs, VS, I&O Ensure crystals, if present, are dissolved before use. Use an in-line filter to administer
Furosemide (Lasix)	Reduces cerebral edema by drawing sodium and water out of brain interstitium	*Post–cardiac arrest cerebral edema:* 40 mg IV over 1-2 min If no response in 1 h, increase to 80 mg or 0.5-1.0 mg/kg IV over 1-2 min If no response, increase dose to 2 mg/kg	Ototoxicity, polyuria, electrolyte disturbances, gastric irritation, muscle cramps, hypotension, dehydration, embolism, vascular thrombosis	Monitor I&O, daily weight, electrolytes, ABGs, VS
Dexamethasone (Decadron)	Steroid that has a stabilizing effect on cell membrane Prevents destructive effect of oxygen free radicals ↓ Inflammation by suppressing WBCs	*Cerebral edema:* 10-20 mg IV loading dose over 1 min 4-10 mg q 6 h Reduce dose after 2-4 days Discontinue gradually over 5-7 days	Flushing, sweating, hypertension, tachycardia, thrombocytopenia, weakness, nausea, diarrhea, GI irritation/hemorrhage, fluid retention, poor wound healing, weight gain, hyperglycemia, muscle wasting, hypokalemia	↑ or ↓ Effects of anticoagulants ↑ Effects of anticonvulsants Adjust dose of antidiabetic agents ↑ Effects of digitalis Monitor glucose, potassium, daily weights, VS Masks signs of infection Taper medication before discontinuing
Methylprednisolone (Solu-Medrol)	An adjunct for SCI management within first 8 h of injury Improves blood flow to injury site, facilitating tissue repair	30 mg/kg IV over 15 min After 45 min, begin maintenance dose infusion of 5.4 mg/kg/h for 23 h	Same as dexamethasone	Same as dexamethasone
Labetalol (Normodyne; Trandate)	Nonselective beta-blocker to decrease BP	10-20 mg IVP over 2 min May repeat with 40-80 mg IVP at 10-min intervals until desired BP is achieved Do not exceed total dose of 300 mg After bolus, may give as continuous infusion at 2-8 mg/min	Hypotension, bradycardia, HF, bronchospasm, ventricular dysrhythmias, diaphoresis, flushing, somnolence, weakness/fatigue	Monitor BP, HR, I&O, daily weight May ↓ glucose May cause further hypotension with nitroglycerin May potentiate with calcium channel blockers Adjust dosage of oral hypoglycemic medications
Enalapril (Vasotec)	ACE inhibitor to decrease BP Used to treat hypertension	0.625-1.25 mg IV q 6 h over 5 min	Headache, hypotension, dysrhythmias, proteinuria, acute kidney injury, neutropenia, angioedema, hyperkalemia	Contraindicated in pregnancy Monitor BP frequently Assess laboratory values: WBCs, electrolytes, renal and liver status Assess ECG rhythm; monitor for edema
Nicardipine (Cardene)	Calcium channel blocker Vasodilatory effect that lowers BP	*Severe hypertension:* 5 mg/h continuous infusion, increase dose by 2.5 mg/h q 15 min until desired BP is reached Not to exceed 15 mg/h When desired BP is reached, wean to 3 mg/h Wean off when continuous IV infusion is no longer required *Cerebral vasospasm:* may be given as an intra-arterial or intraventricular dose of 1-2 mg	Headache, confusion, hypotension, nausea and vomiting, tachycardia ECG changes (e.g., atrioventricular block, ST-segment depression, inverted T wave) May develop hypersensitivity reaction	Monitor BP continuously Lower doses and slower titration required for persons with HF or impaired hepatic or renal function
Phenytoin (Dilantin)	Depresses seizure activity by altering ion transport in motor cortex	*Status epilepticus:* 10-20 mg/kg IV in 0.9% NS only Administer over 20-30 min Do not exceed a total dose of 1.5 g If seizure not terminated, consider other antiepileptic drugs, barbiturates, or anesthesia Follow with maintenance dose of 100 mg IV over 2 min q 6-8 h	Bradycardia, hypotension, nystagmus/ataxia, gingival hyperplasia, agranulocytosis, rash, Stevens-Johnson syndrome, lymphadenopathy, nausea, cardiac arrest, heart block	Slow infusion rate if bradycardia, hypotension, or cardiac dysrhythmias occur Monitor ECG, BP, pulse, and respiratory function Dilute with 0.9% NS only Assess oral hygiene Assess for rash Monitor renal, hepatic, and hematological status Interacts with many medications

TABLE 14.9 PHARMACOLOGY—cont'd

Frequently Used Medications in Nervous System Alterations

Medication	Actions/Use	Dose/Route	Side Effects	Nursing Implications
Fosphenytoin (Cerebyx)	Depresses seizure activity by altering ion transport in motor cortex	*Status epilepticus loading dose:* 15-20 mg PE/kg IV Administer each 100-150 mg PE over a minimum of 1 min If full effect is not immediate, may be necessary to use with benzodiazepine *Nonemergency loading dose:* 10-20 mg PE/kg IV *Maintenance dose:* 4-6 mg PE/kg/24 h	Transient ataxia, dizziness, headache, nystagmus, paresthesia, pruritus, somnolence, hypotension, bradycardia, heart block, respiratory arrest, ventricular fibrillation, tonic seizures, nausea/vomiting, lethargy, hypocalcemia, metabolic acidosis, rash	Slow infusion rate or temporarily stop infusion for bradycardia, hypotension, burning, itching, numbness, or pain along injection site Assess neurological, respiratory, and cardiovascular status Assess seizure activity Monitor renal, hepatic, and hematological status Interacts with many medications
Levetiracetam (Keppra)	Depresses seizure activity Mechanism of action unknown May inhibit intracellular sodium influx in motor cortex	500 mg IV bid, titrate by 1000 mg/day q 2 wk for seizure control Maximum 3000 mg/day in divided doses	Suicidal ideation, muscle weakness, dizziness, psychosis, decreased RBCs, hemoglobin, hematocrit	Adjust dose with acute kidney injury Monitor CBC Monitor for adverse changes in mental status
Diazepam (Valium)	Depresses subcortical areas of CNS Antiepileptic, sedative-hypnotic Antianxiety Adjunct medication to depress seizure activity	*Status epilepticus:* 5-10 mg IV Give 5 mg over 1 min. May be repeated q 10-15 min for a total dose of 30 mg May repeat in 2-4 h; or 0.2-0.5 mg/kg q 15-30 min for 2-3 doses Some specialists suggest 20 mg and titrate total dose over 10 min or until seizures stop Maximum dose in 24 h is 100 mg	Respiratory depression, hypotension, drowsiness, lethargy, bradycardia, cardiac arrest, hypoglycemia	Monitor respiratory status, BP, HR Assess blood glucose Assess IV site for phlebitis
Lorazepam (Ativan)	Depresses subcortical areas of CNS Antiepileptic Sedative-hypnotic Antianxiety	*Status epilepticus:* 4 mg IV over 1 min as initial dose May repeat once in 10-15 min if seizure continues; or 0.05 mg/kg to a total of 4 mg Do not exceed 8 mg in 12 h	Airway obstruction, apnea, blurred vision, confusion, excessive drowsiness, hypotension, bradycardia, respiratory depression, somnolence	Same as diazepam
Pentobarbital sodium (Nembutal sodium)	Barbiturate; sedative; hypnotic agent; antiepileptic for control of increased ICP	100 mg IV initially; give over 2 min; additional doses in increments of 25-50 mg IV; give 50 mg over 1 min; maximum dose 200-500 mg IV *Barbiturate coma:* loading dose 3-10 mg/kg over 3 min to 3 h *Maintenance dose:* 1.5-2 mg/kg IV q 2 h or an infusion of 0.5-3 mg/kg/h; adjust to maintain pentobarbital blood level between 110 and 177 mmol/L (25-40 mg/dL) or ICP <25 mm Hg	Hypotension; myocardial or respiratory depression; thrombocytopenia purpura *Overdose:* apnea, coma, cough reflex depression, flat EEG, hypotension, sluggish or absent reflexes, pulmonary edema	Monitor ICP, CPP, VS, and hemodynamic responses Monitor pentobarbital levels Patient response is variable
Nimodipine	Calcium channel blocker given to prevent vasospasm; reduces neurological deficits after SAH	60 mg PO or via NG tube q 4 h for 21 days; start within 96 h of SAH	Hypotension, peripheral edema, ECG abnormalities, nausea/vomiting, diarrhea, altered liver function, HF, cough, dyspnea	Assess neurological status Monitor VS, I&O, daily weight Observe for signs of HF

ABGs, Arterial blood gases; *ACE,* angiotensin-converting enzyme; *bid,* twice daily; *BP,* blood pressure; *CBC,* complete blood count; *CNS,* central nervous system; *CPP,* cerebral perfusion pressure; *ECG,* electrocardiogram; *EEG,* electroencephalogram; *GI,* gastrointestinal; *HF,* heart failure; *HR,* heart rate; *I&O,* intake & output; *ICP,* intracranial pressure; *IVP,* intravenous push; *NG,* nasogastric; *NS,* normal saline; *PE,* phenytoin equivalent; *PO,* orally; *q,* every; *RBCs,* red blood cells; *SAH,* subarachnoid hemorrhage; *SCI,* spinal cord injury; *VS,* vital signs; *WBCs,* white blood cells.
Data from Gahart B, Nazareno A. *Gahart's 2019 Intravenous Medications.* 35th ed. St. Louis, MO: Elsevier; 2019.

Adequate oxygenation. The goal is to maintain a PaO_2 above 80 mm Hg and to ensure that oxygen delivery to the brain exceeds oxygen consumption. A PaO_2 below 50 mm Hg can precipitate increased ICP. For many patients with increased ICP, short-term management of the airway is accomplished by an endotracheal tube and mechanical ventilation. Positive end-expiratory pressure may be added to facilitate oxygenation; however, it must be used with extreme caution because it may prevent venous outflow and further increase ICP.[35] A tracheostomy tube may be required for long-term ventilatory management.[35] In addition, adequate hematocrit and hemoglobin levels are maintained to promote oxygenation.

Management of carbon dioxide. Hyperventilation decreases $PaCO_2$, which causes vasoconstriction of the cerebral arteries and a reduction of CBF. In the past, hyperventilation was commonly used to manage ICP, but hyperventilation may cause neurological damage by decreasing cerebral perfusion. Hyperventilation is used to decrease ICP for short periods when acute neurological deterioration is occurring (i.e., herniation) and other methods to reduce ICP have failed. If the $PaCO_2$ level is purposefully lowered to less than 35 mm Hg for an extended period, oxygen delivery at the cellular level should be evaluated with the use of a jugular bulb or cerebral tissue oxygen monitor.[6,27,28] It is recommended that the $PaCO_2$ be kept within a normal range, 35 to 45 mm Hg. Hyperventilation should also be avoided when providing manual ventilation via a bag-valve-mask device.[12]

Diuretics. Osmotic and loop diuretics are administered to reduce cerebral brain volume by removing fluid from the brain's extracellular compartment. *Osmotic diuretics,* such as mannitol or hypertonic saline (in solutions ranging from 1.5% to 24% normal saline), draw water from the extracellular space to the plasma by creating an osmotic gradient, thereby decreasing ICP.[7,29] The effects of decreasing ICP and increasing CPP occur within minutes after the infusion. Side effects of osmotic diuretics include hypotension, electrolyte disturbances, and rebound increased ICP. If mannitol is used, the patient must have adequate intravascular volume to prevent hypotension and secondary brain injury. Mannitol is contraindicated in patients with acute kidney injury because it is not metabolized and is excreted unchanged in the urine. *Loop diuretics* (furosemide, torsemide, bumetanide, ethacrynic acid) decrease ICP by removing sodium and water from injured brain cells. These agents also decrease CSF formation (see Table 14.9).

Optimal fluid administration. Fluid administration is provided to optimize MAP, maintain intravascular volume, and normalize CPP. Normal saline solution, an isotonic solution, is recommended for volume resuscitation in acute brain injury. Hypotonic solutions are avoided to prevent an increase in cerebral edema. Strict measurement of intake and output while monitoring serum sodium, potassium, and osmolarity is required. The goal is to keep serum osmolality at less than 320 mOsm/L.[30] If needed, colloids or blood products are administered to restore volume and maintain adequate hematocrit and hemoglobin levels. Hemodynamic monitoring may be used to optimize fluid administration.

Blood pressure management. BP must be carefully controlled in a patient with increased ICP. The MAP is usually kept between 70 and 90 mm Hg; however, it is critical to monitor the ICP and MAP collectively to sustain an adequate CPP of at least 70 mm Hg.[1,28] Hypotension decreases CBF, which leads to cerebral ischemia. When hypotension occurs or ICP cannot be reduced, manipulating the systolic BP with fluids and vasopressor medications may be necessary to achieve an adequate CPP.

Hypertension (>160 mm Hg systolic) can worsen cerebral edema by increasing microvascular pressure. However, hypertension may be necessary for adequate cerebral perfusion. If necessary, systolic BP is lowered with antihypertensive medications (e.g., beta-blockers such as labetalol). Beta-blockers decrease the sympathetic response and catecholamine release associated with neurological injury. Some antihypertensive medications (nitroprusside, nitroglycerin) and some calcium channel blockers (verapamil, nifedipine) cause cerebral vasodilation, which increases CBF and causes increased ICP. Administration of these medications is avoided in patients with poor intracranial compliance. Nicardipine is a calcium channel blocker medication that does not affect cerebral vasculature; it is very effective in providing faster and tighter control of BP than other antihypertensive medications (see Table 14.9).

Reducing metabolic demands. Several therapies may be required to reduce metabolic demands. These include temperature control, sedation, seizure prophylaxis, neuromuscular blockade, and barbiturate therapy.

Temperature control. Targeted temperature management (TTM) incorporates lowering body temperature to normal from a hyperthermic state, decreases cerebral metabolism, blood flow, and volume, thereby decreasing ICP.[31] Body temperature may be controlled noninvasively with the use of a cooling blanket or skin pads placed in direct contact with the skin (external cooling) or invasively by using a catheter placed in a large vein (intravascular cooling). Target temperatures for TTM range from 34°C to 35°C; these temperatures are maintained for at least 24 hours, followed by gradual rewarming.[29] Temperature values differ from those recommended post cardiac arrest. TTM has many potential adverse effects, including coagulopathies and fluid and electrolyte disturbances (see Chapter 11). Current research supports the use of TTM in the post–cardiac arrest patient, but more research is required to determine the long-term outcomes among patients with elevated ICP.[20]

Sedation. Administer analgesia and sedation for the patient with an elevated ICP in an effort to reduce pain, agitation, restlessness, or resistance to mechanical ventilation. Analgesics (e.g., morphine, fentanyl) can be administered in a low-dose continuous infusion or in small, frequent IV boluses for analgesia and sedation, or analgosedation. Common sedatives administered are benzodiazepines and propofol. Benzodiazepines do not affect CBF or ICP and propofol, a sedative-hypnotic medication, reduces cerebral metabolism and ICP. Propofol is a short-acting medication with a rapid onset administered by continuous infusion. Though these are common medications used in this population, the pain and sedation regimen must be tailored based on the patient's history and physical assessment. Refer to Chapter 6 for further information on comfort and sedation. Blood pressure must be closely monitored when sedation is used, as hypotension is common. Patients should be normovolemic before starting sedation, with additional fluids and vasopressor medications used if needed.

Seizure prophylaxis. Patients with a brain disorder or injury are prone to seizures. Seizure activity is associated with high metabolic demands. Typically, seizure prophylaxis is initiated only in high-risk situations because adverse effects can occur from prophylactic medications. For example, phenytoin can impair cognition, and carbamazepine can decrease sodium level and white blood cell count.

Neuromuscular blockade and barbiturate therapy. Neuromuscular blockade is considered for patients unresponsive to other treatments. Barbiturates are given selectively to reduce ICP refractory to other treatments. Pentobarbital is the most common medication used. Patients receiving neuromuscular blockade or barbiturate therapy require arterial pressure monitoring, mechanical ventilation, and intensive nursing management.

Surgical Interventions. Surgical intervention may be required to remove a mass or lesion that is causing the increased ICP. Surgery may involve the removal of infarcted areas or hematomas (epidural, subdural, or intracerebral). Decompressive hemicraniectomy is occasionally performed for severe brain injury or large-volume stroke. The cranial bone is removed, and the dura is opened to create more space for edematous tissue. Protection of the patient's brain from trauma is imperative when there is missing bone.[1,12]

Psychosocial Support. Neurological insults usually occur without warning and may be severe. This places the family in a state of shock and disbelief. In addition, the patient has suffered an insult to the nervous system and may respond inappropriately or uncharacteristically or may not be able to respond to the family at all. Neurological insults cause uncertainty regarding the patient's physical and mental outcomes. The personality and mental changes associated with brain insults can be devastating to the family. The family is supported by providing information and psychosocial support to reduce their anxiety.

STUDY BREAK

3. Which of the following activities may help decrease increased intracranial pressure?
   A. Frequent suctioning
   B. Head elevation to 30 degrees
   C. Pressure on the abdomen while coughing
   D. Valsalva maneuver

TRAUMATIC BRAIN INJURY

TBI is a common occurrence in the United States and is the leading cause of trauma-related deaths among persons younger than 45 years of age. Each year, 1.1 million TBIs occur, resulting in 50,000 immediate deaths and hospitalization of 235,000 individuals. Males are 1.5 times as likely as females to sustain a TBI. The highest incidences of TBI occur in children younger than 4 years of age and in persons ages 15 to 19 years. Survival

after TBI is dependent on prompt emergency treatment and focused management of primary and secondary injuries.[5,12]

Pathophysiology

Traumatic injury can result in damage to the scalp, skull, meninges, and brain, including neuronal pathways, cranial nerves, and intracranial vessels. The extent of TBI can range from mild to severe. Injuries may be open or closed. With an open injury, the scalp is torn or a fracture extends into the sinuses or middle ear. The meninges can also be penetrated. A closed TBI occurs when there is no break in the scalp. Acceleration-deceleration is a common mechanism for TBI. With this injury, the movement of the head follows a straight line, and the moving head (acceleration) hits a stationary object (deceleration). Rotation or a twisting of the brain within the cranial vault adds to the insult. Genetics may play a role in both injury and recovery (see Genetics box).

Scalp Lacerations. Scalp lacerations are common in traumatic injury and are often associated with skull fracture. The scalp offers some resistance to compression and absorbs mild blows by distributing forces over the entire area of the scalp. The scalp is very vascular and can be the source of significant blood loss. The wound is cleansed, debrided, and inspected for a depressed skull fracture, then sutured closed. Inattention to these details can lead to infection.

Skull Fractures. The skull has high compressive strength and is somewhat elastic. After impact, there is an in-bending of the skull at the point of impact and an out-bending at the vertex. The area of out-bending of tensile stresses creates a fracture line that moves toward the base of the skull. There are several types of skull fractures—linear, depressed, and comminuted—and various locations of the fractures (Fig. 14.14).

Linear skull fracture. A linear fracture is the most common type of skull fracture. This fracture usually does not lead to significant complications unless there is an extension of the fracture to the orbit, to the sinus, or across a vessel. If there is extension of the fracture, the patient is admitted for observation of signs of intracranial bleeding and epidural hematoma.

Linear fractures at the skull base are termed *basilar fractures*. This type of fracture is difficult to confirm on a skull radiographic study and is diagnosed clinically. Battle sign (bruising behind the ear) and the presence of "raccoon eyes" (bilateral periorbital edema and bruising) may be indicative of a basilar skull fracture (Fig. 14.15). Dural tears are very common with a basilar skull fracture and may lead to meningitis. Drainage of CSF from the nose (rhinorrhea), postnasal drainage, or drainage of CSF from the ear (otorrhea) may indicate a dural tear. Blood encircled by a yellowish stain on a dressing or bed linens, called the *halo sign*, usually indicates CSF. If CSF is suspected in the drainage, a sample of the drainage is sent to the laboratory for analysis. In the event of a CSF leak, it is important to allow the CSF to flow freely. Nothing should be placed in the nose or ear, although small bandages under the nose or around the ear can be used to collect the drainage. Instruct the patient to avoid blowing the nose. Insert tubes (e.g., gastric tubes, suction catheters, endotracheal tubes) through the mouth rather than through the nose to avoid penetrating the brain as a result of the dural tear.

🧬 GENETICS

Traumatic Brain Injury

The National Institutes of Health (NIH) has sponsored a Precision Medicine Initiative to translate research into practice.[3] Precision medicine focuses on identifying effective approaches to care based on genetic, environmental, and lifestyle or behavioral factors. The interaction of genes with the environment and lifestyle are complex and referred to as multifactorial disorders. The multiplicity of candidate genes and the contributing factors of the environment and lifestyle involved with brain injury and recovery suggest that traumatic brain injury (TBI) is a multifactorial disorder. For example, a mild brain injury is called a concussion, but it manifests in various symptoms, and the trajectory of recovery is variable and unpredictable.[2,7] Risky behaviors, such as driving an automobile at excessive speed, are lifestyle behaviors that, in this example, increase the occurrence of a motor vehicle crash and associated TBI. Some genetic variants are associated with risky lifestyle behaviors. Precision medicine looks globally at these gene-gene and gene-environment-lifestyle interactions to build knowledge around TBI. Other investigations in precision medicine focus on vulnerability to secondary injury after TBI.[2] Secondary brain injury includes damage to brain tissue from hypoperfusion and hypoxia. Some genes are protective, whereas other genes increase vulnerability to neuronal injury in the presence of hypoxemia or hypoperfusion. Gene-gene and gene-environment-lifestyle appear to influence the symptoms, severity, and recovery from TBI.

The genetics of TBI fall into two categories: (1) neuroinflammatory alterations that contribute to secondary injury and (2) neuroregenerative alterations that contribute to repair and recovery.[1] Both categories are considered multifactorial in regulating the brain's response to injury and recovery. Following TBI, the initial neuroinflammatory response can promote secondary neuronal injury or hinder repair mechanisms. Genes that influence neuroinflammation include the pro- and antiinflammatory cytokines. For example, single nucleotide polymorphism (SNP) in the promoter region of the tumor necrosis factor alpha (TNF-α) gene can enhance inflammation and is associated with poor outcomes following TBI.[1] Alternatively, excess production of interleukin-6 (IL-6), another proinflammatory cytokine, following TBI is associated with improved outcomes.[1]

The second genetic category, neuroregenerative alterations, affect the repair and plasticity or growth of neurons and supporting glial cells. Apolipoprotein E (APOE) is the most studied in this category. Patients with an *APOE-4* allele are more likely to have an unfavorable outcome after severe TBI. Patients can be hetero- or homozygous with this allele, and patients who are homozygous for *APOE-4* have the greatest disability following TBI.[3] The *APOE-4* allele is also associated with prolonged complications from concussions and chronic traumatic encephalopathy (CTE).[1]

Mitochondrial DNA (mtDNA) analysis adds insight to our ability to diagnose and treat all categories of TBI. Mitochondria generate cell energy, regulate the cell cycle and differentiation, support and provide cell signaling and calcium storage, and signal apoptosis. Disturbance in the mitochondrial network is implicated in many neurodegenerative diseases. Mitochondrial dysfunction following TBI may be sex-linked. Women may have variations in mtDNA that are protective in TBI.[4] It may be that the changes in energy substrates—small molecules produced by mitochondria and other cells—mitigate or enhance secondary brain injury after trauma.[5] The study of these small molecules that result from metabolism is called metabolomics and represents the newest branch of genomic study.[8]

Many of the genetic studies in TBI have led to proteomic investigations—the study of proteins produced when TBI occurs. The identification of these proteins has helped establish biomarkers with potential to accurately identify TBI severity.[9] The pathological disruption of the blood-brain barrier following injury allows proteins in the cerebrospinal fluid to transfer into the plasma. Serum biomarkers are particularly helpful in diagnosis of mild TBI because imaging is unlikely to demonstrate structural abnormalities.[6] Additional biomarkers for moderate and severe TBI may provide new opportunities to evaluate treatment, prognosticate, and establish precision medicine for this multifactorial condition.

Genetic terms: *promoter region, single nucleotide polymorphism, mitochondrial DNA, apoptosis, allele, proteomics, metabolomics, precision medicine, multifactorial.*

References

1. Bennett ER, Reuter-Rice K, Laskowitz DT. Genetic influences in traumatic brain injury. In: Laskowitz D, Grant G, eds. *Translational Research in Traumatic Brain Injury*. Boca Raton, FL: CRC Press; 2015.
2. Centers for Disease Control and Prevention. *Heads Up*. https://www.cdc.gov/headsup/index.html. Reviewed March 5, 2019. Accessed March 13, 2019.
3. Collins FS, Varmus H. A new initiative on precision medicine. *New Engl J Med.* 2015;372(9):793–795.
4. Conley YP, Okonkwo DO, Deslouches S, et al. Mitochondrial polymorphisms impact outcomes after severe traumatic brain injury. *J Neurotrauma.* 2014;31(1):34–41.
5. Fiandaca MS, Gross TJ, Johnson TM, et al. Potential metabolomic linkage in blood between Parkinson's disease and traumatic brain injury. *Metabolites.* 2018;8(3):e1–e20.
6. Kim HJ, Tsao JW, Stanfill AG. The current state of biomarkers of mild traumatic brain injury. *JCI Insight.* 2018;3(1):e1–e10.
7. Maserati M, Alexander SA. Genetics and genomics of acute neurologic disorders. *AACN Adv Crit Care.* 2018;29(1):57–75.
8. Wolahan SM, Hirt D, Braas D, Glenn TC. Role of metabolomics in traumatic brain injury research. *Neurosurg Clin N Am.* 2016;27(4):465–472.
9. Zhang J, Puvenna V, Janigro D. Biomarkers of traumatic brain injury and their relationship to pathology. In: Laskowitz D, Grant G, eds. *Translational Research in Traumatic Brain Injury.* Boca Raton, FL: CRC Press; 2015.

Depressed skull fracture. A depressed skull fracture occurs when the outer table of the skull is depressed below the inner table of the surrounding intact skull. The dura may be intact, bruised, or torn. If the scalp is lacerated and the dura is torn, there is direct communication between the brain and the environment, and meningitis can occur. In addition, the compressed and bruised brain beneath the depressed bone or bone lodged in brain parenchyma is the source of focal neurological deficit and may become a seizure focus.

Comminuted skull fracture. A comminuted skull fracture occurs when there are multiple linear fractures with a depressed area at the site of impact. The fracture radiates away from the impact site. A comminuted skull fracture is referred to as an "eggshell fracture" because of the appearance of the skull. Risks are similar to those occurring with a depressed fracture.

Brain Injury. TBI is classified as primary or secondary. Primary brain injury can be further divided into focal lesions (contusions, hematomas, penetrating injuries) and diffuse lesions (diffuse axonal injury).

Primary brain injury. Primary brain injury is a direct injury that occurs to the brain from an impact. With impact, the semisolid brain moves around inside the skull. The area under the direct impact is injured *(coup injury)*. Injury distal to the site of impact can occur as the brain moves inside the skull *(contrecoup injury)*. The stretching, shearing, rotational, and tearing forces that result from impact interrupt normal neuronal pathways. Concussion, contusion, penetrating injuries, and diffuse axonal injury are all types of primary brain injury. Intracranial bleeding can occur as a complication of the primary injury. Secondary brain injury may occur because of biochemical consequences of the primary injury (Fig. 14.16).

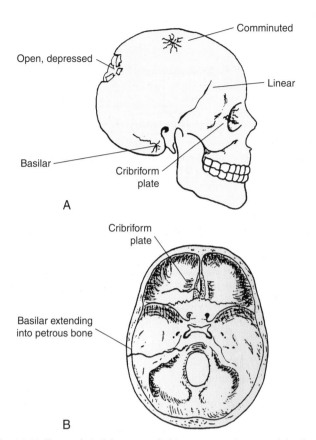

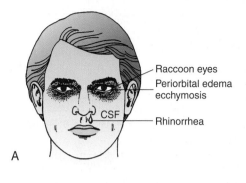

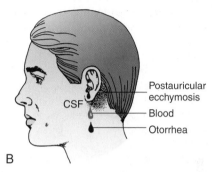

Fig. 14.14 Types of skull fractures. **A,** Linear; open, depressed; basilar; and comminuted fractures. **B,** View of the base of skull with fractures. (From Baker E. *Neuroscience Nursing: A Spectrum of Care.* 3rd ed. St. Louis, MO: Mosby; 2008.

Fig. 14.15 **A,** Raccoon eyes, rhinorrhea. **B,** Battle sign with otorrhea. *CSF,* Cerebrospinal fluid. (From Barker E. *Neuroscience Nursing: A Spectrum of Care.* 3rd ed. St. Louis, MO: Mosby; 2008.)

Concussion. Concussion occurs when a mechanical force of short duration is applied to the skull. This injury results in the temporary failure of impulse conduction. The neurological deficits are reversible and are generally mild. Patients may lose consciousness for a few seconds at the time of injury, but lasting effects are not common.

Contusion. Contusion is the result of coup and contrecoup injuries accompanied by bruising and bleeding into brain tissue. Lacerations of the cortical surface associated with contrecoup injuries may be greater than those seen directly under the point of impact. Signs and symptoms are variable, depending on the location and extent of bleeding.

Diffuse axonal injury. A more global brain injury is diffuse axonal injury. With this injury, widespread white matter axonal damage occurs secondary to rotational and shearing forces. This type of injury is associated with disruption of axons in the cerebral hemispheres, diencephalon, and brainstem. This injury results in vasodilation and increased CBV that precipitates increased ICP. Signs and symptoms are variable, and prognosis is poor.

Penetrating injury. Penetrating injuries are the result of low- or high-velocity forces such as gunshots, knives, or sharp objects. With this type of injury, there is a deep laceration of brain tissue and possible damage to the ventricular system. A low-velocity (stabbing) injury is limited to the tract of entry,

and the greatest concern is bleeding and infection. A high-velocity (gunshot) injury causes extensive damage because of the entry of bone fragments at the site. In addition, because bullets spin irregularly, they create many paths and shock waves that cause extensive brain damage.

Hematoma. Acute hematomas can be life-threatening. There are three types of hematomas: epidural, subdural, and intracerebral (Fig. 14.17).

Epidural hematoma. Collection of blood in the potential space between the inner table of the skull and the dura causes an *epidural hematoma.* This hematoma is typically associated with a linear fracture of the temporal bone and results from tearing of the middle meningeal artery. Arterial blood accumulates rapidly in this space. The patient typically experiences a brief loss of consciousness followed by a lucid period before neurological deterioration. The lucid period can last for a few hours to 48 hours. As the patient's condition deteriorates, the LOC decreases, contralateral deficits appear, and the pupil on the side of the lesion *(ipsilateral)* becomes fixed and dilated.[23]

Subdural hematoma. Collection of blood in the subdural space causes a *subdural hematoma.* It occurs when a surface vein is torn around the cerebral cortex. There are three kinds of subdural hematomas: acute, subacute, and chronic. *Acute subdural hematoma* occurs within 48 hours of an injury. It is almost always seen with cortical or brainstem injury and represents a mass lesion. The risk of death is high because of injury to brain tissue and the mass effect caused by an expanding hematoma. Surgical intervention occurring within 4 hours after the injury improves the mortality risk.[5,12,23] Symptoms of a *subacute subdural hematoma* occur anywhere from 48 hours to 2 weeks after an injury. The onset of symptoms is later because the hematoma grows slowly. A

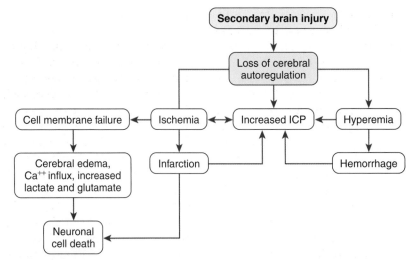

Fig. 14.16 Pathophysiology of secondary brain injury. *Ca++,* Calcium; *ICP,* intracranial pressure.

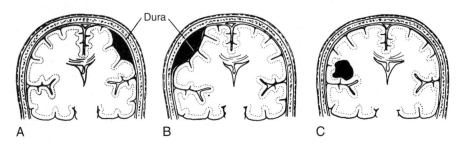

Fig. 14.17 Types of hematomas. **A,** Subdural (takes on contour of brain). **B,** Epidural. **C,** Intracerebral. (From Barker E. *Neuroscience Nursing: A Spectrum of Care.* 3rd ed. St. Louis, MO: Mosby; 2008.)

chronic subdural hematoma occurs as a result of a low-velocity impact. Symptoms occur from 2 weeks to several months after an injury. A higher incidence of chronic subdural hematomas is seen in the elderly, chronic alcohol abusers, and those taking anticoagulants such as warfarin, antiplatelet aggregants, or aspirin.[1] Because symptoms are often subtle, the diagnosis of chronic subdural hematoma is frequently missed.

Intracerebral hematoma. A traumatic intracerebral hematoma is a hemorrhage into brain tissue that creates a mass lesion. This lesion can occur anywhere in the brain. It can be caused by penetrating injuries, deep depressed skull fractures, or extension of a contusion. Signs and symptoms vary according to the location of the lesion and extent of hemorrhage.

Secondary brain injury. Secondary brain injury occurs as a consequence of the initial trauma and is characterized by an inflammatory response and release of cytokines from macrophages that cause increased vascular permeability of the blood vessel wall, leading to vasogenic cerebral edema. A series of biochemical events also contributes to the overproduction of free oxygen radicals that disrupt the cellular membrane, impair cellular metabolism, and cause neuronal deterioration (see Fig. 14.16). Decreased cerebral perfusion from numerous causes, hypoxia, infection, and/or fluid and electrolyte imbalances contributes to secondary brain injury. These insults add to the degree and extent of cellular dysfunction after TBI, increase the extent of brain damage, and affect functional recovery. Proper management minimizes the effects of secondary brain injury.

Assessment

The GCS (see Fig. 14.7) is used as a guide in assessing a patient with a TBI. The assessment is supplemented with a thorough neurological examination specific to the area of the brain involved. Assessment of airway and oxygenation status is essential to ensure adequate oxygenation and CBF. Report and document abnormal respiratory patterns because pattern changes usually indicate deterioration in neurological status. Additional assessment data include ICP, CPP, and hemodynamic monitoring. A patient with a TBI requires the same laboratory and diagnostic studies as a patient with increased ICP.[29,30]

Patient Problems. The same collaborative care plan is applicable for a patient with TBI as for a patient with increased ICP (see Plan of Care for the Patient With Traumatic Brain Injury, Increased Intracranial Pressure, or Acute Stroke earlier in the chapter and Collaborative Plan of Care for the Critically Ill Patient in Chapter 1). These patient problems cover both primary and secondary head injuries. Additional patient problems include dysphagia and potential for aspiration, fever, headache, constipation, potential for fluid imbalance, altered functional ability, and potential for communication barriers.

Management

Medical (Nonsurgical) Interventions. The nonsurgical treatment of a patient with a TBI is the same as for a patient with increased ICP. The emphasis is on reducing ICP, maintaining the airway, providing oxygenation, maintaining cerebral perfusion, and preventing secondary TBI. Although evidence continues to evolve, induced hypothermia may be implemented to protect the injured brain.[5,14] Hypothermia decreases the cerebral metabolic rate and oxygen consumption, lowers levels of glutamate and IL-1, decreases ICP, and increases CPP. Protecting the brain by inducing hypothermia may improve outcomes in persons with TBI.[14] Several strategies are available to induce hypothermia, including external cooling systems, hypothermia blankets, endovascular or endonasal cooling devices, antipyretics, sponging with cold water, and applying ice packs. If available, monitoring the brain temperature to thermoregulate the patient is an optimal choice because the actual brain temperature may be higher than the blood temperature. Adverse effects of hypothermia are assessed; they include dysrhythmias (atrial fibrillation), electrolyte imbalances, acidosis, shivering, and coagulopathies.

Nutritional support after TBI is essential. Hypermetabolism, accelerated catabolism, and excess nitrogen losses are responses to TBI. These responses result in depletion of energy stores, loss of lean muscle mass, reduced protein synthesis, loss of gastrointestinal mucosal integrity, and immune compromise. Nutritional support decreases susceptibility to infections, promotes wound healing, and facilitates weaning from mechanical ventilation.[30]

Surgical Interventions. Various surgical procedures exist to treat TBI. A depressed skull fracture may require surgery to elevate and repair or remove bone fragments. Acute subdural hematomas are usually evacuated via burr holes and epidural hematomas via craniotomy to prevent herniation. Penetrating wounds to the skull and brain may necessitate a craniotomy to explore the pathway of the missile, repair lacerations of intracranial vessels and brain tissue, remove bone fragments, or retrieve a foreign body such as a bullet.

Postoperative care is directed at the several interventions. Important goals are maintaining normal ICP and CPP, maintaining the airway and ventilation, preventing fluid and electrolyte imbalances, preventing complications of immobility, avoiding nutritional deficits, and reducing the incidence of infection.

The craniotomy dressing is assessed for drainage, including color, odor, and amount. Once the dressing is removed, assess the incision for swelling, redness, drainage, and tenderness. Persistent CSF drainage from the wound after surgery may indicate a dural tear and may require a lumbar drain or ventriculostomy for several days to decrease pressure at the fistula site and to aid in healing. A craniotomy may be necessary to repair the dura if leakage persists. Patients with penetrating wounds to the brain are at high risk for the development of infections and brain abscesses.

ACUTE STROKE

Stroke is a major public health problem. It is the fifth leading cause of death in the United States, the most frequent cause of adult disability, and the leading cause of long-term care. Although many strokes are preventable by controlling major risk factors such as hypertension, more than 610,000 new strokes and 185,000 recurrent strokes occur each year in the United States. More than 4 million people are stroke survivors.[33] Persons who have had a stroke have a 10- to 20-fold increased risk of having another stroke. The cost of hospitalization, rehabilitation, long-term care, and lost wages from stroke is estimated at $34 billion annually. Stroke, also known as "brain attack," results in infarction of a focal area of the brain. Early recognition of the signs and symptoms is essential to preserve blood flow to the brain (i.e., facial droop, arm weakness, speech difficulties). A stroke should be assessed and treated as a life-threatening emergency because optimal early treatment improves long-term outcome.[1,26]

The hallmark of stroke is the sudden onset of focal neurological symptoms associated with changes in blood flow to the brain resulting from either a blockage of flow or hemorrhage. Stroke can manifest with maximal focal neurological deficits or as stroke in evolution, in which symptoms evolve over several hours. The definition of stroke includes neurological deficits lasting 24 hours or longer. Although symptoms may completely resolve, CT or MRI will show evidence of permanent damage to the cerebral tissue.

Pathophysiology

Stroke occurs when the blood supply to the brain is disturbed by occlusion (ischemia) or hemorrhage. Brain cells survive only about 3 to 4 minutes when deprived of blood and oxygen. Normal CBF is 50 mL/100 g of brain tissue/min. When CBF drops to 25 mL/100 g/min, neurons become electrically silent but remain potentially viable for several hours. The region of brain with this level of CBF is known as the *ischemic penumbra* (Fig. 14.18). If CBF falls to less than the critical level of 10 mL/100 g/min or the penumbra is not reperfused, irreversible damage occurs. A cascade of metabolic disturbances follows, including lactic acidosis, glutamate release, depletion of ATP, and entry of sodium and calcium into the cells, leading to cytotoxic cerebral edema and mitochondrial failure.

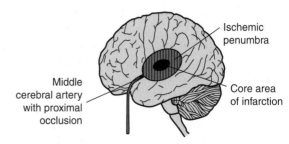

Fig. 14.18 Proximal occlusion of left middle cerebral artery with infarction. Ischemic penumbra represents regional blood flow at about 25 mL/100 g/min. Ischemic penumbra is the area where acute therapies for stroke are targeted.

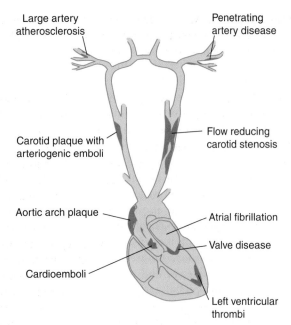

Fig. 14.19 Common arterial and cardiac abnormalities causing ischemic stroke. (From Albers GW, Easton JD, Sacco RL, et al. Antithrombotic and thrombolytic therapy for ischemic stroke. *Chest.* 1998;114[Suppl 5]:683S–698S.)

Ischemic Stroke. *Ischemic stroke* is caused by large artery atherosclerosis, cardioembolic events (Fig. 14.19), or small artery occlusive disease (lacunar stroke); in some cases, the cause is unknown (cryptogenic stroke). Approximately 87% of all strokes in the United States are ischemic.[22,33]

Large artery atherosclerosis. *Large artery atherosclerosis* is the result of stenosis in the large arteries of the head and neck; it is caused by a cholesterol plaque or a thrombus superimposed on plaque. Blood flow may be greatly reduced (stenosis), causing ischemia, or occluded completely, causing a stroke. Hypertension, diabetes, smoking, obesity, and hyperlipidemia are risk factors for this type of stroke.

Cardioembolic stroke. Low-flow states or stasis of blood within the cardiac chambers may result in blood clot formation. An embolism occurs when a blood clot or plaque fractures, breaks off, and travels to the brain. The most common causes of *cardioembolic stroke* are atrial fibrillation, rheumatic heart disease, acute myocardial infarction, endocarditis, mitral valve stenosis, and prosthetic heart valves. Because a cardiac abnormality is the source of the cerebral emboli, it is important to treat the underlying cardiac problem, as well as the neurological problem.

Lacunar stroke. *Lacunar stroke* (small vessel occlusive disease) is caused by chronic hypertension, hyperlipidemia, obesity, and diabetes. These disease states cause lipid material to coat the small cerebral arteries within deep structures of the brain. This process leads to a thickening of the arterial walls, decreased blood flow, and, ultimately, a stroke. The characteristic locations of lacunar infarcts are the basal ganglia, subcortical white matter, thalamus, cerebellum, and brainstem. The recurrence rate of these strokes is about 10- to 12-fold compared with other types of stroke. This type of stroke causes not only physical impairment but also cognitive impairment such as vascular dementia. Patients can have pure motor, pure sensory, or both motor and sensory features of stroke.

Cryptogenic stroke. The *cryptogenic* subtype refers to a stroke of unknown origin.

Hemorrhagic Stroke. *Hemorrhagic strokes* account for approximately 13% of all strokes in the United States.[33] Hemorrhagic stroke occurs when there is bleeding into the brain substance (intracerebral) or subarachnoid space (on the surface of the brain or into the ventricle), or a combination of the two.

Intracerebral hemorrhage. The most common cause of intracerebral hemorrhage (ICH) is uncontrolled hypertension.[13] Another cause of ICH is cerebral amyloid angiopathy. This condition is the result of abnormal amyloid protein deposits in the cerebral blood vessels. As a result, the cerebral blood vessels become friable and prone to spontaneous rupture, even in patients without hypertension.[13] When a blood vessel ruptures, the escaped blood forms a mass that displaces and compresses brain tissue. The severity of the symptoms depends on the location and amount of the hemorrhage. If the hemorrhage is large enough, herniation may result. Secondary causes include excessive anticoagulation, inappropriate use of thrombolytics (recombinant tissue plasminogen activator [rt-PA or Alteplase]), vasopressor medications, drug abuse (cocaine), and coagulopathies. A sudden and often severe motor deficit or loss of consciousness is seen with ICH, although a small ICH may manifest as a headache. Patients with ICH may continue to bleed; therefore close neurological monitoring is necessary.

Hemorrhagic stroke due to ruptured cerebral aneurysm. *Cerebral aneurysm* is a localized dilation of the cerebral artery wall that causes the artery to weaken and become susceptible to rupture. Most aneurysms develop at the bifurcation of large arteries at the base of the brain (circle of Willis). Not all aneurysms rupture; some aneurysms are found incidentally when imaging is done for other reasons. Patients with cerebral aneurysms are asymptomatic before the rupture unless they experience a warning "leak" or sentinel bleeding. Aneurysms most commonly rupture into the subarachnoid space at the basal cisterns. Less commonly, an aneurysm can rupture into the brain parenchyma or ventricle, or a combination of these locations. Bleeding into the subarachnoid space causes increased ICP, impaired cerebral autoregulation, reduced CBF, and irritation of the meninges. The bleeding generally stops through the formation of a fibrin plug and platelet aggregation within the ruptured artery.

After an aneurysm rupture, the patient can develop cardiac dysrhythmias, rebleeding, hydrocephalus, seizures, and cerebral vasospasm. Cardiac dysrhythmias occur as a result of sympathetic nervous system stimulation. Increased sympathetic tone can cause elevated T waves, prolonged QT intervals, and ST abnormalities. Rebleeding after the initial aneurysm rupture may occur before the aneurysm is secured. The mechanism causing the rebleeding is increased tension on the artery from hypertension, or normal breakdown of the clot, which occurs 7 to 10 days after the initial hemorrhage. Early endovascular or surgical intervention is recommended to prevent rebleeding.[13]

Hydrocephalus can occur after SAH through two mechanisms. Bleeding into the intraventricular space can block the flow of CSF and cause acute obstructive hydrocephalus. As blood enters the subarachnoid space, an inflammatory response is triggered that causes fibrosis and thickening of the arachnoid villi, thereby preventing reabsorption of CSF and producing communicating hydrocephalus.

Seizures can occur at SAH onset because of the initial hemorrhage, or within the first 12 hours after rupture, due to increased ICP or rebleeding of the aneurysm. Seizures occurring later are more likely due to ischemic damage secondary to vasospasm. Because of the adverse effects of medications, seizure prophylaxis is not recommended unless seizures occur beyond the first 12 hours after hemorrhage.

Cerebral vasospasm is a narrowing of arteries adjacent to the aneurysm that results in ischemia and infarction of brain tissue if it progresses. It is the leading cause of death after aneurysmal SAH. The usual period for vasospasm to occur is between 3 and 14 days after the rupture. The exact mechanism for vasospasm is unknown, but some factors that contribute to vasospasm are structural changes in the adjacent cerebral arteries, denervation of adjacent arteries, generation of oxygen free radicals, and release of vasoactive substances (serotonin, catecholamines, prostaglandins) that initiate vasospasm, the inflammatory response, and calcium influx.

Hemorrhagic stroke due to arteriovenous malformation. An arteriovenous malformation (AVM) is a congenital anomaly that forms an abnormal communication network between the arterial and venous systems in the brain.[37] Arterial blood under pressure is directly shunted into the venous system without a capillary network. This predisposes the vessels to rupture into the ventricular system or subarachnoid space, causing SAH, or into the brain parenchyma, causing intracranial hemorrhage. Impaired perfusion of the cerebral tissue adjacent to the AVM also occurs. The size and location of AVMs differ. Some AVMs do not hemorrhage but rather cause varying degrees of ischemia, scarring of brain tissue with seizures, abnormal tissue development, compression, or hydrocephalus. AVMs are more prevalent in males and are commonly diagnosed after the patient has had a seizure. Headache is another common manifestation of AVM.

Assessment

Early identification of a stroke is imperative so that rapid treatment can be initiated. The public must be educated on the symptoms of a brain attack because early intervention can minimize stroke deficit. Patients at high risk of stroke are taught risk reduction, the signs and symptoms of stroke, and to seek medical attention immediately (Box 14.1). Specialized stroke centers improve patient outcomes. The stroke center concept is designed to expedite evaluation and management of suspected ischemic stroke, transient ischemic attack (TIA), and ICH. A stroke center is equipped with an emergency department; a stroke team of physicians, nurses, and allied professionals with stroke-specific training; treatment protocols; emergent neuroradiology services; and access to neurosurgical services. Assessment in the emergency department includes an eyewitness description of symptoms, identification of the exact time at which symptoms started, and a neurological assessment.

The neurological examination includes evaluation of mental status (LOC, arousal, orientation), cranial nerve function, motor strength, sensory function, neglect, coordination, and deep tendon reflexes. The National Institutes of Health Stroke Scale (NIHSS; Table 14.10) is used to assess the severity of the presenting signs and symptoms, especially if the patient is a candidate for thrombolytic therapy.

BOX 14.1 Signs and Symptoms of Stroke

- Weakness or numbness of one side of the body (face, arm, leg, or any combination of these)
- Slurred speech or an inability to comprehend what is being said
- Visual disturbance, such as transient loss of vision in one or both eyes, double vision, or a visual field deficit
- Dizziness, incoordination, ataxia, or vertigo
- Sudden-onset severe headache ("worst headache of my life")

TABLE 14.10 National Institutes of Health Stroke Scale

Instructions	Scale	Definition
1a. Level of Consciousness (LOC): The investigator must choose a response if a full evaluation is prevented by such obstacles as an endotracheal tube, language barrier, or orotracheal trauma or bandages.	0	**Alert;** keenly responsive
	1	**Not alert** but arousable by minor stimulation
	2	**Not alert;** requires repeated stimulation to attend
	3	**Responds** only with reflex motor or autonomic effects, or totally unresponsive, flaccid, and areflexic
1b. LOC Questions: The patient is asked the month and his or her age. The answer must be correct—there is no partial credit for being close.	0	**Answers** both questions correctly
	1	**Answers** one question correctly
	2	**Answers** neither question correctly
1c. LOC Commands: The patient is asked to open and close the eyes and then to grip and release the nonparetic hand. Substitute another one-step command if the hands cannot be used.	0	**Performs** both tasks correctly
	1	**Performs** one task correctly
	2	**Performs** neither task correctly
2. Best Gaze: Only horizontal eye movements are tested. Voluntary or reflexive (oculocephalic) eye movements are scored, but caloric testing is not done.	0	**Normal**
	1	**Partial gaze palsy;** gaze is abnormal in one or both eyes
	2	**Forced deviation,** or total gaze paresis not overcome by the oculocephalic maneuver

Continued

TABLE 14.10 National Institutes of Health Stroke Scale—cont'd

Instructions	Scale	Definition
3. **Visual:** Visual fields (upper and lower quadrants) are tested by confrontation, using finger counting or visual threat as appropriate.	0 1 2 3	**No visual loss** **Partial hemianopia** **Complete hemianopia** **Bilateral hemianopia** (blind)
4. **Facial Palsy:** Ask—or use pantomime to encourage—the patient to show teeth or raise eyebrows and close eyes.	0 1 2 3	**Normal** symmetric movements **Minor paralysis** (asymmetry on smiling) **Partial paralysis** (total or near-total paralysis of lower face) **Complete paralysis** of one or both sides
5. **Motor Arm:** The limb is placed in the appropriate position: extend the arms (palms down) 90 degrees if sitting or 45 degrees if supine. Drift is scored if the arm falls before 10 seconds. 5a. Left arm 5b. Right arm	0 1 2 3 4 UN	**No drift;** limb holds position for 10 seconds **Drift;** limb holds position but drifts down before full 10 seconds **Some effort against gravity;** limb cannot get to or maintain position, drifts down to bed, has some effort against gravity **No effort against gravity;** limb falls **No movement** **Amputation** or joint fusion
6. **Motor Leg:** The limb is placed in the appropriate position: hold the leg at 30 degrees (always tested supine). Drift is scored if the leg falls before 5 seconds. 6a. Left leg 6b. Right leg	0 1 2 3 4 UN	**No drift;** leg holds position for full 5 seconds **Drift;** leg falls by the end of the 5-sec period but does not hit bed **Some effort against gravity;** leg falls to bed. By 5 seconds, has some effort against gravity **No effort against gravity;** leg falls to bed immediately **No movement** **Amputation** or joint fusion
7. **Limb Ataxia:** The finger-nose-finger and heel-shin tests are performed on both sides with eyes open.	0 1 2 UN	**Absent** **Present in one limb** **Present in two limbs** **Amputation** or joint fusion
8. **Sensory:** Sensation or grimace to pinprick when tested, or withdrawal from noxious stimulus in the obtunded or aphasic patient	0 1 2	**Normal;** no sensory loss **Mild to moderate sensory loss;** feels that pinprick is less sharp or is dull on the affected side, or there is a loss of superficial pain with pinprick but awareness of being touched **Severe to total sensory loss;** patient is not aware of being touched in the face, arm, and leg
9. **Best Language:** Using items from the published scale, patient is asked to describe what is happening in a picture, to name the items on a naming sheet list, and to read from a set of sentences. Comprehension is judged from responses as well as responses to all of the commands in the preceding general neurological examination.	0 1 2 3	**No aphasia;** normal **Mild to moderate aphasia;** some obvious loss of fluency or facility of comprehension, without significant limitation on ideas **Severe aphasia;** all communication is through fragmentary expression; great need for inference, questioning, and guessing by the listener **Mute, global aphasia;** no usable speech or auditory comprehension
10. **Dysarthria:** An adequate sample of speech must be obtained by asking the patient to read or repeat words from the published list	0 1 2 UN	**Normal** **Mild to moderate dysarthria;** patient slurs some words; can be understood with some difficulty **Severe dysarthria;** patient's speech is so slurred as to be unintelligible; or patient is mute/anarthric **Intubated** or other physical barrier
11. **Extinction and Inattention (Formerly Neglect):** Sufficient information to identify neglect may have been obtained during prior testing. If the patient has a severe visual loss preventing visual bilateral simultaneous stimulation and the cutaneous stimuli are normal, the score is normal.	0 1 2	No abnormality **Visual, tactile, auditory, spatial, or personal inattention** or extinction to bilateral simultaneous stimulation in one of the sensory modalities **Profound hemi-inattention or extinction to more than one modality;** does not recognize own hand or orients to only one side of space

LOC, Level of consciousness.
From National Institute of Neurological Disorders and Stroke, National Institutes of Health. NIH Stroke Scale. http://www.nihstrokescale.org/. Published 1999. Accessed March 11, 2019.

Assessment and stabilization of the airway, breathing, and circulation are a priority. Vital signs are monitored, usually every 15 minutes for the first 6 hours. BP elevations are common in these patients. Because reducing the BP can decrease blood flow and oxygenation to the ischemic brain tissue, a gradual 20% lowering of the hypertensive BP is recommended to prevent enlargement of the infarcted area and worsening of the neurological deficit. The goal for ischemic stroke is to keep the systolic BP at less than 220 mm Hg and the diastolic BP at less than 120 mm Hg.[11] In hemorrhagic stroke, the goal is a MAP less than 130 mm Hg.[4,11]

Monitor the respiratory pattern because changes can indicate that the stroke is extending and more neurological damage is occurring. Hypoxemia after a stroke is common as a result of concurrent medical conditions such as aspiration, pneumonia, hypoventilation, atelectasis, and pulmonary embolism.[1] Obtain a baseline SpO_2 while the patient is breathing room air, and provide supplemental oxygen when the SpO_2 is less than 95%.

Cardiac assessment, including the presence of cardiac dysrhythmias, is important to determine whether the stroke was potentially caused by a cardioembolic event. IV access is obtained, and normal saline infusions are started; hypertonic solutions are avoided. Laboratory studies include electrolytes, cardiac enzymes, complete blood count, urinalysis, and coagulation studies. Obtain a serum glucose level because many patients who present with stroke are hyperglycemic, and up to 20% of patients with stroke are diabetic.[1] Several studies have indicated that individuals with hyperglycemia have poorer outcomes after stroke compared with normoglycemic patients, even without a history of diabetes. The hyperglycemia seems to increase neuronal injury.[1,4]

Once the patient has been transferred to the critical care unit, assessments are compared with the baseline assessments performed in the emergency department. Hemodynamic instability is common in acute stroke because of cardiac disorders and the sympathetic response; therefore assessment of the airway, vital signs, and fluid and electrolyte status continues to be a priority. Elderly patients with stroke often are dehydrated. Dehydration is caused by inadequate water intake, drowsiness, dysphagia, possible infection, diuretic use, and uncontrolled diabetes.[6] Dehydration after a stroke can cause an increased hematocrit and a reduced BP that can worsen the ischemic process.[1,4] In a patient with an acute stroke, monitor neurological status, blood pressure, laboratory values, and cardiac function. Ongoing assessments are similar to those in patients with increased ICP.

Patients with SAH have a different presentation than those with ischemic stroke. When arterial blood enters the subarachnoid space, its presence is irritating to the meninges. The patient may complain of a localized headache, stiff neck (*nuchal rigidity*), pain above and behind the eye, and photophobia. Patients with SAH are often anxious and agitated as a result of pain, altered LOC, and cognitive changes.[1] If conscious, the patient may complain of "the worst headache of my life." Vomiting and decreased LOC are commonly seen. Neurological assessment includes LOC, motor and sensory deficits, and pupillary response. Assessment findings may range from mental status changes and subtle focal deficits to coma or severe neurological deficits.

Diagnostic Tests

Diagnostic tests are performed to differentiate ischemic from hemorrhagic stroke and to establish baseline parameters to monitor the effects of treatment.[1,4] Common diagnostic tests are summarized in Box 14.2.

Management

A patient with stroke has a similar collaborative care plan to those of patients with increased ICP and TBI. Refer to Plan of Care for the Patient with Traumatic Brain Injury, Increased Intracranial Pressure, or Acute Stroke earlier in the chapter.

BOX 14.2   Diagnostic Testing for Stroke

Initial Diagnostic Testing
- Emergency CT scan without contrast
- 12-Lead electrocardiogram
- Review of time of onset and inclusion criteria for patients eligible for rt-PA, including NIHSS assessment
- **Complete blood count:** red blood cells, hemoglobin, hematocrit, platelet count
- **Coagulation studies:** prothrombin time, activated partial thromboplastin time, INR
- Serum electrolytes and glucose
- Urinalysis
- Troponin and cardiac enzymes, to rule out myocardial infarction

Additional Diagnostic Testing
- **MRI with diffusion and perfusion images:** detects ischemia, altered CBF, and cerebral blood volume
- **Arteriography:** detects shallow ulcerated plaques, thrombus, aneurysms, dissections, multiple lesions, AVM, and collateral blood flow
- **MRA images:** detects carotid occlusion and intracranial stenosis or occlusions
- **CT perfusion images:** detects altered CBF and cerebral blood volume
- **CT angiography images:** detects carotid occlusion and intracranial stenosis or occlusions
- **Digital subtraction angiography:** detects carotid occlusion and intracranial stenoses or occlusions
- **Doppler carotid ultrasound:** detects stenosis or occlusions of the carotid arteries
- **Transcranial Doppler ultrasound:** detects stenosis or occlusion of the circle of Willis, vertebral arteries, and basilar artery
- **Transthoracic echocardiography:** detects cardioembolic abnormalities
- **Transesophageal echocardiography:** detects cardioembolic abnormalities; more sensitive than transthoracic echocardiography

AVM, Arteriovenous malformation; *CBF,* cerebral blood flow; *CT,* computed tomography; *INR,* international normalized ratio; *MRA,* magnetic resonance angiography; *MRI,* magnetic resonance imaging; *NIHSS,* National Institutes of Health Stroke Scale; *rt-PA,* recombinant tissue plasminogen activator.

Ischemic Stroke

Candidates for thrombolysis. Early thrombolysis is recommended; rt-PA is the only approved therapy for acute ischemic stroke and must be given within 3 hours after symptom onset.[26] Administration after 3 hours has not been shown to be beneficial and increases the risk for hemorrhagic transformation of the infarct. Only about 5% of eligible patients actually receive rt-PA.[26] This thrombolytic medication does not affect the infarcted area, but by lysing the clot it revitalizes the ischemic penumbra and improves overall neurological function. Careful assessment of patients who are potentially eligible for thrombolytic therapy must be made (Box 14.3).

Before the administration of rt-PA, insert two peripheral IV lines—one for the administration of rt-PA and one for fluids. If possible, place any catheters that are needed (e.g., urinary catheters, nasogastric tubes) before rt-PA is administered to reduce the risk for bleeding. After the administration of rt-PA, invasive procedures may be performed, but the risk of bleeding is higher. Anticoagulants, such as heparin or warfarin, and antiplatelet aggregates, such as aspirin, are withheld for 24 hours after administration of rt-PA to prevent bleeding complications.

Symptomatic hemorrhage is the most common complication after rt-PA administration, with an incidence of 6.4%.[11,26] The highest risk for hemorrhage is within the first 36 hours after administration. Hemorrhage usually occurs into the area of infarct; this is known as hemorrhagic transformation. The incidence of hemorrhagic transformation may be reduced by ensuring that rt-PA is given within 3 hours after symptom onset and by maintaining the systolic BP at less than 185 mm Hg and the diastolic BP at less than 110 mm Hg. Antihypertensive agents are administered as needed to control the BP.

Signs and symptoms of ICH manifest as neurological deterioration, increased ICP, or cerebral herniation. If ICH is suspected, the rt-PA infusion is stopped, an emergency noncontrast CT scan of the head is obtained, and fresh frozen plasma or platelets are administered. Systemic bleeding can also occur. Signs and symptoms include hypotension, tachycardia, pallor, restlessness, or low back pain. Monitor stool, urine, and gastric secretions for the presence of blood. Assess IV sites and gums for signs of external bleeding. Compare baseline coagulation studies with current studies.

Perform neurological assessment (LOC; language, motor, and sensory testing; pupillary response) and vital signs every 15 minutes for the first 2 hours, every 30 minutes for the next 6 hours, and every hour for 16 hours. Record accurate intake and output. Continuous cardiac monitoring is done throughout the hyperacute phase (first 24 to 72 hours). Administer oxygen to maintain the SpO_2 at 95%. Pneumonia is a common complication after stroke; frequent patient repositioning and nebulizer therapy may be indicated.[1]

Nonthrombolytic candidates. For a patient with stroke who is not a candidate for thrombolytic therapy, interventions include neurological, respiratory, and cardiac assessments. Perform these assessments and obtain vital signs every 1 to 2 hours during the first 24 hours after stroke. Control BP to prevent bleeding while maintaining an adequate CPP. For patients with uncontrolled hypertension, BP is managed carefully with IV medications such as labetalol, nitroprusside, or nicardipine. Rapid drops in BP can cause further neurological deterioration by decreasing cerebral perfusion and extending the area of cerebral ischemia. Laboratory tests (complete blood count, blood chemistries, urinalysis, coagulation studies, cardiac enzymes) are performed to identify the causes of the stroke.

Other interventions include the administration of medications to decrease ICP and maintenance of hemodynamic stability. The incidence of cerebral herniation peaks at about 72 hours after the stroke. Because hyperglycemia may exacerbate the extent of neurological injury, glycemic control is advocated (see Chapter 19). Hyponatremia due to cerebral salt wasting may occur; sodium and fluid replacement are necessary to maintain a normal sodium level.

Anticoagulants, such as warfarin, low-molecular-weight heparinoids, or factor Xa inhibitors such as rivaroxaban, may be used to prevent secondary cardioembolic stroke, whereas antiplatelet aggregates, such as aspirin, combination aspirin/dipyridamole (Aggrenox), clopidogrel (Plavix), prasugrel (Effient), and ticagrelor (Brilinta), may be given for prevention of secondary ischemic stroke. Some patients require antihypertensive agents or antiepileptic medications. Maintain adequate fluid balance to ensure proper hydration. Maintain

---

BOX 14.3 Administration of Tissue Plasminogen Activator for Acute Ischemic Stroke

Inclusion Criteria
- Onset of stroke symptoms less than 3 hours
- Clinical diagnosis of ischemic stroke with a measurable deficit using the NIHSS
- Age greater than 18 years
- CT scan consistent with ischemic stroke

Exclusion Criteria
- Stroke symptoms more than 3 hours after symptom onset
- Rapidly improving minor or major stroke (i.e., transient ischemic attack)
- Current intracranial hemorrhage
- Subarachnoid hemorrhage
- Active internal bleeding
- Recent (within 3 months) intracranial or intraspinal surgery or serious head trauma
- Presence of intracranial conditions that may increase the risk of bleeding (e.g., some neoplasms, AVM, or aneurysms)
- Bleeding diathesis
- Current severe uncontrolled hypertension

Administration
- rt-PA dosing: 0.9 mg/kg IV up to maximum of 90 mg
- Give bolus of 10% of total calculated dose IV over 1 minute
- Administer the remaining 90% over the next 60 minutes

AVM, Arteriovenous malformation; *NIHSS,* National Institutes of Health Stroke Scale; *rt-PA,* recombinant tissue plasminogen activator.
Modified from Bader MK, Littlejohns L, Olson D. *AANN Core Curriculum for Neuroscience Nursing.* 6th ed. Chicago, IL: American Association of Neuroscience Nurses; 2016; and Activase (alteplase) [package insert]. South San Francisco, CA: Genentech; https://www.gene.com/download/pdf/activase_prescribing.pdf. 2018.

normothermia to reduce the metabolic needs of the brain. Direct injury or bleeding into the hypothalamus may alter the hypothalamic set point that regulates body temperature, resulting in hyperthermia. Systemic infection or drug reactions may result in fever due to pyrogens increasing body temperature above the hypothalamic set point. Implement aspiration precautions, including elevating the head of the bed and maintaining nothing-by-mouth status, until a swallow screening or formal study rules out dysphagia.

Other Ischemic Events

Transient ischemic attacks. A TIA is defined as the sudden onset of a temporary focal neurological deficit caused by a vascular event. During a TIA, a transient decrease in CBF occurs, but the patient does not experience any permanent deficits.

A TIA is commonly caused by stenosis of the carotid arteries. A common presentation of a TIA is amaurosis fugax (monocular blindness), a transient occlusion of the central retinal artery. Although symptoms of a TIA mimic those of stroke, by definition TIA symptoms last for 24 hours or less.[1] In general, patients with symptoms of TIA should receive a complete stroke workup to determine the cause of TIA. Patients may be managed with anticoagulants or antiplatelet therapy depending on the etiology of the symptoms.

It is important that preventive measures be initiated for people with TIAs to avoid stroke. People experiencing a TIA often ignore the symptoms because they are painless and short-lived, usually about 5 to 10 minutes. Within a year after having a TIA, many persons have a stroke and sustain permanent neurological deficits.[1]

Patients experiencing TIAs with carotid stenosis are evaluated for carotid endarterectomy or carotid angioplasty and stenting. If a patient has carotid stenosis greater than 69% on the symptomatic side, carotid endarterectomy is recommended.[1] Carotid angioplasty with stenting is also an accepted method of treating carotid stenosis for selected patients.[1]

Hemorrhagic Stroke

Intracerebral hemorrhage. Control of BP is important to prevent recurrent hemorrhage. The optimal threshold for BP is unknown. Elevations in BP are not usually treated unless the MAP is greater than 130 mm Hg or the patient has a history of heart failure. If treatment is required, BP is lowered cautiously to prehemorrhage levels. Recombinant factor VIIa may be used to prevent extension of the hemorrhage, but it is effective only if used within 6 hours after onset.

Medical assessment focuses on determining the size and location of the ICH and whether it is amenable to surgical intervention. Small clots usually resolve without surgery. In these instances, more aggressive BP management may be indicated. Surgical resection, although controversial, may be considered for patients who have hematomas larger than 3 cm or who are deteriorating neurologically.[16] Recently a minimally invasive approach to ICH removal has been made available.[8] This approach involves an approved device that is placed into the area of hemorrhage via a minimally invasive approach, and the blood clot is flushed out. Comatose patients with large lesions usually have poorer outcomes regardless of treatment.[16]

Subarachnoid Hemorrhage due to Ruptured Aneurysm. Early diagnosis of the cause of SAH helps to guide treatment. Although a CT scan helps differentiate an aneurysm from an AVM, definitive diagnosis of an aneurysm is determined by digital subtraction or CT angiography. Early surgical or endovascular intervention (within 24 hours after admission) is recommended for patients in good neurological condition whose aneurysm is accessible by surgical or endovascular approaches. The goal is to secure the aneurysm before any episodes of rebleeding or vasospasm occur.[4,13]

A ruptured aneurysm is secured through surgical or endovascular intervention.[4,13] Surgery involves occluding the neck of the aneurysm with a metal clip; reinforcing the sac by wrapping it with muscle, fibrin foam, or solidifying polymer; or proximally ligating a feeding vessel. If the neck of the aneurysm is narrow and accessible, use of a metal clip is desirable. If the neck of the aneurysm is too broad, reinforcing the aneurysmal sac is the goal of surgery. Proximal ligation may be preferred if the aneurysm is directly fed by the internal carotid artery; the disadvantage of this procedure is the potential for stroke should collateral circulation fail.

Endovascular therapy with coils, stents, or a combination of the two may be used to occlude the aneurysm. This therapy consists of navigating a microcatheter through the femoral artery to the aneurysm and placing platinum coils into the aneurysm sac or a stent to cover the opening. Thrombosis occurs, occluding the aneurysm from the feeder vessel. If endovascular attempts fail to obliterate the aneurysm, surgical treatment may be required. Incomplete surgical obliteration may require additional endovascular treatment. Patients with severe neurological compromise after a ruptured aneurysm may benefit from emergency ventriculostomy. The ventriculostomy assists in treating the hydrocephalus associated with the bleeding. It also allows the clinician to monitor ICP and remove CSF to lower ICP if needed. If possible, ventriculostomy is not performed until after the aneurysm has been secured because changing the ICP can contribute to rebleeding.

BP control is an important component of aneurysmal SAH management.[4,10] Administer medications to reduce BP before the aneurysm is secured to prevent rebleeding. After the aneurysm is secured, BP is allowed to rise to prevent vasospasm.[8] If vasospasm occurs, BP may be purposely increased with fluids and medications to augment CBF. Assess neurological status frequently by using the GCS, and monitor for focal deficits and pupillary changes. Monitor temperature because persons with SAH often have a fever, which is associated with worse neurological outcome.[4,10] Elevate the head of the bed to reduce ICP. A feeding tube may be required for nutritional support. Initiate measures for venous thromboembolism prevention. Other important interventions include providing analgesia and bed rest.

Monitor for signs of vasospasm because early intervention results in better patient outcomes.[4] Nimodipine, a neurospecific calcium channel blocker, reduces the incidence and severity of deficits associated with SAH.[4] The recommended dosage is 60 mg every 4 hours for 21 days. Vasospasm is often treated with volume expansion to increase CPP. The modalities used are hypervolemia and hypertension. Hypervolemia refers to increasing the blood volume by using crystalloids, colloids, albumin, plasma protein fraction, or blood. Systolic BP is maintained between 150 and 160 mm Hg (and sometimes higher). The increase in volume and BP forces blood through the vasospastic area at higher pressure. If the patient's BP cannot be maintained at the increased level required, vasoactive medications such as dopamine, dobutamine, or phenylephrine may be warranted. Monitor hemoglobin to assure adequate oxygen carrying capacity.

Therapies for the treatment of symptomatic vasospasm include papaverine, nicardipine, and angioplasty. Intraarterial papaverine application increases the diameter of the vasospastic blood vessel but lasts less than 24 hours. Intraarterial or intraventricular administration of nicardipine, a calcium channel blocker, has a vasodilatory effect. The clinical indications for nicardipine are similar to those for papaverine; however, nicardipine is effective for 2 to 5 days. Cerebral angioplasty is indicated for vasospasm if pharmacological therapy has failed. Risks of angioplasty include perforation or rupture, cerebral artery thrombosis, recurrent vasospasm, and transient neurological deficits.

Arteriovenous Malformation. Spontaneous bleeding from an AVM can occur into the ventricular system, intracerebral tissue, or subarachnoid space. Hemorrhage from an AVM is usually low-pressure bleeding, and the mortality from such a hemorrhage is lower than that from a ruptured aneurysm. The rebleeding rate is also much lower than for an aneurysm. AVMs may also cause symptoms due to ischemia or act as a space-occupying lesion, similar to a tumor.

Treatment interventions for an AVM include embolization, surgery, radiotherapy, or a combination of all three.[38] Surgery for removal of an AVM is done as a single step or in multiple stages. Postoperatively, the major problem is breakthrough bleeding from cauterized vessels. Rapid increases in BP during recovery from anesthesia are avoided, and BP must be tightly controlled during the first 48 hours after resection to prevent bleeding. Embolization is not a curative approach to most AVMs; rather, it is used as preparation for surgery. Embolization may occur in a single setting or may be staged in several procedures over days to weeks. Radiotherapy may be performed alone or for residual AVM after surgery; results are manifested over years.

Postoperative Neurosurgical Care for Intracranial Surgery

The postoperative care of a patient who has undergone a neurosurgical procedure involves frequent and ongoing BP, respiratory, metabolic, and neurological assessments. Neurological assessments are done every 15 to 30 minutes for the first 2 to 12 hours postoperatively, then every hour while the patient is in the critical care unit. Oxygenation and tissue perfusion are monitored. Chest radiographs, CT scans, EEGs, and other diagnostic tests may be necessary to monitor progress.

The position of the head of the bed depends on the specific surgical procedure, the patient's condition, and the physician's preference. Unless they are intubated, unconscious patients are never positioned flat because the tongue can slip backward and obstruct the airway. Unconscious patients may be positioned in a lateral position with the head of the bed flat. Always maintain the neck in a neutral position.

The most common postoperative complications are infection, cerebral hemorrhage, increased ICP, hydrocephalus, and seizures.[1] Intracerebral hemorrhage is detected by a decline in neurological status, signs of increasing ICP, and new or worsened focal deficits (i.e., hemiparesis/hemiplegia, aphasia). It is confirmed by CT scan. Treatment depends on CT findings and may require emergency surgery.

Hydrocephalus can develop any time during the postoperative course as a result of edema or bleeding into the subarachnoid space. Treatment may include placement of a ventriculostomy to drain CSF temporarily. If the hydrocephalus does not resolve, a surgical shunting procedure may be indicated to relieve the brain of excessive CSF.

Seizures can occur at any time but are most common within the first 7 days after surgery. Focal seizures in the form of twitching of selected muscles, particularly of the face and hand, are often seen. Patients may receive postoperative antiepileptic drugs, levetiracetam or phenytoin, if concern for seizures is high. Serum phenytoin levels are monitored to maintain a therapeutic range.

STUDY BREAK

4. The nurse caring for a patient with an acute ischemic stroke anticipates:
   A. Holding blood pressure medications to promote cerebral perfusion so that blood pressure can increase to greater than 200 mm Hg
   B. Planning for inducing hyperthermia to protect ischemic brain
   C. Preparing the patient for emergency surgery
   D. Identifying the precise time of stroke symptom onset when possible

---

SEIZURES AND STATUS EPILEPTICUS

A seizure is an abnormal electrical discharge in the brain that can be caused by a variety of neurological disorders, systemic diseases, and metabolic disorders. Seizures consist of repetitive depolarization of hyperactive, hypersensitive cells that cause an altered state of brain function. In 2017 the International League Against Epilepsy (ILAE) revised its classification of seizures (Table 14.11). The new classification system is based on three key features: where seizures begin in the brain, level of awareness during a seizure, and other features of seizures.[9]

Pathophysiology of Status Epilepticus

When seizures occur in close proximity to each other, they have the potential to lead to a life-threatening medical emergency known as *status epilepticus* (SE). SE can occur with any type of seizure. By definition, SE is present when

TABLE 14.11 Classification of Seizures

Location of Seizure

Focal	Starts in an area on one side of brain *Focal motor:* twitching, jerking, stiffening, rubbing hands, walking, running *Focal non-motor:* changes in sensorium, emotions, or thinking occur first *Auras:* symptoms felt at start of seizure
Generalized	Involves an area on both sides of the brain at the onset *Generalized motor:* stiffening (tonic) and jerking (clonic) *Generalized non-motor:* brief periods of awareness, staring, repeated movements (lipsmaking)
Unknown onset	Onset of seizure unknown
Focal to bilateral	Starts on one side of brain and spreads to both sides

Level of Awareness

Focal aware	Awareness remains intact even if person unable to talk or respond
Focal impaired awareness	Awareness impaired
Awareness unknown	Unknown if person is aware or not if person lives alone or has seizures only at night

Adapted from Fisher RS. The new classification of seizures by the International League Against Epilepsy. *Curr Neurol Neurosci Rep.* 2017;17(6): 48-53.

seizure activity lasts for 30 minutes or longer or when two or more sequential seizures occur without full recovery of consciousness between seizures.[1] SE is more likely to occur with tonic-clonic seizures that have a specific causative factor than with idiopathic seizures. The most frequent precipitating factors for SE are irregular intake of antiepileptic drugs, withdrawal from habitual use of alcohol or sedative drugs, electrolyte imbalance, azotemia, head trauma, infection, and brain tumor.

Physiological changes that occur during SE are divided into two phases. During *phase 1*, cerebral metabolism is increased and compensatory mechanisms (increased CBF and catecholamine release) prevent cerebral damage from hypoxia or metabolic injury. However, these changes can lead to other problems. Hyperglycemia occurs from release of epinephrine and activation of hepatic gluconeogenesis. Hypertension occurs due to increased CBF. Hyperpyrexia results from excessive muscle activity and catecholamine release. Lactic acidosis occurs from anaerobic metabolism. Elevated epinephrine and norepinephrine levels and acidosis contribute to cardiac dysrhythmias. Autonomic dysfunction causes excessive sweating and vomiting, leading to dehydration and electrolyte loss.

Phase 2 begins 30 to 60 minutes after phase 1. Decompensation occurs because the increased metabolic demands cannot be met. This causes decreased CBF, systemic hypotension, increased ICP, and failure of cerebral autoregulation. The patient develops metabolic and respiratory acidosis from hypoxemia and hypoglycemia from depleted energy stores. The lack of oxygen and glucose results in cellular injury. Pulmonary edema is common, and aspiration can occur from decreased laryngeal reflex sensitivity. Cardiac dysrhythmias and heart failure result from hypoxemia, hyperkalemia caused by increased muscle activity, and metabolic acidosis. Acute kidney injury may result from rhabdomyolysis and acute myoglobinuria. Myoglobin is released secondary to excessive muscle activity from prolonged skeletal muscle contraction and traumatic injury during the seizure.

Death from SE is more likely to occur when an underlying disease is responsible for the seizure or from the acute illness that precipitated the seizure. Generalized seizures that last for 30 to 45 minutes can result in neuronal necrosis and permanent neurological deficits. Prompt diagnosis and treatment are important because seizure duration is an important prognostic factor.

Assessment

Assessment during SE incorporates the neurological, respiratory, and cardiovascular systems. Identify characteristics of the seizure and the neurological state before, between, and after seizures. Collect information, including precipitating factors, preceding aura, type of movement observed, automatisms, changes in size of pupils or eye deviation, responsiveness to auditory or tactile stimuli, LOC throughout the seizure, urinary or bowel incontinence, behavior after the seizure, weakness or paralysis of extremities after the seizure, injuries caused by the seizure, and duration of the seizure.[1] Assess respiratory status and SpO_2 to ensure adequate oxygenation. Because decompensation can result in pulmonary edema, observe for the onset of fine basilar crackles and have suction equipment and oxygen readily available. Cardiac monitoring is necessary to assess for dysrhythmias. Assess blood glucose because hypoglycemia is an important cause of SE.

Diagnostic Tests

Laboratory studies for a patient with SE include serum electrolytes, liver function studies, serum medication levels, and blood and urine toxicology screens. Measurements of cardiac enzymes and arterial blood gases assist in assessing the effect of the seizure on other body systems. Patient monitoring includes ECG, continuous EEG, noninvasive BP, and pulse oximetry.

Radiological studies are performed to rule out pathology that may be responsible for the episode of SE. These may include CT or MRI, with or without contrast. Additional studies may be done as needed.

Management

Patient Problems. In addition to the patient problems stated in the Collaborative Plan of Care for the Critically Ill Patient in

Chapter 1, other patient problems relevant to the patient experiencing SE include:

- Impaired tissue perfusion (cerebral and cardiopulmonary)
- Decreased gas exchange
- Ineffective airway clearance
- Disturbed thought process related to the postictal state
- Need for health teaching

Nursing and Medical Interventions. Management during SE includes maintaining a patent airway, providing adequate oxygenation, maintaining vascular access for the administration of medications and fluids, administering appropriate medications, and maintaining seizure precautions. Facilitate a patent airway by positioning the patient appropriately; use of an oral or nasal airway or endotracheal tube may be necessary. Do not place padded tongue blades between the clenched teeth of a patient undergoing a seizure; patients have inadvertently been injured from aspirating teeth that were loosened during forceful attempts to insert a padded tongue blade between their teeth. Suction as needed to remove secretions that collect in the oropharynx. Administer supplemental oxygen to improve oxygenation. Neuromuscular blocking medications may be used to facilitate intubation but will not be effective in halting neuronal firing; attention to seizure control is necessary, even if the patient is paralyzed. A nasogastric tube with intermittent suction may be needed to ensure that the airway is not compromised by aspiration.

Maintain vascular access to provide a route for the administration of medications. If IV access cannot be established, some antiepileptic medications can be administered rectally. The specific medication given to arrest the seizure depends on its type and duration (see Table 14.9). It is essential to monitor BP and to administer volume replacement and vasoactive medications as necessary. IV dextrose is administered unless the blood glucose level is known to be normal or high. Thiamine may also be given prior to glucose if Wernicke's encephalopathy is suspected.

Seizure precautions are continued during SE. They include padding the side rails on the patient's bed and making sure that the bed has full-length side rails. Keep the bed in a low position with side rails up except when providing direct nursing care. If the patient is in a chair when a seizure begins, lower the patient to the floor and place a soft object under the patient's head. Remove the patient's restrictive clothing and jewelry while always maintaining the patient's privacy. Do not restrain the patient because forceful tonic-clonic movements can traumatize the patient.

SE must be treated immediately. Ensure a patent airway and maintain breathing and circulation. Administer medications with a sequential approach that progressively uses more potent medications to control the seizure. The first-line medication is a benzodiazepine, usually IV lorazepam (Ativan). If lorazepam fails to stop seizure activity within 10 minutes, or if intermittent seizures persist for longer than 20 minutes, levetiracetam (Keppra), phenytoin (Dilantin), fosphenytoin (Cerebyx), lamotrigine (Lamictal) or lacosamide (Vimpat) may be administered.[1,15] Phenytoin is mixed only with normal saline and is stable in solution for up to 4 hours. After clearing the IV line with saline, administer phenytoin slowly by IV push (25 to 50 mg/min, not to exceed 50 mg/min). Phenobarbital may be used as an additional medication to control SE, but its utility in SE is lessened by the length of time required to achieve a therapeutic effect. Other medications that have been used in SE include midazolam, clonazepam, lamotrigine, lacosamide, topiramate, and valproic acid (see Table 14.9).[1]

If SE continues despite initial medication administration, propofol (Diprivan) is given; pentobarbital or thiopental may also be used. Propofol is a general anesthetic and sedative-hypnotic agent. Patients may require intubation and mechanical ventilation if inefficient ventilation results. Pentobarbital may also be considered. Assess the patient for hypotension.

> **❓ CRITICAL REASONING ACTIVITY**
>
> Mr. B. is an 18-year-old patient who was admitted in generalized convulsive status epilepticus. Describe the appropriate nursing and medical interventions.

CENTRAL NERVOUS SYSTEM INFECTIONS

The brain and spinal cord are relatively well protected from infective agents by the bones of the skull and vertebral column, the meninges, and the blood-brain barrier. However, infective agents can enter the CNS through the air sinuses, the middle ear, or blood. Injuries and treatments that disrupt the dura (e.g., basilar skull fractures, missile injuries, neurosurgical procedures) also increase the risk for infection. *Meningitis* (infection of the meninges) may be caused by bacteria, viruses, fungi, parasites, or other toxins. These infections are classified as acute, subacute, or chronic. The pathophysiology, clinical presentation, and management differ for each type of microorganism. Box 14.4 lists common organisms that cause meningitis.

Bacterial Meningitis

Bacterial meningitis is a neurological emergency that can lead to substantial morbidity and mortality.[3,18] Approximately 3000 cases occur in the United States each year, and more than 300 people die, with a significant fatality rate among adolescents.[18] Meningitis affects the very young, the very old, and immunosuppressed individuals. Because of its high mortality rate, vaccination against bacterial meningitis is recommended.

Pathophysiology. Bacterial meningitis is an infection of the pia mater and arachnoid layers of the meninges and the CSF in the subarachnoid space. Bacteria gain access in one of three ways: (1) via the blood or through the spread of nearby infection, such as sinusitis; (2) by CSF contamination through surgical procedures or catheters; or (3) through the skull. Airborne droplets can be passed from infected individuals through sneezing, coughing, or kissing, and droplets can be passed through saliva and transmitted via drinks, cigarettes, or utensils. Bacteria enter through the choroid plexuses, multiply in the subarachnoid space, and irritate the meninges. An exudate forms that thickens the CSF and alters CSF flow through and around the brain and spinal cord, resulting in obstruction, interstitial edema, and further inflammation.

BOX 14.4 Causes of Meningitis

Bacterial
- *Streptococcus pneumoniae* (pneumococcus)
- *Neisseria meningitidis* (meningococcus)
- *Haemophilus influenzae* type B (Hib)
- Staphylococci *(Staphylococcus aureus)*
- Gram-negative bacilli *(Escherichia coli, Enterobacter, Serratia)*

Viral
- Echovirus
- Coxsackievirus
- Mumps virus
- Herpes simplex virus types 1 and 2
- St. Louis encephalitis virus
- Colorado tick fever virus
- Epstein-Barr virus
- West Nile virus
- Influenza virus types A and B

Fungal
- *Histoplasma*
- *Candida*
- *Aspergillus*

Assessment. A thorough history and neurological assessment are completed for patients with bacterial meningitis. Patients often are seen in the emergency department with an acute onset of symptoms (e.g., headache, fever, stiff neck, vomiting) that developed over 1 to 2 days. There may be a recent history of infection (ear, sinus, or upper respiratory tract), foreign travel, or illicit drug use. The clinical presentation often reveals signs of systemic infection, including fever (temperature as high as 39.5°C), tachycardia, chills, and petechial rash. Initially the rash may be macular, but it progresses to petechiae and purpura, mainly on the trunk and extremities. Meningeal irritation produces a throbbing headache, photophobia, vomiting, and nuchal rigidity. A positive *Kernig sign* (pain in the neck when the thigh is flexed 90 degrees and the leg extended at the knee) and a positive *Brudzinski sign* (involuntary flexion of the hips when the neck is flexed toward the chest) may be present. The patient's condition can quickly deteriorate to hypotension, shock, and sepsis.

Assess the patient's LOC, motor response, and cranial nerves. Confusion and decreasing LOC are evidence of cortical involvement. Focal neurological deficits may be seen, including hemiparesis, hemiplegia, and ataxia, as well as seizure activity and projectile vomiting. Irritation and damage to cranial nerves occur as a result of inflamed sheaths. As ICP increases, unconsciousness may occur.

Diagnostic Tests. The gold standard for the diagnosis of meningitis is examination of the CSF. A sample may be obtained by lumbar puncture or by aspiration from a ventricular catheter. Diagnosis can also be based on a nasopharyngeal smear and antigen tests. Blood and urine cultures are obtained before antibiotics are started. A CT scan, MRI study, or both may be beneficial in diagnosing bacterial meningitis to exclude other neurological pathological conditions such as cerebral edema, hydrocephalus, fractures, inner ear infection, or mastoiditis. Do not delay the lumbar puncture procedure to obtain scans if the patient has significant neurological deficits.[18]

Collaborative Management

Patient problems. The following patient problems may be applicable to a patient with a CNS infection, including bacterial meningitis:
- Fever
- Potential for injury from seizures
- Potential for decreased cerebral perfusion
- Pain

Nursing and medical management. Antibiotics are started as soon as possible once the diagnosis is suspected because of the rapid progression of the disease process.[18] After administration of antibiotic therapy, the search begins for the offending organism based on patient history, physical examination, CSF cultures, and blood cultures. Droplet isolation is maintained for 24 hours after the initiation of antibiotic therapy. Unusual bacteria and other microorganisms are increasingly responsible for meningitis. Identification of the offending organism or organisms may take time, and final culture results may redirect treatment.

Place the patient in a private room and dim the lighting. Implement seizure precautions. Assess temperature and manage fever with antipyretics and cooling devices. As the acute inflammatory period subsides, monitor the patient closely to prevent secondary complications. These include seizures, increased ICP, syndrome of inappropriate antidiuretic hormone secretion (SIADH), cerebral infarction, gastric bleeding, venous thromboembolism, pneumonia, and sepsis.

⚠ CLINICAL ALERT

Meningitis Care and Precautions

Haemophilus influenzae type B and *Neisseria meningitidis* are common bacteria that cause meningitis. These bacteria are easily spread by droplets generated by coughing, sneezing, or talking and during invasive respiratory procedures. Any patient with suspected meningitis should be placed on droplet precautions. Once these bacteria have been ruled out as the source of infection, or after effective antibiotic therapy has been instituted for 24 hours, droplet precautions may be discontinued.

During the acute phase of bacterial meningitis, the patient requires close monitoring. Increased intracranial pressure may occur, requiring administration of mannitol or hypertonic saline, placement of a ventriculostomy catheter to drain cerebrospinal fluid, or both. Maintain bed rest with the head of the bed elevated 30 to 40 degrees. Continue IV antibiotic therapy to treat the specific organism identified. IV corticosteroids may reduce mortality, hearing loss, and neurological sequelae by decreasing meningeal inflammation.[18] Current practice guidelines recommend that dexamethasone (Decadron) 10 mg be initiated before or with the first dose of antibiotics and then every 6 hours for 4 days in adult patients with suspected bacterial meningitis.[3]

STUDY BREAK

5. A patient is admitted to the critical care unit with a diagnosis of possible meningitis. Actions the nurse anticipates include all of the following except:
   - A. Placing the patient on contact precautions
   - B. Obtaining blood and urine cultures
   - C. Administering antibiotics as soon as possible
   - D. Preparing the patient for lumbar puncture

SPINAL CORD INJURY

Approximately 200,000 people in the United States are living with SCI. Each year, about 11,000 additional individuals sustain SCI. Most SCIs occur in individuals between the ages of 16 and 30 years.[7] The most common causes of SCI are motor vehicle crashes, falls, acts of violence (primarily gunshot wounds), sports injuries, and diving accidents.[7] TBI often occurs with SCI; therefore SCI should be considered a possibility in all unconscious patients.[24] Providing emergency intervention at the scene by skilled providers, decreasing transport time to the hospital, and implementing evidence-based SCI guidelines improve a patient's outcome.

Pathophysiology

SCI occurs with or without associated vertebral injury and results in complex and multifaceted biochemical changes in the spinal cord.[32] An inflammatory reaction creates spinal cord edema, which compresses tissue and blood vessels. Cord edema can ascend or descend from the level of injury. Vascular changes also occur. Microscopic hemorrhages occur in the central gray matter of the spinal cord with extension into surrounding white matter. Hemorrhage exacerbates edema and further decreases blood flow, resulting in ischemia. If the ischemia is not reversed, axonal degeneration and conduction failure of the neurons occur. Eventually, cell death occurs, with permanent loss of function (Fig. 14.20).

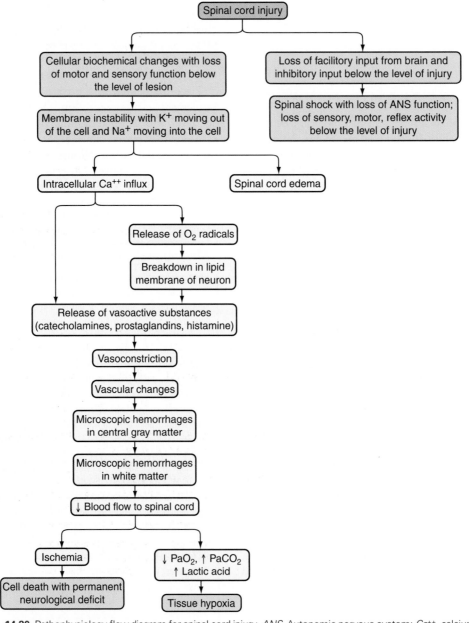

Fig. 14.20 Pathophysiology flow diagram for spinal cord injury. *ANS,* Autonomic nervous system; *Ca++,* calcium; *K+,* potassium; *Na+,* sodium; *O₂,* oxygen; *PaCO₂,* partial pressure of arterial carbon dioxide; *PaO₂,* partial pressure of arterial oxygen.

SCI produces two types of shock. *Spinal shock* is an electrical silence of the cord below the level of injury that causes complete loss of motor, sensory, and reflex activity. It begins within minutes after an injury and lasts for up to 6 weeks. Often the permanence of injury is not known until spinal shock resolves. Resolution is signaled by the return of deep tendon reflexes; rarely, motor or sensory function may return. *Neurogenic shock* occurs from disruption of autonomic pathways; it results in temporary loss of autonomic function below the level of the injury. Sympathetic input is lost, causing vasodilation and distributive shock, which manifests as hypotension, bradycardia, and hypothermia. Bradycardia may be so severe that a temporary pacemaker is required. Duration of neurogenic shock is variable; resolution is signaled by return of sympathetic tone.

SCI can result in a complete or incomplete lesion (Fig. 14.21). A *complete lesion* causes total, permanent loss of motor and sensory function below the level of injury. An incomplete lesion is more common and results in the sparing of some motor and sensory function below the level of injury. The three types of *incomplete lesions* are the *central cord, anterior cord,* and *Brown-Séquard* syndromes. The clinical presentation of each syndrome is based on damage to spinal cord organization and crossing of tracts. Many patients present with a picture of a complete lesion until spinal shock resolves; those with an incomplete lesion show a mixed pattern of motor and sensory function and have a potential for at least partial recovery.

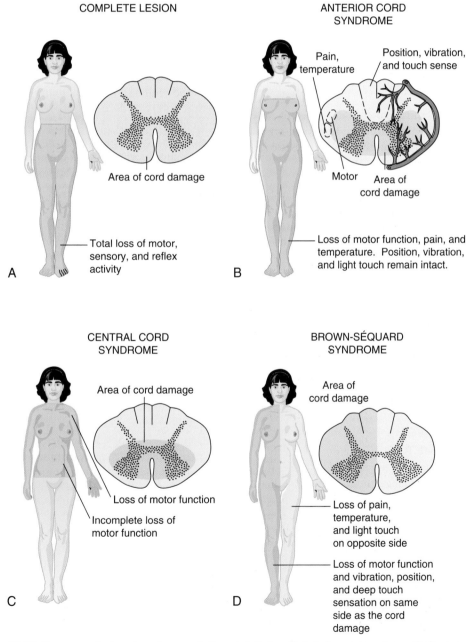

Fig. 14.21 Common spinal cord syndromes. **A,** Complete lesion. **B,** Anterior cord syndrome. **C,** Central cord syndrome. **D,** Brown-Séquard syndrome. (Modified from Ignatavicius DD, Workman ML. *Medical-Surgical Nursing: Patient-Centered Collaborative Care.* 7th ed. Philadelphia, PA: Saunders; 2013.)

Assessment

Airway and Respiratory Assessment.
Assessment of respiratory and neurological status is the first priority for the critical care nurse.[36] Respiratory problems are common with cervical and thoracic SCI. Ineffective breathing patterns are caused by paralysis of the diaphragm or the intercostal muscles or both. Baseline arterial blood gas measurements are obtained on admission. Ongoing assessment of the adequacy of the airway and ventilation, including continuous monitoring of SpO_2, is essential. Emergent treatment, including endotracheal intubation and mechanical ventilation, may be needed.

Respiratory impairment varies with the level and type of injury (complete or incomplete). Complete lesions are associated with the following[1,36]:
- C1-C3: ventilator dependency
- C4-C5: phrenic nerve impairment that may be treated with a phrenic nerve pacemaker
- Cervical injury below C5-T6: intact diaphragmatic breathing, with varying impairment of intercostal and abdominal muscle function

Those with incomplete spinal cord lesions present with varying degrees of respiratory impairment, depending on the level of the lesion and whether the respiratory muscles are impaired.

Neurological Assessment.
All components of the neurological examination are performed for the patient with an SCI, with an emphasis on motor, reflex, and sensory responses. An assessment of the major muscle groups (see Table 14.4) and sensory level (see Fig. 14.6) is completed to determine the level of injury.

A patient with neurogenic shock (injury at T6 and higher) is unable to regulate body temperature; body temperature accommodates to the environmental temperature. The inability to adequately autoregulate body temperature is called *poikilothermia*. Closely monitor temperature, regulate the room temperature to avoid hypothermia, and keep the patient warm with blankets as needed. Hyperthermia can occur quickly if the patient is excessively warmed and should also be avoided, as the goal is normothermia.

Hemodynamic Assessment.
Patients with an SCI are often managed in a critical care unit for the first 7 days after injury to allow early detection and management of unstable heart rate and blood pressure.[25,38] Decreases in heart rate may be associated with hypothermia and hypoxemia, as well as neurogenic shock. Venous stasis occurs as a result of loss of vasomotor tone and paralysis, increasing the risk of venous thromboembolism.

Bowel and Bladder Function.
Spinal shock results in atony of the bowel and bladder. The bladder does not contract, and the detrusor muscle does not open. Urinary retention occurs, and an indwelling urinary catheter is required to prevent damage to the bladder wall. Initiate a bladder program with the resolution of spinal shock; however, it is dependent on the patient's level of injury and functional recovery. Loss of peristaltic movement increases the risk of paralytic ileus. The patient may require gastrointestinal decompression and is assessed for return of bowel sounds, flatus, and bowel movement. A bowel program is initiated as soon as bowel sounds are present.

Skin Assessment.
Because of impaired circulation and immobility, the patient with SCI is at risk for skin breakdown. A complete assessment of all skin surfaces is done every 4 hours. If halo traction or cervical tongs are used to stabilize a cervical fracture, carefully inspect the skin around pin sites and under traction devices. Observe the site for redness, swelling, drainage, and pain. If a cervical collar is in place, assess skin integrity with an emphasis on pressure points (occipital, chin, and sternal regions).

Psychological Assessment.
A psychological assessment is important during the acute phase of SCI. Initially, the patient is concerned with surviving the injury and does not realize the extent of injury or disability. The patient's perceptions are also impaired by medications and the physiological effects of injury. Patients often experience denial, anger, and depression. As the patient gains insight into the situation, include the patient in care planning and give the patient choices because feelings of powerlessness are common.

Family members also go through a similar experience. First, they experience shock related to the injury itself and the seriousness of the patient's condition. During that time, family members need support and answers to their questions.[1] Consultation with a psychiatric or mental health nurse or a psychiatrist may be indicated.[32] Involve the patient and family early in plans for rehabilitation.

Diagnostic Studies

Baseline laboratory studies include electrolytes, complete blood count, prothrombin time, aPTT, platelet count, and arterial blood gases. Common diagnostic studies to confirm the extent of vertebral and cord injury include anteroposterior and lateral spine radiographic studies, chest radiographic studies, CT scan, MRI, and myelography. Somatosensory-cortical evoked potentials may be performed to determine whether sensory pathways between the site of stimulation and the site of recording are intact.

Management

Nursing Interventions.
Nursing interventions are focused on maintaining stabilization of the spinal alignment, preserving the airway and respiratory status, and preventing complications associated with immobility and the SCI (see Plan of Care for the Patient With Spinal Cord Injury and the Collaborative Plan of Care for the Critically Ill Patient in Chapter 1). Once neurogenic shock has resolved, the patient with a complete SCI above T6 must be observed for autonomic dysreflexia (see Clinical Alert box).

◎ PLAN OF CARE

For the Patient With Spinal Cord Injury

Patient Problem

Decreased Functional Ability. Risk factors include muscle weakness or paralysis and spinal immobilization.

Desired Outcomes
- Consequences of immobility minimized (i.e. pressure injury, VTE, pneumonia).
- Maintenance of vertebral alignment.
- Absence of progressive neurologic dysfunction.
- Improved sensory, motor, and reflex function.

Nursing Assessments/Interventions	Rationales
• Perform neurologic assessments (motor, reflex, and sensory).	• Assess subtle changes indicating neurologic deterioration or improvement.
• Report progression of deficits from baseline (difficulty with swallowing or coughing, respiratory stridor, sternal retraction, bradycardia, fluctuating BP, and motor and sensory loss at a higher level than the initial findings).	• Detect worsening of symptoms that indicate need for interventions (e.g., airway management and ventilation).
• Administer steroids (e.g., methylprednisolone) as ordered within the first 8 hours on injury.	• May improve spinal cord function; decreases ischemia and prevents secondary cord injury.
• Institute measures to prevent consequences of immobility: frequent repositioning, use of heel and elbow protectors, passive range of motion and daily evaluation of lower extremities for signs of VTE.	• Promote blood flow to lungs and ventilation efforts; improve pulmonary function; minimize risk for skin breakdown; prevent muscle breakdown and promote venous return from lower extremities.
• Maintain halo or tong traction for immobilization.	• Maintain alignment and prevent complications.
• Perform tong insertion site care (pin care) per routine.	• Prevent infection at the pin site.
• Evaluate pin sites for redness, pain, drainage suggestive of possible infection.	
• If skeletal traction slips or is accidentally removed, maintain the patient's head in a neutral position.	• Maintain alignment and prevent further damage.
• Turn, lift, and transfer the patient using at least three people, with one at head to stabilize neck and to coordinate the move (log roll).	• Maintain the spinal cord in alignment to prevent further trauma to the spinal cord.

Patient Problem

Impaired Temperature Regulation. Risk factors include the body's inability to adapt to environmental temperature changes and the absence of sweating below the level of injury.

Desired Outcomes
- Normothermia within 2-4 hours of diagnosis.
- Normothermia maintained.

Nursing Assessments/Interventions	Rationales
• Monitor temperature at least every 4 h.	• Assess need for intervention.
• Assess for signs of ineffective thermoregulation (skin warm above level of injury or cool below; complaints of being too cold or warm, pilomotor erection).	• Identify need for intervention to maintain normothermia.
• Implement measures to attain normothermia (warm or cool as indicated; adjust ambient room temperature).	• Maintain normothermia; prevent complications.

Patient Problem

Decreased Cerebral and Cardiac Perfusion. A risk factor is the loss of vasomotor tone and subsequent hypovolemia.

Desired Outcomes
- Adequate cardiac output.
- Orientation to name, place, time.
- SBP > 90 mm Hg or within 20 mm Hg of baseline.
- HR 60-100 beats/min, ECG shows NSR.

Nursing Assessments/Interventions	Rationales
• Monitor symptoms of low CO: hypotension, lightheadedness, confusion.	• Identify low CO to provide prompt interventions.
• Monitor hemodynamic measurements; administer fluids.	• Provide objective data to guide and monitor treatment.
• Continuously assess the ECG.	• Identify dysrhythmias associated with low CO.
• Implement measures to prevent orthostatic hypotension: change position slowly; apply antiembolic hose; apply abdominal binder.	• Prevent orthostatic hypotension.

Continued

⊚ PLAN OF CARE—cont'd
For the Patient With Spinal Cord Injury

Patient Problem

Potential for Infection and Pressure Injury. Risk factors include immobilization, surgical intervention, and presence of invasive devices.

Desired Outcomes
- Absence of skin breakdown and pressure injury.
- Absence of infection at tong insertion site, surgical incision sites, or from an IV catheter and urinary catheter.

Nursing Assessments/Interventions	Rationales
• Assess insertion sites and incisions for signs of infection.	• Identify risk and signs of infection.
• Perform tong insertion site care (pin care)	• Prevent infection.
• Reposition frequently, avoiding pressure on bony prominences.	• Decrease risk for pressure injury.
• Assess all skin surfaces every 4 h.	

Patient Problem

Constipation. Risk factors include immobility, atonic bowel, loss of sensation and voluntary sphincter.

Desired Outcome
- Soft, formed bowel movement within 48 hours of initiating a bowel program.

Nursing Assessments/Interventions	Rationales
• Monitor for nausea, vomiting, abdominal distension, malaise, and the presence of a hard fecal mass on digital examination.	• Assess constipation and fecal impaction.
• Monitor the patient's bowel sounds.	• Assess bowel function.
• Administer stool softeners.	• Promote adequate bowel movement.
• Document the patient's bowel movements.	• Assess effectiveness of bowel management program.

BP, Blood pressure; *CO,* cardiac output; *ECG,* electrocardiogram; *HR,* heart rate; *IV,* intravenous; *NSR,* normal sinus rhythm; *SBP,* systolic blood pressure; *SCI,* spinal cord injury; *VTE,* venous thromboembolism; *WBC,* white blood cell count.
Adapted from Swearingen PLW, J.D. *All-in-One Nursing Care Planning Resource.* 5th ed. St. Louis: Elsevier; 2019.

⚠ CLINICAL ALERT
Autonomic Dysreflexia

Medical Emergency: Can Result in Stroke, Seizures, or Other Complications
- Occurs with injury at T6 or above, after spinal shock has resolved
- Characterized by exaggerated response of the sympathetic nervous system

Triggered by a Variety of Stimuli
- Bladder—kinked indwelling catheter, distension, infection, calculi, cystoscopy
- Bowel—fecal impaction, rectal examination, insertion of suppository
- Skin—tight clothing, irritation from bed linens, temperature extremes

Common Signs and Symptoms
- Sudden, severe, pounding headache
- Elevated, uncontrolled blood pressure
- Bradycardia
- Nasal congestion
- Blurred vision
- Profuse diaphoresis above the level of injury
- Flushing above the level of injury
- Pallor, chills, and pilomotor erection below the level of the injury
- Anxiety

Treatment
- Find and remove the cause of stimulation.
- Elevate the head of bed.
- Remain calm and supportive.
- If symptoms persist, give vasodilators to decrease blood pressure.
- Teach patient to recognize and report symptoms.

Nursing and Medical Interventions. Maintaining a patent airway and respiratory function is a priority. Endotracheal intubation and mechanical ventilation are often required, especially in high cervical spine injuries. Care must be taken to prevent neck hyperextension during endotracheal intubation. Patients with complete cervical injury may be placed on a bed that provides side to side rotation (e.g., RotoRest, ArjoHuntleigh, Addison, IL) to optimize pulmonary function. Assess skin regularly for signs of breakdown.

Immobilization of the spinal cord must occur at the scene to prevent further injury. A rigid cervical collar with supporting blocks on a rigid backboard is recommended.[1,7] Once the patient has been hospitalized, external stabilization of a fracture or dislocation is often accomplished by use of a cervical collar, skeletal traction (cervical tongs), a halo vest, or a brace (Fig. 14.22). The halo vest offers many advantages, such as easy access to the neck for diagnostic procedures and surgery, early mobilization, and ambulation. Surgical stabilization of vertebral instability may be required and is usually performed within 24 hours of the injury.

Maintaining perfusion to the spinal cord is crucial. Maintain the MAP at 85 to 90 mm Hg for the first 7 days after the SCI.[25] Avoid a systolic BP less than 90 mm Hg; hypotension contributes to secondary injury by decreasing spinal cord blood flow and perfusion, leading to ischemia and neurological deficit. Fluid volume administration and vasopressor medications may be needed to sustain the BP.[25] Vasopressor response can vary widely because of autonomic instability. A

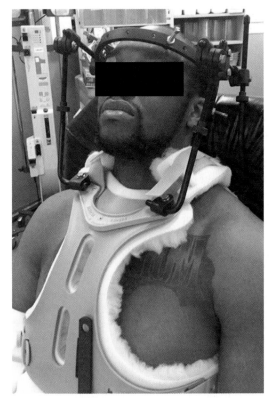

Fig. 14.22 Bremer Halo vest. (From Garfin, SR, Eismont, F.J., Bell, GR, et al. Rothman-Simeone and Herkowitz's The spine. 7th ed. Philadelphia: Elsevier; 2018.)

pulmonary artery catheter may be used to determine the need for fluids accurately.

Acute management of SCI often includes administration of glucocorticoids. Management guidelines recommend treatment with high-dose methylprednisolone (Solu-Medrol), to be started within the first 8 hours after injury as an option for the patient with SCI (see Table 14.9).[7,32] The high-dose therapy requires astute monitoring for adverse effects.

During the first 72 hours after SCI, a nasogastric tube is inserted for gastric decompression until bowel sounds return. This also helps prevent vomiting and possible aspiration and improves pulmonary function. Stress ulcers can occur as a result of ischemia of gastric mucosa and excess gastric acid production. Administration of steroids also increases the risk of ulcer formation. Histamine (H_2)–receptor antagonists or proton pump inhibitors are given to prevent stress ulcers. Institute a bowel care program as soon as bowel sounds return.

Keep the skin clean and dry at all times. Various skin protection devices may be required, including therapeutic beds, mattress overlays, boots, and skin barrier creams. Insert an indwelling urinary catheter immediately on admission to prevent bladder distension; institute an intermittent catheterization program on resolution of spinal shock.

Because of the limited mobility of patients with SCI, measures to prevent venous thromboembolism are started immediately on admission.[1,32] Intermittent pneumatic compression devices are commonly ordered. Heparin prophylaxis may be initiated if the risk of intramedullary or epidural hemorrhage into the spine is low. If the patient is

not a candidate for anticoagulation, a vena cava filter may be considered; however, its effectiveness is controversial. Because metabolic demands are initially increased, adequate nutrition must also be provided.

Surgical Intervention. SCIs may require surgical intervention to achieve greater neurological recovery and restore spinal stability. Surgery is indicated for neurological deterioration, unstable fractures, cord compression in the presence of an incomplete injury, and gross spinal misalignment. Surgery may involve the placement of plates or rods and a bone graft to fuse the spine. Depending on the injury, bone fragments may be removed or the spine may need to be realigned. The issue of when surgery should be performed is controversial.[36] External immobilization devices, such as cervical traction or a halo vest, may also be used.

STUDY BREAK

6. Which of the following assessment findings indicate that the patient with an acute cervical spinal cord injury is experiencing neurogenic shock?
   A. Heart rate of 112 and temperature of 38.7°C
   B. Absence of deep tendon reflexes in the lower extremities
   C. Blood pressure of 84/56 mm Hg and heart rate of 41 beats/min
   D. Inability to sense pain in the lower extremities

CASE STUDY

Ms. J. is a 45-year-old patient with a subarachnoid hemorrhage who underwent clipping of an aneurysm 5 days ago. At present, she is receiving mechanical ventilation and has a pulmonary artery catheter, arterial catheter, and ventriculostomy in place. Nimodipine was started on admission. Cerebral angiography performed today indicates that she is experiencing cerebral vasospasm. Initial treatments include fluid administration (hypervolemia) and medications to increase the blood pressure (hypertension).

Questions

1. When is a patient at greatest risk for developing vasospasm?
2. What effects does vasospasm have on cerebral function?
3. Discuss the benefits of administering nimodipine and achieving hypervolemia and hypertension.
4. Explain the purpose of a ventriculostomy in this patient.

REFERENCES

1. Bader MK, Littlejohns L, Olson D. *A Core Curriculum for Neuroscience Nursing.* 6th ed. Chicago, IL: American Association of Neuroscience Nurses; 2016.
2. Boss, BJ and Huether, SE. Alterations in cognitive systems, cerebral hemodynamics, and motor function. In: McCance KL, Huether SE. *Pathophysiology: The biologic basis for disease in adults and children.* 8th ed. St. Louis, MO: Elsevier; 2019.
3. Brouwer MC, McIntyre P, de Gans J, et al. Corticosteroids for acute bacterial meningitis. *Cochrane Database Syst Rev.* 2015; 9:CD004405.
4. Burns SK, Brewer KJ, Jenkins C, et al. Aneurysmal subarachnoid hemorrhage and vasospasm. *AACN Adv Crit Care.* 2018;29(2): 163–174.

5. Carney N, Totten AM, O'Reilly C, et al. Guidelines for the management of severe traumatic brain injury, fourth edition. *Neurosurgery*. 2018;80(1):6–15.

6. Fan J, Kirkness C, Vicini P, et al. Intracranial pressure waveform morphology and intracranial adaptive capacity. *Am J Crit Care*. 2008;17(6):545–554.

7. Fehlings MG, Wilson JR, Tetreault LA, et al. A clinical practice guideline for the management of patients with acute spinal cord injury: Recommendations on the use of methylprednisolone sodium succinate. *Global Spine J*. 2017;7(Suppl 3):203S–211S.

8. Fiorella D, Arthur AS, Mocco J. The INVEST trial: A randomized, controlled trial to investigate the safety and efficacy of image-guided minimally invasive endoscopic surgery with Apollo vs best medical management for supratentorial intracerebral hemorrhage. *Neurosurgery*. 2016;63:187.

9. Fisher RS. The new classification of seizures by the International League Against Epilepsy. *Curr Neurol Neurosci Rep*. 2017;17(6): 48-53.

10. Francoeur CL, Mayer SA. Management of delayed cerebral ischemia after subarachnoid hemorrhage. *Crit Care*. 2016;20(1):277–282.

11. Gorelick PB, Aiyagari V. The management of hypertension for an acute stroke: What is the blood pressure goal? *Current Cardiol Rep*. 2013;15(6):366-372.

12. Grandhi R, Bonfield CM, Newman WC. Surgical management of traumatic brain injury: A review of guidelines, pathophysiology, neurophysiology, outcomes, and controversies. *J Neurosurg Sci*. 2014;58(4):249-259.

13. Grasso G, Alafaci C, Macdonald RL. Management of aneurysmal subarachnoid hemorrhage: State of the art and future perspectives. *Surg Neurol Int*. 2017;8:11-17.

14. Griesdale DE, Ortenwall V, Norena M, et al. Adherence to guidelines for management of cerebral perfusion pressure and outcome in patients who have severe traumatic brain injury. *J Crit Care*. 2015;30(1):111–115.

15. Grover EH, Nazzal Y, Hirsch LJ. Treatment of convulsive status epilepticus. *Curr Treat Options Neurol*. 2016;18(3):11–15.

16. Hemphill JC, Greenberg SM, Anderson CS, et al. Guidelines for the management of spontaneous intracerebral hemorrhage: A guideline for healthcare professionals. *Stroke*. 2018;49: 2032-2060.

17. Kocak Y, Ozturk S, Ege F, et al. A useful new coma scale in acute stroke patients: FOUR score. *Anaesth Intensive Care*. 2012;40(1):131-136.

18. Koedel U, Klein M, Pfister H. New understandings on the pathophysiology of bacterial meningitis. *Curr Opin Infect Dis*. 2010;23(3):217-223.

19. Ledwith MB, Bloom S, Maloney-Wilensky E, et al. Effect of body position on cerebral oxygenation and physiologic parameters in patients with acute neurological conditions. *J Neurosci Nurs*. 2010;42(5):280-287.

20. Madden LK, Hill M, May TL, et al. The implementation of targeted temperature management: an evidence-based guideline from the Neurocritical Care Society. *Neuro Crit Care*. 2017; 27:468-487.

21. McNett M, Moran C, Janki C, et al. Correlations between hourly pupillometer readings and intracranial pressure values. *J Neurosci Nurs*. 2018;49(4):229–234.

22. Mozaffarian D, Benjamin EJ, Go AS, et al. AHA statistical update. *Circulation*. 2015;131:434-441.

23. Nasi D, Iaccarino C, Romano A, et al. Surgical management of traumatic supra and infratentorial extradural hematomas: Our experience and systematic literature review. *Neurosurg Rev*. 2019. doi:10.1007/s10143-019-01083-7. [Epub ahead of print]

24. Nguyen R, Fiest KM, McChesney J, et al. The international incidence of traumatic brain injury: A systematic review and meta-analysis. *Can J Neurol Sci*. 2016;43(6):774-785.

25. Ploumis A, Yadlapalli N, Fehlings MG, et al. A systematic review of the evidence supporting a role for vasopressor support in acute SCI. *Spinal Cord*. 2010;48(5):356-362.

26. Rabinstein AA, Ackerson T, Adeoye OM, et al. 2018 guidelines for the early management of patients with acute ischemic stroke: A guideline for healthcare professionals from the American Heart Association/American Stroke Association. *Stroke*. 2018;49:e46–e110.

27. Riker RR, Fugate JE; Participants in the International Multi-Disciplinary Consensus Conference on Multimodality Monitoring. Clinical monitoring scales in acute brain injury: Assessment of coma, pain, agitation, and delirium. *Neurocrit Care*. 2014;21(Suppl 2):S27–S37.

28. Rivera LL, Püttgen HA. Multimodality monitoring in the neurocritical care unit. *Continuum*. 2018;24(6):1776–1788.

29. Sacco TL, Davis JG. Management of intracranial pressure part I: Pharmacologic interventions. *Dimen Crit Care Nurs*. 2018;37(3): 120-129.

30. Sacco TL, Davis JG. Management of intracranial pressure part II: Nonpharmacologic interventions. *Dimen Crit Care Nurs*. 2019;38(2):61-69.

31. Sadaka F, Veremakis C. Therapeutic hypothermia for the management of intracranial hypertension in severe traumatic brain injury: A systematic review. *Brain Inj*. 2012;26(7–8):899-908.

32. Stauber MA. Not all spinal cord injuries involve a fracture. *Adv Emerg Nurs J*. 2011;33(3):226-231.

33. Centers for Disease Control and Prevention. *Stroke Facts*. https://www.cdc.gov/stroke/facts.htm. Reviewed September 6, 2017. Accessed March 10, 2019.

34. Topbaş E. Diagnosis and monitoring of neurological changes in intensive care. *Emerg Med Crit Care*. 2018;2(1):10–19.

35. Young N, Rhodes J, Mascia L, et al. Ventilatory strategies for patients with acute brain injury. *Curr Opin Crit Care*. 2010;16(1):45–52.

36. Yue JK, Chan AK, Winkler EA, et al. A review and update on the guidelines for the acute management of cervical spinal cord injury—Part II. *J Neurosurg Sci*. 2016;60(3):367–384.

37. Zacharia BE, Vaughan KA, Jacoby A, et al. Management of ruptured brain arteriovenous malformations. *Curr Atheroscler Rep*. 2012;14(4):335–342.

Acute Respiratory Failure

Jenny Lynn Sauls, PhD, MSN, RN, CNE

Many additional resources, including self-assessment exercises, are located on the Evolve companion website at http://evolve.elsevier.com/Sole/.
- Animations
- Clinical Skills: Critical Care Collections
- Student Review Questions
- Video Clips

INTRODUCTION

Acute respiratory failure (ARF) is the most common admitting diagnosis in critical care units, resulting in significant cost and in-hospital mortality of 20% to 50%, depending on severity.[74] It may occur as the primary problem or secondary to other conditions. This chapter includes a review of the pathophysiology, as well as common causes, symptoms, medical management, and nursing care involved in the treatment of patients with ARF.

ACUTE RESPIRATORY FAILURE

Definition

ARF is defined as an inability of the respiratory system to provide oxygenation and/or to remove carbon dioxide from the body. ARF is classified as oxygenation failure resulting in hypoxemia without a rise in carbon dioxide levels or ventilation failure resulting in hypercapnia and hypoxemia. Oxygenation failure, also known as hypoxemic or type 1 ARF, is characterized by a partial pressure of arterial oxygen (PaO_2) lower than 60 mm Hg with normal to decreased levels of carbon dioxide. Ventilation failure, also known as hypercapnic or type 2 ARF, is characterized by a partial pressure of arterial carbon dioxide ($PaCO_2$) greater than 50 mm Hg. These values are based on arterial blood levels with the patient breathing room air. ARF differs from chronic respiratory failure in that it evolves rapidly over minutes to hours, providing little time for physiological compensation. Chronic respiratory failure develops over time and allows the body's compensatory mechanisms to activate. ARF and chronic respiratory failure are not mutually exclusive. ARF may occur when a person who has chronic respiratory failure develops a respiratory infection or is exposed to other types of stressors, creating an increased demand or decreased supply of oxygen (O_2) that overwhelms the already compromised respiratory system. This is referred to as *acute-on-chronic* respiratory failure.

Pathophysiology

Failure of Oxygenation. Oxygenation failure occurs when the PaO_2 cannot be adequately maintained; it is the most commonly occurring type of ARF. Five generally accepted mechanisms that reduce PaO_2 and create a state of hypoxemia are hypoventilation, intrapulmonary shunting, ventilation-perfusion mismatching, diffusion defects, and decreased barometric pressure (Fig. 15.1). Decreased barometric pressure, which occurs at high altitudes, is not addressed in this text. Nonpulmonary conditions such as decreased cardiac output and low hemoglobin level may also result in tissue hypoxia.

Hypoventilation. Alveolar ventilation refers to the amount of gas that enters the alveoli per minute. In the normal lung, the partial pressure of alveolar oxygen (PAO_2) is approximately equal to the PaO_2. If the alveolar ventilation is reduced because of hypoventilation, the PAO_2 and the PaO_2 are both reduced. Factors that can lead to hypoventilation include a drug overdose that causes central nervous system (CNS) depression, neurological disorders that cause a decrease in the rate or depth of respirations, and abdominal or thoracic surgery leading to shallow breathing patterns secondary to pain on inspiration. Hypoventilation also produces an increase in the alveolar carbon dioxide (CO_2) level because the CO_2 that is produced in the tissues is delivered to the lungs but is not released from the body.

Intrapulmonary shunting. In normally functioning lungs, a small amount of blood returns to the left side of the heart without engaging in alveolar gas exchange. This is referred to as the *physiological shunt*. If, however, a larger amount of blood returns to the left side of the heart without participating in gas exchange, the shunt becomes pathological, and a decrease in the PaO_2 occurs. A pathological shunt exists when areas of the lung

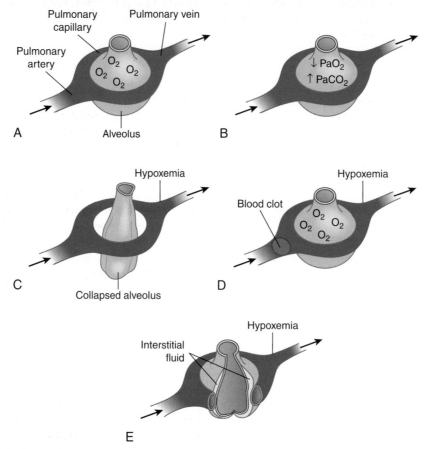

Fig. 15.1 Pulmonary causes of hypoxemia. **A,** Normal alveolar-capillary unit. **B,** Hypoventilation causes an increased partial pressure of carbon dioxide *(PaCO₂)* and a decreased partial pressure of arterial oxygen *(PaO₂)*. **C,** Shunt. **D,** Ventilation-perfusion mismatch resulting from pulmonary embolus. **E,** Diffusion defect due to increased interstitial fluid. *O₂,* Oxygen.

that are inadequately ventilated are adequately perfused (see Fig. 15.1), causing the blood to shunt past the lung and return unoxygenated to the left side of the heart. Common causes of shunting leading to hypoxemia include atelectasis, pneumonia, and pulmonary edema.

As the shunt worsens, the PaO_2 continues to decrease. This cause of hypoxemia cannot be treated effectively solely by increasing the fraction of inspired oxygen (FiO_2) because the increased O_2 is unable to reach the alveoli. Treatment is directed toward opening the alveoli and improving ventilation.

Ventilation-perfusion mismatch. Gas exchange in the lungs is dependent on the balance between ventilated areas of the lung (ventilation) receiving blood flow (perfusion). The rate of ventilation ($\dot{V}$) usually equals the rate of perfusion ($\dot{Q}$), resulting in a ventilation-to-perfusion ratio ($\dot{V}/\dot{Q}$) of 1.0. If ventilation exceeds blood flow, the $\dot{V}/\dot{Q}$ ratio is greater than 1.0; if ventilation is less than blood flow, the $\dot{V}/\dot{Q}$ ratio is less than 1.0. $\dot{V}/\dot{Q}$ mismatch can occur in conditions such as pneumonia or pulmonary edema when obstructed airways inhibit ventilation (and perfusion is normal) or in the case of pulmonary embolism when a clot in the pulmonary circulation obstructs perfusion.

Diffusion defects. Diffusion is the movement of gas from an area of high concentration to an area of lower concentration. In the lungs, O_2 and CO_2 move between the alveoli and the blood by diffusing across the alveolar-capillary membrane. The alveolar-capillary membrane has six barriers to the diffusion of O_2 and CO_2: surfactant, alveolar epithelium, interstitial fluid, capillary endothelium, plasma, and red blood cell membrane. Under normal circumstances, O_2 and CO_2 diffuse across the alveolar-capillary membrane in 0.25 second. The distance between an alveolus and a pulmonary capillary is usually only one or two cells thick. This narrowness of space facilitates efficient diffusion of O_2 and CO_2 across the cell membrane.

In respiratory failure, the distance between the alveoli and the capillaries may be increased by accumulation of fluid in the interstitial space (see Fig. 15.1). Changes in capillary perfusion pressure, leakage of plasma proteins into the interstitial space, and destruction of the capillary membrane contribute to the buildup of fluids around the alveolus. Fibrotic changes in the lung tissue itself, such as those seen in chronic obstructive pulmonary disease (COPD), can also contribute to a reduction in the diffusion capacity of the lungs. As diffusion capacity is reduced, reductions in PaO_2 occur first, resulting in hypoxemia. Because CO_2 is more readily diffusible than O_2, hypercapnia is a late sign of diffusion defects.

Low cardiac output. Adequate tissue oxygenation depends on a balance between O_2 supply and demand. The mechanism for delivering O_2 to the tissues is cardiac output. A normal cardiac output results in the delivery of 600 to 1000 mL/min of O_2, which generally exceeds the normal amount of O_2 needed by the tissues. If the cardiac output decreases, less oxygenated blood is delivered. To maintain normal aerobic metabolism in low cardiac output states, the tissues must extract increasing amounts of O_2 from the blood. When this increase in extraction can no longer compensate for the decreased cardiac output, the cells convert to *anaerobic metabolism*. This results in the production of lactic acid, which depresses the function of the myocardium and further lowers cardiac output.

Low hemoglobin level. Between 96% and 100% of the body's O_2 is transported to the tissues bound to hemoglobin. Each gram of hemoglobin can carry 1.34 mL of O_2 when all of its O_2 binding sites are completely filled. Arterial oxygen saturation (SaO_2) refers to the percentage of O_2 binding sites on each hemoglobin molecule that are filled with O_2 (normally 96% to 100%). If a patient's hemoglobin level is lower than normal, the O_2 supply to the tissues may be impaired and tissue hypoxia can occur. An alteration in hemoglobin function (e.g., carbon monoxide poisoning, sickle cell disease) can also decrease O_2 delivery to the tissues.

Tissue hypoxia. The final step in oxygenation is the use of O_2 by the tissues. Anaerobic metabolism occurs when the tissues cannot obtain adequate O_2 to meet metabolic needs. Anaerobic metabolism is inefficient and results in the accumulation of lactic acid. The point at which anaerobic metabolism begins to occur is not known and may vary with different organ systems. The effects of tissue hypoxia vary with the severity of hypoxia but may result in cellular death and subsequent organ failure.

Failure of Ventilation. $PaCO_2$ is the variable used to evaluate ventilation. When ventilation is reduced, $PaCO_2$ is increased (hypercapnia). When ventilation is increased, $PaCO_2$ is reduced (hypocapnia). Hypoventilation and $\dot{V}/\dot{Q}$ mismatching are the two mechanisms responsible for hypercapnia. Hypercapnia significantly increases cerebral blood flow, causing the patient to appear restless and anxious. As intracranial pressure rises, the level of consciousness (LOC) decreases, progressing to coma if effective treatment does not occur.

Hypoventilation. Hypoventilation is the cause of respiratory failure that occurs in patients with CNS abnormalities, neuromuscular disorders, drug overdoses, and chest wall abnormalities (see Fig. 15.1). In hypoventilation, CO_2 accumulates in the alveoli and is not blown off. Respiratory acidosis occurs rapidly, before renal compensation can occur. Mechanical ventilation may be necessary to support the patient until the initial cause of the hypoventilation can be corrected.

Ventilation-perfusion mismatch. Because the upper and lower airways do not participate in gas exchange, the volume of inspired gas that fills these structures is referred to as physiological *dead space*. This dead space normally accounts for 25% to 30% of the inspired volume. A major mechanism for the elevation of $PaCO_2$ is an increase in the volume of dead space in relation to the total tidal volume (V_T). Dead space increases when an area that is well ventilated has reduced perfusion and no longer participates in gas exchange.

Assessment

Respiratory assessment and evaluation of gas exchange are discussed in depth in Chapter 10. Changes in mental status resulting from hypoxemia and hypercapnia begin with anxiety, restlessness, and confusion and may deteriorate to lethargy, severe somnolence, and coma if respiratory failure is not resolved.

Observe the rate, depth, and pattern of respiration. In response to hypoxemia, compensatory mechanisms produce tachypnea and an increase in V_T (hyperventilation). As these compensatory mechanisms fail, respirations become shallow. Bradypnea is an ominous sign. Use of accessory muscles and intercostal retractions are also cause for concern because they indicate respiratory muscle fatigue. By auscultation, assess the adequacy of airflow and the presence of adventitious breath sounds. Also note the presence of a cough and the amount and characteristics of any sputum production.

A thorough cardiac assessment provides information about the heart's ability to deliver O_2 to the tissues and cells. Monitor for changes in blood pressure (BP), heart rate, and cardiac rhythm. ARF initially causes tachycardia and increased BP. Worsening of ARF can result in dysrhythmias, angina, bradycardia, hypotension, and cardiac arrest. Evaluate peripheral perfusion by palpating pulses for strength and bilateral equality, and assess the skin for a decrease in temperature and the presence of cyanosis or pallor.

Because nutritional status is an important factor in maintaining respiratory muscle strength, assess for recent weight loss, muscle wasting, nausea, vomiting, abdominal distension, and skin turgor quality.

The psychosocial status of the patient can also affect outcomes; therefore identify the patient's significant others and their roles in the family structure. An understanding of the patient's educational level, socioeconomic background, spiritual beliefs, and cultural or ethnic practices is important in determining an educational plan for discharge and future self-care.

Serial chest radiographs and pulmonary function tests provide important assessment information. Laboratory studies that are essential for the patient with respiratory failure include the following: electrolytes, which determine adequate muscle function; hemoglobin and hematocrit, to evaluate the blood's O_2 carrying capacity; and arterial blood gas (ABG) measurements, to assess gas exchange and acid-base balance. Noninvasive monitoring of oxygenation, such as pulse oximetry (SpO_2), provides information about the patient's oxygenation, whereas continuous end-tidal CO_2 monitoring provides information about the patient's ventilation.

Physiological changes with aging may make identifying the signs and symptoms of ARF more difficult in older adults. The most common early sign of hypoxemia in the older adult is a change in mental status, such as confusion or agitation. These changes are often mistaken for dementia or a normal sign of advancing age.[14] See the Lifespan Considerations box for additional information.

❓ CRITICAL REASONING ACTIVITY

Mr. R. is a 66-year-old man who has smoked 1.5 packs of cigarettes per day for 40 years (60 pack-years). He is admitted with an acute exacerbation of COPD. His baseline ABGs drawn in the clinic 2 weeks ago showed the following: pH, 7.36; $PaCO_2$, 55 mm Hg; PaO_2, 69 mm Hg; bicarbonate, 30 mEq/L; SaO_2, 92%. In the critical care unit, Mr. R. has coarse crackles in his left posterior lower lung and a mild expiratory wheeze bilaterally. His cough is productive of thick yellow sputum. His skin turgor is poor; he is febrile, tachycardic, and tachypneic. Currently, Mr. R.'s ABGs while receiving O_2 at 2 L/min via a nasal cannula are as follows: pH, 7.32; $PaCO_2$, 64 mm Hg; PaO_2, 50 mm Hg; bicarbonate, 30 mEq/L; SaO_2, 86%.

1. What is your interpretation of Mr. R.'s baseline ABG findings from the clinic?
2. What is the probable cause of Mr. R.'s COPD exacerbation, and what treatment is indicated at this time?
3. What ABG changes would indicate that Mr. R.'s respiratory status is deteriorating from baseline?

ABGs, Arterial blood gases; *COPD,* chronic obstructive pulmonary disease; *O_2,* oxygen; *$PaCO_2$,* partial pressure of arterial carbon dioxide; *PaO_2,* partial pressure of arterial oxygen; *SaO_2,* arterial oxygen saturation.

👤 LIFESPAN CONSIDERATIONS

Older Adults

- Rib ossification results in decreased compliance of thorax.
- Decreased vital capacity and ventilator reserve, and increased residual volume are associated with decreased chest wall mobility.
- Loss of alveolar wall tissue and capillaries decreases surface area for gas exchange, resulting in decreased partial pressure of arterial oxygen (PaO_2), which reduces exercise tolerance.
- Decline in muscle mass contributes to respiratory muscle fatigue and decreased endurance.
- Decreased compensatory response to hypoxemia and hypercapnia occurs; feelings of dyspnea remain intact and may be enhanced despite the decline in the compensatory response; there is a greater risk for respiratory depression caused by medications.
- Decreased effectiveness of the immune system increases susceptibility to infection.
- Because of age-related decreases in chemoreceptor and central nervous system (CNS) function, older adults have a lower ventilatory response to hypoxia and hypercapnia. In addition, hypoxia in the elderly may not produce the same compensatory increases in heart rate, stroke volume, and cardiac output that are seen in younger adults.
- Increasing age can lead to a slower response to oxygen (O_2) therapy.

- PaO_2 levels decrease with age, but aging does not produce significant alterations in pH or partial pressure of arterial carbon dioxide ($PaCO_2$). For this reason, hypercapnia and a falling pH are causes for concern.

Pregnant Women

- Advanced stages of pregnancy challenge pulmonary mechanics through elevation of the diaphragm and altered thoracic configuration, resulting in increased negative pleural pressures, reducing functional residual capacity (FRC) and expiratory reserve volume (ERV) as well as shortened chest height.
- Oxygen consumption and basal metabolic rate (BMR) increase, which lowers oxygen reserve.
- Dyspnea and breathlessness are commonly reported by healthy pregnant women starting from the first trimester.
- Due to physiological changes in pregnancy, monitor ventilation and oxygenation frequently.

References

Brashers VL. Structure and function of the pulmonary system. In: McCance KL, Huether SE. *Pathophysiology: The Biologic Basis for Disease in Adults and Children.* 8th ed. St. Louis, MO: Elsevier; 2019:1143–1158.

LoMauro A, Aliverti A. Respiratory physiology of pregnancy. *Breathe.* 2015;11(4):297–301.

Interventions

The goals for treating patients with ARF include maintaining a patent airway, optimizing O_2 delivery, minimizing O_2 demand, treating the cause of ARF, and preventing complications.

Maintain a Patent Airway. Some causes of ARF, such as COPD, cardiogenic pulmonary edema, pulmonary infiltrates in immunocompromised patients, and palliation in the terminally ill, may be effectively treated with noninvasive positive-pressure ventilation (NPPV).[8,54,75] However, if a patient is unable to maintain a patent airway or if NPPV does not improve ventilation or oxygenation, intubation and mechanical ventilation may be indicated. (Refer to Chapter 10 for nursing care related to NPPV and mechanical ventilation.)

Optimize Oxygen Delivery. Strategies for optimizing O_2 delivery depend on the needs of the patient. Initially provide supplemental O_2 via nasal cannula or face mask to maintain the PaO_2 higher than 60 mm Hg or the SaO_2 higher than 90%. If supplemental O_2 is ineffective in raising PaO_2 levels, high-flow nasal cannula[23] or noninvasive mechanical ventilation may be

considered. Invasive mechanical ventilation is the next step (see Clinical Alert box).

Patients are positioned for ease of breathing and to enhance $\dot{V}/\dot{Q}$ matching. Other methods to optimize O_2 delivery include red blood cell transfusion to ensure adequate hemoglobin levels for transport of O_2, and enhancing cardiac output and BP to deliver sufficient O_2 to the tissues. Refer to the Plan of Care for the Patient With Acute Respiratory Failure for detailed interventions and rationales for optimizing oxygenation.

Minimize Oxygen Demand. Decreasing the patient's O_2 demand begins with providing adequate rest. Avoid unnecessary physical activity. Agitation, restlessness, pain, fever, sepsis, and patient-ventilator dyssynchrony must be addressed because they all contribute to increased O_2 demand and consumption.

Treat the Cause of Acute Respiratory Failure. While the patient is being treated for hypoxemia, efforts must be made to identify and reverse the cause of ARF. Specific interventions for acute respiratory distress syndrome (ARDS), COPD, asthma, pneumonia, and pulmonary embolism are detailed later in the chapter.

! CLINICAL ALERT

Acute Respiratory Failure

Concern	Symptoms	Nursing Actions
Respiratory muscle fatigue	Diaphoresis Nasal flaring Tachycardia Abdominal paradox Muscle retractions • Intercostal • Suprasternal • Supraclavicular Central cyanosis	**Improve oxygen (O_2) delivery:** • Administer O_2 • Ensure adequate cardiac output and blood pressure • Correct low hemoglobin • Administer bronchodilators **Decrease O_2 demand:** • Provide rest • Reduce fever • Relieve pain and anxiety • Position patient for optimum gas exchange and perfusion • Prepare for possible intubation and mechanical ventilation
Cerebral hypoxia and carbon dioxide (CO_2) narcosis from increased CO_2 retention	Lethargy Somnolence Coma Respiratory acidosis	**Maintain airway patency** • Prepare for possible intubation and mechanical ventilation

Prevent Complications. Finally, be alert to the potential complications that the patient with ARF may encounter. Implement measures to prevent complications of immobility, adverse effects from medications, fluid and electrolyte imbalances, development of gastric ulcers, and hazards of mechanical ventilation.

Patient Problems

Several problems are considered in the care of a patient with ARF (see Plan of Care for the Patient With Acute Respiratory Failure), depending on the etiology and other comorbidities. Expected outcomes include adequate organ and tissue oxygenation, effective breathing, and adequate gas exchange.

◎ PLAN OF CARE

For the Patient With Acute Respiratory Failure[a]

Patient Problem
Decreased Gas Exchange. Risk factors include ventilation-perfusion mismatch, diffusion abnormality, alveolar-capillary membrane changes, decreased hemoglobin-carrying capacity, decreased cardiac output.

Desired Outcomes
• PaO_2 80 to 100 mm Hg.
• $PaCO_2$ 35 to 45 mm Hg or within patient's expected range.
• SaO_2 or SpO_2 greater than 92% or within patient's expected range.
• Alert and oriented to person, place, and time, or no further decline in LOC.
• Color pink or absence of cyanosis.
• Heart rate less than 100 beats/min.
• RR 24 breaths/min or less.

Nursing Assessments/Interventions	Rationales
• Monitor SpO_2 continuously and report values ≥92%.	• Assess response to oxygen therapy. • Values ≥92% can indicate need for increase in supplemental O_2.
• Review ABGs when available. Report critical values to the provider: (PaO_2 <80 mm Hg, SaO_2 <90%, and/or $PaCO_2$ >45 mm Hg). • Monitor heart rate. • Monitor for signs and symptoms of respiratory distress and report promptly: restlessness, anxiety, change in mental status, shortness of breath, tachypnea, and use of accessory muscles.	• Assess values indicative of respiratory failure and response to treatment. • Tachycardia indicates a compensatory mechanism for hypoxemia. • Allows for early identification and treatment.
• Position patient to facilitate comfort and respiratory excursion (usually semi-Fowler's). • Position patient with good lung down when side lying.	• Promote comfort and diaphragmatic descent; maximize inhalation; decrease WOB; and promote $\dot{V}/\dot{Q}$ matching. • Facilitate $\dot{V}/\dot{Q}$ matching.

Continued

⊙ PLAN OF CARE—cont'd

For the Patient With Acute Respiratory Failure[a]

Nursing Assessments/Interventions	Rationales
• Administer supplemental oxygen to achieve oxygen saturation ≥92%. Begin with lower concentrations of FiO_2; if SpO_2 does not rise to ≥92%, increase FiO_2 in small increments while monitoring SpO_2 or ABG values; notify provider promptly of the need for significant increases in FiO_2.	• Support perfusion of tissues and organs.
• Prepare for use of NPPV with a CPAP mask, or intubation and mechanical ventilation.	• NPPV may prevent the need for intubation; mechanical ventilation may be indicated to achieve oxygenation and ventilation goals.

Patient Problem

Dyspnea. Risk factors include ineffective inspiration and expiration.

Desired Outcomes

- Absence of dyspnea or use of accessory muscles.
- Symmetrical chest wall movement with midline trachea.
- Respirations unlabored at a rate of 12 to 16 breaths/min.
- Patient verbalizes ability to breathe comfortably.

Nursing Assessments/Interventions	Rationales
• Assess respiratory status every 2 h: rate, rhythm, and depth; use of accessory muscles; intercostal retractions; nasal flaring.	• Guide early identification of respiratory distress and initiate immediate intervention.
• Assess position assumed for breathing.	• Three-point position for breathing (bending forward with hands on knees) indicates increasing respiratory distress.
• Consider prone positioning if unable to optimize oxygenation.	• May improve oxygenation in ARDS for patients on mechanical ventilation when used for periods >12 h/day.
• Encourage slow, deep breathing and/or teach pursed-lip breathing technique to achieve an I:E ratio of 1:2 or 1:3.	• Facilitate controlled breathing pattern and maintain a positive pressure in the airways.
• Provide pain relief.	• Prevent splinting and hypoventilation.
• If patient has lung pathology, position for maximal gas exchange; place the "good" lung down.	• Increase perfusion to the good lung and facilitate gas exchange.
• Assist with and pace activities; provide patient with periods of rest.	• Reduce oxygen consumption and demands.
• Administer $beta_2$-agonist drugs by metered-dose inhaler or nebulizer to increase airflow as prescribed; evaluate their effectiveness.	• Decrease airway resistance secondary to bronchoconstriction.
• Administer corticosteroids as indicated (see Table 15.2).	• Decrease inflammation and edema to improve airflow in narrowed airways.
• Prepare for chest tube insertion for pneumothorax, hemothorax, or flail chest; connect to drainage system.	• Remove air or blood from pleural space and promote reexpansion of lung.
• Anticipate the need for intubation and mechanical ventilation.	• Early intubation and ventilation can prevent deterioration of respiratory function or respiratory arrest.
• If patient is mechanically ventilated, sedate according to goals for patient; avoid oversedation.	• Facilitate gas exchange and mechanical ventilation; promote earlier weaning and extubation.

Patient Problem

Insufficient Airway Clearance. Risk factors include the inability to cough, presence of endotracheal tube, thick secretions.

Desired Outcomes

- Ability to cough effectively to clear secretions.
- Tolerates suctioning to clear secretions while maintaining an SpO_2 greater than 92%.
- Breath sounds clear after cough or suctioning.

Nursing Assessments/Interventions	Rationales
• Auscultate anterior and posterior bilateral breath sounds every 1-2 h, after coughing or suctioning, and otherwise as needed.	• Presence of crackles or rhonchi indicates fluid accumulation; presence of wheezes indicates bronchoconstriction. • Fine crackles should clear with deep breathing. • Coarse crackles require deep cough and/or suctioning.
• Assess sputum characteristics: amount, color, consistency, odor. Document findings and culture as appropriate.	• Provide assessment data about the cause of respiratory failure: colored sputum, infection; thick tenacious sputum, dehydration; frothy sputum, pulmonary edema.
• Change patient's position every 2 h.	• Mobilize secretions.
• Encourage patient to cough and deep breathe at least every 2 h.	• Improve lung capacity, clear secretions, and facilitate gas exchange.
• Assess the need for hyperinflation therapy. Encourage patient to slowly and deeply inhale approximately twice the normal V_T, hold the breath for 5 sec, and exhale; repeat 10 times every hour.	• Inability to take deep breaths indicates a need for hyperinflation therapy to maximize alveolar expansion and mobilize secretions.

⊚ PLAN OF CARE—cont'd

For the Patient With Acute Respiratory Failure[a]

Nursing Assessments/Interventions	Rationales
• Suction (nasotracheal or endotracheal) as determined by patient assessment.	• Prevent unnecessary suctioning and reduce complications associated with suctioning.
• Provide adequate humidification with supplemental oxygen or mechanical ventilation.	• Prevent drying of secretions and facilitate secretion removal.
• When not contraindicated, encourage fluid intake of at least 2.5 L/day.	• Reduce viscosity of secretions and promote expectoration.

[a]See Collaborative Plan of Care for the Critically Ill Patient (Chapter 1) and Plan of Care for the Mechanically Ventilated Patient (Chapter 10).
ABGs, Arterial blood gases; *ARDS,* acute respiratory distress syndrome; *CPAP,* continuous positive airway pressure; *I:E ratio,* inspiratory-to-expiratory ratio; *FiO_2,* fraction of inspired oxygen; *LOC,* level of consciousness; *NPPV,* noninvasive positive-pressure ventilation; *O_2,* oxygen; *PaCO_2,* partial pressure of arterial carbon dioxide; *PaO_2,* partial pressure of arterial oxygen; *RR,* respiratory rate; *SaO_2,* arterial oxygen saturation; *SpO_2,* pulse oximetry; $\dot{V}/\dot{Q}$, ventilation/perfusion; *WOB,* work of breathing.
Adapted from Swearingen PL, Wright JD. *All-in-One Nursing Care Planning Resource.* 5th ed. St. Louis, MO: Elsevier; 2019.

RESPIRATORY FAILURE IN ACUTE RESPIRATORY DISTRESS SYNDROME

Definition

ARDS, the most severe form of ARF, was originally described in 1967 as an acute illness manifested by dyspnea, tachypnea, decreased lung compliance, and diffuse alveolar infiltrates on chest radiographic studies. The syndrome was observed in young adult patients after trauma who developed shock or required excessive fluid administration, or both. Autopsy results revealed that pathological heart and lung findings were similar to those described in infant respiratory distress syndrome.

Although mortality attributed to ARDS has trended downward over the past several decades, death rates vary depending on ARDS definition, disease severity, study site, age, body mass index (BMI), geographical location, race, gender, and season.[20,60,82] National ARDS-related mortality over a 15-year period between 1999 and 2013 decreased from 13,612 to 9762 or approximately 30%.[20,60] Average annual in-hospital case mortality has been reported at 47% using a nationwide sample.[43]

The current definition of ARDS known as the Berlin criteria was revised in 2012. Criteria for ARDS include (1) acute onset within 1 week after clinical insult; (2) bilateral pulmonary opacities not explained by other conditions; and (3) altered PaO_2/FiO_2 ratio. Severity is determined by the PaO_2/FiO_2 ratio when the patient is treated with positive end-expiratory pressure (PEEP) or continuous positive airway pressure (CPAP) of 5 cm H_2O or higher: mild ARDS, 200 mm Hg to 300 mm Hg; moderate ARDS, 100 mm Hg to 200 mm Hg; and severe ARDS, less than 100 mm Hg.[79]

Etiology

Several possible causes of ARDS are listed in Box 15.1; they are categorized into direct and indirect factors. However, certain risk factors such as pneumonia, sepsis, aspiration, and trauma have a higher associated frequency of ARDS, and the presence of two or more factors increases the risk.[82,83]

As more individuals survive ARDS, prevention of long-term disabilities is a priority of care. Survivors report ongoing concerns regarding physical well-being, mental health, and social health, all

---

BOX 15.1   Possible Causes of Acute Respiratory Distress Syndrome

Direct Causes
- Aspiration of gastric contents
- Fat embolism
- Inhalation of toxic gases
- Multisystem trauma (chest and/or lung injury)
- Near-drowning
- Pneumonia

Indirect Causes
- Burns
- Cardiopulmonary bypass
- Drug overdose
- Fractures, especially of the pelvis or long bones
- Multiple transfusions
- Multisystem trauma (without chest and/or lung injury)
- Pancreatitis
- Sepsis

---

having a tremendous effect on quality of life. Reports of weakness, mobility issues, breathing problems, nausea, swallowing difficulties, fatigue, problems with memory, anxiety, and depression are commonly reported.[25,26,42] Fifty-nine percent of survivors suffer some combination of general anxiety, depression, and posttraumatic stress for as long as 2 years. As physical functioning improves, overall improvement in psychosocial well-being occurs.[9] Physical therapy for critically ill patients while in the critical care unit can improve mobility and strength, but use of a physical therapist (PT) to provide therapy is infrequent.[45] Greater strength at discharge can improve long-term survival and quality of life.[25]

The critical care nurse can have a positive impact on in-hospital outcomes by collaborating with attending physicians to request PT-provided mobility for patients with ARF. The critical care nurse can also have a positive effect on quality of life after discharge of ARDS patients and families by providing information on community resources, support groups, and respite care. It is also important to educate the patient and family about what to expect after discharge and to help them develop coping strategies to manage these stressors.

💡 **CRITICAL REASONING ACTIVITY**

Ms. T. is a 41-year-old woman who was admitted to the critical care unit and mechanically ventilated for acute asthma. She was extubated yesterday and will be transferred out of the critical care unit tomorrow. What are the important points you must cover in your teaching with Ms. T.?

Pathophysiology

ARDS is characterized by acute and diffuse injury to the lungs leading to respiratory failure. A cell-mediated, overly aggressive immune response results in alveolar-capillary membrane damage and massive fluid leakage throughout the body, producing edema. Alveolar flooding leads to noncardiogenic pulmonary edema, shunting, $\dot{V}/\dot{Q}$ mismatch, decreased compliance, and hypoxemia. ARDS occurs in three phases: the acute exudative or inflammatory phase, the proliferative phase, and the fibrotic phase.[12]

The *acute phase* is characterized by uncontrolled inflammation, which produces excessive amounts of inflammatory mediators that damage the pulmonary capillary endothelium, activating massive aggregation of platelets and formation of intravascular thrombi. The platelets release serotonin and a substance that activates neutrophils. Other inflammatory factors, such as endotoxin, tumor necrosis factor, and interleukin-1, are also activated. Neutrophil activation causes release of inflammatory mediators such as proteolytic enzymes, toxic O_2 products, arachidonic acid metabolites, and platelet-activating factors. These mediators damage the alveolar-capillary membrane, which leads to increased capillary membrane permeability. Fluids, protein, and blood cells leak from the capillary beds into the alveoli, resulting in pulmonary edema. Pulmonary hypertension occurs secondary to vasoconstriction caused by the inflammatory mediators. The pulmonary hypertension and pulmonary edema lead to $\dot{V}/\dot{Q}$ mismatching. The production of surfactant is stopped, and the surfactant that is present is inactivated.[12]

During the acute phase of ARDS, damage to the alveolar epithelium and the vascular endothelium occurs. The damaged cells become susceptible to bacterial infection and pneumonia. The lungs become less compliant, resulting in decreased ventilation. A right-to-left shunt of pulmonary blood develops, and hypoxemia refractory to O_2 supplementation becomes profound. The work of breathing increases.[12]

The *proliferative phase* of ARDS, which overlaps with the fibrotic phase, occurs between 1 and 3 weeks after onset. During this phase, pulmonary edema resolves, and a fibrin matrix (hyaline membrane) forms, resulting in progressive hypoxemia.[12]

The final phase of ARDS, the *fibrotic phase*, occurs 2 to 3 weeks after the initial insult. During this phase, fibrosis obliterates the alveoli, bronchioles, and interstitium. The lungs become fibrotic, with decreased functional residual capacity and severe right-to-left shunting. The inflammation and edema become worse with narrowing of the airways. Resistance to airflow and atelectasis increase.[12]

The inflammatory mediators responsible for alveolar-capillary membrane damage cause similar damage to capillaries throughout the body, resulting in widespread edema and multiple organ failure or multiple organ dysfunction syndrome (MODS; see Chapter 12). Cause of death may not be related to ARF but more likely to MODS related to ARDS.[12] The pathophysiology of ARDS is outlined in Fig. 15.2.

Assessment

Assessment of a patient with ARDS is collaborative. A key clinical finding of ARDS is respiratory distress with dyspnea, tachypnea, and hypoxemia that does not respond to supplemental O_2 therapy (refractory hypoxemia). Hypoxemia triggers hyperventilation, resulting in respiratory alkalosis. Initial signs of ARDS may also include fine crackles, restlessness, disorientation, and change in the LOC. Pulse and temperature may be increased. Chest radiographic studies show interstitial and alveolar infiltrates over the first 24 to 48 hours after onset.[12]

As ARDS progresses and the PaO_2 decreases, dyspnea becomes severe. Intercostal and suprasternal retractions are often present, with a significant increase in work of breathing. Other signs may include tachycardia and central cyanosis. As pulmonary edema develops, the lungs become noncompliant, making ventilation increasingly difficult, resulting in hypoventilation and respiratory acidosis. For patients who are already intubated, peak inspiratory pressures will be elevated as an indicator of decreased static compliance. Patients developing ARDS frequently require noninvasive supplemental O_2 at the maximum level, with little effect on the PaO_2. Metabolic acidosis caused by lactic acid buildup often results and is confirmed by serum lactate level determinations.

Once ARDS is diagnosed, important assessment data that are used to guide treatment include hemodynamic measurements, ABGs, mixed venous blood gases, serial chest radiographic studies, computed tomography (CT), echocardiography, bronchoscopy, and plasma brain natriuretic peptide (BNP) levels.[37] Nutritional needs and psychosocial needs of the patient and family also must be assessed. There is some evidence to suggest that esophageal pressure measurements are beneficial in evaluating pleural pressure and lung compliance, which could assist in a more tailored approach to ventilator strategies such as levels of PEEP.[39]

STUDY BREAK

1. The Berlin criteria for acute respiratory distress syndrome (ARDS) include:
   A. Acute onset within 1 week after clinical insult
   B. Bilateral pulmonary opacities not explained by other conditions
   C. Altered partial pressure of arterial oxygen/fraction of inspired oxygen (PaO_2/FiO_2) ratio
   D. All the above

Interventions

Achieving adequate oxygenation is the primary goal in the treatment of ARDS. This can be accomplished with the use of NPPV in some patients,[65] but many patients require endotracheal intubation and mechanical ventilation.[7] Early recognition of the need for intubation is essential in preventing increased

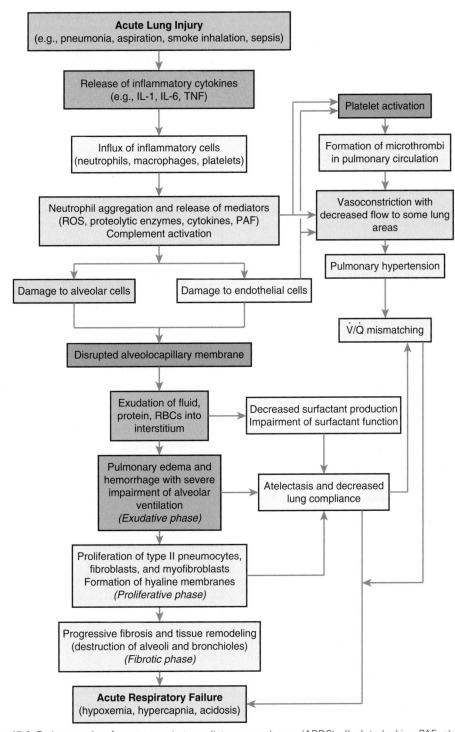

Fig. 15.2 Pathogenesis of acute respiratory distress syndrome (ARDS). *IL,* Interleukin; *PAF,* platelet-activating factor; *RBCs,* red blood cells; *ROS,* reactive oxygen species; *TNF,* tumor necrosis factor; $\dot{V}/\dot{Q}$, ventilation/perfusion. (From Brashers VL, Huether SE. Alterations of pulmonary function. In: McCance KL, Huether SE, eds. *Pathophysiology: The Biologic Basis for Disease in Adults and Children.* 8th ed. St. Louis, MO: Elsevier; 2019.)

morbidity and mortality.[30,60] Lung-protective ventilation strategies have proven to be effective with use of lower tidal volumes, some measure of PEEP, and permissive hypoxemia. Other treatments currently being researched are extracorporeal membrane oxygenation (ECMO), corticosteroid therapy, prone positioning, and therapeutic hypothermia. Other treatments are primarily supportive, providing an opportunity for the body to heal itself.

Oxygenation. Patients with ARDS usually require intubation and mechanical ventilation to meet oxygenation needs. Selection of ventilator settings is based on lung-protective strategies that attempt to achieve adequate oxygenation while minimizing the risks of ventilator-associated complications such as oxygen toxicity, barotrauma, and volutrauma. Lung-protective strategies consist of low V_T (4 to 8 mL/kg of predicted ideal body weight [IBW]), low end-inspiratory plateau pressure (<30 cm H_2O), FiO_2 at nontoxic levels (<0.60), and PEEP. Actual body weight should not be used to calculate V_T. The body weight may change secondary to accumulation of body fluid, but the size of the lungs does not change. Large clinical trials have shown reduced mortality and complications with the use of low V_T and low plateau pressure.[27,31] These lower volumes and plateau pressures prevent the alveoli from overdistending and minimize shearing. Despite extensive research supporting the use of low tidal volume for improving outcomes, use of this strategy has been much less than optimal, indicating a need for an intervention to improve the implementation of this treatment option.[86] The optimal PEEP to treat ARDS and improve outcomes needs further study, although current clinical guidelines include the use of higher levels of PEEP for patients with moderate to severe disease.[27,46]

Patients with ARDS require significant support to achieve and maintain arterial oxygenation. High levels of FiO_2 may be required for short periods while aggressive work is done to reduce the FiO_2 to the lowest level that maintains the PaO_2 higher than 60 mm Hg. To prevent O_2 toxicity and increased mortality, the goal is to maintain the PaO_2 with levels of FiO_2 at 0.50.[2]

Ventilatory support for patients with ARDS typically includes PEEP to restore functional residual capacity, open collapsed alveoli, prevent collapse of unstable alveoli, and improve arterial oxygenation.[50] Despite numerous studies involving the use of PEEP, findings are inconclusive regarding the levels that are most efficacious. When using high levels of PEEP, assess for potential adverse effects (see Chapter 10). PEEP increases intrathoracic pressure, potentially leading to decreased cardiac output. Excessive pressure in stiff lungs increases peak inspiratory and plateau pressures, which may result in barotrauma and pneumothorax. Treatment of a pneumothorax requires prompt insertion of a chest tube. Monitor patients receiving high levels of PEEP therapy every 2 to 4 hours, and after every adjustment in the PEEP setting, for changes in respiratory status such as increased respiratory rate, worsening adventitious breath sounds, decreased or absent breath sounds, decreased SpO_2, and increasing dyspnea.

Although not considered standard of care, a few nontraditional modes of mechanical life support are used in some patients to treat ARDS with hypoxemia refractory to standard modes. These include ECMO and pressure-controlled, inverse-ratio ventilation. These modes may offer improved alveolar ventilation and arterial oxygenation while decreasing the risk of lung injury in select patients. None has been successful enough to be considered part of current clinical practice guidelines[1,27,61,69] (see Chapter 10). Ongoing studies on the use of ECMO show promise, but evidence is inconclusive at this time (see Evidence-Based Practice box).

EVIDENCE-BASED PRACTICE

Extracorporeal Membrane Oxygenation in Acute Respiratory Distress Syndrome

Problem
Patients with acute respiratory distress syndrome (ARDS) require mechanical ventilation and other support to ensure adequate oxygenation and ventilation.

Clinical Question
What is best practice for extracorporeal membrane oxygenation (ECMO) in patients with ARDS?

Evidence
In this systematic review and meta-analysis, the authors analyzed 27 studies including data collected on 1674 patients. They compared outcomes of ECMO with low-tidal-volume ventilation versus low tidal volume (V_T) alone in mechanically ventilated adults diagnosed with severe ARDS as related to hospital mortality. Findings indicated that although hospital mortality risks are not significantly different in the two groups (ECMO: 33.3% to 86%, low V_T: 36.3% to 71.2%), lower mortality was observed in two studies favoring ECMO over low V_T alone. However, the lack of studies with appropriate control groups leads to questions regarding the strength of the evidence. More studies are needed to determine the role of ECMO as a strategy for the treatment of ARDS.

Implications for Nursing
Nurses must collaborate with respiratory therapists and intensivists to provide the safest and most effective management strategy for each patient. Protocols that include nontraditional modes of mechanical ventilation such as ECMO may be effective for improving outcomes for select patients with ARDS. Assessment for tolerance, improvement in oxygenation, and adverse effects is essential for optimal outcomes.

Level of Evidence
A—Meta-analysis

Reference
Tillmann BW, Klingel ML, Iansavichene AE, et al. Extracorporeal membrane oxygenation (ECMO) as a treatment strategy for severe acute respiratory distress syndrome (ARDS) in the low tidal volume era: A systematic review. *J Crit Care*. 2017;41:64–71.

Pharmacological Treatment. Despite clinical studies of various medications, no pharmacological agents are considered standard therapy for ARDS. The use of corticosteroid therapy for the treatment of ARDS has been debated for many years, and research has failed to produce strong enough results to document the use of these drugs as standard of care,[6,51] although there is ongoing research in this area that suggests improved outcomes for some patients with ARDS.[6,28,33,58]

Critical illness–related corticosteroid insufficiency (CIRCI) in critically ill patients is believed to be a problem that occurs in ARDS.[6] Although a task force of experts in critical care medicine was convened in 2008 to explore this concept, it is only recently that adequate evidence enabled established guidelines for the diagnosis and treatment of this phenomenon that is also believed to occur in other critical illnesses such as sepsis, septic shock, severe community-acquired pneumonia, cardiac arrest, and trauma.

Sedation and Comfort. Patients with ARDS routinely receive sedation to promote comfort, rest, and sleep; alleviate anxiety; prevent self-extubation or harm; and ensure adequate ventilation. Undersedation may result in breathing dyssynchrony between the patient and the ventilator, which causes inadequate gas exchange and increases the risk for ventilator-induced lung injury. Adapting ventilator settings to the patient's respiratory efforts can be effective in alleviating dyssynchrony. Light sedation with propofol and opioids, such as fentanyl or morphine can be safely given to promote comfort and decrease anxiety associated with intubation and ventilation and to control dyssynchrony.[24,49]

Oversedation can lead to long-term sequelae such as delirium, resulting in an increase in ventilator days, prolonged lengths of stay, and worse outcomes. The amount of sedation used must be monitored carefully with validated sedation and delirium scales to achieve predetermined end points or goals for each individual patient situation[11,24,76] (see Chapter 6).

Therapeutic paralysis with a neuromuscular blocking agent may be required to completely control ventilation and promote adequate oxygenation. Additional benefits may include decreased work of breathing, improvement in ventilator dyssynchrony, and decreased mortality. Early short-term administration of neuromuscular blocking agents in patients with severe ARDS may improve survival without increasing muscle weakness.[80] Current clinical practice guidelines for use of neuromuscular blockade suggest an early course of a continuous infusion of cisatracurium for 48 hours in severe ARDS.[59]

Prone Positioning. Patients with severe ARDS may benefit from prone positioning when it is used early and along with other protective ventilation strategies. Placing the patient in the prone position for more than 12 hours has been shown to decrease mortality in those with moderate to severe ARDS when used with lower V_T ventilation[27] (see Evidence-Based Practice box). Turning the patient to the prone position (*proning*) alters the $\dot{V}/\dot{Q}$ ratio by maintaining posterior perfusion while allowing optimal ventilation in the larger, dorsal portion of the lungs. Placing the patient prone removes the weight of the heart and abdomen from the lungs, facilitates removal of secretions, improves oxygenation, and enhances recruitment of airways.

Turning the patient to the prone position is a procedure that requires several healthcare professionals to ensure the patient's safety. Care must be taken to avoid dislodging the endotracheal tube (ETT) and other tubes and lines. Several commercial devices and pronation beds are available to assist in turning the patient. Potential complications from the prone position are accidental dislodgement of tubes and lines, gastric aspiration, peripheral nerve injury, pressure ulcers, corneal ulceration, facial edema, and agitation. Administer promotility agents or postpyloric feedings to minimize the risk of vomiting and enhance emptying of gastric contents. Maintain proper body alignment while the patient is in the prone position to decrease the risk of nerve damage. Use pillows and foam support equipment to prevent overextension or flexion of the spine and reduce weight bearing on bony prominences. Place hydrocolloid or silicone dressing on chest, pelvis, elbows, and knees to maintain skin integrity. To avoid peripheral nerve injury and contractures of the shoulders, position the arms carefully and reposition them often. Reposition the head hourly to reduce facial edema and decrease ocular pressure. Provide frequent oral care and suctioning as needed. Apply moisture barrier to the patient's entire face to protect the skin from the massive amount of drainage from the mouth and nose. Lubricate the eyes to prevent corneal drying and abrasions. Assess the patient frequently for tolerance of proning. Patient and family education regarding the use of pronation is essential in decreasing anxiety.[84]

EVIDENCE-BASED PRACTICE

Prone Positioning in Acute Respiratory Distress Syndrome

Problem
Prone positioning is sometimes used as a treatment for ARDS that is refractory to conventional mechanical ventilation.

Clinical Question
What outcomes are associated with prone positioning for moderate to severe ARDS as compared to traditional ventilatory management?

Evidence
In this systematic review and meta-analysis, the authors analyzed eight randomized controlled trials (RCTs) including data collected on 2129 patients. They compared outcomes of prone positioning versus traditional ventilation in the supine position in adults diagnosed with ARDS. Findings indicated that although mortality risks were not different between the two groups, lower mortality occurred when 12 hours or more of prone positioning was implemented for patients with moderate to severe ARDS. When compared with supine positioning, prone positioning was associated with greater risk of endotracheal tube obstruction and pressure injury.

Implications for Nursing
Nurses are responsible for the positioning and mobility of critically ill patients and must collaborate with other healthcare providers to provide the safest and most effective treatment for each individual. Positioning protocols for patients with moderate to severe ARDS may include pronation to improve outcomes. Assessment for tolerance, improvement in oxygenation, and adverse effects is essential for optimal outcomes. Nurses can also implement strategies to reduce complications such as pressure injury.

Level of Evidence
A—Meta-analysis

Reference
Munshi L, Del Sorbo L, Adhikari NKJ, et al. Prone position for acute respiratory distress syndrome: A systematic review and meta-analysis. *Ann Am Thorac Soc.* 2017;14(Suppl 4):S280–S288.

Fluids and Electrolytes. Conservative fluid management, including diuresis, is the goal for patients with ARDS. Successful fluid management results in reduced mortality, shorter length of mechanical ventilation, and fewer critical care unit days. Patients who are hypotensive or hypovolemic should receive aggressive fluid resuscitation initially and then conservative fluid management after resolution of shock. This strategy is associated with a lower mortality rate.[36]

Nutrition. The goal of nutritional support is to provide adequate nutrition that is tolerated to meet the patient's level of metabolism and reduce morbidity (see Chapter 7).[72] It is generally recommended to begin enteral nutrition at 25 to 30 kilocalories per kilogram of IBW within 48 hours for critically ill adults.[57] However, delivering higher calories to those with ARDS results in an increased likelihood of mortality.[66] Current opinion supports withholding feeding for ARDS patients in the most acute phase of the illness.

Psychosocial Support. The onset of ARDS and its long recovery phase result in stress and anxiety for both the patient and the family. The patient may also experience feelings of isolation and dependence because of impaired communication and a prolonged recovery phase. Always remember to provide a warm, nurturing environment in which the patient and family can feel safe. Providing a therapeutic environment includes taking the time to explain procedures, equipment, changes in the patient's condition, and outcomes to the patient and family members. Encourage family presence and allow the patient and family to participate in the planning of care and to verbalize fears and questions.

STUDY BREAK

2. Lung-protective ventilation strategies include:
   A. Tidal volume (V_T) calculated according to current patient weight
   B. V_T at 4 to 8 mL/kg predicted ideal body weight
   C. Consistent use of 100% fraction of inspired oxygen (FiO_2)
   D. Positive end-expiratory pressure (PEEP) levels of 30 cm H_2O for 8 hours each day

---

ACUTE RESPIRATORY FAILURE IN CHRONIC OBSTRUCTIVE PULMONARY DISEASE

Pathophysiology

COPD is a progressive yet preventable disease characterized by airflow limitations that are not fully reversible. These airflow limitations are associated with an abnormal inflammatory response to noxious particles or gases. COPD is a disease of the small airways and the lung parenchyma that results in chronic bronchitis and emphysema. Its incidence and effect on chronic morbidity and mortality are increasing. COPD is the third leading cause of death in the United States after cardiac disease and cancer. The primary cause of COPD is tobacco smoke, and smoking cessation is the most effective intervention to reduce the risk of developing COPD and stop disease progression. Other contributing factors to the development of COPD include air pollution, occupational exposure to dust or chemicals, age and female sex, and the genetic abnormality alpha$_1$-antitrypsin deficiency.[12,35]

The primary pathogenic mechanism in COPD is chronic inflammation, which may directly injure the airway and lead to systemic effects. Exposure to inhaled particles leads to airway inflammation and injury. The body repairs this injury through the process of airway remodeling, which causes scarring, narrowing, and obstruction of the airways. Destruction of alveolar walls and connective tissue results in permanent enlargement of air spaces. Increased mucus production results from enlargement of mucus-secreting glands and an increase in the number of goblet cells. Areas of cilia are destroyed, contributing to the patient's inability to clear thick, tenacious mucus. Structural changes in the pulmonary capillaries thicken the vascular walls and inhibit gas exchange. Systemic inflammation also causes direct effects on peripheral blood vessels and may be a concomitant factor in the association of cardiovascular disease with COPD.[12] Table 15.1 outlines the physiological changes that result from COPD.

ARF can occur at any time in a patient with COPD. These patients normally have little respiratory reserve, and any condition that increases the work of breathing worsens $\dot{V}/\dot{Q}$ mismatching. Common causes of ARF in patients with COPD are acute exacerbations, heart failure, dysrhythmias, pulmonary edema, pneumonia, dehydration, and electrolyte imbalances.

Assessment

The hallmark symptoms of COPD are progressive dyspnea, chronic cough, and sputum production. The diagnosis is confirmed by post bronchodilator spirometry that documents irreversible airflow limitations. These pulmonary function tests show an increase in total lung capacity and a reduction in forced expiratory volume over 1 second (FEV_1) with a FEV_1/forced vital capacity (FVC) ratio less than 0.70.[35] Functional residual capacity is increased as a result of air trapping.

? CRITICAL REASONING ACTIVITY

Mr. B. has just been intubated for acute respiratory failure (ARF). Currently, he is agitated and very restless. What contributing factors are associated with Mr. B.'s agitation? What nursing actions are indicated in this situation?

TABLE 15.1 Pathological and Physiological Changes in Chronic Obstructive Pulmonary Disease

Pathological Changes	Physiological Changes
Mucus hypersecretion	Sputum production
Ciliary dysfunction	Retained secretions Chronic cough
Chronic airway inflammation	Expiratory airflow limitation
Airway remodeling	Terminal airway collapse Air trapping Lung hyperinflation
Thickening of pulmonary vessels	Poor gas exchange with hypoxemia and hypercapnia Pulmonary hypertension Cor pulmonale (right ventricular enlargement and heart failure)

By the time the characteristic physical findings of COPD are evident on physical examination, a significant decline in lung function has occurred. The chest is often overexpanded or barrel shaped because the anterior-posterior diameter increases in size. Assess for use of accessory muscles and pursed-lip breathing. Clubbing of the fingers indicates long-term hypoxemia. Lung auscultation usually reveals diminished breath sounds, prolonged exhalation, wheezing, and crackles. ABG results show mild hypoxemia in the early stages of the disease and worsening hypoxemia and hypercapnia as the disease progresses. Over time, as a compensatory mechanism, the kidneys increase bicarbonate production and retention (metabolic alkalosis) in an attempt to keep the pH within normal limits.

Exacerbation of COPD often results in a change in the patient's baseline dyspnea and an increase in sputum volume. Assess for changes in the character of the sputum, which may signal the development of a respiratory infection. Assess for additional symptoms, which may include anxiety, wheezing, chest tightness, tachypnea, tachycardia, fatigue, malaise, confusion, fever, and sleeping difficulties. Wheezing indicates narrowing of the airways. Retraction of intercostal muscles may occur with inspiration, and exhalation is prolonged through pursed lips. The patient is typically more comfortable in the upright position. Tachycardia and hypotension may result from reduced cardiac output.

Life-threatening ARF is indicated by tachypnea of more than 30 breaths/min, accessory muscle use, acute decline in mental status, hypoxemia that does not improve with supplemental oxygen via Venturi mask with FiO_2 greater than 40%, $PaCO_2$ greater than 60 mm Hg or pH less than 7.25.[35]

Know the patient's baseline ABG values to detect changes that indicate ARF. At baseline, the patient with COPD usually has ABG results that show a normal pH, a moderately low PaO_2 in the range of 60 to 65 mm Hg, and an elevated $PaCO_2$ in the range of 50 to 60 mm Hg (compensated respiratory acidosis).

! CLINICAL ALERT

Indications of Impending Acute Respiratory Failure Requiring Noninvasive Ventilation

- Severe dyspnea with respiratory muscle fatigue and/or increased work of breathing (WOB)
- Hypoxemia not responsive to supplemental oxygen
- Respiratory acidosis (pH ≤7.35)

Interventions

Box 15.2 outlines the care of patients with stable COPD. These interventions are individualized to reduce risk factors, manage symptoms, limit complications, and enhance quality of life. When a patient has an acute exacerbation, the goals of therapy are to provide support during the episode of acute failure, treat the triggering event, and return the patient to the previous level of functioning.

BOX 15.2 Treatment of Stable Chronic Obstructive Pulmonary Disease

- Reduce exposure to airway irritants
- Counseling or treatment for smoking cessation
- Remain in an air-conditioned environment during times of high air pollution
- Influenza and pneumococcal vaccinations
- Inhaled bronchodilators (short-acting, long-acting, or combination)
- Inhaled glucocorticosteroids for severe disease and repeated exacerbations
- Pulmonary rehabilitation program with exercise training
- Long-term administration of oxygen for more than 15 h/day for severe disease

---

Oxygen. The most important intervention for an acute exacerbation of COPD is to correct hypoxemia. O_2 is administered to achieve a SaO_2 of 88% to 92%. A Venturi mask delivers more precise oxygen concentrations than nasal prongs but may not be tolerated as well. High-flow oxygen therapy by nasal cannula may be better tolerated and has been shown to effectively oxygenate some COPD patients with ARF. When delivering high concentrations of O_2, be aware of the possibility that it can blunt the COPD patient's hypoxic drive, which can diminish respiratory efforts and further increase CO_2 retention. Titrate oxygen slowly and incrementally and reevaluate ABGs frequently after the initiation of therapy to monitor both O_2 and CO_2 levels.[35]

Bronchodilator Therapy. The use of short-acting inhaled beta$_2$-agonists with or without short-acting anticholinergics is recommended for treating an acute exacerbation.[35] Table 15.2 lists commonly administered bronchodilator agents. Short-acting, inhaled beta$_2$-agonists cause bronchial smooth muscle relaxation that reverses bronchoconstriction. They are primarily administered via a nebulizer or a metered-dose inhaler with a spacer. The dosage and frequency vary, depending on the delivery method and the severity of bronchoconstriction. Adverse effects are dose related and are more common with oral or IV administration than with inhalation. Adverse effects include tachycardia, dysrhythmias, tremors, hypokalemia, anxiety, bronchospasm, and dyspnea.

Corticosteroids. Administration of systemic corticosteroids improves lung function, recovery time, oxygenation, and length of stay. Prednisone, 40 mg/day for 5 days, is the recommended regimen. Nebulizer treatment with budesonide alone can be an effective alternative to oral prednisone for some patients.[35] Common adverse effects of steroid therapy include hyperglycemia and an increased risk of infection.

Antibiotics. Administration of antibiotics to patients with COPD exacerbation improves survival for those who are moderately or severely ill. Antibiotic therapy, preferably by the oral route, is recommended for a period of 5 to 7 days in patients with increased dyspnea and increased sputum volume and purulence or if mechanical ventilation is required. Antibiotic selection should be based on local bacterial resistance patterns; however, initial therapy often begins with an aminopenicillin alone or in

TABLE 15.2   PHARMACOLOGY

Bronchodilators

Medication	Action/Use	Dose/Route	Side Effects	Nursing Implications
Beta$_2$-agonists (short-acting) Albuterol Levalbuterol	Bronchial smooth muscle relaxation Used for relief of acute symptoms or prevention of exercise-induced asthma	Refer to drug guide for specific information related to each medication	Tremor, anxiety, bronchospasm, dyspnea, tachycardia, dysrhythmias, palpitations, hypertension, hypokalemia, throat irritation, refractory asthma	Assess respiratory and cardiac status. Monitor response to treatment within 1 h. Teach correct use of inhaler and spacer (specific to metered-dose inhaler medications). Teach proper use of medication for acute exacerbations and prevention.
Beta$_2$-agonists (long-acting) Salmeterol Formoterol	Bronchial smooth muscle relaxation; used for long-term prevention of symptoms	Refer to drug guide for specific information related to each medication	Same as for short-acting beta$_2$-agonists	Do not use to treat acute exacerbations. Assess respiratory and cardiac status. Provide teaching.
Anticholinergics Ipratropium bromide (SAMA) Tiotropium bromide (LAMA)	Inhibit action of acetylcholine, causing bronchial smooth muscle relaxation; used to treat or prevent bronchospasm in COPD	Generally given via inhalation; refer to drug guide for specific information related to each medication	Dry mouth, bitter taste, dizziness, bronchoconstriction, palpitations; lower incidence of tachycardia than for beta$_2$-agonists	Monitor respiratory status and response to treatment. Avoid contact with eyes, and report changes in vision. Provide relief of dry mouth (hard candy, liquids, sugarless gum).

COPD, Chronic obstructive pulmonary disease; *LAMA,* long-acting muscarinic antagonist; *SAMA,* short-acting muscarinic antagonist.

---

conjunction with a clavulanic acid, macrolide, or tetracycline antibiotic. For patients with severe disease or frequent exacerbations, sputum cultures are advised, as gram-negative or resistant pathogens may not be sensitive to the above-mentioned antibiotics.[35]

Ventilatory Assistance. Patients with ARF from a COPD exacerbation may require positive-pressure ventilation with or without intubation. Early treatment with NPPV improves outcomes in 85% of patients, resulting in decreased mortality and a reduced intubation rate.[75] See Clinical Alert box for indications for noninvasive ventilation (NIV), which assists the patient's respiratory efforts by delivering positive airway pressure through a nasal, oronasal, or full face mask[35] (see Chapter 10).

Intubation and invasive mechanical ventilation are indicated in those patients for whom trials of NPPV have failed. Other indications include persistent or worsening hypoxemia, respiratory or cardiac arrest, decreased LOC, aspiration, inability to remove secretions, hemodynamic instability, or life-threatening ventricular dysrhythmias.[35] Long-term morbidity for COPD patients requiring intermittent mandatory ventilation (IMV) is significant.[32]

In the late stages of severe COPD, patients often report that their quality of life deteriorates because of severe activity limitations and comorbid conditions. Decisions regarding intubation, mechanical ventilation, cardiopulmonary resuscitation, and other forms of life support should be made by the patient in conjunction with the patient's family and physician before ARF occurs. Critical care nurses are in an ideal position to facilitate discussions about advance directives and to answer questions.

> **STUDY BREAK**
> 3. Possible treatments for acute respiratory failure (ARF) in the patient with chronic obstructive pulmonary disease (COPD) include:
>   A. Noninvasive ventilation
>   B. Bronchodilators
>   C. Corticosteroids
>   D. All the above

ACUTE RESPIRATORY FAILURE IN ASTHMA

Pathophysiology

Asthma is a chronic inflammatory disorder of the airways. The inflammation causes the airways to become hyperresponsive when the patient inhales allergens, viruses, or other irritants (Box 15.3). Episodic airflow obstruction results because these irritants cause bronchoconstriction, airway edema, mucus plugging, and airway remodeling (Fig. 15.3). Air trapping, prolonged exhalation, and $\dot{V}/\dot{Q}$ mismatching with an increased intrapulmonary shunt occur. The airflow limitations in asthma are largely reversible. When asthma is controlled, symptoms and exacerbations should be infrequent.[12]

Assessment

Initial clinical manifestations of asthma exacerbation include expiratory wheezing, dyspnea, chest tightness, prolonged expiration, tachycardia, tachypnea, and nonproductive cough. The patient initially hyperventilates, producing respiratory alkalosis. As the airways continue to narrow, it becomes more difficult for the patient to exhale. Peak expiratory flow (PEF) readings will be less than 50% of the patient's normal values. The patient may exhibit inspiratory and expiratory wheezing, agitation, use of accessory muscles, and suprasternal retractions.

BOX 15.3 Asthma Triggers

Inhalant Allergens
- Animals
- Cockroaches
- House-dust mites
- Indoor fungi
- Outdoor allergens

Occupational Exposures
- Chemical agents
- Fumes
- Organic and inorganic dusts

Irritants
- Fumes: perfumes, cleaning agents, sprays
- Indoor or outdoor pollution
- Tobacco smoke

Other Factors Influencing Asthma Severity
- Exercise
- Gastroesophageal reflux disease
- Rhinitis and sinusitis
- Sensitivity: aspirin, other nonsteroidal antiinflammatory drugs, sulfites
- Topical and systemic beta-blockers
- Viral respiratory infections

! CLINICAL ALERT

Asthma

Signs of impending acute respiratory failure (ARF) requiring intubation and ventilation in asthma exacerbation:
- "Silent" chest
- Breathlessness at rest and the need to sit hunched forward
- Single-word responses
- Agitation, confusion, drowsiness
- Respiratory rate (RR) greater than 30 breaths/min; heart rate (HR) greater than 120 beats/min; oxygen saturation (SpO_2) greater than 90%
- Peak expiratory flow (PEF) 50% or less than predicted or personal best

Interventions

Mild exacerbations of asthma can be managed by the patient at home with the use of inhaled short-acting beta$_2$-agonists to treat bronchoconstriction and inhaled low-dose corticosteroid for inflammation (see Table 15.2). Treatment of acute, severe exacerbations of asthma requires O_2 therapy to maintain SpO_2 of 93% to 95% (94% to 98% for children 6 to 11 years of age), repeated administration of rapid-acting inhaled bronchodilators, and systemic steroid administration for adults and children (Table 15.3). Adding a short-acting anticholinergic to the regimen initially may prevent the need for hospitalization and improve lung function but does not prove helpful in decreasing length of stay for children hospitalized for asthma exacerbation.[34]

Most patients respond well to treatment, but some may need intubation and mechanical ventilation. Precise management of mechanical ventilation is required to enhance outcomes and prevent complications. In cases that are refractory to standard treatment, oxygenation may be improved by delivering a mixture of helium and O_2 (heliox) to the lungs. Because helium is less dense than O_2, it enhances gas flow through the constricted airways and may improve oxygenation.[34]

During a patient's recovery from a severe asthmatic event, focus efforts on teaching the patient asthma management techniques to achieve control. Teach the patient to implement environmental controls to prevent symptoms, understand the differences between medications that relieve and those that control symptoms, properly use inhaler devices, monitor the level of asthma control, and schedule a follow-up visit with the healthcare provider within 1 week. A written action plan and goals of treatment mutually determined by the patient and the healthcare provider helps patients achieve asthma control and assists with early identification and treatment of exacerbations.[34]

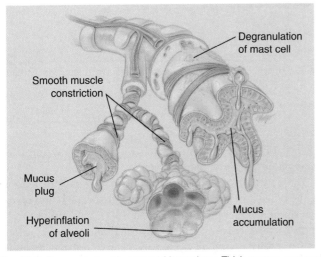

Fig. 15.3 Airway obstruction caused by asthma. Thick mucus, mucosal edema, and smooth muscle spasm cause obstruction of small airways in bronchial asthma. (Modified from Des Jardins T, Burton GC. *Clinical manifestations and assessment of respiratory disease.* 3rd ed. St. Louis, MO: Mosby; 1995.)

Labels in figure: Degranulation of mast cell; Smooth muscle constriction; Mucus plug; Hyperinflation of alveoli; Mucus accumulation

ACUTE RESPIRATORY FAILURE RESULTING FROM PNEUMONIA

Definition and Etiology

Pneumonia is the leading cause of death from infection in the United States and a common cause of ARF. Pneumonia is a lower respiratory tract infection with a variety of risk factors, with the elderly being particularly vulnerable, as incidence and mortality are highest in this population. Other risk factors

A severe asthma exacerbation, *status asthmaticus,* occurs when the bronchoconstriction does not respond to bronchodilator therapy, and ARF ensues, resulting in respiratory acidosis and severe hypoxemia. Auscultation of a "silent" chest, indicating complete absence of air movement, is an ominous sign indicating impending medical emergency requiring prompt intervention to preserve life (see Clinical Alert box).

TABLE 15.3 Emergency Treatment of Severe Asthma

Therapy	Purpose	Goals
Oxygen via nasal cannula or face mask	Correct hypoxemia	Maintain SpO_2 at 93%-95%
Inhaled rapid-acting beta$_2$-agonists via nebulizer (continuous), followed by intermittent on-demand therapy	Relieve airway obstruction caused by bronchoconstriction	Achieve PEF >60% of predicted or personal best; normalize or improve ABGs; respiratory rate <30 breaths/min without use of accessory muscles
Inhaled anticholinergics (added to beta$_2$-agonist therapy)	Relieve bronchoconstriction	Relieve sensation of dyspnea; patient able to complete full sentences without breathlessness
Systemic corticosteroids within 1 hour (orally)	Reverse airway inflammation	Improve lung sounds; prevent intubation

ABGs, Arterial blood gases; *PEF,* peak expiratory flow; *SpO2,* arterial oxygen saturation.

TABLE 15.4 Pneumonia Definitions and Common Infectious Causes

Type	Criteria	Infectious Causes
Community-acquired pneumonia (CAP)	Pneumonia that develops outside a healthcare facility.	*Streptococcus pneumoniae* *Haemophilus influenza* *Staphylococcus aureus* *Mycoplasma pneumoniae* *Chlamydophila pneumonia* *Moraxella catarrhalis* *Legionella pneumophila* *Influenza* *Rhinovirus* *Coronavirus*
Health care–associated pneumonia (HCAP); Hospital acquired pneumonia (HAP); Ventilator-associated pneumonia (VAP)	Pneumonia that develops in individuals with recent hospitalization, nursing home or extended care stays, home infusion therapy, long-term dialysis, home wound care, as well as those who are non-ambulatory, those with tube feedings, and those taking gastric acid reducing agents.	*Staphylococcus aureus* *Pseudomonas aeruginosa* *Enterobacter species* *Klebsiella pneumoniae*

From Brashers VL, Huether SE. Alterations of pulmonary function. In: McCance KL, Huether SE. *Pathophysiology: The Biologic Basis for Disease in Adults and Children.* 8th ed. St. Louis, MO: Elsevier; 2019.

include those with compromised immunity, COPD, alcoholism, altered LOC, chest trauma, impaired swallowing, malnutrition, endotracheal intubation, immobilization, heart disease, and liver disease.[5] Nursing home residents and smokers are also at an increased risk for developing pneumonia.[12]

Pathophysiology

For pneumonia to occur, enough organisms must accumulate in the lower respiratory tract to overwhelm the patient's defense mechanisms. The lower respiratory tract is usually a sterile environment. It is protected by the warming and filtering of air as it passes through the upper airway; closure of the epiglottis; cough and sneezing reflexes; mucociliary clearance; and alveolar macrophages. The major routes of entry for these organisms are aspiration of gastric or oropharyngeal secretions (most common), inhalation of aerosols or particles, and hematogenous spread from another infected site into the lungs. The normal bronchomucociliary clearance mechanism is overwhelmed by the infective organism, causing a large influx of phagocytic cells along with exudate into the airways and alveoli. This inflammatory response leads to

a ventilation-perfusion mismatch resulting in dyspnea, hypoxemia, fever, and leukocytosis.[12]

The pathogens responsible for pneumonia vary depending on the type (community versus hospital-associated) and on the environmental factor or cause (Table 15.4). The pathogens include bacteria, viruses, fungi, protozoa, and parasites, along with multidrug-resistant organisms such as methicillin-resistant *Staphylococcus aureus* (MRSA). Fungal causes of pneumonia are uncommon unless the patient is immunocompromised.

Prevention of pneumonia is a priority. The most common bacterial cause of community-acquired pneumonia is streptococcal or pneumococcal infection, which may be prevented by receiving the pneumococcal vaccination (Box 15.4). The Centers for Disease Control and Prevention (CDC) recommends that adults 65 years of age or older receive two vaccines, beginning with the conjugate dose (PCV13), followed by the polysaccharide dose (PPSV23) at least 1 year later.[18] Influenza is a common cause of viral pneumonia. An annual influenza vaccine is recommended for all persons of at least 6 months of age (with rare exceptions), pregnant women, those with chronic health conditions, and those at high risk for complications of influenza.[19]

BOX 15.4 Pneumococcal Vaccine Recommendations for Prevention of Pneumococcal Disease

- **Pneumococcal conjugate vaccine (PCV13)** is recommended for all children younger than 2 years, all adults 65 years or older, and people 2 through 64 years of age with certain risk factors (i.e., chronic heart disease, chronic lung disease, diabetes, CSF leaks, cochlear implants, sickle cell disease, congenital or acquired asplenia or splenic dysfunction, HIV infection, chronic renal failure or nephrotic syndrome, and diseases treated with immunosuppressive medications or radiation such as malignant neoplasm, leukemia, lymphoma, Hodgkin's disease, and solid organ transplantation).
- **Pneumococcal polysaccharide vaccine (PPSV23)** is recommended for all adults 65 years or older. People 2 through 64 years old who are at high risk of pneumococcal disease or those who smoke should also receive PPSV23. These include long-term health problems such as heart disease, lung disease, sickle cell disease, diabetes, alcoholism, cirrhosis, CSF leaks, or cochlear implant. Vaccination is also recommended for those with increased risk for infection such as Hodgkin's disease; lymphoma or leukemia; kidney failure; multiple myeloma; nephrotic syndrome; HIV infection or AIDS; damaged spleen, or no spleen; organ transplant as well as those taking immunosuppressant medications.

CSF, Cerebrospinal fluid.
From Centers for Disease Control and Prevention. Vaccines and Preventable Diseases: Pneumococcal Vaccination. https://www.cdc.gov/vaccines/vpd/pneumo/hcp/who-when-to-vaccinate.html. Updated December 6, 2017. Accessed March 4, 2019.

Assessment

The clinical presentation for pneumonia commonly begins with fever, cough (often productive), and dyspnea. Other symptoms may include chills, malaise, and pleuritic chest pain. Older adult patients may present with nonspecific symptoms such as changes in mental status with hypothermia. Physical findings may include crackles, increased tactile fremitus, egophony, and whispered pectoriloquy. Recommended diagnostic studies include a chest radiograph, which may show local or diffuse infiltrates depending on the severity and distribution of the infection, white blood cell count, and procalcitonin or C-reactive protein level. Obtain blood and sputum cultures before antibiotic administration without delaying implementation of antibiotic therapy. Abnormal laboratory results include an elevated white blood cell count; serum procalcitonin or C-reactive protein levels, which are used to differentiate between bacterial and viral source; and ABG results demonstrating hypoxemia and hypocapnia.[12]

Initial management of pneumonia requires establishing adequate ventilation and oxygenation, adequate hydration, pulmonary hygiene, and antibiotic administration within 4 hours of presentation for bacterial cause.

VENTILATOR-ASSOCIATED PNEUMONIA AND EVENTS

One of the complications of mechanical ventilation is ventilator-associated pneumonia (VAP), which significantly increases ventilator time, length of stay, cost of care, and ultimately mortality. VAP is defined as pneumonia that develops in a patient who is intubated and ventilated at the time of or within 48 hours prior to the onset of the event[44] and is now included as one of several problems of oxygenation in the broad category of ventilator-associated events (VAEs) as defined by the National Healthcare Safety Network.[16] Because limited research has been completed to validate this recent classification, most of the literature still refers to the condition as VAP. VAP is a preventable hospital-acquired infection affecting an average of 15% to 70% of critically ill individuals,[55,70] and it complicates the course of illness for these patients, who require invasive mechanical ventilation. The longer the requirement for mechanical ventilation, the greater the likelihood that the patient will contract VAP. The crude mortality rate for VAP ranges from 14% to 59%.[38,53,55,70]

Pathophysiology

The pathogenesis of VAP is depicted in Fig. 15.4. Patients with an ETT are at increased risk for aspiration of oral and gastric secretions. The ETT is inserted into the trachea past the vocal cords, thereby holding the glottis in the open position and compromising its ability to prevent aspiration. Sources of exogenous pathogens include contamination from healthcare personnel, ventilator and respiratory equipment, and the biofilm coating on the ETT.

Assessment

VAP has traditionally been diagnosed with clinical criteria including a new or progressive pulmonary infiltrate along with fever, leukocytosis, and purulent tracheobronchial secretions. However, these criteria lack objectivity, specificity, and sensitivity, making surveillance for VAP a long-standing challenge that has implications for prevention and outcomes for mechanically ventilated individuals.[16,17] Lung ultrasound, a noninvasive bedside approach, is currently being researched as an alternative to chest x-ray for critically ill individuals and has shown promising results.[85] Mini bronchoalveolar lavage fluid amylase level also shows promise as a diagnostic tool for diagnosing VAP.[70,77]

Because of the difficulty in accurately diagnosing VAP, in 2011 the CDC convened a work group of experts who developed a new approach for monitoring VAEs, including VAP. The VAE surveillance standards (Fig. 15.5) are based on objective criteria for several complications that can occur in patients who require mechanical ventilation.

Interventions

The interventions for VAP are aimed at prevention and treatment.[78] Because VAP has been identified as the most prevalent infection acquired by critically ill patients requiring mechanical ventilation, prevention of VAP is a major focus. The Institute for Healthcare Improvement endorses a "bundle of care" to improve overall care of mechanically ventilated patients. Bundles are evidence-based interventions that are grouped together to improve outcomes. Components of the ventilator bundle include head of bed (HOB) elevation to at least 30 degrees, daily awakening ("sedation vacation") with assessment of need for continuing mechanical ventilation, prophylaxis for stress ulcers and deep venous thrombosis, and regular antiseptic oral

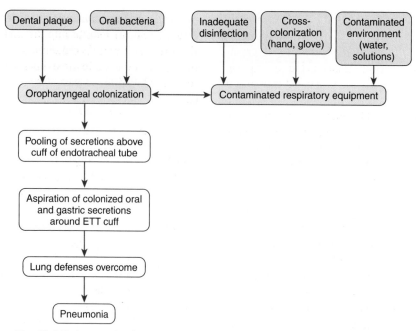

Fig. 15.4 Pathogenesis of ventilator-associated pneumonia. *ETT,* Endotracheal tube.

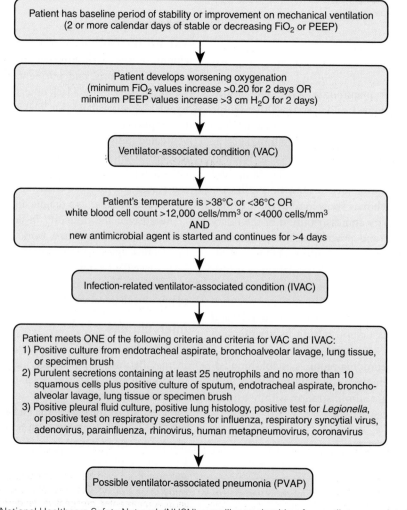

Fig. 15.5 National Healthcare Safety Network (NHSN) surveillance algorithm for ventilator-associated events. *FiO₂,* Fraction of inspired oxygen; *PEEP,* positive end-expiratory pressure. (Modified from Centers for Disease Control and Prevention. Device-Associated Module VAE. http://www.cdc.gov/nhsn/PDFs/pscManual/10-VAE_FINAL.pdf. Published January 2015. Accessed March 2019.)

care to include chlorhexidine.[41] Implementation of the ventilator bundle is an effective prevention strategy for decreasing the occurrence of VAP.[67]

Currently being researched is a bundle that includes seven mandatory components and three highly recommended components that shows significant and sustained reduction in the incidence of VAP. Mandatory strategies include (1) education in airway management; (2) hand hygiene with alcohol prior to airway management; (3) controlled cuff pressure; (4) chlorhexidine for oral care; (5) HOB elevation; (6) protocols to avoid or reduce duration of intubation/ventilation; and (7) protocols to avoid elective exchange of ventilator circuits, humidifiers, and ETT. Three highly recommended strategies are (1) selective oropharyngeal or gastrointestinal (GI) decontamination; (2) continuous aspiration of subglottic secretions; and (3) two to three doses of antibiotic during intubation of those with previous decreased LOC.[4]

Also showing promise for improved compliance with evidence-based interventions and a decrease in VAEs, infection-related ventilator-associated complications, and probable VAP is a large clinical trial that included education to improve evidence-based practice, implementation of a comprehensive unit-based safety program, and measurement and feedback of performance. Interventions used for prevention included HOB elevation, use of ETT with subglottic suctioning, oral care six times per day (every 4 hours), spontaneous awakening trials, and spontaneous breathing trials.[68]

Another investigation of prevention strategies included hand hygiene, HOB elevation, oral hygiene three times per day with chlorhexidine, maintaining ETT cuff pressures at 25 cm H_2O or more, daily sedation vacation and readiness for extubation trials, and daily active mobilization. Continuous aspiration

of subglottic secretions was an added intervention 2 months into the trial. Six months into the trial, researchers added selective oropharyngeal decontamination (SOD) with colistin, tobramycin, and nystatin three times per day for individuals likely to be intubated for at least 48 hours. This preventive program showed sustained decreased incidence of VAP, with SOD providing additional value.[53]

Some evidence supports administration of probiotics to decrease the risk of VAP, but further research is needed.[52] Antioxidants are also being explored as a treatment to reduce oxidative stress.[40] Subglottic secretion drainage is also an effective strategy for prevention of VAP.[87]

The critical care nurse is primarily responsible for providing these preventive interventions. Nurses are more likely to adhere to established guidelines if they understand and support the standards. For this reason, it is important that the critical care nurse be involved in the development and implementation of guidelines and standards of care, working collaboratively with physicians and other healthcare personnel to prevent VAP and VAE. Strategies for prevention of VAP are summarized in Box 15.5, and an example of an oral care protocol is described in Box 15.6.

STUDY BREAK

4. Evidence-based interventions for the prevention of ventilator-associated pneumonia (VAP) include:
   A. Head of bed (HOB) flat with patient supine
   B. Readiness-to-wean trials every other day
   C. Regular antiseptic oral care
   D. Deep vein thrombosis (DVT) prophylaxis on select patients

---

BOX 15.5 Prevention of Ventilator-Associated Pneumonia

1. Implement effective infection control measures, including staff education and hand hygiene with alcohol
2. Conduct surveillance of VAE
3. Implement components of IHI ventilator bundle:
   - Maintain head-of-bed elevation at least 30 degrees
   - Daily sedation interruptions and daily assessment of readiness to wean from ventilator
   - Deep vein thrombosis prophylaxis
   - Peptic ulcer disease prophylaxis
   - Daily oral care with chlorhexidine
4. Prevent transmission of microorganisms:
   - Use sterile water in, and for cleaning of, respiratory equipment
   - Change the ventilator circuit only when it is visibly soiled
   - Drain condensate in ventilator circuits away from the patient
   - Do not instill normal saline into the ETT
5. Modify host risk for infections:
   - Avoid intubation and reintubation; use noninvasive ventilation if possible
   - Intubate patients orally

- Control cuff pressures at 25 cm H_2O or more
- Use orogastric tubes
- If available, use an ETT that allows continuous aspiration of subglottic secretions
- Oropharyngeal/GI decontamination with colistin, tobramycin, and nystatin for those likely to be intubated for at least 48 hours
- Two to three doses of antibiotic during intubation of those with previous decreased LOC
- Use sedation and weaning protocols
- Daily active mobilization

6. Other prevention strategies:
   - Enteral nutrition is preferred over parenteral
   - Develop and implement an early mobilization program
   - Administer IV fluids to avoid fluid overload; monitor intake and output
   - Administer analgesics and sedatives using protocols and sedation scales
   - Use lung-protective strategies for mechanical ventilation
   - Discontinue mechanical ventilation as soon as possible

ETT, Endotracheal tube; *GI,* gastrointestinal; *IHI,* Institute for Healthcare Improvement; *LOC,* level of consciousness; *VAE,* ventilator-associated event.

Data from Alvarez-Lerma F, Palomar-Martinez M, Sanchez-Garcia M, et al. Prevention of ventilator-associated pneumonia: The multimodal approach of the Spanish ICU "pneumonia zero" program. *Crit Care Med.* 2018;46(2):181–189; Klarin B, Adolfsson A, Torstensson A, et al. Can probiotics be an alternative to chlorhexidine for oral care in the mechanically ventilated patient? A multicenter, prospective, randomized controlled open trial. *Crit Care.* 2018;22(272):1–10; Landell C, Boyer V, Abbas M, et al. Impact of a multifaceted prevention program on ventilator-associated pneumonia including selective oropharyngeal decontamination. *Intensive Care Med.* 2018;44:1777–1786; Rawat N, Yang T, Ali K, et al. Two-state collaborative study of a multifaceted intervention to decrease ventilator-associated events. *Crit Care Med.* 2017;45(7):1208–1215.

BOX 15.6 Example of an Oral Care Protocol

Equipment
1. Oral suction catheter
2. Soft toothbrush or suction toothbrush
3. Toothettes, oral swab, or suction swab
4. Hydrogen peroxide (1.5%) mouth rinse or toothpaste
5. Water-based mouth moisturizer
6. Oral chlorhexidine gluconate (0.12%) rinse
7. Suction source and tubing

Interventions
1. Assess intubated patients every 2 hours, before repositioning or deflating the endotracheal tube, and as needed to determine the need for removal of oropharyngeal secretions. Suction as needed.
2. Brush teeth, gums, and tongue twice a day using a soft pediatric or adult toothbrush with toothpaste or cleaning solution.
3. Swab oral chlorhexidine gluconate (0.12%) over all oral surfaces for 30 seconds twice a day; suction excess.
4. Avoid brushing teeth or oral intake for 2 hours after chlorhexidine use.
5. Apply moisturizer to oral mucosa and lips every 2 to 4 hours.

Treatment. VAP is associated with a high risk of mortality (20% to 50%) or, at best, results in a significant increase in ventilator days and length of hospital stay. Current guidelines recommend that hospitals develop antibiograms that target their usual pneumonia population to assist in correct antibiotic selection to prevent exposure to unnecessary antibiotics and decrease the occurrence of antibiotic-resistant organisms. Recommendations also support short-course antibiotic regimen (7 days) when possible and antibiotic deescalation.[48]

Empiric antibiotics for individuals with suspected VAP should cover *S. aureus, Pseudomonas aeruginosa,* and other gram-negative bacilli. This regimen includes gram-positive antibiotics such as vancomycin or linezolid; gram-negative antibiotics such as piperacillin, cefepime, or imipenem; and gram-negative antibiotics such as ciprofloxacin, gentamicin, or colistin. Antibiotics are subsequently adjusted based on culture results, but initial treatment should not be delayed while awaiting culture results.[48] Current evidence suggests that aerosolized colistin[81] and amikacin[38] may be useful for improving outcomes for patients with VAP.

ACUTE RESPIRATORY FAILURE RESULTING FROM PULMONARY EMBOLISM

Definition and Classification

An embolus is a clot or plug of material that travels from one blood vessel to another, smaller vessel. The clot lodges in the smaller vessel and obstructs blood flow. When an embolus lodges in the pulmonary vasculature, it is called a pulmonary embolism (PE). The embolus may be a clot that has broken off from a deep vein thrombosis (DVT), a globule of fat from a long bone fracture, septic vegetation, or an iatrogenic catheter fragment. In pregnancy, amniotic fluid can be the cause of a PE. Most PEs originate from DVT of the lower extremities.[63,64] PE and DVT are the two components of the disease process known as venous thromboembolism (VTE).

Prognosis for individuals depends on the size of the PE, prompt diagnosis and treatment, and underlying disease. A *massive* PE manifests as systolic hypotension (<90 mm Hg), and the associated mortality rate is 30% to 80%. A *nonmassive* PE manifests with a systolic BP of at least 90 mm Hg and results in a 5% mortality. This is the most commonly occurring PE.[63]

Etiology

The three main mechanisms that favor the development of VTE, often referred to as Virchow's triad, are (1) venous stasis, (2) hypercoagulability of blood, and (3) damage to the vessel walls. Specific risk factors for VTE are listed in Box 15.7.

PE is present in approximately 40% of patients who have DVT, but it goes undetected in many cases because approximately half of these patients present no signs or symptoms. Approximately 200,000 individuals develop DVT each year, 50,000 of which are complicated by PE. DVT is the underlying cause for 90% of PE, causing approximately 25,000 deaths per year.[64] After sudden cardiac death, massive PE is the second leading cause of mortality.[63] Critically ill patients are at high risk for VTE, and DVT prophylaxis is considered a standard of care for these patients.

Pathophysiology

The pulmonary circulation has an enormous capacity to compensate for a PE. This compensatory mechanism results from the lung vasculature that is necessary to accommodate

---

BOX 15.7 Risk Factors for Venous Thromboembolism

Hereditary
- Antithrombin deficiency
- Factor V Leiden
- Protein C deficiency
- Protein S deficiency
- Prothrombin mutations

Acquired
- Acute infectious disease
- Acute myocardial infarction
- Age greater than 75 years
- Burns
- Cancer
- Heart failure
- Heparin-induced thrombocytopenia
- History of previous venous thromboembolism
- Immobility for longer than 3 days
- IV drug abuse
- Lower extremity fractures
- Major surgery in previous 4 weeks
- Multiple trauma
- Nephrotic syndrome
- Oral contraceptives
- Plane or car trip longer than 4 hours in previous 4 weeks
- Pregnancy/postpartum period
- Sepsis
- Spinal cord injury
- Stroke
- Systemic lupus erythematosus (SLE)
- Ulcerative colitis

increased blood flow during exercise, and it is the reason many patients do not initially decompensate from a massive PE. An embolus that lodges in the pulmonary vasculature completely or partially occludes a pulmonary artery or one of its branches, impeding the forward flow of blood. Blood flow to the alveoli beyond the occlusion is eliminated,[12] which results in pulmonary infarction in approximately 10% of patients.[63] The result is a lack of perfusion to ventilated alveoli, an increase in dead space, a $\dot{V}/\dot{Q}$ mismatch, and a decrease in CO_2 tension in the embolized lung zone. Gas exchange cannot occur (see Fig. 15.1).[12]

Reaction to the mechanical obstruction causes the release of a number of inflammatory mediators such as prostaglandins, serotonin, and histamine. The ensuing inflammation causes constriction of bronchi and widespread vasoconstriction, resulting in poor pulmonary perfusion and increased dead space. The lack of blood flow to the lung also contributes to inadequate production of surfactant, resulting in atelectasis, which contributes further to hypoxemia. Pulmonary artery constriction leads to increased right ventricular afterload and may eventually cause right ventricular failure.[12]

PE remains the third leading cause of in-hospital mortality.[63] Prognosis for the patient with a PE depends on the size of the PE, prior underlying disease, and prompt diagnosis and treatment. An estimated 10% of patients with PE die within the first few hours, and 30% die later as a result of a recurring PE. Mortality is reduced to less than 5% with adequate anticoagulation.

Assessment

Because the presenting signs and symptoms for PE are relatively vague, it is important for the critical care nurse to recognize those who have an increased risk. Classic presentation includes sudden onset of pleuritic chest pain, shortness of breath, and hypoxemia. Suspect a PE in any patient who has respiratory distress that cannot be explained by other diagnosis. Assess for the following physical findings that are present in about half of those with PE: tachypnea, crackles, accentuated S_2, tachycardia, and fever. Less common potential findings include diaphoresis, S_3 or S_4 gallop, evidence of thrombophlebitis, edema of the lower extremities, heart murmur, and cyanosis.[63]

Diagnosis

D-Dimer Assay. D-Dimers are fibrin degradation products or fragments produced during fibrinolysis. A positive test indicates thrombus formation. A positive D-dimer assay also can occur in many other conditions, such as infection, cancer, surgery, pregnancy, heart failure, and kidney failure. Because D-dimer is nonspecific, it is not recommended for use in diagnosing PE but may be safely used to rule out PE in young, healthy individuals; its use is not well established in children.[63]

Ventilation-Perfusion Scan. A $\dot{V}/\dot{Q}$ scan is a noninvasive nuclear medicine procedure that calculates pulmonary airflow and blood flow. A $\dot{V}/\dot{Q}$ scan may detect dead space from impaired perfusion of ventilated alveoli. Results of $\dot{V}/\dot{Q}$ scans are reported as low, medium, or high probability; however, results are not confirmatory. $\dot{V}/\dot{Q}$ scanning may be used if CT scanning is unavailable or contraindicated.[63]

Duplex Ultrasonography (Compression Ultrasound). Duplex ultrasonography is a noninvasive imaging study that is useful in detecting lower-extremity DVT. When evaluating for DVT, the blood flow is assessed as the vessel is compressed. It has a high sensitivity and specificity for DVT in the leg above the knee, but it is not accurate in detecting DVT in pelvic vessels or small vessels in the calf.[63]

High-Resolution Multidetector Computed Tomography Angiography. High-resolution multidetector CT angiography (MDCTA), also called spiral CT, is the preferred tool for detecting a PE. It is highly accurate for direct visualization of large emboli in the main and lobar pulmonary arteries. MDCTA does not always visualize small emboli in distal vessels, but a pulmonary angiogram has the same limitation.[63]

Pulmonary Angiography. Pulmonary angiography provides direct anatomical visualization of the pulmonary vasculature and provides close to 100% certainty of an obstruction when performed correctly, but it is an invasive procedure and difficult to perform. For these reasons, this diagnostic procedure is recommended only if CT scanning is unavailable. MDCTA is now replacing pulmonary angiography as the standard of care because it is noninvasive, cheaper, widely available, and has a high level of sensitivity and specificity.[63]

> ### ❓ CRITICAL REASONING ACTIVITY
>
> Mr. C., age 27 years, was hospitalized 3 days ago after fracturing his femur in a snow-skiing accident. He has just been admitted to the critical care unit with a pulmonary embolism (PE) and is orally intubated and receiving mechanical ventilation. What actions would you take to decrease Mr. C.'s risk of developing ventilator-associated pneumonia (VAP)?

Prevention

The best therapy for VTE and subsequent PE is prevention with thorough nursing assessment and identification of critically ill patients who are at risk followed by nursing interventions to decrease the occurrence of VTE and PE. Box 15.8 outlines some nursing interventions to prevent VTE.

Treatment

Current recommendations from the American College of Chest Physicians permit at-home treatment or early discharge treatment for low-risk PE patients such as nonpregnant adults with suspected PE, pregnant women with suspected PE, and adult cancer patients with suspected PE.[47] For hospitalized critically ill patients, anticoagulation therapy with heparin begins immediately for the initial management of acute PE with low-molecular-weight heparin (LMWH) or IV unfractionated heparin (UFH). For VTE prevention, LMWH or UFH is recommended, without mechanical prophylaxis. If pharmacological prophylaxis is contraindicated, pneumatic compression devices or graduated compression stockings are recommended for VTE prophylaxis.[71] An oral anticoagulant, such as warfarin, is started at the time of PE diagnosis and continued for at least 3 months. Direct thrombin inhibitors

BOX 15.8 Nursing Measures to Prevent Venous Thromboembolism

1. Assess patient on admission to unit for risk for VTE and anticipate prophylaxis orders.
2. Review daily with healthcare team:
   - Current VTE risk factors
   - Necessity for central venous catheter
   - Current VTE prophylaxis
   - Risk for bleeding
   - Response to treatment
3. Implement prescribed prophylactic regimen:
   - Pharmacological prophylaxis
     - *Recommend* UFH or LMWH
     - *Suggest* LMWH or fondaparinux over UFH
     - *Suggested* over mechanical prophylaxis
   - Nonpharmacological (mechanical) prophylaxis for patients not receiving pharmacological prophylaxis
     - *Suggests* intermittent pneumatic compression device or graduated compression stockings
     - *Suggests* pharmacological *or* mechanical VTE prophylaxis alone over mechanical combined with pharmacological
4. Document implementation, tolerance, and complications of prophylaxis.
5. Assess extremities on a regular basis:
   - Pain or tenderness
   - Unilateral edema
   - Erythema
   - Warmth
6. Implement a mobility program.
7. Monitor for low-grade fever.
8. Encourage fluids to prevent dehydration:
   - Administer IV fluids as prescribed; maintain accurate intake and output records.
9. Avoid adjusting the knee section of the bed or using pillows under knees.
10. Provide patient education regarding prevention.

LMWH, Low-molecular-weight heparin; *UFH,* unfractionated heparin; *VTE,* venous thromboembolism.

such as dabigatran or factor Xa inhibitors such as apixaban may be used as an alternative to warfarin for prophylaxis and treatment of PE. LMWH or UFH is continued until international normalized ratio (INR) levels remain at 2.0 for 24 hours but is not discontinued sooner than 5 days after initiation of therapy.[63] Anticoagulants work with the body's inherent fibrinolytic system to prevent further clotting and relieve the thromboembolic burden.

Use of thrombolytic medication is based on severity of the PE, risk of bleeding, and prognosis. Thrombolytic therapy is indicated for the treatment of acute PE accompanied by hypotension (systolic BP <90 mm Hg) in the absence of a high risk for bleeding. It may also be considered for those patients receiving anticoagulation who are at risk of developing hypotension and have a low risk of bleeding. Because of increased risk for major bleeding and lack of demonstration of sustained benefits of reducing mortality when compared to anticoagulation therapy alone, thrombolysis is not recommended for most patients.[3,63]

While the patient is on anticoagulant therapy, regularly monitor the laboratory values and assess the patient for any signs or symptoms of bleeding or heparin-induced thrombocytopenia (HIT). HIT is a complication of LMWH and UFH. It is caused by antibodies that activate platelets, leading to thrombocytopenia. HIT syndrome, sometimes referred to as heparin-induced thrombocytopenia and thrombosis (HITT), results in thromboembolism such as DVT or PE. To detect this problem, observe the patient for decreasing platelet count, skin lesions at the injection site, and systemic reactions such as fever and chills. The presence of HIT dictates discontinuation of heparin products. Direct thrombin inhibitors such as lepirudin, argatroban, or danaparoid are alternatives for patients who have developed or have a history of HIT.[63]

Surgical embolectomy or catheter embolectomy involves manual removal of the thrombus from the pulmonary artery; it is an option for adult patients with massive PE and those who have contraindications for fibrinolytic therapy or do not respond favorably to those medications. Vena cava filters may be placed in the inferior vena cava to prevent recurrence of PE by capturing clots that are migrating from the lower extremities. Both permanent filters and temporary retrievable filters are available. Permanent vena cava filters are rarely used and have many associated complications. Temporary retrievable vena cava filters are used to prevent PE in patients who have contraindications for anticoagulation therapy, major bleeding during anticoagulation therapy, or recurring PE. These devices can be removed by a minimally invasive technique under fluoroscopy. The routine use of these filters is not recommended, as serious complications can occur.[10,63]

Other treatments focus on maintaining the airway, breathing, and circulation. Supplemental O_2 may be administered to maintain SpO_2 at greater than 90%. If the location of the PE is known, positioning the patient with the "good" lung in the dependent position is warranted. Analgesics are given to alleviate pain and anxiety. If the patient is hemodynamically unstable, inotropic or vasopressor support may be required.

STUDY BREAK

5. Patients at risk for the development of deep vein thrombosis (DVT) may include:
   A. Those older than 75 years
   B. Those who are immobile for longer than 3 days
   C. Pregnant women
   D. Patients with burn injury
   E. All the above

ACUTE RESPIRATORY FAILURE IN ADULT PATIENTS WITH CYSTIC FIBROSIS

Definition

Cystic fibrosis (CF) is a genetic disorder (see Genetics box) that results from defective chloride ion transport, which leads to the formation of thick mucus. The thick, sticky mucus obstructs glands of the lungs, pancreas, liver, salivary glands, and testes, causing organ dysfunction. Although CF is a multisystem disease, it has its greatest effect on the lungs, with respiratory failure being the primary cause of death. The thick mucus narrows the airways and reduces airflow. The constant presence of thick mucus provides an excellent breeding ground for bacteria, leading to chronic lower respiratory tract bacterial infections. The mucus-producing cells in the lungs increase in number and size over time, resulting in mucus plugging. Respiratory complications of CF include pneumothorax, arterial erosion, hemorrhage, chronic bacterial infection, and respiratory failure.[13,21] Respiratory or cardiorespiratory events cause the greatest number of deaths.[22]

Etiology

CF affects primarily whites but is occasionally seen in other races. For many years, CF was considered a disease of children. Because of significant improvements in care, currently more than half of those with CF are adults with a median age of 19.3 years. The median predicted survival of those born in 2017 was 46.2 years, meaning that half of these persons will live to that age. This is up from the median predicted survival of 43.6 years for those born between 2013 and 2017. Survival of CF individuals has steadily increased over the past 3 decades.[22]

Most children now undergo newborn screening for CF, so the diagnosis is typically made early in life (75% by age 2 years), but a few patients are diagnosed as adults. Diagnostic testing is a multiple-step process that includes sweat chloride test (gold standard), a genetic or carrier test, and clinical evaluation at a center accredited by the Cystic Fibrosis Foundation. Sweat test levels of 60 mmol/L or greater indicate that CF is likely. Levels between 30 and 59 mmol/L indicate that additional testing is in order. Being tested as a carrier is a personal preference, but the American College of Obstetricians and Gynecologists suggests that anyone considering having a child be offered the testing opportunity.[21]

Assessment

Individuals with CF may experience a variety of symptoms, including salty-tasting skin, persistent cough (productive at times), frequent lung infections, wheezing, shortness of breath, poor growth despite eating well, fatty bulky stools, difficulty eliminating, and infertility in males. Assessment of respiratory status, nutritional status, and elimination are routine.

Interventions

Because CF is a complicated and chronic disease, outcomes are best when CF patients are cared for by experts in an environment in which efforts are comprehensive and coordinated in partnership with CF care teams. Respiratory failure is the cause of death for 63% of patients with CF.[22] As the disease process progresses, patients develop increased ventilator requirements, air trapping, and respiratory muscle weakness. All of these conditions are complicated by chronic bacterial infections that can quickly become overwhelming. In the past, mechanical ventilation was not considered a treatment option because patient outcomes were poor. During the past 20 years, the standard of care for ARF in CF has been revisited because of improved ventilator modalities, more aggressive pharmacological therapy, and the option of lung transplantation. Lung transplantation provides the opportunity for a tremendous improvement in the quality of life, but acute exacerbations of respiratory failure must be overcome during the wait for a transplant (see Transplant Considerations box).

🧬 GENETICS

Cystic Fibrosis

Cystic fibrosis (CF) is an autosomal recessive disease, meaning that both parents must be carriers of a variant gene. As with all autosomal recessive conditions, each child of two-parent carriers has a 25% chance of being born with two variant genes (i.e., homozygous).[5] The disease is most common among whites of northern European descent, Latinos, and Pueblo and Zuni American natives. Newborn screening for CF occurs in all 50 US states and uses a combination of a biochemical marker and genetic assays.

A defect in the chloride ion channel from a mutation in the cystic fibrosis transmembrane conductance regulator (CFTR) gene results in CF. Note that all genes are conventionally identified in italics, so the gene that codes the CFTR channel is identified as *CFTR*. The *CFTR* codes a variety of proteins used to build chloride channels across a cell membrane. There are more than 2000 polymorphisms in this gene, but not all variations result in symptomatic CF.[6] To illustrate, one genetic variation prevents the CFTR protein from folding properly so that the chloride channel does not reach the cell surface. A different genetic polymorphism, less common and associated with less severe symptoms, results in a functional pump but a "sticky" gate slowing chloride entry into the channel.

The defects in transporting chloride into and out of cells—CFTR dysfunction—results in thick mucus that is difficult to clear. This mucus interferes with normal organ function, particularly in lungs, the gastrointestinal (GI) tract, and pancreas. Thick mucus production in the lungs interferes with gas exchange, leading to chronic hypoxemia. Lung disease from CF can lead to chronic respiratory insufficiency that results in morbidity and erodes quality of life. Mucus production in the GI tract blocks intestinal fluids, causing GI obstruction and impaired absorption of nutrients. Thick mucus is more likely to colonize microorganisms, contributing to infection and inflammation with subsequent adverse and irreversible changes in these organs. Dysfunction of the CFTR channel results in thick pancreatic mucus that blocks the ducts and prevents digestive enzymes from reaching the small intestine. This results in reduced ability to absorb nutrients in many patients with a diagnosis of CF. Signs and symptoms are typically seen when CFTR function is less than 10%.[8] Patients with the most severe symptoms have less than 1% CFTR activity and manifest the full spectrum of disease involvement, including pancreatic insufficiency; recurrent, severe pulmonary infections; GI obstruction; and congenital absence of the vas deferens.[8] Improved care focuses on nutritional strategies, use of devices to assist clearance of respiratory mucus, prevention of infection, and implementation of rapidly emerging therapies to restore chloride transport affect the pathobiology of CF.

New medications target the defective chloride channel as CFTR modulators that stabilize the protein fold of the dysfunctional channel, facilitate protein maturation to repair the chloride channel, and move the channel to the surface of the cellular membrane.[4] Treatment has expanded from a single medication targeting one rare CF mutation to using combinations of medications, ultimately improving or even restoring CFTR function in different genetic mutations.[7]

Continued

GENETICS—cont'd

Cystic Fibrosis

People with one copy of the CFTR mutation are heterozygous carriers. Because more than 10 million individuals in the United States are estimated to have a single gene for CF, genetic testing for all couples who are at high risk for carrier status because of their ethnicity or family history is recommended.[3] Initially, testing is performed on one future parent; if that person is a carrier, the other future parent is tested to calculate the risk that the children of those two parents will have CF. It is not possible to test for all variations of the *CFTR* in a single genetic test; testing typically identifies 90 common mutations.[3] Therefore a negative screen does not guarantee that an individual is not a carrier or does not have a *CFTR* mutation that causes CF symptoms. The clinician individualizes advice to people seeking CF genetic testing. Manifestations of CF can be mild, and not all potential parents perceive the diagnosis of CF as a serious disorder. The clinician also individualizes interventions to manage CF based on genotype. For example, some medications to correct the CFTR channel defect are not useful in all cystic fibrosis genotypes. Not all patients will have severe pulmonary or pancreatic symptoms and need intensive therapy. The Cystic Fibrosis Foundation has links to information and support groups for families in which CF is a potential or actual condition.[2] A referral to a genetic counselor can occur before genetic testing to educate patients and families about risk and the nuances around CF as an inheritable condition. Genetic counselors can also facilitate testing and interpretation and help integrate genetic information into treatment options.[1]

Genetic terms: *single gene trait, autosomal recessive, genetic testing, carrier, homozygous, heterozygous, genetic counseling*

References

1. Braverman G, Shapiro ZE, Bernstein JA. Ethical issues in contemporary clinical genetics. *Mayo Clin Proc Innov Qual Outcomes.* 2018;2(2):81–90.
2. Foundation for Cystic Fibrosis. *Carrier Testing for Cystic Fibrosis.* https://www.cff.org/What-is-CF/Testing/Carrier-Testing-for-Cystic-Fibrosis/. Accessed February 12, 2019.
3. Gregg AR. Expanded carrier screening. *Obstet Gynecol Clin North Am.* 2018;45(1):103–112.
4. Harutyunyan M, Huang Y, Mun KS, et al. Personalized medicine in CF: From modulator development to therapy for cystic fibrosis patients with rare CFTR mutations. *Am J Physiol Lung Cell Mol Physiol.* 2018;314(4):L529–L543.
5. Jorde LB. Genes and genetic disease. In: McCance S, Huether K, eds. *Pathophysiology.* 8th ed. Philadelphia, PA: Elsevier; 2019.
6. Katkin JP. Cystic Fibrosis. *UpToDate.* http://www.uptodate.com/contents/cystic-fibrosis-clinical-manifestations-and-diagnosis. Published November 1, 2018. Accessed February 19, 2019.
7. Kym PR, Wang X, Pizzonero M, Van der Plas SE. Recent progress in the discovery and development of small-molecule modulators of CFTR. *Prog Med Chem.* 2018;57(1):235–276.
8. Rowe SM, Hoover W, Slomon GM, et al. Cystic fibrosis. In: Broaddus VC, Mason RJ, Ernst JD, et al., eds. *Murray and Nadel's Textbook of Respiratory Medicine.* Philadelphia, PA: Elsevier; 2015:822–852.

The goals of care for a patient with CF focus on nutrition and fitness, airway clearance, antibiotic therapy, and CFTR modulator therapies.[29] For those suffering an exacerbation that requires admission to a critical care unit, a multidisciplinary approach includes a PT who specializes in CF to evaluate airway clearance and adjust regimens as appropriate, a dietitian to evaluate caloric needs and any needed adjustments in nutritional requirements, and a pharmacist as well as an infectious disease specialist to evaluate antibiotic selection.[15]

Antibiotic Therapy. Antibiotic selection is based on the patient's most recent sputum bacterial isolates. *Pseudomonas aeruginosa* is the most common pathogen found in adult patients with CF. Guidelines developed by the European Cystic Fibrosis Society recommend a combination of two or more IV antibiotics for 14 days for *P. aeruginosa,* with reevaluation of lung function at that time to determine whether further treatment is needed. In general, an exacerbation requires antibiotics that may be given orally, by inhalation, and/or intravenously.[15] Chronic infection with MRSA is associated with worsening pulmonary function and is therefore currently under investigation for appropriate treatment. In the meantime, rifampin is the recommended medication if tolerated by the patient.[73]

Airway Clearance. Mucolytic agents are routinely administered to facilitate clearance of mucus. Recombinant human DNase (Pulmozyme) is the drug of choice.[15] It decreases the viscosity of sputum by catalyzing extracellular DNA into smaller fragments. Chest physiotherapy is used to increase airway clearance and should be based on individual preference, as little evidence supports the use of one or the other.[18] Hydrators, such as hypertonic saline (7%), which increase airway surface liquid, have been shown to improve lung function and decrease exacerbations. Mannitol is also a hydrator that shows promise. Because both hydrators act as irritants, they require pretreatment with a bronchodilator to improve tolerance.[18] Bronchodilators are routinely prescribed and administered before chest physiotherapy as well to increase airway clearance. Other techniques recommended to facilitate airway clearance include percussion and postural drainage, positive expiratory pressure (PEP) devices, active cycle of breathing technique, autogenic drainage, oscillatory PEP devices, high-frequency chest compression devices, and exercise.[21] A new drug for CF was recently approved (Box 15.9).

BOX 15.9 Applying Genetics in Pharmacologic Management of Cystic Fibrosis

- Trikafta was recently approved to treat CF
- It is a combination of three drugs that target the defective CFTR gene
- Trikafta helps the protein made by the CFTR gene mutation to function more effectively
- Trikafta treats the mutation that affects 90% of the population with CF
- Trikafta increased the percent predicted forced expiratory volume in one second, (FEV1) in clinical trials

Nutritional Support. Enteral nutrition with high caloric content and pancreatic enzyme supplements, if needed, is started early in the course of treatment. Dietary supplements of salt may be required with perfuse diaphoresis, as well as fat-soluble vitamins. Antioxidants and vitamin D supplementation are also needed in some patients. Insulin may be required to manage cystic fibrosis–related diabetes (CFRD).[21, 62]

Cystic Fibrosis Transmembrane Conductance Regulator Modulators. These medications are designed to target the underlying cause of CF by correcting the malfunctioning protein made by the *CFTR* gene. Ivacaftor (Kalydeco), lumacaftor/ivacaftor (Orkambi), and tezacaftor/ivacaftor (Symdeko) are approved for use in people with CF who are have specific CF mutations. Individuals who are homozygous (i.e., have two copies) or heterozygous (i.e., have one copy) for specific CFTR variants experience reduced symptoms from CF after administration of these drugs, which bind directly to certain formations of defective chloride channels, improving function by opening the gate to allow transport of chloride. Ivacaftor is the first CF drug that treats the underlying pathology of CF rather than symptoms. Clinical trials are underway and currently showing promising results for next-generation triple-combination modulators that have the potential to address the underlying cause of CF for more than 90% of individuals who suffer from this disease.[21]

Ventilatory Support. If ventilator support is necessary, noninvasive mechanical ventilation is the first line of therapy. Endotracheal intubation with mechanical ventilation is the next step. The goal of mechanical ventilation is the same as for any patient with ARF. Adult patients with CF are at high risk for pneumothorax and massive hemoptysis.[13] The critical care nurse must be aware of these life-threatening complications, constantly monitor for them, and respond quickly.

 TRANSPLANT CONSIDERATIONS

Lung Transplantation

Criteria for Transplant Recipients
Criteria for placement on the waiting list for lung transplantation include a life expectancy of less than 24 to 36 months, significant effect of the lung disease on other organ systems, and the effects of the disease process on quality of life. Time on the waitlist is also considered. Multiple data are evaluated to determine priority status for transplant: (1) waiting list survival probability during the next year, (2) waitlist urgency measure, (3) survival probability during the first posttransplant year, (4) posttransplant survival measure, and (5) raw allocation score, which is used to calculate a normalized score weighing probability of survival and anticipated benefit.[3] Contraindications for lung transplantation include current steroid use of more than 20 mg daily, significant coronary artery disease, cachexia or obesity, active alcohol or drug abuse, cigarette smoking, active infection, previous cardiothoracic surgery, ventilation dependency, and hepatitis B virus antigen positive.[1,4]

Patient Management
Antirejection medications are needed after organ transplantation. Maintenance therapy consists of medications that inhibit T-cell proliferation and differentiation, deplete lymphocytes, and inhibit macrophages. Immunosuppressive medications consist of triple therapy: a calcineurin inhibitor (tacrolimus [Prograf] or cyclosporine [Neoral]), a corticosteroid (prednisone), and mycophenolate mofetil (CellCept). Complications associated with immunosuppressive therapy include nephrotoxicity, hypertension, hyperlipidemia, bone loss, new-onset diabetes mellitus, and infection.[2]

Complications
Primary graft dysfunction is a major cause of morbidity and mortality and is comparable to acute respiratory distress syndrome. Patients present with malaise, increased work of breathing, activity intolerance, and oxygen desaturation. Management includes supplemental oxygen, positive-pressure ventilation, and aggressive pulmonary hygiene. Mechanical ventilation, nitric oxide inhalation, or extracorporeal membrane oxygenation may be indicated. Large-airway and vascular anastomosis complications may occur, potentially requiring reanastomoses or stenting if granulomatous tissue threatens airway obstruction. Urgent relisting for lung transplantation may be required.[3,4]

Infection is one of the major complications after transplantation. The lung is the most common site and is the leading cause of death. Bacterial and fungal infections occur most frequently in the first months; viral infections, especially cytomegalovirus, are more prevalent in the months after transplantation. Other complications include inadequate bronchial anastomosis, pneumothorax, pleural effusions, and gastroesophageal reflux disease (GERD).

Preventing Rejection
Compliance with immunosuppressive medication is essential to avoid or decrease the incidence of rejection episodes. *Hyperacute rejection* occurs within minutes or hours of transplantation and is caused by humoral or antibody-mediated B-cell production against the transplanted organ.[2] It may present as acute desaturation and tissue hypoxia or by radiographic changes. *Acute* or *cellular-mediated rejection* usually occurs within the first 12 weeks after transplant. Symptoms include fatigue, dyspnea, fever, hypoxemia, pulmonary infiltrates, or pleural effusions. To differentiate rejection from infection, a biopsy may be indicated. Management includes high-dose corticosteroids and optimizing maintenance immunosuppression.

Recurrent acute rejection has been associated with the development of *chronic rejection* or obliterative bronchiolitis (OB) in which inflammation and fibrosis of small airways occur. More than 40% of lung transplant recipients develop OB by 5 years after transplant.[2] Symptoms include progressive shortness of breath, decreased exercise tolerance, airflow limitation, and progressive decline in pulmonary function. Management is individualized and includes aggressively managing acute rejection and infection and optimizing the immunosuppression regimen.[2,4]

References
1. Bittle GJ, Sanchez PG, Kon ZN, et al. The use of lung donors older than 55 years: A review of the United Network of Organ Sharing database. *J Heart Lung Transplant.* 2013;32(8): 760–768.
2. Costa J, Benvenuto LJ, Sonnett JR, et al. Long-term outcomes and management of lung transplant recipients. *Best Pract Res Clin Anaesthesiol.* 2017;31(2):285–297.
3. Organ Procurement and Transplantation Network. LAS Calculator. https://optn.transplant. hrsa.gov/resources/allocation-calculators/las-calculator. Accessed December 28, 2018.
4. Snell GI, Levvey BJ, Westall GP. The changing landscape of lung donation for transplantation. *Am J Transplant.* 2015;15:859–860.

CASE STUDY

Mrs. P. is a 57-year-old woman who was admitted to the critical care unit after a motor vehicle crash. She sustained multiple long bone fractures and a chest contusion and experienced an episode of hypotension in the emergency department. She received 3 units of red blood cells and 2 L of IV fluid in the emergency department. Within 12 hours, she became short of breath, with an increase in respiratory rate requiring high levels of supplemental oxygen. She was electively intubated and placed on volume-control mechanical ventilation with a positive end-expiratory pressure (PEEP) of 5 cm H_2O. Continuous IV analgesia and sedation infusions were started. The decision was made to titrate the infusion to keep her calm and comfortable. During the next 8 hours, her oxygen saturation (SpO_2) steadily deteriorated, and the high-pressure alarms on the ventilator activated frequently. The nurse noted steadily rising peak airway pressures. The fraction of inspired oxygen (FiO_2) had to be increased to 0.80 and the PEEP increased to 14 cm H_2O to maintain her partial pressure of arterial oxygen (PaO_2) at 60 mm Hg. Her chest radiograph showed bilateral infiltrates with normal heart size. The sedation infusion required frequent upward titrations to maintain the desired goal of light sedation. The diagnosis of acute respiratory distress syndrome (ARDS) was made.

During the next 6 hours, Mrs. P. steadily became more hypoxemic. She was changed to pressure-controlled ventilation with a PEEP of 20 cm H_2O. The FiO_2 had to be increased to 1.0 (100%) to maintain a PaO_2 greater than 60 mm Hg. She was extremely restless, with tachycardia, diaphoresis, and a labile arterial oxygen saturation (SaO_2). The decision was made to start a neuromuscular blocking agent with continuous analgesia and sedation. During the next few hours her general condition continued to deteriorate. Her SaO_2 ranged from 85% to 87%. Her chest radiographic findings were worse and revealed a complete whiteout. The nurses and physicians decided to turn her to the prone position in an effort

to improve oxygenation. An hour after she was turned to the prone position, her SpO_2 began to slowly rise. After 2 hours in the prone position, her SpO_2 stabilized at 93%. Slowly, the FiO_2 was decreased to 0.60, with a stable SpO_2 of 92%. After 18 hours, she was returned to the supine position. Her SpO_2 decreased to 90% and remained stable. She was weaned off the neuromuscular blocking agent, and the sedation level was reduced to reach a goal of feeling calm and comfortable.

Mrs. P. slowly improved over the next week. Her ventilator settings were changed from pressure-control to assist-control, and then to pressure support. The PEEP was decreased to a physiological level. The sedation was interrupted on a daily basis for weaning parameters and spontaneous breathing trials. She was extubated on the seventh day, and the next day she was transferred to the general orthopedic nursing unit on 4 L of oxygen per nasal cannula.

Questions

1. Identify the risk factors Mrs. P. had for ARDS.
2. The American-European Consensus Conference recommended three criteria for diagnosing ARDS in the presence of a risk factor. List these criteria.
3. Explain the use of the high PEEP level and the nursing monitoring responsibilities.
4. Explain the rationale for the use of analgesia, sedation, and neuromuscular blocking agents and what nursing interventions should occur when these agents are used.
5. Explain the rationale for treating patients with moderate to severe ARDS with mechanical ventilation and prone positioning, and identify nursing interventions to reduce complications associated with proning.

REFERENCES

1. Abrams D, Brodie D. Extracorporeal membrane oxygenation is first-line therapy for acute respiratory distress syndrome. *Crit Care Med.* 2017;45(12):2070–2076.
2. Aggarwal NR, Brower RG, Hager, DN, et al. Oxygen exposure resulting in arterial oxygen tensions above protocol goal was associated with worse clinical outcomes in acute respiratory distress syndrome. *Crit Care Med.* 2018;48(4):517–524.
3. Aggarwal V, Nicolais CD, Lee A, et al. Acute Management of Pulmonary Embolism—American College of Cardiology. https://www.acc.org/latest-in cardiology/articles/2017/10/23/12/12/acute-management-of-pulmonary-embolism. Published 2017.
4. Alvarez-Lerma F, Palomar-Martinez M, Sanchez-Garcia M, et al. Prevention of ventilator associated pneumonia: The multimodal approach of the Spanish ICU "pneumonia zero" program. *Crit Care Med.* 2018;46(2):181–189.
5. American Thoracic Society, Infectious Diseases Society of America. Guidelines for the management of adults with hospital-acquired, ventilator-associated, and healthcare-associated pneumonia. *Am J Respir Crit Care Med.* 2005;171:388–416.
6. Annane D, Pastores SM, Arlt W, et al. Critical illness–related corticosteroid insufficiency (CIRCI): A narrative review from a multi-specialty task force of the Society of Critical Care Medicine (SCCM) and the European Society of Intensive Care Medicine (ESICM). *Crit Care Med.* 2017;45(12):2089–2098.
7. Bellani G, Laffey JG, Pham T, et al; LUNG SAFE Investigators; ESICM Trial Group. Noninvasive ventilation of patients with acute respiratory distress syndrome: Insights from the LUNG SAFE study. *Am J Respir Crit Care Med.* 2017;195:67–77.
8. Bhavani MR, Sushm J, Prathyusha M, et al. Effectiveness of noninvasive positive pressure ventilation for acute exacerbation of chronic obstructive pulmonary disease. *IJCT.* 2018;5(2):102–106.
9. Bienvenu OJ, Colantuoni E, Mendez-Tellez PA, et al. Cooccurrence of and remission from general anxiety, depression, and posttraumatic stress disorder symptoms after acute lung injury: A two-year longitudinal study. *Crit Care Med.* 2015;43(3):642–652.
10. Bikdeli B, Wang Y, Jimenez D, et al. Association of inferior vena cava filter use with mortalitiy rates in older adults with acute pulmonary embolism. *JAMA Intern Med.* 2019;179(2):263–265.
11. Borkowska M, Labeau S, Schepens T, et al. Nurses' sedation practices during weaning of adults from mechanical ventilation in an intensive care unit. *AJCC.* 2018;27(1):32–42.
12. Brasher VL, Huether SE. Alterations of pulmonary function. In: McCance KL, Huether SE, eds. *Pathophysiology: The Biologic Basis for Disease in Adults and Children.* 8th ed. St. Louis, MO: Elsevier; 2019:1176–1190.
13. Brasher VL, Huether SE. Alterations of pulmonary function in children. In: McCance KL, Huether SE, eds. *Pathophysiology: The Biologic Basis for Disease in Adults and Children.* 8th ed. St. Louis, MO: Elsevier; 2019:1220–1222.
14. Brashers VL. Structure and function of the pulmonary system. In: McCance KL, Huether SE, eds. *Pathophysiology: The Biologic Basis for Disease in Adults and Children.* 8th ed. St. Louis, MO: Elsevier; 2019:1143–1158.
15. Castellani C, Duff AJA, Bell SC, et al. ECFS best practice guidelines: The 2018 revision. *J Cystic Fibro.* 2018;17:153–178.
16. Centers for Disease Control and Prevention. Device-Associated Module PNEU. http://www.cdc.gov/nhsn/PDFs/pscManual/6pscVAPcurrent.pdf. Published January 2019. Accessed March 5, 2019.
17. Centers for Disease Control and Prevention. Device-Associated Module VAE. http://www.cdc.gov/nhsn/PDFs/pscManual/10-VAE_FINAL.pdf. Published January 2019. Accessed March 5, 2019.

18. Centers for Disease Control and Prevention. Pneumonia Can Be Prevented—Vaccines Can Help. https://www.cdc.gov/pneumonia/prevention.html. Published October 18, 2018. Accessed March 4, 2019.

19. Centers for Disease Control and Prevention. Prevent Seasonal Flu: Who Should Get Vaccinated This Season? https://www.cdc.gov/flu/consumer/vaccinations.htm. Updated August 31, 2018. Accessed March 4, 2019.

20. Cochi SH, Kempker JA, Annangi S, et al. Mortality trends of acute respiratory distress syndrome in the United States from 1999–2013. *Ann Am Thorac Soc.* 2016;13(10):1742–1751.

21. Cystic Fibrosis Foundation. About Cystic Fibrosis. https://www.cff.org/What-is-CF/About-Cystic-Fibrosis/. Accessed March 6, 2019.

22. Cystic Fibrosis Foundation. Patient Registry: Annual Date Report. https://www.cff.org/Research/Researcher-Resources/Patient-Registry/2017-Patient-Registry-Annual-Data-Report.pdf. Published 2017. Accessed March 6, 2019.

23. Delorme M, Bouchard PA, Simon M, et al. Effects of high-flow nasal cannula on the work of breathing in patients recovering from acute respiratory failure. *Crit Care Med.* 2017;45(12):1981–1988.

24. Devlin JW, Yoanna S, Celine G. et al. Clinical practice guidelines for the prevention and management of pain, agitation/sedation, delirium, immobility, and sleep disruption in adult patients in the ICU. *Crit Care Med.* 2018;46(9):1–45.

25. Dinglas VD, Friedman LA, Colantuoni E, et al. Muscle weakness and 5-year survival in acute respiratory distress syndrome survivors. *Crit Care Med.* 2017;45(3):446–453.

26. Eakin MN, Patel Y, Mendez-Tellez P. et al. Patients' outcomes after acute respiratory failure: A qualitative study with the PROMIS framework. *AJCC.* 2017;26(6):456–465.

27. Fan E, Del Sorbo L, Goligher EC, et al. An official American Thoracic Society/European Society of Intensive Care Medicine/Society of Critical Care Medicine Clinical Practice Guideline: Mechanical ventilation in adult patients with acute respiratory distress syndrome. *Am J Respir Crit Care Med.* 2017;195(9):1253–1263.

28. Festic E, Carr GE, Cartin-Ceba R, et al. Randomized clinical trial of a combination of an inhaled corticosteroid and beta agonist in patients at risk of developing the acute respiratory distress syndrome. *Crit Care Med.* 2017;45(5):798–805.

29. Flume PA, Robinson KA, O'Sullivan BP, et al; Clinical Practice Guidelines for Pulmonary Therapies Committee. Cystic fibrosis pulmonary guidelines: Airway clearance therapies. *Respir Care.* 2009;54(4):522–537.

30. Frat JP, Ragot S, Coudroy R, et al. Predictors of intubation in patients with acute hypoxemic respiratory failure treated with a noninvasive oxygenation strategy. *Crit Care Med.* 2018;46(2):208–215.

31. Fuller BM, Ferguson IT, Mohr NM, et al. A quasi-experimental, before-after trial examining the impact of an emergency department mechanical ventilator protocol on clinical outcomes and lung-protective ventilation in acute respiratory distress syndrome. *Crit Care Med.* 2017;45(4):645–652.

32. Gadre SK, Duggal A, Mireles-Cabodevila E, et al. Acute respiratory failure requiring mechanical ventilation in severe chronic obstructive pulmonary disease (COPD). *Medicine.* 2018;97(17):1–5.

33. Gerard L, Bidoul T, Castanares-Zapatero D, et al. Open lung biopsy in nonresolving acute respiratory distress syndrome commonly identifies corticosteroid-sensitive pathologies, associated with better outcome. *Crit Care Med.* 2018;46(6):907–914.

34. Global Initiative for Asthma (GINA). Global Strategy for Asthma Management and Prevention. http://www.ginasthma.org/. Published 2018. Accessed February 2, 2019.

35. Global Initiative for Chronic Obstructive Lung Disease (GOLD). Global Strategy for the Diagnosis, Management, and Prevention of Chronic Obstructive Pulmonary Disease. http://www.gold-copd.org/. Published 2019. Accessed February 2, 2019.

36. Grissom CK, Hirshberg EL, Dickerson JB, et al. Fluid management with a simplified conservative protocol for the acute respiratory distress syndrome. *Crit Care Med.* 2015;43(2):288–295.

37. Harman EH, Pinsky MR. Acute Respiratory Distress Syndrome. https://emedicine.medscape.com/article/165139. Updated October 17, 2018. Accessed December 28, 2018.

38. Hassan N, Awdallah F, Abbassi M, et al. Nebulized versus IV amikacin as adjunctive antibiotic for hospital and ventilator-acquired pneumonia postcardiac surgeries: A randomized controlled trial. *Crit Care Med.* 2018;46(1):45–52.

39. Hoffman G, Haan L, Anderson J. Esophageal pressure measurements in patients with acute respiratory distress syndrome. *Crit Care Nurse.* 2016;36(5):27–36.

40. Howe K, Clochesy J, Goldstein L, et al. Mechanical ventilation antioxidant trial. *AJCC.* 2015;24(5):440–445.

41. *How-To Guide: Prevent Ventilator-Associated Pneumonia.* Cambridge, MA: Institute for Healthcare Improvement; 2012. (Available at http://www.ihi.org). Accessed March 6, 2019.

42. Huang M, Parker AM, Bienvenu OJ, et al. Psychiatric symptoms in acute respiratory distress syndrome survivors: A 1-year national multicenter study. *Crit Care Med.* 2016;44(5):954–965.

43. Ike JD, Kempker JA, Kramer MR, et al. The association between acute respiratory distress syndrome hospital case volume and mortality in a US cohort, 2002–2011. *Crit Care Med.* 2018;46(5):764–773.

44. Institute for Healthcare Improvement. Ventilator Associated Pneumonia. http://www.ihi.org/Topics/VAP/Pages/default.aspx. Published 2019. Accessed March 5, 2019.

45. Jolley SE, Moss M, Needham DM, et al. Point prevalence study of mobilization practices for acute respiratory failure patients in the United States. *Crit Care Med.* 2017;45(2):205–215.

46. Kacmarek RM, Villar J, Sulemanji D, et al. Open lung approach for the acute respiratory distress syndrome: A pilot, randomized controlled trial. *Crit Care Med.* 2016;44(1):32–42.

47. Kaiser Permanente. Pulmonary Embolism Diagnosis and Treatment Guideline. https://wa.kaiserpermanente.org/static/pdf/public/guidelines/pulmonary-embolism.pdf. Published 2017. Accessed March 11, 2019.

48. Kalil AC, Metersky ML, Klompas M, et al. Management of adults with hospital-acquired and ventilator-associated pneumonia: 2016 Clinical practice guidelines by the Infectious Diseases Society of America and the American Thoracic Society. *Clin Infect Dis.* 2016;63(5):e61–e111.

49. Kallet RH, Zhuo H, Yip V, et al. Spontaneous breathing trials and conservative sedation practices reduce mechanical ventilation duration in subjects with ARDS. *Resp Care.* 2018;63(1):1–10.

50. Kangelaris KN, Ware LB, Wang CY, et al. Timing of intubation and clinical outcomes in adults with acute respiratory distress syndrome. *Crit Care Med.* 2016;44(1):120–129.

51. Kido T, Muramatsu K, Asakawa T, et al. The relationship between high-dose corticosteroid treatment and mortality in acute respiratory distress syndrome. *BMC Pulm Med.* 2018;18(1);28.

52. Klarin B, Adolfsson A, Torstensson A, et al. Can probiotics be an alternative to chlorhexidine for oral care in the mechanically ventilated patient? A multicenter, prospective, randomized controlled open trial. *Crit Care*. 2018;22(272):1–10.

53. Landell C, Boyer V, Abbas M, et al. Impact of a multifaceted prevention program on ventilator-associated pneumonia including selective oropharyngeal decontamination. *Intens Care Med*. 2018;44:1777–1786.

54. Lari S, Attaran D, Vakillia F, et al. Early effectiveness of noninvasive positive pressure ventilation on right ventricular function in chronic obstructive pulmonary disease subjects with acute hypercapnic respiratory failure. *JCTM*. 2017;5(2):558–563.

55. Magill SS, Li Q, Gross C, et al. Incidence and characteristics of ventilator-associated events reported to the national healthcare safety network in 2014. *Crit Care Med*. 2016;44(12); 2154–2162.

56. Mandell LA, Wunderkink RG, Anzueto A, et al. Infectious Disease Society of America/American Thoracic Society consensus guidelines on the management of community-acquired pneumonia in adults. *Clin Infect Dis*. 2007;44:S27–S72.

57. McClave SA, Taylor BE, Marindale RG, et al. Guidelines for the provision and assessment of nutrition support therapy in the adult critically ill patient: Society of Critical Care Medicine (SCCM) and American Society for Parenteral and Enteral Nutrition (ASPEN). *J Parenter Enteral Nutr*. 2016;40:159–211.

58. Medura GU, Bridges L, Siemienuik RAC, et al. An exploratory reanalysis of the randomized trial on efficacy of corticosteroids as rescue therapy for the late phase of acute respiratory distress syndrome. *Crit Care Med*. 2018;46(6):884–899.

59. Murray MJ, DeBlock H, Erstand B, et al. Clinical practice guidelines for sustained neuromuscular blockade in the adult critically ill patient. *Crit Care Med*. 2016;44(11):2079–2103.

60. Ni YN, Luo J, Yu H, et al. Can body mass index predict clinical outcomes for patients with acute lung injury/acute respiratory distress syndrome? *Crit Care*. 2017;21(1):36.

61. Nigoghossian CD, Dzierba A, Etheridge J, et al. Effect of extracorporeal membrane oxygenation use on sedative requirements in patient with severe acute respiratory distress syndrome. *Pharmacotherapy*. 2016;36(6):607–616.

62. Nutrition in Children and Adults Clinical Care Guidelines. CFF. org. https://www.cff.org/Care/Clinical-Care-Guidelines/Nutrition-and-GI-Clinical-Care-Guidelines/Nutrition-in-Children-and-Adults-Clinical-Care-Guidelines/. Accessed March 9, 2019.

63. Ouellette DR. Pulmonary Embolism. http://emedicine.medscape.com/article/300901. Updated June 21, 2018. Accessed December 28, 2018.

64. Patel K. Deep Venous Thrombosis (DVT). https://jemedicine.medscape.com/article/1911303. Updated July 5, 2017. Accessed December 28, 2018.

65. Patel BK, Wolfe KS, MacKenzie EL, et al. One-year outcomes in patients with acute respiratory distress syndrome enrolled in a randomized clinical trial of helmet versus facemask noninvasive ventilation. *Crit Care Med*. 2018;46(7):1078–1084.

66. Peterson SJ, Lateef OB, Freels S, et al. Early exposure to recommended calorie delivery in the intensive care unit is associated with increased mortality in patients with acute respiratory distress syndrome. *J Parenter Enteral Nutr*. 2018;42(4):739–747.

67. Pileggi C, Mascaro V, Bianco A, et al. Ventilator bundle and its effects on mortality among ICU patients: A meta-analysis. *Crit Care Med*. 2018;46(7):1167–1175.

68. Rawat N, Yang T, Ali K, et al. Two-state collaborative study of a multifaceted intervention to decrease ventilator-associated events. *Crit Care Med*. 2017;45(7):1208–1215.

69. Sahetya S, Brower RG, Stephens S. Survival of patients with severe acute respiratory distress syndrome treated without extracorporeal membrane oxygenation. *AJCC*. 2018;27(3): 220–227.

70. Samanta S, Poddar B, Azim A, et al. Significance of mini bronchoalveolar lavage fluid amylase level in ventilator-associated pneumonia: A prospective observational study. *Crit Care Med*. 2018;46(1):71–78.

71. Schunemann HJ, Cushman M, Burnett AE, et al. American Society of Hematology 2018 guidelines for management of venous thromboembolism: Prophylaxis for hospitalized and nonhospitalized medical patients. *Blood Adv*. 2018;2(22): 3198–3225.

72. Shirai K, Yoshida S, Matsumaru N, et al. Effect of enteral diet enriched with eicosapentaenoic acid, gamma-linolenic acid, and antioxidants in patients with sepsis-induced acute respiratory distress syndrome. *J Intensive Care*. 2015;3(24):1–10.

73. Simon RH. Cystic Fibrosis: Antibiotic Therapy for Chronic Pulmonary Infection. https://www.uptodate.com/contents/cystic-fibrosis-antibiotic-therapy-for-chronic-pulmonary-infection?topicRef=110933. Updated January 30, 2019. Accessed March 8, 2019.

74. Society of Critical Care Medicine. Critical Care Statistics. http://www.sccm.org/Communications/Critical-Care-Statistics. Accessed November 23, 2018.

75. Stefan MS, Pekow, PS, Shieh MS, et al. Hospital volume and outcomes of noninvasive ventilation in patients hospitalized with an acute exacerbation of chronic obstructive pulmonary disease. *Crit Care Med*. 2017;45(1):20–27.

76. Stephens RJ, Dettmer MR, Roberts BW, et al. Practice patterns and outcomes associated with early sedation depth in mechanically ventilated patients: A systematic review and meta-analysis. *Crit Care Med*. 2018;46(3):471–481.

77. Sukhen S, Poddar B, Azim A, et al. Significance of mini bronchoalveolar lavage fluid amylase level in ventilator-associated pneumonia: A prospective observational study. *Crit Care Med*. 2018;46(1):71–78.

78. Tablan OC, Anderson LJ, Besser R, et al. Guidelines for Preventing Health-Care-Associated Pneumonia. https://www.cdc.gov/infectioncontrol/guidelines/pdf/guidelines/healthcare-associated-pneumonia.pdf. Updated October 18, 2016. Accessed March 5, 2019.

79. The ARDS Definition Task Force. Acute respiratory distress syndrome: The Berlin definition. *JAMA*. 2012;307(23):2526–2533.

80. Torbic H, Duggal A. Neuromuscular blocking agents for acute respiratory distress syndrome. *J Crit Care*. 2019;49: 179–184.

81. Valachis A, Samonis G, Kofteridis DP. The role of aerosolized colistin in the treatment of ventilator-associated pneumonia: A systematic review and metaanalysis. *Crit Care Med*. 2015;43(3):527–533.

82. Villar J, Ambros A, Soler JA, et al. Age, PaO_2/FiO_2, and plateau pressure score: A proposal for a simple outcome score in patients with the acute respiratory distress syndrome. *Crit Care Med*. 2016;44(7):1361–1369.

83. Villar J, Martin-Rodriguez C, Dominguez-Berrot AM, et al. A quantile analysis of plateau and driving pressures: Effects on

mortality in patients with acute respiratory distress syndrome receiving lung-protective ventilation. *Crit Care Med.* 2017;45(5): 843–850.

84. Vollman KM, Dickinson S, Powers J. Pronation therapy. In: Wiegand DL, ed. *AACN Procedure Manual for Critical Care.* 7th ed. St. Louis, MO: Mosby; 2019:142–167.

85. Wang G, Ji X, Xu Y, et al. Lung ultrasound: A promising tool to monitor ventilator-associated pneumonia in critically ill patients. *Crit Care.* 2016;20:320.

86. Weiss CH, Baker DW, Weiner S, et al. Low tidal volume ventilation use in acute respiratory distress syndrome. *Crit Care Med.* 2016;44(8):1515–1522.

87. Wen Z, Zhang H, Ding J, et al. Continuous versus intermittent subglottic secretion drainage to prevent ventilator-associated pneumonia: A systematic review. *Crit Care Nurse.* 2017;37(5): e10–e17.

16

Acute Kidney Injury

Kathleen G. Kerber, MSN, APRN-CNS, CCRN, CNRN

Many additional resources, including self-assessment exercises, are located on the Evolve companion website at http://evolve.elsevier.com/Sole/.
- Animations
- Clinical Skills: Critical Care Collections
- Student Review Questions
- Video Clips

INTRODUCTION

The kidney is the primary regulator of the body's internal environment. With sudden cessation of renal function, all body systems are affected by the diminished ability to maintain fluid and electrolyte balance and the disruption of metabolic waste and toxin elimination. Kidney injury is common in the critically ill; almost two-thirds of patients experience some degree of renal dysfunction.[9]

Acute kidney injury (AKI) is the internationally recognized term for renal dysfunction in acutely ill patients.[11] In contrast to acute renal failure, AKI encompasses the range of renal dysfunction from mild impairment to complete cessation of renal function. AKI that progresses to chronic renal failure is associated with increased morbidity and mortality and reduced quality of life.[9,11,15] Nurses play a pivotal role in promoting positive outcomes in patients with AKI. Recognition of high-risk patients, preventive measures, sharp assessment skills, and supportive nursing care are fundamental to ensure delivery of high-quality care to these challenging and complex patients. This chapter discusses the pathophysiology, assessment, and collaborative management of AKI.

REVIEW OF ANATOMY AND PHYSIOLOGY

The kidneys are a pair of highly vascularized, bean-shaped organs that are located retroperitoneal on each side of the vertebral column, adjacent to the first and second lumbar vertebrae. The right kidney sits slightly lower than the left kidney because the liver lies above it. An adrenal gland sits on top of each kidney and is responsible for the production of aldosterone, a hormone that influences sodium and water balance. Each kidney is divided into two regions: an outer region called the *cortex* and an inner region called the *medulla.*

The *nephron* is the basic functional unit of the kidney. A nephron is composed of a renal corpuscle (glomerulus and Bowman's capsule) and a tubular structure, as depicted in Fig. 16.1. Approximately 1 million nephrons exist in each kidney, and approximately 85% of these nephrons are found in the cortex of the kidney and have short loops of Henle.[8] The remaining 15% of nephrons are called *juxtamedullary nephrons* because of their location just outside the medulla. Juxtamedullary nephrons have long loops of Henle and, along with the vasa recta (long capillary loops), are primarily responsible for concentration of urine. The number of functioning nephrons decreases with age, and after the age of 40 years, the number of functioning nephrons decline by 10% with each decade of life.[8] Nephrons cannot be regenerated, so injured nephrons will not be replaced.

The kidneys receive approximately 20% to 25% of the cardiac output, which amounts to about 1100 mL of blood per minute.[8] Blood enters the kidneys through the renal artery, travels through a series of arterial branches, and reaches the glomerulus by way of the afferent arteriole (*afferent* meaning "to carry toward"). The glomerulus is a tuft of capillaries that filter blood by using the hydrostatic pressure created by the afferent and efferent arterioles. This hydrostatic pressure pushes filtrate into the tubular system. In the tubular region of the nephron, selective absorption and secretion occurs. Blood leaves the glomerulus through the efferent arteriole (*efferent* meaning "to carry away from"), which divides into two extensive capillary networks called the *peritubular capillaries* and the *vasa recta.* These capillaries then rejoin to form venous branches by which blood eventually exits the kidney via the renal vein.

The kidneys perform numerous functions that are essential for the maintenance of a stable internal environment. The following text provides a brief overview of key roles the kidneys perform in maintaining homeostasis. Box 16.1 lists functions of the kidney.

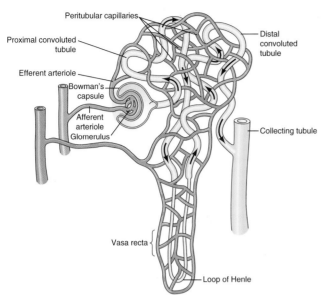

Fig. 16.1 Anatomy of the nephron, the functional unit of the kidney. (From Banasik J. Renal function. In: Banasik J, Copstead L, eds. *Pathophysiology*. 6th ed. Philadelphia, PA: Elsevier; 2019.)

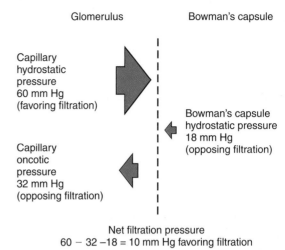

Fig. 16.2 Average pressures involved in filtration from the glomerular capillaries.

BOX 16.1 Functions of the Kidney

- Regulation of fluid volume
- Regulation of electrolyte balance
- Regulation of acid-base balance
- Regulation of blood pressure
- Excretion of nitrogenous waste products
- Regulation of erythropoiesis
- Metabolism of vitamin D

Regulation of Fluid and Electrolytes and Excretion of Waste Products

As blood flows through each glomerulus, water, electrolytes, and waste products are filtered out of the blood across the glomerular membrane and into Bowman's capsule, to form what is known as *filtrate*. The glomerular capillary membrane is approximately 100 times more permeable than other capillaries. It acts as a high-efficiency sieve and normally allows only substances below a certain molecular weight to cross. Normal glomerular filtrate is basically protein free and contains electrolytes and nitrogenous waste products, such as creatinine, urea, and uric acid, in amounts similar to those in plasma.[8] Red blood cells, albumin, and globulin are too large to pass through a healthy glomerular membrane.

Glomerular filtration occurs as the result of a pressure gradient, which is the difference between the forces that favor filtration and the pressures that oppose filtration. The capillary hydrostatic pressure favors glomerular filtration, whereas the colloid osmotic pressure and the hydrostatic pressure in Bowman's capsule oppose filtration (Fig. 16.2). Under normal conditions, the capillary hydrostatic pressure is greater than the two opposing forces, and glomerular filtration occurs. A mean arterial pressure of at least 60 mm Hg is necessary to maintain capillary hydrostatic pressue.[8] If capillary hydrostatic pressure decreases, glomerular filtration will decrease.

At a normal glomerular filtration rate (GFR) of 80 to 125 mL/min, the kidneys produce 180 L/day of filtrate. As the filtrate passes through the various components of the nephron's tubules, 99% is reabsorbed into the peritubular capillaries or vasa recta. *Reabsorption* is the movement of substances from the filtrate back into the capillaries. A second process that occurs in the tubules is *secretion,* or the movement of substances from the peritubular capillaries into the tubular network. Various electrolytes are reabsorbed or secreted at numerous points along the tubules, thus helping to regulate the electrolyte composition of the internal environment.

Aldosterone and antidiuretic hormone (ADH) are involved in water reabsorption in the distal convoluted tubule and collecting duct. Aldosterone also plays a role in sodium reabsorption and promotes the excretion of potassium. Eventually the remaining filtrate (1% of the original 180 L/day) is excreted as urine, for an average urine output of 1 to 2 L/day.

STUDY BREAK

1. Glomerular filtration rate is directly influenced by
   A. Antidiuretic hormone (ADH) secretion
   B. Mean arterial pressure
   C. Serum sodium
   D. Serum osmolality

Regulation of Acid-Base Balance

The kidneys help maintain acid-base equilibrium in three ways: reabsorbing filtered bicarbonate in the proximal and distal tubules, producing new bicarbonate, and excreting lesser amounts of hydrogen ions (acid) buffered by phosphates and ammonia.[8] The tubular cells can generate ammonia to help with excretion of hydrogen ions. This ability of the kidney to assist with ammonia production and excretion of hydrogen ions (in exchange for sodium) is the predominant adaptive response by the kidney during acidosis. When alkalosis is present, increased amounts of bicarbonate are excreted in the urine and cause the serum pH to return toward normal.

Regulation of Blood Pressure

Specialized cells in the afferent and efferent arterioles and the distal tubule are collectively known as the *juxtaglomerular apparatus*. These cells are responsible for the production of a hormone called *renin*, which plays a role in blood pressure regulation. Renin is released whenever blood flow through the afferent and efferent arterioles decreases. A decrease in the sodium ion concentration of the blood flowing past these specialized cells (e.g., hypovolemia) also stimulates the release of renin. Renin activates the renin-angiotensin-aldosterone cascade, as depicted in Fig. 16.3, which ultimately results in the production of angiotensin II. Angiotensin II causes vasoconstriction and release of aldosterone from the adrenal glands, thereby raising blood pressure and flow and increasing sodium and water reabsorption in the distal tubule and collecting ducts.

Regulation of Erythrocyte Production

Erythropoietin is secreted by the kidneys to stimulate production of red blood cells in the bone marrow. Severe anemia can develop in persons with advanced kidney disease as a consequence of reduced erythropoietin production.

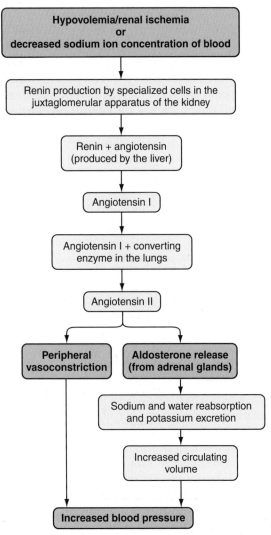

Fig. 16.3 The renin-angiotensin-aldosterone cascade.

Regulation of Vitamin D₃ Production

The kidneys produce the active form of vitamin D known as calcitriol. Calcitriol is important for calcium and phosphate regulation, influencing calcium deposition in the bone and reabsorption in the gastrointestinal tract.[8]

STUDY BREAK

2. Acid-base regulation of the kidney is performed primarily in which section of the nephron?
   A. Bowman's capsule
   B. Glomerulus
   C. Afferent arteriole
   D. Proximal and distal tubules

PATHOPHYSIOLOGY OF ACUTE KIDNEY INJURY

Definition

The Kidney Disease Improving Global Outcomes (KDIGO) is an international work group of the National Kidney Foundation. In 2012 the KDIGO Clinical Practice Guidelines for Acute Kidney Injury were published, focusing on the prevention, recognition, and management of AKI.[11] These guidelines define AKI as a sudden decline in kidney function that causes disturbances in fluid, electrolyte, and acid-base balances because of a loss in small solute clearance and decreased GFR.[11] The cardinal features of AKI are azotemia and oliguria. Azotemia refers to increases in blood urea nitrogen (BUN) and serum creatinine. Oliguria is defined as urine output of less than 0.5 mL/kg/h. These guidelines define three stages of AKI, which reflect changes in serum creatinine and urine output and provide a model for early recognition and stage-based management of AKI (Table 16.1).[11]

TABLE 16.1 Kidney Disease Improving Global Outcomes (KDIGO) Criteria for the Diagnosis of Acute Kidney Injury

Stage	Serum Creatinine	Urine Output Criteria
1	1.5-1.9 times baseline OR ≥0.3 mg/dL (≥26.5 μmol/L) increase	<0.5 mL/kg/h for 6-12h
2	2.0-2.9 times baseline	<0.5 mL/kg/h for ≥12h
3	3.0 times baseline OR Increase in serum creatinine to ≥4.0 mg/dL (≥353.6 μmol/L) OR Initiation of renal replacement therapy OR In patients <18 yr., decrease in eGFR to <35 mL/min/1.73 m²	<0.3 mL/kg/h for ≥24h OR Anuria for ≥12h

eGFR, Estimated glomerular filtration rate.
From Kidney Disease Improving Global Outcomes (KDIGO). Acute Kidney Injury Work Group: KDIGO clinical practice guidelines for acute kidney injury. *Kidney Int Suppl*. 2012;2(1):1–138.

Etiology

Although sepsis is the most common cause of AKI, its etiology in critically ill patients is often multifactorial and develops from a combination of hypoperfusion, direct nephron injury, and tubular obstruction.[14] The causes of AKI are categorized by *where* the precipitating factor exerts a pathophysiological effect on the formation of urine. The formation of urine proceeds in three steps: (1) delivery of blood for ultrafiltration (prerenal), (2) processing of ultrafiltrate by tubular secretion and reabsorption (intrarenal), and (3) excretion of kidney waste products through the ureters, bladder, and urethra (postrenal). Three mechanisms contribute to the development of AKI (Fig. 16.4): (1) alterations in renal blood flow (prerenal), (2) renal tubular injury (intrarenal), and (3) bilateral obstrucion to urine flow (postrenal).

Prerenal Causes of Acute Kidney Injury. Conditions that result in AKI by interfering with renal perfusion are classified as *prerenal*. A mean arterial pressure of at least 60 mm Hg is necessary to maintain glomerular filtration.[8] Most prerenal causes of AKI are related to conditions that reduce blood flow to the glomerulus,

including intravascular volume depletion, decreased cardiac output, renal vasoconstriction, or pharmacological agents that impair autoregulation and GFR (Box 16.2).[13] For example, major abdominal surgery can cause hypoperfusion of the kidney because of blood loss during surgery or excessive vomiting or nasogastric suction during the postoperative period.

Abdominal compartment syndrome, an intraabdominal pressure of 20 mm Hg or greater (see Chapter 20), is another prerenal cause of AKI. It is an increased pressure in the abdomen that is a complication of abdominal surgery, abdominal trauma, pancreatitis, or liver disease.[8] As abdominal pressure increases, there is compression on the renal vasculature, activation of the sympathetic and renin-angiotensin systems, and reduced cardiac output leading to reduced kidney perfusion and the development of AKI.

In prerenal AKI, the body attempts to normalize renal perfusion by reabsorbing sodium and water. If adequate blood flow is restored to the kidney, normal renal function resumes. Most forms of prerenal AKI can be reversed by treating the cause. However, if the prerenal situation is prolonged or severe, it can progress to intrarenal damage, acute tubular necrosis (ATN), or acute cortical necrosis.[13] Implementation of preventive measures, recognition of the condition, and prompt treatment of prerenal conditions are extremely important in preventing the progression to ATN.

Intrarenal Causes of Acute Kidney Injury. Conditions that produce AKI by directly acting on functioning kidney tissue (either the glomerulus or the renal tubules) are classified as *intrarenal*. The most common intrarenal condition is ATN.[9]

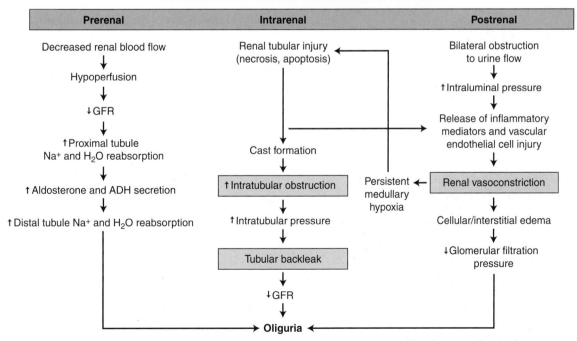

Fig. 16.4 Mechanisms that contribute to oliguria. *ADH,* Antidiuretic hormone; *GFR,* glomerular filtration rate. (From McCance K, Huether S. *Pathophysiology: The Biologic Basis for Disease in Adult and Children.* 8th ed. St. Louis, MO: Elsevier; 2019.)

BOX 16.2 Prerenal Causes of Acute Kidney Injury

Intravascular Volume Depletion
- Hemorrhage
- Trauma
- Surgery
- Intraabdominal compartment syndrome
- Gastrointestinal loss
- Renal loss
- Diuretics
- Osmotic diuresis
- Diabetes insipidus
- Volume shifts
- Burns

Vasodilation
- Sepsis
- Anaphylaxis
- Medications (antihypertensives, afterload-reducing agents)
- Anesthesia

Decreased Cardiac Output
- Heart failure
- Myocardial infarction
- Cardiogenic shock
- Dysrhythmias
- Pulmonary embolism
- Pulmonary hypertension
- Positive-pressure ventilation
- Pericardial tamponade

Medications That Impair Autoregulation and Glomerular Filtration
- Angiotensin-converting enzyme (ACE) inhibitors in renal artery stenosis
- Inhibition of prostaglandins by nonsteroidal antiinflammatory medication use during renal hypoperfusion
- Norepinephrine
- Ergotamine
- Hypercalcemia

[handwritten: → right fluid, wrong place]
[handwritten: → NSAIDS]

BOX 16.3 Intrarenal Causes of Acute Kidney Injury

Glomerular, Vascular, or Hematological Problems
- Glomerulonephritis (poststreptococcal)
- Vasculitis
- Malignant hypertension
- Systemic lupus erythematosus
- Hemolytic uremic syndrome
- Disseminated intravascular coagulation
- Scleroderma
- Bacterial endocarditis
- Hypertension of pregnancy
- Thrombosis of renal artery or vein

Tubular Problems (Acute Tubular Necrosis or Acute Interstitial Nephritis)
- Ischemia
- Causes of prerenal azotemia (see Box 16.2)
- Hypotension from any cause
- Hypovolemia from any cause
- Obstetrical complications (hemorrhage, abruptio placentae, placenta previa)
- Medications (see Box 16.5)
- Radiocontrast media (large volume; multiple procedures)
- Transfusion reaction causing hemoglobinuria
- Tumor lysis syndrome
- Rhabdomyolysis
- Preexisting renal impairment
- Diabetes mellitus
- Hypertension
- Volume depletion
- Severe heart failure
- Advanced age
- Miscellaneous: heavy metals (mercury, arsenic), paraquat, snake bites, organic solvents (ethylene glycol, toluene, carbon tetrachloride), pesticides, fungicides

This condition may occur after prolonged ischemia (prerenal), exposure to nephrotoxic substances, or a combination of these. Contrast media and heme pigment substances are also considered nephrotoxic.

Ischemic ATN usually occurs when perfusion to the kidney is considerably reduced. The renal ischemia overwhelms the normal autoregulatory defenses of the kidneys, thereby initiating cell injury that may lead to cell death. Some patients have ATN after only several minutes of hypotension or hypovolemia, whereas others can tolerate hours of renal ischemia without any apparent tubular damage.

Nephrotoxic medications (particularly aminoglycosides and radiographic contrast media) damage the tubular epithelium by direct drug toxicity, intrarenal vasoconstriction, and intratubular obstruction. AKI does not occur in all patients who receive nephrotoxic medications; however, predisposing factors such as advanced age, diabetes mellitus, and dehydration enhance susceptibility to intrinsic damage.[10,23] Other intrarenal causes of AKI are listed in Box 16.3.

Multiple mechanisms are involved in the pathophysiology of ATN. Fig. 16.5 is a detailed diagram showing some of the mechanisms that play a role in the ATN cascade resulting in a reduced GFR. Mechanisms include alterations in renal hemodynamics, tubular function, and tubular cellular metabolism. Decreases in cardiac output, intravascular volume, or renal blood flow activate the renin-angiotensin-aldosterone cascade. Angiotensin II causes further renal vasoconstriction and decreased glomerular capillary pressure, resulting in a decreased GFR. The decreased GFR and renal blood flow lead to tubular dysfunction. In addition, administration of medications that cause vasoconstriction of the renal vessels, including nonsteroidal antiinflammatory drugs (NSAIDs), angiotensin-converting enzyme (ACE) inhibitors, angiotensin II receptor blockers (ARBs), cyclosporine, and tacrolimus, can precipitate ATN.[10,20] The renal tubules in the medulla are very susceptible to ischemia. The medulla receives only 20% of the renal blood flow but is very sensitive to any reduction in blood flow. When the tubules are damaged, necrotic endothelial cells and other cellular debris accumulate and can obstruct the lumen of the tubule. This intratubular obstruction increases the intratubular pressure, which decreases the GFR and leads to tubular dysfunction. In addition, the tubular damage often produces

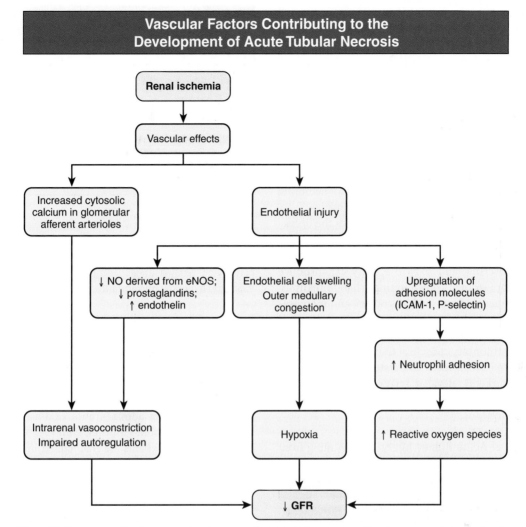

Fig. 16.5 Factors contributing to the development of acute tubular necrosis. Renal vasoconstriction and endothelial injury promote renal ischemia and tubular injury. *eNOS,* Endothelial nitric oxide synthase; *GFR,* glomerular filtration rate; *ICAM-1,* intercellular adhesion molecule 1; *NO,* nitric oxide. (From Haseley L, Jefferson JA. Pathophysiology and etiology of acute kidney injury. In: Feehally J, Floege J, Tonelli M, Johnson R, eds. *Comprehensive Clinical Nephrology.* 6th ed. St. Louis, MO: Elsevier; 2019.)

alterations in the tubular structure that permit the glomerular filtrate to leak out of the tubular lumen and back into the plasma, resulting in oliguria.[13]

Ischemic episodes result in decreased energy supplies, including adenosine triphosphate (ATP). Oxygen deprivation results in a rapid breakdown of ATP. The proximal tubule is very dependent on ATP, which explains why it is the most commonly injured portion of the renal tubule. Without ATP, the sodium-potassium ATPase of the cell membrane is not able to effectively transport electrolytes across the membrane. This leads to increased intracellular calcium levels, free radical formation, and breakdown of cell structures. Cellular edema occurs, which further decreases renal blood flow, damages the tubules, and ultimately leads to tubular dysfunction and oliguria.[13]

Contrast-induced acute kidney injury. Although the administration of contrast media is generally considered safe for individuals with normal kidney function, contrast-induced acute kidney injury (CI-AKI) is a leading cause of AKI in the hospitalized patient.[11,24] Critically ill patients are at increased risk for CI-AKI because of hemodynamic instability, volume depletion, multiple organ dysfunction, and the administration of nephrotoxic medications.[10,23]

Two pathological mechanisms contribute to the development of CI-AKI. The first mechanism is the direct toxic effect of the contrast media on the cells lining the renal tubule.[13] The second mechanism of injury is the result of reduced medullary blood flow.[13]

Contrast agents are suspected to initiate vasodilation of renal blood vessels, followed by an intense and persistent vasoconstriction.[13] Oxygen delivery to the renal cells is reduced, precipitating cell injury. In addition, contrast agents stimulate the influx of extracellular calcium, which may lead to a loss of medullary autoregulation and may also have a direct toxic effect on the renal tubules.[13] Patients with chronic renal insufficiency are at the greatest risk for developing CI-AKI.[11] Other risk factors include diabetes, dehydration, advanced age, heart failure, ongoing treatment with nephrotoxic medications, and vascular disease.[11] Many studies have been conducted to evaluate interventions to prevent CI-AKI; however, results have been inconsistent.[11,24] Hydration is the intervention that has consistently demonstrated benefit in randomized controlled trials. The KDIGO Guidelines recommend intravascular volume expansion with isotonic saline (0.9%) or bicarbonate solutions before aministration of contrast (see Evidence-Based Practice box).[11]

Heme pigment–induced kidney injury. Heme pigment–induced injury occurs in the renal tubules because of the degradation of myoglobin and hemoglobin. The heme pigment, which is a product of degradation, is toxic to the lining of the tubules. Under normal conditions, the kidney can handle the amount of heme pigment that is produced by the body. However, in situations where the heme pigment load is great, such as in rhabdomyolysis or hemolytic transfusion reaction, the risk of tubular injury is increased.

Rhabdomyolysis is a syndrome that occurs with the breakdown of skeletal muscle. Muscle injury can be related to trauma, burns, or compression. Involuntary muscle activity such as rigors, shivering, and seizure activity can produce skeletal muscle breakdown precipitating rhabdomyolysis. Illicit use of serotonergic drugs such as cocaine and methamphetamines can trigger hypertonicity, seizure activity, and agitation, leading to muscle breakdown. Rhabdomyolysis may be seen with voluntary muscle activity such as running or physical training but is usually associated with concurrent dehydration. A markedly elevated serum creatinine kinase level and the presence of tea-colored urine are findings suggestive of rhabdomyolysis.[8,16]

Postrenal Causes of Acute Kidney Injury. AKI resulting from obstruction of the flow of urine is classified as *postrenal* or obstructive renal injury. Obstruction can occur at any point along the urinary system (Box 16.4). With postrenal conditions, increased intratubular pressure results in a decrease in the GFR and abnormal nephron function. The presence of hydronephrosis on renal ultrasonography or a postvoid residual volume greater than 100 mL suggests postrenal obstruction. The location of the obstruction in the urinary tract determines the method by which the obstruction is treated. Treatment may include bladder catheterization, ureteral stenting, or placement of nephrostomy tubes.

Course of Acute Kidney Injury

The patient with AKI progresses through three phases of the disease process: the initiation phase, the maintenance phase, and the recovery phase.[8]

Initiation Phase. The initiation phase is the period that elapses from the occurrence of the precipitating event to the beginning of the change in urine output. This phase spans several hours to 2 days, during which time the normal renal processes begin to deteriorate, but kidney cell death has not yet occurred. The patient is unable to compensate for the diminished renal function and exhibits clinical signs and symptoms of AKI. Kidney injury is potentially reversible during the initiation phase.

Maintenance Phase. During the maintenance phase, intrinsic renal damage is established, and the GFR stabilizes at approximately 5 to 10 mL/min. Urine volume is usually at its lowest point during the maintenance phase; however, patients may have urine outputs

---

BOX 16.4 Postrenal Causes of Acute Kidney Injury

- Benign prostatic hypertrophy
- Blood clots
- Renal stones or crystals
- Tumors
- Postoperative edema
- Medications
- Tricyclic antidepressants
- Ganglionic blocking agents
- Foley catheter obstruction
- Ligation of ureter during surgery

---

greater than 400 mL in 24 hours. This phase usually lasts 8 to 14 days but may last up to 11 months. The longer a patient remains in this stage, the slower the recovery and the greater the chance of permanent renal damage. Complications resulting from uremia, including hyperkalemia and infection, occur during this phase.

Recovery Phase. The recovery phase is the period during which the renal tissue recovers and repairs itself. A gradual increase in urine output and an improvement in laboratory values occur. Some patients experience diuresis during this phase. This diuresis reflects excretion of salt and water accumulated during the maintenance phase, the osmotic diuresis induced by filtered urea and other solutes, and the administration of diuretics to enhance salt and water elimination. However, with early and aggressive use of dialysis, many patients are maintained in a relative "dry" or volume-depleted state and do not have a large post-ATN diuresis. Recovery may take as long as 4 to 6 months.

ASSESSMENT

Patient History

It is important to obtain a thorough patient history. Kidney-related symptoms provide valuable clues to assist the clinician in focusing the assessment. For example, dysuria, increased frequency, incontinence, nocturia, pyuria, or hematuria can be indicative of urinary tract infection. The history provides clues about comorbidities that predispose the patient to AKI, including diabetes mellitus, hypertension, immunological diseases, and any hereditary disorders such as polycystic disease. Review the medical record to identify additional risk factors, such as recent transfusions, surgery, or radiographic procedures. Information on exposure to potential nephrotoxins, such as aminoglyocides, is important. Risk factors for development of aminoglycoside nephrotoxicity include volume depletion, prolonged use of the drug (>10 days), hypokalemia, sepsis, preexisting renal disease, high trough concentrations, concurrent use of other nephrotoxic drugs, and older age (see Lifespan Considerations box).[9,10] Symptoms of AKI are usually seen about 1 to 2 weeks after exposure. In addition, a history of over-the-counter medication use, including NSAIDs, is important. Box 16.5 lists medications that are associated with AKI. Recreational drug use (cocaine, methamphetamines, "bath salts") has been associated with the development of rhabdomyolysis and subsequent AKI.[18,21]

LIFESPAN CONSIDERATIONS

Older Adults

- The most important renal physiological change that occurs with aging is a decrease in the glomerular filtration rate (GFR). Atherosclerosis and hypertension can impair autoregulation and limit the kidneys' capacity to maintain GFR.[19] With advancing age, there is also a decrease in renal mass, the number of glomeruli, and peritubular density.[8] Serum creatinine levels may remain the same in the elderly patient even with a declining GFR because of decreased muscle mass, which leads to decreased creatinine production.

- The ability to concentrate and dilute urine is impaired because of an inability of the renal tubules to maintain the osmotic gradient in the medullary portion of the kidney. This tubular change affects the countercurrent mechanism and significantly alters sodium conservation, especially if a salt-restricted diet is being followed. There is a diminished ability to excrete medications, including radiocontrast dyes used in diagnostic testing and antibiotics, which necessitates a decrease in medication dosing to prevent nephrotoxicity.[10]

- Age-related changes in renin and aldosterone levels can lead to fluid and electrolyte abnormalities. Renin levels are decreased in older adults, resulting in less angiotensin II production and lower aldosterone levels.[19]

- Older adults are prone to development of volume depletion (prerenal conditions) because of a decreased ability to concentrate urine and conserve sodium. Volume status is difficult to assess because of altered skin turgor and decreased skin elasticity, decreased baroreceptor reflexes, and mouth dryness caused by mouth breathing. Urinary indices are of limited value in assessment of older adults because of their impaired ability to concentrate urine.

- Older patients tend to exhibit uremic symptoms at lower levels of serum blood urea nitrogen (BUN) and creatinine than do younger patients. The typical signs and symptoms of AKI may be attributed to other disorders associated with aging, delaying prompt diagnosis and treatment. Atypical signs and symptoms of uremia may be seen, such as an unexplained exacerbation of well-controlled heart failure, unexplained mental status changes, or personality changes.[13]

Morbid Obesity

- Morbid obesity is defined as a body mass index (BMI) greater than 40 kg/m². [5] The increase in body mass can result in functional and structural nephron changes, including glomerular hyperfiltration, glomerulomegaly, and glomerulosclerosis.[5]

- Detection of acute kidney injury (AKI) is complicated because weight-based formulas for creatinine clearance have not been validated for this population. Whereas the incidence of AKI among morbidly obese patients is unknown, the comorbidities associated with obesity, which include chronic kidney disease, diabetes mellitus, sleep-disordered breathing, heart failure, and hypertension, are known to increase the risk of AKI.[14,15]

- In obese patients, medication dosing based on actual weight may result in nephrotoxicity. The use of adjusted body weight (ABW) is recommended for lipophilic nephrotoxic medications, including aminoglycosides.[4,10] Pharmacists use multiple adjusted and ideal weight formulas based on a medication's pharmacokinetics to calculate ideal dosages.

Pregnant Women

- Although the incidence of pregnancy-related AKI is low, it is associated with maternal and fetal mortality.[2] Risk factors for the development of AKI include intravascular volume depletion related to nausea and vomiting and urinary tract infection.[2] The kidneys enlarge and the urine collection system dilates to accommodate an increased vascular volume during pregnancy. These changes can lead to the development of hydronephrosis and increased risk for urinary tract infection.[2]

- Additional conditions associated with the development of pregnancy-related AKI include a type of severe preeclampsia known as the HELLP syndrome (*h*emolysis, *e*levated *l*iver enzymes, and *l*ow *p*latelets), as well as septic abortion and sepsis.[17]

- Early detection of pregnancy-related AKI can be challenging because the GFR increases by 50% during pregnancy.[17] This normal renal response facilitates the elimination of metabolic wastes, including creatinine, and should be considered when laboratory parameters are used in the diagnosis of pregnancy-related AKI.[2,17]

EVIDENCE-BASED PRACTICE

Prevention of Contrast-Induced Acute Kidney Injury (CI-AKI)

Problem

Acute kidney injury is a recognized complication associated with the administration of IV contrast material. Hydration is the intervention that has demonstrated consistent benefit in randomized controlled trials. Although isotonic saline is recognized as effective for hydration, IV administration of a 154 mEq/L solution of sodium bicarbonate is used as an alternative solution. Data are controversial on which IV fluid is best for hydration.[11] The oral administration of acetylcysteine in addition to hydration is also used, yet the evidence does not demonstrate efficacy.

Question

Which prevention protocol results in the lowest incidence of CI-AKI: hydration with isotonic saline, hydration with sodium bicarbonate solution, or the addition of oral acetylcysteine to hydration?

Evidence

This double-blind, placebo and comparator drug randomized controlled study compared IV sodium bicarbonate with IV sodium chloride and oral acetylcysteine with oral placebo for the prevention of AKI in high-risk patients undergoing coronary and noncoronary angiography. The sample size was 4993 patients, with 2511 patients receiving sodium bicarbonate and 2482 receiving sodium chloride infusions. All patients were randomly assigned to receive acetylcysteine or placebo in addition to the assigned hydration fluid. The researchers concluded that there was no benefit of IV sodium bicarbonate over IV sodium chloride or of oral acetylcysteine over placebo for the prevention of CI-AKI.

Implications for Nursing

Hydration is an evidence-based intervention to minimize the risk of CI-AKI. Nurses advocate for patients by ensuring that hydration is ordered and administered. Nurses have a critical role in reducing the incidence of CI-AKI.

Level of Evidence

B—Randomized Controlled Study

Reference

Weisbord SD, Gallagher M, Jneid H, et al. Outcomes after angiography with sodium bicarbonate and acetylcysteine. *N Engl J Med*. 2018;378(7):603–614.

BOX 16.5 Common Nephrotoxic Medications

- Aminoglycosides
- Amphotericin B
- Acyclovir
- Angiotensin-converting enzyme (ACE) inhibitors
- Angiotensin receptor blockers (ARBs)
- Adefovir
- Cephalosporins
- Cyclosporine
- Cisplatin
- Daptomycin
- Fluorouracil (5-FU)
- Fluoroquinolones
- Famotidine
- Interferon
- Indinavir
- Methotrexate
- Nonsteroidal antiinflammatory drugs (NSAIDs)
- Penicillin
- Pentamidine
- Rifampin
- Ritonavir
- Tacrolimus
- Vancomycin

Vital Signs

Changes in blood pressure are common in AKI. Patients with kidney injury from prerenal causes may become hypotensive and experience tachycardia because of volume deficits. ATN, particularly if associated with oliguria, often causes hypertension. Patients may hyperventilate as the lungs attempt to compensate for the metabolic acidosis often seen in AKI. Body temperature may be decreased because of the antipyretic effect of the uremic toxins, normal, or increased because of infection.

Physical Assessment. Assess the patient's general appearance for signs of *uremia* (retention of nitrogenous substances normally excreted by the kidneys) such as malaise, fatigue, disorientation, and drowsiness. Assess the skin for color, texture, bruising, petechiae, and edema. Assess the patient's hydration status. Evaluate current and admission body weight and intake and output information. Skin turgor, mucous membranes, breath sounds, presence of edema, neck vein distension, and vital signs (blood pressure and heart rate) are all key indicators of fluid balance. An oliguric patient with weight loss, tachycardia, hypotension, dry mucous membranes, flat neck veins, and poor skin turgor may be volume depleted (prerenal cause). Weight gain, edema, distended neck veins, and hypertension in the presence of oliguria suggest an intrarenal cause. Table 16.2 summarizes the systemic manifestations of AKI according to body system and lists the pathophysiological mechanisms involved.

Evaluation of Laboratory Values

Creatinine is a byproduct of muscle metabolism and is produced at a relatively constant rate. When kidney function is decreased, creatinine levels rise rapidly, indicating a decline in function or a decrease in the GFR. Serial changes in serum creatinine and urine output are evidence-based markers for the identification of AKI.[11] However, the value of serum creatinine in predicting kidney cell injury is limited, as serum creatinine levels are influenced by muscle mass, age, hydration status, and medications (see Clinical Alert box).

! CLINICAL ALERT

Serum Creatinine

The same serum creatinine level can reflect very different glomerular filtration rates (GFRs) in patients because of differences in muscle mass. For example, a 25-year-old man weighing 220 lb with a serum creatinine level of 1.2 mg/dL has an estimated GFR of 133 mL/h (normal), whereas a 75-year-old woman weighing 121 lb with the same serum creatinine level of 1.2 mg/dL has an estimated GFR of 35 mL/h (markedly decreased).

BUN is a blood test associated with kidney function but is not considered a reliable indicator of kidney function. Urea is a byproduct of protein metabolism. Extrarenal factors, including dehydration, a high-protein diet, starvation, and blood in the gastrointestinal tract, can elevate the BUN level. For example, with gastrointestinal bleeding, the blood in the gut breaks down, resulting in an increased protein load and an elevated BUN level.

The BUN/creatinine ratio can be useful in differentiating the type of AKI. The normal BUN/creatinine ratio ranges from 10:1 to 20:1 (e.g., BUN is 20 mg/dL and creatinine is 1.0 mg/dL). If the ratio is greater than 20:1 (e.g., BUN is 60 mg/dL and creatinine level is 1.0 mg/dL), problems other than kidney injury should be suspected. In prerenal conditions, an increased BUN/creatinine ratio is typically noted. There is a decrease in the GFR and a reduction in urine flow through the renal tubules. This allows more time for urea to be reabsorbed from the renal tubules back into the blood. Creatinine is not readily reabsorbed; therefore the serum BUN level rises out of proportion to the serum creatinine level. A normal BUN/creatinine ratio is present in ATN, where there is actual injury to the renal tubules and a rapid decline in the GFR; urea and creatinine levels both rise proportionally from increased reabsorption and decreased clearance.

Historically, the measurement of creatinine clearance over 24 hours has been considered a reliable estimate of GFR. Timed urine collections are cumbersome, and they are susceptible to multiple errors in collection. To measure creatinine clearance accurately, a precise collection procedure is required:

1. The bladder is emptied, the exact time is recorded, and the specimen is discarded.
2. All urine for the next 24 hours is saved in a container and stored in a refrigerator.
3. Exactly 24 hours after the start of the procedure, the patient voids again, and the specimen is saved.
4. The serum creatinine level is assessed at the end of 24 hours.
5. The 24-hour urine collection is sent to the laboratory for testing. (Urine can also be obtained from an indwelling urinary catheter.)

TABLE 16.2	**Systemic Manifestations of Acute Kidney Injury**	
System	**Manifestation**	**Pathophysiological Mechanism**
Cardiovascular	Heart failure	Fluid overload and hypertension
	Pulmonary edema	↑ Pulmonary capillary permeability
		Fluid overload
		Left ventricular dysfunction
	Dysrhythmias	Electrolyte imbalances (especially hyperkalemia and hypocalcemia)
	Peripheral edema	Fluid overload
		Right ventricular dysfunction
	Hypertension	Fluid overload
		↑ Sodium retention
Hematological	Anemia	↓ Erythropoietin secretion
		Loss of RBCs through gastrointestinal tract, mucous membranes, or dialysis
		↓ RBC survival time
		Uremic toxin interference with folic acid secretion
Electrolyte imbalances	Alterations in coagulation	Platelet dysfunction
	Susceptibility to infection	↓ Neutrophil phagocytosis
	Metabolic acidosis	↓ Hydrogen ion excretion
		↓ Bicarbonate ion reabsorption and generation
		↓ Excretion of phosphate salts or titratable acids
		↓ Ammonia synthesis and ammonium excretion
Respiratory	Pneumonia	Thick, tenacious sputum from ↓ oral intake
		Depressed cough reflex
		↓ Pulmonary macrophage activity
	Pulmonary edema	Fluid overload
		Left ventricular dysfunction
		↑ Pulmonary capillary permeability
Gastrointestinal	Anorexia, nausea, vomiting	Uremic toxins
		Decomposition of urea, releasing ammonia that irritates mucosa
	Stomatitis and uremic halitosis	Uremic toxins
		Decomposition of urea releasing ammonia that irritates oral mucosa
	Gastritis and bleeding	Uremic toxins
		Decomposition of urea releasing ammonia that irritates mucosa, causing ulcerations and increased capillary fragility
Neuromuscular	Drowsiness, confusion, irritability, and coma	Uremic toxins produce encephalopathy
		Metabolic acidosis
		Electrolyte imbalances
	Tremors, twitching, and convulsions	Uremic toxins produce encephalopathy
		↓ Nerve conduction from uremic toxins
Psychosocial	Decreased mentation, decreased concentration, and altered perceptions	Uremic toxins produce encephalopathy
		Electrolyte imbalances
		Metabolic acidosis
		Tendency to develop cerebral edema
Integumentary	Pallor	Anemia
	Yellowness	Retained urochrome pigment
	Dryness	↓ Secretions from oil and sweat glands
	Pruritus	Dry skin
		Calcium and/or phosphate deposits in skin
		Uremic toxins' effect on nerve endings
	Purpura	↑ Capillary fragility
		Platelet dysfunction
	Uremic frost (rarely seen)	Urea or urate crystal excretion
Endocrine	Glucose intolerance (usually not clinically significant)	Peripheral insensitivity to insulin
		Prolonged insulin half-life from ↓ renal metabolism
Skeletal	Hypocalcemia	Hyperphosphatemia from ↓ excretion of phosphates
		↓ Gastrointestinal absorption of vitamin D
		Deposition of calcium phosphate crystals in soft tissues

RBCs, Red blood cells.

If a reliable 24-hour urine collection is not possible, an estimate of GFR can be made using a serum creatinine value in an evidence-based equation for GFR estimation. Three common equations are the Cockcroft-Gault, Modification of Diet in Renal Disease (MDRD), and Chronic Kidney Disease Epidemiology Collaboration (CKD-EPI) equations. Each of these equations uses serum creatinine values, but they apply different correction factors to address the effects of nutritional state, age, gender, and muscle mass on serum creatinine values.

Several urinary and serum proteins are used for early detection of AKI.[3,8] Serum cystatin C is a protein marker of kidney function that is less influenced by muscle mass and diet.[3,8] It is filtered by the glomerulus and catabolized in the tubules. Serum levels can be used as an alternative measurement of GFR, and the presence of urinary cystatin C in the tubules is a marker for tubular injury.[3,11] Because of inconclusive trials comparing serum cystatin C with serum creatinine in the detection of AKI and differences among assays to measure cystatin C, serum creatinine measurement is recommended by the KDIGO Guidelines to evaluate kidney function.[11]

Other laboratory tests include neutrophil gelatinase-associated lipocalin (NGAL, lipocalin-2), which can be measured in blood or urine samples. Levels rise within 2 hours of injury.[3,16]

Tissue inhibitor of metalloproteinase-2 (TIMP-2) and insulin-like growth factor–binding protein 7 (IGFBP7) are cell cycle arrest markers.[3] Their presence in urine is indicative of tubular injury.[3] Table 16.3 summarizes these tests.

Analyses of urinary sediment and electrolyte levels are helpful in distinguishing among the various causes of AKI. Inspect the urine for the presence of cells, casts, and crystals. In prerenal conditions, the urine typically has no cells but may contain hyaline casts. Casts are cylindrical bodies that form when proteins precipitate in the distal tubules and collecting ducts. Red blood cell casts indicate bleeding into the tubules or red blood cells passing through the glomerulus. White blood cell casts indicate an inflammatory process. Coarse, muddy-brown, granular casts are classic findings in ATN.[13] Postrenal conditions may manifest with stones, crystals, sediment, bacteria, or clots from obstruction.

Urine electrolyte levels help discriminate between prerenal causes and ATN. Obtain urine samples (often called spot urine levels) for electrolyte determinations before diuretics are administered because these medications alter the urine results for up to 24 hours. Urinary sodium concentrations of less than 10 mEq/L are seen in prerenal conditions because the kidneys attempt to conserve sodium and water to compensate for the hypoperfusion state. Urine sodium concentrations are greater than 40 mEq/L in ATN because of impaired reabsorption in the diseased tubules.[13]

The fractional excretion of sodium (FE_{Na}) is a useful test for assessing how well the kidney can concentrate urine and conserve sodium. In prerenal conditions, the FE_{Na} is less than 1%, whereas ATN presents with an FE_{Na} greater than 1%.[13] Table 16.4 summarizes laboratory data that are useful in differentiating among the three categories of AKI.

Urine specific gravity and osmolality have a limited role in the diagnosis of AKI, especially in older adults, because the body's ability to concentrate urine decreases with age.[19] In general, prerenal conditions cause concentrated urine (high specific gravity and osmolality), whereas intrinsic azotemia causes dilute urine (low specific gravity and osmolality). The volume of urine output is also not a good indicator of renal function. Although patients with nonoliguric AKI excrete large volumes of fluid with little solute, they still have renal dysfunction and azotemia.

TABLE 16.3 Acute Kidney Injury: Selected Laboratory Findings

Laboratory Test	Normal Range	Critical Value[a]	Significance
Creatinine	Male 0.6-1.2 mg/dL Female 0.5-1.1 mg/dL	>4 mg/dL	Released by muscle Eliminated by glomerular filtration and is therefore considered a GFR marker
Creatinine clearance	Male 107-139 mL/min Female 87-107 mL/min Values decrease 6.5 mL/min with each decade of life past 40 years of age	A decrease in creatinine clearance after correction for age represents decline in kidney function	Measure of GFR
Blood urea nitrogen (BUN)	10-20 mg/dL	>100 mg/dL	Urea is product of protein metabolism. Elevation can indicate renal impairment
Serum cystatin C	Investigational use only	Investigational use only	GFR marker
Urine cystatin C	Not present	Indicative of tubule injury	Tubular injury marker
Neutrophil gelatinase-associated lipocalin (NGAL, lipocalin-2)	No rise in NGAL from baseline; results vary according to testing methods	Rise from baseline indicative of renal tubular injury	Tubular injury marker
Tissue inhibitor of metalloproteinase-2 (TIMP-2)	Not present in urine	Presence in urine	Cell cycle arrest marker Appears in urine after kidney injury
Insulin-like growth factor–binding protein 7 (IGFBP7)	Not present in urine	Presence in urine	Cell cycle arrest marker Appears in urine after kidney injury

[a]Critical value may vary depending on the laboratory performing the test.

GFR, Glomerular filtration rate.

Data from Chen LX, Koyner JL. Biomarkers in acute kidney injury. *Crit Care Clin.* 2015;31(4):633–647; Pagana KD, Pagana TJ, Pagana TN. *Mosby's Manual of Diagnostic and Laboratory Test Reference.* 13th ed. St. Louis, MO: Elsevier; 2017.

TABLE 16.4   Urine Findings Useful in Differentiating Causes of Acute Kidney Injury

Type of Injury	Specific Gravity	Urine Osmolality	Urine Sodium	Microscopic Examination	BUN/CR Ratio	FENa
Prerenal	>1.020	>500 mOsm/L	<10 mEq/L	Few hyaline casts possible	Elevated	<1%
Intrarenal	1.010	<350 mOsm/L	>20 mEq/L	Epithelial casts, red blood cell casts, pigmented granular casts	Normal	>1%
Postrenal	Normal to 1.010	Variable	Normal to 40 mEq/L	May have stones, crystals, sediment, clots, or bacteria	Normal	>1%

BUN, Blood urea nitrogen; *CR,* creatinine; *FENa,* fractional excretion of sodium.

TABLE 16.5   Diagnostic Procedures for Assessing the Renal System

Procedure	Purpose	Potential Problems
Renal ultrasonography	To obtain information on size, shape, and position of the kidneys	Minimal risk, noninvasive without contrast media
Computed tomography	To visualize the renal parenchyma to obtain data on the size, shape, and presence of lesions, cysts, masses, calculi, obstructions, congenital anomalies, and abnormal accumulation of fluid	Hypersensitivity reaction to contrast media (if used)
Renal angiography	To visualize the arterial tree, capillaries, and venous drainage of the kidneys to obtain data on the presence of tumors, cysts, stenosis infarction, aneurysms, hematomas, lacerations, and abscesses	Hypersensitivity reaction to contrast media Hemorrhage or hematoma at the catheter insertion site Acute kidney injury
Magnetic resonance imaging (MRI)	To visualize renal anatomy	Minimal risk, noninvasive, without contrast media
Renal biopsy	To obtain data for making a histological diagnosis to determine the extent of pathology, appropriate therapy, and possible prognosis	Hemorrhage Postbiopsy hematoma

---

STUDY BREAK

4. Which one of the following common diagnostic tests is most accurate in assessing kidney function?
   A. Specific gravity of urine
   B. Blood urea nitrogen (BUN)
   C. Serum creatinine
   D. Creatinine clearance

DIAGNOSTIC PROCEDURES

Various diagnostic procedures are used to evaluate renal function. Noninvasive procedures are usually performed before any invasive procedures are conducted. Noninvasive diagnostic procedures that assess the renal system include radiography of the kidneys, ureters, and bladder (KUB); renal ultrasonography; and magnetic resonance imaging (MRI). KUB radiography delineates the size, shape, and position of the kidneys. It may also detect abnormalities such as calculi, hydronephrosis (dilation of the renal pelvis), cysts, or tumors. Renal ultrasonography is helpful in evaluating for obstruction, which is manifested by hydronephrosis or hydroureter (dilation of the ureters). Ultrasound studies can also document the size of the kidneys, which may be helpful in differentiating acute and chronic renal conditions. The kidneys are often small in chronic kidney disease. Real-time ultrasound is used during renal biopsy and during placement of percutaneous nephrostomy tubes (which are often placed for hydronephrosis). MRI provides anatomical information about renal

structures. Invasive diagnostic procedures for assessing the renal system include renal angiography and renal biopsy. Diagnostic procedures are summarized in Table 16.5.

As with all diagnostic procedures, instruct the patient, assist with the procedure, and monitor the patient after the procedure. When evaluation for AKI is performed, it is important to assess for allergies to contrast media and to provide appropriate fluids to the patient to maintain hydration before and after the procedure. Urinary output is closely monitored after the procedure.

 CRITICAL REASONING ACTIVITY

Identify two strategies that the critical care nurse can use to help prevent acute kidney injury (AKI).

PATIENT PROBLEMS

Nursing care of the patient with AKI is complex. The Plan of Care for the Patient With Acute Kidney Injury addresses patient problems, nursing interventions, and expected outcomes. See also the Collaborative Plan of Care for the Critically Ill Patient in Chapter 1.

NURSING INTERVENTIONS

Accurate measurement of intake and output and determination of daily weights are two vital nursing interventions. A urine meter or other type of accurate measuring device is

◎ PLAN OF CARE

For the Patient With Acute Kidney Injury

Patient Problem
Potential for Fluid, Electrolyte, and Acid Imbalance. A risk factor is the kidney's inability to maintain biochemical homeostasis.

Desired Outcomes
- Body weight within patient's normal range.
- Breath sounds clear.
- Hemodynamic parameters within normal limits.
- Electrolytes within normal limits.
- Absence of peripheral edema.

Nursing Assessments/Interventions	Rationales
• Weigh patient daily and report weight gain of 0.5-1.0 kg in 24 h.	• Weight change from the previous 24 h is a sensitive indicator of fluid loss or gain.
• Measure intake and output hourly during critical phase. Report new onset of urine output less than 0.5 mL/kg/h.	• Provide early indication of fluid imbalances.
• Monitor respiratory status for development of adventitious breath sounds, tachypnea and increased work of breathing.	• The lungs are one of the first organs to be affected by fluid overload; increased work of breathing and tachypnea are early signs of fluid overload.
• Assess hemodynamic response to fluid management interventions.	• Guide fluid management strategies for AKI.
	• Postural hypotension, tachycardia, and hypotension indicate low preload, whereas jugular vein distension, elevated central venous pressures, and hypertension indicate volume overload.
• Monitor cardiac rhythm.	• Altered levels of potassium, sodium, calcium, and magnesium occur in AKI and are associated with cardiac rhythm disturbances.
• Monitor electrolyte values, especially potassium level.	• Hyperkalemia can cause life-threatening cardiac rhythm disturbances; elevated T waves and widening QRS complexes indicate elevated potassium levels.
• Assess patient for signs and symptoms of uremia: confusion and increased bleeding.	• Assess indicators of uremia.
• Institute safety measures.	• Prevent infection, falls, and pressure ulcers associated with elevated levels of uremic waste.

AKI, Acute kidney injury.
Adapted from Swearingen PL, Wright JD. *All-in-One Nursing Care Planning Resource.* 5th ed. St. Louis, MO: Elsevier; 2019.

essential for recording urinary output. Normal urine output is 0.5 to 1 mL/kg/h. Oral fluid intake must also be carefully monitored. Fluid intake levels are often restricted to the amount of urine output in a 24-hour period plus insensible loss (approximately 600 to 1000 mL/day).[23] Administer IV fluids as prescribed before procedures in which radiocontrast media will be used.[11,24]

Assessment of daily weights is one of the most useful noninvasive diagnostic tools. The daily weight is used to validate intake and output measurements. A 1-kg gain in body weight is equal to a 1000-mL fluid gain. Record the weight at the same time each day and with the same scale. Many critical care beds have built-in scales, which simplify the procedure. When the patient is weighed, ensure that the scale is properly calibrated and that the same number of bed linens and pillows are weighed with the patient each time. Recognize signs and symptoms of fluid volume overload, which can lead to pulmonary edema and severe respiratory distress (see Clinical Alert box).

Infection is the most common and serious complication of AKI.[7,23] Nurses play a key role in preventing infections. Indwelling urinary catheters are not routinely inserted because they increase the risk of infection, and many patients remain oliguric for 8 to 14 days. Strict aseptic technique with all IV lines (central and peripheral), including temporary access devices used for dialysis, is also of extreme importance, both at the time of insertion and during daily maintenance.

Another key role of the nurse in preventing AKI, as well as delaying its progression, is monitoring *trough* blood medication levels. Nurses are responsible for scheduling and obtaining the trough blood levels at the appropriate times to ensure accurate results. Medication dosage adjustments must be made to prevent accumulation of the medication and toxic side effects. For example, aminoglycoside doses are based on medication levels and the patient's estimated creatinine clearance.[4] A *trough blood level* is drawn just before the next dose is given and is an indicator of how well the body has cleared the medication.

⚠ CLINICAL ALERT

Fluid Volume Overload

Signs and symptoms of fluid volume overload include hypertension, edema, crackles, dyspnea, neck vein distension, weight gain, decreased urine output, decreased hematocrit, and presence of an S_3 heart sound.

❓ CRITICAL REASONING ACTIVITY

Describe factors in elderly patients that increase susceptibility to the development of acute kidney injury (AKI).

MEDICAL MANAGEMENT OF ACUTE KIDNEY INJURY

Prerenal Causes

AKI from prerenal conditions is usually reversible if renal perfusion is quickly restored; therefore early recognition and prompt treatment are essential. However, prevention of prerenal conditions is just as important as early recognition and aggressive management. Prompt replacement of extracellular fluids and aggressive treatment of shock may help prevent AKI. Hypovolemia is treated in numerous ways, depending on the cause. Blood loss may necessitate blood transfusions, whereas patients with pancreatitis or peritonitis are usually treated with isotonic solutions, such as normal saline. Hypovolemia resulting from large urine or gastrointestinal losses often requires the administration of a hypotonic solution, such as 0.45% saline. Patients with cardiac instability usually require positive inotropic medications, antidysrhythmic medications, preload- or afterload-reducing medications, or a mechanical cardiac assist device. Hypovolemia from intense vasodilation may require vasoconstrictor medications, isotonic fluid replacement, and antibiotics (if the patient has sepsis) until the underlying problem has been resolved. Invasive hemodynamic monitoring with a central venous catheter or pulmonary artery catheter may be considered in the management of fluid balance.

Intrarenal Causes: Acute Tubular Necrosis

Common interventions for the patient with ATN include medication therapy, dietary management such as protein and electrolyte restrictions, management of fluid and electrolyte imbalances, and renal replacement therapies such as intermittent hemodialysis or continuous renal replacement therapy (CRRT).

Considering the detrimental effect of AKI, the focus is on prevention. The most important preventive strategies are identification of patients at risk and elimination of potential contributing factors. Aggressive treatment must begin at the earliest sign of renal dysfunction.

Postrenal Causes

Postrenal obstruction should be suspected whenever a patient has an unexpected decrease in urine volume. Postrenal conditions are usually resolved with the insertion of an indwelling bladder catheter, either transurethral or suprapubic. Occasionally, a ureteral stent may be placed if the obstruction is caused by calculi or carcinoma.

In general, maintenance of cardiovascular function and adequate intravascular volume are the two key goals in the prevention of AKI. Box 16.6 summarizes important measures for preventing AKI.

Pharmacological Management Considerations

Fluid imbalances, retention of toxins, electrolyte disturbances, and metabolic acidosis are the physiological consequences of AKI. Management of AKI includes careful selection of medications to treat the physiological consequences of AKI and protect the kidney from additional injury.

> **BOX 16.6 Measures to Prevent Acute Kidney Injury**
>
> **Avoid Nephrotoxins**
> - Use iso-osmolar radiocontrast media.
> - Limit contrast volume to less than 100 mL.
> - Use antibiotics cautiously with appropriate dose modification.
> - Monitor medication levels (aminoglycosides).
> - Stop certain medications (NSAIDs, ACE inhibitors, ARBs) before high-risk procedures.
>
> **Optimize Volume Status Before Surgery or Invasive Procedures**
> - Aim for urinary output greater than 40 mL/h.
> - Keep mean arterial pressure greater than 70 mm Hg.
> - Hydrate with normal saline before and after procedures requiring radiocontrast media.
> - Hold diuretics on the day before and the day of procedures.
>
> **Reduce Incidence of Nosocomial Infections**
> - Use indwelling urinary catheters judiciously.
> - Remove indwelling urinary catheters when no longer needed.
> - Use strict aseptic technique with all IV lines.
>
> **Implement Tight Glycemic Control in the Critically Ill**
>
> **Aggressively Investigate and Treat Sepsis**

ACE, Angiotensin-converting enzyme; *ARBs,* angiotensin receptor blockers; *NSAIDs,* nonsteroidal antiinflammatory drugs.

Diuretics. Diuretics are prescribed to increase urine output, thereby increasing the elimination of fluid and urinary solutes. The mechanism of action for most diuretics is to decrease the reabsorption of sodium in the renal tubules. Water remains with sodium in the tubules and is eliminated as urine. Other solutes, including potassium, chloride, calcium, and magnesium, are also influenced by sodium reabsorption rates. Urinary excretion of these electrolytes is typically increased with the administration of diuretics.[8] Table 16.6 lists diuretic classes and mechanisms of action.

IV Fluid Replacement. Fluid volume replacement is indicated for the management of sepsis and other prerenal causes of AKI. Solutions such as isotonic saline and Lactated Ringer's (LR) solution are considered balanced, as these solutions have an ion concentration like plasma. Ion balance is important, as low-ion-balance solutions may affect acid-base balance as hydrogen and chloride ions shift.[6] The ability to correct ion balance is impaired in AKI. Hyperchloremic acidosis can result because of chloride ion excess. Alternation of normal saline and LR has been shown to benefit patients at risk for AKI.[25]

Medication therapy for the patient with AKI poses a challenge because most medications or their metabolites are eliminated from the body by the kidneys.[20] Medication dose adjustments are often necessary to prevent toxic levels and adverse reactions. Assessment of renal function by creatinine clearance is often used to assist with medication dosing. The pharmacokinetic characteristics of the medication to be given, the route of elimination, and the extent of protein binding are also considered. Clinical pharmacists assist in determining optimal medication dosages for critically ill patients.

TABLE 16.6 Diuretic Class and Mechanism of Action

Diuretic Class	Mechanism of Action
Loop diuretics (furosemide, bumetanide)	Inhibit sodium, potassium, and chloride ion transport across the tubule membrane
Thiazide diuretics (hydrochlorothiazide, chlorthalidone)	Inhibit sodium and chloride transport across the tubule membrane
Carbonic anhydrase inhibitors (acetazolamide)	Inhibit hydrogen ion secretion and bicarbonate reabsorption, which reduces sodium reabsorption in the proximal tubules
Aldosterone antagonists (spironolactone)	Inhibit action of aldosterone in the tubules, decrease sodium reabsorption, and decrease potassium secretion in the collecting tubules
Sodium channel blockers (triamterene, amiloride)	Block entry of sodium ion into sodium channel, decrease sodium ion reabsorption, and decrease potassium secretion in the collecting tubules

Many medications are removed by dialysis, and extra medication doses are often required to avoid suboptimal medication levels. Medications that are primarily water soluble, such as vitamins and phenobarbital, should be administered after dialysis. Medications that become bound to proteins or lipids or are metabolized by the liver are not removed by dialysis and can be given at any time.

Dietary Management

Dietary management in patients with AKI is important. Energy expenditure in catabolic patients with AKI is much higher than normal. Dialysis also contributes to protein catabolism. The loss of amino acids and water-soluble vitamins in the dialysate solution constitutes another drain on the patient's nutritional stores. The overall goal of dietary management for AKI is provision of adequate energy, protein, and micronutrients to maintain homeostasis in patients who may be extremely catabolic. Nutritional recommendations include[11]:

- Caloric intake of 25 to 35 kcal/kg of ideal body weight per day
- Protein intake of no less than 0.8 g/kg. Patients who are extremely catabolic should receive 1.5 to 2.0 g/kg of ideal body weight per day—75% to 80% of which contains all of the required essential amino acids.
- Sodium intake of 0.5 to 1.0 g/day
- Potassium intake of 20 to 50 mEq/day
- Calcium intake of 800 to 1200 mg/day
- Fluid intake equal to the volume of the patient's urine output plus an additional 600 to 1000 mL/day

In addition, patients undergoing dialysis usually receive multivitamins, folic acid, and occasionally an iron supplement to replace the water-soluble vitamins and other essential elements lost during dialysis. If the patient is unable to ingest or tolerate an adequate oral nutritional intake, enteral feedings or total parenteral nutrition is prescribed. Nutritional support must supply the patient with sufficient nonprotein glucose calories, essential amino acids, fluids, electrolytes, and essential vitamins. Adequate nutrition not only prevents further catabolism, negative nitrogen balance, muscle wasting, and other uremic complications but also enhances the patient's tubular regenerating capacity, resistance to infection, and ability to combat other multisystem dysfunctions (see Chapter 7). The physician may also prescribe early renal replacement therapy to treat the increased fluid volume from enteral or total parenteral nutrition.

Management of Fluid, Electrolyte, and Acid-Base Imbalances

Fluid Imbalance. Volume overload is managed by dietary restriction of salt and water and administration of diuretics. In addition, dialysis or other renal replacement therapies may be indicated for fluid control.

Electrolyte Imbalance. Common electrolyte imbalances in AKI are listed in the Laboratory Alert box. Hyperkalemia is common in AKI, especially if the patient is hypercatabolic. Hyperkalemia occurs when potassium excretion is reduced because of the decrease in GFR. Sudden changes in the serum potassium level can cause dysrhythmias, which may be fatal.[8,23] Fig. 16.6 shows the electrocardiographic changes commonly seen in hyperkalemia.

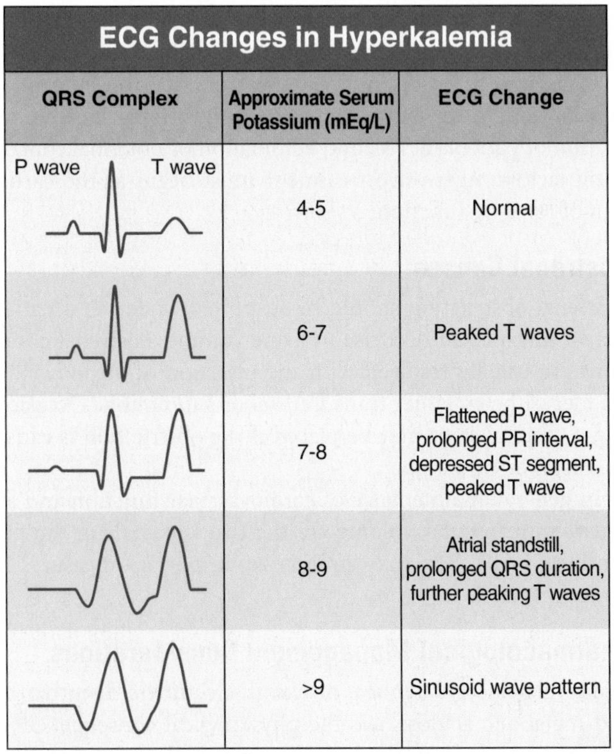

ECG Changes in Hyperkalemia

QRS Complex	Approximate Serum Potassium (mEq/L)	ECG Change
P wave T wave	4-5	Normal
	6-7	Peaked T waves
	7-8	Flattened P wave, prolonged PR interval, depressed ST segment, peaked T wave
	8-9	Atrial standstill, prolonged QRS duration, further peaking T waves
	>9	Sinusoid wave pattern

Fig. 16.6 Electrocardiographic (ECG) changes seen in hyperkalemia. (From Weiner D, Linas S, Wingo C. Disorders of potassium metabolism. In: Feehally J, Floege J, Tonelli M, Johnson R, eds. *Comprehensive Clinical Nephrology.* 6th ed. St. Louis, MO: Elsevier; 2019.)

Three approaches are used to treat hyperkalemia: (1) reduce the body potassium content, (2) shift the potassium from outside the cell to inside the cell, and (3) antagonize the membrane effect of the hyperkalemia. Only dialysis and administration of cation exchange resins (sodium polystyrene sulfonate [Kayexalate]) reduce plasma potassium levels and total body potassium content in patients with renal dysfunction. In the past, sorbitol was combined with sodium polystyrene sulfonate powder for administration; however, because their concomitant use has been implicated in cases of colonic intestinal necrosis, this combination is not recommended.[20] Other treatments only "protect" the patient for a brief time until dialysis or cation exchange resins can be instituted. Table 16.7 summarizes medications used in the treatment of hyperkalemia.

Hyponatremia generally results from water overload. However, as nephrons are progressively damaged, the ability to conserve sodium is lost, and major salt-wasting states can develop, causing hyponatremia. Hyponatremia is treated with fluid restriction, specifically restriction of free water intake. Alterations in serum calcium and phosphorus levels occur frequently in AKI because of abnormalities in excretion, absorption, and metabolism of the electrolytes. Mild degrees of hypermagnesemia are common in AKI secondary to decreased renal excretion.

! LABORATORY ALERT

Acute Kidney Injury

Laboratory Test	Normal Range	Critical Value[a]	Significance
Potassium (K^+)	3.5-5 mEq/L	>6.5 mEq/L	**Hyperkalemia:** potential for heart blocks, asystole, ventricular fibrillation; may cause muscle weakness, diarrhea, and abdominal cramps
Sodium (Na^+)	136-145 mEq/L	<120 mEq/L	**Hyponatremia:** potential for lethargy, confusion, coma, or seizures; may cause nausea, vomiting, and headaches
Total calcium (Ca^{++})	9.0-10.5 mg/dL	<6.0 mg/dL	**Hypocalcemia:** potential for seizures, muscle cramps, laryngospasm, stridor, tetany, heart blocks, and cardiac arrest; may see positive Chvostek's or Trousseau's sign
Magnesium (Mg^{++})	1.3-2.1 mEq/L	>3.0 mg/dL	**Hypermagnesemia:** potential for bradycardia and heart blocks, lethargy, coma, hypotension, hypoventilation, weak-to-absent deep tendon reflexes, nausea, and vomiting

[a]Critical values may vary by facility and laboratory.
Data from Pagana KD, Pagana TJ. *Mosby's Manual of Diagnostic and Laboratory Tests.* 6th ed., St. Louis, MO: Elsevier; 2018.

TABLE 16.7 PHARMACOLOGY

Medications to Treat Hyperkalemia

Medication	Action/Use	Dosage/ Route	Side Effects	Nursing Implications
Sodium polystyrene sulfonate (Kayexalate)	↑ Fecal excretion of potassium by exchanging sodium ions for potassium ions	*Oral:* 15 g 1-4 times daily *Rectal:* 30-50 g via enema q 1-2 h initially prn then q6h prn	Constipation, hypokalemia, hypernatremia, nausea and vomiting, fecal impaction in the elderly	Available as a powder or suspension Mix powder with full glass of liquid and chill to increase palatability Do not mix oral powder with orange juice Do not mix with sorbitol
Insulin and dextrose	Shifts potassium temporarily from the extracellular fluid (blood) into the intracellular fluid; dextrose helps prevent hypoglycemia	*IV:* Initial dose 5-10 units regular insulin and 50 mL of 50% dextrose IV push Continuous infusion: 10% dextrose with regular insulin 20 units/L	Hyperglycemia, hypoglycemia, hypokalemia	If the serum glucose level is >300 mg/dL, the physician may order only the insulin
Sodium bicarbonate	Shifts potassium temporarily from the extracellular fluid (blood) to the intracellular fluid	*IV:* 50-100 mEq/L push	Hypernatremia, hypokalemia, pulmonary edema	Do not mix with any other medications to prevent precipitation Helpful if patient has a severe metabolic acidosis
Albuterol	Adrenergic agonist ↑ plasma insulin concentration; shifts potassium to intracellular space	*Inhalation:* 10-20 mg over 15 min	Tachycardia, angina, palpitations, hypertension, nervousness, irritability	Note that the dose used is much higher than that used in treating pulmonary conditions Use concentrated form (5 mg/mL) to minimize the volume to be inhaled
Calcium gluconate	Emergent management of life-threatening hyperkalemia, stabilizes cardiac cell	*IV:* 5-8 mL of 10% solution (500-800 mg) max 3 g IV, slow injection	Bradycardia, hypotension, syncope, necrosis if infiltrated	Has no effect on lowering serum potassium Has an almost immediate effect on ECG appearance Be sure IV is patent to prevent extravasation
Calcium chloride	Emergent management of life-threatening hyperkalemia, stabilizes cardiac cell membrane	*IV:* 5-10 mL of 10% solution (500-1000 mg) slow injection	Bradycardia, hypotension, syncope, necrosis if infiltrated	Has no effect on lowering serum potassium Has an almost immediate effect on ECG appearance Be sure IV is patent; prevent extravasation

ECG, Electrocardiogram; *PO,* by mouth; *q,* every; *qid,* 4 times a day.
Data from Gahart B, Nazareno AR, Ortega M. *Gahart's 2019 Intravenous Medications: A Handbook for Nurses and Health Professionals.* St. Louis, MO: Elsevier; 2019; Skidmore-Roth R. *Mosby's 2019 Nursing Drug Reference.* 32nd ed. St. Louis, MO: Elsevier; 2019.

STUDY BREAK
5. Upon admission to the critical care unit, the patient's serum potassium is 8.1 mEq/L. Tall peaked T waves, prolonged QRS duration, and bradycardia are noted. Which pharmacological intervention would be most appropriate for this situation?
   A. Regular insulin 10 units subcutaneous administered with 50 mL dextrose 50% IV
   B. Kayexalate enema
   C. Calcium chloride 5 to 10 mL of a 10% solution given by slow IV injection
   D. Albuterol 10 to 20 mg administered by nebulizer over 20 minutes

Acid-Base Imbalance. Metabolic acidosis is the primary acid-base imbalance seen in AKI. Box 16.7 summarizes the etiology and signs and symptoms of metabolic acidosis in AKI. Treatment of metabolic acidosis depends on its severity. In mild metabolic acidosis, the lungs compensate by excreting carbon dioxide. Patients with a serum bicarbonate level of less than 15 mEq/L and a pH of less than 7.20 are usually treated with IV sodium bicarbonate. The goal of treatment is to raise the pH to a value greater than 7.20. Rapid correction of the acidosis should be avoided, however, because tetany may occur due to hypocalcemia. The pH determines how much ionized calcium is present in the serum; the more acidic the serum, the more ionized calcium is present. If the metabolic acidosis is rapidly corrected, the serum ionized calcium level decreases as the calcium binds with albumin and other substances such as phosphate and sulfate. For this reason, IV calcium gluconate may be prescribed. Renal replacement therapies also may correct metabolic acidosis because they remove excess hydrogen ions, and bicarbonate is added to the dialysate and replacement solutions.

Renal Replacement Therapy

Renal replacement therapy is the primary treatment for the patient with AKI. The decision to initiate renal replacement therapy is a clinical decision based on the fluid, electrolyte, and metabolic status of each patient. Renal replacement therapy options include intermittent hemodialysis, CRRT, and peritoneal dialysis.

BOX 16.7 Metabolic Acidosis in Acute Kidney Injury

Etiology
- Inability of kidney to excrete hydrogen ions; decreased production of ammonia by the kidney (normally assists with hydrogen ion excretion)
- Retention of acid end products of metabolism, which use available buffers in the body; inability of kidney to synthesize bicarbonate

Signs and Symptoms
- Low pH of arterial blood (pH <7.35)
- Low serum bicarbonate
- Increased rate and depth of respirations to excrete carbon dioxide from the lungs (compensatory mechanism); known as Kussmaul respiration
- Low partial pressure of carbon dioxide ($PaCO_2$)
- Lethargy and coma if severe

Definition. *Dialysis* is defined as the separation of solutes by differential diffusion through a porous or semipermeable membrane that is placed between two solutions. The various dialysis methods are distinguished by the type of semipermeable membrane and the two solutions that are used.

Indications for Dialysis. The most common reasons for initiating dialysis in AKI are acidosis, hyperkalemia, volume overload, and uremia. Dialysis is usually started early during the renal dysfunction, before uremic complications occur.

Principles and Mechanisms. Dialysis therapy is based on two physical principles that operate simultaneously: diffusion and ultrafiltration. *Diffusion* (or clearance) is the movement of solutes such as urea from the patient's blood to the dialysate cleansing fluid, across a semipermeable membrane (the hemofilter). Substances such as bicarbonate may also cross in the opposite direction, from the dialysate through the semipermeable membrane into the patient's blood. Movement of solutes across the semipermeable membrane depends on the following:
- The number of solutes on each side of the semipermeable membrane; typically, the patient's blood has larger amounts of solutes such as urea, creatinine, and potassium
- The surface area of the semipermeable membrane (the size of the hemofilter)
- The permeability of the semipermeable membrane
- The size and charge of the solutes
- The rate of blood flowing through the hemofilter
- The rate of dialysate cleansing fluid flowing through the hemofilter

Ultrafiltration is the removal of plasma water and some low-molecular-weight particles by using a pressure or osmotic gradient. Ultrafiltration is primarily aimed at controlling fluid volume, whereas dialysis is aimed at decreasing waste products and treating fluid and electrolyte imbalances.[8]

Vascular Access. An essential component of all renal replacement therapies is adequate, easy access to the patient's bloodstream. Several types of vascular access (Fig. 16.7 and 16.8), including percutaneous venous catheters, arteriovenous fistulas, and arteriovenous grafts, are used for hemodialysis.

Temporary percutaneous catheters are commonly used in patients with AKI because they can be used immediately. The typical catheter has a double lumen and a wide bore (11.5 to 13.5 French) and is 15, 20, or 24 cm long. Three-lumen catheters are also available to provide access for infusions and central venous pressure measurement. The internal jugular vein is preferred for insertion of these catheters due to optimal blood flow with less risk of a pneumothorax, followed by the femoral vein.[12] The subclavian site is not recommended because of the risk of subclavian vein stenosis.[12] Routine replacement of hemodialysis catheters to prevent infection is not recommended, and the decision to remove or replace the catheter is based on clinical need and/or signs and symptoms of infection.[12]

An *arteriovenous fistula* is an internal, surgically created communication between an artery and a vein. The most

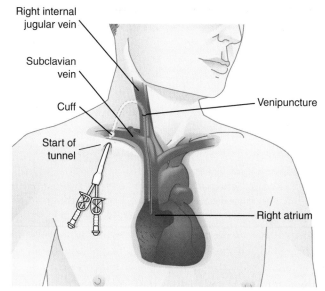

Fig. 16.7 Central venous catheter used for hemodialysis. (From Headley CM. Acute kidney injury and chronic kidney disease. In: Lewis SL, Dirksen SR, Heitkemper MM, et al., eds. *Medical-Surgical Nursing: Assessment and Management of Clinical Problems.* 9th ed. St. Louis, MO: Mosby; 2014.)

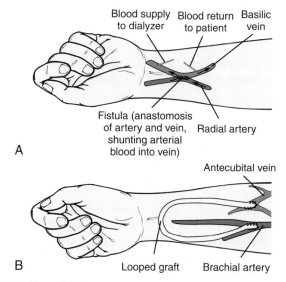

Fig. 16.8 Hemodialysis access devices. **A,** Arteriovenous fistula. **B,** Arteriovenous graft. (From Headley CM. Acute kidney injury and chronic kidney disease. In: Lewis SL, Dirksen SR, Heitkemper MM, et al., eds. *Medical-Surgical Nursing: Assessment and Management of Clinical Problems.* 9th ed. St. Louis, MO: Mosby; 2014.)

frequently created fistula anastomoses the radial artery and the cephalic vein in a side-to-side or end-to-side manner. The anastomosis permits blood to bypass the capillaries and flow directly from the artery into the vein. The vein is forced to dilate to accommodate the increased pressure that accompanies the arterial blood. This method produces a vessel that is easy to cannulate but requires 4 to 6 weeks before it is mature enough to use.

Arteriovenous grafts are created with the use of several types of prosthetic materials. Most commonly, polytetrafluoroethylene

(Teflon) grafts are placed under the skin and are surgically anastomosed between an artery (usually brachial) and a vein (usually antecubital). The graft site usually heals within 2 to 4 weeks.

Nursing care of arteriovenous fistula or graft. Protect the vascular access site. Auscultate an arteriovenous fistula or graft for a bruit and palpate for the presence of a thrill or buzz every 8 hours. Do not use the extremity that has a fistula or graft for drawing blood specimens, obtaining blood pressure measurements, or administering IV therapy or intramuscular injections. Such activities produce pressure changes within the altered vessels that could result in clotting or rupture. Alert other healthcare personnel of the presence of the fistula or graft by posting a large sign at the head of the patient's bed that indicates which arm should be used. Evaluate the presence and strength of the pulse distal to the fistula or graft at least every 8 hours. Inadequate collateral circulation past the fistula or graft may result in loss of this pulse. Notify the physician immediately if no bruit is auscultated, no thrill is palpated, or the distal pulse is absent.

Nursing care of percutaneous catheters. Strict aseptic technique must be applied to any percutaneous catheter placed for dialysis. Transparent, semipermeable polyurethane dressings are recommended because they allow continuous visualization for assessment of signs of infection.[7] Replace transparent dressings on temporary percutaneous catheters every 7 days or per institution protocol and no more than once a week for percutaneous catheters unless the dressing is soiled or loose.[7] Monitor the catheter site visually when changing the dressing or by palpation through an intact dressing. Tenderness at the insertion site, swelling, erythema, or drainage is reported to the physician. To prevent accidental dislodgement, minimize manipulation of the catheter. Do not use the catheter to administer fluids or medications or to sample blood unless a specific order is obtained. Three-lumen catheters permit infusions, medication administration, and blood sampling through the specified lumen not dedicated to renal replacement therapy. Dialysis personnel may instill medication in the catheter to maintain patency and clamp the catheter when not in use.

Hemodialysis. Intermittent hemodialysis is the most frequently used renal replacement therapy for treatment of AKI.[11] Hemodialysis consists of simply cleansing the patient's blood through a hemofilter using diffusion and ultrafiltration. Water and waste products of metabolism are easily removed. Hemodialysis is efficient and corrects biochemical disturbances quickly. Treatments are typically 3 to 4 hours long and are performed in the critical care unit at the patient's bedside. Patients with AKI may be hemodynamically unstable and unable to tolerate intermittent hemodialysis. In those instances, other methods of renal replacement therapy, such as peritoneal dialysis or CRRT, are considered.

Complications. Several complications are associated with hemodialysis. Hypotension is common and is usually the result of preexisting hypovolemia, excessive amounts of fluid removal, or excessively rapid fluid removal.[8] Other factors that contribute to hypotension include left ventricular dysfunction from preexisting heart disease or medications, autonomic dysfunction resulting from medication or diabetes, and inappropriate vasodilation resulting from sepsis or antihypertensive medication therapy. Dialyzer membrane incompatibility may also cause hypotension.

Dysrhythmias may occur during dialysis. Causes of dysrhythmias include a rapid shift in the serum potassium level, clearance of antidysrhythmic medications, preexisting coronary artery disease, hypoxemia, or hypercalcemia from rapid influx of calcium from the dialysate solution.

Muscle cramps may occur during dialysis, but they occur more commonly in chronic renal failure. Cramping is thought to be caused by ischemia of the skeletal muscles resulting from aggressive fluid removal. The cramps typically involve the legs, feet, and hands and occur most often during the last half of the dialysis treatment.

A decrease in the arterial oxygen content of the blood can occur in patients undergoing hemodialysis. Usually, the decrease ranges from 5 to 35 mm Hg (mean, 15 mm Hg) and is not clinically significant except in the unstable critically ill patient. Several theories have been offered to explain the hypoxemia, including leukocyte interactions with the hemofilter and a decrease in carbon dioxide levels resulting from either an acetate dialysate solution or a loss of carbon dioxide across the semipermeable membrane.

Dialysis disequilibrium syndrome often occurs after the first or second dialysis treatment or in patients who have had sudden, large decreases in BUN and creatinine levels because of the hemodialysis. Because of the blood-brain barrier, dialysis does not deplete the concentrations of BUN, creatinine, and other uremic toxins in the brain as rapidly as it decreases those substances in the extracellular fluid. An osmotic concentration gradient established in the brain allows fluid to enter until the concentration levels equal those of the extracellular fluid. The extra fluid in the brain tissue creates a state of cerebral edema for the patient, which results in severe headaches, nausea and vomiting, twitching, mental confusion, and occasionally seizures. The incidence of dialysis disequilibrium syndrome may be decreased using shorter, more frequent dialysis treatments.

Infectious complications associated with hemodialysis include vascular access infections and hepatitis C. Vascular access infections are usually caused by a break in sterile technique, whereas hepatitis C is usually acquired through transfusion.

Hemolysis, air embolism, and hyperthermia are rare complications of hemodialysis. Hemolysis can occur when the patient's blood is exposed to incorrectly mixed dialysate solution. An air embolism can occur when air is introduced into the bloodstream through a break in the dialysis circuit. Hyperthermia may result if the temperature control devices on the dialysis machine malfunctions. Complications of hemodialysis are summarized in Box 16.8.

Nursing care. The patient receiving hemodialysis requires specialized monitoring and interventions by the critical care nurse. Monitor laboratory values and report abnormal results

---

BOX 16.8 **Complications of Dialysis**

- Hypotension
- Cramps
- Bleeding or clotting
- Dialyzer reaction
- Hemolysis
- Dysrhythmias
- Infections
- Hypoxemia
- Pyrogen reactions
- Dialysis disequilibrium syndrome
- Vascular access dysfunction
- Technical errors (incorrect dialysate mixture, contaminated dialysate, air embolism)

---

to the nephrologist and dialysis staff. Weigh the patient daily to monitor fluid status. On the day of dialysis, do not administer dialyzable (water-soluble) medications until after treatment. Consult the dialysis nurse or pharmacist to determine which medications to withhold or administer. Supplemental doses are administered as ordered after dialysis. Administration of antihypertensive medications is avoided for 4 to 6 hours before treatment. Doses of other medications that lower blood pressure (narcotics, sedatives) are reduced, if possible. Assess the percutaneous catheter, fistula, or graft frequently; report unusual findings such as loss of bruit, redness, or drainage at the site. After dialysis, assess the patient for signs of bleeding, hypovolemia, and dialysis disequilibrium syndrome.

Continuous Renal Replacement Therapy. CRRT is a continuous extracorporeal blood purification system managed by the bedside critical care nurse. It is like conventional intermittent hemodialysis in that a hemofilter is used to facilitate the processes of ultrafiltration and diffusion. It differs in that CRRT provides a slow removal of solutes and water rather than the rapid removal of water and solutes that occurs with intermittent hemodialysis.

Indications. The clinical indications for CRRT are like those for intermittent hemodialysis, including volume overload, hyperkalemia, acidosis, and uremia. It is frequently selected for patients with AKI because of the ability to provide a gentle correction of uremia and fluid imbalances while minimizing hypotension.

Principles. The first CRRT systems were introduced in the 1970s. The extracorporeal circuit consisted of an arterial access catheter, hemofilter, and venous return catheter. The patient's blood pressure determined the flow rate through the circuit. Arteriovenous systems are no longer used because of therapy limitations related to patient-dependent blood flow and concern for complications related to arterial cannulation. Venovenous circuits are currently the standard for renal replacement therapy.[1] Improvements in dual-lumen venous catheters, mechanical blood pumps, and user-friendly renal

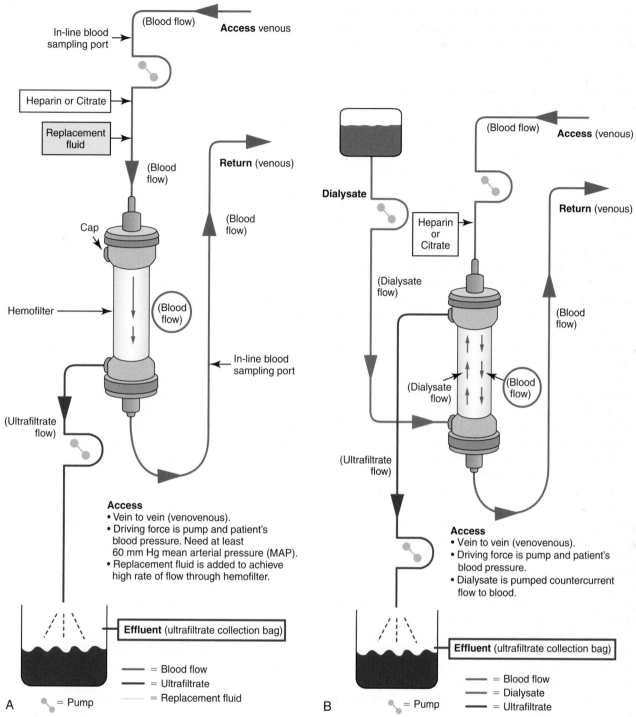

Fig. 16.9 A, Schematic diagram of continuous venovenous hemofiltration (CVVH). **B,** Schematic diagram of continuous venovenous hemodialysis (CVVHD). (From Urden L, Lough M, Stacy K, eds. *Critical Care Nursing: Diagnosis and Management.* 8th ed. St. Louis, MO: Mosby; 2018.)

replacement therapy cassette circuits and monitors have increased the safety and efficiency of venovenous replacement therapies. In venovenous therapy, two venous accesses or a dual-lumen venous catheter is used. Blood is pulled from the access port of the dual-lumen dialysis catheter or from one of two single-lumen venous catheters by the negative pressure gradient created by a blood pump. The blood travels through the hemofilter and returns to the patient via the return port of the dual-lumen venous dialysis catheter or via a second venous catheter (Fig. 16.9).

Four types of continuous venovenous replacement therapies are used (Table 16.8):
1. Slow continuous ultrafiltration (SCUF)
2. Continuous venovenous hemofiltration (CVVH)

TABLE 16.8 Continuous Renal Replacement Therapies

Modality	Name	Purpose	Vascular Access Required	Description
SCUF	Slow continuous ultrafiltration	Fluid removal	Dual-lumen venous catheter or two large venous catheters	Venous blood is circulated through a hemofilter and returned to the patient through a venous catheter; ultrafiltrate (fluid removed) is collected in a drainage bag as it exits the hemofilter
CVVH	Continuous venovenous hemofiltration	Fluid and some uremic waste product removal	Dual-lumen venous catheter or two large venous catheters	Venous blood is circulated through a hemofilter and returned to the patient through a venous catheter; replacement fluid is used to increase flow through the hemofilter; ultrafiltrate (fluid removed) is collected in a drainage bag as it exits the hemofilter
CVVHD	Continuous venovenous hemodialysis	Fluid and maximal uremic waste product removal	Dual-lumen venous catheter or two large venous catheters	Venous blood is circulated through a hemofilter (surrounded by a dialysate solution) and returned to the patient through a venous catheter; replacement solution may be used to improve convection; ultrafiltrate (fluid and waste products removed) is collected in a drainage bag as it exits the hemofilter
CVVHDF	Continuous venovenous hemodiafiltration	Maximal fluid and uremic waste product removal	Dual-lumen venous catheter or two large venous catheters	Venous blood is circulated through a hemofilter (surrounded by a dialysate solution) and returned to the patient through a venous catheter; replacement solution is used to maintain fluid balance; ultrafiltration (fluid and waste products removed) is collected in a drainage bag as it exits the hemofilter

3. Continuous venovenous hemodialysis (CVVHD)
4. Continuous venovenous hemodiafiltration (CVVHDF)

Slow continuous ultrafiltration (SCUF), also known as isolated ultrafiltration, is used to remove plasma water in cases of volume overload. SCUF can remove 3 to 6 L of ultrafiltrate per day. Solute removal is minimal and therefore is not indicated for patients with conditions requiring removal of uremic toxins and correction of acidosis.

Continuous venovenous hemofiltration (CVVH) is used to remove fluids and solutes through the process of convection, which is the transfer of solutes across the semipermeable membranes of the hemofilter. As plasma moves across the membrane (ultrafiltration), it carries solute molecules. Increasing the volume of plasma water that crosses the hemofilter membranes increases the amount of solute removed. Replacement solution is added to replenish plasma water and electrolytes lost because of the high ultrafiltration rate. Replacement solutions typically are commercially prepared and contain electrolytes and a bicarbonate or lactate base. Calcium and magnesium are not present in bicarbonate-based replacement solutions because they will form precipitates; these two electrolytes must be administered separately. Replacement solutions can be administered before the hemofilter (predilution) or after the hemofilter (post dilution).

Continuous venovenous hemodialysis (CVVHD) is like CVVH in that ultrafiltration removes plasma water. It differs in that dialysate solution is added around the hemofilter membranes to facilitate solute removal by the process of diffusion. Because the dialysate solution is constantly refreshed around the hemofilter membranes, the solute clearance is greater with this therapy, and therefore it can be used to treat both volume overload and azotemia.

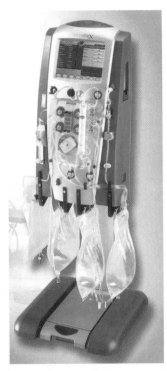

Fig. 16.10 Prismaflex continuous renal replacement therapy system. (Courtesy Baxter, Deerfield, IL.)

Continuous venovenous hemodiafiltration (CVVHDF) combines ultrafiltration, convection, and dialysis to maximize fluid and solute removal. It is useful for the management of volume overload associated with high solute removal requirements.

Automated devices are marketed to facilitate delivery of the various CRRT therapies (Fig. 16.10).

Anticoagulation. The efficiency of the hemofilter can decline over time or fail suddenly because of clogging or clotting. Clogging results from the accumulation of protein and blood cells on the hemofilter membrane.[22] Filter clotting is the result of progressive loss of the hollow fibers within the hemofilter.[22] In most situations, CRRT requires some form of intervention to prevent clogging and clotting.

During CRRT, the patient's blood comes in contact with the extracorporeal circuit, which causes activation of the coagulation cascade. Heparin is used frequently in CRRT to inhibit coagulation and extend the life of the hemofilter. However, heparin may be contraindicated if there is a risk of bleeding or heparin-induced thrombocytopenia.

An alternative to heparin during CRRT is citrate. Citrate chelates calcium in the serum and inhibits activation of the coagulation cascade.[22] Systemic anticoagulation is minimal because the liver quickly converts citrate to bicarbonate. Citrate is infused into the circuit above the filter. Close monitoring of serum ionized calcium levels and calcium replacement through a separate venous line are required. Metabolic alkalosis is a concern with this therapy. Bicarbonate-based replacement solutions should not be used with citrate therapy.

Nursing care. The critical care nurse is responsible for monitoring the patient receiving CRRT. In many critical care units, the CRRT system is set up by the dialysis staff but maintained by critical care nurses with additional training. Monitor the patient's hemodynamic status hourly, including fluid intake and output.[1] Monitor temperature because significant heat can be lost when blood is circulating through the extracorporeal circuit. Specialized devices are available to warm the dialysate or replacement fluid or to rewarm the blood returning to the patient.

Assess ultrafiltration volume hourly and administer replacement fluid per protocol. Assess the hemofilter every 2 to 4 hours for clotting (as evidenced by dark fibers or a rapid decrease in the amount of ultrafiltration without a change in the patient's hemodynamic status). If clotting is suspected, flush the system with 50 to 100 mL of normal saline and observe for dark streaks or clots. If clots are present, the system may have to be changed. Monitor results of serum chemistries, clotting studies, and other tests. Assess the CRRT system frequently to ensure that the filter and lines are visible always, kinks are prevented, and the blood tubing is warm to the touch. Assess the ultrafiltrate for blood (pink-tinged to frank blood), which is indicative of membrane rupture. Use sterile technique during vascular access dressing changes.

Peritoneal Dialysis.
Peritoneal dialysis is the removal of solutes and fluid by diffusion through a patient's own semipermeable membrane (the peritoneal membrane) with a dialysate solution that has been instilled into the peritoneal cavity. The peritoneal membrane surrounds the abdominal cavity and lines the organs inside the abdominal cavity. This renal replacement therapy is not commonly used for the treatment of AKI because of its comparatively slow ability to alter biochemical imbalances.

Indications. Clinical indications for peritoneal dialysis include acute and chronic kidney injury, severe water intoxication, electrolyte disorders, and drug overdose. Advantages of peritoneal dialysis include easy and rapid assembly of the equipment, relatively inexpensive cost, minimal danger of acute electrolyte imbalances or hemorrhage, and easily individualized dialysate solutions. In addition, automated peritoneal dialysis systems are available. Disadvantages of peritoneal dialysis are that it requires at least 36 hours for a therapeutic effect to be achieved, biochemical disturbances are corrected slowly, access to the peritoneal cavity is sometimes difficult, and the risk of peritonitis is high.

Complications. Although rare, many complications can result from peritoneal dialysis. Complications can be divided into three categories: mechanical problems, metabolic imbalances, and inflammatory reactions. Potential complications resulting from mechanical problems include perforation of the abdominal viscera during insertion of the catheter, poor drainage in or out of the abdominal cavity because of catheter blockage, patient discomfort from the pressure of the fluid within the peritoneal cavity, and pulmonary complications because of the pressure of the fluid in the peritoneal cavity. Metabolic imbalances include hypovolemia and hypernatremia from excessively rapid removal of fluid, hypervolemia from impaired drainage of fluid, hypokalemia from the use of potassium-free dialysate, alkalosis from the use of an alkaline dialysate, disequilibrium syndrome from excessively rapid removal of fluid and waste products, and hyperglycemia from the high glucose concentration of the dialysate. Inflammatory reactions include peritoneal irritation produced by the catheter and peritonitis from bacterial infection.

Nursing care. Use aseptic technique when handling the peritoneal catheter and connections. Observe for peritonitis, the most common complication of peritoneal dialysis. Peritonitis is manifested by abdominal pain, cloudy peritoneal fluid, fever and chills, nausea and vomiting, and difficulty in draining fluid from the peritoneal cavity.

Transplantation.
Kidney transplantation is a therapeutic option for patients with end-stage kidney disease. Refer to the Transplant Considerations box for criteria and patient management after kidney transplantation.

? CRITICAL REASONING ACTIVITY

Describe factors that increase the risk for contrast-induced acute kidney injury and discuss interventions that may be used to decrease the risk.

TRANSPLANT CONSIDERATIONS

Kidney Transplantation

Criteria for Transplant Recipients

Usually the recipient is younger than age 70 years, has an estimated life expectancy of 2 years or more, and is expected to have an improved quality of life after transplantation. Patients with active substance abuse or poor treatment compliance and who lack psychosocial support before and after transplant are not considered good transplant candidates. Infection and active malignancy are absolute contraindications to transplantation.

Patient Management

The kidney from a living donor functions almost immediately after transplantation; however, a cadaver kidney may not function immediately, and temporary hemodialysis may be needed. Careful monitoring of fluid and electrolyte balance is imperative, often every 4 to 6 hours in the immediate postoperative period.[1] Fluid balance may be determined by clinical assessment and hemodynamic monitoring. Chronic anemia is a consequence of end-stage renal disease (ESRD) and may limit tissue oxygen delivery; therefore hemoglobin and hematocrit levels are monitored closely.

Maintenance immunosuppression therapy consists of medications that inhibit T-cell proliferation and differentiation, deplete lymphocytes, and inhibit macrophages. A lymphocyte-depleting agent such as basiliximab, an interleukin-2 receptor blocking antibody, is often used. Maintenance immunosuppressive medications generally consist of triple therapy: a calcineurin inhibitor (tacrolimus [Prograf] or cyclosporine [Neoral]), a corticosteroid (prednisone), and mycophenolate mofetil (CellCept). Complications associated with immunosuppressive therapy include nephrotoxicity, hypertension, hyperlipidemia, bone loss, new-onset diabetes mellitus, and infection.[2] Potential kidney recipients at high immunological risk may receive plasmapheresis to decrease rejection risk with human leukocyte antigen (HLA) incompatibility.[3]

Complications

Complications seen in the postoperative phase of care may be classified as *surgical* or *physiological*. Surgical-related complications include urine leak and arterial and venous bleeding caused by anastomotic failure. This may require reoperation for surgical repair or placement of a stent. Physiological complications include infection and acute tubular necrosis. Arterial or venous thrombosis and renal artery stenosis may also occur.

The patient and family must be knowledgeable of the signs and symptoms of infection. Common signs of infection include low-grade fever, malaise, fatigue, nausea, and possibly decreased urine output. One of the most common infections is cytomegalovirus, which presents as a fall in white blood cell count, fatigue, and fever.

A common cause of death after a kidney transplant is cardiovascular disease. Immunosuppressants, especially corticosteroids and calcineurin inhibitors, can contribute to development of hypertension and diabetes mellitus, playing a role in the development and progression of atherosclerosis and lipid disorders.[3]

Preventing Rejection

Compliance with immunosuppressive medication is essential. *Hyperacute rejection* occurs within minutes or hours of transplantation and is caused by humoral or antibody-mediated B-cell production against the transplanted organ. *Accelerated rejection* occurs 24 hours to 5 days after transplantation and is due to presensitization from prior exposure to one or more of the donor's antigens. *Acute rejection* occurs days to 3 months after transplantation and involves the activation and proliferation of T cells with destruction of renal tissue. Acute rejection accounts for approximately 90% of all rejection episodes. Acute rejection is diagnosed based on clinical presentation and biopsy findings. Symptoms of rejection include fever, edema, gross hematuria, pain, increased blood urea nitrogen and creatinine, weight gain, elevated blood pressure, and decreased urine output. Management includes high-dose "pulse" steroid therapy with methylprednisolone, thymoglobulin, and muromonab-CD3.[2] Chronic rejection occurs months to years after transplantation and is caused by chronic kidney allograft dysfunction. This is often consequent to fibrosis and intimal hyperplasia within vessels in the transplanted organ. Risk factors include frequency of acute rejection episodes, hyperlipidemia, hypertension, hyperglycemia, and frequency of infection. During posttransplant follow-up, serum levels of immune-modulating agents are closely monitored to allow drug titration and maintenance of therapeutic levels.

References

1. Baker RJ, Mark PB, Patel RL, et al. Renal association clinical practice guideline in postoperative care in the kidney transplant recipient. *BMC Nephrol.* 2017;18(1):174.
2. Enderby C, Keller CA. An overview of immunosuppression in solid organ transplantation. *Am J Manag Care.* 2015;21(Suppl 1):S12–S23.
3. Wang JH, Skeans MA, Israni AK. Current status of kidney transplant outcomes: Dying to survive. *Adv Chronic Kidney Dis.* 2016:23(5):281–286.

CASE STUDY

Mr. B. age 32 years, was admitted to the critical care unit from the emergency department after successful cardiopulmonary resuscitation. Prior to admission, a family member placed an emergency call after Mr. B. failed to report to work. Upon arrival, emergency responders found Mr. B. unresponsive and in a contorted position on his back with his lower legs flexed underneath his buttocks. A syringe and tourniquet were noted nearby. Agonal respirations were present, and Mr. B. was intubated and manual bag ventilation begun. During transport to the emergency department, chest compressions were initiated for the onset of pulseless electrical activity. While in the emergency department, return of spontaneous circulation was achieved after 2 L of normal saline, IV epinephrine 1 mg every 4 minutes during chest compressions, and multiple administrations of naloxone. Mechanical ventilation was initiated and an indwelling, temperature-sensing urinary catheter was placed. The preliminary toxicology screen report was positive for opiates and cocaine. The findings of the computed tomography (CT) scan of the head were consistent with anoxic injury.

Upon arrival to the critical care unit, a central line catheter for central venous pressure measurement was placed, and targeted temperature management was initiated with a programmable cooling/warming system. Infusions of norepinephrine and normal saline fluid boluses were required to achieve and maintain a mean arterial pressure of 65 mm Hg. An echocardiogram indicated global hypokinesis with a preliminary diagnosis of stress-induced cardiomyopathy. Life-threatening serum laboratory values were present, including potassium 8.5 mEq/L, lactate 11.8 mmol/L, and creatinine 4.71 mg/dL.

IV insulin and dextrose was administered for the emergent management of hyperkalemia. Urine output was less than 0.3 mL/kg/h, and a temporary dialysis catheter was placed for the initiation of continuous venovenous hemofiltration (CVVH).

Purple discoloration and edema were present on the thighs extending to the lower legs. Feet were blue with blistering evident. Posterior tibial and dorsalis pedis pulses were absent. Emergent compartment fasciotomies were performed 24 hours after admission. Seventy-two hours after admission, bilateral transfemoral amputations were performed.

CASE STUDY—cont'd

Deep tissue injury was present on buttocks and sacrum at the time of admission. Despite aggressive pressure injury management strategies, the patient subsequently developed a stage III pressure injury.

After 2 weeks, Mr. B. transitioned from CVVH to hemodialysis 3 days per week and was transferred to a rehabilitation center for brain injury recovery and mobility assistance after his double amputations.

Questions

1. What factors predisposed Mr. B. to acute kidney injury?
2. What clinical findings assisted in the diagnosis of acute kidney injury for this patient?
3. At time of admission, Mr. B. received IV insulin and dextrose for the management of life-threatening hyperkalemia. What is the mechanism of action for this pharmacological intervention?
4. On day 2 of hospitalization, a temporary dialysis catheter was placed in the right internal jugular vein. Why is this the preferred site for placement?

REFERENCES

1. Astle S. Continuous renal replacement therapies. In: Wiegand DLM, ed. *AACN Procedure Manual for Critical Care*. 7th ed. Philadelphia, PA: Saunders; 2017:1054-1066.
2. Balofsky A, Fedarau M. Renal failure in pregnancy. *Crit Care Clin*. 2016;31(1):73-83.
3. Chen LX, Koyner JL. Biomarkers in acute kidney injury. *Crit Care Clin*. 2015;31(4):633-647.
4. Gahart B, Nazareno AR, Ortega M. *Gahart's 2019 Intravenous Medications: A Handbook for Nurses and Health Professionals*. St. Louis, MO: Elsevier; 2019.
5. Gameiro J, Goncalves M, Pereira M, et al. Obesity, acute kidney injury and mortality in patients with sepsis: A cohort analysis. *Ren Fail*. 2018;40(1):120-126.
6. Glassford NJ, Belllomo R. Does fluid type and amount affect kidney function in critical illness? *Crit Care Clin*. 2018;34(2):279-298.
7. Gould CV, Umscheid CA, Argarwal RK, et al. Guideline for Prevention of Catheter-Associated Urinary Tract Infections 2009. http://www.cdc.gov/infectioncontrol/guidelines/cauti. Updated February 15, 2017. Accessed January 31, 2019.
8. Hall J. *Guyton and Hall Textbook of Medical Physiology*. 13th ed. Philadelphia, PA: Elsevier; 2016.
9. Hoste EA, Bagshaw SM, Cely CM, et al. Epidemiology of acute kidney injury in critically ill patients: The multinational AKI-EPI study. *Int Care Med*. 2015;41(8):1411-1423.
10. Kane-Gill SL, Goldstein SL. Drug-induced acute kidney injury. *Crit Care Clin*. 2015;31(4):675–684.
11. Kidney Disease Improving Global Outcomes (KDIGO) Acute Injury Work Group. KDIGO clinical practice guideline for acute kidney injury. *Kidney Int*. 2012;2(1):1–138.
12. Marschall J, Mermel DO, Fakih M. Strategies to prevent central line–associated bloodstream infections in acute care hospitals: 2014 update. *Infect Control Hosp Epidemiol*. 2014;35(7):753-771.
13. Huether S. Alterations of renal and urinary tract function, In McCance K, Huether S. *Pathophysiology: The Biologic Basis for Disease in Adult and Children*. 8th ed. St. Louis, MO: Elsevier; 2019:1246-1277.
14. Mehta RL, Burdmann EA, Cerda J, et al. Recognition and management of acute kidney injury in the International Society of Nephrology Oby25 Global Snapshot: A multinational cross-sectional study. *Lancet*. 2016;387(10032):2017-2025.
15. Mehta RL, Cerda J, Burdmann EA, et al. International Society of Nephrology Oby25 initiative for acute kidney injury (zero preventable deaths by 2025): A human rights case for nephrology. *Lancet*. 2015;385(9987):2616-2643.
16. Pagana KD, Pagana TJ, Pagana TN. *Mosby's Diagnostic and Laboratory Test Reference*. 13th ed. St. Louis, MO: Elsevier; 2017.
17. Parfitt SE, Hering SL. Recognition and management of sepsis in the obstetrical patient. *AACN Adv Crit Care*. 2018;29(3): 303-315.
18. Rasimas JJ, Sinclair CM. Assessment and management of toxidromes in the critical care unit. *Crit Care Clin*. 2017;33(3): 521-541.
19. Rosner M. Acute kidney injury in the elderly. *Clin Geriatr Med*. 2013;29(3):565-578.
20. Skidmore-Roth R. *Mosby's 2019 Nursing Drug Reference*. 32nd ed. St. Louis, MO: Elsevier; 2019.
21. Srisung W, Faisal J, Prabhakar S. Synthetic cannabinoids and acute kidney injury. *Bayl Univ Med Cent Proc*. 2015;28(4): 457-477.
22. Thompson A, Li F, Gross AK. Considerations for medication management and anticoagulation during continuous renal replacement therapy. *AACN Adv Crit Care*. 2017;28(1):51–63.
23. Vanmassenhove J, Kielstein J, Jorres A, et al. Management of patients at risk of acute kidney injury. *Lancet*. 2017;389(10084): 2139-2151.
24. Weisbord SD, Gallagher M, Jneid H, et al. Outcomes after angiography with sodium bicarbonate and acetylcysteine. *N Engl J Med*. 2018;378(7):603-614.
25. Zampieri FG, Ranzani OT, Azevedo LC, et al. Lactated Ringer is associated with reduced mortality and less acute kidney injury in critically ill patients: A retrospective cohort analysis. *Crit Care Med*. 2016;44(12):2163-2170.

Hematological and Immune Disorders

Karen Baker Sovern, MSN, RN

Many additional resources, including self-assessment exercises, are located on the Evolve companion website at http://evolve.elsevier.com/Sole/.
- Animations
- Clinical Skills: Critical Care Collections
- Student Review Questions
- Video Clips

INTRODUCTION

Hematological and immunological functions are necessary for gas exchange, tissue perfusion, nutrition, acid-base balance, protection against infection, and hemostasis. These complex, integrated responses are easily disrupted because most critically ill patients experience some abnormalities in hematological and immune function. This chapter provides a general overview of the pertinent anatomy and physiology of these organ systems and the typical alterations in red blood cells (RBCs), immune activity, and coagulation function. Table 17.1 defines key terms used in this chapter. Guidelines are also presented for assessment and plans for care, including strategies that are needed by novice critical care nurses who care for patients at risk for these disorders.

REVIEW OF ANATOMY AND PHYSIOLOGY

Hematopoiesis

Hematopoiesis is defined as the formation and maturation of blood cells. The primary site of hematopoietic cell production is the bone marrow; secondary hematopoietic organs that participate in this process include the spleen, liver, thymus, lymphatic system, and lymphoid tissues. Negative feedback mechanisms within the body induce the bone marrow's pluripotent hematopoietic stem cells to differentiate into one of the three blood cell types (Fig. 17.1): erythrocytes (RBCs), leukocytes (white blood cells, or WBCs), or thrombocytes (platelets).[5]

In infancy, most bones are filled with blood-forming red marrow; in adulthood, productive bone marrow is found in the vertebrae, skull, mandible, thoracic cage, shoulder, pelvis, femora, and humeri.[12] Hematopoietic and immunological organs and their key functions are summarized in Fig. 17.2.

Lifespan Considerations

Aging affects several aspects of both hematological and immune systems. For example, elderly individuals have a greater risk of infection related to alterations in immunoglobulin levels. Changes in bone marrow reserve, immune function, lean body mass, hepatic function, and renal function contribute to the challenges of caring for this rapidly expanding, vulnerable population. Consideration should also be given to other populations with specific lifespan-related changes, such as pregnant women. These changes and implications are described in the Lifespan Considerations box.

Components and Characteristics of Blood

Blood was recognized as being essential to life as early as the 1600s, but the specific composition and characteristics of blood were not defined until the 20th century. Blood has four major components: (1) a fluid component called *plasma*, (2) *circulating solutes* such as ions, (3) *serum proteins*, and (4) *cells*. Plasma makes up about 55% of blood volume and is the transportation medium for important serum proteins, such as albumin, globulin, fibrinogen, prothrombin, and plasminogen. The hematopoietic cells make up the remaining 45% of blood volume. Characteristics of blood and potential alterations that may occur in critically ill patients are shown in Table 17.2.[12]

Hematopoietic Cells

Erythrocytes. *Erythrocytes* (RBCs) are flexible, biconcave disks without nuclei whose primary function is to deliver an oxygen-carrying molecule called hemoglobin throughout the body. This physiological configuration permits RBCs to travel at high speeds and to navigate small blood vessels, exposing more surface area for gas exchange. In each cubic millimeter (mm^3) of blood, there are approximately 5 million RBCs.[12]

RBCs are generated from precursor *stem cells* under the influence of a growth factor called *erythropoietin*. Erythropoietin is secreted by the kidney in response to a perceived decrease in perfusion or tissue hypoxia. Maturation of RBCs

TABLE 17.1   Hematology and Immunology Key Terms

Term	Definition
Active immunity	A term used when the body actively produces cells and mediators that result in the destruction of the antigen
Anemia	A reduction in the number of circulating red blood cells or hemoglobin that leads to inadequate oxygenation of tissues; subtypes are named by etiology (e.g., aplastic anemia means "without cells") or by cell appearance (e.g., macrocytic anemia has large cells)
Antibody	Immune globulin that is created by specific lymphocytes and designed to immunologically destroy a specific foreign antigen
Anticoagulants	Factors inhibiting the clotting process
Antigen	Any substance that is capable of stimulating an immune response in the host
Autoimmunity	Situation in which the body abnormally sees self as nonself and an immune response is activated against those self tissues
Bone marrow transplantation	Replacement of defective bone marrow with marrow that is functional; described in terms of the source of the transplant (e.g., autologous comes from self, allogeneic comes from another person)
Cellular immunity	Production of cytokines in response to foreign antigen
Coagulation pathway	A predetermined cascade of coagulation proteins that is stimulated by production of the platelet plug and occurs progressively, producing a fibrin clot; there are two pathways (intrinsic and extrinsic) triggered by different events that merge into a single sequence of events leading to a fibrin clot; clotting may be initiated by either or both pathways
Coagulopathy	Disorder of normal clotting mechanisms; most often used to describe inappropriate bleeding but can also refer to clotting
Cytokines	Cell-killer substances or mediators secreted by white blood cells; when secreted by a lymphocyte, they are called lymphokines, and secretions from monocytes are called monokines
Disseminated intravascular coagulation	Disorder of hemostasis characterized by exaggerated microvascular coagulation and intravascular depletion of clotting factors, with subsequent bleeding; also called consumption coagulopathy
Ecchymosis	Blue or purplish hemorrhagic spot on skin or mucous membrane; round or irregular, nonelevated
Epistaxis	Bleeding from the nose
Erythrocyte	Red blood cell
Fibrinolysis	Breakdown of fibrin clots that naturally occurs 1-3 days after clot development
Hemarthrosis	Blood in a joint cavity
Hematemesis	Bloody emesis
Hematochezia	Blood in stool; bright red
Hematoma	Raised, hardened mass indicative of blood vessel rupture and clotting beneath the skin surface; if subcutaneous, it appears as a blue-purple or purple-black area; may occur in spaces such as the pleural or retroperitoneal area
Hematopoiesis	Development of the early blood cells (erythrocytes, leukocytes, thrombocytes), encompassing their maturation in the bone marrow or lymphoreticular organs
Hematuria	Blood in the urine
Hemoglobinuria	Hemoglobin in the urine
Hemoptysis	Coughing up blood from the airways or lungs
Hemorrhage	Copious, active bleeding
Hemostasis	A physiologic process involving hematologic and nonhematologic factors that lead to formation of a platelet or fibrin clot to control the loss of blood
HIV	A retrovirus that transcribes its RNA-containing genetic material into DNA of the host cell nucleus; this virus has a propensity for the immune cells, replacing the RNA of lymphocytes and macrophages and causing an immunodeficient state
Humoral immunity	Production of antibodies in response to foreign proteins
Immunocompromised	Quantitative or qualitative defects in white blood cells or immune physiology; may be congenital or acquired and may involve a single element or multiple processes; immune incompetence leads to lack of normal inflammatory, phagocytic, antibody, or cytokine responses
Immunoglobulin	A specific type of antibody named by its molecular structure (e.g., immunoglobulin A)
Leukocyte	General term for white blood cells; there are three major subtypes: granulocytes (neutrophils, basophils, eosinophils), lymphocytes, and monocytes
Lymphoreticular system	Cells and organs containing immunologically active cells
Macrophage	Differentiated monocyte that migrates to lymphoreticular tissues of the body
Melena	Blood pigments in stool; dark or black
Menorrhagia	Excessive bleeding during menstruation
Neutropenia	Serum neutrophil count lower than normal; predisposes patients to infection
Passive immunity	A situation in which antibodies against a specific disease are transferred from another person
Petechiae	Small, red or purple, nonelevated dots indicative of capillary rupture; often located in areas of increased pressure (e.g., feet or back) or on the chest and trunk

Continued

TABLE 17.1   Hematology and Immunology Key Terms—cont'd

Term	Definition
Primary immunodeficiency	Congenital disorders in which some part of the immune system fails to develop
Procoagulants	Factors enhancing clotting mechanisms
Purpura	Large, mottled bruises
Reticulocytes	Slightly immature erythrocytes that are able to continue some essential functions of red blood cells
Secondary or acquired immunodeficiency	Immune disorder resulting from factors outside the immune system and involving the loss of a previously functional immune defense
Thrombocyte	Platelet
Thrombocytopenia	Serum platelet count lower than normal; predisposes individuals to bleeding as a result of inadequate platelet plugs
Thrombosis	Creation of clots; usually refers to excess clotting
Tissue anergy	Absence of a "wheal" tissue response to antigens and evidence of altered antibody capabilities
Tolerance	The body's ability to recognize self as self and therefore mount a rejection response against nonself but not self tissues
Transfusion	IV infusion of blood or blood products

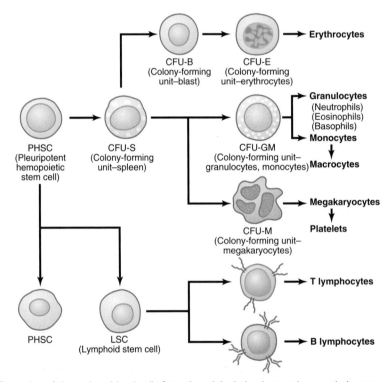

Fig. 17.1 Formation of the various blood cells from the original pleuripotent hemopoietic stem cell (PHSC) in the bone marrow. (From Hall J. *Guyton and Hall Textbook of Medical Physiology.* 13th ed. Philadelphia, PA: Saunders; 2015.)

takes 4 to 5 days, and their lifespan is about 120 days. *Reticulocytes* are immature RBCs that are released when there is a demand for RBCs that exceeds the number of available mature cells. Reticulocytes are active but less effective than mature cells and circulate about 24 hours before maturing. The spleen and liver are important for removal and clearance of senescent RBCs.[24]

The RBC contains *hemoglobin*, which binds with oxygen in the lungs and transports it to the tissues. The rate of erythrocyte production increases when oxygen transport to tissues is impaired, and it decreases when tissues are hypertransfused or exposed to high oxygen tension. The oxygen affinity for hemoglobin is modulated primarily by the concentration of 2,3-diphosphoglycerate (2,3-DPG) and depends on the blood pH and body temperature. Erythrocytes are also vital for maintenance of acid-base balance because they transport carbon dioxide away from the tissues.[8]

Platelets. *Platelets*, or *thrombocytes*, are the smallest of the formed elements of the blood. A normal platelet count ranges from 150,000 to 400,000 per mm³ of blood. Platelets are created by hematopoietic stem cells in response to hormonal stimulation. Platelets have a lifespan of 8 to 12 days, but they may be used more rapidly if there are vascular injuries or clotting stimuli. Two-thirds of the platelets circulate in the blood. The spleen stores the remaining one-third and may become enlarged if excess or rapid platelet removal occurs. In patients who have had a splenectomy, 100% of the platelets remain in circulation.[4,15]

Platelets are the first responders in the clotting response, and they form a platelet plug that temporarily repairs an injured vessel. Platelets also release mediators that are necessary for completion of clotting. These mediators include histamine and serotonin, which contribute to vasospasm; adenosine diphosphate, which assists platelet adhesion and aggregation; and calcium and phospholipids, which are necessary for clotting.[4,20] During circulation, platelets also may adhere to roughened or sheared surfaces, such as blood vessel walls or indwelling catheters.

Leukocytes. *Leukocytes* (WBCs) are larger and less numerous than RBCs, and they have nuclei. The average number of WBCs ranges from 5000 to 10,000 per mm³ in the adult. Leukocytes are derived from hematopoietic stem cells that are stimulated by a triggering mechanism within the immunological response. Cells vary in appearance, function, storage site, and lifespan. Specific characteristics of WBC development and life cycle are shown in Table 17.3.

Leukocytes are released into the bloodstream for transport to the tissues, where they perform specific functions.[7] WBCs play a key role in the defense against infectious organisms and foreign antigens. They produce and transport factors such as antibodies that are vital in maintaining immunity. Numbers of WBCs are increased in circumstances of inflammation, tissue injury, allergy, or invasion with pathogenic organisms. Their numbers are diminished in states of malnutrition, advancing age, and immune disease.[25]

WBCs are classified according to their structure (granulocytes or agranulocytes), their function (phagocytes or

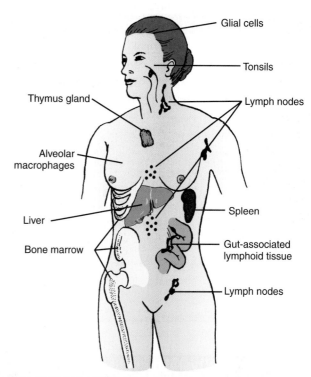

Organ	Key Functions
Bone marrow	Site of production for all hematopoietic cells.
Liver	The liver produces clotting factors, produces bile from RBC breakdown, and detoxifies many substances in the blood; its proper functioning is essential for normal hemostasis and metabolism. The liver filters and stores blood in addition to its many other metabolic functions.
Lymph nodes	Storage site for lymphocytes. Part of the continuous lymphatic system that filters foreign matter.
Spleen	The spleen is a highly vascular organ involved in the production of lymphocytes; the filtering and destruction of erythrocytes; the filtering and trapping of foreign matter, including bacteria and viruses; and the storage of blood. Although it is not necessary for survival, the spleen plays an important role in hemostasis and protection against infection.
Thymus gland	The thymus gland and lymph nodes are also part of the hematopoietic system; they are primarily involved in immunologic functions.
Tonsils, glial cells, alveolar macrophages, gut-associated lymphoid tissue	Lymphoid tissue responsive to antigens passing the initial barrier defenses, and possessing some inflammatory properties.

Fig. 17.2 Hematopoietic organs and their functions. *RBC,* Red blood cell. (Modified from Black JM, Hawks JH, eds. *Medical-Surgical Nursing: Clinical Management for Positive Outcomes.* 8th ed. Philadelphia, PA: Saunders; 2009.)

immunocytes), and their affinity for certain dyes. The *granulocytes* (or *polymorphonuclear leukocytes*) include neutrophils, basophils, and eosinophils, all of which function in phagocytosis.[2] The *agranulocytes* consist of *monocytes* (phagocytes) and *lymphocytes* (immunocytes).[6]

TABLE 17.2 Characteristics of Blood

Characteristic	Normal	Alterations
Color	*Arterial:* bright red *Venous:* dark red or crimson	Hypochromic (light color) in anemia Lighter color in dilution
pH	*Arterial:* 7.35-7.45	<7.35: acidosis >7.45: alkalosis
Specific gravity	*Plasma:* 1.026 *Red blood cells:* 1.093	— —
Viscosity	3.5-4.5 times that of water	Loss of plasma volume or increased cell production increases viscosity. Abnormal immunoglobulin (e.g., in multiple myeloma) increases viscosity.
Volume	*Plasma volume:* 45 mL/kg *Cell volume:* 30 mL/kg *Average male:* about 5000 mL	Fat tissue contains little water, so total blood volume best correlates to lean body mass. Women have more fat, and therefore blood volume is usually lower than in men. Plasma volume rises with progression of pregnancy. Volume increases with immobility and decreases with prolonged standing; this may be the result of changes in pressure in the glomerulus and glomerular filtration rate. Blood volume is highest in neonates and lowest in the elderly. Lack of nutrients causes decreased red blood cell and plasma formation. Increased environmental temperature increases blood volume.

TABLE 17.3 Overview of Leukocytes

Cell Type	Characteristics	Development and Migration	Lifespan
Granulocytes			
Polymorphonuclear leukocytes (polys)	Large granules and horseshoe-shaped nuclei that differentiate and become multilobed	Mature in the bone marrow Maturing granulocytes that are no longer dividing accumulate as a reserve in the bone marrow Normally about a 5-day supply is present in the bone marrow	Average of 12 h in the circulation About 2-3 days in the tissues
Neutrophils	Have small, fine, light pink or lilac acidophilic granules on staining and a segmented, irregularly lobed, purple nucleus		4 days
Band neutrophils	Less well defined because they are slightly immature forms of the same cell	Normally takes about 14 days for development	
Eosinophils	Have large, round granules that contain red-staining basic mucopolysaccharides and multilobed purple-blue nuclei		Unknown
Basophils	Coarse blue granules conceal the segmented nucleus Granules contain histamine, heparin, and acid mucopolysaccharides		Unknown
Agranulocytes			
Lymphocytes	Small cells with a large, round, deep-staining, single-lobed nucleus and very little cytoplasm Cytoplasm is slightly basophilic and stains pale blue	T lymphocytes constantly circulate, following a path from the blood, to the lymphatic tissue, through the lymphatic channels, and back to the blood through the thoracic duct B lymphocytes are largely noncirculating; they remain mainly in the lymphoid tissue and may differentiate into plasma cells	Lifespan varies Small populations of memory lymphocytes survive for many years Most T lymphocytes of the peripheral lymphatic tissue recirculate about every 10 h Mature plasma cells have a survival time of 2-3 days
Monocytes	Large cells with a prominent, multishaped nucleus that is sometimes kidney shaped Chromatin in the nucleus looks like lace, with small particles linked together in strands Blue-gray cytoplasm filled with many fine lysozymes that stain pink with Wright's stain	Monocytes spend less time in the bone marrow pool than granulocytes	Circulation time is about 36 h After the monocyte is transformed into a macrophage in the tissues, its lifespan ranges from months to years

Granular leukocytes.

Neutrophils. Neutrophils are the most numerous of the granulocytes, constituting 54% to 62% of the WBC differential count.[6] The *differential count* measures the percentage of each type of WBC present in the venous blood sample. These cells are divided into segmented neutrophils, in which filaments in the cell give the nuclei an appearance of having lobes, and band neutrophils, which are immature and have a thicker or U-shaped nucleus. Normally band neutrophils constitute only about 3% to 5% of WBCs.[15] The phrase *a shift to the left* refers to an increased number of "bands," or band neutrophils, compared with mature neutrophils on a complete blood count (CBC) report. This finding generally indicates an acute bacterial infectious process that draws on the WBC reserves in the bone marrow and causes less mature forms to be released. Similarly, a *shift to the right* indicates an increased number of circulating mature cells and may be associated with liver disease, Down's syndrome, or megaloblastic or pernicious anemia.[15]

The survival time of neutrophils is short. Once released from the bone marrow, they circulate in the blood for less than 24 hours before migrating to the tissues, where they live for another few days. When serious infection is present, neutrophils may live only hours as they phagocytize infectious organisms.[6] Because of this short lifespan, medications that affect rapidly multiplying cells (e.g., chemotherapeutic agents) quickly decrease the neutrophil count and alter the patient's ability to fight infection.

Eosinophils. Eosinophils are larger than neutrophils and make up 1% to 3% of the WBC count.[6,15] They are important in the defense against allergens and parasites and are thought to be involved in the detoxification of foreign proteins. Eosinophils are found largely in the tissues of the skin, lungs, and gastrointestinal tract. Eosinophils respond to chemotactic mechanisms that trigger them to participate in phagocytosis, but they also contain bactericidal substances and lysosomal enzymes that aid in the destruction of invading organisms.[6]

Basophils. The third type of granulocyte is the basophil, which has large granules that contain heparin, serotonin, and histamine. They participate in the body's inflammatory and allergic responses by releasing these substances. Basophils, which constitute less than 1% of the WBC differential, play an important role in acute systemic allergic reactions and inflammatory responses.[6]

Nongranular leukocytes (agranulocytes).

Monocytes. Monocytes are the largest of the leukocytes and constitute 3% to 7% of the WBC differential.[15] Once they migrate from the bloodstream into the tissues, monocytes mature into tissue macrophages, which are powerful phagocytes. In the lung, these tissue macrophages are alveolar macrophages; in the liver, Kupffer cells; and in connective tissue, histiocytes. In addition to *phagocytosis* ("eating" large foreign particles and cell fragments), macrophages are vital in the phagocytosis of necrotic tissue and debris. Like eosinophils, macrophages contain lysosomal enzymes and bactericidal substances. When activated by antigens, macrophages secrete substances called monokines that act as chemical communicators between the cells involved in the immune response. Although monocytes may circulate for only 36 hours, they can survive for months or even years as tissue macrophages.[6]

Lymphocytes. In the adult, approximately 25% to 33% of the total WBCs are lymphocytes.[15] Lymphocytes circulate in and out of tissues and may live for days or years, depending on their type. They contribute to the body's defense against microorganisms, but they are also essential for tumor immunity (surveillance for abnormal cells), delayed hypersensitivity reactions, autoimmune diseases, and foreign tissue rejection. Lymphocytes are responsible for specific immune responses and participate in two types of immunity: *humoral immunity,* which is mediated by B lymphocytes; and *cellular immunity,* which is mediated by T lymphocytes.

B lymphocytes, or B cells, originate in the bone marrow and are thought to mature there. B cells perform in antibody production. T cells are produced in the bone marrow, but they migrate to the thymus for maturation; then most travel to and reside in lymphoid tissues throughout the body. T-cell functions include delayed hypersensitivity, graft rejection, graft-versus-host reaction, defense against intracellular organisms, and defense against neoplasms.[6] T cells live longer than B cells and participate in long-term immunity. The natural killer cell is a third type of lymphocyte. It is responsible for surveillance and destruction of virus-infected and malignant cells.

STUDY BREAK

1. An immunocompromised patient has a high risk of developing a life-threatening infection. An awareness of abnormal laboratory results can be key to early detection and intervention. The term *shift to the left* is indicative of an acute bacterial infection and observed with the following laboratory results:

   A. Decreased number of basophils

   B. Increased number of band neutrophils compared to mature neutrophils

   C. Decreased number of eosinophils

   D. Increased number of mature neutrophils compared to band neutrophils

---

Immune Anatomy

Immune activity involves an integrated, multilevel response against invading pathogens. It requires both WBCs of the hematopoietic system and the secondary hematopoietic organs, termed the *lymphoreticular system.* The lymphoreticular system consists of lymphoid tissue, lymphatic channels and nodes, and phagocytic cells that engulf and process foreign materials (see Fig. 17.2).

The body's ability to resist and fight infection is called *immunity.* The human body is constantly exposed to normal and unusual microorganisms that are capable of causing disease. The healthy person's immune system recognizes potential pathogens and destroys them before tissue invasion occurs; however, the person with a dysfunctional immune system is at risk of overwhelming, life-threatening infection.

Immune Physiology

The immune response protects the body from disease by recognizing, processing, and destroying foreign invaders. It aids in the removal of damaged cells and defends the body against the proliferation of abnormal or malignant cells.

The recognition of nonself molecules called *antigens* is the key triggering activity of the immune system. Microorganisms (e.g., bacteria, viruses, fungi, parasites), abnormal or mutated cells, transplanted cells, nonself protein molecules (e.g., vaccines), and nonhuman molecules (e.g., penicillin) can act as antigens. These antigens are detected by the body as foreign, or nonself, and are destroyed by immunological processes. The body's response to an antigen is determined by factors such as genetics, amount of antigen, and route of exposure. In autoimmunity, the body abnormally sees self as nonself, and an immune response is activated against those tissues. Autoimmunity can result from injury to tissues, infection, or malignancy, although in many cases the cause is not known. An example of an autoimmune disease is systemic lupus erythematosus.[11]

An intact and healthy immune system consists of both natural (nonspecific) defenses and acquired (specific) defenses. The nonspecific defenses are the first line of protection and include the processes of inflammation and phagocytosis. When nonspecific mechanisms fail to protect the body from invasion, the specific defenses of humoral and cellular immunity are put into action. *Active immunity* is a term used when the body actively produces cells and mediators that result in destruction of the antigen. *Passive immunity* is that which is transferred from another person, as when maternal antibodies are transferred to the newborn through the placenta.[19]

Nonspecific Defenses. The body's nonspecific defenses consist of the physical and chemical barriers to invasion, the protective and repairing processes of inflammation and phagocytosis, and other substances that stimulate the body to fight back. The body's first line of defense against infection consists of physical and chemical barriers.

Epithelial surfaces. The epithelial surfaces are those that are exposed to the environment. Intact skin and mucous membranes provide a protective covering; they also secrete substances that have antimicrobial effects. For example, sweat glands produce a lysozyme, which is an antimicrobial enzyme; and sebaceous glands secrete sebum, which has antimicrobial and antifungal properties. The skin constantly exfoliates, a process that sloughs off bacterial and chemical hazards. These same epithelial surfaces are colonized by "normal" bacterial flora that protect the body from microorganisms by occupying space on the epithelium, preventing pathogen attachment.

Epithelial surfaces also have unique physical and chemical properties that protect them from pathogen invasion. For example, mucus and cilia work together to trap and remove harmful substances in the respiratory tract. The motility of the intestines maintains an even distribution of bacterial flora, thereby preventing overgrowth or invasion of pathogens, and promotes evacuation of harmful microbes. Chemical barriers to pathogenic entry include the unique pH of the skin and mucosa of the gastrointestinal and urinary tracts. This pH inhibits the growth of many microorganisms. Immunoglobulin A (IgA, also called *secretory IgA*) and phagocytic cells are biological factors present in respiratory and gastrointestinal secretions. They are essential for destruction of particular pyogenic bacteria.[6,17]

Inflammation and phagocytosis. The second line of defense involves the processes of inflammation and phagocytosis. Inflammation is initiated by cellular injury, is necessary for tissue repair, and is harmful when uncontrolled. When cellular injury occurs, a process called *chemotaxis* generates both a mediator and a neutrophil response. Mediator substances (histamine, serotonin, kinins, lysosomal enzymes, prostaglandin, platelet-activating factor, clotting factors, and complement proteins) are released at the site of injury. These mediators cause vasodilation, increase blood flow, induce capillary permeability, and promote chemotaxis and phagocytosis by neutrophils. Inflammatory symptoms such as redness, heat, pain, and swelling are sequelae of these responses. *Complement* proteins enhance the antibody activity, phagocytosis, and inflammation.[6,17]

Neutrophils are attracted to, and migrate to, areas of inflammation or bacterial invasion, where they ingest and kill invading microorganisms by phagocytosis. The inflammatory response is a rapid process initiated by granulocytes and macrophages. Granulocytes arrive within minutes after cellular injury. Once phagocytes have been attracted to an area by the release of mediators, a process called *opsonization* occurs, in which antibody and complement proteins attach to the target cell and enhance the phagocyte's ability to engulf the target cell. Once the bacteria have been engulfed, they are killed and digested within the cell by lysosomal enzymes. Exudate formation at the inflammatory site has three functions: dilute the toxins produced, deliver proteins and leukocytes to the site, and carry away toxins and debris.[6]

Infectious organisms that escape the local phagocytic responses may be engulfed and destroyed in a similar fashion by tissue macrophages within the lymphoreticular organs. The portal circulation of the spleen and liver filters most of the blood, removing infectious organisms before they infect tissues. In the lymphatic system, pathogenic substances are filtered by the lymph nodes and are phagocytized by tissue macrophages. Here they may also stimulate immune responses by the lymphoid cells.

Other nonspecific defenses. Another nonspecific defensive activity is the release from WBCs of cytokines and chemokines, which are either proinflammatory, antiinflammatory, or both. These naturally occurring biological response modifiers, which include interleukins (ILs), tumor necrosis factor (TNF), colony-stimulating factors, monoclonal antibodies, and interferons (IFNs), mediate various interactions among immune system cells.[17]

At least 30 human ILs exist. An example of an interleukin is IL-1. IL-1, a proinflammatory cytokine, is an endogenous pyrogen that increases body temperature in infection, thereby inhibiting the growth of temperature-sensitive pathogens. IL-1 also activates phagocytes and lymphocytes and acts as a growth factor for many cells. The IFNs have antitumor and antiviral activity and include 20 subtypes of IFN-alpha, 2 subtypes of IFN-beta, and IFN-gamma.

Through recombinant DNA technology, IFNs and other naturally occurring substances can be produced synthetically for the treatment of many disorders. IFNs, colony-stimulating factors, and monoclonal antibodies are some examples of biological therapies currently approved for the treatment of certain malignant disorders.[18]

? CRITICAL REASONING ACTIVITY

What disorders are associated with anemia in the critically ill patient?

Specific Defenses. *Specificity* refers to the finding that an immune response stimulates cells to develop immunity for a specific antigen. Two types of specific immune responses exist: humoral immunity and cell-mediated immunity. They are not mutually exclusive but act together to provide immunity.

Humoral immunity. Humoral immunity is mediated by B lymphocytes and involves the formation of antibodies (immunoglobulins) in response to specific antigens that bind to their receptor sites. Antigen binding activates the differentiation of B lymphocytes into plasma cells that produce specific antibodies in response to those antigens. Five classes of immunoglobulins exist: IgG, IgM, IgA, IgD, and IgE. The clinical features and abnormalities associated with these immunoglobulins are described in Table 17.4.[17]

Once antibodies have been synthesized and released, they bind to their specific antigen and form an antigen-antibody complex that activates phagocytosis and complement proteins. This humoral response is regulated by the activity of T lymphocytes. Helper T cells promote B-lymphocyte activity and the production of antibodies, whereas suppressor T cells reduce the humoral response.

The body generates both primary and secondary humoral responses. In the *primary response,* antigens that have evaded the nonspecific defenses are engulfed and processed by macrophages. The macrophages then present the processed antigens to the lymphocytes, which proliferate, differentiate, and produce antibodies. In this first exposure, antibodies of the IgM subtype appear first and predominate, and IgG immunoglobulins appear later. During this primary response, the immunoglobulins develop an immunological memory for antigens. Then, when any subsequent exposure to the antigen occurs, a quicker, stronger, and longer-lasting IgG-mediated *secondary response* occurs. IgG antibodies predominate and may be detectable in the serum for decades.[17]

Cell-mediated immunity. Cellular immunity is mediated by T lymphocytes. Cell-mediated immunity is a more delayed reaction than the humoral response and occurs only when there is direct contact with sensitized lymphocytes. It is important in viral, fungal, and intracellular infections and is the mechanism involved in transplant rejection and recognition of neoplastic cells.

Cell-mediated immunity is initiated by macrophage recognition of nonself foreign materials. The macrophages trap, process, and present such materials to T lymphocytes, which then migrate to the site of the antigen, where they complete antigen destruction. Once contact is made with a specific antigen, the T lymphocytes differentiate into helper/inducer T cells, suppressor T cells, and cytotoxic killer cells. Although these T cells are microscopically identical, they can be distinguished by proteins present on the cell surface, called clusters of differentiation (CDs). Helper T cells (also known as CD4 cells because they carry a CD4 marker) enhance the humoral immune response by stimulating B cells to differentiate and produce antibodies.[7] Suppressor T cells reduce and suppress the humoral and cell-mediated responses. The ratio of helper to suppressor T cells is normally 2:1, and an alteration in this ratio may cause disease.[15] For example, a depressed ratio (a decrease of helper T cells in relation to suppressor T cells) is found in AIDS, whereas a higher ratio (a decrease in suppressor T cells in relation to helper T cells) is a feature of an autoimmune disease.

Cytotoxic or killer T cells (CD8 marker) participate directly in the destruction of antigens by binding to and altering the intracellular environment, which ultimately destroys the cell. Killer cells also release cytotoxic substances into the antigen cell that cause cell lysis. Killer T cells additionally provide the body with immunosurveillance capabilities that monitor for abnormal cells or tissue. This mechanism is responsible for the rejection of transplanted tissue and the destruction of single malignant cells.[13]

TABLE 17.4 Immunoglobulins

Antibody	Description	Normal Value
IgG	Most abundant immunoglobulin Major influence with bacterial disease Crosses the placenta Coats microorganisms to enhance phagocytosis Activates complement	75% of total 500-1600 mg/dL
IgM	Primary immunoglobulin response to antigen, with levels increased by 7 days after exposure Present mostly in the intravascular space Causes antigenic agglutination and cell lysis via complement activation	10% of total 60-280 mg/dL
IgA	Found on mucosal surfaces of respiratory, GI, and GU systems, preventing antigen adherence Influential with bacteria and some viral organisms First antibody formed after exposure to antigen but rapidly diminishes as IgG increases Does not cross the placenta but passes to newborn through colostrum and breast milk Deficiency caused by congenital autosomal dominant or recessive disease or related to anticonvulsant use Deficiency (<5 mg/dL) manifests as chronic sinopulmonary infection	15% of total 90-450 mg/dL
IgD	Activates B lymphocytes to become plasma cells, which are the key immunoglobulin-producing cells	1% of total 0.5-3.0 mg/dL
IgE	Attaches to mast cells and basophils on epithelial surfaces and enhances release of histamine and other vasoactive mediators responsible for the "wheal and flare" reaction Important for allergic responses, inflammatory reactions, and parasitic infections	0.002% of total 0.01-0.04 mg/dL

GI, Gastrointestinal; GU, genitourinary.

Hemostasis

Hemostasis is a physiological process involving platelets, blood proteins (clotting factors), and the vasculature. This process involves the formation of blood clots to stop bleeding from injured vessels and natural anticoagulant and fibrinolytic systems to limit clot formation. Many substances that may activate the clotting system, including collagen, proteases, and bacterial endotoxins, are released during tissue destruction. The three physiological mechanisms that trigger clotting in the body are tissue injury, vessel injury, and the presence of a foreign body in the bloodstream. When one of these trigger factors is present, a series of physical events occurs that results in a fibrin clot.

Although the events of hemostasis are sequential, they require integration of components from the hematopoietic and coagulation systems. Within seconds after injury, platelets are attracted and adhere to the site of injury. The activated platelets then undergo changes in shape to expose receptors on their surfaces. RBCs increase the rate of platelet adherence by facilitating migration of platelets to the site and by liberating adenosine diphosphate (ADP), which enables platelets to stick to the exposed tissue (collagen). The exposed receptors on the activated platelet surfaces are capable of binding fibrinogen, an essential component underlying platelet aggregation. Serotonin and histamine are released by the adhered platelets and cause immediate constriction of the injured vessel to lessen bleeding. Vasoconstriction is followed by vasodilation, bringing the necessary cellular products of the inflammatory response to the site. With minor vessel injury, *primary hemostasis* is temporarily achieved with platelet plugs, usually within seconds. During *secondary hemostasis*, the platelet plug is solidified with fibrin, an end product of the coagulation pathway, and requires several minutes to reach completion (Fig. 17.3).[6,10]

Coagulation Pathway.

In the classic theory, coagulation is viewed as occurring through two distinct pathways, *intrinsic* and *extrinsic*, that share a common "final" pathway, the formation of insoluble fibrin.[10,16] The in vitro model (Fig. 17.4A) illustrates the classic theory of coagulation.

Both pathways begin with an initiating event and involve a cascading sequence of clotting factor activation precipitated by a preceding reaction. The soluble clotting factors become insoluble fibrin. When blood is exposed to subendothelial collagen or is "injured," factor XII is activated, which initiates coagulation via the *intrinsic pathway*. In the *extrinsic pathway*, tissue injury precipitates release of a substance known as *tissue factor*, which activates factor VII. Factor VII is key in initiating blood coagulation, and the two pathways intersect at the activation of factor X.[10,16] Both coagulation pathways lead to a *final common pathway* of clot formation, retraction, and fibrinolysis.

In patients, coagulation occurs via the in vivo model (see Fig. 17.4B). In patients, tissue factor is the major factor for initiating coagulation (see Fig. 17.4B).

The coagulation factors are plasma proteins that circulate as inactive enzymes, and most are synthesized in the liver. Vitamin K is necessary for synthesis of factors II, VII, IX, and X and proteins C and S (anticoagulation factors). For this reason, liver disease and vitamin K deficiency are commonly associated with impaired hemostasis.[4,24]

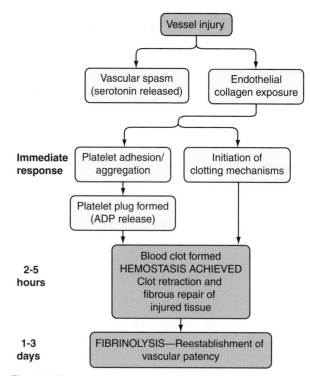

Fig. 17.3 Coagulation physiology. *ADP,* Adenosine diphosphate.

Coagulation Antagonists and Clot Lysis.

Activation of the clotting factors, inhibition of these activated clotting factors, and production of circulating anticoagulant proteins maintain the balance of the coagulation processes. Normal vascular endothelium is smooth and intact, preventing the collagen exposure that initiates the intrinsic clotting pathway. Rapid blood flow dilutes and disperses clotting factors. Clotting factors that are not contained within a formed clot are filtered and removed from circulation by the liver. Several plasma proteins, including antiplasmin and antithrombin III, are present to localize clotting at the site of injury. When coagulation protein levels are deficient, clotting may become inappropriately widespread, such as in disseminated intravascular coagulation (DIC). The most potent anticoagulant forces are the fibrin threads, which absorb 85% to 90% of thrombin during clot formation, and antithrombin III, which inactivates thrombin that is not contained within the clot. Heparin, which is produced in small quantities by basophils and tissue mast cells, acts as a potent anticoagulant. Heparin combines with antithrombin III to increase the effectiveness of the latter. This complex removes several of the activated coagulation factors from the blood.[4]

Once blood vessel integrity has been restored via hemostasis, blood flow must be reestablished. This goal is accomplished by the fibrinolytic system, which breaks down clots (*lysis*) and removes them. *Fibrinolysis* occurs 1 to 3 days after clot formation and is mediated by plasmin, an enzyme that digests fibrinogen and fibrin (Fig. 17.5). The plasma protein plasminogen is the inactive form of plasmin. It is incorporated into the blood clot as the clot forms and cannot initiate clot lysis until it is activated. Substances capable of activating plasminogen include tissue plasminogen activator, thrombin, fibrin, factor XII, lysosomal enzymes, and urokinase.[4] Thrombin and plasmin are key for maintaining the balance between coagulation and lysis.

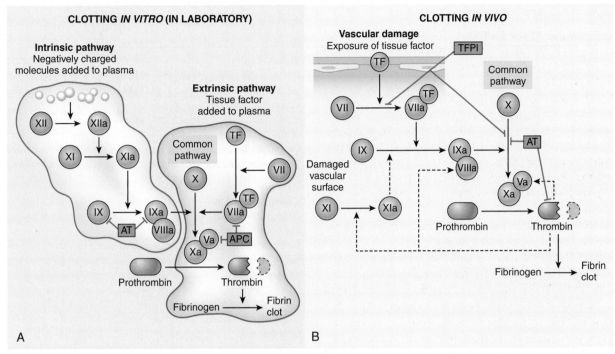

Fig. 17.4 Coagulation pathways. **A,** Classic theory of coagulation in vitro illustrating separate intrinsic and extrinsic pathways. **B,** Coagulation in vivo; clotting initiated by release of tissue factor (TF). *APC,* Antigen-presenting cell; *AT,* antithrombin; *TFPI,* tissue factor pathway inhibitor. (From McCance KL. Structure and function of the hematological system. In: McCance KL, Huether SE, eds. *Pathophysiology: The Biologic Basis for Disease in Adults and Children.* 8th ed. St. Louis, MO: Mosby; 2019:890–925.)

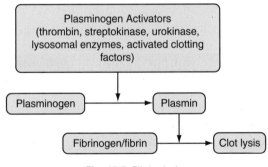

Fig. 17.5 Fibrinolysis.

Fibrinolysis is active within the microcirculation, where it maintains the patency of the capillary beds. Larger vessels contain less plasminogen activator, a characteristic that may predispose them to clot formation.

When plasmin digests fibrinogen, fragments known as *fibrin split products,* or *fibrin degradation products,* are produced and function as potent anticoagulants. In cases of excessive clotting and clot lysis, these molecules contribute to the coagulopathy. Fibrin split products are not normally present in the circulation but are seen in some hematological disorders and with thrombolytic therapy.

FOCUSED ASSESSMENT OF HEMATOLOGICAL AND IMMUNOLOGICAL FUNCTION

An understanding of both normal and disrupted hematological and immunological system activities is paramount to good assessment skills and use of therapeutic interventions. Nursing assessment involves evaluation of risk factors for hematological and immunological alterations, assessment of the patient's concerns, performance of a focused physical examination, and interpretation of pertinent laboratory tests.

Past Medical History

A complete health history includes an assessment of prior medical and surgical problems, allergies, use of medication or homeopathic remedies, and family history. Conditions that may indicate hematological or immunological disorders are presented in Box 17.1.

Evaluation of Patient Concerns and Physical Examination

Inspect the patient's general appearance and assess for signs of fatigue, acute illness, or chronic disease. The most common manifestations of either hematological or immunological disease include indicators of altered oxygenation, bleeding or clotting tendencies, and infection or accentuated immunological activity. The most important assessment parameters for detection of anemia, bleeding, and infection are shown in Table 17.5. Transplantation may be indicated for a variety of hematological or immunological disorders (see Transplant Considerations box).

TRANSPLANT CONSIDERATIONS

Hematopoietic Stem Cell

Indications

Hematopoietic stem cell transplantation (HSCT) may be considered as treatment for a variety of hematological or immunological diseases in which the stem cells do not function properly. These include conditions of abnormal red blood cell (RBC) production (e.g., sickle cell disease), hematological malignancies (e.g., leukemia, lymphoma, myeloma, myelodysplastic syndrome), lack of normal blood cell production (e.g., aplastic anemia), and immune system disorders (e.g., severe combined immunodeficiency syndrome). Transplantation of stem cells may help correct the underlying physiological problem. HSCT is classified by the source of the donor stem cells: bone marrow, peripheral blood stem cells, or umbilical cord blood.

Categories

Allogeneic transplant: patient receives stem cells from a sibling, parent, or unrelated donor (not immunologically identical)

Autologous transplant: patient receives his or her own stem cells after treatment with chemotherapy or radiation

Syngeneic transplant: patient receives stem cells from his or her identical twin (immunologically identical match)

Minitransplant: lower doses of chemotherapy or radiation are administered in preparation for transplantation

Tandem transplant: high-dose chemotherapy and transplantation are performed in two sequential courses

Tissue Typing

Proteins on the surface of leukocytes, called human leukocyte antigens (HLAs), are present on both donor and recipient cells. HLA-matching between donor and recipient is essential for determining an appropriate donor. If the donor's cells are not an adequate match, they will recognize the patient's organs and tissues as foreign and destroy them in a process known as graft-versus-host disease (GVHD). In addition, the patient's immune system may recognize the donor stem cells as foreign and destroy them; this is known as graft rejection. The higher the number of matching HLAs, the greater the chance that the transplantation will be successful.

Complications

Patients receiving HSCT are susceptible to severe infections because of their profoundly immunocompromised state resulting from disease, bone marrow ablation in preparation for transplantation, and the use of immunosuppressive therapy after transplantation to prevent GVHD and graft rejection. Engraftment occurs after transplantation when stem cells repopulate the bone marrow and are able to reconstitute the immune system. Complications occur at any time during the HSCT continuum: from the pre-engraftment stage to day 30 after transplantation; early after engraftment, usually between days 30 and 100; and late after transplantation, more than 100 days after transplantation of donor stem cells.

Complications include bacterial, fungal, protozoal, or viral infections; bleeding; sepsis; GVHD (acute or chronic); hepatic veno-occlusive disease (weight gain, painful hepatomegaly, and jaundice); and respiratory complications. Short-term side effects include nausea, vomiting, fatigue, anorexia, mucositis, alopecia, and skin reactions. Potential long-term risks related to pretransplantation chemotherapy and radiation include infertility, cataracts, new cancers, and damage to major organs.

Data from Antin JH, Raley DY. *Manual of Stem Cell and Bone Marrow Transplantation.* 2nd ed. Cambridge, UK: Cambridge University Press; 2013; National Cancer Institute, National Institutes of Health. Blood-Forming Stem Cell Transplants. https://www.cancer.gov/about-cancer/treatment/types/stem-cell-transplant/stem-cell-fact-sheet. Last reviewed August 2013. Accessed July 4, 2019; and Soiffer RJ. *Hematopoietic Stem Cell Transplantation.* Totowa, NJ: Springer Science & Business Media; 2009.

BOX 17.1   Conditions That May Indicate Hematologic or Immunological Problems[a]

Hematologic Disorders
- Alcohol consumption, excess
- Allergies
- Anemia of any kind
- Benzene exposure (gasoline, dry cleaning chemicals)
- Blood clots
- Delayed wound healing
- Excess bleeding
- Jaundice
- Liver disease
- Medications: allopurinol, antibiotics, anticoagulants, anticonvulsants, antidiabetics, antidysrhythmics, antiinflammatory agents, aspirin derivatives, chemotherapy, histamine blockers
- Neoplastic disease
- Pertinent surgical procedures: hepatic resection, partial or total gastric resection, splenectomy, tumor removal, valve replacement
- Pesticide exposure
- Poor nutrition
- Previous transfusion of blood or blood products
- Radiation: occupational, environmental
- Recurrent infection
- Renal disease
- Substance abuse

Immunological Disorders
- Alcohol consumption, excess
- Allergies
- Anorexia or weight loss
- Bone tenderness or joint pain
- Delayed wound healing
- Diabetes mellitus
- Diarrhea
- Fever
- Liver disease
- Lymphadenopathy
- Medications: antibiotics, antiinflammatory agents, corticosteroids, chemotherapy, immunosuppressives
- Nausea and vomiting
- Neoplastic disease
- Night sweats
- Pertinent surgeries: hepatic resection, lung resection, small bowel resection, splenectomy, tumor removal
- Pesticide exposure
- Poor nutrition
- Previous transfusion of blood or blood products
- Radiation: occupational, environmental
- Recurrent infections
- Renal disease
- Substance abuse

[a]This chart does not correlate specific risks with particular disease conditions because many overlap. History information should be supplemented with physical examination and laboratory test information.

TABLE 17.5 Physical Assessment for Hematological and Immune Disorders

Body System	Anemia	Bleeding	Infection[a]
Neurological	Difficulty concentrating Dizziness Fatigue Somnolence Vertigo	*Bleeding into brain (cerebrum, cerebellum):* alteration in level of consciousness, focal deficits such as unequal pupils or motor movement, headache Bleeding into potential spaces	*Encephalitis:* confusion, lethargy, difficulty arousing, headache, visual difficulty or photosensitivity, nausea, hypertension *Meningitis:* lethargy and somnolence, confusion, nuchal rigidity
Head and neck	Headache Tinnitus	*Bleeding into eye:* visual disturbances, frank hemorrhagic conjunctiva, bloody tears *Bleeding into nasopharyngeal area:* nasal stuffiness, epistaxis *Oral bleeding:* petechiae of buccal mucosa or gums, hemorrhagic oral lesions *Bleeding into subcutaneous tissue of head or neck:* enlarged, bruised areas, raccoon's eyes, bruising	*Conjunctivitis:* reddened conjunctiva, excess tearing of eye, puslike exudates from eye, blurred vision, swelling of eyelid, eye itching *Otitis media:* earache, difficulty hearing, itching inner ear, ear drainage *Sinusitis:* discolored nasal mucus, nasal congestion, face pain, eye pain, blurred vision *Oropharyngeal:* oral ulcerations or plaques, halitosis, reddened gums, abnormal papillae of the tongue, sore throat, difficulty swallowing *Lymphadenitis:* swollen neck lymph glands, tender lymph glands, a lump left when patient swallows
Pulmonary	Air hunger Anxiety Dyspnea Tachypnea	*Alveolar bleeding:* crackles on breath sound assessment, alveolar fluid on radiography, low oxygen saturation *Upper airway bleeding (e.g., trachea, bronchi):* hemoptysis *Pleural space bleeding:* decreased breath sounds, unequal chest excursion	*Bronchitis:* persistent cough, sputum production, gurgles in upper airways, wheezes in upper airways, hypoxemia and/or hypercapnia *Pneumonia:* chest discomfort pronounced with inspiration, persistent cough, sputum production, diminished breath sounds, crackles or gurgles, asymmetrical chest wall movement, labored breathing, nasal flaring with breathing, hypoxemia *Pleurisy:* chest discomfort pronounced with inspiration, sides of chest more painful, usually unilateral discomfort, splinting with deep breaths
Cardiovascular	Clubbing of digits Heart murmur Hypotension Nail beds pale Capillary refill slow Peripheral pulses weak and thready Tachycardia	*Pericardial bleeding:* dyspnea, chest discomfort, hypotension, narrow pulse pressure, muffled heart sounds, increased jugular venous distension *Vascular bleeding:* visible blood, hematoma, or bruising of subcutaneous tissue	*Myocarditis:* dysrhythmias, murmurs or gallops, elevated jugular venous pulsations, weak thready pulses, hypotension, point of maximal impulse shifted laterally *Pericarditis:* constant aching discomfort in the chest unrelieved by rest or nitrates; pericardial rub; muffled heart sounds
Gastrointestinal	Abdominal pain Constipation Splenic enlargement, tenderness	*Upper GI bleeding:* hematemesis, vomiting (coffee-ground appearance) *Lower GI bleeding:* melena *Hepatic or splenic rupture:* acute abdominal pain, abdominal distension, rapid-onset hypotension with hematocrit and hemoglobin *Hemorrhagic pancreatitis:* acute abdominal pain, abdominal distension, hypotension with hematocrit and hemoglobin	*Gastritis:* nausea, vomiting within 30 min after eating, heme-positive emesis, gastric pain that is initially improved by eating *Infectious diarrhea:* more than six loose stools per day, clay-colored or foul-smelling stools, abdominal cramping or distension *Cholelithiasis/pancreatitis:* epigastric pain, intolerance to high-fat meal, clay-colored stools, nausea and vomiting, hyperglycemia, hypocalcemia, ↓ albumin, ↑ lipase and amylase *Hepatitis:* jaundice, right upper quadrant discomfort, hepatomegaly, elevated transaminases and bilirubin, fatty food intolerances, nausea and vomiting, diarrhea
Genitourinary	—	Bladder spasms with distended bladder Hematuria	*Urethritis:* painful urination, difficulty urinating, genitourinary itching *Cystitis:* small frequent urination, feeling of bladder fullness *Nephritis:* flank discomfort, oliguria, protein in urine *Vaginitis:* itching or vaginal discharge
Musculoskeletal	Muscle fatigue Muscle weakness	Altered joint mobility Painful or swollen joints Warm, painful, swollen muscles	*Arthritis:* joint discomfort, swollen and warm joints *Myositis:* aching muscles, weakness

Continued

TABLE 17.5   Physical Assessment for Hematological and Immune Disorders—cont'd

Body System	Anemia	Bleeding	Infection[a]
Dermatological	Cyanosis Jaundice (hemolytic anemia) Pallor Poor skin turgor Skin cool to touch	Bleeding from line insertion sites, puncture wounds, skin tears Ecchymosis Petechiae	*Superficial skin infection:* rashes, itching, raised and/or discolored skin lesions, open-draining skin lesions *Cellulitis:* redness, warmth and swelling of subcutaneous tissue area, radiating pain from area toward middle of body
Hematological/ immunological	—	—	*Bacteremia:* positive blood culture

[a]Signs and symptoms presented in this chart are unique features of each process and do not include the common constitutional signs and symptoms seen with all infections, such as fever, chills, malaise, leukocytosis, positive tissue culture for microorganisms, or increased erythrocyte sedimentation rate.
GI, Gastrointestinal.

Diagnostic Tests

Hematological and immunological abnormalities are usually diagnosed by using the patient's clinical profile in conjunction with a few key laboratory tests. The most invasive microscopic examinations of the bone marrow or lymph nodes are done only if laboratory tests are inconclusive or an abnormality in cellular maturation is suspected (i.e., aplastic anemia, leukemia, or lymphoma).

The first screening diagnostic tests performed are a CBC with differential and a coagulation profile. The CBC evaluates the cellular components of blood.[2,15] The CBC reports the total RBC count and RBC indices, hematocrit, hemoglobin, WBC count and differential, platelet count, and cell morphologies. A summary of common hematological diagnostic laboratory tests, their normal values, and general implications of abnormal findings is shown in Table 17.6 (RBCs and WBCs) and Table 17.7 (coagulation).

SELECTED ERYTHROCYTE DISORDERS

Many pathological conditions affect the erythrocytes, ranging from mild anemias to life-threatening RBC lysis. A decrease in functional RBCs with a resulting oxygenation deficit is termed *anemia;* it is a common problem in critically ill patients. *Polycythemia,* a disorder in which the number of circulating RBCs is increased, is seen less often but can affect hypoxic patients (e.g.,

in chronic obstructive pulmonary disease). It leads to increased blood viscosity and thrombotic complications.

Anemia

Pathophysiology. The term *anemia* refers to a reduction in the number of circulating RBCs or hemoglobin that leads to inadequate oxygenation of tissues. Although symptoms vary depending on the type, cause, and severity of the anemia, the basic clinical findings are the same. As oxygenation delivery is decreased, tissues become hypoxic and 2,3-DPG increases, causing hemoglobin to release oxygen. Blood flow is redistributed to areas where oxygenation is most vital, such as the brain, heart, and lungs. Anemia is described as mild, moderate, or severe based on symptoms, irrespective of actual RBC serum values. Patients are able to adjust and compensate to lower RBC levels when the condition is chronic or slow in onset.

Anemia is classified by its origin or by the microscopic appearance of the RBCs. Hematologists typically use the microscopic classifications (e.g., microcytic, hypochromic), but critical care nurses best plan the nursing care by using the etiological classifications. Causes of anemia include (1) blood loss (acute or chronic), (2) impaired production, (3) increased RBC destruction, or (4) a combination of these.[2] Iron deficiency anemia is the most common type of anemia.[2] The types of anemia are described in Table 17.8.

TABLE 17.6   Functions and Normal Values of Blood Cells

Test	Reason Evaluated	Normal Value	Alterations
RBCs			
Erythrocyte (RBC)	Respiration Oxygen transport Acid-base balance	5 million/mm³	↑ In polycythemia, dehydration ↓ In anemia, fluid overload, hemorrhage
Mean corpuscular volume (MCV)	Average size of each RBC; reflects maturity	80-100/femtoliter	↑ In nutrition deficiency ↓ In iron deficiency
Mean corpuscular hemoglobin (MCH)	Average amount of hemoglobin in each RBC	26-34 picograms	↓ In disorders of hemoglobin production
Mean corpuscular hemoglobin concentration (MCHC)	Average concentration of hemoglobin within a single RBC	31%-38%	↓ In cells with hemoglobin deficiency
Reticulocyte count	Immature RBCs released when suddenly in demand	1%-2% of total RBC count	↑ In recent blood loss or with chronic hemolysis

TABLE 17.6 Functions and Normal Values of Blood Cells—cont'd

Test	Reason Evaluated	Normal Value	Alterations
RBCs—cont'd			
Serum folate	Amount of available vitamin for RBC development	95-500 mcg/mL	↓ In malnutrition or folic acid deficiency
Serum iron level	Iron stores within the body	40-160 mcg/dL	↓ With inadequate iron intake or inadequate absorption (e.g., gastric resection)
Total iron binding capacity (TIBC)	Reflection of liver function and nutrition	250-400 mcg/dL	↓ In chronic illness (e.g., infection, neoplasia, cirrhosis)
Ferritin level	Precursor to iron; reflects body's ability to create new iron stores	15-200 ng/mL	↓ Levels demonstrate inability to regenerate iron stores and hemoglobin
Transferrin level	Protein that binds to iron for removal or recirculation after RBCs are hemolyzed	200-400 mg/dL	↓ With excess hemolysis
Haptoglobin level	Protein that binds with heme for removal or recirculation after RBCs are hemolyzed	40-240 mg/dL	↓ With excess hemolysis
WBCs			
Leukocytes (WBCs)	Inflammatory and immune responses Defend against infection, foreign tissue	4500-11,000/ mm³	↑ In inflammation, tissue necrosis, infection, hematological malignancy ↓ In bone marrow depression (e.g., radiation, immune disorders), chronic disease
Granular Leukocytes			
Neutrophils	Polymorphonuclear neutrophils Phagocytosis of invading organisms	50%-70% of WBCs	↑ In inflammation, infection, surgery, myocardial infarction ↓ In aplastic anemia, in hepatitis, with some pharmacological agents
Eosinophils	Defend against parasites; detoxification of foreign proteins Phagocytosis	1%-5% of WBCs	↑ In allergic attacks, autoimmune diseases, parasitic infections, dermatological conditions ↓ In stress reactions, severe infections
Basophils	Release heparin, serotonin, and histamine in allergic reactions; inflammatory response	0-1% of WBCs	↑ After splenectomy and with hemolytic anemia, radiation, hypothyroidism, leukemia, chronic hypersensitivity ↓ In stress reactions
Nongranular Leukocytes			
Monocytes	Mature into macrophages; phagocytosis of necrotic tissue, debris, foreign particles	1%-8% of WBCs	↑ In bacterial, parasitic, and some viral infections; chronic inflammation ↓ In stress reactions
Lymphocytes	Defend against microorganisms	20%-40% of WBCs	↑ In bacterial and viral infections, lymphocytic leukemia ↓ In immunoglobulin deficiency
B lymphocytes	Humoral immunity and production of antibodies	270-640/mm³	↑ In bacterial and viral infections, lymphocytic leukemia ↓ In immunoglobulin deficiency, stress
T lymphocytes	Cell-mediated immunity	500-2400/mm³	↓ With chemotherapy, immunodeficiencies, HIV disease, end-stage renal disease, immunosuppressive medications
Platelets			
Thrombocytes (platelets)	Blood clotting; hemostasis	150,000-400,000/mm³	↑ In polycythemia vera, after splenectomy, with certain cancers ↓ In leukemia, bone marrow failure, DIC, hemorrhage, hypersplenism, radiation exposure, large foreign bodies in blood (e.g., aortic balloon pump), hypothermia, hyperthermia, severe infection

DIC, Disseminated intravascular coagulation; *RBCs*, red blood cells; *WBCs*, white blood cells.

TABLE 17.7 Common Coagulation Profile Studies

Test	Normal Value	Critical Value	Comments
Activated clotting time (ACT)	70-120 sec Therapeutic range for anticoagulation: 150-600 sec	Not specified	Used to monitor heparin therapy and detect clotting factor deficiencies.
Activated partial thromboplastin time (aPTT)	30-40 sec	>70 sec	Used to monitor heparin therapy and detect clotting factor deficiencies. ↑ With anticoagulation therapy, liver disease, vitamin K deficiency, DIC
Prothrombin time (PT) International normalized ratio (INR)	11-12.5 sec 0.8-1.1 INR Therapeutic range for anticoagulation: 1.5-2.0 times control value	PT >20 sec INR >5	Evaluates extrinsic pathway; used to monitor oral anticoagulant therapy ↑ With warfarin therapy, liver disease, vitamin K deficiency, obstructive jaundice
Fibrinogen level	200-400 mg/dL	<100 mg/dL associated with spontaneous bleeding	↓ In DIC and fibrinogen disorders ↑ In acute infection, in hepatitis, with oral contraceptive use
Fibrin degradation products (FDPs)	<10 mcg/mL	>40 mcg/mL	Evaluates hematologic disorders ↑ In DIC, fibrinolysis, thrombolytic therapy
Fibrin D-dimer	<0.4 mcg/mL	Not specified	Presence diagnostic for DIC
Platelet count	150,000-400,000/mm³	<20,000/mm³	Measures number of circulating platelets ↓ In thrombocytopenia
Platelet aggregation test	Varies; 3-5 min	Not specified	Measure of platelet function and aids in evaluation of bleeding disorders Prolonged in von Willebrand disease, acute leukemia, idiopathic thrombocytopenic purpura, liver cirrhosis, aspirin use
Calcium Ionized calcium	9-10.5 mg/dL 4.5-5.6 mg/dL	<6.0 mg/dL <2.2 mg/dL	↓ With massive transfusions of stored blood

DIC, Disseminated intravascular coagulation.
From Pagana KD, Pagana TJ. *Mosby's Manual of Diagnostic and Laboratory Test.* 6th ed. St. Louis, MO: Elsevier; 2018.

Assessment and Clinical Manifestations. Signs and symptoms of anemia begin gradually and initially include fatigue, weakness, and shortness of breath.[2,21] Signs and symptoms are related to three physiological effects of reduced RBCs: (1) decreased circulating volume caused by loss of RBC mass, (2) decreased oxygenation of tissues resulting from reduced hemoglobin binding sites, and (3) compensatory mechanisms implemented by the body in its attempt to improve tissue oxygenation. Decreased circulating volume is manifested by clinical findings reflective of low blood volume (e.g., low right atrial pressure) and the effects of gravity on the lack of volume (e.g., orthostasis). Tissue hypoxia from inadequate oxygen delivery results in compensatory activities, including an increased depth and rate of respiration to increase oxygen availability, tachycardia to increase oxygen delivery, and the shunting of blood away from nonvital organs to perfuse the vital organs.[2,21] Inadequate oxygenation of the tissues leads to organ dysfunction.

In addition to the general symptoms of anemia, unique disorders have their own classic clinical features. The patient with *aplastic anemia* may have bruising, nosebleeds, petechiae, and a decreased ability to fight infections. These effects result from thrombocytopenia and decreased WBC counts, which occur when the bone marrow fails to produce blood cells. Assessment of the patient with *hemolytic anemia* may reveal jaundice, abdominal pain, and enlargement of the spleen or liver. These findings result from the increased destruction of RBCs, their sequestration (abnormal distribution in the spleen and liver,[24]

and the accumulation of breakdown products. Patients with *sickle cell anemia* may have joint swelling or pain and delayed physical and sexual development. In crisis, the sickle cell patient often has decreased urine output, peripheral edema, and signs of uremia because renal tissue perfusion is impaired because of sluggish blood flow.

Laboratory findings in anemia include a decreased RBC count and decreased hemoglobin and hematocrit values. The reticulocyte count is usually increased, indicating a compensatory increase in RBC production with release of immature cells. Patients with hemolytic anemia also have an increased bilirubin level. In sickle cell disease, a stained blood smear reveals sickled cells. In aplastic anemia, the reticulocyte, platelet, RBC, and WBC counts are decreased because the marrow fails to produce any cells.

Medical Interventions. Medical treatment is focused on identifying and treating the cause of the anemia. Supplemental oxygen and blood component therapy may be required to support the cardiovascular system. In anemia associated with blood loss, initial treatment is with IV administration of volume expanders (crystalloid or colloid) and/or transfusion of packed RBCs. Products that stimulate erythropoietin production may be ordered. For certain types of anemia, cause-specific interventions may be indicated. Splenectomy may be performed for hemolytic anemia, and bone marrow transplantation (BMT) may be preferred for refractory aplastic anemia. In sickle cell disease,

TABLE 17.8 Anemias

	Marrow Failure to Produce RBCs Aplastic Anemia	Hemolytic Anemia	Sickle Cell Anemia (Hemolytic Subtype)	Vitamin B₁₂ Deficiency	Folic Acid Deficiency	Iron Deficiency
Pathophysiology	Disorder or bone marrow toxin damages the erythrocyte precursors, leading to ↓ RBC production	Stimulus causes extrasplenic destruction of the RBC, leading to hemolyzed RBC fragments in the circulating bloodstream; cell fragments ↑ blood viscosity and slow blood flow, leading to ischemia and/or infarction. Extrasplenic hemolysis also leads to ↑ levels of circulating bilirubin and unbound iron.	Presence of abnormal Hgb causes RBCs to assume a sickle or crescent shape. Sickling alters the blood viscosity, leading to microvascular occlusion; sickling crisis leads to hypoxia, thrombosis, and infarction in tissues and organs.	Pernicious anemia is caused by decreased gastric production of HCl and intrinsic factor, which play a role in vitamin B₁₂ absorption.	Malabsorption of dietary folic acid results from lack of intake or absorption.	Body's iron stores are inadequate for RBC development; Hgb-deficient RBCs result.
Etiology	Disorder or bone marrow toxin damages hematopoietic stem cells and results in ↓ production of RBCs, WBCs, and platelets.	*Abnormal RBC membrane or Hgb:* Anemia of chronic disease Hereditary RBC shape disorders Paroxysmal nocturnal hemoglobinuria Porphyria Sickle cell disease G6PD deficiency Thalassemias *Immune reaction:* Autoimmune hemolytic syndrome BMT hemolytic transfusion reaction Autoimmune diseases *Physical damage to RBCs:* Blunt trauma Extracorporeal circulation Prosthetic heart valves Thermal injury *Unknown:* IgA deficiency Cocaine use Snake or spider bite	Hereditary hemolytic anemia caused by abnormal amount of hemoglobin S in relation to hemoglobin A	Familial incidence related to autoimmune response with gastric mucosal atrophy Higher incidence in autoimmune disorders: SLE, myxedema, Graves disease Common in Northern Europeans; rare in children and black and Asian populations Occurs postoperatively with gastric surgery	Common in infants, adolescents, pregnant and lactating women, alcoholic patients, older adults, cancer, intestinal disease (jejunitis, small bowel resection), prolonged use of anticonvulsants or estrogens, excessive cooking of foods	Present in 10%-30% of all American adults; primarily from dietary deficiency Also in pregnant and lactating women, infants, adolescents Malabsorption such as diarrhea, gastric resection, blood loss, or intravascular hemolysis
	Disorders: Bone metastases *Medications:* Chemotherapy agents Antiretroviral agents *Toxic exposures:* Radiation to long bones					
	Disorders: Immune suppression Transplantation Pregnancy Vitamin B₁₂ deficiency *Viral infection:* EBV, CMV *Medications:* Anticonvulsants Antidysrhythmics Antiinflammatory agents Chloramphenicol Quinines *Toxic exposures:* Benzene Arsenic Herbicides, insecticides Lacquers; paint thinners Radiation exposure Toluene (glue)					
Nursing Implications	Monitor diet and medications that interfere with marrow production of cells[22] High risk of infection and bleeding; implement bleeding precautions Administer transfusions cautiously; exposure to antigens may enhance rejection if BMT is required later.	Begin plasma reinfusion at a rate of 25 mL/h for 15 min, then 100 mL/h. Assess for hypersensitivity. Assess for fluid shifts into the interstitial spaces during infusion or within 6-12 h after infusion. Monitor for vomiting, pain at infusion site, diarrhea.	Incurable, although severity remains consistent throughout lifetime Common cause of death is intracranial thrombosis or hemorrhage.	Lifetime treatment requires ongoing patient teaching. Heart failure prevention Special oral hygiene Monitor for persistent neurological deficits.	Foods high in folic acid: beef, liver, peanut butter, red beans, oatmeal, asparagus, broccoli	Monitor for allergic reactions to iron. Give oral supplements with straw to prevent staining teeth; causes skin irritation and iron deposits.

Continued

TABLE 17.8 Anemias—cont'd

	Marrow Failure to Produce RBCs / Aplastic Anemia	Hemolytic Anemia	Sickle Cell Anemia (Hemolytic Subtype)	Vitamin B12 Deficiency	Folic Acid Deficiency	Iron Deficiency
Clinical Presentation	$\downarrow$ Production of cells in the earliest phase: bone marrow failure resulting in low RBC count Signs and symptoms are those common in profound anemia	Symptoms of infection, bleeding, and anemia occur simultaneously; earliest symptoms are usually the result of WBC dysfunction. Platelet production abnormalities lead to bleeding symptoms within 7-10 days, followed by symptoms of anemia.	Rapid hemolysis of RBCs leads to spleen uptake with enlarged and tender spleen; metabolism of RBCs often leads to excess bilirubin with jaundice and itching.	Hyperviscosity and poor perfusion (e.g., altered mentation, hypoxemia) sickled cells removed from circulation, causing enlarged and tender spleen; long-term sickling and thrombosis causes $\downarrow$ joint mobility, gut dysfunction, cardiac failure, and risk for stroke	Inhibited growth of all cells: anemia, leukopenia, thrombocytopenia Demyelination of peripheral nerves to spinal cord Triad: weakness, sore tongue, paresthesias	Similar to vitamin B12 deficiency but without neurological symptoms *Signs:* poor oxygenation, dizziness, irritability, dyspnea, pallor, headache, oral ulcers, tachycardia	Classic: "pica" (desire to eat nonfood items), ice or dirt cravings *Cardiovascular/respiratory compromise:* hypoxia, fatigue, headache, cracks in mouth corners, smooth tongue, paresthesias, neuralgias
Diagnostic Tests	CBC used as screening test Bone marrow aspiration and biopsy confirm maturation failure	CBC used as screening test Bone marrow aspiration and biopsy reflect absence of precursor or stem cells	Reticulocytes usually ≥4% total RBC count ↑ Total bilirubin ↑ Direct bilirubin ↓ Transferrin ↓ Haptoglobin	Hgb electrophoresis abnormality	Schilling test ↓ Hgb and RBC ↑ MCV ↓ MCHC ↓ WBC ↓ Platelets ↑ LDH	Macrocytosis Serum folate <4 mg/dL Abnormal platelet appearance ↑ Reticulocyte count	↓ Hct and Hgb ↓ Iron level with ↑ binding capacity ↓ Ferritin level ↓ RBC with hypochromia and microcytes ↓ MCHC
Management	Erythropoietin per dosing guidelines (Procrit, Aranesp)	Eliminate cause Bone marrow stimulants Corticosteroids Immunosuppressive agents for autoimmune process Chelating (iron binding) agents Limit transfusions when possible to ↓ risk of rejection Allogeneic BMT	Staphylococcal protein A is capable of trapping IgG complexes that are thought to cause RBC autoantibodies. If autoantibodies are present, give immunosuppressive agents. Administer antiplatelet medications (e.g., salicylic acid).	Administer large volumes of IV fluids to dilute viscous blood. Oxygen therapy reduces sickling. Treat infections early. Manage extreme pain (result of ischemia); Gene transplants used experimentally	Vitamin B12 30 mcg IM or deep SC for 5-10 days then 100-200 mcg IM or deep SC every month	Folic acid 0.25-1 mg/day PO	Ferrous sulfate 325 mg PO tid and ascorbic acid to aid absorption

BMT, Bone marrow transplantation; *CBC,* complete blood count; *CMV,* cytomegalovirus; *EBV,* Epstein-Barr virus; *G6PD,* glucose-6-phosphate dehydrogenase; *HCl,* hydrochloride; *Hct,* hematocrit; *Hgb,* hemoglobin; *IgA,* immunoglobulin A; *IgG,* immunoglobulin G; *IM,* intramuscular; *LDH,* lactate dehydrogenase; *MCHC,* mean corpuscular hemoglobin concentration; *MCV,* mean corpuscular volume; *PO,* orally; *RBCs,* red blood cells; *SC,* subcutaneously; *SLE,* systemic lupus erythematosus; *tid,* three times daily; *WBCs,* white blood cells.

oxygenation and correction of dehydration are important for the prevention or reversal of erythrocyte sickling.

Nursing Care. Nurses address problems common to the anemic patient. Problems vary and may include low cardiac output, decreased tissue perfusion, and altered gas exchange; risk for bleeding; fatigue and decreased exercise tolerance; pain; and skin alterations.

The patient problems and interventions from the Collaborative Plan of Care for the Critically Ill Patient in Chapter 1 apply and are tailored to the patient with anemia.

Nursing management of anemia is based on a continuous, thorough nursing assessment and the prescribed medical treatment. Monitor vital signs, the electrocardiogram, hemodynamic parameters, heart and lung sounds, and peripheral pulses to assess tissue perfusion and gas exchange. In addition, assess mental status, urine output, and skin color and temperature. Be alert for tachycardia and orthostatic hypotension, indicators that the patient's cardiovascular system is not adequately compensating for the anemia. Provide comfort measures to prevent or treat pain, and monitor closely for signs of infection. Institute bleeding precautions if the patient is at risk for further blood loss.

Interventions for patients at risk for bleeding or infection are discussed later in this chapter. Carefully monitor laboratory results, such as the CBC. Other vital nursing interventions include promoting rest and oxygen conservation; administering blood components, medication therapy, and IV fluids; and monitoring the patient's responses to the therapy. The desired goal of treatment and nursing intervention is optimal tissue perfusion, oxygenation, and gas exchange.

 CRITICAL REASONING ACTIVITY

Why is the critical care unit often a dangerous place for the immunosuppressed patient?

WHITE BLOOD CELL AND IMMUNE DISORDERS

Many pathological conditions are classified as WBC or immune disorders. They may involve the WBCs themselves or other complementary immune processes. The immune system can fail to develop properly, lose its ability to react to invasion by pathogens, overreact to harmless antigens, or turn immune functions against self. Regardless of the cause, WBC and immune disorders or their treatments suppress the mechanisms needed for inflammation and combating infection. Because the clinical features and complications are similar among a variety of disorders, this first section addresses general causes, signs and symptoms, and management of immunological suppression. This is followed by in-depth discussions of specific WBC and immune disorders.

The Immunocompromised Patient

Pathophysiology. The *immunocompromised* patient is one who has defined quantitative or qualitative defects in WBCs or immune physiology. The defect may be congenital or acquired,

and it may involve a single element or multiple processes. Regardless of the cause, the physiological outcome is immune incompetence—lack of normal inflammatory, phagocytic, antibody, or cytokine responses. Immune incompetence is often asymptomatic until pathogenic organisms invade the body and create infection. Infection is the leading cause of death in immunocompromised patients.

Assessment and Clinical Manifestations. The risk for infection is the primary clinical problem for those with immune compromise. A detailed database containing the patient's history, physical examination findings, and laboratory studies is paramount for rapid detection of infection.

Immunocompromise in the critically ill is caused by many factors. In addition to existing immunodeficiency disease and life-threatening illness, immune defenses are altered by invasive procedures, inadequate nutrition, and the presence of opportunistic pathogens. Many of the medications and treatments administered in critical care depress the patient's immune system. Evaluate the patient's medical and social history, current medications, and risk factors for infection (Table 17.9). Immunosuppressed patients do not respond to infection with typical signs and symptoms of inflammation (see Clinical Alert box).

CLINICAL ALERT

Infection in Immunocompromised Patients

Immunocompromised patients do not have typical signs and symptoms of infection.
- Erythema, swelling, and exudate formation are usually not evident.
- Symptoms of infection may be absent, masked, or present atypically.
- Fever is considered the cardinal and sometimes the only symptom of infection. However, some patients with infection do not have a fever.
- Patients are also more likely to describe pain at the site of infection, although physical inflammatory signs may be absent.

Laboratory results that reflect leukopenia, low CD4 counts, and decreased immunoglobulin levels may demonstrate disorders of immune components.[2] A common test of the humoral (antibody) response to antigens is a skin test with intradermal injection of typical pathogens capable of initiating an antibody response. Absence of a "wheal" tissue response to the antigens (called tissue *anergy*) is evidence of altered antibody capabilities.

Patient Problem. The primary problem for the immunocompromised patient is decreased immunity with potential for systemic and local infection.

Medical Interventions. In *primary immunodeficiencies*, B-cell and T-cell defects are treated with specific replacement therapy or BMT. These treatments aim to reverse the cause of the immune dysfunction and prevent infectious complications. If the serum IgG level is less than 300 mg/dL, an infusion of immunoglobulin may be ordered to reverse the cause of the immune dysfunction. Gene replacement therapy is an emerging treatment for selected disorders.

TABLE 17.9 Risk Factors for Infection in the Immunocompromised Patient

Patient Characteristic	Physiological Mechanism of Risk of Infection
Host Characteristics	
Alcoholism	↓ Neutrophil activity Hepatic/splenic congestion also slows phagocytic response
Abuse of IV drugs	Chronic altered barrier defense leads to reduced WBCs and slowed phagocytic responses Constant viral exposure may also alter T-cell function
Aging	*Slowed phagocytosis:* bacterial infection, more rapid dissemination of infection *Slowed macrophage activity:* more fungal infection, more visceral infection *Atrophy of thymus:* ↑ risk of viral illness ↓ *Antigen-specific immunoglobulins:* diminished immune memory
Frequent hospitalizations	Frequent exposure to environmental organisms other than own normal flora Potential exposure to resistant organisms and other people's organisms through cross-contamination.
Malnutrition	*Inadequate WBC count:* infection ↓ *Neutrophil activity:* bacterial infection, at risk of infection *Impaired phagocytic function:* bacterial infection *Impaired integumentary/mucosal barrier:* general infection risk ↓ *Macrophage mobilization:* risk of fungal or rapidly disseminating infection ↓ *Lymphocyte function:* ↑ risk of viral and opportunistic infection Thymus and lymph node atrophy with iron deficiency
Stress	Induces ↑ release of adrenal hormones (cortisol), which causes ↓ circulating eosinophils and lymphocytes
Immune Defects and Disorders	
Lymphopenia	↓ Antibody response to previously exposed antigens ↓ Recognition and destruction of viral and opportunistic organisms
Macrophage dysfunction or destruction	Altered response to fungi Inadequate antigen-antibody response Greater potential for visceral infection
Neutropenia	Inadequate neutrophils to combat pathogens (especially bacteria)
Splenectomy	Inability to recognize and remove encapsulated bacteria (e.g., streptococcus) Compromised reticuloendothelial system and ↓ antibodies lead to frequent and early bacteremia
Disease Processes	
Burns	Physiological stressor thought to ↓ phagocytic responses Altered barrier defenses allowing pathogen entry Protein loss through skin leads to malnutrition-related immunocompromise
Cancer	Structural disruption may lead to bone marrow or lymphatic abnormalities Certain cancers have specific immune defects (e.g., diminished phagocytic activity, T-cell defects) Radiation therapy destroys lymphocytes and causes shrinkage of lymphoid tissue Chemotherapy causes ↓ lymphocytes and alters proliferation and differentiation of stem cells
Cardiovascular disease	Inadequate tissue perfusion slows WBC response to tissue with pathogenic organism
Diabetes mellitus	↓ Numbers of neutrophils Hyperglycemia causes ↓ phagocytic activity and immunoglobin defects Vascular insufficiency leads to slowed phagocytic response to pathogens Neuropathy and glycosuria predispose to ↓ bladder emptying and urinary tract infections
Gastrointestinal disease	↓ Bowel motility allows normal flora to translocate across the gastrointestinal wall to the bloodstream
Hepatic disease	↓ Neutrophil count
Infectious diseases	↓ Phagocytic activity Hypermetabolism with infection accelerates phagocytic cell use and death Certain viral and opportunistic infections ↓ bone marrow production of WBCs
Pulmonary disease	Inadequate oxygenation suppresses neutrophil activity
Renal disease	↓ Neutrophil activity caused by uremic toxins ↓ Immunoglobulin activity
Traumatic injuries	Altered barrier defenses allowing pathogen entry Type of infection depends on source and severity of injury (e.g., soil or water contamination, skin flora)

TABLE 17.9 Risk Factors for Infection in the Immunocompromised Patient—cont'd

Patient Characteristic	Physiological Mechanism of Risk of Infection
Medications and Treatments	
Antibiotics	Normal flora destroyed, enhanced resistant organism growth, fungal superinfection
Immunosuppressive agents and corticosteroids	↓ Phagocytic activity Altered T-cell recognition of pathogens, especially viruses ↓ Interleukin-2 production leads to increased risk of malignancy ↓ IgG production Lack of immune memory to recall antibodies to previously encountered pathogens
Invasive devices	Altered barrier defenses allowing entry of pathogens, especially skin organisms
Surgical procedures/wounds	Normal flora may be translocated by surgical procedure Altered barrier defenses caused by surgical entry Stress of surgery and anesthetic agents reduces neutrophil activity
Transfusion of blood products	Risk of transfusion-transmitted infections undetected by donor screening: cytomegalovirus, hepatitis, HIV Exposure to foreign antigens in blood products causes T-lymphocytic immune suppression and increases risk of infection

IgG, Immunoglobulin G; *WBC,* white blood cell.

In *secondary immunodeficiencies,* the underlying causative condition is treated. For example, malnutrition is corrected, or doses of immunosuppressive medications are adjusted. Risk factors for infection are carefully assessed and avoided. For example, assess the need for invasive lines and use meticulous sterile technique when managing lines. Prophylactic antimicrobial agents are ordered during the period of highest risk for infection. For example, patients receiving bone marrow–suppressing cancer chemotherapy receive broad-spectrum antimicrobials when their WBC count is lowest. Patients who have HIV infection or are recovering from organ transplantation have defined CD4 or immune suppression levels that place them at risk for specific infections.[9] These patients often receive antimicrobial prophylaxis against infections with herpes simplex, *Candida albicans, Pneumocystis jirovecii, Mycobacterium avium-intracellulare, Mycobacterium tuberculosis,* and cytomegalovirus.

Nursing Intervention. Nursing interventions focus on protecting the patient from infection. Provide a protective environment to reduce the risk of infection. High-efficiency particulate air (HEPA) filtration of the air and laminar airflow in single-patient rooms is recommended to prevent infection with airborne microorganisms.

Hand washing is paramount for staff, patients, and visitors. Nursing staff members play an important role in ensuring skin integrity and sterile technique when procedures are unavoidable. Other important hygiene measures include general bathing with antimicrobial soaps, oral care, and perineal care.

General health promotion including adequate fluid, nutrition, and sleep is important in bolstering the patient's defenses against infection. Dietary restriction, such as prohibiting raw fruits and vegetables, is controversial and not standardized.[23]

Nursing interventions are presented in the Plan of Care for the Immunocompromised Patient.

Neutropenia

Pathophysiology. Neutropenia is defined as an absolute neutrophil count of less than 1500 cells/mm^3 of blood. Neutropenia occurs as a result of inadequate production or excess destruction of neutrophils. Patients with low neutrophil counts are predisposed to infections because of the body's reduced phagocytic ability.[2,6] Neutropenia is classified based on the patient's predicted risk for infection: mild (1000 to 1500 cells/mm^3), moderate (500 to 1000 cells/mm^3), and severe (<500 cells/mm^3).[2]

Assessment and Clinical Manifestations. Obtain a thorough medical and social history to identify risk factors for neutropenia. Common causes include acute or overwhelming infections, radiation exposure, exposure to chemicals and medications, or other disease states (Box 17.2).

No specific signs or symptoms indicate a low neutrophil count; therefore it is essential to evaluate the patient carefully for risk factors for neutropenia and clinical findings consistent with infection. Many patients describe fatigue or malaise that coincides with the drop in counts and precedes infectious signs and symptoms.

Examine every body system for physical findings of infection. Typical signs may not be evident. Pain such as sore throat or urethral discomfort may be indicative of an infected site. Areas of heavy bacterial colonization (e.g., oral mucosa, perineal area, venipuncture and catheter sites) have the highest risk of infection; however, the most common clinical infections are sepsis and pneumonia. Additional signs or symptoms of systemic infection include a rise in temperature from its normal set point, chills, and accompanying tachycardia.

◎ PLAN OF CARE

For the Immunocompromised Patient

Patient Problem

Decreased Immunity/Potential for Systemic and Local Infection. Risk factors include immunocompromise or immunosuppression, invasive procedures, and presence of opportunistic pathogens.

Desired Outcomes
- Absence of fever, redness, swelling, pain, and heat.
- WBC and differential, urinalysis, and cultures within normal limits.
- Chest radiographic study without infiltrates.
- Absence of adventitious breath sounds.

Nursing Assessments/Interventions	Rationales
• Establish baseline assessment with documented history, physical examination, and laboratory study results.	• Establish trends to guide and monitor treatment.
• Follow universal precautions, including hand hygiene.	• Decrease risk of infection.
• Plan nurses' assignments to reduce the possibility of infection spread between patients.	• Decrease spread of infection.
• Be careful handling secretions and excretions that are known to be infected.	• Prevent cross-contamination.
• Monitor visitors for any recent history of communicable diseases.	• Prevent infection.
• Clean all multipurpose equipment (e.g., oximeter probes, noninvasive BP cuffs, bed scale slings, electronic thermometers) between uses.	• Prevent cross-contamination.
• Assess patient for signs and symptoms of infection.	• Guide early recognition and treatment
• Monitor vital signs and temperature at least every 4 hours; report and investigate any elevation in temperature; rectal temperatures are not recommended.	• Assess for infection.
• Monitor laboratory results: WBC and differential, blood, urine, sputum, wound, and throat cultures.	• Assess for infection.
• Report abnormal results.	
• Note the presence of chills, tachycardia, oliguria, or altered mentation that may indicate sepsis; report subtle changes to physician.	• Assess for infection.
• Encourage incentive spirometry and change of position every 1-2 hours.	• Prevent atelectasis.
• Avoid breaks in the skin and mucous membranes:	• Maintain intact skin—the first line of defense.
• Change position every 2 hours; avoid wetness.	
• Provide skin lubricants and moisture barriers as indicated.	
• Provide meticulous oral and bathing hygiene.	
• Use strict aseptic technique for dressing changes.	• Prevent infection.
• Avoid stopcocks in IV systems; use closed injection of site systems.	• Stopcocks can harbor bacteria and are an entry site for any infectious agent.
• Limit invasive devices and procedures whenever possible.	• Decrease risk for infection.
• Use private room; limit visitors; limit fresh flowers and standing water.	• Fresh flowers have a potential to introduce pathogenic organisms.
• Ensure that sleep needs are being met.	• Enhance resistance to infection and aid in healing.
• Control glucose levels.	• Hyperglycemia compromises phagocytic activity.
• Change oxygen setups with humidification (e.g., nasal cannula) every 24 hours.	• Prevent bacterial growth.
• Obtain cultures for first fever (38.0°C; temperature measured twice, 4 hours apart) and for new fever (38.3°C) after 72 hours on an antimicrobial regimen:	• Identify site(s) of infections and guide antimicrobial treatment.
• Blood cultures from two different sites.	
• Blood cultures from existing venous/arterial access devices.	
• Urine culture.	
• Sputum culture, if obtainable.	
• Stool culture, if obtainable.	
• Culture of open lesions or wounds.	
• Administer antimicrobial therapy as ordered.	• Treat infection and assess effectiveness of antibiotics.
• Measure antimicrobial peak and trough levels as ordered.	
• Be alert to superinfection with fungal flora any time 7-10 days after initiation of antibiotics.	• Assess complications of antibiotic therapy; oral or topical nystatin may be indicated.

⊚ PLAN OF CARE—cont'd

For the Immunocompromised Patient

Patient Problem

Weight Loss. Risk factors include NPO status; anorexia, nausea, and vomiting; and painful oral mucosa.

Desired Outcomes

- Adequate caloric and protein intake.
- Ideal or stable body weight.
- Laboratory values remain within normal limits (total protein, serum albumin, electrolytes, hemoglobin, and hematocrit).

Nursing Assessments/Interventions	Rationales
• Assess baseline nutritional status:	• Obtain baseline assessment.
• Height and weight	
• BMI	
• Laboratory values	
• Assess presence of weakness	
• Fatigue	
• Infection	
• Other signs of malnutrition	
• Obtain dietary consultation to determine nutrients and intake required.	• Optimize nutritional therapy to reduce risks.
• Administer enteral or parenteral nutritional therapy as ordered and observe response.	
• Establish food preferences, encourage meals from home, and provide relaxed atmosphere during meals.	• Tailor nutritional support based on patient's preferences.
• Determine deterrents to adequate intake:	• Assess risks for decreased nutrition.
• Fasting (NPO) status	
• Presence of anorexia, nausea, vomiting, stomatitis.	
• Monitor daily weight, laboratory values, protein and caloric intake, and I&O.	• Monitor nutritional status.
• Encourage small, frequent, high-calorie, and high-protein meals.	• Promote adequate intake.
• Provide meticulous mouth care before and after meals.	• Maintain oral mucosa and facilitate oral intake.
• Administer antiemetics as needed, 30 min before meals.	• Encourage adequate intake.

BMI, Body mass index; *BP,* blood pressure; *I&O,* intake and output; *NPO,* nothing by mouth; *WBC,* white blood cell.
Adapted from Swearingen PL, Wright JD. *All-in-One Nursing Care Planning Resource.* 5th ed. St. Louis, MO: Elsevier; 2019.

BOX 17.2 Causes of Neutropenia

Malnutrition
- Calorie deficiency
- Deficiency of iron, protein, and/or Vitamin B

Health States
- Addison disease
- Anaphylactic shock
- Brucellosis
- Chronic fever or illness
- Cirrhosis
- Diabetes mellitus
- Older age
- Hypothermia
- Infection (any severe bacterial or viral disease)
- Renal trauma

Medications and Substances
- Alcohol
- Alkylating agents, antineoplastic and immunosuppressive (e.g., cyclophosphamide)
- Allopurinol (Zyloprim)
- Anticonvulsants (e.g., phenytoin)
- Antidysrhythmics (e.g., procainamide, quinidine)
- Antimicrobials (e.g., aminoglycosides, chloramphenicol, sulfonamides, trimethoprim-sulfamethoxazole)
- Antiretroviral agents (e.g., zidovudine)
- Antitumor antibiotics (e.g., bleomycin, doxorubicin [Adriamycin])
- Arsenic
- Phenothiazines (e.g., prochlorperazine)

Absolute neutrophil count. The diagnostic test indicated when neutropenia is suspected is the WBC count with differential. The differential demonstrates the percentage of each type of WBC circulating in the bloodstream. Calculate the absolute neutrophil count by multiplying the total WBC count (without a decimal point) times the percentages (with decimal points) of polymorphonuclear leukocytes (polys; also called segs or neutrophils) and bands (immature neutrophils):

$$WBC \times (segs + bands) \times 100$$

This gives a number that is translated into the categories of mild, moderate, or severe neutropenia.

Patient Problem. The specific problem related to all patients with neutropenia is potential for systemic and local infection.

Medical Intervention. Medical treatment of neutropenia is aimed at preventing and treating infection while reversing the cause of the neutropenia. Patients with anticipated neutropenia, such as those receiving antineoplastic or antiretroviral therapy, may be given bone marrow growth factors. Also known as *colony-stimulating factors* (CSFs), these agents enhance bone marrow regeneration of granulocyte colony-stimulating factor (G-CSF), macrophage colony-stimulating factor (M-CSF), or both cell lines (GM-CSF).[2,11]

Prophylactic antiinfective agents may be ordered to prevent infection, and potent broad-spectrum antimicrobial agents are ordered when there is evidence of infection. In sepsis accompanying neutropenia, granulocyte transfusions are occasionally used to supplement phagocytosis.

Nursing Intervention. Nursing care of patients with neutropenia is the same as for all immunocompromised patients (see Plan of Care for the Critically Ill Patient with Potential for Decreased Immunity or Infection in Chapter 1). Desired patient outcomes related to medical and nursing interventions include absence of infection, negative cultures, and an absolute neutrophil count of 1500 cells/mm³ or higher.

Malignant White Blood Cell Disorders: Leukemia, Lymphoma, and Multiple Myeloma

Pathophysiology. Malignant diseases involving WBCs are termed leukemia, lymphoma, or plasma cell neoplasm (multiple myeloma). They are differentiated by the cell type affected and by the stage of cell development when malignancy occurs. Regardless of the specific neoplastic disorder, deficiency of functional WBCs is a common problem. The unique pathophysiological and clinical characteristics of these disorders are described in Table 17.10. Despite normal serum cell counts, WBC activity is always impaired, and infection is the most common complication in all these disorders.

Assessment and Clinical Manifestations. Malignant hematological diseases have common risk factors such as genetic mutations (see Genetics box); viral infection (especially retroviral); exposure to radiation, carcinogens, benzene derivatives, or pesticides; and T-lymphocyte immune suppression (e.g., high-dose steroids, immunosuppressive medications after transplantation). Other risk factors that are unique to specific malignancies are included in Table 17.10.

Assessment findings common to all malignant WBC disorders involve alterations in the immunological response to injury or microbes. As in other disorders affecting WBC function, minimized inflammatory reactions and responses to pathogens are typical. Fever is particularly difficult to interpret; it may be a manifestation of the disease process or may accompany an infectious complication. General signs and symptoms such as fatigue, malaise, myalgia, activity intolerance, and night sweats are nonspecific indicators of immune disease. Each malignant WBC disorder is also associated with signs and symptoms representative of the cell line and location of the malignancy. For example, bone pain is common in multiple myeloma, whereas lymph node enlargement is more representative of lymphoma.[18] When symptoms overlap into more than one component of the immune system, it is often difficult to differentiate among these disorders.

Knowledge of oncological emergencies associated with these malignant diseases is also important. Oncological emergencies may be a consequence of the cancer itself or of a specific treatment plan (see Table 17.10). These complications are likely to precipitate admission to the critical care unit and are associated with significant morbidity and mortality.

Patient Problems. The patient problems associated with hematological malignancies vary. Common problems include an increased risk for infection, decreased tissue perfusion, and risk for bleeding.

Medical Intervention. Each major subtype of hematological malignancy is associated with slightly different presenting symptoms, prognostic variables, and treatment implications. The treatment plan is based on the stage of the definitive diagnosis established by histopathology.

Therapy commonly includes chemotherapy and biotherapy. BMT is used in selected cases. Surgery may be performed to establish a pathological diagnosis by excisional or incisional biopsy, but it has no other significant role in the management of hematological malignancies. Radiation may be used to treat lymphoma if the disease is limited to a single node or node group.

The complexity of treatment is illustrated in the following examples. Leukemia is considered a *systemic* disease at diagnosis. Treatment of acute leukemia requires a complex chemotherapy treatment plan called *induction* chemotherapy, and it is associated with a period of severe cytopenia that requires supportive care and transfusion therapy. The management of chronic myelogenous leukemia has been improved with the development of imatinib mesylate (Gleevec), an oral agent that results in high remission rates.[14] Therapy for multiple myeloma involves careful staging and a choice of induction chemotherapy plans, leading to autologous stem cell transplantation for most patients. Radiation therapy is used palliatively to control the pain associated with bone lesions. Because of the rapid application of advances in molecular biology, there has been a dramatic improvement in remission and cure rates for most hematological malignancies.

Nursing Intervention. The care of patients with hematological malignancies is similar to that for all immunocompromised patients; however, specialized management of cancer therapies must be incorporated into the individual care plan. Oncology nursing references for chemotherapy administration guidelines, management of nausea and vomiting related to acute therapy, and oncological treatment modalities are available from the Oncology Nursing Society (ONS) at https://www.ons.org/.

? CRITICAL REASONING ACTIVITY

How can therapeutic choices such as interventions and medications worsen the hematological or immunological compromise of critically ill patients?

🧬 GENETICS

Factor V Leiden: An Inherited Clotting Disorder

Thrombophilia describes an increased tendency to form abnormal blood clots within blood vessels. Abnormal clotting leads to venous thromboembolism (VTE) or deep vein thrombosis (DVT) and pulmonary embolism (PE). The most common inherited thrombophilia is factor V Leiden, an autosomal dominant disorder.[2]

The genetic variation in coagulation factor V Leiden is a missense mutation.[4] A missense mutation results in *F5* coding for a substitute amino acid during the translation of DNA to a protein. Although 12 mutations for factor V have been identified, only 8 are considered pathological.[8] People with factor V Leiden thrombophilia have a greater risk of developing VTE. Women with factor V Leiden are more likely to experience miscarriage because of thrombophilia, particularly during the second or third trimester.

Factor V is a clotting factor, essential in the conversion of prothrombin to thrombin in the clotting cascade. The clotting cascade has proteins that not only start the clotting process but also slow or stop the process so that clots do not grow large or abnormally. Activated protein C inactivates factor V. Among people with factor V Leiden thrombophilia, the genetic defect results in an inability to stop factor V–induced clotting.[4] When prolonged clotting continues, abnormal blood clots form. Increasing age, obesity, injury, smoking, surgery, pregnancy, and estrogen-based medications can enhance the risk of developing abnormal blood clots in people with factor V Leiden thrombophilia. The interaction of a genetic polymorphism with other factors as with factor V Leiden thrombophilia is an example of multifactorial genetic conditions—the gene-environment interactions—that can influence the onset, severity, or manifestations of a genetic condition. To illustrate, there is a 30-fold increased risk for VTE among women who use hormonal contraceptives or hormone replacement therapy or who are pregnant when they have factor V thrombophilia.[1]

Factor V Leiden disease leads to a gain in function; clotting is enhanced. Individuals with two copies of the *F5* gene—a homozygous inheritance—experience a 10-fold decrease in the inactivation of factor V. Reduced inactivation of factor V results in persistent procoagulation signaling. Compared to noncarriers, heterozygous inheritance (a single copy of the gene) leads to a three- to fivefold increased risk of VTE throughout the lifespan.

Like most inherited diseases, assessing genetic risk starts with obtaining a personal and family history. If two or more first-degree relatives were diagnosed with unprovoked VTE in a three-generation family tree, consider this a significant indicator of *F5* genetic disease. An unprovoked VTE (i.e., *not* associated with cancer, immobility, surgery, or trauma) should lead to further serum analysis such as prothrombin time, activated partial thromboplastin time, antithrombin activity, protein C activity, and free protein S.[6] The incidence of factor V Leiden mutation occurs too infrequently to recommend routine genetic screening.[2]

There is no test of routine serum factors to identify the presence of factor V Leiden disease, since the condition occurs only when factor V is activated. Prothrombin genotyping may be done simultaneously with the factor V Leiden

genotyping to identify the etiology of unprovoked VTE.[1,4] Genotypic tests, completed with serum analyses of clotting-related factors, are sometimes labeled a thrombotic screen. A positive genetic test for factor V Leiden has several clinical implications. Clinicians may offer long-term anticoagulation to reduce future thrombotic events, although there is limited evidence to support the exact duration of therapy.[7] Managing thrombophilia during pregnancy requires specialized knowledge and close monitoring.

Clinicians need to be aware of the legal and ethical implications of offering a genetic test.[3] In the United States, the Genetic Information Nondiscrimination Act (GINA) bans genetic discrimination related to health insurance eligibility and coverage, regulating employers.[3] The Affordable Care Act also prevents insurers from declining coverage based on preexisting genetic conditions in most employees.[3] The results of an individual genetic test shared with relatives can have an impact on relationships and perception of health. Uncertainty around the risk versus manifestation of a condition can be confusing and fraught with misinterpretation by patients, their family members, and clinicians. Direct-to-consumer genetic testing is widely available (e.g., 23andMe, Ancestry).[5] However, the nuances around interpretation of genetic results and meaningful support for decisions to seek treatment are not generally provided by commercial self-pay services. Nurses and advanced practice nurses need to build and use knowledge of genomic testing for a variety of conditions to counsel patients and advocate for clear communication about genomic, personalized health care.

Genetic terms: *missense, translation, heterozygous, homozygous, autosomal recessive, genotype, multifactorial, gain in function mutation, legal and ethical implications of genetic testing, GINA*

References
1. Applegate JS, Gronefeld D. Factor V Leiden. *Radiol Technol.* 2019;90(3):259–273.
2. Carroll BJ, Piazza G. Hypercoagulable states in arterial and venous thrombosis: When, how, and who to test? *Vasc Med.* 2018;23(4):388–399.
3. Lough ME, Seidel GD. Legal and clinical issues in genetics and genomics. *CNS.* 2015;29(2):68–70.
4. McCance KL, Rate NS. Alterations of erythrocyte, platelet, and homostatic function. In: McCance KL, Huether SE, eds. *Pathophysiology.* 8th ed. St. Louis, MO: Elsevier; 2019:926–962.
5. National Human Genome Institute. Direct-to-Consumer Genomic Testing. https://www.genome.gov/27570940/april-20-directtoconsumer-genomic-testing/. Published February 13, 2019. Accessed February 27, 2019.
6. Pagana KD, Pagana TJ. *Mosby's Manual of Diagnostic and Laboratory Tests.* St. Louis, MO: Elsevier; 2018.
7. Prandoni P, Barbar S, Milan M, et al. Optimal duration of anticoagulation: Provoked versus unprovoked VTE and role of adjunctive thrombophilia and imaging tests. *Thromb Haemost.* 2015;113(6):1210–1215.
8. US National Library of Medicine. Genetics Home Reference Factor V Leiden Thrombophilia. http://ghr.nlm.nih.gov/condition/factor-v-leiden-thrombophilia. Published March 5, 2019. Accessed February 27, 2019.

SELECTED IMMUNOLOGICAL DISORDERS

Primary Immunodeficiency

In primary immunodeficiencies, the dysfunction exists in the immune system. Most primary immunodeficiencies are congenital disorders related to a single gene defect. The onset of symptoms may occur within the first 2 years of life or in the second or third decade of life. These defects of the immune system typically result in frequent or recurrent infections and sometimes predispose the affected individual to unusual or severe infections.[17] Disorders are grouped by the specific immunological disruption.

Secondary Immunodeficiency

Secondary or acquired immunodeficiencies result from factors outside the immune system; they are not related to a genetic defect and involve loss of a previously functional immune defense system. AIDS is the most notable secondary immunodeficiency disorder caused by an infection. Aging, dietary insufficiencies, malignancies, stressors (emotional, physical), immunosuppressive therapies, and certain diseases such as diabetes or sickle cell disease are additional conditions that may be associated with acquired immunodeficiencies. Risk factors for infections in immunocompromised patients are described in Table 17.9.

TABLE 17.10 Malignant White Blood Cell Disorders

Leukemia	Lymphoma	Multiple Myeloma
Pathophysiology		
Cancer involving any of the WBCs during the early phase of maturation within the bone marrow	Cancer affecting the lymphocytes after their bone marrow maturation, when they reside within the lymph node	Cancer involving the mature and differentiated immunoglobulin-producing macrophage called a plasma cell; the malignancy is primarily manifested by excess abnormal immunoglobulin
Classification		
Acute leukemia: excess proliferation of immature cells *Chronic leukemia:* excess proliferation of mature cells Leukemias are further classified according to whether they originate in the lymphocyte cell line or are nonlymphocytic.	Hodgkin and non-Hodgkin subtypes have more sub-classifications denoting the maturity of the cell involved and the aggressiveness of the malignancy.	Disease is classified as limited or extensive depending on plasma viscosity, bone manifestations, presence of hypercalcemia, and renal involvement.
Risk Factors		
Chromosomal abnormalities Viral infection Radiation Herbicides and pesticides Benzene and toluene Immunosuppressive therapy	Chromosomal abnormalities Alkylating agents Viral infection Radiation Herbicides and pesticides Benzene and toluene Immunosuppressive therapy Alkylating agents Autoimmune disease	Older age Male gender African American descent Chronic hypersensitivity reactions Autoimmune diseases
Clinical Manifestations		
Fever *Constitutional symptoms:* fatigue, malaise, weakness, night sweats Easy bruising and bleeding from mucous membranes (e.g., gums) Bone pain	Enlarged (>2 cm), nontender lymph node(s) Usually immovable and irregularly shaped Masses in body cavities or other organs (e.g., peritoneal cavity, lungs)	*Thrombotic events:* deep vein thrombosis, pulmonary embolism, cerebral infarction Bone pain Renal failure
Acute Complications		
Leukostasis DIC Tumor lysis syndrome	Airway obstruction Superior vena cava syndrome Bowel obstruction Neoplastic tamponade Pleural effusion	Hyperviscosity Renal failure Hypercalcemia
Staging		
All patients are viewed as having systemic disease or late-stage disease.	Classified by number of lymph nodes involved, number of lymph node groups, whether involved nodes are only above the diaphragm or on both sides of the diaphragm, and how many extranodal sites are involved	Disease is classified as limited when there are only elevated abnormal immunoglobin levels; it is described as extensive when there are bone lesions, hypercalcemia, or renal dysfunction
Diagnostic Tests		
CBC shows either ↓ WBCs or large number of immature WBCs (blasts), ↓ RBCs, ↓ platelets Bone marrow aspiration and biopsy	Lymph node biopsy CT scans Chemistry: alkaline phosphatase	Bence Jones protein in urine Immunoglobulin electrophoresis Plasma viscosity

TABLE 17.10 Malignant White Blood Cell Disorders—cont'd

Leukemia	Lymphoma	Multiple Myeloma
Medical Management		
Systemic chemotherapy BMT	Radiation therapy for single node or node group if above the diaphragm for control or remission Radiation used if palliation of tumor is the goal of therapy Systemic chemotherapy for multinode involvement, aggressive tumor subtypes Autologous BMT for patients with high risk of relapse Allogeneic BMT for patients with residual disease, especially involving bone marrow	Systemic chemotherapy provides an average of only 14-36 months of remission BMT or "double" BMT may increase survival Radiation therapy used to palliatively treat bone lesions
Nursing Care Issues		
Infection control practices Bleeding precautions	Infection control practices Edema management Monitoring for lymphoma masses compressing body organs	Infection control practices Safe mobility Thrombosis precautions Aspiration precautions if hypercalcemic

BMT, Bone marrow transplant; *CBC*, complete blood count; *CT*, computed tomography; *DIC*, disseminated intravascular coagulation; *RBCs*, red blood cells; *WBCs*, white blood cells.

AIDS and HIV

Pathophysiology. HIV is a retrovirus that transcribes its RNA-containing genetic material into the DNA of the host cell nucleus by using an enzyme called reverse transcriptase.[9] HIV causes AIDS by depleting helper T cells, CD4 cells, and macrophages.[1]

Seroconversion is manifested by the presence of HIV antibodies and usually occurs 2 to 4 weeks after the initial infection.[9] Seroconversion is associated with flulike symptoms such as fever, sore throat, headache, malaise, and nausea that usually last 1 to 2 weeks.[2] This is followed by a decrease in the HIV antibody titer as infected cells are sequestered in the lymph nodes. The earlier stages of HIV infection may last for as long as 10 years and may produce few or no symptoms, although viral particles are actively replacing normal cells. This phenomenon is evident through the decreasing CD4 cell count as the disease progresses.[2] As the CD4 cell count decreases, the patient becomes more susceptible to opportunistic infections, malignancies, and neurological disease. AIDS is the final stage of HIV infection. Fig. 17.6 shows the progression of disease and common clinical manifestations. It is estimated that 99% of untreated HIV-infected individuals will progress to AIDS.[2] Treatment with combined antiviral medication regimens can control the progression to AIDS, which is now considered, for many infected individuals, a chronic disease.

HIV is transmitted through exposure to infected body fluids, blood, or blood products.[9] Common modes of transmission include rectal or vaginal intercourse with an infected person; IV drug use with contaminated equipment; transfusion with contaminated blood or blood products; and accidental exposure through needlesticks, breaks in the skin, and gestation or childbirth (transmission from mother to fetus). Risk of transmission is more likely when the infected person has advanced disease, although transmission of HIV can occur at any time or during any stage of infection. Since the 1980s, all blood products are screened for HIV, hepatitis virus, and human T-cell lymphotropic virus. The risk of HIV transmission to healthcare workers is low.

Assessment and clinical manifestations. The initial phase of HIV disease may be asymptomatic or may manifest as an acute seroconversion syndrome with symptoms similar to those of mononucleosis. This is followed by asymptomatic disease as HIV progressively destroys immune cells.[9] AIDS is defined by the presence of a CD4 count lower than $200/mm^3$ and the presence of an indicator condition2 (see Fig. 17.6).

Diagnosis of HIV infection is based on the presence of one of the core antigens of HIV or the presence of antibodies to HIV. Core antigens are tested through protein electrophoresis. HIV antibodies are detected by enzyme-linked immunosorbent assay (ELISA) and are confirmed by the Western blot test and polymerase chain reaction (PCR).[15] Positive antibody test results are accurate for the presence of HIV infection, although a negative test result does not rule out HIV infection. Additional laboratory findings in AIDS may include an abnormal helper-to-suppressor T-cell ratio (<1.0), leukopenia, and thrombocytopenia.

Patient problems. Nursing care of the patient with AIDS is complex, and nursing care is tailored to the clinical manifestations of the disease. Patient problems commonly associated with AIDS may include decreased gas exchange, decreased immunity and potential for systemic infection, diarrhea, weight loss, delirium or decreased memory, acute and chronic pain, fatigue, and need for health teaching.

Medical intervention. Medical treatment consists of primary control of HIV invasion of CD4 cells through antiretroviral therapy. Antiretroviral medications are categorized as nucleoside reverse transcriptase inhibitors, nonnucleoside reverse transcriptase inhibitors, and protease inhibitors. The specific agents used and the most appropriate strategies of combination therapy are a rapidly evolving field.

Equally important to quality of life are prevention and management of opportunistic infections. Antimicrobials are administered to prevent high-risk opportunistic infections when predefined CD4 levels are reached. Additional treatment

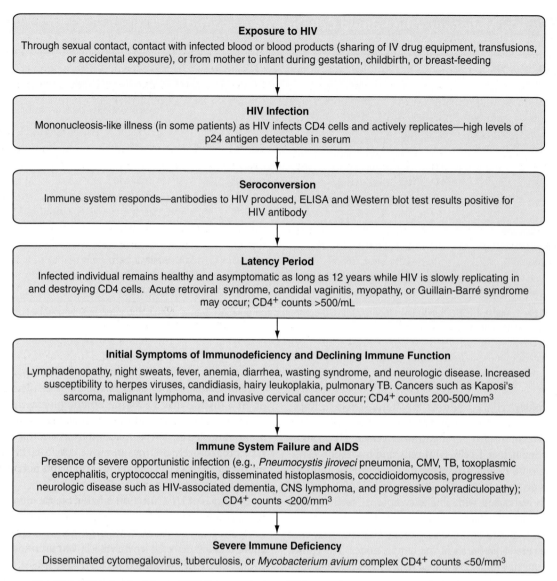

Exposure to HIV
Through sexual contact, contact with infected blood or blood products (sharing of IV drug equipment, transfusions, or accidental exposure), or from mother to infant during gestation, childbirth, or breast-feeding

HIV Infection
Mononucleosis-like illness (in some patients) as HIV infects CD4 cells and actively replicates—high levels of p24 antigen detectable in serum

Seroconversion
Immune system responds—antibodies to HIV produced, ELISA and Western blot test results positive for HIV antibody

Latency Period
Infected individual remains healthy and asymptomatic as long as 12 years while HIV is slowly replicating in and destroying CD4 cells. Acute retroviral syndrome, candidal vaginitis, myopathy, or Guillain-Barré syndrome may occur; CD4$^+$ counts >500/mL

Initial Symptoms of Immunodeficiency and Declining Immune Function
Lymphadenopathy, night sweats, fever, anemia, diarrhea, wasting syndrome, and neurologic disease. Increased susceptibility to herpes viruses, candidiasis, hairy leukoplakia, pulmonary TB. Cancers such as Kaposi's sarcoma, malignant lymphoma, and invasive cervical cancer occur; CD4$^+$ counts 200-500/mm^3

Immune System Failure and AIDS
Presence of severe opportunistic infection (e.g., *Pneumocystis jiroveci* pneumonia, CMV, TB, toxoplasmic encephalitis, cryptococcal meningitis, disseminated histoplasmosis, coccidioidomycosis, progressive neurologic disease such as HIV-associated dementia, CNS lymphoma, and progressive polyradiculopathy); CD4$^+$ counts <200/mm^3

Severe Immune Deficiency
Disseminated cytomegalovirus, tuberculosis, or *Mycobacterium avium* complex CD4$^+$ counts <50/mm^3

Fig. 17.6 HIV pathophysiology. *CMV,* Cytomegalovirus; *CNS,* central nervous system; *ELISA,* enzyme-linked immunosorbent assay; *TB,* tuberculosis.

may include respiratory support, nutritional support, administration of blood products or IV fluids, administration of analgesics, and physical therapy.

Nursing interventions. Nursing care of patients with HIV infection requires complex assessment and intervention skills. Evaluate the neurological status, mouth, respiratory status, abdominal symptoms, and peripheral sensation. As with all immunosuppressed patients, protect those with HIV infection from infection with other pathogens (see Plan of Care for the Immunocompromised Patient). These patients provide additional clinical challenges because of their multisystem clinical complications. Carefully monitor response to medications; persons with HIV infection have a higher propensity for adverse medication reactions than other patient groups.

Desired patient outcomes of medical treatment and nursing interventions include absence of infection, adequate oxygenation, adequate nutrition and hydration, skin integrity, and absence of pain. Complications such as diarrhea and seizures

are controlled. Last, reinforce the understanding the patient has of disease transmission; the course of the disease; and symptoms of opportunistic infections, treatments, and medications.

BLEEDING DISORDERS

Patients with abnormal hemostasis often require critical care treatment. A general approach to assessing and managing the bleeding patient is included, followed by a more thorough discussion of thrombocytopenia and DIC.

The Bleeding Patient

Pathophysiology. Bleeding disorders, also referred to as *coagulopathies,* are caused by abnormalities in one of the stages of clotting. Disorders may be inherited (e.g., hemophilia, von Willebrand disease) or acquired (e.g., vitamin K deficiency, DIC).[16] Coagulopathies induce bleeding manifestations, and many care principles are universal. This section addresses the universal care of patients with disorders of coagulation.

Assessment and Clinical Manifestations. A patient with abnormal bleeding requires a careful medical and social history. Assess for medical disorders and medications known to interfere with platelets, coagulation proteins, or fibrinolysis. Disruptions in hemostasis commonly occur with renal disease, hepatic or gastrointestinal disorders, or malnutrition. Medications that may alter hemostasis include aminoglycosides, anticoagulants, antiplatelet agents, cephalosporins, histamine blockers, nitrates, sulfonamides, sympathomimetics, and vasodilators.

The physical examination is extremely important. Although many patients with bleeding disorders demonstrate active bleeding from body orifices, mucous membranes, and open lesions or IV line sites, equal numbers of patients have less obvious bleeding. The most susceptible sites for bleeding are existing openings in the epithelial surface. Mucous membranes have a low threshold for bleeding because the capillaries lie close to the membrane surface, and minor injury may damage and expose vessels. Substantial blood loss can occur in any coagulopathy, resulting in hypovolemic shock. A general overview of assessment findings that indicate bleeding is included in Table 17.5.

Diagnostic tests are performed to evaluate the cause of the bleeding disorder and the extent of blood loss.[2] The CBC provides quantitative values for RBCs and platelets. When the disorder arises from coagulation protein or clot lysis abnormalities, screening coagulation tests for fibrinogen level, prothrombin time (PT), and activated partial thromboplastin time (aPTT) are usually ordered. Point-of-care tests for hemoglobin, hematocrit, and aPTT are important resources to obtain immediate feedback on the patient's status. In certain disease states, the results of additional specialized tests, such as bleeding time and level of fibrin degradation products, are monitored.

A thromboelastogram (TEG) is a newer non-invasive that quantitatively measures the ability of the blood to form a clot. The test is done to identify hypercoagulable states, identify accelerated fibrinolysis, and to assess function of platelets and coagulation factors.[15] Results may be used to guide treatment. Table 17.11 provides information about TEG.

Patient Problems. A patient with a hemostatic disorder can have bleeding in any body system. The major patient problems include potential for bleeding and hypovolemic shock, potential for skin and tissue breakdown, and acute pain (see Plan of Care for the Patient With a Bleeding Disorder in this chapter and Plan of Care for the Patient in Shock in Chapter 12).

Medical Intervention. Medical treatment for bleeding patients depends on the suspected cause. Component-specific replacement transfusions are preferred over whole blood because they provide more targeted treatment of the bleeding disorder. Transfusion thresholds are established based on laboratory values and patient-specific variables. In general, the threshold for RBC transfusion is a hematocrit of 28% to 31%, based on the patient's cardiovascular tolerance (see Evidence-Based Practice box). If angina or orthostasis is present, a higher threshold may be maintained. The threshold for transfusing platelets is usually between 20,000 and 50,000/mm^3 of blood. Cryoprecipitate is usually infused if the fibrinogen level is lower than 100 mg/dL.[15] Fresh frozen plasma is used to correct a prolonged PT and aPTT or a specific factor deficiency.[15] A summary of blood product components, clinical indications, and nursing implications is included in Table 17.12.

When the cause of bleeding is unknown or multifactorial, nonspecific interventions aimed at stopping bleeding are used. These include local and systemic procoagulant medications and therapies. Local therapies to stop bleeding are used when systemic anticoagulation is necessary for treatment of another health condition (e.g., myocardial infarction, ischemic stroke, pulmonary embolism). Local procoagulants act by direct tissue contact and initiation of a surface clot.

Systemic procoagulant medications may be used judiciously to enhance vasoconstriction (e.g., vasopressin), enhance clot formation (e.g., somatostatin), or prevent fibrinolysis (e.g., aminocaproic acid). Each agent has significant adverse effects that must be considered before implementation. All may enhance clot production and induce thrombotic vascular or neurological events. They may be contraindicated if the patient has simultaneous procoagulant risk factors.

TABLE 17.11 Thromboelastogram (TEG) Parameters

Parameter	Clotting Phase Assessed	Normal Values	Implications
Reaction time (R)	Activation—time to activate the intrinsic pathway and initiate clot (amplitude 2 mm)	5-10 min	Dependent on clotting factors Prolonged R time may indicate need for FFP
Kinetics (K)	Amplification—time to form a clot with a certain level of strength (amplitude 20 mm)	1-3 min	Dependent on fibrinogen Prolonged time may indicate need for FFP or cryoprecipitate
Alpha angle (A)	Propagation—characterization of maximal speed of thrombus generation, fibrin deposition, and coss-linking)	53-72 degrees	Dependent on fibrinogen Narrow angle may indicate need for cryoprecipitate and/or platelets
Maximum amplitude (MA)	Termination—maximal strength of the clot; measures amplitude of TEG curve	50-70 min	Dependent on platelets and interaction of fibrin with clotting factors GPIIb/IIa Low amplitude may indicate need for platelets
Lysis at 30 min (A30 or LY30)	Fibrinolytic—speed of fibrinolysis	0-8%	Represents fibrinolysis Higher percentage may indicate need for tranexamic acid

FFP, Fresh frozen plasma.

Adapted from Shaydakov M, Blebea J. Thromboelastography (TEG). *Stat Pearls.* Treasure Island, FL: Stat Pearls Publishing, 2020 (https://www.ncbi.nlm.nih.gov/books/NBK537061/).

Nursing Intervention. Patients with bleeding disorders often have multisystem manifestations. Administration of fluids and blood products is a priority nursing intervention that requires careful consideration of the patient's specific coagulation defect. If the patient's blood does not clot because of thrombocytopenia, administration of RBCs before platelets will result in RBC loss from disrupted vascular structures.

Additional nursing interventions specific to the patient with a coagulopathy include weighing dressings to assess blood loss, assessing fluids for occult blood, observing for oozing and bleeding from skin and mucous membranes, and leaving clots undisturbed. Precautions such as limiting invasive procedures (including indwelling urinary catheters and rectal temperature measurement) are also important.

◎ PLAN OF CARE

For the Patient with a Bleeding Disorder

Patient Problem
Potential for Bleeding/Hemorrhage due to depletion of clotting factors or platelets.

Desired Outcomes
- Absence of bleeding.
- Stable vital signs.
- Oriented to person, place, and time; no changes in mental status.

Nursing Assessments/Interventions	Rationales
• Regularly assess LOC and monitor vital signs.	• Changes in mentation and vital signs can indicate hemorrhage.
• Prevent excess pressure when taking BP.	• Frequent BP readings can cause bleeding under the cuff.
• Assess for abdominal pain and distension.	• May indicate GI bleeding.
• Assess stool, urine, vomitus, and nasogastric drainage for occult blood.	• Bleeding initially may be undetectable.
• Regularly assess puncture sites.	• May detect external bleeding.
• Post "bleeding precautions" sign.	• Alert all caregivers to the potential for bleeding to use caution when implementing care and treatments.
• Ensure no administration of rectal medications, IM injections, or flossing of teeth.	• Prevent disruption in skin and mucous membranes.
• Recognize signs and symptoms of subcutaneous bleeding (e.g., oozing, ecchymoses, hematomas).	• Assess for bleeding disorders.
• Administer blood products as ordered.	• Correct deficiencies.
• Administer procoagulants (e.g., somatostatin, estrogen) as ordered.	• Promote clotting and decrease bleeding.
• Administer topical hemostatic agents if indicated.	• Decrease bleeding from skin lesions.

Patient Problem
Potential for Skin and Tissue Breakdown due to altered circulation.

Desired Outcome
- Skin and tissue remain intact.

Nursing Assessments/Interventions	Rationales
• Regularly assess skin and mucous membranes for changes.	• Changes in color, sensation, and temperature may occur.
• Reposition patient every 2 hours; provide good skin and oral care.	• Promote circulation.
• Keep extremities warm.	• Prevent tissue hypoxia and improve circulation.
• Elevate any limb that is bleeding.	• Reduce blood flow to the area to prevent further blood loss.
• Use alternatives to tape for dressings.	• Tape can damage fragile skin.

BP, Blood pressure; *GI,* gastrointestinal; *IM,* intramuscular; *LOC,* level of consciousness.
Data from Swearingen PL, Wright JD. *All-in-One Nursing Care Planning Resource.* 5th ed. St. Louis, MO: Elsevier; 2019.

TABLE 17.12 Summary of Blood Products and Administration

Blood Component	Description	Actions	Indications	Administration	Complications
Whole blood	RBCs, plasma, and stable clotting factors	Restores oxygen-carrying capacity and intravascular volume	Symptomatic anemia with major circulating volume deficit Massive hemorrhage with shock	Donor and recipient must be ABO and Rh compatible Use microaggregate filter *Rate of infusion:* 2-4 units/h but more rapid in cases of shock	Hemolytic reaction Allergic reaction Hypothermia Electrolyte disturbances Citrate intoxication Infectious diseases

TABLE 17.12 Summary of Blood Products and Administration—cont'd

Blood Component	Description	Actions	Indications	Administration	Complications
RBCs	RBCs centrifuged from whole blood	Restores oxygen-carrying capacity and intravascular volume	Symptomatic anemia when patient is at risk for fluid overload Acute hemorrhage	Donor and recipient must be ABO and Rh compatible Use microaggregate filter *Rate of infusion:* 2-4 units/h but more rapid in cases of shock	Infectious diseases Hemolytic reaction Allergic reaction Hypothermia Electrolyte disturbances Citrate intoxication
Leukocyte-poor cells or washed RBCs	RBCs from which leukocytes and plasma proteins have been reduced	Restores oxygen-carrying capacity and intravascular volume	Symptomatic anemia with patient history of repeated, febrile, nonhemolytic transfusion reactions Acute hemorrhage	Donor and recipient must be ABO and Rh compatible Use microaggregate filter *Rate of infusion:* 2-4 units/h but more rapid in cases of shock	Allergic reaction Hemolytic reaction Hypothermia Electrolyte disturbances Citrate intoxication Infectious diseases
Fresh frozen plasma	Plasma rich in clotting factors with platelets removed	Replaces clotting factors	Deficit of coagulation factors as in DIC, liver disease, and massive transfusions Major trauma with signs or symptoms of hemorrhage	Donor and recipient must be ABO compatible, but it is not necessary to be Rh compatible *Rate of infusion:* 10 mL/min	Allergic reaction Febrile reactions Circulatory overload Infectious diseases
Platelets	Removed from whole blood	Increases platelet count and improves hemostasis	Thrombocytopenia Platelet dysfunction (prophylactically for platelet counts 10,000-20,000/mm³), evidence of bleeding with platelet count <50,000/mm³	Do not use microaggregate filter; use component filter obtained from blood bank ABO testing is not necessary but is usually done Usually 6 units are given at one time	Infectious diseases Allergic reactions Febrile reactions
Cryoprecipitate antihemophilic factor	Coagulation factor VIII with 250 mg of fibrinogen and 20%-30% of factor XIII	Replaces selected clotting factors	Hemophilia A, von Willebrand disease Hypofibrinogenemia Factor XIII deficiency Massive transfusions	Repeat doses may be necessary to attain desired serum level *Rate of infusion:* approximately 10 mL of diluted component per minute	Allergic reactions Infectious diseases
Albumin	Prepared from plasma	Expands intravascular volume by increasing oncotic pressure	Hypovolemic shock Liver failure	Special administration set *Rate of infusion:* over 30-60 min	Circulatory overload Febrile reaction
Granulocytes	Prepared by centrifugation or filtration leukopheresis, which removes granulocytes from whole blood	Increases the leukocyte level	Decreased WBCs usually from chemotherapy or radiation	Must be ABO and Rh compatible *Rate of infusion:* 1 unit over 2-4 h; closely observe for reaction	Rash Febrile reaction Hepatitis
Plasma proteins	Pooled from human plasma	Expands intravascular volume by increasing oncotic pressure	Hypovolemic shock	ABO compatibility not necessary *Rate of infusion:* over 30-60 min	Circulatory overload Febrile reaction

DIC, Disseminated intravascular coagulation; *RBCs,* red blood cells; *WBCs,* white blood cells.

Thrombocytopenia

Pathophysiology. A quantitative deficiency of platelets is called *thrombocytopenia.* By definition, this is a platelet count of less than 150,000/mm³.[10,15] A value of 30,000/mm³ is considered critically low, and spontaneous bleeding may occur.[15] Fatal hemorrhage is a great risk when the count is lower than 10,000/mm³.[3] The pathophysiology may be related to decreased production of platelets by the bone marrow, increased destruction of platelets, or sequestration of platelets (abnormal distribution).[10,21]

Assessment and Clinical Manifestations. Many critical care therapies and medications interfere with platelet production and cause thrombocytopenia. A thorough medical, social, and medication history can help identify factors that can cause thrombocytopenia (Box 17.3). Heparin-induced thrombocytopenia (HIT) can occur and is described in Box 17.4.[2,10]

Clinically, the presenting symptoms of thrombocytopenia are petechiae, purpura, and ecchymosis, with oozing from mucous membranes. The patient may also have melena, hematuria, or epistaxis.

EVIDENCE-BASED PRACTICE

Red Blood Cell Transfusion

Problem

Transfusion of red blood cells (RBCs) is not a benign procedure. It is associated with complications, including transfusion reactions and acute lung injury. Determining clinical indicators for transfusion, including thresholds, is important.

Clinical Question

What outcomes are associated with RBC transfusions? What clinical indicators and thresholds should be used to trigger transfusion orders?

Evidence

The systematic review by Carson and colleagues evaluated 31 trials involving 12,587 patients across clinical specialties. About half used a 7 g/dL threshold, and the others used a transfusion threshold range of 8 to 9 g/dL. Participants who were assigned to receive blood at lower blood counts were 43% less likely to receive a blood transfusion than those who were given blood at higher thresholds. The risk of dying within 30 days of the transfusion did not differ between groups.

The authors concluded that it was not harmful to the participants' health status to give blood at lower or higher blood counts. The amount of blood patients received and the risk of patients receiving blood transfusions unnecessarily would be substantially reduced. Because transfusions can have harmful effects, the safety implications are appreciated.

Implications for Nursing

The transfusion of RBCs can be avoided in most patients with hemoglobin above 7 to 8 g/dL. The safety of transfusion in certain clinical subgroups, including those with acute coronary syndrome, myocardial infarction, neurological injury or traumatic brain injury, acute neurological disorders, stroke, thrombocytopenia, cancer, hematological malignances, and bone marrow failure, is unknown. Blood is a limited source, and the procedure itself comes with potential risk. Thus evaluating clinical need may decrease the incidence of posttransfusion issues, including infection (pneumonia, wound infection, blood poisoning); heart attacks, strokes, and problems with blood clots. The patient's underlying comorbidities must be considered in decision making. Monitor serial hemoglobin levels and assess patients for signs and symptoms related to lower hemoglobin and hematocrit levels.

Level of Evidence

A—Systematic Review

Reference

Carson JL, Stanworth SJ, Rouginian N, et al. Transfusion thresholds and other strategies for guiding allogeneic red blood cell transfusion. *Cochrane Database Syst Rev.* 2018; 10:CD002042.

BOX 17.3 Causes of Thrombocytopenia

Bone Marrow Suppression
- Aplastic anemia
- Burns
- Cancer chemotherapy
- Exposure to ionizing radiation
- Nutritional deficiency (vitamin B_{12}, folate)

Interference With Platelet Production (Other Than Nonspecific Marrow Suppression)
- Alcohol
- Histamine$_2$-blocking agents
- Histoplasmosis
- Hormones
- Thiazide diuretics

Platelet Destruction Outside the Bone Marrow
- Artificial heart valves
- Cardiac bypass machine
- Heat stroke
- Heparin
- Infections: severe or sepsis
- Intraaortic balloon pump
- Large-bore IV lines
- Splenic sequestration of platelets
- Sulfonamides
- Transfusions
- Trimethoprim-sulfamethoxazole

Immune Response Against Platelets
- Idiopathic thrombocytopenic purpura
- Mononucleosis
- Thrombotic thrombocytopenic purpura
- Vaccinations
- Viral illness

Interference With Platelet Function
- Cirrhosis
- Diabetes mellitus
- Hypothermia
- Malignant lymphomas
- Nonsteroidal antiinflammatory agents
- Omega 3 (fish oil)
- Sarcoidosis
- Scleroderma
- Systemic lupus erythematosus
- Thyrotoxicosis
- Uremia

Medications
- Aminoglycosides
- Dextran
- Diazepam
- Digitoxin
- Dopamine
- Epinephrine
- Loop diuretics
- Nonsteroidal antiinflammatory agents
- Omega 3 (fish oil)
- Phenothiazines
- Phenytoin
- Salicylate derivatives
- Tricyclic antidepressants
- Vitamin E

BOX 17.4 Heparin-Induced Thrombocytopenia

Definition

Heparin-induced thrombocytopenia (HIT) is defined as a decrease of 50% or more from the highest platelet count after heparin has been initiated to nadir of approximately 20×10^9/L. It usually occurs 5 to 10 days after the start of heparin therapy. However, delayed-onset HIT can develop after heparin has been discontinued, and spontaneous (autoimmune) HIT can develop in the absence of exposure to heparin; however, the timing may be unclear. Heparin binds to platelet factor 4 (PF4), forming an antigenic complex on the surface of the platelets. Some patients develop an antibody to this complex, which stimulates removal of platelets by splenic macrophages, and thrombocytopenia develops. The primary complication of HIT is not bleeding, but hypercoagulability and thrombosis.

Risks

The risk for HIT is 10-fold higher among those receiving unfractionated heparin as opposed to low-molecular-weight heparin (LMWH). HIT also occurs more frequently in patients who have had major surgery. The 4Ts score for estimating the pretest probability of HIT is calculated including the categories: thrombocytopenia (acute), timing of fall in platelet count or other sequelae, thrombosis or other sequelae, and other cause for thrombocytopenia. The pretest probability score of 6-8 is high; 4-5 is intermediate; and 0-3 is low.

Complications

Major complications are thromboembolic in nature. These include deep vein thrombosis, pulmonary embolism, myocardial infarction, thrombotic stroke, arterial occlusion in limbs, and disseminated intravascular coagulation.

Diagnosis

HIT usually develops 5 to 10 days after initiation of heparin therapy; however, rapid-onset HIT can occur within the first hours after heparin exposure. Clinical criteria include a 50% decrease from the highest level after heparin is started and a new thrombosis or anaphylactoid reaction after heparin bolus. PF4-heparin antibody tests are done if clinical criteria are present.

Treatment

HIT is treated by discontinuing all heparin products, including heparin flushes and heparin-coated infusion catheters. Treatment focuses on administration of medications that inhibit thrombin formation or cause direct thrombin inhibition: argatroban (Novastan), danaparoid (Orgaran), fondaparinux (Arixtra), or bivalirudin (Angiomax). Treatment with warfarin, LMWH, aminocaproic acid, or platelets is avoided because these agents may exacerbate the prothrombotic state.

From Greinacher A, Selleng S. Thrombocytopenia. In: Vincent JL, Abraham E, Moore FA, et al., eds. *Textbook of Critical Care.* 7th ed. Philadelphia, PA: Elsevier; 2017:79–83.e1.

Patient Problems. Patients with thrombocytopenia have many of the same problems as listed under the care of the bleeding patient. An additional problem is altered body due to petechiae and ecchymosis (see Clinical Alert box).

! CLINICAL ALERT

Bleeding Disorders

Inspect all body surfaces for overt bleeding, such as bruising or petechiae, which indicates subcutaneous bleeding. Internal bleeding is more difficult to recognize because it may occur even without a known injury and symptoms are often subtle.

Medical Intervention. Medical treatment of thrombocytopenia includes infusions of platelets. Patients who require multiple platelet transfusions are evaluated for infusion of single-donor platelet products, which permits administration of 6 to 10 units of platelets with exposure to the antigens of only one person. For every unit of single-donor platelets, the platelet count is expected to increase by 5000 to 10,000/mm^3. Patients who receive many platelet transfusions can become refractory, or alloimmunized, to the different platelet antigens and may benefit from receiving platelets that are a match for their own HLA type. After multiple platelet transfusions, febrile and allergic transfusion reactions are common; they can be reduced by administration of acetaminophen and diphenhydramine before transfusion.

Thrombopoietin, a platelet-stimulating cytokine, is being investigated as an alternative to platelet transfusion. Some thrombocytopenias are autoimmune induced and may respond to filtration of antibodies via plasmapheresis or immune suppression with corticosteroids. When the spleen is enlarged and tender and these other supportive therapies are unsuccessful, splenectomy can alleviate the autoimmune reaction.

Nursing Intervention. Nursing interventions for the patient with thrombocytopenia are similar to those listed for the bleeding patient. Recognize and limit factors that can deplete or shorten the lifespan of platelets. For example, high fever and high metabolic activity (e.g., seizures) prematurely destroy platelets.

Desired patient outcomes include adequate tissue perfusion, skin integrity, prompt recognition and treatment of bleeding, and absence of pain.

STUDY BREAK

2. When the patient's hematological and immunological systems are compromised, it is not uncommon to require transfusions of several different types of blood products. What patient condition would warrant the administration of platelets as the first consideration?
   A. Anemia
   B. Thrombocytopenia
   C. Vitamin K deficiency
   D. Neutropenia

Disseminated Intravascular Coagulation

Pathophysiology. DIC is a serious disorder of hemostasis that is characterized by exaggerated microvascular coagulation, depletion of clotting factors, and subsequent bleeding.[12] Because clotting factors are used up in the abnormal coagulation process, this disorder is also called *consumption coagulopathy.*

The clinical course of DIC ranges from an acute, life-threatening process to a chronic, low-grade condition. Sepsis is the most common cause of acute DIC.[10,20] Acute DIC develops rapidly and is the most serious form of acquired coagulopathy. Patients with chronic DIC may have more subtle clinical and laboratory findings.

Whatever the initiating event in DIC, procoagulants that cause diffuse, uncontrolled clotting are released. The coagulation pathways are activated by release of tissue factor due to endothelial damage (intrinsic pathway) or direct tissue damage (extrinsic pathway). Large amounts of thrombin are produced, resulting in deposition of fibrin in the microvasculature, consumption of available clotting factors, and stimulation of fibrinolysis.

Clotting in the microvasculature of the patient with DIC causes organ ischemia and necrosis. The skin, lungs, and kidneys are most often damaged. Thrombophlebitis, pulmonary embolism, cerebrovascular accident, gastrointestinal bleeding, and renal failure may result from thrombosis. In addition, microvasculature thrombosis may result in cyanosis of the fingers and toes; purpura fulminans; or infarction and gangrene of the digits, the tip of the nose, or the penis.[21]

The fibrinolysis that ensues results in release of *fibrin degradation products,* which are potent anticoagulants that interfere with thrombin, fibrin, and platelet activity. RBCs are damaged as they try to pass through the blocked capillary beds, leading to excess hemolysis. The lack of available clotting factors coupled with the anticoagulant forces results in an inability to form clots when needed and predisposes the patient with DIC to hemorrhage (Fig. 17.7).

Assessment and Clinical Manifestations. DIC is always a secondary complication of excessive clotting stimuli and may be triggered by vessel injury caused by disease states, tissue injury, or a foreign body in the bloodstream. Sepsis, multisystem trauma, and burns are the main risk factors for DIC.[2] Recognition of potential risk factors and conscientious monitoring of the high-risk patient can facilitate early intervention (see Table 17.13 for a summary of common risk factors for DIC).

Clinically, the patient with DIC first develops microvascular thrombosis. Thrombosis leads to organ ischemia and necrosis that may be manifested as changes in mental status, angina, hypoxemia, oliguria, or nonspecific hepatitis. Cyanosis and infarction of the fingers, toes, and tip of the nose may occur if the DIC is severe. After a thrombotic phase of hours to a few days, depletion of clotting factors and clot lysis cause excessive bleeding. Early signs may include occult blood in the stool, emesis, and urine. Capillary fragility and depleted clotting factors often appear early as mucosal or subcutaneous tissue bleeding, seen as gingival bleeding, petechiae, or ecchymosis. Overt bleeding ranges from mild oozing from venipuncture sites to massive hemorrhage from all body orifices. Occult bleeding into body cavities, such as the peritoneal and retroperitoneal spaces, is detected by changes in vital signs or other classic signs of blood loss.[2,10]

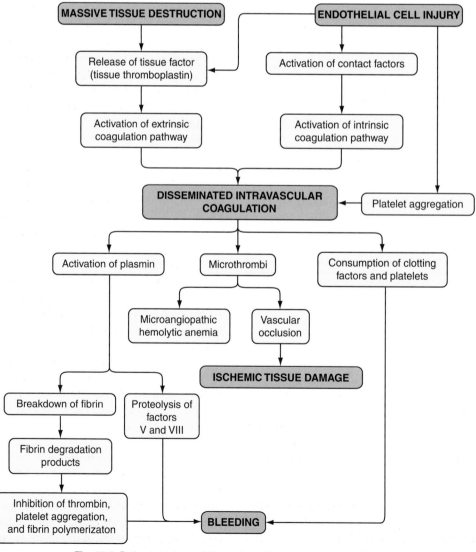

Fig. 17.7 Pathophysiology of disseminated intravascular coagulopathy.

TABLE 17.13 Causes of Disseminated Intravascular Coagulation

Cause	Examples
Infections	Bacterial (especially gram-negative), fungal, viral, mycobacterial, protozoan, rickettsial
Trauma	Burns; crush or multiple injuries; snakebite; severe head injury
Obstetric causes	Abruptio placentae, placenta previa, amniotic fluid embolism, retained dead fetus, missed abortion, eclampsia, hydatidiform mole, septic abortion
Hematologic/immunologic disorders	Transfusion reaction, transplant rejections, anaphylaxis, acute hemolysis, transfusion of mismatched blood products, autoimmune disorders, sickle cell crisis
Oncologic disorders	Carcinomas, leukemias, metastatic cancer
Miscellaneous	Extracorporeal circulation, pulmonary or fat embolism, anoxia, acidosis, hyperthermia or hypothermia, hypovolemic shock, ARDS, sustained hypotension, shock

ARDS, Acute respiratory distress syndrome.
From Marti-Carvajal AJ, Anand V, Ivan S. Treatment for disseminated intravascular coagulation in patients with acute and chronic leukemia. *Cochrane Database Syst Rev.* 2015;15(6):CD008562.

Diagnosis of DIC is based on recognition of pertinent risk factors, clinical symptoms, and the results of laboratory studies. Evidence of factor depletion in the form of thrombocytopenia and low fibrinogen levels is seen in the early phase; however, definitive diagnosis is based on evidence of excess fibrinolysis detectable by elevated fibrin degradation products, an increased D-dimer level, or a decreased antithrombin III level.[2,10] Altered laboratory values in DIC are described in the Laboratory Alert box.

! LABORATORY ALERT

Disseminated Intravascular Coagulation

Test	Normal Value[a]	Alteration
Platelet count	150,000-400,000/mm³	Decreased
Prothrombin time (PT)	11-16 sec	Prolonged
Activated partial thromboplastin time (aPTT)	30-45 sec	Prolonged
Thrombin time (TT)	10-15 sec	Prolonged
Fibrinogen	150-400 mg/dL	Decreased
Fibrin degradation products	<10 mcg/mL	Increased
Antithrombin III	>50% of control (plasma)	Decreased
D-Dimer assay	<100 mcg/L	Increased
Protein C	71%-142% of normal activity	Decreased
Protein S	61%-130% of normal activity	Decreased

[a]Critical values vary by facility and laboratory.

Patient Problems. The patient with DIC is likely to involve multiple systems that encompass both thrombotic and hemorrhagic manifestations. Patient problems may include potential for bleeding or hemorrhage, decreased peripheral tissue perfusion, fluid volume deficit, excessive clotting, impaired skin integrity, and acute pain.

Medical Intervention. Medical treatment of DIC is aimed at identifying and treating the underlying cause, stopping the abnormal coagulation, and controlling the bleeding. Correction of hypotension, hypoxemia, and acidosis is vital, as is treatment of infection if it is the triggering factor. If the cause is obstetrical, evacuation of the uterus for retained fetal tissue or other tissue must be performed. Blood volume expanders and crystalloid IV fluids, such as Lactated Ringer's solution or normal saline, are given to counteract hypovolemia caused by blood loss (see Chapter 12).

Blood component therapy is used to replace deficient platelets and clotting factors and to treat hemorrhage. Platelet infusions are usually necessary because of consumptive thrombocytopenia. Administration of platelets is the highest priority for transfusion because platelets provide the clotting factors needed to establish an initial platelet plug at any bleeding site. Fresh frozen plasma is administered for fibrinogen replacement. It contains all clotting factors and antithrombin III; however, factor VIII is often inactivated by the freezing process, necessitating administration of concentrated factor VIII in the form of cryoprecipitate.[2,10,21] Transfusions of packed RBCs are given to replace cells lost through hemorrhage.

Heparin is a potent thrombin inhibitor and may be administered, in low doses, to block the clotting process that initiates DIC. Heparin is given to prevent further clotting and thrombosis that may lead to organ ischemia and necrosis. Although heparin's antithrombin activity prevents further clotting, it may increase the risk of bleeding and can cause further problems. Its use in patients with DIC is controversial.[2,21]

Other pharmacological therapy in DIC includes the administration of synthetic antithrombin III, which also inhibits thrombin.[2,10] Antithrombin III concentrates may shorten the course of the disease and may increase the survival rate. Administration of aminocaproic acid (Amicar) inhibits fibrinolysis by interfering with plasmin activity. Fibrinolytics should be given only if other treatments have been unsuccessful and hemorrhage is life-threatening; there is no clear evidence of risk versus benefit with their use.[2]

Nursing Intervention. Nursing care of the patient with DIC is aimed at prevention and recognition of thrombotic and hemorrhagic events. Assessment for complications facilitates prompt and aggressive interventions. Few patients who survive DIC are without some functional deficit caused by ischemia or hemorrhage. Psychosocial support for the patient and family is critical in these circumstances.

Pain relief and promotion of comfort are important nursing priorities. Assess the location, intensity, and quality of the patient's pain, along with the patient's response to discomfort. Optimize care to prevent vasoconstriction, which contributes to tissue ischemia and its associated discomfort. Relief of discomfort also reduces oxygen consumption, which is important for these patients with limited circulatory flow. Administer pain medication as ordered and before painful procedures. Positioning, with support and proper body alignment and frequent changes, also enhances the patient's level of comfort.

Monitor the results of coagulation laboratory studies for evidence of disease resolution. As fewer clots are created, the platelet count and fibrinogen level are among the first laboratory values to return to normal. The levels of fibrin degradation products and D-dimer fall, and antithrombin III levels rise, as fibrinolysis slows. Other coagulation tests are less sensitive and are not usually assessed.

STUDY BREAK

3. Which of the following medical conditions is least likely to predispose a patient to disseminated intravascular coagulation (DIC)?
   A. Gram-negative bacterial infections
   B. Abruptio placentae
   C. Transfusion reaction
   D. Acute renal failure

CASE STUDY

Mr. F. is a 62-year-old man with acute myelogenous leukemia diagnosed 15 months ago. He received induction (high-dose) chemotherapy, which resulted in disease remission. He received additional chemotherapy over the next 4 months and underwent an allogeneic peripheral blood stem cell transplant (identical-matched donor; his sister). He was started on standard immunosuppressive medications to prevent graft-versus-host disease (GVHD). Forty-three days after his transplant, Mr. F. was diagnosed with acute GVHD (skin changes on arms and palms of hands). During a routine follow-up visit, Mr. F. complains of mucositis and xerostomia, photosensitivity, dry and irritated eyes, joint pain, a rash on his arms, and an 8-lb weight loss since his last visit 1 month ago.

Questions

1. What risk factors are associated with developing chronic GVHD?
2. What are possible signs and symptoms of chronic GVHD?
3. What is the priority of care for the patient experiencing chronic GVHD?
4. What are key nursing interventions for the patient with chronic GVHD?

❓ CRITICAL REASONING ACTIVITY

What criteria are used to prioritize nursing and medical interventions for the bleeding patient?

REFERENCES

1. Centers for Disease Control and Prevention. *HIV Surveillance Report.* Vol. 29. http://www.cdc.gov/hiv/library/reports/hiv-surveillance.html. Published November 2018. Accessed June 21, 2019.

2. Ferri FF. *Ferri's Clinical Advisor.* Philadelphia, PA: Elsevier; 2019.

3. Greinacher A, Selleng S. Thrombocytopenia. In: Vincent JL, Abraham E, Moore FA, et al., eds. *Textbook of Critical Care.* 7th ed. Philadelphia, PA: Elsevier; 2017:79-83.e1.

4. Hall JE. Hemostasis and blood coagulation. In: Hall JE, ed. *Guyton and Hall Textbook of Medical Physiology.* 13th ed. Philadelphia, PA: Saunders; 2015:451-461.

5. Hall JE. Red blood cells, anemia, and polycythemia. In: Hall JE, ed. *Guyton and Hall Textbook of Medical Physiology.* 13th ed. Philadelphia, PA: Saunders; 2015:413-422.

6. Hall JE. Resistance of the body to infection: I. Leukocytes, granulocytes, the monocyte-macrophage system, and inflammation. In: Hall JE, ed. *Guyton and Hall Textbook of Medical Physiology.* 13th ed. Philadelphia, PA: Saunders; 2015:423-432.

7. Hall JE. Resistance of the body to infection: II. Immunity and the allergy innate immunity. In: Hall JE, ed. *Guyton and Hall Textbook of Medical Physiology.* 13th ed. Philadelphia, PA: Saunders; 2015:433-444.

8. Hall JE. Transport of oxygen and carbon dioxide in blood and tissue fluids. In: Hall JE, ed. *Guyton and Hall Textbook of Medical Physiology.* 13th ed. Philadelphia, PA: Saunders; 2015:495-504.

9. Kwong J. Infection and human immunodeficiency virus infection. In: Lewis SL, Bucher L, Heitkemper MM, Harding MM, et al., eds. *Medical-Surgical Nursing: Assessment and Management of Clinical Problems.* 10th ed. St. Louis, MO: Elsevier; 2017:213-233.

10. Lewis AJ, Rosengart MR. Coagulopathy in the ICU. In: Vincent JL, Abraham E, Moore FA, et al., eds. *Textbook of Critical Care.* 7th ed. Philadelphia, PA: Elsevier; 2017:84-87.e1.

11. Lewis SL. Genetics and genomics. In: Lewis SL, Bucher L, Heitkemper MM, Harding MM, et al., eds. *Medical-Surgical Nursing: Assessment and Management of Clinical Problems.* 10th ed. St. Louis, MO: Elsevier; 2013:178-190.

12. Marti-Carvajal AJ, Anand V, Ivan S. Treatment for disseminated intravascular coagulation in patients with acute and chronic leukemia. *Cochrane Database Syst Rev.* 2015;15(6):CD008562.

13. McGloughlin SA, Paterson DL. Infections in the immunocompromised patient. In: Vincent JL, Abraham E, Moore FA, et al., eds. *Textbook of Critical Care.* 7th ed. Philadelphia, PA: Elsevier; 2017:889-895.e1.

14. National Comprehensive Cancer Network (NCCN). *Guidelines for Patients: Chronic Myeloid Leukemia.* Plymouth Meeting, PA: National Comprehensive Cancer Network Foundation; 2018.

15. Pagana KD, Pagana RJ, Pagana TN. *Diagnostic and Laboratory Test Reference.* 14th ed. St. Louis, MO: Elsevier; 2019.

16. Patton KT, Thibodeau GA. Blood. In: Patton KT, Thibodeau GA, eds. *Anatomy and Physiology.* 10th ed. St. Louis, MO: Elsevier; 2019:606-633.

17. Patton KT, Thibodeau GA. Innate immunity. In: Patton KT, Thibodeau GA, eds. *Anatomy and Physiology.* 10th ed. St. Louis, MO: Elsevier; 2019:746-758.

18. Polek C. Cancer. In: Lewis SL, Bucher L, Heitkemper MM, Harding MM, et al., eds. *Medical-Surgical Nursing Assessment and Management of Clinical Problems.* 10th ed. St. Louis, MO: Elsevier; 2017:234-269.

19. Roberts D. Arthritis and connective tissue diseases. In: Lewis SL, Bucher L, Heitkemper MM, Harding MM. et al., eds. *Medical-Surgical Nursing: Assessment and Management of Clinical Problems.* 9th ed. St. Louis, MO: Elsevier; 2017:1517-1551.

20. Rome SI. Assessment of hematologic system. In: Lewis SL, Bucher L, Heitkemper MM, Harding MM. et al., eds. *Medical-Surgical Nursing: Assessment and Management of Clinical Problems.* 10th ed. St. Louis, MO: Elsevier; 2017:587-605.

21. Rome SI. Hematologic problems. In: Lewis SL, Bucher L, Heitkemper MM, Harding MM, et al., eds. *Medical-Surgical Nursing: Assessment and Management of Clinical Problems*. 10th ed. St. Louis, MO: Elsevier; 2017:606-655.

22. Sonbol MB, Firwana B, Diab M, Witzig TE. Evaluating the effect of neutropenic diet on infection and mortality rate in cancer patients: Meta-analysis. *J Clin Oncol*. 2015;33(15):9619.

23. Swearingen PL, Wright JD. *All-In-One Nursing Care Planning Resource*. 5th ed. St. Louis, MO: Elsevier; 2019.

24. Wu KH. Liver, pancreas, and biliary tract problems. In: Lewis SL, Bucher L, Heitkemper MM, Harding MM, et al., eds. *Medical-Surgical Nursing: Assessment and Management of Clinical Problems*. 10th ed. St. Louis, MO: Elsevier; 2017:974-1013.

25. Yeager JJ. Infection and inflammation. In: Meiner SE, Yeager JJ, eds. *Gerontologic Nursing*. 6th ed. St. Louis, MO: Elsevier; 2019:230-240.

18

Gastrointestinal Alterations

Katherine F. Alford, PhD, RN, CPHQ, CPPS

Many additional resources, including self-assessment exercises, are located on the Evolve companion website at http://evolve.elsevier.com/Sole/.
- Animations
- Clinical Skills: Critical Care Collections
- Student Review Questions
- Video Clips

INTRODUCTION

Body cells require water, electrolytes, and nutrients (carbohydrates, fats, and proteins) to obtain the energy necessary to fuel body functions. The primary function of the alimentary tract (oropharyngeal cavity, esophagus, stomach, and small and large intestines) and accessory organs (pancreas, liver, and gallbladder) is to provide the body with a continual supply of nutrients. In addition, food must move through the system at a rate slow enough for digestive and absorptive functions to occur but also fast enough to meet the body's needs. Meeting these goals requires the appropriate and timely movement of nutrients through the gastrointestinal (GI) tract *(motility)*, the presence of specific enzymes to break down nutrients *(digestion)*, and the existence of transport mechanisms to move the nutrients into the bloodstream *(absorption)*. Each part is adapted for specific functions, including food passage, storage, digestion, and absorption.

This chapter provides a brief physiological review of each section of the GI system and of the general assessment of the GI system. This provides the foundation for the discussion of GI disorders commonly encountered in the critical care setting: acute upper GI bleeding, acute pancreatitis, and liver failure. Assessment, treatment, and nursing care for common GI disorders are discussed.

REVIEW OF ANATOMY AND PHYSIOLOGY

Gastrointestinal Tract

The anatomical structure of the GI system is shown in Fig. 18.1. It comprises the alimentary canal (beginning at the oropharynx and ending at the anus) and the accessory organs (pancreas, liver, and gallbladder) that empty their products into the canal at certain points. A review of the anatomy of the gut wall is provided as an introduction to this section because it is the foundation for the understanding of absorption of nutrients and GI protective mechanisms.

Gut Wall. The GI tract begins in the esophagus and extends to the rectum. It is composed of multiple tissue layers.

Mucosa. The innermost layer, the mucosa, is the most important physiologically. This layer is exposed to food substances and therefore plays a role in nutrient metabolism. The mucosa is also protective. The cells in this layer are connected by tight junctions that produce an effective barrier against large molecules and bacteria. They also protect the GI tract from bacterial colonization. The goblet cells in the mucosa secrete mucus, which provides lubrication for food substances and protects the mucosa from excoriation.

In the stomach, the special architecture of cells of the mucosa and the mucus that is secreted are known as the *gastric mucosal barrier.* This physiological barrier is impermeable to hydrochloric acid, which is normally secreted in the stomach, but it is permeable to other substances, such as salicylates, alcohol, steroids, and bile salts. Disruption of this barrier by these types of substances plays a role in ulcer development. In addition, these cells have a special feature—they regenerate rapidly. Because of this characteristic, disruptions in the mucosa can be quickly healed.

Submucosa. The second layer of the gut wall, the submucosa, is composed of connective tissue, blood vessels, and nerve fibers. The muscular layer follows this layer and is the major layer of the wall. The serosa is the outermost layer.

Beneath the mucosa, submucosa, and muscular layer are various nerve plexuses that are innervated by the autonomic nervous system. Disturbances in these neurons in a given segment of the GI tract cause a lack of motility.

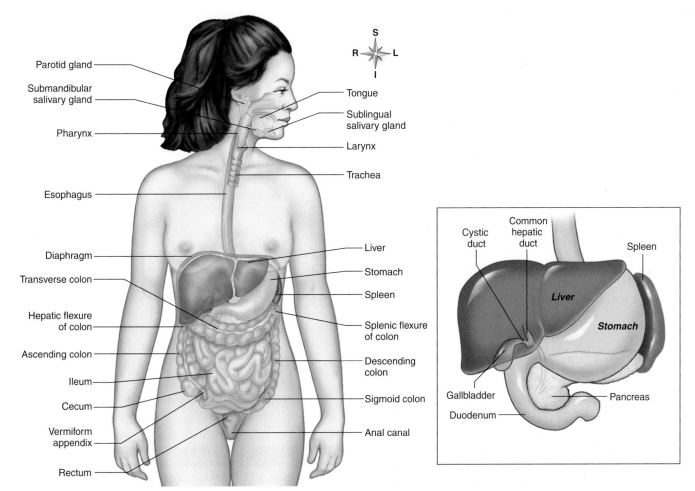

Fig. 18.1 The gastrointestinal system. (From Patton KT, Thibodeau GA. *Anthony's Textbook of Anatomy and Physiology*. 20th ed. St. Louis, MO: Mosby; 2013.)

Oropharyngeal Cavity

Mouth. Swallowing is a complex mechanism involving oral, pharyngeal, and esophageal stages. Food substances are ingested into the oral cavity primarily by the intrinsic desire for food called *hunger*. Food in the mouth is initially subject to mechanical breakdown by the act of chewing *(mastication)*. Chewing of food is important for digestion of all foods, but particularly for digestion of fruits and raw vegetables, because they require the cellulose membranes around their nutrients to be broken down. The muscles used for chewing are innervated by the motor branch of the fifth cranial nerve.

Salivary glands. Saliva is the major secretion of the oropharynx. It is produced by three pairs of salivary glands: submaxillary, sublingual, and parotid. Saliva is rich in mucus, which lubricates food. Salivary amylase, a starch-digesting enzyme, is also secreted. Stimuli such as sight, smell, thoughts, and taste of food stimulate salivary gland secretion. Parasympathetic stimulation promotes a copious secretion of watery saliva. Conversely, sympathetic stimulation produces a scant output of thick saliva. The normal daily secretion of saliva is 1200 mL.

Pharynx. The role of the pharynx in swallowing is a complex process, as the pharynx serves several other functions, the most important of which is respiration. The pharynx participates in the function of swallowing for only a few seconds at a time to aid in the propulsion of food, which is triggered by the presence of fluid or food in the pharynx. Box 18.1 outlines the three broad stages of swallowing.

Esophagus. Once fluid or food enters the esophagus, it is propelled through the lumen by the process of *peristalsis,* which involves relaxation and contraction of esophageal muscles that are stimulated by the bolus of food. This process occurs repeatedly until the food reaches the lower esophageal sphincter,

---

BOX 18.1 **Stages of Swallowing**

Oral: Voluntary
- Initiation of the swallowing process, usually stimulated by a bolus of food in the mouth near the pharynx

Pharyngeal: Involuntary
- Passage of food through the pharynx to the esophagus

Esophageal: Involuntary
- Promotes passage of food from the pharynx to the stomach

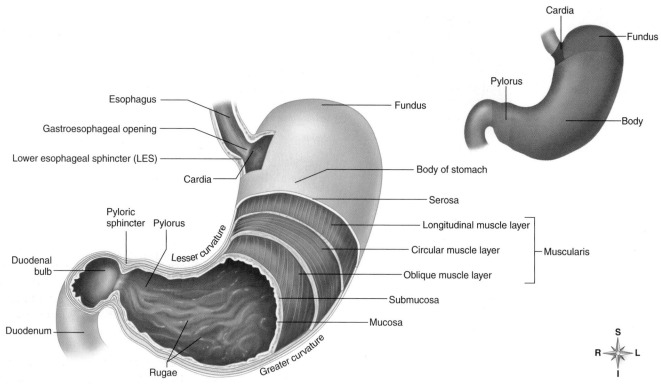

Fig. 18.2 The stomach. (From Patton KT, Thibodeau GA. *Anthony's Textbook of Anatomy and Physiology.* 20th ed. St. Louis, MO: Mosby; 2013.)

which is the last centimeter of the esophagus. This area is normally contracted, thus preventing reflux of gastric contents into the esophagus, a phenomenon that would damage the esophageal lining by exposure to gastric acid and enzymes. Waves of peristalsis cause this sphincter to relax and allow food to enter the stomach. Mucosal layers in the esophagus secrete mucus, which protects the lining from damage by gastric secretions or food and serves as a lubricant.

Stomach. The stomach is located at the distal end of the esophagus. It is divided into four regions: the *cardia*, the *fundus,* the *body,* and the *antrum* (Fig. 18.2). The muscular walls form multiple folds that allow for greater expansion of the stomach. The motor functions of the stomach include storing food until it can be accommodated by the lower GI tract, mixing food with gastric secretions until it forms a semifluid mixture called *chyme*, and slowly emptying the chyme into the small intestine at a rate that allows for proper digestion and absorption. Motility is accomplished through peristalsis. The distal end of the stomach opens into the small intestine; this opening is surrounded by the pyloric sphincter, which prevents duodenal reflux.

Gastric secretions are produced by mucus-secreting cells that line the inner surface of the stomach and by two types of tubular glands: oxyntic (gastric) glands and pyloric glands. Table 18.1 summarizes the major gastric secretions.

An oxyntic gland is composed of three types of cells: mucous neck cells, peptic (chief) cells, and oxyntic (parietal) cells. *Mucous cells* secrete a viscid and alkaline mucus that coats the stomach mucosa, thereby providing protection and lubrication

TABLE 18.1	Gastric Secretions
Gland/Cells	**Secretion**
Cardiac gland	Mucus
Fundic (gastric) gland	Mucus
Mucous neck cells	Mucus
Pyloric gland	Mucus
Parietal cells	Water
	Hydrochloric acid
	Intrinsic factor
Chief cells	Pepsinogen
	Mucus

for food transport. *Parietal cells* secrete hydrochloric acid solution, which begins the digestion of food in the stomach. Hydrochloric acid is very acidic (pH, 0.8). Stimulants of hydrochloric acid secretion include vagal stimulation, gastrin, and the chemical properties of chyme. Histamine, which stimulates the release of gastrin, also stimulates the secretion of hydrochloric acid. The acidic environment of the stomach promotes the conversion of pepsinogen, a proteolytic enzyme secreted by *gastric chief cells*, to pepsin. Pepsin begins the initial breakdown of proteins. Pepsin is active only in a highly acidic environment (pH <5); therefore hydrochloric acid secretion is essential for protein digestion.

An essential protein secreted only by the stomach's parietal cells is *intrinsic factor*. Intrinsic factor is necessary for the absorption of vitamin B_{12} in the ileum. Vitamin B_{12} is critical for

TABLE 18.2 Electrolyte and Acid-Base Disturbances Associated With the Gastrointestinal Tract

Fluid Loss	Imbalances
Gastric juice	Metabolic alkalosis Potassium deficit Sodium deficit Fluid volume deficit
Small intestine juice/large intestine juice (recent ileostomy)	Metabolic acidosis Potassium deficit Sodium deficit Fluid volume deficit
Biliary or pancreatic fistula	Metabolic acidosis Sodium deficit Fluid volume deficit

TABLE 18.3 Pancreatic Enzymes and Their Actions

Enzyme	Action
Carboxypolypeptidase[a]	Digests proteins
Cholesterol esterase	Digests fats
Chymotrypsin[a]	Digests proteins
Deoxyribonuclease	Digests proteins
Pancreatic amylase	Digests carbohydrates
Pancreatic lipase	Digests fats
Ribonuclease	Digests proteins
Trypsin[a]	Digests proteins

[a]Activated only after it is secreted into the intestinal tract.

the formation of red blood cells (RBCs), and a deficiency in this vitamin causes anemia.

The stomach also secretes fluid that is rich in sodium, potassium, and other electrolytes. Loss of these fluids via vomiting or gastric suction places the patient at risk for fluid and electrolyte imbalances and acid-base disturbances (Table 18.2).

Small Intestine. The segment spanning the first 10 to 12 inches of the small intestine is called the *duodenum.* This anatomical area is physiologically important because pancreatic juices and bile from the liver empty into this structure. The duodenum also contains an extensive network of mucus-secreting glands called *Brunner glands.* The function of this mucus is to protect the duodenal wall from digestion by gastric juice. Secretion of mucus by Brunner glands is inhibited by sympathetic stimulation, which leaves the duodenum unprotected from gastric juice. This inhibition is one of the reasons why this area of the GI tract is the site for more than 50% of peptic ulcers.

The segment spanning the next 7 to 8 feet of the small intestine is called the *jejunum,* and the remaining 10 to 12 feet comprise the *ileum.* The opening into the first part of the large intestine is protected by the *ileocecal valve,* which prevents reflux of colonic contents back into the ileum.

The movements of the small intestine include mixing contractions and propulsive contractions. The chyme in the small intestine takes 3 to 5 hours to move from the pylorus to the ileocecal valve, although this activity is greatly increased after meals. Digestion and absorption of foodstuffs occur primarily in the small intestine. The anatomical arrangement of villi and microvilli in the small intestine greatly increases the surface area in this part of the intestine and accounts for its substantial digestive and absorptive capabilities. Located on the entire surface of the small intestine are small pits called *crypts of Lieberkühn,* which produce intestinal secretions at a rate of 2000 mL/day. These secretions are neutral in pH and supply the watery vehicle necessary for absorption.

In the small intestine, digestion of carbohydrates, fats, and proteins begins with degradation by pancreatic enzymes that are secreted into the duodenum. Pancreatic juice contains enzymes necessary for digesting all three of these major nutrients (Table 18.3). It also contains large quantities of bicarbonate ions, which play an important role in neutralizing the acidic chyme that is emptied from the stomach into the duodenum. Pancreatic juice is secreted primarily in response to the presence of chyme in the duodenum.

The small intestine also handles absorption of water, electrolytes, and vitamins. Up to 10 L of fluid enter the GI tract daily, but the fluid composition of stool is only about 200 mL. Sodium is actively reabsorbed in the small intestine. In the ileum, chloride is absorbed and sodium bicarbonate is secreted. Potassium is absorbed and secreted in the GI tract. Vitamins, with the exception of B_{12}, and iron are absorbed in the upper part of the small bowel. Vitamin B_{12} is absorbed in the terminal ileum in the presence of intrinsic factor.

Large Intestine. The large intestine, or colon, is anatomically divided into the ascending colon, transverse colon, descending colon, and rectum (Fig. 18.3). The functions of the colon are absorption of the water and electrolytes from the chyme and storage of fecal material until it can be expelled. The proximal half of the colon performs primarily absorptive activities, whereas the distal half performs storage activities. The characteristic contractile activity in the colon is called *haustration;* it propels fecal material through the tract. A mass movement moves feces into the rectal vault, and then the urge to defecate is elicited. The mucosa of the large intestine is lined with crypts of Lieberkühn, but the cells contain very few enzymes. Rather, mucus is secreted, which protects the colon wall against excoriation and serves as a medium for holding fecal matter together.

Accessory Organs

Pancreas. The pancreas is located in both upper quadrants of the abdomen, with the *head* in the upper right quadrant and the *tail* in the upper left quadrant. The head and tail are separated by a midsection called the *body of the pancreas* (Fig. 18.4). Because the pancreas lies retroperitoneally, it cannot be palpated; this characteristic also explains why diseases of the pancreas can cause pain that radiates to the back. In addition, a well-developed pancreatic capsule does not exist, and this may explain why inflammatory processes of

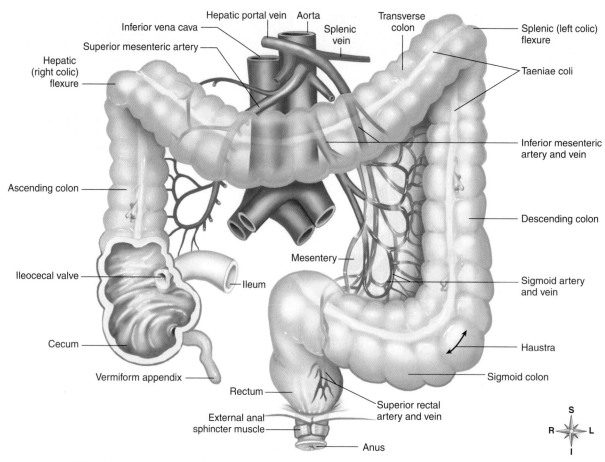

Fig. 18.3 The large intestine. (From Patton KT, Thibodeau GA. *Anthony's Textbook of Anatomy and Physiology.* 20th ed. St. Louis, MO: Mosby; 2013.)

the pancreas can freely spread and affect the surrounding organs (stomach and duodenum).

The pancreas has both *exocrine* functions (production of digestive enzymes) and *endocrine* functions (production of insulin and glucagon). The cells of the pancreas, called *acini*, secrete the major pancreatic enzymes that are essential for normal digestion (see Table 18.3). Trypsinogen and chymotrypsinogen are secreted in an inactive form so that autodigestion of the gland does not occur. Bicarbonate is also secreted by the pancreas and plays an important role in enabling the pancreatic enzymes to work to break down foodstuffs. After breakdown by pancreatic enzymes, food is further digested by enzymes in the small intestine and is absorbed into the bloodstream. The presence of acid in the stomach stimulates the duodenum to produce the hormone secretin, which stimulates pancreatic secretions. Protein substances in the duodenum stimulate the production of cholecystokinin.

The endocrine functions of the pancreas are accomplished by groups of alpha and beta cells that compose the islets of Langerhans. *Beta cells* secrete insulin, and *alpha cells* secrete glucagon. Both are essential to carbohydrate metabolism. When beta cells are affected by disease, blood glucose levels can increase.

The exocrine and endocrine functions of the pancreas are essential to digestion and carbohydrate metabolism, respectively. Pancreatic dysfunction can predispose the patient to malnutrition and accounts for many clinical problems.

The pancreatic response to low-flow states (i.e., decreased cardiac output) or hypotension is often ischemia of the pancreatic cells. This ischemia plays a role in the release of cardiotoxic factors (myocardial depressant factor), which decrease cardiac output. Pancreatic ischemia can also result in acute pancreatitis, which is discussed later in the chapter.

Liver. The liver is the largest internal organ of the body; it is located in the right upper abdominal quadrant. The basic functional unit of the liver is the liver lobule (Fig. 18.5). Hepatic cells are arranged in cords that radiate from the central vein into the periphery. Blood from portal arterioles and venules empties into channels called *sinusoids*. Lining the walls of the sinusoids are specialized phagocytic cells called *Kupffer cells*. These cells remove bacteria and other foreign material from the blood.

The liver has a rich blood supply. It receives blood from both the hepatic artery and the portal vein, which drains structures of the GI tract. The blood supplied to the liver by these two vessels accounts for approximately 25% of the cardiac output.

The liver performs more than 400 functions. The following discussion of hepatic functions is based on the classification by Guyton and Hall[31] and includes vascular, secretory, metabolic, and storage functions. These actions are summarized in Box 18.2.

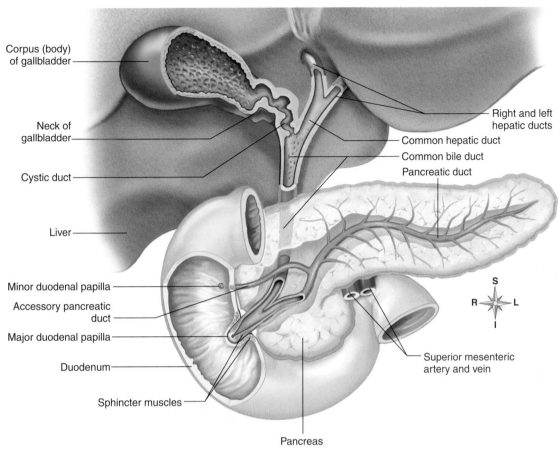

Fig. 18.4 The pancreas and gallbladder. (From Patton KT, Thibodeau GA. *Anthony's Textbook of Anatomy and Physiology.* 20th ed. St. Louis, MO: Mosby; 2013.)

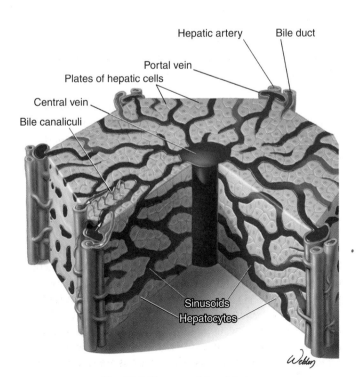

Fig. 18.5 The normal liver lobule.

BOX 18.2 Functions of the Liver

Metabolic Functions
- Carbohydrate, fat, and protein metabolism
- Synthesis of prothrombin (factor I), fibrinogen (factor II), and factors VII, IX, and X
- Removal of activated clotting factors
- Detoxification of medications, hormones, and other substances

Vascular Functions
- Blood storage
- Blood filtration

Secretory Functions
- Production of bile
- Secretion of bilirubin
- Conjugation of bilirubin

Storage Functions
- Blood
- Glucose
- Vitamins (A, B$_{12}$, D, E, K)
- Fat

Metabolic functions.

Carbohydrate metabolism. The liver plays an important role in the maintenance of a normal blood glucose concentration. When the concentration of glucose increases to greater than normal levels, it is stored as glycogen (*glycogenesis*). When blood glucose levels decrease, glycogen stored in the liver is split to form glucose (*glycogenolysis*). If blood glucose levels decrease to less than normal and glycogen stores are depleted, the liver can make glucose from proteins and fats (*gluconeogenesis*).

Fat metabolism. Almost all cells in the body are capable of lipid metabolism; however, the liver metabolizes fats so rapidly that it is the primary site for these functions. The liver is also the primary site for the conversion of excess carbohydrates and proteins to triglycerides.

Protein metabolism. All nonessential amino acids are produced in the liver. Amino acids must be deaminated (cleared of ammonia) to be used for energy by cells or converted into carbohydrates or fats. Ammonia is released and removed from the blood by conversion to urea in the liver. The urea that is secreted by the liver into the bloodstream is excreted by the kidneys.

With the exception of gamma globulins, the liver also produces all plasma proteins in the blood. The major types of plasma proteins are albumins, globulins, and fibrinogen. *Albumin* maintains blood oncotic pressure and prevents plasma loss from the capillaries. *Globulins* are essential for cellular enzymatic reactions. *Fibrinogen* helps to form blood clots.

Production and removal of blood clotting factors. The liver synthesizes fibrinogen (factor I), prothrombin (factor II), and factors VII, IX, and X. Vitamin K is essential for the synthesis of other clotting factors. The liver also removes active clotting factors from the circulation, which prevents clotting in the macrovasculature and microvasculature.

Detoxification. The liver detoxifies medications, hormones, and other toxic substances into inactive forms for excretion. This process is usually accomplished by conversion of the fat-soluble compounds to water-soluble compounds that are excreted via the bile or the urine.

Vascular functions.

Blood storage. Resistance to blood flow in the liver (hepatic vascular resistance) is normally low. Any increase in pressure to the veins of the liver causes blood to accumulate in the sinusoids, which can store up to 400 mL of blood. This blood volume serves as a compensatory mechanism in cases of hypovolemic shock; blood from the liver is shunted into the circulation to increase blood volume.

Blood filtration. Kupffer cells line the sinusoids. They cleanse the blood of bacteria and foreign material that have been absorbed through the GI tract. These cells are extremely phagocytic and normally prevent almost all bacteria from reaching the systemic circulation.

Secretory functions.

Bile production. The secretion of bile is a major function of the liver. Bile is composed of water, electrolytes, bile salts, phospholipids, cholesterol, and bilirubin. Approximately 500 to 1000 mL of bile is produced daily. Bile salts emulsify fats and foster their absorption. The bile salts are reabsorbed in the terminal portion of the ileum and are then transported back to the liver, where they can be used again. Bile travels to the gallbladder via the common bile duct, where it is stored and concentrated.

Bilirubin metabolism. Bilirubin, a physiologically inactive pigment, is a metabolic end product of the degradation of hemoglobin (Hgb). Bilirubin enters the circulation bound to albumin and is *unconjugated.* This portion of the bilirubin is reflected in the *indirect* serum bilirubin level. Accumulation of unconjugated bilirubin is toxic to cells. In the liver, bilirubin is *conjugated* with glucuronic acid. Conjugated bilirubin is soluble and is excreted in bile. Some conjugated bilirubin returns to the blood and is reflected in the *direct* serum bilirubin level.

Excess bilirubin accumulation in the blood results in *jaundice.* Jaundice has several categories, including hepatocellular, hemolytic, and obstructive. Viral hepatitis is the most common cause of *hepatocellular jaundice* (jaundice caused by hepatic cell damage). Cirrhosis and liver cancer also decrease the liver's ability to conjugate bilirubin. *Hemolytic jaundice* results from increased RBC destruction, such as that resulting from blood incompatibilities or sickle cell disease. *Obstructive jaundice* is usually caused by gallbladder disease (e.g., gallstones).[51,52]

Storage functions.

Storage, synthesis, and transport of vitamins and minerals. The liver plays a central role in the storage, synthesis, and transport of various vitamins and minerals. It functions as a storage depot principally for vitamins A, D, and B_{12}, accumulating, respectively, up to 3-, 10-, and 12-month supplies of these nutrients to prevent deficiency states.

Gallbladder. The gallbladder is a saclike structure that lies beneath the right lobe of the liver. Its primary function is the storage and concentration of bile. The gallbladder holds approximately 70 mL of bile. Bile salts are secreted into the duodenum when nutrients are ingested. The gallbladder is connected to the duodenum by the common bile duct. Bile flow is controlled by contraction of the gallbladder and relaxation of the sphincter of Oddi, which is located at the junction of the common bile duct and the duodenum. Contraction of the gallbladder is controlled by hormonal (*cholecystokinin*) and central nervous system signals and is initiated by the presence of food in the duodenum. Bile salts emulsify fats and assist in the absorption of fatty acids.

Neural Innervation of the Gastrointestinal System

Functions of the GI system are influenced by neural and hormonal factors. The autonomic nervous system exerts multiple effects. Parasympathetic cholinergic fibers, or medications that mimic parasympathetic effects, stimulate GI secretion and motility. Sympathetic stimulation, or medications with adrenergic effects, tends to be inhibitory. Parasympathetic and sympathetic fibers also innervate the gallbladder and the pancreas. Other neural regulators of gastric secretions are stimulated by sight, smell, and thoughts of food and by the presence of food in the mouth. In this phase (cephalic), the brain centers reflexively cause parasympathetic stimulation of gastric secretions by chief and parietal cells.

Hormonal Control of the Gastrointestinal System

The GI tract is considered to be the largest endocrine organ in the body. Hormones that influence GI function include those produced by specialized cells in the GI tract and those produced by other endocrine organs (i.e., pancreas and gallbladder). GI hormones modulate motility, secretion, absorption, and maturation of GI tissues. Table 18.4 summarizes the common GI hormones and their actions.

TABLE 18.4 Actions of Gastrointestinal Hormones

Action	Gastrin	Cholecystokinin	Secretin	Gastric Inhibitory Peptide
Acid secretion	Stimulates	Stimulates	Inhibits	Inhibits
Gastric motility	Stimulates	Stimulates	Inhibits	—
Gastric emptying	Inhibits	Inhibits	Inhibits	Inhibits
Intestinal motility	Stimulates	Stimulates	Inhibits	—
Mucosal growth	Stimulates	Stimulates	Inhibits	—
Pancreatic HCO_3^- secretion	Stimulates	Stimulates	Stimulates	0
Pancreatic enzyme secretion	Stimulates	Stimulates	Stimulates	0
Pancreatic growth	Stimulates	Stimulates	Stimulates	—
Bile HCO_3^- secretion	Stimulates	Stimulates	Stimulates	0
Gallbladder contraction	Stimulates	Stimulates	Stimulates	—

0, No effect; —, not yet tested; *HCO_3^-*, bicarbonate.

Blood Supply of the Gastrointestinal System

The blood supply to organs within the abdomen is referred to as the *splanchnic circulation*. The GI system receives the largest percentage of the cardiac output. Approximately one-third of the cardiac output supplies these tissues. The superior and inferior mesenteric and celiac arteries supply the stomach, small and large intestines, pancreas, and gallbladder. The liver has a dual blood supply and receives part of its supply from the hepatic artery. Circulation to the GI system is unique in that venous blood draining the system empties into the portal vein, which perfuses the liver. The portal vein supplies 70% to 75% of liver blood flow.

STUDY BREAK

1. What is responsible for maintaining the body's oncotic pressure?
   A. Fibrinogen
   B. Albumin
   C. Globulin
   D. Collagen

A large percentage of cardiac output perfuses the GI tract; therefore the GI tract is a major source of blood flow during times of increased need, such as during exercise or as a compensatory mechanism in hemorrhage. Conversely, prolonged occlusion or hypoperfusion of a major artery supplying the GI tract can lead to mucosal ischemia and eventually necrosis. Necrosis of intestinal villi can destroy the GI tract's barrier to harmful toxins and bacteria. These bacteria can then enter the blood supply and cause septic shock.

Lifespan Considerations

Several changes occur in the GI system as a result of the aging process and pregnancy. Changes related to the aging process include decreased salivation, or xerostomia (dry mouth syndrome), which may change the patient's taste perception; delayed esophageal and bowel emptying; increased bowel emptying, which may lead to anxiety about incontinence; decreased thirst sensation, which may lead to a reduction of fluid intake; decreased gastric secretions; and altered drug metabolism.[19] The most common GI disorders in elderly patients are functional bowel disorders such as chronic constipation, irritable bowel syndrome,[1] peptic ulcer disease (PUD),[24,26,28] and neoplasms.[41] Upper abdominal discomfort in an elderly patient may be associated with coronary artery disease.[31]

Elderly patients are at risk for malnutrition[19] or undernutrition[56] and for vitamin and mineral deficiencies due to a reduction of olfactory, gustatory, and visual food perception that can lead to a decrease in appetite. Malnutrition is one of the most relevant conditions that negatively influence the health of older people. Malnourished patients have an increased hospital length of stay and are more susceptible to infections. Oral nutritional support is important to correct malnutrition and for patients at risk for malnutrition. Oral nutritional supplements (ONSs) may be used as an adjunct in a patient's nutritional management.[19] ONS is defined as the supplementary oral intake of dietary food for special medical purposes in addition to normal foods. ONSs are usually liquid, but they are also available in other forms such as powders, dessert-style servings, or bars. Use of ONSs has been shown to decrease hospital complications and readmission, increase protein intake, and improve weight in the elderly.[19]

GI discomforts that frequently occur during pregnancy include nausea and vomiting, gastroesophageal reflux disease (GERD), hemorrhoids,[65] and pelvic floor disorders, including constipation[10] and fecal incontinence.[59] Nausea and vomiting during pregnancy may be caused by gastric motility disturbances and pregnancy-associated alterations as a result of differing reactions to taste and smell and involvement of behavioral and psychological factors. GERD, which is the abnormal reflux of gastric contents into the esophagus, is experienced by 30% to 80% of pregnant women, and about one-third of pregnant women complain of hemorrhoids.[65] GERD symptoms are similar to those of heartburn. In pregnant women, contributing factors include obesity, increased intraabdominal pressure, and a decrease in lower esophageal sphincter pressure.[68] Constipation is a common symptom experienced by pregnant women in the first trimester, and it affects up to 25% of pregnant women for up to 3 months after

GENETICS

Cytochrome P450 Enzymes and the Patient's Response to Medications

Pharmacogenomics is the study of the whole genome, the proteins (e.g., RNA, enzymes, drug receptors), and the technology used to guide medication development and testing. *Pharmacogenetics* refers to individual genetic profiles and how one's genetic profile influences the response to medications.[1]

Enzymes produced by the cytochrome P450 (CYP450) genes are the source of 70% to 80% of enzymes involved in the metabolism of medications. The word *cytochrome,* meaning "colored cell," refers to the red heme molecule in CYP450 enzymes. The P450 portion of the name is derived from the wavelength of light absorbed in mass spectrography (450 nanometers).[4] The name of each CYP450 gene begins with CYP followed by a number associated with a specific group within the CYP genes, a letter representing the gene's subgroup, and a number assigned to the gene within the subgroup. To illustrate, the gene that is in group 2, subgroup D, gene 6 is labeled *CYP2D6.*

CYP450 enzymes also break down toxins produced by normal cell functions, detoxify ingested procarcinogens such as nitrates, and alter harmful substances such as hydrocarbons from cigarette smoke. The CYP450 enzymes also synthesize fatty acids, cholesterol, prostaglandins, and hormones.

The CYP450 enzymes are abundant in the liver and are also found in intestines, lungs, and other tissues. A polymorphism is a genetic variation, and some CYP450 enzymes have heritable polymorphisms. Common gene polymorphisms in the CYP450 genes affect the function of enzymes. Typically, the polymorphism is a single nucleotide polymorphism (SNP). For example, an individual may inherit low-, normal-, or high-functioning enzymes and be genotyped as poor (slow), intermediate, extensive (normal), and ultra-rapid metabolizers.

When a polymorphism results in reduced volume or function of a CYP450 enzyme (i.e., a slow metabolizer), a medication that is metabolized by that enzyme may undergo reduced inactivation. For medications that are prodrugs like codeine and clopidogrel, slow-metabolizing CYP450 enzymes may mean that the medication is not converted to an active form and therapeutic blood levels are not achieved. When the CYP450 enzyme group is genotyped as ultra-rapid, rapid metabolism leads to rapid medication clearance and ineffective treatment. Toxic effects may manifest early or with greater severity due to either poor or ultra-rapid metabolism.

Foods, body temperature, pH, medications, and environmental factors affect the activity of most CYP enzymes. For example, grapefruit reduces the function of CYP450 enzymes in the gastrointestinal tract, resulting in greater serum levels of some oral medications when taken following a meal with this citrus fruit. Medications can also induce (increase activity) and inhibit (reduce activity) of families of CYP450 enzymes.

Each person inherits two genes (i.e., two alleles) for CYP450 enzymes, and both genes contribute to CYP enzyme function. Polymorphisms of CYP2C9, CYP2C19, CYP2D6, and CYP3A5 affect clinical decisions when prescribing medications metabolized by these enzymes.[7] CYP1A2, CYP2A6, CYP2B6, CYP2C8, and CYP3A4 all show variability that affects medication metabolism, but the evidence for significant clinical effects is limited.[7] To illustrate, *CYP2D6* polymorphisms result in a phenotypic continuum able to metabolize medications: intermediate, extensive, and ultra-fast metabolizers. For the CYP2D6 inheritance patterns, *extensive metabolizers* are considered normal or "wild type." *Intermediate metabolizers* have less enzymatic activity, resulting in high serum medication concentrations with standard doses or therapeutic failure when a prodrug is not converted to an active form. About 10% of white Europeans, and as many as 50% of Asians, inherit alleles resulting in a slow metabolic response.[6] Populations with a North African inheritance have more ultra-fast metabolic alleles compared with other people.[4] Nurses need to consider ethnicity and race in recommending and interpreting pharmacogenetic testing.

The CYP2D6 enzymes metabolize many beta-blockers, antidysrhythmics, antiplatelets, antipsychotics, and selective serotonin reuptake inhibitors.[1] Clopidogrel,

a prodrug, requires activation by several CYP450 enzymes to reduce platelet activity. Intermediate metabolizers experience reduced medication effectiveness with potential for new cardiovascular events. Reduced function of CYP2D6 is linked to increased incidence of bradycardia from some beta-blockers and dysrhythmias from lengthening of the QTc interval with the use of antipsychotics.[7] CYP2D6 function may explain ineffective treatment of bipolar disease.[9]

The CYP2D6 enzymes have specific clinical implications for codeine administration. Patients with inherited low CYP2D6 enzymatic activity cannot convert codeine to its active form; therefore codeine provides no pain relief for them, and adjusting the dose does not change this response. Conversely, individuals who inherit a genotype that results in ultra-rapid metabolism experience a quick conversion of codeine into morphine, causing unanticipated respiratory depression and sedation. In oncology and palliative care, pharmacogenetic testing may be indicated when opioids are used to manage pain. Persistent pain, serious adverse effects at low doses, and breakthrough pain with more than four episodes per day should be considered the criteria for CYP450 screening.[10] Clinical genotyping can limit trial-and-error dosing and avoid adverse effects from a dose that is too high or too low based on the individual's metabolic genetic profile. Genotyping results are not affected by underlying disease or co-administration of other medications and do not change over time.

The US Food and Drug Administration (FDA) lists medications for which pharmacogenetic biomarkers are relevant.[5] (http://www.fda.gov/drugs/sciencere-search/researchareas/pharmacogenetics/ucm083378.htm). The Clinical Pharmacogenetics Implementation Consortium lists indications for genetic testing for more than 350 drugs (https://cpicpgx.org/genes-drugs/).[3] Pharmacogenetic testing to personalize treatment is increasing. However, clinicians, including nurses, often do not have the knowledge and skills to interpret tests and guide patients.[2,8] Individuals have access to pharmacogenetic testing outside of healthcare settings. The clinical implications of a commercial test are not always clear to patients who may decide to stop a medication based on testing. Genomic literacy is essential to providing the benefits of genetic testing and precision medicine.

Genetic terms: *pharmacogenomics, pharmacogenetics, polymorphism, allele, single nucleotide polymorphism (SNP), phenotype, genotype, precision medicine.*

References

1. Brazeau D. Basics of pharmacogenetics. In: Lea DH, Cheek D, Brazeau D, et al., eds. *Mastering Pharmacogenomics: A Nurse's Handbook for Success.* Indianapolis, IN: Sigma Theta Tau; 2015:35–58.
2. Calzone KA, Kirk M, Tonkin E, et al. The global landscape of nursing and genomics. *J Nurs Scholarsh.* 2018;50(3):249–256.
3. Clinical Pharmacogenetics Implementation Consortium (CPIC). Genes-Drugs. 2019. https://cpicpgx.org/genes-drugs/. Published March 5, 2019. Accessed February 19, 2019.
4. Correia MA. Drug biotransformation. In: Katzung BG, ed. *Basic and Clinical Pharmacology.* 14th ed. New York, NY: McGraw-Hill; 2018:56–73.
5. US Federal Drug Administration. Table of Pharmacogenomic Biomarkers in Drug Labeling. https://www.fda.gov/Drugs/ScienceResearch/ucm572698.htm. Published August 3, 2018. Accessed February 19, 2019.
6. Giarelli E. Integrating pharmacogenomics into healthcare. In: Lea DH, Cheek D, Brazeau D, et al., eds. *Mastering Pharmacogenomics: A Nurse's Handbook for Success.* Indianapolis, IN: Sigma Theta Tau; 2015:59–78.
7. Hibma JE, Giacomini KM. Pharmacogenomics. In: Katzung BG, ed. *Basic and Clinical Pharmacology.* New York, NY: McGraw-Hill; 2018:74–88.
8. Paul JL, Leslie H, Trainer AH, Gaff C. A theory-informed systematic review of clinicians' genetic testing practices. *Eur J Hum Genet.* 2018;26(10):1401–1416.
9. Seripa D, Lozupone M, Miscio G, et al. CYP2D6 genotypes in revolving door patients with bipolar disorders: A case series. *Medicine (Baltimore).* 2018;97(37):e11998.
10. Vieira CMP, Fragoso RM, Pereira D, Medeiros R. Pain polymorphisms and opioids: An evidence based review. *Mol Med Rep.* 2019;19(3):1423–1434.

delivery.[70] Hyperemesis gravidarum, which is defined as persistent nausea and vomiting after 6 to 8 weeks of gestation, occurs in less than 1% of pregnant women. Severe nausea and vomiting from hyperemesis gravidarum can lead to dehydration, postural hypotension, tachycardia, electrolyte imbalances, ketosis, muscle wasting, and weight loss.[10]

Pica, the compulsive consumption of nonfood items, can also occur during pregnancy. The etiology of pica is not well understood. It has been suggested that mineral deficiencies (e.g., iron, zinc) may be a contributing factor. The most common cravings are for dirt (*geophagia*), ice (*pagophagia*), and laundry or corn starch (*amylophagia*). Cravings for cigarette ashes, burnt matches, stones, coffee grounds, paint chips, clay, baking soda, lead-based paint, and sand have also been reported.[68]

Other, less common pregnancy GI disorders reported in the literature include obstetric cholestasis, acute fatty liver, diarrhea, inflammatory bowel diseases such as Crohn's disease and ulcerative colitis, irritable bowel syndrome, appendicitis, gallbladder disease, pancreatitis,[10] cirrhosis, and hepatitis.[65] The Lifespan Considerations box highlights these changes and related nursing implications.

LIFESPAN CONSIDERATIONS

Older Adults

- Provide oral care to keep mucous membranes moist due to decreased salivation.
- Elderly patients may experience delayed esophageal emptying. Symptoms include complaints of bloating or regurgitation when drinking a large amount of fluids with meals.
- Dysphagia increases the risk for aspiration, especially during meals. Elevate the patient's head of bed during mealtime or feedings.
- Assess for problems during feeding such as tremors, dementia, and functional impairments.[48]
- Due to decreased senses of taste, sight, and smell, providing adequate nutrition to those receiving oral feedings is challenging. Obtain dietary consultation to assist with meal planning and administer oral nutritional supplements as ordered.[20]
- Decreased gastric acid secretion may result in anemia, which can lead to hypoxemia. Assess the patient's complete blood count, arterial blood gases, and pulse oximetry values, as appropriate.
- Elderly patients are at higher risk for complications of gallbladder disease, such as pancreatitis, due to an increased incidence of gallstones. Assess for signs and symptoms of cholecystitis.
- Blood flow to the liver decreases by almost one-half by age 85, which may lead to an impaired medication metabolism. Assess the patient for medication toxicity and consult with the clinical pharmacist to identify the need for adjusting medication dosages.
- Some medications (i.e., nifedipine and verapamil) cause rectosigmoid dysmotility and severe constipation.[28] Assess need for medication and provide interventions to prevent or treat constipation.
- The elderly may also experience diarrhea due to increased bowel emptying. Use of laxatives and nonsteroidal antiinflammatory drugs (NSAIDs) can cause bowel disturbances. Assess bowel function and medication side effects.

Pregnant Women

- Pregnancy can cause decreased gastric motility, resulting in nausea and vomiting. Assess the patient for signs and symptoms of dehydration and complications. Administer recommended first-line therapy for nausea as prescribed (doxylamine succinate and vitamin B_6).[6,65]
- Pregnancy increases levels of female sex hormones, which in turn can decrease lower esophageal sphincter pressure resulting in heartburn, regurgitation, and/or gastroesophageal reflux disease (GERD). Assess nutritional status, diet, and physical activity.[69] Instruct the patient to avoid lying in a supine position after meals, consider nonpharmacological remedies that are safe in pregnancy (e.g., ginger root), administer first-line medications of antacids and sucralfate, and consider alginate preparations if antacids do not provide relief.[10]

- Constipation may occur due to decreased colonic motility and increased pressure on the rectosigmoid colon. Assess the patient's fluid and fiber intake and administer laxatives and bulking agents, as prescribed. Do not discontinue oral iron.[10]
- Weight gain and increased pelvic pressure can cause engorgement of rectal veins, inflammation of the anal mucosa, varicose veins of the anus and rectum, and hemorrhoids. Prevent constipation and obtain nutritional consultation for dietary changes to increase fluids and fiber. Administer supplemental fiber as prescribed.[69] Apply warm soaks, witch hazel pads, and topical creams such as hydrocortisone-pramoxine to provide pain relief.
- Diarrhea or having frequent stools may also occur during pregnancy, particularly at term when labor is near. However, diarrhea can also be a symptom of a more serious disease. Monitor stool frequency and other symptoms accompanied with diarrhea such as fever or severe abdominal pain lasting for more than 48 hours, as these can be signs of an illness caused by infective agents such as bacteria, viruses, and protozoa. Assess the onset of the diarrhea, stool frequency, patient's recent travel history, recent antibiotic use, employment history, food and water intake, and contact with ill family members. Anticipate obtaining stool cultures. Instruct the patient on hand washing and avoidance of contaminated foods. Other nonpharmacological treatments include oral hydration with salt- or sugar-containing fluids and consuming bland foods or a BRAT diet (bananas, rice, applesauce, and toast). Instruct the patient to avoid milk and high-fat foods. Loperamide (Imodium) can be used in pregnancy in the absence of bloody diarrhea. Antibiotics may be indicated for infectious diarrhea.[69]
- Pica, or compulsion to consume nonfood items, may occur in pregnancy. Treatment of pica is tailored to the patient and the nonfood item consumed.
- Assess the patient for anemia. Obtain laboratory tests to determine the underlying cause.[69]
- Pregnant women are more vulnerable to hepatitis E virus (HEV). In HEV, there is no apparent increase in mortality rate and no reports of fetal transmission.
- In pregnant women who are positive for hepatitis B surface antigen with viral DNA present in the serum, the risk of transmission to the neonate is high during delivery. Routine screening for hepatitis B virus (HBV) infection is warranted to minimize the transmission risk. Pregnant patients, in their third trimester of pregnancy, may be treated with lamivudine (Epivir) to decrease HBV transmission.[65]
- Because anal sphincter weakness may occur during and after pregnancy, fecal incontinence has been reported as early as 12 weeks' gestation. Treatment includes dietary modification and fiber supplementation. Loperamide (Imodium) may be given as a pharmacological intervention. Pelvic floor muscle training may alleviate symptoms of fecal incontinence. Surgical intervention is typically reserved for women when other options have failed.[59]

CRITICAL REASONING ACTIVITY

The nurse is caring for a patient who is admitted with acute abdominal pain and vomiting. His admission vital signs and laboratory values include the following:

Blood pressure	94/72 mm Hg
Heart rate	114 beats/min
Respiratory rate	32 breaths/min
Potassium	3.0 mEq/L
Calcium	7.0 mg/dL
Arterial oxygen saturation	88%
Serum amylase	280 IU/L
Serum lipase	320 IU/L

1. What is the suspected medical diagnosis?
2. What are the priority nursing and medical interventions?

GENERAL ASSESSMENT OF THE GASTROINTESTINAL SYSTEM

A comprehensive assessment of the abdomen includes a history, inspection, auscultation, percussion, and palpation. Use the four-quadrant method (right upper, right lower, left upper, and left lower) to map the abdomen for descriptive purposes by drawing imaginary lines crossing at the umbilicus. Use these landmarks to describe symptoms, such as pain.

History

Unless an emergency situation requires immediate intervention, begin assessment of the GI system by obtaining a history. Question the patient about past problems with indigestion, difficulty swallowing (dysphagia), pain on swallowing, nausea and vomiting, heartburn, belching, abdominal distension or bloating, diarrhea, constipation, and bleeding. Note that problems such as anorexia, fatigue, and headache may relate to specific GI ailments. Explore symptoms in terms of when they became apparent, any precipitating factors, what treatment was sought, factors that relieved or made the symptoms worse, and whether the symptom is current. Obtain a weight history that includes usual and ideal body weight along with a history of fluctuations, acute weight loss, and interventions or treatments for weight loss.

Pain assessment is challenging. Pain receptors in the abdomen are less likely to be localized and are mediated by common sensory structures projected to the skin. Therefore it is often difficult to distinguish the pain of a peptic ulcer or cholecystitis from that of a myocardial infarction. Abdominal pain is often caused by engorged mucosa, pressure in the mucosa, distension, or spasm. Visceral pain is likely to cause pallor, perspiration, bradycardia, nausea and vomiting, weakness, and hypotension. Increasing intensity of pain, especially after surgery or other intervention, is always significant and usually signifies complicating factors such as inflammation, gastric distension, hemorrhage into tissue or the peritoneal space, or peritonitis. Obtain a description of the location and the type of pain in the patient's own words.

Obtain a history of any GI surgical procedures, including the specific types and dates. Also, record a list of current medications because many medications have GI side effects.

Inspection

Inspect the abdomen, focusing on the following characteristics: skin color and texture, symmetry and contour of the abdomen, masses and pulsations, and peristalsis and movement. Record findings.

Skin Color and Texture. Observe for pigmentation of skin (jaundice), lesions, discolorations, old or new scars, and vascular and hair patterns. Assess general nutrition and hydration status.

Symmetry and Contour of Abdomen. Note the size and shape of the abdomen and the presence of visible protrusions and adipose distribution. Always investigate abdominal distension, particularly in the presence of pain, because it usually indicates trapped air or fluid within the abdominal cavity.

Masses and Pulsations. Look for any obvious abdominal masses, which are best observed on deep inspiration. Pulsations, if they are seen, usually originate from the aorta.[35]

Peristalsis and Movement. Motility of the stomach may be reflected in movement of the abdomen in lean patients, and this is a normal sign. However, strong contractions are abnormal and indicate the presence of disease.

Auscultation

Auscultation of bowel sounds is a noninvasive and simple method to assess GI motility and function, and it is valuable in the examination of patients with acute abdominal pain.[21,31] Bowel sounds are high-pitched, gurgling sounds caused by air and fluid as they move through the GI tract. Auscultate bowel sounds before palpation. However, if no bowel sounds are audible on the initial assessment, auscultation can be done after palpation because palpation may stimulate peristalsis.[7] Position the patient for proper auscultation. A supine position with the patient's arms at the sides or folded at the chest is usually recommended. Place a pillow under the patient's knees to relax the abdominal wall.

Bowel sounds are best heard with the diaphragm of the stethoscope and are systematically assessed in all four quadrants of the abdomen. Assess the frequency and character of the sounds. The frequency of bowel sounds has been estimated at 5 to 35 per minute, and the sounds are usually irregular. The amount of time required for bowel sounds to be auscultated ranges from 30 seconds to 7 minutes. Therefore assess for bowel sounds for at least 5 minutes before determining that bowel sounds are absent.[7] Box 18.3 reviews common causes of increased and decreased bowel sounds as they relate to acute illness.

When a patient's bowel sounds are diminished or absent, bowel obstruction, intestinal ischemia, paralytic ileus, or

BOX 18.3 Causes of Changes in the Frequency of Bowel Sounds

Causes of Decreased Bowel Sounds
- Gangrene
- Late bowel obstruction
- Peritonitis
- Reflux ileus
- Surgical manipulation of bowel

Causes of Increased Bowel Sounds
- Bleeding esophageal varices
- Bleeding ulcers or electrolyte disturbances
- Diarrhea
- Early pyloric or intestinal obstruction
- Subsiding ileus

peritonitis can be considered. When a patient's bowel sounds are increased, consider GI bleeding or bowel obstruction.[7,31] Vascular sounds such as bruits may be heard; they indicate dilated, tortuous, or constricted vessels. Venous hums are normally heard from the inferior vena cava. A hum in the periumbilical region in a patient with cirrhosis indicates obstructed portal circulation. Peritoneal friction rubs may be heard and may indicate infection, abscess, or tumor.[35]

Percussion

Percussion provides information about the structure of abdominal organs and tissues and is aimed at detecting fluid, gaseous distension, and masses. Because of the presence of gas within the GI tract, percussed tympany predominates. Solid masses are dull on percussion. Differences from normal sensation may be related to fluid in an area that does not normally contain fluid. For example, a collapsed lung changes the percussion note, as does a solid mass in the abdomen. Percussion that produces a dull note in the midline of the lower abdomen in a male patient most likely represents a distended urinary bladder. Organ borders of the liver, spleen, and stomach may also be ascertained with the use of percussion.

Palpation

Palpation is the use of touch to determine the characteristics of an area of the body, including skin elevation or depression, warmth, tenderness, pulses, and crepitus. Palpation is also used to evaluate the major organs with respect to shape, size, position, mobility, consistency, and tension. Perform palpation last because it often elicits pain or muscle spasm. Deep abdominal tenderness and rebound tenderness must be differentiated. Rebound tenderness occurs when pain is elicited after deep palpation when the examiner's hand is quickly released. Rigidity or guarding of the abdomen is also noted. Masses in the liver, spleen, kidneys, gallbladder, or descending colon can be palpated. When palpating the gallbladder in a thin, elderly female patient, palpate the right lower abdominal quadrant in addition to the right upper abdominal quadrant. A pulsatile mass palpated in the abdomen might be an abdominal aneurysm, and an acutely tender mass that descends with inspiration in the right upper quadrant might be an inflamed gallbladder.

STUDY BREAK

2. An elderly patient presented to a hospital's emergency department with a chief complaint of constipation for 1 week. The patient had a medical history of hypertension, diabetes, and hyperlipidemia. The patient had been taking calcium supplements for a year. What should the nurse perform first?
   A. Ask the physician to discontinue the patient's calcium supplements.
   B. Instruct the patient and family member to increase the patient's fluid intake.
   C. Assess the patient for abdominal pain and usual diet.
   D. Administer a stool softener, as ordered.

ACUTE GASTROINTESTINAL BLEEDING

Pathophysiology

Many causes of acute GI bleeding necessitate admission of a patient to the critical care unit. Box 18.4 reviews the most common causes of this emergency condition.

Peptic Ulcer Disease. PUD is characterized by a break in the mucosa that extends through the entire mucosa and into the muscle layers, damaging blood vessels and causing hemorrhage or perforation into the GI wall (Fig. 18.6).[31] Duodenal and gastric ulcers are the most common types of PUD, and the most common causes of upper GI bleeding. The ulcer in PUD is a crater surrounded by acutely or chronically inflamed cells. Over time, the inflamed tissue is replaced by necrotic tissue, then by granulation tissue, and finally by scar tissue.[36]

BOX 18.4 Causes of Gastrointestinal Bleeding

Causes of Upper Gastrointestinal Bleeding
- Duodenal ulcer
- Esophageal or gastric varices
- Gastric ulcer
- Mallory-Weiss tear

Causes of Lower Gastrointestinal Bleeding
- Cancer
- Diverticulosis
- Hemorrhoids
- Inflammatory disease
- Polyps
- Vascular ectasias

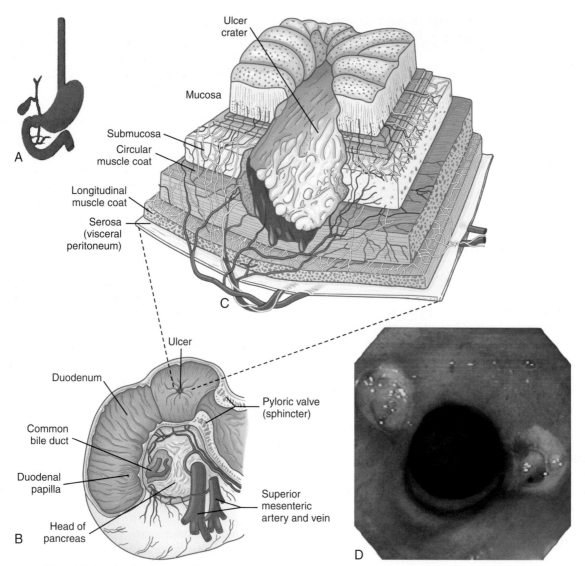

Fig. 18.6 Duodenal ulcer. **A,** Location of the ulcer in the gastrointestinal tract, location noted via the *red dot.* **B,** Placement of the ulcer from outside the gastrointestinal lumen. **C,** Deep ulceration in the duodenal wall extending as a crater through the entire mucosa and into the muscle layers. **D,** Bilateral duodenal ulcers in person using nonsteroidal antiinflammatory drugs. (**A, C, D,** from Huether S, McCance K. *Understanding Pathophysiology.* 6th ed. St. Louis, MO: Elsevier; 2017. **B,** Courtesy David Bjorkman, MD, University of Utah School of Medicine, Department of Gastroenterology, Salt Lake City, UT.)

The secretion of acid is important in the pathogenesis of ulcer disease. Acetylcholine (a neurotransmitter), gastrin (a hormone), and secretin (a hormone) stimulate the chief cells, which stimulate acid secretion. Parietal cell mass in people with PUD is 1.5 to 2 times greater than in people without the disease. Complications of PUD include bleeding, perforation, gastric outlet obstruction, and gastric cancer.[24] Risk factors for the development of PUD are presented in Box 18.5. Contributing factors in ulcer formation are shown in Box 18.6. Infection with *Helicobacter pylori (H. pylori)* bacteria is a major cause of duodenal ulcers.[16] Chronic use of NSAIDs is also a contributing cause of PUD in patients with *H. pylori*

infection. Treatment choices include standard triple therapy, sequential therapy, quadruple therapy, and levofloxacin-based triple therapy.[24] Selected studies of GI function are reviewed in Table 18.5. Characteristics of gastric and duodenal ulcers are presented in Table 18.6.

Stress-Related Mucosal Bleeding or Stress Ulcers. Stress-related mucosal bleeding, or stress ulcers, are an acute form of peptic ulcer that often accompanies severe illness, systemic trauma, or neurological injury.[30] Ischemia is the prior etiology associated with stress ulcer formation. Ischemic ulcers develop within hours after an event such as hemorrhage, multisystem

BOX 18.5 Risk Factors for Peptic Ulcer Disease

- Alcohol consumption
- *Helicobacter pylori* infection: elevates levels of gastrin and pepsinogen and releases toxins and enzymes that promote inflammation and ulceration
- Nonsteroidal antiinflammatory drugs (NSAIDs): inhibit prostaglandins
- Smoking: stimulates acid secretion

BOX 18.6 Contributing Factors to Ulcer Formation

- Increased number of parietal cells in the gastric mucosa
- Gastrin levels that remain higher for longer after eating
- Gastrin levels that continue to stimulate secretion of acid and pepsin
- Failure of feedback mechanism
- Rapid gastric emptying that overwhelms buffering capacity
- Association of *Helicobacter pylori* with mucosal epithelial cell necrosis
- Decreased muscosal bicarbonate secretion

trauma, severe burns, heart failure, or sepsis.[30] The shock, anoxia, and sympathetic responses decrease mucosal blood flow, leading to ischemia. Stress ulcers that develop as a result of burn injury are often called *Curling ulcers*. Stress ulcers associated with severe head trauma or brain surgery are called *Cushing ulcers*. The decreased mucosal blood flow and hypersecretion of acid caused by overstimulation of the vagal nuclei are associated with Cushing ulcers.[30]

Administration of antacids, histamine receptor (H₂-receptor) antagonists, and proton pump inhibitors (PPIs) may be an effective form of therapy. A meta-analysis showed that critically ill patients at risk for the development of stress-related mucosal bleeding benefited from administration of PPI prophylaxis, which significantly decreased the rate of bleeding compared with H₂-receptor antagonists.[9] However, there is conflicting evidence that use of PPIs in critically ill patients was associated with increased risk of GI bleeding when compared with H₂-receptor antagonists.[44] PUD prophylactic measures are still currently recommended by the Institute for Healthcare Improvement as part of a "bundle" of best practices for care of the critically ill adult, specifically in PUD prophylaxis for prevention of ventilator-associated pneumonia or ventilator-associated events.[34,49,57]

Mallory-Weiss Tear. A Mallory-Weiss tear is an arterial hemorrhage resulting from an acute longitudinal tear in the gastroesophageal mucosa. Mallory-Weiss tears account for 10% to 15% of upper GI bleeding episodes. They are associated with long-term use of NSAIDs or aspirin and with excessive alcohol intake. The upper GI bleeding usually occurs after episodes of forceful retching. Bleeding usually resolves spontaneously; however, lacerations of the esophagogastric junction may cause massive GI bleeding, requiring surgical repair.

Esophageal Varices. In chronic liver failure, liver cell structure and function are impaired, resulting in increased portal venous pressure, called *portal hypertension* (see later discussion of Hepatic Failure). As a result, part of the venous blood in the splanchnic system is diverted from the liver to the systemic circulation by the development of connections to neighboring low-pressure veins. This phenomenon is called *collateral circulation*. The most common sites for the development of these collateral channels are the submucosa of the esophagus and rectum, the anterior abdominal wall, and the parietal peritoneum. Fig. 18.7 shows a liver with collateral circulation. The normal portal venous pressure is 2 to 6 mm Hg. As these veins experience increases in pressure, they become distended with blood, the vessels enlarge, and varices develop when the pressure exceeds 10 mm Hg. The varices tend to bleed when the portal venous pressures reach 12 mm Hg. The most common sites for development of these varices are the esophagus and the upper portion of the stomach.[68]

Assessment

Clinical Presentation. Patients manifest blood loss from the GI tract in several ways. Vomiting or drainage from a nasogastric tube that yields blood or coffee grounds–like material is

TABLE 18.5 Selected Studies of Gastrointestinal Function

Test	Normal Findings	Clinical Significance
Stool studies	*Fat:* 2-6 g/24 h	Steatorrhea can result from intestinal malabsorption or pancreatic insufficiency
	Occult blood: none	Positive test is associated with bleeding
Gastric acid stimulation	11-20 mEq/h after stimulation	Increased with duodenal ulcers Decreased with gastric atrophy or gastric carcinoma
Glucose breath test or D-xylose	Negative for hydrogen and CO_2	May indicate intestinal bacterial overgrowth
Urea breath test	Negative for isotopically labeled CO_2	Presence of *Helicobacter pylori* infection

CO_2, Carbon dioxide.
Modified from Huether SE. Structure and function of the digestive system. In: McCance KL, Huether SE, eds. *Pathophysiology: The Biologic Basis for Disease in Adults and Children.* 8th ed. St. Louis, MO: Elsevier; 2019.

TABLE 18.6 Characteristics of Gastric and Duodenal Ulcers

Characteristic	Gastric Ulcer	Duodenal Ulcer
Incidence		
Age at onset	50–70 yr	20–50 yr
Family history	Usually negative	Positive
Gender prevalence	Equal in women and men	Equal in women and men
Stress factors	Increased	Average
Ulcerogenic medications	Normal use	Increased use
Cancer risk	Increased	Not increased
Pathophysiology		
Abnormal mucus	May be present	May be present
Parietal cell mass	Normal or decreased	Increased
Acid production	Normal or decreased	Increased
Serum gastrin	Increased	Normal
Serum pepsinogen	Normal	Increased
Associated gastritis	More common	Usually not present
Helicobacter pylori	May be present (60%–80%)	Often present (95%–100%)
Clinical Manifestations		
Pain	Upper abdomen	Upper abdomen
	Intermittent	Intermittent
	Pain–antacid–relief pattern	Pain–antacid or food–relief pattern
	Food-pain pattern	Nocturnal pain common
Clinical course	Chronic ulcer without pattern of remission and exacerbation	Pattern of remissions and exacerbations for years

From Huether SE. Alterations of digestive function. In: McCance KL, Huether SE, eds. *Pathophysiology: The Biologic Basis for Disease in Adults and Children.* 8th ed. St. Louis, MO: Elsevier; 2019.

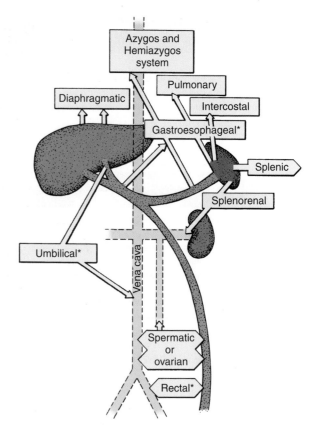

Fig. 18.7 The liver and collateral circulation. *Indicates most common sites.

associated with upper GI bleeding. However, blood or coffee grounds–like contents may not be present if bleeding has ceased or if the bleeding arises beyond a closed pylorus. Upper GI bleeding commonly manifests with *hematemesis,* which is bloody vomitus that is either bright red, indicating fresh blood, or has the appearance of coffee grounds, resulting from older blood that has been in the stomach long enough for the gastric juices to act on it. Blood may also pass via the colon. *Melena* is shiny, black, foul-smelling stool that results from the degradation of blood by stomach acids or intestinal bacteria. Bright red or maroon blood *(hematochezia)* is usually a sign of a lower GI source of bleeding, but it may be observed with massive upper GI bleeding (>1000 mL). Often GI blood loss is occult (not visible) and is detected only by testing the stool with a chemical reagent *(guaiac).* Stool and nasogastric drainage can test positive with guaiac for up to 10 days after a bleeding episode. Hematemesis and melena indicate an episode of acute upper GI bleeding. Upper GI bleeding may also

be accompanied by mild epigastric pain or abdominal distress. Pain arises from the acid bathing the ulcerated crater.

Finally, patients with acute upper GI bleeding may manifest clinical signs and symptoms of blood loss (see Clinical Alert box). Rapidly assess for hemodynamic stability associated with bleeding and collaborate with the multiprofessional team to determine whether the bleeding is acute or chronic in etiology. Patients with acute upper GI bleeding commonly have signs or symptoms of hypovolemic shock. Fig. 18.8 describes the pathophysiology of acute upper GI bleeding.

> **! CLINICAL ALERT**
>
> ### *Clinical Signs and Symptoms of Upper Gastrointestinal Bleeding*
>
> - Abdominal discomfort
> - Hematemesis
> - Hematochezia
> - Melena
> - Signs and symptoms of hypovolemic shock
>   - Change in level of consciousness
>   - Cool, clammy skin
>   - Decreased gastric motility
>   - Decreased urine output
>   - Hypotension
>   - Tachycardia

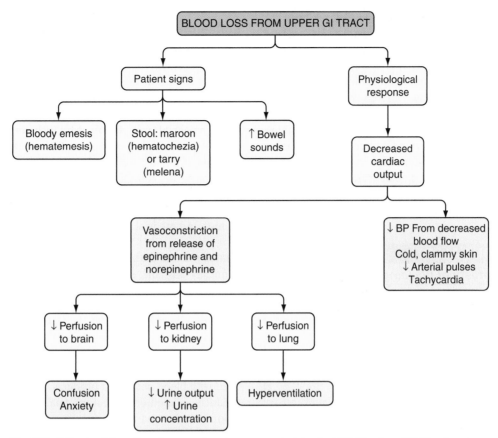

Fig. 18.8 Pathophysiology flow diagram of acute upper gastrointestinal (GI) bleeding. *BP*, Blood pressure.

Assess for comorbid conditions in the older adult. Conditions such as chronic hypertension or cardiovascular disease often mask signs of shock and make resuscitative attempts difficult.

Nursing Assessment. Initial evaluation of the patient with upper GI bleeding involves rapid assessment of the severity of blood loss, hemodynamic stability, and the necessity for fluid resuscitation. Monitor signs of hypovolemic shock (see Chapter 12). Changes in blood pressure and heart rate depend on the amount of blood loss, the suddenness of the blood loss, and the degree of cardiac and vascular compensation. Monitor vital signs at least every 15 minutes. As blood loss exceeds 1000 mL, the shock syndrome progresses, causing decreased blood flow to the skin, lungs, liver, and kidneys.

Hypotension is an advanced sign of shock. As a rule, a systolic pressure of less than 100 mm Hg, a postural decrease in blood pressure of greater than 10 mm Hg, or a heart rate of greater than 120 beats/min reflects a blood loss of at least 1000 mL—25% of the total blood volume.

Hypertension is a common comorbid condition in those at risk of GI bleeding. In the chronically hypertensive patient, normal values for predicting perfusion do not apply; therefore assess other parameters, such as level of consciousness and urinary output. Decreasing blood pressure is often associated with increasing blood loss.

Hemodynamic monitoring (see Chapter 9) may be initiated to evaluate the patient's hemodynamic response to the blood loss. An electrocardiogram may show ST-segment depression or flattening of the T waves, both of which indicate decreased coronary blood flow resulting in ischemia.

Abdominal assessment may reveal a soft or distended abdomen. Bowel sounds most often are hyperactive as a result of the sensitivity of the bowel to blood.

In addition to the physical examination, obtain a history to identify whether there have been previous episodes of bleeding or surgery for bleeding; a family history of bleeding; or a current illness or disease that may lead to bleeding, such as a coagulopathy, cancer, or liver disease. Also assess patterns of drug or alcohol ingestion and other risk factors.

Medical Assessment

Laboratory studies. The common laboratory studies ordered for a patient with acute upper GI bleeding are listed in the Laboratory Alert box. Although a complete blood count is always ordered, the hematocrit (Hct) value does not change substantially during the first few hours after an acute bleeding episode. During this time, do not underestimate the severity of the bleeding. Only when extravascular fluid enters the vascular space to restore volume does the Hct value decrease. This effect is further complicated by fluids and blood products that are administered during the resuscitation period. Platelet and white blood cell (WBC) counts may be increased, reflecting the body's attempt to restore homeostasis. An electrolyte profile is also indicated. Decreases in levels of potassium and sodium are common as a result of the accompanying vomiting. Later, serum sodium levels may increase as a result of the loss of vascular volume. The glucose level is often increased related to the stress response. Increases in the levels of blood urea nitrogen (BUN) and creatinine reflect decreased perfusion to the liver and kidneys. Liver function tests, clotting profiles, and serum ammonia levels are ordered to rule out preexisting liver disease. An arterial blood gas analysis is ordered to evaluate the patient's acid-base and oxygenation status. Respiratory alkalosis is common with GI bleeding due to patient anxiety and the effects of the sympathetic nervous system. As shock progresses, the patient may develop metabolic acidosis as a result of anaerobic metabolism. Hypoxemia may also be present as a result of decreased circulating Hgb levels.

! LABORATORY ALERT

Upper Gastrointestinal Bleeding

Arterial Blood Gases
Metabolic acidosis
Respiratory alkalosis

Complete Blood Count
Hematocrit: Normal, then ↓
Hemoglobin: Normal, then ↓
Platelet count: Initially ↑, then ↓
White blood cell count: ↑

Gastric Aspirate for pH and Guaiac
Guaiac positive
Possibly acidotic pH

Hematology Profile
Prothrombin time, partial thromboplastin time: Usually ↑
Serum enzyme levels: ↓

Serum Electrolyte Panel
Ammonia: Possibly ↑
Blood urea nitrogen, creatinine: ↑
Calcium: Normal or ↓
Glucose: Hyperglycemia common
Lactate: ↑
Potassium: ↓, then ↑
Sodium: ↓

Endoscopy and barium study. Endoscopy is the procedure of choice for the diagnosis and treatment of active upper GI bleeding and for the prevention of rebleeding. Endoscopy allows for direct mucosal inspection with the use of a flexible, fiberoptic scope. The procedure can be done at the bedside, which is an advantage when caring for a critically ill patient. Endoscopic evaluation of the source of the bleeding usually is not undertaken until the patient is hemodynamically stable. Barium studies can be performed to help define the presence of peptic ulcers, the sites of bleeding, the presence of tumors, and the presence of inflammatory processes.[33]

Patient Problems

The patient problems most commonly seen in patients with acute GI bleeding are related to hypovolemia due to volume loss (see Chapter 12).

Collaborative Management: Nursing and Medical Considerations

The management of acute GI bleeding initially consists of treatment to restore hemodynamic stability, followed by diagnosis of the cause of bleeding and initiation of specific and supportive therapies (Box 18.7). The nurse's role during the initial management of acute GI bleeding includes assessment, carrying out prescribed medical therapy, monitoring the patient's physiological and psychosocial responses to the interventions, monitoring for complications of the disease process or treatment regimen, and providing supportive care. In addition, the nurse supports the patient and family and explains the diagnostic tests and medical therapies.

Hemodynamic Stabilization. For patients who are hemodynamically unstable, establish immediate venous access using a large-bore IV catheter and begin fluid administration (see Chapter 12). For the restoration of vascular volume, infuse fluids as rapidly as the patient's cardiovascular status allows and until vital signs return to baseline.

Patients who continue to bleed, or who have an excessively low Hct value (<25%) and clinical symptoms, may be resuscitated with blood and blood products. The decision to use blood products is based on laboratory data and clinical examination. Blood is transfused to improve oxygenation (by increasing the number of RBCs) or to improve coagulation (by replacing platelets and plasma). The Hct value may not initially reflect actual blood volume during the first 24 to 72 hours after a hemorrhage and until vascular volume is restored. A reasonable goal for blood transfusions is a Hct of 30%, but this goal is individually determined based on clinical assessments. One unit of packed RBCs usually increases the Hgb value by 1 g/dL and the Hct value by 2% to 3%, but this effect is influenced by the patient's intravascular volume status and whether the patient is actively bleeding. Carefully monitor the patient for complications of blood transfusion therapy: hypocalcemia, hyperkalemia, infection, increased ammonia levels, hypothermia, and anaphylactic reactions.

Gastric Lavage. Gastric lavage may be performed to reduce bleeding and to evaluate whether the bleed is coming from the

---

BOX 18.7 Management of Upper Gastrointestinal Bleeding

Hemodynamic Stabilization
- Colloids
- Crystalloids
- Blood or blood products

Definitive and Supportive Therapies
- Gastric lavage
- Pharmacological therapies
  - Antacids
  - H₂-histamine blockers
  - Proton pump inhibitors
  - Mucosal barrier enhancers
- Endoscopic therapies
  - Sclerotherapy
  - Heater probe
  - Laser
- Surgical therapies

upper GI tract.[15] Large-volume gastric lavage before endoscopy for acute upper GI bleeding is safe and provides better visualization of the gastric fundus. Insert a large-bore nasogastric tube and connect it to suction. If lavage is ordered, instill 1000 to 2000 mL of room-temperature normal saline via the nasogastric tube and gently remove the gastric contents by intermittent suction or gravity until the secretions are clear. Iced lavage is used in some centers, although the evidence for this use is not well documented. After lavage, the nasogastric tube may be removed or left in place. Nasogastric tubes left in place can increase hydrochloric acid secretion in the stomach and cause increased bleeding. Of all upper GI hemorrhages, 80% to 90% are self-limited and stop with lavage therapy alone or on their own. Carefully document the nature of the nasogastric secretions or vomitus, such as color, amount, and pH.[55]

Pharmacological Therapy. Pharmacological agents are given to decrease gastric acid secretion or to reduce the effects of acid on the gastric mucosa. The agents most commonly used are antacids, histamine antagonists (H_2-receptor blockers), PPIs, and mucosal barrier enhancers. Antibiotics may also be ordered. Table 18.7 describes the treatments commonly used to decrease gastric acid secretion or reduce the effects of acid on the gastric mucosa (see Evidence-Based Practice box).

Antibiotics. *H. pylori* infection is often associated with PUD. Triple-agent therapy with a PPI and two antibiotics for 14 days is the recommended treatment for eradication of *H. pylori*. The first-line treatment for *H. pylori* infection consists of triple therapy with a PPI (e.g., esomeprazole, omeprazole, pantoprazole, rabeprazole) plus the antibiotics amoxicillin and clarithromycin.[22] In case first-line therapy fails, a bismuth-based quadruple therapy has proved effective in 76% of patients. This second-line therapy consists of a PPI or H_2-receptor antagonist, bismuth, metronidazole, and a tetracycline. Alternatively, a 10-day course of levofloxacin may be administered as a second-line therapy for *H. pylori* infections.[45] If the infection is resistant to clarithromycin, quadruple therapy should be used.[22]

Endoscopic Therapy. Endoscopy is the treatment of choice for upper GI bleeding, and several endoscopic therapies have been developed. Endoscopy is performed only after the patient is stabilized hemodynamically but within 24 hours after manifestation of the GI bleeding.[15] The advantage of endoscopic therapies is that they can be applied during the diagnostic procedure. *Sclerotherapy* involves injecting the bleeding ulcer with a necrotizing agent. The agents most commonly used are morrhuate sodium, ethanolamine, and tetradecyl sulfate. These agents work by traumatizing the endothelium, causing necrosis and eventually

TABLE 18.7 PHARMACOLOGY

Pharmacological Treatments to Decrease Gastric Acid Secretion and/or Reduce Acid Effects on Gastric Mucosa

Medication	Action/Use	Dose/Route	Side Effects	Nursing Implications
Histamine Blockers	Block all factors that stimulate the parietal cells in the stomach to secrete hydrochloric acid		Most H_2 blockers do not have any side effects. Some have the side effects of diarrhea, headache, dizziness, rash, and tiredness	Watch for a worsening of symptoms: vomiting of blood, blood in stools, unintentional weight loss, difficulty swallowing, persistent abdominal pain. Many require renal dosing adjustments
Cimetidine		Upper GI bleeding prophylaxis: 50 mg/h; lowered in renal disease/IV infusion Duodenal ulcer prophylaxis: 400 mg qHS or 300 mg bid/PO		
Famotidine		20 mg bid/PO or IV		
Nizatidine		150-300 mg daily Not available IV		
Ranitidine		50 mg q6-8h; unlabeled/IM or IV		
Proton Pump Inhibitors	Inhibit gastric acid secretion by specific inhibition of the hydrogen-potassium–adenosine triphosphatase enzyme system		Constipation, diarrhea, flatulence, headaches, nausea, abdominal pain, and vomiting	Monitor for presence of blood in vomit or stool, unintentional weight loss, difficulty swallowing, abdominal pain, or persistent vomiting
Esomeprazole		20-40 mg daily, up to 10 days/IV		
Lansoprazole		30 mg daily/PO		
Omeprazole		20-40 mg daily/PO Not available IV		
Pantoprazole		40 mg daily/PO or IV		
Mucosal Barrier Enhancers	Reduce the effects of acid secretion; promote healing		Constipation, dizziness, lightheadedness, severe allergic reactions	Assess for presence of dizziness
Sucralfate		1 g QID, 1 h AC and qHS/PO		May have sensitivity to the aluminum in it

Continued

TABLE 18.7 PHARMACOLOGY—cont'd

Pharmacological Treatments to Decrease Gastric Acid Secretion and/or Reduce Acid Effects on Gastric Mucosa

Medication	Action/Use	Dose/Route	Side Effects	Nursing Implications
Antacids	Direct alkaline buffer to control the pH of the gastric mucosa		Cause a laxative effect; dangerous when used with renal failure; nausea, vomiting, abdominal pain, diarrhea	Assess for allergies; patients with heart failure or hypertension should use low-sodium medications; monitor for side effects. Often given q1-2h to maintain gastric pH >5
Aluminum hydroxide		500-1500 mg 3-6 times daily/PO	Constipation	
Calcium carbonate		80-140 mEq q3-6h/PO	Produces gas and belching	
Magnesium hydroxide		400-1200 mg QID PRN/PO	Diarrhea	
Magnesium oxide		400 mg BID/PO	Diarrhea	

AC, Before meals; *BID,* twice a day; *H₂,* histamine; *PO,* by mouth; *q,* every; *qHS,* every hour of sleep; *QID,* four times a day; *PRN,* as needed.
From Skidmore-Roth L. *Mosby's 2019 Nursing Drug Reference.* 32nd ed. St. Louis, MO: Elsevier; 2019.

EVIDENCE-BASED PRACTICE

Preventing Upper Gastrointestinal Bleeding in Critically Ill Patients

Problem
There is evidence to support that upper gastrointestinal (GI) bleeding due to stress ulcers contributed to increased morbidity and mortality in critically ill patients. However, the incidence of stress-induced GI bleeding in critical care units has decreased, and not all critically ill patients may need prophylactic treatment. In addition, stress ulcer prophylaxis may be associated with negative effects, such as or ventilator-associated pneumonia (VAP).

Clinical Questions
How effective are prophylactic interventions in decreasing upper GI bleeding risk compared to placebo or no prophylaxis?

Evidence
Toews and colleagues reviewed 106 studies, which involved a total of 15,027 critically ill patients, to investigate whether GI prophylaxis was effective in reducing the occurrence of upper GI bleeding risk when compared to placebo or no prophylaxis. In comparison with placebo or no treatment, several medications resulted in lower rates of upper GI bleeding: H₂-receptor antagonists, 11% lower; antacids, 9% lower; and sucralfate, 5% lower. Proton pump inhibitors were no more effective in preventing upper GI bleeding when compared to placebo or no treatment. Low-quality evidence suggested that proton pump inhibitors may be more effective than H₂-receptor antagonists. Any treatment and the

incidence of nosocomial pneumonia was associated with both benefits and harms. Larger, high-quality randomized controlled trials (RCTs) are needed to confirm these findings.

Implications for Nursing
Critically ill patients may benefit from stress ulcer prophylaxis to prevent upper GI bleeding; however, assess for complications of administering H₂-receptor antagonists, antacids, sucralfate, and proton pump inhibitors in critically ill patients. In addition to hospital-acquired pneumonia or VAP, patients may exhibit symptoms of thrombocytopenia, interstitial nephritis, and confusion with H₂-receptor antagonist use. Proton pump inhibitors are associated with increased *Clostridium difficile* diarrhea. Antacids may cause diarrhea or constipation, and sucralfate may cause constipation and interfere with the absorption of certain antibacterial agents.

Level of Evidence
A—Systematic review

References
Toews I, George AT, Peter JV, et al. Interventions for preventing upper gastrointestinal bleeding in people admitted to intensive care units. *Cochrane Database Syst Rev.* 2018;6:CD008687.

sclerosis of the bleeding vessel. Thermal methods of endoscopic therapy include use of the heater probe, laser photocoagulation, and electrocoagulation to tamponade the vessel. Endoclipping—band dilators and hemoclips—may be used to provide hemostasis and to decrease the incidence of rebleeding.[15]

During endoscopy, assist with procedures and monitor for untoward effects. Maintain the airway and observe the patient's breathing during endoscopy. Assist in positioning the patient in a left lateral reverse Trendelenburg position to help prevent respiratory complications. Other common complications of sclerotherapy include fever and oozing from the bleeding site.

Surgical Therapy. Surgery may be considered for patients who have massive GI bleeding. The patient is usually admitted to a critical care unit for initial management and stabilization in preparation for emergency surgery. The most common reason for emergency surgery is massive rebleeding that occurs within 8 hours of admission. Patients may also become surgical candidates if they continue to bleed despite aggressive medical intervention. Criteria for delayed surgery vary, but it is usually considered in those patients who require more than 8 units of blood within a 24-hour period.

Surgical therapies for PUD include gastric resection (antrectomy, gastrectomy, gastroenterostomy, vagotomy) and combined operations to restore GI continuity (Billroth I, Billroth II) or to prevent complications of the surgery (vagotomy and pyloroplasty). An *antrectomy* may be performed for duodenal ulcers to decrease the acidity of the duodenum by removing the antrum, which secretes gastric acid. A *vagotomy* decreases acid secretion in the stomach by dividing the vagus nerve along the esophagus. A *pyloroplasty* may be performed in conjunction with a vagotomy to prevent stomach atony, a common complication of the vagotomy procedure. A *Billroth I* procedure involves vagotomy, antrectomy, and anastomosis of the stomach to the duodenum. A *Billroth II* procedure involves vagotomy, resection of the antrum, and anastomosis of the stomach to the jejunum (Fig. 18.9). A perforation can be treated by simple closure with the use of a patch to cover the gastric mucosal hole (omental patch) or by excision of the ulcer and suturing of the surrounding tissue.

Impaired emptying of solids or liquids from the stomach into the small intestine (gastric outlet obstruction) may also necessitate surgical intervention. The major symptoms of obstruction are vomiting and continued pain that is localized in the epigastrium.

Postoperative nursing care is focused on preventing and monitoring potential complications. Fluid and electrolyte imbalances are common from loss of fluids during the surgical procedure, surgical drains, and a nasogastric tube that may be left in place to decompress the stomach. In addition, the GI system may not function normally after surgery, with resulting nausea, vomiting, ileus, or diarrhea. Providing adequate nutrition is important to promote wound healing. In cases of prolonged ileus after surgery, total parenteral nutrition may be considered. Monitor for signs and symptoms of wound infection: erythema, swelling, tenderness, drainage, fever, and increased WBC count. A systemic infection may result from peritonitis if perforation has allowed stomach or intestinal contents to spill into the peritoneum. Postoperative rupture of the anastomosis may also lead to this complication.

Pain is an important postoperative nursing concern. Abdominal incisions are associated with postoperative discomfort because of their anatomical location. Implement incentive spirometry and other pulmonary hygiene measures to reduce the risk of postoperative lung infections. Pulmonary infections are common because incisional pain impairs the ability to cough and breathe deeply.

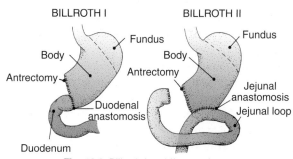

Fig. 18.9 Billroth I and II procedures.

Patient Problems. Several patient problems are associated with the postoperative care of the patient with upper GI bleeding. These problems include Potential Infection; Acute Pain; Potential for Fluid, Electrolyte, and Acid-Base Imbalances; Potential for Impaired Nutrition; Potential for Decreased Multisystem Tissue Perfusion; and Decreased Gas Exchange (see Collaborative Plan of Care for the Critically Ill Patient in Chapter 1).

Recognition of Potential Complications. Perforation of the gastric mucosa is the major GI complication of PUD (see Clinical Alert box). The most common signs of perforation are an abrupt onset of abdominal pain followed rapidly by signs of peritonitis. Emergent surgery is indicated for treatment. Fluid and electrolyte resuscitation and treatment of any immediate complication are the priorities. These patients almost always have nasogastric tubes placed for gastric decompression. Broad-spectrum antibiotics are also usually prescribed before surgery. Antacids and histamine blockers may or may not be indicated, depending on the cause of the upper GI bleeding. Mortality rates for patients with perforation range from 10% to 40%, depending on the age and condition of the patient at the time of surgery.

> **! CLINICAL ALERT**
> ### *Acute Gastric Perforation*
> - Abdominal tenderness
> - Abrupt onset of severe abdominal pain
> - Boardlike abdomen
> - Leukocytosis
> - Presence of free air on radiography
> - Usually absent bowel sounds

Treatment of Variceal Bleeding

Bleeding esophageal or gastric varices are usually a medical emergency because they cause massive upper GI blood loss. The patient typically develops hemodynamic instability and signs and symptoms of shock. Often the cause of the bleeding is unknown unless the patient has a history of cirrhosis or has previously bled from varices. Initial treatment of esophageal and gastric varices is the same. Top priorities include hemodynamic stabilization and establishment of a patent airway. Gastric lavage may be used to clear the stomach and to document the amount of blood loss. Diagnosis of the cause of the bleeding through endoscopy is a priority before definitive treatment for the varices can be started.[58]

Somatostatin or Octreotide. Somatostatin or octreotide (a long-acting somatostatin) is ordered to slow or stop bleeding. These medications decrease splanchnic blood flow and reduce portal pressure and have minimal adverse effects. Octreotide is given to stabilize patients before definitive treatment is performed. Octreotide is recommended for patients with variceal upper GI bleeding, and it can be used as adjunctive therapy for nonvariceal upper GI bleeding.[15] Octreotide is given as an

BOX 18.8 Vasopressin (Pitressin) Therapy

Mechanism of Action

Vasoconstrictor: constricts the splanchnic vascular bed, contracts intestinal smooth muscle, and lowers portal vein pressure

Dose

Given by IV, although it may be given intraarterially. IV infusion is started at 0.2-0.4 unit/min and increased by 0.2 unit/min each hour until hemorrhage is controlled, to a maximum dose of 0.8 unit/min. (The medication may also be given by body weight: initial dose of 0.002-0.005 unit/kg/min IV titrated to a maximum dose of 0.01 unit/kg/min.) Continued for at least 24 h after bleeding is controlled. Wean slowly.

Side Effects

- *Gastrointestinal:* cramping, nausea, vomiting, diarrhea
- *Cardiovascular:* dizziness, diaphoresis, hypertension, cardiac dysrhythmias, exacerbation of heart failure
- *Neurologic:* tremors, headache, vertigo, decreased level of consciousness
- *Integumentary:* pallor, localized gangrene

Nursing Considerations

- Monitor for angina and dysrhythmias.
- Infuse through a central line.
- Assess serum sodium.
- Assess neurologic status.

From Gahart BL, Nazareno AR. *2019 Intravenous Medications: A Handbook for Nurses and Health Professionals.* 35th ed. St. Louis, MO: Elsevier; 2019.

IV bolus of 25 to 100 mcg followed by an infusion of 25 to 50 mcg/h for 1 to 5 days. Postprandial hyperglycemia may occur in nondiabetic patients receiving octreotide. Monitor for both hypoglycemia and hyperglycemia.[32]

Vasopressin. Vasopressin (Pitressin) (Box 18.8) is a synthetic antidiuretic hormone. Vasopressin lowers portal pressure by vasoconstriction of the splanchnic arteriolar bed. Ultimately, it decreases pressure and flow in liver collateral circulation channels to decrease bleeding. However, vasopressin does not improve survival rates from active variceal bleeding and is rarely used because of its adverse effects.[15]

Endoscopic Procedures. *Sclerotherapy* is another option in the treatment of bleeding varices. After the varices are identified, the sclerosing agent is injected into the varix and the surrounding tissue. Usually, several applications of the sclerosing agent several days apart are needed to decompress the bleeding varix.

Endoscopic band ligation is another treatment for varices.[15] Under endoscopy, a rubber band is placed over the varix. This treatment results in thrombosis, sloughing, and fibrosis of the varix.

Transjugular Intrahepatic Portosystemic Shunt. *Transjugular intrahepatic portosystemic shunting (TIPS)* is a nonsurgical treatment for recurrent variceal bleeding after sclerotherapy. TIPS has been used primarily to treat the major consequences of portal hypertension, such as bleeding and ascites, or as a bridge to liver transplantation in a cirrhotic patient.[42] Placement of the shunt is performed with the use of fluoroscopy. A stainless steel stent is placed between the hepatic and portal veins to create a portosystemic shunt in the liver and decrease portal pressure.[15] A lower portal pressure decreases pressure within the varix, thereby decreasing the risk of acute hemorrhage.

Approximately 10% to 20% of patients do not stop bleeding after endoscopic treatment combined with somatostatin infusion, and others rebleed within the first couple of days after cessation of the initial bleed. After a second unsuccessful endoscopic attempt, the TIPS procedure is used as a treatment option. Although TIPS is also commonly used for other indications, such as Budd-Chiari syndrome, acute variceal bleeding, and hepatic hydrothorax, the best available evidence supports the use of TIPS in secondary prevention of variceal bleeding and in refractory ascites.[25,53] Early preemptive TIPS can be the first choice for high-risk patients such as those with uncontrolled variceal bleeding,[42] severe portal hypertension,[29] a Child-Pugh score of B with active bleeding, or a Child-Pugh score of C up to 13 points.[5]

✳ QSEN EXEMPLAR

Safety and Quality Improvement

The surgeon informed the critical care nurse that the operating room was not available, and an abdominal washout needed to be done immediately at the patient's bedside. The nurse gathered the necessary equipment for the procedure and checked the patient's orders. The surgeon recently placed an order for two units of fresh frozen plasma (FFP) to be administered during the washout. The nurse informed the surgeon that the FFP would be delayed by 2 hours because the patient's type and screen was expired, and the patient needed a new type and screen per hospital policy. The blood bank also needed time to prepare the FFP. These circumstances necessitated that the procedure be delayed. The surgeon blamed the intensivists for not placing the order for FFP. When the FFP arrived, the patient's nurse verified the FFP with another registered nurse and a time-out was called before the procedure. During the time-out, the nurse checked the patient's informed consent. The nurse informed the surgeon that the patient did not have a consent for the abdominal washout on the electronic health record (EHR), and the procedure was stopped. The surgeon called the patient's legal proxy, and obtained phone consent. After the procedure, the nurse wrote an incident report about the event. A root cause analysis (RCA) revealed that the surgeon did not relay the plans for the abdominal washout to the intensivists during morning rounds. A communication breakdown occurred between the intensivists and the surgeon. To prevent future communication gaps, the nurse added the item "discussion during morning rounds" on the bedside shift report and performed an in-service about the hospital policy on time-outs and bedside procedures in collaboration with the quality management clinician. The RCA team recommended an EHR visual alert for patients with expired type and screens.

Esophagogastric Tamponade. If bleeding continues despite therapy, esophagogastric balloon tamponade therapy may provide temporary control. Inflation of the balloon ports applies pressure to the vessels supplying the varices to decrease blood flow, thereby stopping the bleeding. Three types of tubes are used for tamponade: Sengstaken-Blakemore, Minnesota, and Linton tubes. The adult *Sengstaken-Blakemore tube* has three lumina: one for gastric aspiration (similar to that in a nasogastric tube), one for inflation of the esophageal balloon, and one for inflation of the gastric balloon (Fig. 18.10). The *Minnesota*

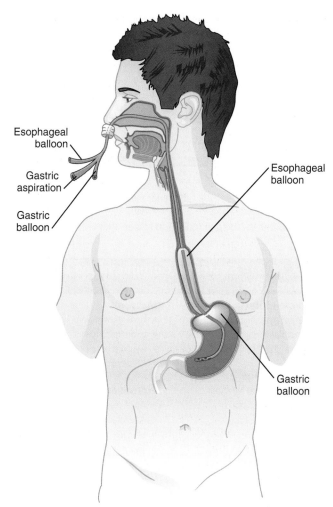

Fig. 18.10 Sengstaken-Blakemore tube. (From Good VS, Kirkwood PL, eds. *AACN Advanced Critical Care Nursing.* 2nd ed. Philadelphia, PA: Saunders; 2017.)

Esophageal balloon

Gastric aspiration

Gastric balloon

Esophageal balloon

Gastric balloon

tube has an additional lumen that allows for aspiration of esophageal secretions. The Minnesota tube is commonly used because it allows for suction of secretions above and below the balloon. The *Linton tube* has a gastric balloon only, with lumens for gastric and esophageal suction; it is reserved for those with bleeding gastric varices.

Regardless of type, the balloon tip is inserted into the stomach, and the gastric balloon is inflated and clamped. The tube is then withdrawn slowly until resistance is met so that pressure is exerted at the gastroesophageal junction. Correct positioning and traction are maintained by the use of an external traction source or a nasal cuff around the tube at the mouth or nose. External traction can be attached to a helmet or to the foot of the bed. Proper amounts of traction are essential because too little traction lets the balloon fall away from the gastric wall, resulting in insufficient pressure on the bleeding vessels, whereas too much traction causes discomfort, gastric ulceration, or vomiting. If bleeding does not stop with inflation of the gastric balloon, the esophageal balloon is inflated and clamped (Sengstaken-Blakemore or Minnesota tube). Normal inflation pressure of the esophageal balloon is 20 to 45 mm Hg.

Monitor balloon lumen pressures and the patency of the system. The gastric balloon port placement below the gastroesophageal junction must be confirmed by radiographic images. Defer to the provider's orders, but typically, deflate the balloon every 8 to 12 hours to decompress the esophagus and gastric mucosa. During this procedure, assess the status of the bleeding and be prepared for hemostasis. Deflate the esophageal balloon before deflating the gastric balloon; otherwise, the entire tube will displace upward and occlude the airway.

Spontaneous rupture of the gastric balloon, upward migration of the tube, and occlusion of the airway are possible complications that need to be assessed. Esophageal rupture may occur and is characterized by the abrupt onset of severe pain. In the event of either of these two life-threatening emergencies, all three lumina are cut and the entire tube is removed. For this reason, ensure that scissors are at the patient's bedside at all times. Endotracheal intubation is strongly recommended to protect the airway if the patient requires balloon tamponade treatment.

Other complications of esophagogastric tamponade include ulcerations of the esophageal or gastric mucosa. In addition, lesions can develop around the mouth and nose as a result of the traction devices. Clean and lubricate the areas around the traction devices to prevent skin breakdown. Suction the nasopharynx frequently because the tube insertion results in an increase in secretions and the patient's swallowing reflex is decreased. Irrigate the nasogastric tube at least every 2 hours to ensure patency and to keep the stomach empty. This measure helps prevent aspiration and prevents accumulation of blood in the stomach, which is especially important in the patient with liver failure. Ammonia is a byproduct of blood breakdown and cannot be detoxified by the patient with liver failure.[18]

Surgical Interventions. Permanent decompression of portal hypertension is achieved only through surgical creation of a *portocaval shunt* that diverts blood around the blocked portal system. In these operations, a connection is made between the portal vein and the inferior vena cava that diverts blood flow into the vena cava to decrease portal pressure. Several variations of this procedure exist, including the end-to-side shunt and the side-to-side shunt (Fig. 18.11). Other surgical techniques for reduction of portal pressure include splenorenal and mesocaval shunting.[67]

Surgical shunts decrease rebleeding but do not improve survival. The procedure is associated with a higher risk of encephalopathy and makes liver transplantation, if needed, more difficult. A temporary increase in ascites occurs after all of these procedures, and careful assessments and interventions are required during the care of these patients (see the later discussion of Hepatic Failure).

ACUTE PANCREATITIS

Acute pancreatitis is an acute inflammatory disease of the pancreas. The intensity of the disease ranges from mild, in which the patient has abdominal pain and elevated blood amylase and lipase levels, to extremely severe, which results in multiple organ failure. In 85% to 90% of patients, the disease is self-limited

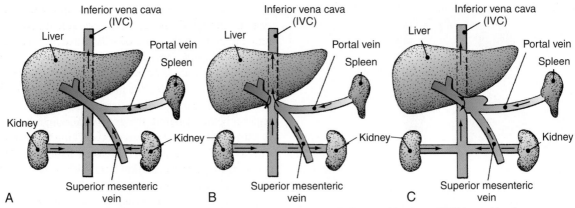

Fig. 18.11 Types of portocaval shunt. **A,** Normal portal circulation. **B,** End-to-side shunt. **C,** Side-to-side shunt.

(mild acute pancreatitis), and patients recover rapidly. However, the disease can run a fulminant course and is associated with high mortality rates. Severe acute pancreatitis develops in 25% of patients with acute pancreatitis. Management of severe pancreatitis requires intensive nursing and medical care.

Pathophysiology

Acute pancreatitis is an inflammation of the pancreas with the potential for necrosis of pancreatic cells resulting from premature activation of pancreatic enzymes. It is one of the most common pancreatic diseases. Each year about 275,000 patients are hospitalized in the United States due to acute pancreatitis.[27] Normally, pancreatic juices are secreted into the duodenum, where they are activated. These enzymes are essential for the metabolism of carbohydrates, fats, and proteins. The most common theory regarding the development of pancreatitis is that an injury or disruption of pancreatic acinar cells allows leakage of pancreatic enzymes into pancreatic tissue. The leaked enzymes (trypsin, chymotrypsin, and elastase) become activated in the tissue and start the process of *autodigestion*. The activated enzymes break down tissue and cell membranes, causing edema, vascular damage, hemorrhage, necrosis, and fibrosis.[32] These now toxic enzymes and inflammatory mediators are released into the bloodstream and cause injury to vessel and organ systems, such as the hepatic and renal systems. Acute pancreatitis starts as a localized pancreatic inflammation and is usually accompanied by a compensatory antiinflammatory response syndrome (CARS). Excessive CARS makes the patient susceptible to infections.[32] Box 18.9 reviews the major systemic complications of acute fulminating pancreatitis.

Acute pancreatitis has numerous causes (Box 18.10), but the most common are alcohol ingestion and biliary disease. Many medications can initiate acute pancreatitis due to ingestion of toxic doses or a medication reaction. Pancreatitis may also develop after blunt or penetrating abdominal trauma and after endoscopic exploration of the biliary tree.

Most patients with mild acute pancreatitis are treated with a short period of bowel rest, simple IV hydration, and analgesia. Severe acute pancreatitis is treated with intensive hemodynamic and pulmonary management, nutrition support, infection control, and pharmacological agents.[32]

Metabolic complications of acute pancreatitis include hypocalcemia and hyperlipidemia, which are related to the areas of

---

BOX 18.9 Systemic Complications of Acute Pancreatitis

Cardiovascular
- Cardiac dysrhythmias
- Hypovolemic shock
- Myocardial depression

Gastrointestinal
- Gastrointestinal bleeding
- Pancreatic abscess
- Pancreatic pseudocyst

Hematologic
- Coagulation abnormalities
- Disseminated intravascular coagulation

Metabolic
- Hyperglycemia
- Hyperlipidemia
- Hypocalcemia
- Metabolic acidosis

Pulmonary
- Acute respiratory distress syndrome
- Atelectasis, pneumonia, pleural effusion
- Hypoxemia

Renal
- Acute renal failure
- Azotemia
- Oliguria

BOX 18.10 Causes of Acute Pancreatitis

- Alcohol consumption
- Biliary disease
  - Common bile duct obstruction
  - ERCP procedure
  - Gallstones
- Heredity
- Hypercalcemia
- Hypertriglyceridemia
- Idiopathic
- Infections
- Medications
  - Azathioprine
  - Corticosteroids
  - Estrogen
  - Furosemide
  - Octreotide
  - Pentamidine
  - Sulfonamides
  - Thiazide diuretics
- Traumatic injury of the pancreas
- Tumors of pancreatic ductal system or metastatic tumors

ERCP, Endoscopic retrograde cholangiopancreatography.

---

fat necrosis. Hypocalcemia is a major complication and usually indicates a more serious manifestation of acute pancreatitis. Various hormone imbalances, particularly parathyroid hormone imbalance, also occur in pancreatitis.[40]

Assessment

History and Physical Examination. A diagnosis of acute pancreatitis is based on clinical examination and the results of laboratory and radiological tests (see Laboratory Alert box).

Nurses conduct initial and ongoing assessments, monitor and report physical and laboratory data, and coordinate the multiprofessional plan of care.

! LABORATORY ALERT

Pancreatitis

Albumin: ↓
Alkaline phosphatase: ↑ with biliary disease
Bilirubin, AST, LDH: ↑
Calcium: ↓
Glucose: ↑ with islet cell damage
Hematocrit: ↑ with dehydration; ↓ with hemorrhagic pancreatitis
Potassium: ↓
Serum and urine amylase: ↑
Serum lipase: ↑
White blood cell count: ↑

AST, Aspartate transaminase; *LDH,* lactate dehydrogenase.

Patients who have organ failure at admission or within 72 hours after onset of the disease have a complicated clinical course with persistence of multisystem dysfunction. Multiorgan dysfunction syndrome triggers additional mechanisms that render translocation of bacteria manifesting as sepsis. Early and persistent organ failure in patients with acute pancreatitis is an indicator of a prolonged hospital stay and an increased risk of mortality.[32]

Most patients with acute pancreatitis develop severe abdominal pain. It is most often epigastric or midabdominal pain that radiates to the back. The pain is caused by edema, chemical irritation and inflammation of the peritoneum, and irritation or obstruction of the biliary tract.[32]

Nausea and vomiting are also common symptoms and are caused by hypermotility or paralytic ileus secondary to the pancreatitis or peritonitis. Abdominal distension accompanies the bowel symptoms, along with accumulation of fluid in the peritoneal cavity.[32] This fluid contains enzymes and kinins that increase vascular permeability and dilate the blood vessels. Hypotension and shock occur from the intravascular volume depletion, leading to myocardial insufficiency. Fever and leukocytosis are also symptoms of the inflammatory process.

Patients with more severe pancreatic disease may have ascites, jaundice, or palpable abdominal masses. Two rare signs that may be present in any disease associated with retroperitoneal hemorrhage result in a bluish discoloration of the flanks *(Grey Turner's sign)* or around the umbilical area *(Cullen's sign),* indicative of blood in these areas.[62,63] Because of the increase in abdominal size, measure and record the abdominal girth at least every 4 hours to detect internal bleeding (see Clinical Alert box).

! CLINICAL ALERT

Signs and Symptoms of Acute Pancreatitis

- Abdominal guarding, distension
- Cullen's sign
- Dehydration
- Fever
- Grey Turner's sign
- Nausea and vomiting
- Pain

Diagnostic Tests. Acute pancreatitis is diagnosed based on clinical findings, the presence of associated disorders, and laboratory testing. Pain associated with acute pancreatitis is similar to that associated with PUD, gallbladder disease, intestinal obstruction, or acute myocardial infarction. This similarity exists because pain receptors in the abdomen are poorly differentiated as they exit the skin surface. Because the clinical history, presenting signs and symptoms, and physical findings mimic those of many other GI and cardiovascular disorders, endoscopic and transabdominal ultrasound studies and computed tomography (CT) scans are performed to determine the extent of involvement and the presence of complications.

Serum lipase and amylase tests are the most specific indicators of acute pancreatitis because these enzymes are released as the pancreatic cells and ducts are destroyed. An elevated serum amylase level is a characteristic diagnostic feature. Amylase levels usually rise within 12 hours after the onset of symptoms and return to normal within 3 to 5 days. Serum lipase levels increase within 4 to 8 hours after clinical symptom onset and then decrease within 8 to 14 days. Serum trypsin levels are very specific for pancreatitis but may not be readily available. Urine trypsinogen-2 and urine amylase levels are also elevated. The C-reactive protein level increases within 48 hours and is a marker of severity. The ratio of amylase clearance to creatinine clearance by the kidney can be diagnostic. Other conditions associated with increased serum amylase levels are listed in Box 18.11.[14]

Other common laboratory abnormalities associated with acute pancreatitis include an elevated WBC count resulting from the inflammatory process and an elevated serum glucose level resulting from beta cell damage and pancreatic necrosis. Hypokalemia may be present because of associated vomiting. Hyperkalemia may be a systemic complication in the presence of acute renal failure. Hypocalcemia is common with severe disease and usually indicates pancreatic fat necrosis. Serum albumin and protein levels may decrease as a result of the movement of fluid into the extracellular space. Increases in serum bilirubin, lactate dehydrogenase, and aspartate transaminase levels and prothrombin time are common in the presence of concurrent liver disease. Serum triglyceride levels may increase dramatically and be a causative factor in the development of the acute inflammatory process. Arterial blood gas analysis often shows hypoxemia and retained carbon dioxide levels, which indicate respiratory failure.[54]

BOX 18.11 Conditions Associated With Increased Serum Amylase Levels

- Acute pancreatitis
- Biliary tract disease
- Burns
- Cerebral trauma
- Chronic alcoholism
- Diabetic ketoacidosis
- Gynecological disorders
- Intraabdominal disease (perforation, obstruction, aortic disease, peritonitis, appendicitis)
- Pneumonia
- Pregnancy
- Prostatic disease
- Renal insufficiency
- Salivary gland disease
- Shock
- Tumors

CT modalities and magnetic resonance imaging are also used to confirm the diagnosis. Contrast-enhanced CT reliably detects pancreatic necrosis located in the parenchyma. It is considered the gold standard for diagnosing pancreatic necrosis and for grading acute pancreatitis.[62,63] The Balthazar CT severity index is a scoring system that ranges from 0 to 10 and is obtained by adding points attributed to the extent of the inflammatory process to the volume of pancreatic necrosis. A higher index is associated with increased severity of disease. Magnetic resonance imaging can better detect necrosis in the peripancreatic collections. However, an acutely ill patient might not be able to tolerate this procedure.[63] Endoscopic retrograde cholangiopancreatography (ERCP) combines radiography with endoscopy and may assist in diagnosis.

Predicting the Severity of Acute Pancreatitis. Patients with acute pancreatitis can develop mild or fulminant disease. The prognosis of pancreatitis is based on classification criteria developed by Ranson[56] (Box 18.12). The number of signs present within the first 48 hours after admission directly relates to the patient's chance of morbidity and mortality. In Ranson's research, patients with fewer than three signs had a 1% mortality rate; those with three or four signs had a 15% mortality rate; those with five or six signs had a 40% mortality rate; and those with seven or more signs had a 100% mortality rate.

The Atlanta Classification is accepted worldwide as the first clinically reliable classification system. This system defines severe acute pancreatitis as the presence of three or more Ranson criteria or a score of 8 or higher on the Acute Physiology and Chronic Health Evaluation (APACHE II) criteria. The Apache III prognostic system is similar to APACHE II with the addition of several variables (e.g., diagnosis and prior treatment location). High APACHE III and five or more Ranson criteria can predict multiple complications or death in critically ill patients.[56] Another scale used to predict multiorgan failure is the Sepsis-Related Organ Failure Assessment (SOFA).[66]

BOX 18.12 Ranson Criteria for Predicting Severity of Acute Pancreatitis[a]

At Admission or on Diagnosis
- Age >55 years (>70 years)
- Leukocyte count >16,000/mm³ (>18,000/mm³)
- Serum AST level >250 IU/L
- Serum glucose level >200 mg/dL (>220 mg/dL)
- Serum LDH level >350 IU/L (>400 IU/L)

During Initial 48 Hours
- Base deficit >4 mEq/L (>5 mEq/L)
- Decrease in hematocrit >10%
- Estimated fluid sequestration >6 L (>4 L)
- Increase in blood urea nitrogen level >5 mg/dL (>2 mg/dL)
- Partial pressure of arterial oxygen <60 mm Hg
- Serum calcium level <8 mg/dL

[a]Criteria values for nonalcoholic acute pancreatitis (shown in parentheses) differ from those in alcohol-related disease.
AST, Aspartate transaminase; *LDH,* lactate dehydrogenase.
Modified from Ranson JC. Risk factors in acute pancreatitis. *Hosp Pract (Off Ed).* 1985;20(4):69–73.

Patient Problems

Actual or potential patient problems associated with acute pancreatitis or with systemic complications of the disease process are found in the Collaborative Plan of Care for the Critically Ill Patient in Chapter 1. These problems include Acute Pain; Decreased Multisystem Tissue Perfusion; Potential for Infection; Potential for Fluid, Electrolyte, and Acid-Base Imbalances; and Potential for Impaired Nutrition. Tailor these problems and nursing interventions to the patient's presentation, such as addressing hemodynamic instability and pain.

Medical and Nursing Interventions

Nursing and medical priorities for the management of acute pancreatitis include several interventions. Managing respiratory dysfunction is a high priority. Replace fluids and electrolytes to maintain or replenish vascular volume and electrolyte balance. Administer analgesics for pain control. Supportive therapies are aimed at decreasing gastrin release from the stomach and preventing the gastric contents from entering the duodenum.

Fluid Replacement. In patients with severe acute pancreatitis, fluid collects in the retroperitoneal space and peritoneal cavity. Patients sequester up to one-third of their plasma volume. Initially, most patients develop some degree of dehydration and, in severe cases, hypovolemic shock. Hypovolemia and shock are major causes of death early in the disease process. Fluid replacement is a high priority in the treatment of acute pancreatitis.

Fluid replacement helps maintain perfusion to the pancreas and kidneys, reducing the potential for complications. The IV solutions ordered for fluid resuscitation are usually colloids or Lactated Ringer's solution; however, fresh frozen plasma and albumin also may be administered. Aggressive IV fluid administration with crystalloids at 5 to 10 mL/kg/h is often required to maintain hemodynamic stability. Vigorous IV fluid replacement at 20 mL/kg/h for 8 to 12 hours is indicated if the patient manifests symptoms of hypotension and tachycardia.[62,63]

Evaluating the effectiveness of fluid replacement includes accurate monitoring of intake and output. A decrease in urine output to less than 50 mL/h is an early and sensitive measure of hypovolemia and hypoperfusion. Monitor vital signs and skin temperature. Although patient responses vary, reasonable goals are to maintain systolic blood pressure at greater than 100 mm Hg without an orthostatic decrease, a mean arterial pressure of greater than 60 mm Hg, and a heart rate of less than 100 beats/min. Warm extremities indicate adequate peripheral circulation.

Patients with severe manifestations of the disease require pulmonary artery pressure monitoring to evaluate fluid status and response to treatment. The pulmonary artery occlusion pressure is the most sensitive measure of adequacy of volume status and left ventricular filling pressure. A pulmonary artery occlusion pressure between 11 and 14 mm Hg is a realistic goal for most patients with pancreatitis.

Patients with severe disease who do not respond to fluid therapy alone may need vasopressors to support blood pressure. Patients with acute hemorrhagic pancreatitis may also need packed RBCs in addition to fluid therapy to restore intravascular volume.

New Modalities. Surgical decompression of *abdominal compartment syndrome* (ACS, also referred to as intraabdominal hypertension) may be used to relieve retroperitoneal edema, fluid collections in the abdomen, ascites, ileus, and overly aggressive use of fluid therapy in patients with severe acute pancreatitis. ACS is defined as intraabdominal pressure greater than 20 mm Hg with new-onset organ failure. ACS is seen early in about 60% of patients with severe acute pancreatitis and is associated with multiple organ dysfunction.

Pentoxifylline has been shown to decrease inflammation, bacterial translocation, and infections. It is a methylxanthine derivative that improves blood flow by increasing erythrocyte and leukocyte flexibility; it also stimulates production of cytokines. Clinical trials for off-label use in pancreatitis are underway.[78]

Electrolyte Replacement. Hypocalcemia (serum calcium level <8.5 mg/dL) is a common electrolyte imbalance. It is associated with a high mortality rate. Calcium is essential for many physiological functions: catalyzing impulses for nerves and muscles, maintaining the integrity of cell membranes and vessels, clotting blood, strengthening bones and teeth, and increasing contractility in the heart. A sign of hypocalcemia on the electrocardiogram is lengthening of the QT interval. Severe hypocalcemia (serum calcium level <6 mg/dL) may cause tetany, seizures, positive Chvostek and Trousseau signs, and respiratory distress. Place patients with severe hypocalcemia on seizure precaution status, and ensure that respiratory support equipment is readily available (e.g., oral airway, suction). Monitor calcium levels, administer replacement as ordered, and monitor the patient's response to calcium replacement. Monitor serum albumin levels because true serum calcium levels can be evaluated only in comparison with serum albumin levels. Also monitor for calcium toxicity, indicated by lethargy, nausea, shortening of the QT interval, and decreased excitability of nerves and muscles. Hypomagnesemia may also be present in patients with hypocalcemia, and magnesium replacement may be required.

Potassium is another electrolyte that may need to be replaced early in the treatment regimen. Hypokalemia is associated with cardiac dysrhythmias, muscle weakness, hypotension, decreased bowel sounds, ileus, and irritability. Potassium must be diluted and administered via an infusion pump according to the unit protocol.

Hyperglycemia is not a common complication of acute pancreatitis because most of the pancreatic gland must be necrosed before the insulin-secreting islet cells are affected. More commonly, hyperglycemia is a result of the body's stress response to acute illness.

Nutrition Support. Nasogastric suction and "nothing by mouth" status have been the classic treatments for patients with acute pancreatitis to suppress pancreatic exocrine secretion by preventing the release of secretin from the duodenum. Because secretin, which stimulates pancreatic secretion production, is stimulated when acid is in the duodenum, gastric suction has been a primary treatment. Nasogastric suctioning may also reduce nausea, vomiting, and abdominal pain. A nasogastric tube is essential in patients with ileus, severe gastric distension, and a decreased level of consciousness to prevent complications resulting from pulmonary aspiration.

However, trends in nutritional management are changing. Early nutritional support may be ordered to prevent atrophy of gut lymphoid tissue, prevent bacterial overgrowth in the intestine, and increase intestinal permeability. Immediate oral feeding in patients with mild acute pancreatitis is safe and may accelerate recovery.[32] The enteral route is still preferred for providing nutrition in patients with severe acute pancreatitis.[4]

STUDY BREAK

3. What medications are prescribed to patients recently diagnosed with peptic ulcer disease (PUD) from *Helicobacter pylori*?
   A. Esomeprazole, amoxicillin, and clarithromycin
   B. Metronidazole, pantoprazole, and amoxicillin
   C. Tetracycline, metronidazole, and levofloxacin
   D. Clarithromycin, bismuth, and tetracycline

Comfort Management. Pain control is a nursing priority in patients with acute pancreatitis, not only because the disorder produces extreme patient discomfort but also because pain increases the patient's metabolism and thus increases pancreatic secretions. The pain of pancreatitis is caused by edema and distension of the pancreatic capsule, obstruction of the biliary system, and peritoneal inflammation from pancreatic enzymes. Pain is often severe and unrelenting and is related to the degree of pancreatic inflammation.

Perform a baseline pain assessment early after the patient's admission. Include information about the onset, intensity, duration, and location (local or diffuse) of the pain. Analgesic administration is a nursing priority. Adequate pain control requires the use of IV opiates, often in the form of a patient-controlled analgesia (PCA) pump. If a PCA pump is not ordered, administer pain medications on a routine schedule, rather than as needed, to prevent uncontrollable abdominal pain. Traditionally, opiate analgesics (e.g., morphine) were considered to cause spasm of the sphincter of Oddi and to exacerbate pain; however, this practice is now questioned. Meperidine (Demerol) may be ordered in place of morphine if pancreatitis occurs secondary to gallbladder disease.[62,63] Insertion of a nasogastric tube connected to low intermittent suction may help ease pain. Depending on the patient's hemodynamic status, position the patient to relieve some of the discomfort.

? CRITICAL REASONING ACTIVITY

A 50-year-old patient is admitted with hematemesis and reports having dark stools for the past 12 hours. Which of the following admission data is the best indicator of the amount of blood lost?

Blood pressure	95/60 mm Hg (supine)
Heart rate	125 beats/min
Respiratory rate	28 breaths/min
Hematocrit	27%
Hemoglobin	14 g/dL

Pharmacological Intervention. Various pharmacological therapies have been researched in the treatment of acute pancreatitis. Medications given to rest the pancreas have been studied—specifically, anticholinergics, glucagon, somatostatin, cimetidine, and calcitonin—but these have not been shown to be effective. Prevention of stress ulcers is achieved through the use of histamine blockers, PPIs, and antacids.

Antibiotics have also been studied in the treatment of inflammation of the pancreas with the idea of preventing pancreatic pseudocysts or abscesses. It is not known whether antibiotics improve survival or merely prevent septic complications.[62,63]

Treatment of Systemic Complications. Multisystemic complications of acute pancreatitis are related to the ability of the pancreas to produce many vasoactive substances that affect organs throughout the body. These complications are summarized in Box 18.9.

Pulmonary complications are common in patients with both mild and severe manifestations of the disease. Arterial hypoxemia, atelectasis, pleural effusions, acute respiratory distress syndrome (ARDS), and pneumonia have been identified in many patients with acute pancreatitis. Accumulation of fluid in the peritoneum causes restricted movement of the diaphragm. Arterial oxygen saturation is continuously monitored, and arterial blood gases are assessed as needed. Treatment of hypoxemia includes supplemental oxygen and vigorous pulmonary hygiene, such as deep breathing, coughing, and frequent position changes. Some patients may need intubation to ensure adequate ventilation; others can be maintained with noninvasive ventilation modes. Pulmonary emboli have also been documented as a complication of acute pancreatitis. Careful fluid administration is necessary to prevent fluid overload and pulmonary congestion. Patients with severe disease may develop acute respiratory failure.

Close monitoring and management of other systemic complications of acute pancreatitis, such as coagulation abnormalities and hemorrhage, cardiovascular failure and dysrhythmias, and acute renal failure, are also important. Coagulation defects in acute pancreatitis are similar to disseminated intravascular coagulation (DIC) and are associated with a high mortality rate. The cardiac depression associated with acute pancreatitis may vary. The presence of hypovolemic shock is a grave presentation; astute cardiovascular monitoring and volume replacement are required to reverse this serious complication. Impaired renal function has been documented in many patients.

GI complications of acute pancreatitis include pancreatic pseudocyst and abdominal abscess. Suspect a pseudocyst in any patient who has persistent abdominal pain with nausea and vomiting, a prolonged fever, and an elevated serum amylase level. CT can be helpful in diagnosing the location and size of the pseudocyst. Early recognition and treatment of a pancreatic pseudocyst are important because this condition is associated with a high mortality rate. Signs and symptoms of an abdominal abscess include an increased WBC count, fever, abdominal pain, and vomiting. CT provides a definitive diagnosis.

Surgical Therapy. Pancreatic resection for acute necrotizing pancreatitis may be performed to prevent systemic complications of the disease process. In this procedure, dead or infected pancreatic tissue is surgically removed while most of the gland is preserved.[62,63] Many surgical treatment modalities, including laparoscopic techniques, are available. The indication for surgical intervention is clinical deterioration of the patient despite conventional treatments or the presence of peritonitis.

Surgery may also be indicated for pseudocysts; however, surgery is usually delayed because some pseudocysts resolve spontaneously. Surgical treatment of a pseudocyst can be performed through internal or external drainage, or needle aspiration. Acute surgical intervention may be required if the pseudocyst becomes infected or perforated.

Surgery may also be performed when gallstones are the cause of the acute pancreatitis. A cholecystectomy is usually performed.

HEPATIC FAILURE

Chronic liver disease, or cirrhosis, is the 12th leading cause of death in the United States, accounting for 36,427 deaths in 2010.[13,37] However, recent data suggest that liver-related mortality is higher than estimated by 121%, making it the 8th leading cause of death in the United States. End-stage liver disease is characterized as deterioration from a compensated to an uncompensated state. Critically ill patients with end-stage liver disease have a mortality rate of 50% to 100%.[43] Hepatic failure also results from chronic liver disease, in which healthy liver tissue is replaced by fibrotic tissue. This form of liver failure is called *cirrhosis*. Finally, liver cells can be replaced by fatty cells or tissue; this is known as *nonalcoholic fatty liver disease.*[15]

Pathophysiology

The normal liver architecture is pictured in Fig. 18.5. The basic functional unit of the liver is called a *lobule*. The liver lobule is uniquely made in that it has its own blood supply, which allows the liver cells *(hepatocytes)* to be exposed continuously to blood. Hepatic failure results when the liver is unable to perform its many functions (see Box 18.2). Liver failure results from necrosis or a decrease in the blood supply to liver cells. This problem is most often caused by hepatitis or inflammation of the liver.

Hepatitis. *Hepatitis* is an acute inflammation of the hepatocytes. This inflammation is accompanied by edema. As the inflammation progresses, blood supply to the hepatocytes is interrupted, causing necrosis and breakdown of healthy cells. Blood may back up in the portal system, causing *portal hypertension.*

Liver cells have the capacity to regenerate. Over time, liver cells that become damaged are removed by the body's immune system and replaced with healthy liver cells. Therefore most patients with hepatitis recover and regain normal liver function.

Hepatitis is most often caused by a virus. Several hepatitis viruses have been identified, and they are termed hepatitis A, B, C, D, E, and G. Researchers continue to study other viruses that may be associated with acute hepatitis. Modes of transmission are summarized in Box 18.13. Characteristics of hepatitis in terms of type, route of transmission, severity, and prophylaxis are presented in Table 18.8.

Assessment. Patients with hepatitis are often asymptomatic. In many patients, prodromal symptoms of anorexia, nausea,

BOX 18.13 Modes of Transmission for Hepatitis

- Contact with:
  - Blood and blood products
  - Saliva
  - Semen
- Direct contact with infected fluids or objects
- Percutaneously through mucous membranes

vomiting, abdominal pain or distension, and fatigue may be present. Symptoms then progress to a low-grade fever, an enlarged and tender liver, and jaundice (see Clinical Alert box).[32]

! CLINICAL ALERT

Signs and Symptoms of Fulminant Hepatic Failure (Acute Liver Failure)

- Chills
- Convulsions
- Decreased level of consciousness, coma
- Hyperexcitability
- Insomnia
- Irritability
- Jaundice
- Lethargy
- Nausea and vomiting
- Sudden onset of high fever

Assessment of risk factors often assists in the diagnosis of hepatitis. Laboratory tests show elevated liver function enzymes. The diagnosis is confirmed by identifying antibodies specific to each type of hepatitis. Recovery from acute hepatitis usually occurs within 9 weeks for hepatitis A or 16 weeks for hepatitis B. Hepatitis B, C, D, and G may progress to chronic forms.[14]

Patient problems. Many patient problems are associated with viral hepatitis. These include Fatigue; Potential for Bleeding; Potential for Infection; Potential for Impaired Nutrition; Nausea; and Potential for Skin Abrasions.

Medical and nursing interventions. No definitive treatment for acute inflammation of the liver exists. Goals for medical and nursing care include providing rest and assisting the patient in obtaining optimal nutrition. Most patients are cared for at home unless the disease becomes prolonged or fulminant failure develops. Medications to help the patient rest or to decrease agitation must be closely monitored because most of these medications require clearance by the liver, which is impaired during the acute phase.

Maintenance of the nutritional status of the patient is a nursing priority. Loss of appetite, nausea, and vomiting may persist for weeks. Administer antiemetics to reduce symptoms. Collaborate with a dietitian to develop a nutritional plan. Offer small, frequent, palatable meals and supplements. Regularly assess intake and output, daily weight, serum albumin level, and nitrogen balance as ongoing nutritional evaluation. Instruct patients to avoid drinking alcohol or taking over-the-counter medications that can cause liver damage.[3,38] Box 18.14 lists common hepatotoxic medications.

Liver transplantation is the standard of care for patients with progressive, irreversible acute or chronic liver disease when there are no other medical or surgical options. The leading indication for liver transplantation is hepatitis C.[23,61] See the Transplantation Considerations box.

BOX 18.14 Common Hepatotoxic Medications

Analgesics
- Acetaminophen (Tylenol)
- Salicylates (aspirin)

Anesthetics
- Halothane (Fluothane)

Anticonvulsants
- Phenytoin (Dilantin)
- Phenobarbital

Antidepressants
- Monoamine oxidase inhibitors

Antimicrobial Agents
- Isoniazid
- Nitrofurantoin (Macrodantin)
- Rifampin
- Silver sulfadiazine (Silvadene)
- Tetracycline

Antipsychotic Medications
- Haloperidol (Haldol)

Cardiovascular Medications
- Quinidine sulfate

Hormonal Agents
- Antithyroid medications
- Oral contraceptives
- Oral hypoglycemics (tolbutamide)

Sedatives
- Chlordiazepoxide (Librium)
- Diazepam (Valium)

Others
- Cimetidine (Tagamet)

TABLE 18.8 Characteristics of Hepatitis

Type	Route of Transmission	Severity	Prophylaxis
Hepatitis A	Fecal-oral, parenteral, sexual	Mild	Hygiene, immune serum globulin, HAV vaccine, Twinrix[a]
Hepatitis B	Parenteral, sexual	Severe, may be prolonged or chronic	Hygiene, HBV vaccine, Twinrix[a]
Hepatitis C	Parenteral	Mild to severe	Hygiene, screening blood, interferon-alpha
Hepatitis D	Parenteral, fecal-oral, sexual	Severe	Hygiene, HBV vaccine
Hepatitis E	Fecal-oral	Severe in pregnant women	Hygiene, safe water
Hepatitis G	Parenteral, sexual	Unknown	Unknown

[a]A bivalent vaccine containing the antigenic components, a sterile suspension of inactivated hepatitis A virus combined with purified surface antigen of the hepatitis B virus.[60]

HAV, Hepatitis A virus; *HBV,* hepatitis B virus.

Modified from Huether SE. Alterations of digestive function. In: McCance KL, Huether SE, eds. *Pathophysiology: The Biologic Basis for Disease in Adults and Children.* 8th ed. St. Louis, MO: Elsevier; 2019.

TRANSPLANT CONSIDERATIONS

Liver

Criteria for Transplant Recipients

Because of the chronic, significant shortage of available organs, optimal patient selection for evaluation and timing of waiting list activation is vital. The patient must not be so critically ill that survival is unlikely but must be acutely ill enough to experience deterioration in quality of life. Contraindications for liver transplantation include active malignancies, active substance abuse, advanced cardiopulmonary disease (such as severe refractory pulmonary hypertension or chronic obstructive pulmonary disease), and uncontrolled or untreated HIV infection. Following extensive transplant evaluation to determine the ability to survive transplantation, compliance with pre- and posttransplant care, and the presence of adequate psychosocial support and financial and insurance clearance, a patient is activated on the liver transplant waiting list. Waiting list placement is determined primarily by the Model for End-Stage Liver Disease (MELD) score. The MELD score is calculated using serum creatinine, serum bilirubin, and international normalized ratio to predict survival.[1]

Patient Management

Maintenance therapy consists of medications that inhibit T-cell proliferation and differentiation, deplete lymphocytes, and inhibit macrophages. Immunosuppressive medications consist of triple therapy—a calcineurin inhibitor (tacrolimus [Prograf] or cyclosporine [Neoral]), a corticosteroid (prednisone), and mycophenolate mofetil (CellCept) or azathioprine (Imuran). Induction immune suppression, if used, may begin in the operating room, often in the anhepatic phase before implantation of the donor liver. The *anhepatic phase* refers to the interval between explantation of the native liver and implantation of the donor liver into the recipient. Agents such as basiliximab (monoclonal antibody) may be used. This is in an effort to delay using calcineurin inhibitors to protect renal function. Immune modulation agents are titrated based on serum levels. Complications associated with immunosuppressive therapy affect all body systems and include nephrotoxicity, hypertension, hyperlipidemia, bone loss, new-onset diabetes mellitus, and increased risk of infection and risk of malignancy.[4]

Complications

Postoperative complications include bleeding, renal failure, infection, pleural effusions, biliary leaks, biliary obstruction or strictures at anastomoses sites, and fluid and electrolyte imbalances. Vascular complications such as portal vein thrombosis and arterial thrombosis may also occur, potentially causing primary liver nonfunction and urgent relisting for liver transplant. Infection is the leading cause of death in the liver transplant patient. Psychosocial issues may occur consequent to posttraumatic stress from acute or critical illness, as well as altered family dynamics and shifting roles. Biliary stones (cast syndrome) and recurrent cholangitis are other possible complications. One to 6 months after transplantation, cytomegalovirus (CMV), Epstein-Barr virus (EBV), *Pneumocystis carinii*, and *Aspergillus* are often seen. After 6 months, the rate of infection is the same as the general population unless the patient requires high doses of immunosuppressive medications.[2]

Preventing Rejection

Compliance with immunosuppressive medication is essential. *Hyperacute rejection* occurs within minutes or hours of transplantation and is caused by humoral or antibody-mediated B-cell production against the transplanted organ. *Acute rejection* occurs days to 3 months after transplantation and involves the activation and proliferation of T cells with destruction of liver tissue. Acute rejection accounts for approximately 40% of all rejection episodes. *Chronic rejection* occurs months to years after transplantation and may lead to the need for retransplantation.[3]

Rejection is suspected if aspartate aminotransferase (AST), alanine aminotransferase (ALT), or bilirubin increases, and this warrants a liver biopsy. Abdominal discomfort, fatigue, fever, jaundice, ascites, dark urine, and loss of appetite may indicate rejection. Most rejection is reversible if diagnosed and treated early; therefore compliance with scheduled laboratory testing is important. Management of acute rejection includes increasing the dosages of current immunosuppressive medications. Managing risk of rejection also includes patient and family education on optimal use of immune suppression medications and strict compliance with dosing schedules.

References

1. Adler JT, Axelrod DA. Regulations' impact on donor and recipient selection for liver transplantation: How should outcomes be measured and MELD exception scores be considered? *AMA J Ethics*. 2016;18(2):133–142.
2. Barnard A, Konyn P, Saab S. Medical management of metabolic complications of liver transplant recipients. *Gastroenterol Hepatol*. 2016;12(10):601–608.
3. Choudhary NS, Saigal S, Bansal RK, et al. Acute and chronic rejection after liver transplantation: What a clinician needs to know. *J Clin Exp Hepatol*. 2017;7(4):358–366.
4. Shanzhou H, Tang Y, et al. Outcomes of organ transplantation from donors with a cancer history. *Med Sci Monit*. 2018;24:997–1007.

Hepatitis can lead to acute hepatic failure. The clinical manifestations of this disorder are discussed later. Special precautions must be taken to prevent spread of the virus when caring for the patient with hepatitis. These include the *universal precautions* while handling all items that are contaminated with the patient's body secretions, including patient care items such as thermometers, dishes, and eating utensils.

Cirrhosis. Cirrhosis causes severe alterations in the structure and function of liver cells. It is characterized by inflammation and liver cell necrosis that may be focal or diffuse. Fat deposits may also be present. The enlarged liver cells cause compression of the liver lobule and lead to increased resistance to blood flow and portal hypertension. Necrosis is followed by regeneration of liver tissue but not in a normal fashion. Fibrous tissue is laid down over time, which distorts the normal architecture of the liver lobule. These fibrotic changes are usually irreversible and result in chronic liver dysfunction. Table 18.9 characterizes the types of cirrhosis.

Nonalcoholic Fatty Liver. The term *fatty liver* refers to an accumulation of excessive fats in the liver; it is morphologically distinguishable from cirrhosis. Alcohol abuse is the most common cause of this disorder. Other causes include obesity, diabetes, hepatic resection, starvation, and total parenteral nutrition. Damage caused by the fat deposits may result in liver dysfunction, failure, and death.[52]

Assessment of Hepatic Failure

Presenting Clinical Signs. Initial clinical signs of hepatic failure are vague and include weakness, fatigue, loss of appetite, weight loss, abdominal discomfort, nausea and vomiting, and change in bowel habits. As destruction in the liver progresses, the systemic effects of the disease become apparent. Impaired liver function results in loss of the normal vascular, secretory, and metabolic functions of the liver (see Box 18.2). The functional sequelae of liver disease are divided into three categories: (1) portal hypertension, (2) impaired liver metabolic processes, and (3) impaired bile formation and flow.

TABLE 18.9	Characteristics of Types of Cirrhosis		
Type	Cause	Consequences	Sequelae
Alcoholic (Laennec's)	Long-term alcohol abuse	Fatty liver Fibrotic tissue replaces liver cells	Acetaldehyde, a toxic metabolite of alcohol ingestion, causes liver cell damage and death
Biliary	Long-term obstruction of bile ducts	Decrease in bile flow	Degeneration and fibrosis of the ducts
Cardiac	Severe long-term right-sided heart failure	Decreased oxygenation of liver cells	Cellular death
Postnecrotic	Exposure to hepatotoxins or chemicals, infection, or metabolic disorder	Massive death of liver cells	Development of liver cancer

These derangements and their clinical manifestations are summarized in Box 18.15.

Portal hypertension. Portal hypertension causes two main clinical problems for the patient: hyperdynamic circulation and development of esophageal or gastric varices. Liver cell destruction causes shunting of blood and increased cardiac output. Vasodilation is also present, which causes decreased perfusion to all body organs, even though the cardiac output is very high. This phenomenon is known as *high-output failure* or *hyperdynamic circulation.* Clinical signs and symptoms are those of heart failure and include jugular vein distension, pulmonary crackles, and decreased perfusion to all organs. Initially, the patient may have hypertension, flushed skin, and bounding pulses. When a patient experiences low blood pressure, dysrhythmias are common. Increased portal venous pressure causes the formation of varices that shunt blood to decrease pressure. These varices can cause massive upper GI bleeding.[64] Splenomegaly is also associated with portal hypertension.

Impaired metabolic processes. The liver is the most complex organ because it carries out many metabolic processes. Liver failure causes altered metabolism of carbohydrates, fats, and proteins; decreased synthesis of blood clotting factors; decreased removal of activated clotting components; decreased metabolism of vitamins and iron; decreased storage functions; and decreased detoxification functions.

Altered carbohydrate metabolism may result in unstable blood glucose levels. The serum glucose level may increase to more than 200 mg/dL. This condition is termed *cirrhotic diabetes.* Altered carbohydrate metabolism may also result in malnutrition and a decreased stress response. Hypoglycemia may also be seen secondary to depletion of hepatic glycogen stores and decreased gluconeogenesis.[31]

Altered fat metabolism may result in a fatty liver. Fat is used by all cells for energy. Altered metabolism may cause fatigue and decreased activity tolerance in many patients. Alterations in skin integrity are common in chronic liver disease and are related to this metabolic dysfunction. Bile salts are not adequately produced, which leads to an inability of the small intestine to metabolize fats. Malnutrition often results.

Protein metabolism, albumin synthesis, and serum albumin levels are decreased. Albumin is necessary for colloid oncotic pressure to hold fluid in the intravascular space and for nutrition. Low albumin levels are also associated with the development of ascites, a complication of hepatic failure. Globulin is another protein that is essential for the transport of substances in the blood. Fibrinogen is an essential protein that is necessary for normal clotting. A low plasma fibrinogen level, coupled with decreased synthesis of many blood clotting factors, predisposes the patient to bleeding. Clinical signs and symptoms range from bruising and nasal and gingival bleeding to frank hemorrhage. Disseminated intravascular coagulation (DIC) may also develop.

Kupffer cells in the liver play an important role in fighting infections throughout the body. Loss of this function predisposes the patient to severe infections, particularly sepsis caused by gram-negative bacteria.

The liver also removes activated clotting factors from the general circulation to prevent widespread clotting in the system. Loss of this function predisposes the patient to clot formation and complications such as pulmonary embolus.

Decreased metabolism and storage of vitamins A, B$_{12}$, and D; iron; glucose; and fat predispose the patient to many nutritional deficiencies. The liver loses the function of detoxifying medications, ammonia, and hormones. Loss of ammonia

BOX 18.15 Clinical Signs and Symptoms of Liver Disease

Cardiac
- Activity intolerance
- Dysrhythmias
- Edema
- Hyperdynamic circulation
- Portal hypertension

Dermatological
- Jaundice
- Pruritus
- Spider angiomas

Electrolytes
- Hypernatremia
- Hypokalemia
- Hyponatremia (dilutional)

Endocrine
- Increased aldosterone
- Increased antidiuretic hormone

Fluid Alterations
- Ascites
- Decreased volume in vascular space
- Water retention

Gastrointestinal
- Abdominal discomfort
- Decreased appetite
- Diarrhea
- Malnutrition
- Nausea and vomiting
- Varices or gastrointestinal bleeding

Hematological
- Anemia
- Disseminated intravascular coagulation
- Impaired coagulation

Immune System
- Increased susceptibility to infection

Neurological
- Hepatic encephalopathy

Pulmonary
- Dyspnea
- Hepatopulmonary syndrome
- Hyperventilation
- Hypoxemia
- Ineffective breathing patterns

Renal
- Hepatorenal syndrome

conversion to urea in the liver is responsible for many of the altered thought processes seen in liver failure because ammonia is allowed to enter the central nervous system directly. These alterations range from minor sensory perceptual changes, such as tremors, slurred speech, and impaired decision making, to dramatic confusion or profound coma.

Hormonal imbalances are common in liver disease. The most important physiological imbalance is the activation of aldosterone and antidiuretic hormone, which contribute to the fluid and electrolyte disturbances commonly found in liver disease. Sodium and water retention and portal hypertension lead to third-spacing of fluid from the intravascular space into the peritoneal cavity *(ascites)*. The resultant decrease in plasma volume causes activation of compensatory mechanisms in the body to release antidiuretic hormone and aldosterone, causing further water and sodium retention. The *renin-angiotensin system* is also activated, which causes systemic vasoconstriction. The kidneys are most severely affected, and urine output decreases because of impaired perfusion. Sexual dysfunction is common in patients with liver disease, and this can lead to self-concept alterations. Dermatological lesions that occur in some patients with liver failure, called *spider angiomas*, are related to an endocrine imbalance. These vascular lesions may be venous or arterial and represent the progression of liver disease.

Impaired bile formation and flow. The liver's inability to metabolize bile is reflected clinically in an increased serum bilirubin level and a staining of tissue by bilirubin (i.e., jaundice). Jaundice is generally present in patients with a serum bilirubin level greater than 3 mg/dL.

Patient Problems

Refer to the Plan of Care for the Patient With Liver Failure for a detailed description of patient problems, specific nursing interventions, and selected rationales. Other interventions are discussed in the Collaborative Plan of Care for the Critically Ill Patient in Chapter 1.

◎ PLAN OF CARE

For the Patient with Liver Failure

Patient Problem
Potential for Delirium. Risk factors include cerebral accumulation of ammonia, medications that require liver metabolism, GI bleeding, and decreased perfusion states.

Desired Outcomes
- Orientation to person, place, and time.
- Free of injury.

Assessments/Interventions	Rationales
• Monitor ammonia levels and conduct ongoing neurological assessments.	• Assess trends in neurological status and response to treatment.
• Determine patient's baseline personality and memory by asking the patient's family and friends.	
• Observe for asterixis and report to the provider.	• May be present in advanced disease states.
• Administer lactulose as indicated and monitor results.	• Reduce ammonia levels and improve neurological status.
• Reduce the risk of stress ulcer–related bleeding through stress ulcer prophylaxis administration.	• Prevent bleeding, which may lead to hepatic encephalopathy.
• Use sedatives and narcotics judiciously.	• Drug metabolism is impaired in hepatic failure.
• Prevent and treat infection, dehydration, and electrolyte or acid-base disturbances.	• Assess for altered mental status associated with elevated ammonia level.
	• Shifting electrolytes may further alter the patient's mental status.
• Reorient the patient and provide safety support during periods of impaired mentation.	• Provide orientation and reduce risk for injury.

Patient Problem
Potential for Bleeding/Hemorrhage. Risk factors include portal hypertension and altered coagulation factors.

Desired Outcomes
- Orientation to person, place, and time.
- Bruising absent.
- Hemoglobin and hematocrit within normal limits for the patient.
- Absent of signs of hypovolemic shock:
  - Systolic blood pressure >90 mm Hg.
  - Heart rate <100 bpm.

Assessments/Interventions	Rationales
• Assess vital signs every 1-2 hours or more frequently if vital signs are abnormal.	• Assess for bleeding and need for prompt treatment; esophageal varices, portal hypertension, gastric or duodenal ulcers, or Mallory-Weiss tears are common in hepatic failure and can lead to significant bleeding.
	• Patients with varices treated with banding or sclerotherapy may require more frequent monitoring given the risk of perforation and subsequent hemorrhage.
• Immediately notify the provider of signs and symptoms of bleeding (i.e., bruising, weakness, pallor, hematemesis, altered vital signs, agitation, mental status changes).	• Assess for hemorrhage and initiate intervention.

◉ PLAN OF CARE—cont'd

For the Patient with Liver Failure

Assessments/Interventions	Rationales
• Reduce the risk of stress ulcer–related bleeding through peptic ulcer prophylaxis administration.	• Reduce risk for gastric and duodenal ulcers. • Reduce the impact of hemodynamic and inflammatory changes, which may damage the gastric mucosa.

Patient Problem

Fluid Overload. Risk factors include portal hypertension and compromised regulatory mechanisms.

Desired Outcomes
- Normal lung sounds (i.e., absence of crackles, rales).
- Respiratory rate <20 breaths/min.
- Edema decreasing or absent.
- Abdominal girth decreasing.

Assessments/Interventions	Rationales
• Monitor and document weight and I&O.	• Output should equal or exceed intake. • Weight loss, especially when using diuretics, should not exceed 0.5 kg/day to prevent electrolyte imbalance.
• Monitor electrolytes, especially Na⁺ and K⁺; report critical values to the provider.	• Hyponatremia associated with water retention occurs in the late stages of hepatic failure. • Hypokalemia is common in chronic alcoholic liver disease.
• Assess for and report dyspnea and bibasilar crackles.	• Indicate pulmonary edema.
• Provide frequent mouth care to minimize thirst.	• Reduce thirst without compounding fluid volume excess.
• Apply compression stockings or sequential compression devices.	• Reduce peripheral edema.
• Monitor skin integrity.	• Edema increases risk for device-related pressure injuries.

bpm, Beats per minute; *GI,* gastrointestinal; *I&O,* intake and output; *K⁺,* potassium; *Na⁺,* sodium.
Adapted from Swearingen PL, Wright JD. *All-in-One Nursing Care Planning Resource.* 5th ed. St. Louis, MO: Elsevier; 2019.

Medical and Nursing Interventions

Nursing and medical management for the patient with liver failure is aimed at supportive therapies and early recognition and treatment of complications associated with the disease process. Management of acute liver failure challenges the best skills of providers, intensivists, and nurses.

Diagnostic Tests. Altered laboratory results in patients with liver disease (see Laboratory Alert box) are a direct result of the destruction of hepatic cells (liver enzymes) or of impaired liver metabolic processes.

⚠ LABORATORY ALERT

Liver Failure

Albumin: ↑	Enzymes
Ammonia: ↑	APT: ↑
Bile pigments	AST: ↑
Total bilirubin: ↑	ALT: ↑
Direct or conjugated bilirubin: ↑	Urine
Cholesterol: ↑	Bilirubin: ↑
Coagulation tests	Urobilinogen: ↑
Prothrombin time: Prolonged	
Partial thromboplastin time:	
Prolonged	

ALT, Alanine transaminase; *APT,* alkaline phosphatase; *AST,* aspartate transaminase.

Parenchymal tests such as liver biopsy can be performed to study the liver cell architecture directly. The liver is characteristically small and has a marked decrease in functioning hepatic cell structures. This characteristic allows for a definitive diagnosis of the cause of the hepatic failure. An ultrasound study may detect impaired bile flow.

Supportive Therapy. Hemodynamic instability and decreased perfusion to core organs are the end result of portal hypertension and hyperdynamic circulation. Invasive monitoring may be used in the critically ill patient, but it must be weighed in terms of the potential for infection in a patient with an impaired immune response. Administration of vasoactive medications and fluids may be ordered to support blood pressure and kidney perfusion and close monitoring by the nurse. Portal hypertension also predisposes the patient to esophageal and gastric varices, which have the potential to bleed.

The patient with liver failure is at risk for bleeding complications because of decreased synthesis of clotting factors. Protect patients who have a prolonged prothrombin time and partial thromboplastin time and a decreased platelet count from injury by padding the side rails and assisting with all activities. Keep venipuncture and other needlesticks to a minimum. Blood products may be ordered in severe cases. Antacids, PPIs, or histamine blockers are ordered to prevent gastritis and bleeding from stress ulcers.

Administration of all medications metabolized by the liver must be restricted. The administration of such medications could cause acute liver failure in a patient with chronic disease.[70]

Support for the Failing Liver. Advances have been made in the development of artificial support of liver function, spurred on by the shortage of donor organs and the high incidence of mortality related to acute or chronic liver failure.[17] Bioartificial liver devices (BLDs) were developed to partially replace the synthetic and regulatory function of the liver besides detoxifying the patient's plasma. BLDs may serve as a bridge to liver transplantation or support liver function long enough to allow regeneration of normal liver function.[47]

Another type of support is the Molecular Adsorbents Recirculating System (MARS), an extracorporeal albumin dialysis technique that uses an albumin-impregnated membrane to remove both protein-bound and water-soluble toxins from the blood.[50] Cytokines are believed to play an important role in acute-on-chronic liver failure. Cytokines can be cleared from plasma by MARS and by another system, known as fractionated plasma separation, adsorption, and dialysis (Prometheus). However, at present, neither of these treatments is able to change serum cytokine levels.

STUDY BREAK

4. Early clinical signs of liver disease include all of the following except:
   A. Pulmonary crackles
   B. Jugular vein distension
   C. Dysrhythmias
   D. Esophageal varices

❓ CRITICAL REASONING ACTIVITY

A 45-year-old business executive is admitted to the telemetry unit. He tells the nurse that he travels a lot for business and recently returned from a trip to Mexico. During your initial assessment, he tells you that he is not married, and he relates stories about some of the women he has met and dated on his many trips. His history includes persistent abdominal pain, nausea with occasional vomiting, fatigue, and decreased appetite. Initial vital signs and laboratory results include the following:

Heart rate	70 beats/min
Urine	Clear and dark yellow
Aspartate transaminase (AST)	20 IU/L
Alanine transaminase (ALT)	70 IU/L
Serum albumin	3.2 mg/dL
Total serum bilirubin	1.5 mg/dL

1. What is the most likely diagnosis?
2. What precautions should the nurse take while caring for this patient?

Treatment of Complications

Ascites. Impaired handling of salt and water by the kidneys and other abnormalities in fluid homeostasis predispose the patient to an accumulation of fluid in the peritoneum, known as *ascites*. Ascites is problematic because as more fluid is retained, it pushes up on the diaphragm, thereby impairing breathing. Regularly assess respiratory rate, breath sounds, and pulse oximetry values. Monitor and record abdominal girth at the level of the umbilicus to assess for increased fluid accumulation. Position the patient in a semi-Fowler's position to promote diaphragm movement. Encourage frequent deep-breathing and coughing exercises and changes in position to facilitate full or optimal breathing. Some patients may require intubation and mechanical ventilation until medical management of the ascites is accomplished. Ascites may also result in *abdominal compartment syndrome.*[39] Box 18.16 lists the physiological effects that can occur with this complication.

Ascites is medically managed through bed rest, a low-sodium diet, fluid restriction, and diuretic therapy. Diuretics must be administered cautiously, however; if the intravascular volume is depleted too quickly, acute renal failure may be induced. Closely monitor the serum creatinine level, the BUN level, and urine output for early detection of renal impairment. Also monitor electrolyte levels, particularly serum potassium and sodium levels, when diuretics are administered.

Paracentesis, in which ascitic fluid is withdrawn through percutaneous needle aspiration, is another medical therapy for ascites. Closely monitor vital signs during this procedure, especially as fluid is withdrawn. Major complications include sudden loss of intravascular pressure (decreased blood pressure) and tachycardia. To prevent these complications, 1 to 2 L of fluid is usually withdrawn at one time. Document the amount, color, and character of peritoneal fluid obtained. Often a specimen of the fluid is sent to the laboratory for analysis. Measure the patient's abdominal girth before and after the procedure. Albumin may be administered to increase colloid osmotic pressure and to decrease loss of fluid into the peritoneal cavity.

Peritoneovenous shunting is a surgical procedure used to relieve ascites resistant to other therapies. The physician may insert a *LeVeen shunt* by placing the distal end of a tube in the peritoneum and tunneling the other end under the skin into the jugular vein or superior vena cava. A valve that opens and closes according to pressure gradients allows ascitic fluid to flow into the superior vena cava. The patient's breathing normally triggers the valve. During inspiration, pressure increases in the peritoneum and decreases in the vena cava, thereby allowing fluid to

---

BOX 18.16   Physiological Effects of Abdominal Compartment Syndrome

Cardiovascular
- Decreased venous return
- Increased systemic vascular resistance and intrathoracic pressure
- Reduction in cardiac output

Gastrointestinal
- Impaired lymphatic, venous, and arterial flow
- Poor healing of anastomoses

Hepatic and Renal
- Decreased blood flow to liver and kidney
- Functional impairment of both organs

Neurological
- Simultaneously increased intracranial pressure from head trauma and from intraabdominal hypertension

Respiratory
- Atelectasis
- Impaired ventilation
- Pneumonia
- Respiratory failure

flow from the peritoneum into the general circulation. Major complications of this therapy include hemodilution, shunt clotting, wound infection, leakage of ascitic fluid from the incision, and bleeding problems.

A variation of this procedure is the *Denver shunt,* which involves placement of a pump in addition to the peritoneal catheter (Fig. 18.12).[11] The Denver shunt is currently being used to treat both cirrhotic and pleural ascites. Fluid is allowed to flow through the pump from the peritoneum into the general circulation at a uniform rate to increase blood volume and renal blood flow; retain nutrients and improve nutritional status; increase diuresis; improve mobility and respiration; and relieve massive, refractory ascites. The popularity and use of the Denver shunt have been limited because it has been associated with adverse events, including shunt occlusion, peritoneal infection, ascitic leak, bleeding, DIC, pneumothorax, and pneumoperitoneum. Strict adherence to shunt placement recommendations and the manufacturer's instruction manual[9] will help avoid the complications.[46]

Portal systemic encephalopathy. *Portal systemic encephalopathy,* commonly known as *hepatic encephalopathy,* is a functional derangement of the central nervous system that causes altered levels of consciousness and cerebral manifestations ranging from confusion to coma. Impaired motor ability is often present as well. *Asterixis,* a flapping tremor of the hand, is an early sign of hepatic encephalopathy that can be assessed by the nurse.

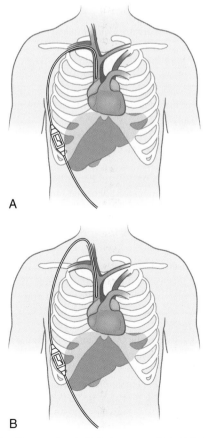

Fig. 18.12 The Denver shunt. Percutaneous placement of the venous and peritoneal catheters of a Denver ascites shunt. The venous catheter may be placed into the subclavian vein **(A)** or the internal jugular vein **(B)**.

The exact cause of hepatic encephalopathy is unknown, but abnormal ammonia metabolism is hypothesized to be the primary cause. Increased serum ammonia levels interfere with normal cerebral metabolism. In acute liver failure, signs and symptoms of this disorder may appear rapidly; in chronic liver failure, they often occur over time. Many conditions precipitate the development of hepatic encephalopathy, including fluid and electrolyte and acid-base disturbances, increased protein intake, portosystemic shunts, blood transfusions, GI bleeding, and many medications such as diuretics, analgesics, narcotics, and sedatives. Progression of hepatic encephalopathy can be divided into stages (Box 18.17).

Management of hepatic encephalopathy involves addressing precipitating factors such as infection, GI bleeding, and electrolyte and acid-base imbalances. Measures for decreasing ammonia production are necessary. Protein intake is limited to 20 to 40 g/day. Lactulose, neomycin, and metronidazole are medications that are ordered to reduce bacterial breakdown of protein in the bowel.[47]

Lactulose is the first-line treatment for hepatic encephalopathy. Lactulose creates an acidic environment in the bowel that causes the ammonia to leave the bloodstream and enter the colon. Ammonia becomes trapped in the bowel. Lactulose also has a laxative effect that allows for elimination of the ammonia. Lactulose is given orally or via a rectal enema.

Neomycin and metronidazole are second-line treatments for hepatic encephalopathy. Neomycin is a broad-spectrum antibiotic that destroys the normal bacteria found in the bowel, thereby decreasing protein breakdown and ammonia production. Neomycin (4-12 grams per day in divided doses) is given orally every 4 to 6 hours. This medication is toxic to the kidneys and cannot be given to patients with renal failure. Daily renal function studies are monitored when neomycin is administered. Metronidazole is given 500-750 mg per day for 1 week.

Metronidazole does not cause diarrhea, and it is not nephrotoxic. Metronidazole may cause epigastric discomfort, which may in turn result in poor compliance with long-term treatment.

Restriction of medications that are toxic to the liver is another important treatment. Collaborate with the clinical pharmacist to review all medications that are metabolized by the liver.

Nursing measures for protecting the patient with an altered mental status from harm are a priority. Many patients with hepatic encephalopathy need to be sedated to prevent them from doing harm to themselves or to others. Diazepam (Valium), or lorazepam (Ativan) must be used judiciously; however, these medications are less dependent on liver function for excretion.

Hepatorenal syndrome. Acute renal failure that occurs with liver failure is called *hepatorenal syndrome.* The pathophysiology

---

BOX 18.17 Stages of Portal Systemic Encephalopathy

Stage 1
- Impaired decision making
- Slurred speech
- Tremors

Stage 2
- Asterixis
- Drowsiness
- Loss of sphincter control

Stage 3
- Dramatic confusion
- Somnolence

Stage 4
- Gastrointestinal alterations
- Profound coma
- Unresponsiveness to pain

of this disorder is not well understood, but it is associated with end-stage cirrhosis and ascites, decreased albumin levels, and portal hypertension. Decreased urine output and an increased serum creatinine level usually occur acutely. The prognosis for the patient with hepatorenal syndrome is generally poor because therapies to improve renal function usually are ineffective.[18] The goals of general medical therapies are to improve liver function while supporting renal function. Fluid administration and diuretic therapy are used to improve urine output. Medications that are toxic to the kidney are discontinued. Occasionally, hemodialysis is used to support renal function if there is a chance for an improvement in liver function. Because of the poor prognosis, it is appropriate for the critical care nurse to begin to address end-of-life decisions with the patient and family.[20] This is done with consideration of the individual nurse's comfort level, as well as the organizational policy and family dynamics.[12]

Hepatopulmonary syndrome. *Hepatopulmonary syndrome* (HPS) is a pulmonary complication that is observed in patients with chronic liver disease, portal hypertension, or both. HPS occurs because of intrapulmonary vascular dilation that may induce severe hypoxemia. HPS is defined as a triad of liver disease, increased alveolar-arterial oxygen gradient, and intrapulmonary vascular dilations. Patients with HPS experience hypoxia due to ventilation-perfusion mismatch, pulmonary capillary vasodilation, and limitation of oxygen diffusion. Pulse oximetry and arterial blood gas measurements are useful screening tools for HPS. Current medical and surgical therapies for HPS include oxygen and TIPS; liver transplantation is the definitive treatment to improve symptoms and survival.[43] The current 1- and 5-year survival rates for patient who received liver transplantation are 86% to 90% and 72% to 80%, respectively.[8]

Patient Outcomes

Outcomes for the patient with liver failure are included in the Plan of Care for the Patient with Liver Failure and the Collaborative Plan of Care for the Critically Ill Patient (see Chapter 1).

CASE STUDY

The critical care nurse receives a report from the emergency department of a patient to be admitted to the unit. Mr. G. is a 47-year-old man with a week-long history of severe abdominal pain that worsens with food intake. The pain is associated with nausea and vomiting. Mr. G. is oriented to person and place; however, he is disoriented to day and time and is described as "lethargic." A nasogastric tube and urinary catheter were placed, and IV access was established in the emergency department.

Vital signs include the following: heart rate, 110 beats/min; respirations, 30 breaths/min; blood pressure, 104/56 mm Hg; and temperature, 38°C.

Laboratory values include the following: white blood cell count, 19,000/mm³; hematocrit, 38%; sodium, 148 mEq/L; potassium, 4.0 mEq/L; chloride, 114 mEq/L; blood urea nitrogen, 25 mg/dL; creatinine, 1.0 mg/dL; glucose, 180 mg/dL; amylase, 500 IU/L; and lipase, 600 IU/L.

Questions
1. What further data should the critical care nurse request from the nurse in the emergency department?
2. In addition to management of shock, what is another priority treatment?
3. What further assessment data would be valuable for long-term management of this patient?

REFERENCES

1. Agarwal A, Khan MH, Whorwell PJ. Irritable bowel syndrome in the elderly: An overlooked problem? *Dig Liver Dis.* 2009;41: 721–724.
2. Ahmed T, Haboubi N. Assessment and management of nutrition in older people and its importance to health. *Clin Interv Aging.* 2010;5:207–216.
3. Al-Khafaji A, Huang DT. Critical care management of patients with end-stage liver disease. *Crit Care Med.* 2011;39(5): 1157–1166.
4. Al-Omran M, AlBalawi ZH, Tashkandi MF, et al. Enteral versus parenteral nutrition for acute pancreatitis. *Cochrane Database Syst Rev.* 2010;1:CD002837.
5. Albrades JG, Tandon P. Therapies: Drugs, scopes, and transjugular intrahepatic portosystemic shunt—When and how? *Dig Dis.* 2015;33(4):524–533.
6. American College of Obstetricians and Gynecologists. ACOG Practice Bulletin No. 189 Summary: Nausea and Vomiting of Pregnancy. *Obstet Gynecol.* 2018;131(1): 190–193.
7. Baid H. A critical review of auscultating bowel sounds. *Br J Nurs.* 2009;18(18):1125–1130.
8. Beilman G, Banton K. Management of the postoperative liver transplant patient. In: Vincent J, Abraham E, Kochanek P, et al., eds. *Textbook of Critical Care.* 8th ed. Philadelphia, PA: Elsevier; 2019:1106–111.
9. Barkun AN, Bardou M, Pham CQ, et al. Proton pump inhibitors vs. histamine 2 receptor antagonists for stress-related mucosal bleeding prophylaxis in critically ill patients: A meta-analysis. *Am J Gastroenterol.* 2012;107(4):507–520.
10. Boregowda G, Shehata HA. Gastrointestinal and liver disease in pregnancy. *Best Pract Res Clin Obstet Gynaecol.* 2013;27: 835–853.
11. Carefusion. About the Denver Shunt. http://www.bd.com. Published 2019. Accessed June 21, 2019.
12. Cawood AL, Elia M, Stratton RJ. Systematic review and meta-analysis of the effects of high protein oral nutritional supplements. *Ageing Res Rev.* 2012;11(2):278–296.
13. Centers for Disease Control and Prevention. Chronic Liver Disease and Cirrhosis. http://www.cdc.gov/nchs/fastats/liver-disease.htm. Accessed June 21, 2019.
14. Centers for Disease Control and Prevention. Viral Hepatitis. http://www.cdc.gov/hepatitis. Accessed June 21, 2019.
15. Chaptini L, Peikin S. Gastrointestinal bleeding. In: Parrillo JE, Dellinger RP, eds. *Critical Care Medicine: Principles of Diagnosis and Management in the Adult.* 5th ed. St. Louis, MO: Elsevier; 2019:1192–1209.
16. Cover TL, Balser MJ. *Helicobacter pylori* and other gastric *Helicobacter* species. In: Bennett JE, Dolin R, Baser MJ, eds. *Mandell, Douglas, and Bennett's Principles and Practice of Infectious Disease.* 9th ed. Philadelphia, PA: Elsevier; 2020:2660–2668.
17. DellaVolpe JD, Garavaglia JM, Huang DT. Management of complications of end-stage liver disease in the intensive care unit. *J Intensive Care Med.* 2016;31(2):94–103.
18. Dhillon A, Ershoff, B. Hepatorenal syndrome. In Vincent J, Abraham E, Kochanek P, et al., eds. *Textbook of Critical Care.* 7th ed. Philadelphia, PA: Elsevier; 2017:657–661.
19. Didier R, Shahar DR, Gille D, et al. Understanding the gastrointestinal tract of the elderly to develop dietary solutions that prevent malnutrition. *Oncotarget.* 2015;6(17):13858–13859.

20. Dundar HZ, Yilmazlar T. Management of hepatorenal syndrome. *World J Nephrol*. 2015;4(2):277–286.

21. Durup-Dickenson M, Christensen MK, Gade J. Abdominal auscultation does not provide clear clinical diagnoses. *Dan Med J*. 2013;60(5):A4620.

22. Ermis F, Tasci ES. Current *Helicobacter pylori* treatment in 2014. *World J Methodol*. 2015;5(2):101–107.

23. Everson GT. Hepatic failure and liver transplantation. In: Goldman L, Shafer AI, eds. *Goldman-Cecil Medicine*. 26th ed. Philadelphia, PA: Elsevier; 2020:998–1004.

24. Fashner J, Gitu AC. Diagnosis and treatment of peptic ulcer disease and *H. pylori* infection. *Am Fam Physician*. 2015;91(4):236–242.

25. Fidelman N, Kwan SW, LaBerge JM, et al. The transjugular intrahepatic portosystemic shunt: An update. *AJR Am J Radiol*. 2012;199:746–755.

26. Franklin LE, Spain MP, Edlund BJ. Pharmacological management of chronic constipation in older adults. *J Gerontol Nurs*. 2012; 38(4):9–15.

27. Forsmark CE, Vege SS, Wilcox CM. Acute pancreatitis. *N Engl J Med*. 2016;375(20):1972–1981.

28. Gallegos-Orozco JF, Foxx-Orenstein AE, Sterler SM, et al. Chronic constipation in the elderly. *Am J Gastroenterol*. 2012;107:18–25.

29. Garcia-Pagan JC, Reverter E, Abraldes JG, et al. Acute variceal bleeding. *Semin Respir Crit Care Med*. 2012;33(1):46–54.

30. Ghassemi KA, Jensen DM. Lower GI bleeding: Epidemiology and management. *Curr Gastroenterol Rep*. 2013;15(7):333.

31. Guyton AC, Hall JE. *Textbook of Medical Physiology*. 13th ed. Philadelphia, PA: Elsevier; 2016.

32. Huether SE. Structure and function of the digestive system. In: McCance KL, Huether SE, eds. *Pathophysiology: The Biologic Basis for Disease in Adults and Children*. 8th ed. St. Louis, MO: Elsevier; 2019:1294–1320.

33. Hwang JH, Shergill AK, Acosta RD, et al. The role of endoscopy in the management of variceal hemorrhage. *Gastrointest Endosc*. 2014;80(2):221–227.

34. Institute for Healthcare Improvement. How-to Guide: Prevent Ventilator-Associated Pneumonia. http://www.ihi.org/resources/Pages/Tools/HowtoGuidePreventVAP.aspx. Updated February 2012. Accessed June 21, 2019.

35. Jarvis C. *Physical Examination and Health Assessment*. 7th ed. Philadelphia, PA: Saunders; 2015.

36. Klein K, Gralnek IM. Acute non-variceal upper gastrointestinal bleeding. *Curr Opin Crit Care*. 2015;21(2):154–162.

37. Kochanek KD, Murphy SL, Xu J. Deaths: Final data for 2011. *Natl Vital Stat Rep*. 2015;63(3):1–120.

38. Krok KL. Care of the patient with end-stage liver disease. In: Lanken PN, Manaker S, Kohl B, et al., eds. *Intensive Care Unit Manual*. 2nd ed. Philadelphia, PA: Elsevier Saunders; 2014:271–277.

39. Liou IW. Management of end-stage liver disease. *Med Clin North Am*. 2014;98(1):119–152.

40. Lipsett PS, Rueda M. Acute pancreatitis. In: Vincent J, Abraham E, Kochanek P, et al., eds. *Textbook of Critical Care*. 7th ed. Philadelphia, PA: Elsevier; 2017:685–691.

41. Leo S, Accettura C, Gnoni A, et al. Systemic treatment of gastrointestinal cancer in elderly patients. *J Gastrointest Cancer*. 2013; 44(1):22–32.

42. Loffroy R, Favelier S, Pottecher P, et al. Transjugular intrahepatic portosystemic shunt for acute variceal gastrointestinal bleeding: Indications, techniques and outcomes. *Diagn Interv Imaging*. 2015;96(7–8):745–755.

43. Lv Y, Fan D. Hepatopulmonary syndrome. *Dig Dis Sci*. 2015;60:1914–1923.

44. Maclaren R, Reynolds PM, Allen RR. Histamine-2 receptor antagonists vs proton pump inhibitors on gastrointestinal tract hemorrhage and infectious complications in the intensive care unit. *JAMA Intern Med*. 2014;174(4):564.

45. Malfertheiner P, Selgrad M. Helicobacter pylori. *Curr Opin Gastroenterol*. 2014;3(6):589–595.

46. Martin LG. Percutaneous placement and management of the Denver shunt for portal hypertensive ascites. *AJR Am J Roentgen*. 2012;119:W449–W453.

47. Martinez-Camacho A, Fortune BE, Everson GT. Hepatic encephalopathy. In: Vincent J, Abraham E, Kochanek P, et al., eds. *Textbook of Critical Care*. 7th ed. Philadelphia, PA: Elsevier; 2017:665–672.

48. Morley JE. Defining undernutrition (malnutrition) in older persons. *J Nutr Health Aging*. 2018;22(3):308–310.

49. Munro N, Ruggiero M. Ventilator-associated pneumonia bundle reconstruction for best care. *AACN Adv Crit Care*. 2014;25(2):163–175.

50. Pares A, Mas A. Extracorporeal liver support in severe alcoholic hepatitis. *World J Gastroenterol*. 2014;20(25):8011–8017.

51. Pawlotsky J-M. Acute viral hepatitis. In: Goldman L, Shafer AI, eds. *Goldman-Cecil Medicine*. 26th ed. Philadelphia, PA: Elsevier; 2020:958–965.e.

52. Pawlotsky J-M. Chronic viral and autoimmune hepatitis. In: Goldman L, Shafer AI, eds. *Goldman-Cecil Medicine*. 26th ed. Philadelphia, PA: Elsevier; 2020:966–972.e2.

53. Qi S, Jia J, Bai M, et al. Transjugular intrahepatic portosystemic shunt for acute variceal bleeding: A meta-analysis. *J Clin Gastroenterol*. 2015;49(6):495–505.

54. Rahimi RS, Rockey DD. Complications and outcomes in chronic liver disease. *Curr Opin Gastroenterol*. 2011;27:204–209.

55. Rajala MW, Ginsberg GG. Tips and tricks on how to optimally manage patients with upper gastrointestinal bleeding. *Gastrointest Endosc Clin North Am*. 2015;25(3):607–617.

56. Ranson JC. Risk factors in acute pancreatitis. *Hosp Pract*. 1985;20(4):69–73.

57. Resar R, Griffin FA, Haraden C, et al. *Using Care Bundles to Improve Health Care Quality: IHI Innovation Series White Paper*. Cambridge, MA: Institute for Healthcare Improvement; 2012.

58. Shah NL, Banaei YP, Hojnowski KL, et al. Management options in decompensated cirrhosis. *Hepat Med*. 2015;2015(7):43–50.

59. Shin GH, Toto EL, Schey R. Pregnancy and postpartum bowel changes: Constipation and fecal incontinence. *Am J Gastroenterol*. 2015;110:521–529.

60. Swearingen PL. *All-in-One Nursing Care Planning Resource*. 5th ed. St. Louis, MO: Elsevier; 2019.

61. Tanaka T, Sugawara Y, Kokudo N. Liver transplantation and autoimmune hepatitis. *Intractable Rare Dis Res*. 2015;4(1):33–38.

62. Talukdar R, Vege SS. Acute pancreatitis. *Curr Opin Gastroenterol*. 2015;31(5):374–379.

63. Talukdar R, Vege SS. Early management of severe acute pancreatitis. *Curr Gastroenterol Rep*. 2011;13:123–130.

64. Toews I, George AT, Peter JV, et al. Interventions for preventing upper gastrointestinal bleeding in people admitted to intensive care units. *Cochrane Database Sys Rev*. 2018;6:CD008687.

65. Van der Woude CJ, Metselaar HJ, Danese S. Management of gastrointestinal and liver diseases during pregnancy. *Gut*. 2014;63:1014–1023.

66. Vincent JL, Moreno R, Takala J, et al. The SOFA (Sepsis-Related Organ Failure Assessment) score to describe organ dysfunctions/failure. *Intensive Care Med.* 1996;22: 707–710.

67. Thomas E, Fair J. Portal hypertension: Critical care considerations. In: Vincent J, Abraham E, Kochanek P, et al., eds. *Textbook of Critical Care.* 7th ed. Philadelphia, PA: Saunders; 2017.

68. Wybourn C, Campbell A. Gastrointestinal bleeding. In: Vincent J, Abraham E, Kochanek P, et al., eds. *Textbook of Critical Care.* 7th ed. Philadelphia, PA: Elsevier; 2017:90–93.

69. Zielinski R, Searing K, Deibel M. Gastrointestinal distress in pregnancy prevalence, assessment, and treatment of 5 common minor discomforts. *J Perinat Neonatal Nurs.* 2015; 29(1):23–31.

Endocrine Alterations

Sharon A. Watts, DNP, FNP-BC, CDE
Marthe J. Moseley, PhD, RN, CCRN-K, CCNS

Many additional resources, including self-assessment exercises, are located on the Evolve companion website at http://evolve.elsevier.com/Sole/.

- Animations
- Clinical Skills: Critical Care Collections
- Student Review Questions
- Video Clips

INTRODUCTION

The endocrine glands form a communication network linking all body systems. Hormones from these glands control and regulate metabolic processes such as energy production, fluid and electrolyte balance, and response to stress. This system is closely linked to and integrated with the nervous system. In particular, the hypothalamus and the pituitary gland play major roles in hormonal regulation. The hypothalamus manufactures and secretes several releasing or inhibiting hormones that are conveyed to the pituitary. The pituitary gland responds to these hormones by increasing or decreasing hormone secretion, thus regulating circulating hormone levels. This system is designed as a feedback control mechanism. Positive feedback stimulates release of a hormone when serum hormone levels are low. Negative feedback inhibits the release of hormones when serum hormone levels are high. Examples of how these feedback systems work to control circulating levels of cortisol are provided in Fig. 19.1. Similar feedback systems control the secretion and inhibition of other hormones outside hypothalamic-pituitary control.

Diseases involving the hypothalamus, the pituitary gland, and the primary endocrine organs (i.e., pancreas, adrenal glands, and thyroid gland) interfere with normal feedback mechanisms and the secretion of hormones. Crisis states occur when these diseases are untreated or undertreated or when the patient is physiologically or psychologically stressed.

The stress of critical illness provokes a significant response by the endocrine system. Excess glucose in the blood occurs as a result of release of *counterregulatory hormones* that promote hepatic gluconeogenesis and decreased peripheral use of glucose, with resulting relative hypoinsulinemia. Adrenal insufficiency can occur as a result of insult or damage to the gland itself (primary); dysfunction of the hypothalamus, pituitary, or both (secondary); or whenever cortisol levels are inadequate for the demand (relative). Thyroid hormone balance is disrupted by changes in peripheral metabolism that cause a decrease in triiodothyronine (T_3) levels. Pituitary and hypothalamus dysfunction as a result of brain tumor, trauma, or surgery can cause significant fluid and electrolyte imbalances that complicate critical illness.

This chapter describes both the endocrine response to critical illness and the crises that occur because of imbalances of hormones from the pancreas, adrenal glands, thyroid gland, and posterior pituitary gland. Older adult patients present diagnostic and treatment challenges due to endocrine disorders. Responses to endocrine dysfunction are blunted, and many of the compensatory mechanisms are lost with advanced age.[2,9] Lifespan Considerations boxes are integrated throughout the chapter to highlight information specific to older adults and pregnant women.

HYPERGLYCEMIA IN THE CRITICALLY ILL PATIENT

Critically ill patients are at high risk for hyperglycemia from many different stressors, including their disease states, illness-related hormonal responses to stress, and the critical care environment. Refer to Box 19.1 for risk factors associated with the development of increased blood glucose levels.

Although stress-induced hyperglycemia is a normal physiological response due to the *fight-or-flight* mode, glucose elevation is associated with poor outcomes in hospitalized patients with and without a formal diagnosis of diabetes. Hyperglycemia in acutely ill patients has been linked to impaired immune function, cerebral ischemia, osmotic diuresis, poor wound healing, decreased erythropoiesis, increased hemolysis, endothelial dysfunction, increased thrombosis, vasoconstriction with resulting hypertension, decreased respiratory muscle function, neuronal damage, and impaired gastric motility.[16] Acute hyperglycemia

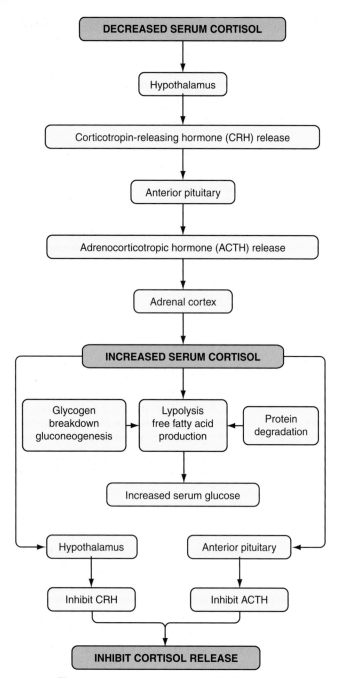

Fig. 19.1 Feedback system for cortisol regulation.

- Preexisting diabetes mellitus, diagnosed or undiagnosed
- Comorbidities such as obesity, pancreatitis, cirrhosis, hypokalemia
- Stress response release of cortisol, growth hormone, catecholamines (epinephrine and norepinephrine), glucagon, glucocorticoids, cytokines (interleukin-1, interleukin-6, and tumor necrosis factor)
- Advanced age
- Lack of muscular activity
- Relative insulin deficiency or insulin resistance
- Administration of exogenous catecholamines, glucocorticoids
- Administration of dextrose solutions, nutritional support
- Medication therapy such as thiazides, beta-blockers, highly-active antiretroviral therapy (HAART), phenytoin, tacrolimus, cyclosporine

injury necessitating dialysis, blood transfusion requirements, and polyneuropathy.[16] Findings of this study led many hospitals to institute tight glycemic control protocols in critically ill patients as a standard of care. Subsequent studies conducted in broader populations have demonstrated higher rates of mortality in nonsurgical populations and significantly higher rates of severe hypoglycemia in patients who were intensively controlled, raising questions about the degree of glycemic control that should be maintained in critically ill individuals.[14,16,17] In response, the American Diabetes Association and the American Association of Clinical Endocrinologists issued a joint statement on inpatient glycemic control. Current guidelines recommend an initial target glucose level of no greater than 180 mg/dL; targets of 140 to 180 mg/dL are appropriate for most critically ill patients once insulin therapy has been initiated.[2] Glycemic targets at the lower end of this range may be most beneficial. Glycemic targets of 110 mg/dL or less are no longer recommended for critically ill individuals.[2,3,16]

Achieving Optimal Glycemic Control

To optimize patient safety, IV delivery of short-acting insulin guided by an evidence-based protocol is the preferred method for treating hyperglycemia to a target range of 140 to 180 mg/dL in critically ill patients.[2,3,16] These nurse-managed protocols include frequent glucose monitoring and insulin dosage adjustments based on patient-specific glucose targets. Frequent blood glucose monitoring, with blood glucose measurements every 30 minutes to 2 hours, is intended to ensure the appropriate insulin dosage and to minimize the incidence of hypoglycemia. The key elements for glycemic control protocols are described in Box 19.2. Systems approaches are required to limit the patient's risk associated with this complex therapy.[16] Computer decision support software is helpful in managing glucose control. Although strict control of insulin delivery is labor intensive, these protocols reduce hospitalization costs due to fewer inpatient complications; reduce critical care and hospital lengths of stay; reduce ventilator days; and reduce charges for radiology, laboratory tests, and pharmaceuticals.[16]

during the course of illness has been associated with poor clinical outcomes, including mortality in critically ill patients who have been treated for myocardial infarction, traumatic brain injury, burns, trauma, subarachnoid hemorrhage, or transplantation.[16]

Effective glycemic control improves patient outcomes, but recommendations regarding target values are changing. In 2001 Van den Berghe and colleagues published a landmark study showing that intensive insulin control of hyperglycemia in a critically ill surgical population decreased mortality and morbidity, including sepsis, acute kidney

BOX 19.2 Key Components of a Glucose Management Protocol

- Frequent plasma blood glucose measurements taking into consideration awareness of previous blood glucose levels, insulin dose adjustments, and individual patient parameters
- Concentration of insulin infusion with the intention of avoiding hypoglycemia
- Initial IV insulin bolus dose if appropriate, accounting for characteristics of individual patients
- Proactive measures for titration to increase or decrease insulin infusion based on glucose levels incorporated into nurse-directed protocols
- Interventions for:
  - Hypoglycemia, should it occur
  - Interruption of feeding, either parenteral or enteral
  - Transport of the patient from the critical care unit for diagnostic testing
  - Discontinuation of the IV insulin infusion
  - Transfer of the patient from the critical care unit

Data from Compton F, Ahlborn R, Weidehoff T. Nurse-directed blood glucose management in a medical intensive care unit. *Crit Care Nurse*. 2017;37(3):30–41.

✳ QSEN EXEMPLAR

Evidence-Based Practice and Quality Improvement

A group of nurses from the critical care unit and an endocrinology advanced practice nurse practitioner noticed that their organization's quality scores for patients with severe hyperglycemia (glucose >300 mg/dL) were above the national aggregate for comparable-size units. The nurses were cognizant that hyperglycemia is associated with increased mortality, morbidity, longer hospital stays, and associated costs. They understood that extreme physiological stress, changes in nutrition, steroid use, and variability in practice patterns all contribute to critical care unit hyperglycemia.

Identified gaps for reducing hyperglycemia in their unit included a need for a more user-friendly insulin infusion titration guides, medical resident resistance to ordering the infusion protocol, lack of education about severe hyperglycemia for the nurses and rotating residents, and a lack of guidance for titration of insulin during steroid use. A 1-year comprehensive audit of hyperglycemia was instituted to screen for hyperglycemia fallouts. Results indicated that while the overall numbers of hyperglycemia were low (n = 50), a potential communication gap existed, as 46% of nurses did not notify a provider when two consecutive hyperglycemic events occurred.

Successful interventions to mitigate severe hyperglycemia by the nurses included:
- Education of medical and nursing staff on diabetes protocols, insulin infusion, and steroid guidance.
- Set expectations for nurses to notify the provider if there are two consecutive blood glucose levels greater than 300 mg/dL in a 12-hour period.
- Staff to report severe hyperglycemia episodes at safety huddles.
- Identify nurse champions to use a generated report to audit hyperglycemic episodes. Data included provider contact, actions taken, documentation, and causes with individual nurse follow-up as needed.
- Monthly review of hyperglycemia audits at staff meetings.

Results indicated that 2 years prior to the intervention, four of the quarterly seven data points on a statistical process control chart for the unit's hyperglycemia were well above the national aggregate. After interventions the hyperglycemia rates were closer to or below the national average. Moreover, the continued vigilance has helped sustain this important nurse-led quality improvement project.

Reference

Neelon L, Basawil K, Whitney L, et al. Critical care nurse–led quality improvement hyperglycemia reduction initiative. *J Nurs Care Qual*. 2019;34(2):91–93.

The transition from IV to subcutaneous insulin therapy must be carefully timed to limit the risk for hyperglycemia. Most patients may be transitioned from IV to subcutaneous insulin when they are eating regular meals or when their clinical condition warrants transfer to a lower intensity level of care.[2,16] Subcutaneous basal insulin should be administered 1 to 2 hours before the insulin infusion is discontinued.[10]

It is recommended that the subcutaneous insulin regimen for a non–critically ill patient include basal, nutritional, and correction insulin components.[2] Protocols are additionally individualized to the patient with regard to weight and renal function. Glycemic protocols typically include a consistent carbohydrate meal plan.[2] Daily insulin dose adjustments, IV fluid changes, and retiming of point-of-care glucose monitoring may be required for significant glucose elevations and to account for significant changes in dietary intake imposed by "nothing by mouth" status or nausea and vomiting. Adjustments to the insulin dose regimen also may be required if the patient is receiving enteral feedings, parenteral nutrition, or high-dose glucocorticoids, or if the patient's blood glucose level falls to less than 100 mg/dL. Effective communication among providers, nursing staff, pharmacists, and clinical dietitians is imperative for safe implementation of basal-nutritional-correction insulin protocols. Insulin regimens that are composed exclusively of sliding-scale insulin have been associated with poor patient outcomes and are no longer recommended as the only method of insulin delivery for hospitalized patients.[2]

Many facilities that use basal-nutritional-correctional insulin protocols discontinue oral medications for the duration of the hospitalization. Metformin is contraindicated in acute renal failure or with the use of contrast dye. Thiazolidinediones, such as pioglitazone, increase the risk of fluid retention and heart failure. Other agents, such as sulfonylureas, may increase the risk for hypoglycemia. Sodium-glucose transport protein 2 (SGLT2) inhibitors and glucagon-like peptide 1 (GLP-1) agonists have the potential to contribute to electrolyte imbalance and are not well studied in the hospitalized population. Dipeptidyl peptidase 4 (DPP-4) inhibitors likewise have not been extensively studied for hospital use. Because many patients experience a significant change in their diabetes treatment regimen during the course of a hospitalization, accurate medication reconciliation and effective discharge education are critical for all hospitalized patients who are being treated for diabetes.

STUDY BREAK

1. The critical care nurse has just completed the second blood glucose bedside assessment. The results of both of the blood glucose values are as follows: 315 mg/dL at 0900 and 350 mg/dL at 1300. What is the priority in terms of nursing actions given the findings?
   A. Plan the next monthly in-service to educate medical and nursing staff on altered blood glucose levels.
   B. Report the hypoglycemia findings at the morning safety huddle, which would be tomorrow morning.
   C. Notify the provider, as two consecutive blood glucose measurements are greater than 300 mg/dL in a 12-hour period.
   D. Determine who is in charge of the monthly review of hyperglycemia audits at the next staff meeting.

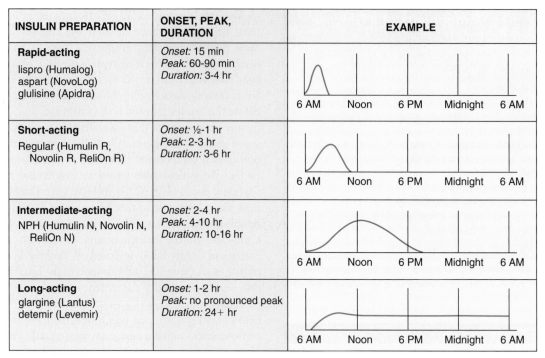

INSULIN PREPARATION	ONSET, PEAK, DURATION	EXAMPLE
Rapid-acting lispro (Humalog) aspart (NovoLog) glulisine (Apidra)	*Onset:* 15 min *Peak:* 60-90 min *Duration:* 3-4 hr	
Short-acting Regular (Humulin R, Novolin R, ReliOn R)	*Onset:* ½-1 hr *Peak:* 2-3 hr *Duration:* 3-6 hr	
Intermediate-acting NPH (Humulin N, Novolin N, ReliOn N)	*Onset:* 2-4 hr *Peak:* 4-10 hr *Duration:* 10-16 hr	
Long-acting glargine (Lantus) detemir (Levemir)	*Onset:* 1-2 hr *Peak:* no pronounced peak *Duration:* 24+ hr	

Fig. 19.2 Commercially available insulin preparations showing onset, peak, and duration of action. (From Dirksen SR. Nursing management of diabetes. In: Lewis SL, Bucher L, Heitkemper MM, et al., eds. *Medical-Surgical Nursing: Assessment and Management of Clinical Problems*. 10th ed. St. Louis, MO: Mosby; 2017.)

Hypoglycemia as a Preventable Adverse Effect of Glucose Management

Intensive insulin therapy is associated with a sixfold increased risk for an episode of severe hypoglycemia (i.e., glucose ≤54 mg/dL).[14] The increased incidence of hypoglycemia in critically ill patients is associated with reduction or discontinuation of nutrition without adjustment of insulin therapy (e.g., interruption of parenteral or enteral feedings during diagnostic examinations); heart failure; kidney disease; liver disease; sepsis; and the use of or change in dosage of inotropic medications, vasopressor support, and glucocorticoid therapy.[3]

Many episodes of hypoglycemia are preventable; therefore ensure that the glucose testing is accurate and consistent. Concurrent and shift-to-shift coordination and adjustment of all medical and nutritional therapies (including increasing, decreasing, or temporarily suspending any of them) is required to prevent hypoglycemia.

Hyperglycemia in the Critically Ill

Stress-induced hyperglycemia affects patients with and without a formal diagnosis of diabetes mellitus (DM). In the critically ill, stress-induced hyperglycemia exacerbates the elevated glucose levels of patients with preexisting diabetes, predisposes them to an even higher incidence of complications and comorbidities, and affects the treatments for all disease states. Individuals with diabetes are hospitalized more frequently, are more prone to complications, and have longer hospital stays and higher hospital costs than patients without diabetes.[3] Therapy aimed at establishing euglycemic levels

contributes to improved patient outcomes. Critically ill patients with diabetes are most effectively managed with insulin therapy regardless of their usual home self-management regimen.[2,16] Fig. 19.2 and Table 19.1 provide a review of the insulin action profiles of various insulin products and common insulin regimens. In addition, Table 19.2 lists oral agents used in the management of type 2 diabetes presented by class, along with information on injectable agents used to regulate blood glucose.

PANCREATIC ENDOCRINE EMERGENCIES

Review of Physiology

DM is a metabolic disease of glucose imbalance resulting from alterations in insulin secretion, insulin action, or both.[1] The number of people with DM has been increasing, with an incidence of more than 422 million worldwide.[20] The two most common types of DM are type 1 and type 2. Type 1 DM is primarily caused by the destruction of pancreatic islet beta cells, which results in an *absolute insulin deficiency* and a tendency to develop ketoacidosis. In most cases, type 1 DM is an autoimmune disorder. A subset of patients, primarily of African American or Asian ancestry, may experience a genetic but non-immunological form of type 1 diabetes.[1]

Type 2 is the most common form of diabetes. It results from the combination of insulin resistance and insulin secretory defects.[1] The net result is a *relative insulin deficiency*. A combination of cardiovascular risk factors, including hypertension, atherogenic dyslipidemia, and hyperglycemia, makes up the *cardiometabolic risk syndrome* and significantly increases the risk of developing type 2 DM. The other causes of DM include

TABLE 19.1 Common Insulin Regimens

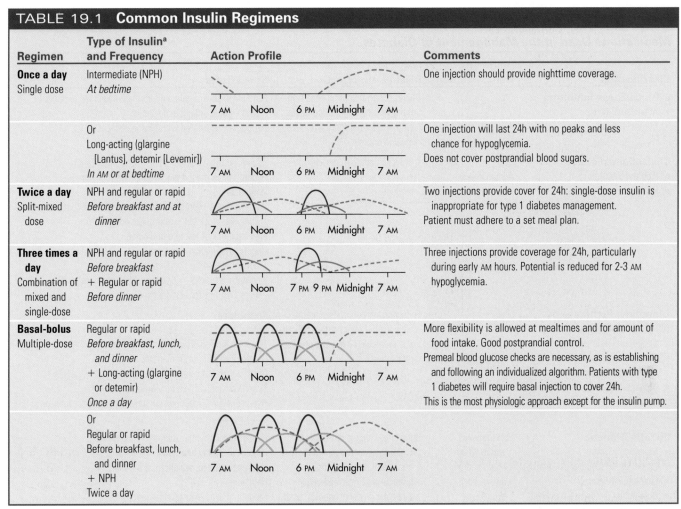

Regimen	Type of Insulin[a] and Frequency	Action Profile	Comments
Once a day Single dose	Intermediate (NPH) *At bedtime*	7 AM Noon 6 PM Midnight 7 AM	One injection should provide nighttime coverage.
	Or Long-acting (glargine [Lantus], detemir [Levemir]) *In AM or at bedtime*	7 AM Noon 6 PM Midnight 7 AM	One injection will last 24h with no peaks and less chance for hypoglycemia. Does not cover postprandial blood sugars.
Twice a day Split-mixed dose	NPH and regular or rapid *Before breakfast and at dinner*	7 AM Noon 6 PM Midnight 7 AM	Two injections provide cover for 24h: single-dose insulin is inappropriate for type 1 diabetes management. Patient must adhere to a set meal plan.
Three times a day Combination of mixed and single-dose	NPH and regular or rapid *Before breakfast* + Regular or rapid *Before dinner*	7 AM Noon 7 PM 9 PM Midnight 7 AM	Three injections provide coverage for 24h, particularly during early AM hours. Potential is reduced for 2-3 AM hypoglycemia.
Basal-bolus Multiple-dose	Regular or rapid *Before breakfast, lunch, and dinner* + Long-acting (glargine or detemir) *Once a day*	7 AM Noon 6 PM Midnight 7 AM	More flexibility is allowed at mealtimes and for amount of food intake. Good postprandial control. Premeal blood glucose checks are necessary, as is establishing and following an individualized algorithm. Patients with type 1 diabetes will require basal injection to cover 24h. This is the most physiologic approach except for the insulin pump.
	Or Regular or rapid Before breakfast, lunch, and dinner + NPH Twice a day	7 AM Noon 6 PM Midnight 7 AM	

[a]Insulin types include rapid-acting (lispro, aspart, glulisine), short-acting (regular), intermediate-acting (NPH), and long-acting (glargine, detemir).

From Dirksen SR. Nursing management: Diabetes mellitus. In: Lewis SL, Bucher L, Heitkemper MM, et al, eds. Medical-Surgical Nursing: Assessment and Management of Clinical Problems. 10th ed. St Louis, MO: Mosby; 2017.

TABLE 19.2 PHARMACOLOGY

Medications Used in the Management of Diabetes

Classification	Route of Administration	Mechanism of Action	Side Effects
Sulfonylureas • Glipizide (Glucotrol, Glucotrol XL) • Glyburide (Micronase, DiaBeta, Glynase) • Glimepiride (Amaryl)	Oral	Stimulates release of insulin from pancreatic beta cells; decreases glycogenesis and gluconeogenesis; enhances cellular sensitivity to insulin; agents are longer-acting	Hypoglycemia Weight gain Photosensitivity Cholestatic jaundice; use with caution in patients with hepatic or renal dysfunction
Meglitinides • Repaglinide (Prandin) • Nateglinide (Starlix)	Oral	Stimulates rapid, short-lived release of insulin from the pancreas; taken within 30 min of meal	Hypoglycemia; medication is held if no meal is taken Weight gain
Biguanide • Metformin (Glucophage, Glucophage XR, Fortamet, Riomet)	Oral	↓ Rate of hepatic glucose production; augments glucose uptake from tissues, especially muscles	Stomach upset—take with meals Diarrhea Lactic acidosis; medication is held before IV contrast procedures and 48h afterward Withhold if eGFR below 45 mL/min/1.73 m^2 not on medication already Or May continue cautiously if eGFR below 30 mL/min/1.73 m^2 currently maintained on the medication May cause vitamin B$_{12}$ deficiency

Continued

TABLE 19.2   PHARMACOLOGY—cont'd

Medications Used in the Management of Diabetes

Classification	Route of Administration	Mechanism of Action	Side Effects
α-Glucosidase Inhibitors • Acarbose (Precose) • Miglitol (Glyset)	Oral	Delays absorption of glucose from the gastrointestinal tract; taken with first bite of food; withheld if meal is missed	Flatulence; abdominal pain; diarrhea; avoid use in patients with chronic intestinal disorders Hypoglycemia treated with glucose only
Thiazolidinediones • Pioglitazone (Actos) • Rosiglitazone (Avandia)	Oral Administered at bedtime	↑ Glucose update in muscle ↓ Endogenous glucose production	Edema; contraindicated in class III/IV heart failure Hypoglycemia if used with insulin or sulfonylureas Weight gain Cardiovascular events such as myocardial infarction and stroke (Avandia: black box warning issued by FDA) Increased risk of fracture in women Hepatic dysfunction—withhold if ALT >2.5 times upper limit of normal Pioglitazone use for >1 year may be associated with increased risk for bladder cancer
Dipeptidyl Peptidase-4 (DPP-4) Inhibitors • Sitagliptin (Januvia) • Saxagliptin (Onglyza) • Linagliptin (Tradjenta) • Alogliptin (Nesina)	Oral	Enhances incretin system; stimulates insulin release from pancreatic beta cells; ↓ hepatic glucose production	Angioedema Pancreatitis Upper respiratory tract infection; sore throat Gastrointestinal upset; diarrhea Dose reduction for renal impairment Hypoglycemia (with sulfonylureas or insulin) Hypersensitivity reactions (anaphylaxis, Stevens-Johnson syndrome)
Incretin Mimetic • Exenatide (Byetta) • Exenatide ER (Bydureon—weekly) • Liraglutide (Victoza) • Dulaglutide (Trulicity—weekly) • Lixisenatide (Adlyxin) • Semaglutide (Ozempic)	Subcutaneous within 60 min of am and pm meals; dose titrated	Stimulates release of insulin; ↓ glucagon secretion; ↑ satiety; ↓ gastric emptying (avoid in patients with gastroparesis); ↓ hepatic gluconeogenesis; used in treatment of type 2 diabetes	Hypoglycemia (with insulin-secreting agents) Pancreatitis (may be fatal) Nausea; vomiting; weight loss; diarrhea Headache Medullary thyroid tumor (liraglutide)
Amylin Analog • Pramlintide (Symlin)	Subcutaneous (abdomen or thigh)	Take with each significant carbohydrate-containing meal. ↑ Glucagon secretion; ↑ satiety; ↓ gastric emptying; ↓ hepatic gluconeogenesis	Hypoglycemia Nausea; vomiting; decreased appetite Headache (May be used in type 1 and type 2 diabetes; held if no significant meal is taken)
Sodium-Glucose Transport Protein 2 (SGLT2) Inhibitors • Canagliflozin (Invokana) • Dapagliflozin (Farxiga) • Empagliflozin (Jardiance) • Ertugliflozin (Steglatro)	Oral	Inhibits action of SGLT2 in the proximal nephron, allowing for excess secretion of glucose in the urine	Hypoglycemia if combined with insulin or secretagogue Polyuria Dehydration Genitourinary tract infections Weight loss Candidiasis UTI DKA Necrotizing fasciitis Decreased eGFR Hypotension
Combination Agents (Variety of combinations available)	Oral	Combine effects of each class	Combine side effects of all medications to obtain complete risk profiles. Combinations of sulfonylureas or meglitinides with other agents may increase the risk for hypoglycemia.

ALT, Alanine aminotransferase; *DKA,* diabetic ketoacidosis; *eGFR,* estimated glomerular filtration rate; *FDA,* US Food and Drug Administration; *UTI,* urinary tract infection.
Modified from Dirksen SR. Nursing management: Diabetes mellitus. In: Lewis SL, Bucher L, Heitkemper MM, et al, eds. *Medical-Surgical Nursing: Assessment and Management of Clinical Problems.* 10th ed. St. Louis, MO: Mosby; 2017; Imam TH. Changes in metformin use in chronic kidney disease. *Clin Kidney J.* 2017;10(3):301–304.

GENETICS

Type 2 Diabetes: Complex Genetics

The causes of type 2 diabetes mellitus (T2DM) are complex, resulting from a combination of genetic and lifestyle factors. T2DM is an example of a multifactorial, polygenic disease. *Multifactorial* means that the disease results from an interaction among genes, lifestyle, and the environment.[6] *Polygenic* means that more than one gene is implicated in the development of the disease and more than 150 DNA variations are associated with the risk of developing T2DM.[1] Most of polymorphisms associated with T2DM act by subtly changing the amount, timing, and location of gene expression.

The condition tends to run in families but does not display a pattern of single gene inheritance. Nonetheless, T2DM is highly associated with inheritance. Offspring of parents with T2DM have a significant risk for a similar diagnosis—as much as a sixfold increase over the general population.[9]

Genome-wide association studies (GWAS) have helped researchers build the long list of polymorphisms that contribute to T2DM.[9] Many of the genetic polymorphisms are linked to insulin secretion and resistance. Several contributing genetic polymorphisms are found in the intron (noncoding) regions of the genome. Lifestyle and environmental factors such as high caloric intake, physical inactivity, smoking, and obesity contribute to the onset and severity of T2DM. There is evidence that implementing lifestyle changes can decrease the occurrence of T2DM despite a genetic predisposition.[8]

Epigenetics may help explain the linkages between genetic risk and lifestyle in the onset and progression of T2D. Epigenetics is the study of changes in gene function that are inheritable but do involve a change in DNA sequence.[3] Changes in gene function may be the result of DNA methylation or histone modifications. For example, epigenetics has demonstrated sustained metabolic tissue derangements in offspring when maternal obesity and diabetes coexist during pregnancy.[1]

Gene function is also altered by endocrine-disrupting chemicals that interfere with hormonal signaling pathways. Chemicals used in manufacturing, resin-based medical supplies, and pesticides have been linked to T2DM.[2] For example, mercury can alter pancreatic beta cell function, inducing hyperglycemia. Mercury contamination can occur from discharge in mining and paper industries. Lifestyle factors that affect the gut microbiome can alter the onset and progression of T2DM.[7] Diet can alter DNA methylation, histone modifications, and expression of microRNA (miRNA), influencing the onset and progression of T2DM.[4]

Epigenetics holds promise for strategies to delay the onset of T2DM and perhaps reduce the severity of its associated complications.[3] Understanding the synthesis of proteins (the proteome) that influence metabolic pathways may yield strategies to prevent and cure this common disease. Metabolomics, the large-scale study of small molecules—metabolites—within a cell, tissue, and organ, is being used to guide treatment. Metabolomics uses technology developed during genomic studies to build knowledge around global biological systems like glucose regulation and use in humans. There are also investigations about environmental influences on the DNA formation of proteins involved in glucose regulation and use; this is the study of epigenetics. Both metabolomics and epigenetics hold promise for new treatments and potentially for prevention of this common condition[5].

Genetic terms: *multifactorial genetic disorders, polygenetic disorders, gene expression, genome-wide association studies (GWAS), intron, deoxynucleic acid (DNA), ribonucleic acid (RNA), epigenetics, translation, transcription, proteomics, metabolomics.*

References

1. Agarwal P, Morriseau TS, Kereliuk SM, et al. Maternal obesity, diabetes during pregnancy and epigenetic mechanisms that influence the developmental origins of cardiometabolic disease in the offspring. *Crit Rev Clin Lab Sci.* 2018;55(2):71–101.
2. Alavian-Ghavanini A, Ruegg J. Understanding epigenetic effects of endocrine disrupting chemicals: From mechanisms to novel test methods. *Basic Clin Pharmacol Toxicol.* 2018;122(1):38–45.
3. Genereux DP. Epigenetics and Disease. In: McCance KD, Huether SE, eds. *Pathophysiology.* St. Louis, MO: Elsevier; 2019:177–189.
4. Huang D, Cui L, Ahmed S, et al. An overview of epigenetic agents and natural nutrition products targeting DNA methyltransferase, histone deacetylases and microRNAs. *Food Chem Toxicol.* 2019;123:574–594.
5. Ingelsson E, McCarthy MI. Human genetics of obesity and type 2 diabetes mellitus: Past, present, and future. *Circ Genom Precis Med.* 2018;11(6):e002090.
6. National Institutes of Health. What Are Complex or Multifactorial Disorders? http://ghr.nlm.nih.gov/handbook/mutationsanddisorders/complexdisorders. Published February 19, 2019. Accessed February 20, 2019.
7. Sharma S, Tripathi P. Gut microbiome and type 2 diabetes: Where we are and where to go? *J Nutr Biochem.* 2019;63:101–108.
8. Standley RA, Vega RB. Furthering precision medicine genomics with healthy living medicine. *Prog Cardiovasc Dis.* 2019;62(1):60–67.
9. Udler MS, Kim J, von Grotthuss M, et al. Type 2 diabetes genetic loci informed by multi-trait associations point to disease mechanisms and subtypes: A soft clustering analysis. *PLoS Med.* 2018;15(9):e1002654.

insulin resistance during pregnancy (gestational diabetes, or GDM), medications such as corticosteroids, genetic disorders such as cystic fibrosis, pancreatic damage, viruses, and disorders of the pituitary and adrenal glands.[1] In addition, polycystic ovary syndrome is strongly associated with the development of obesity and insulin resistance and places a woman at significant risk for development of GDM and type 2 DM later in life.[1]

Genetic factors have a strong role in the development of type 1 DM (see Genetics box). For example, rates of type 1 DM are particularly high in Scandinavia. Genetic alterations may play a role in the development of type 2 DM and related conditions, such as obesity and the cardiometabolic risk syndrome. The incidence of type 2 DM in the United States is higher among Hispanics or Latinos, African Americans, Native Americans, Alaska Natives, Asian Americans, and Pacific Islanders.[1]

Hyperglycemic Crises

Pathogenesis. Diabetic ketoacidosis (DKA) and hyperosmolar hyperglycemic state (HHS) are endocrine emergencies. The underlying mechanism for both DKA and HHS is a reduction in the net effective action of circulating insulin coupled with a concomitant elevation of counterregulatory hormones (Fig. 19.3). Together, this hormonal mix leads to increased hepatic and renal glucose production and decreased use of glucose in the peripheral tissues.

Historically, DKA was described as the crisis state in type 1 DM, whereas HHS was thought to occur in type 2 DM. Now, DKA and HHS are increasingly being seen concurrently in the same patient.8

Etiology of diabetic ketoacidosis. Numerous factors precipitate DKA (Box 19.3). In many patients, DKA is the initial indication of previously undiagnosed type 1 DM. In the critically ill, the presence of coexisting autoimmune disorders of the

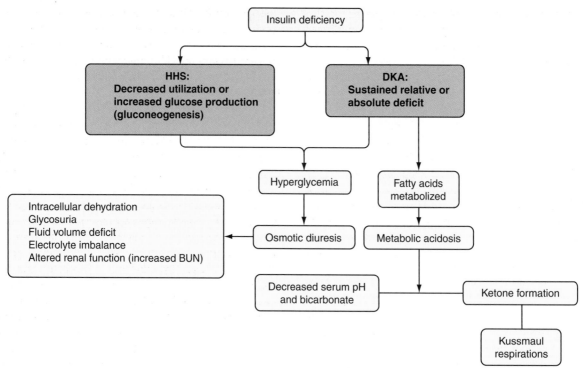

Fig. 19.3 Pathophysiology of diabetic ketoacidosis (DKA) and hyperosmolar hyperglycemic state (HHS). *BUN,* Blood urea nitrogen.

BOX 19.3 **Factors Leading to Diabetic Ketoacidosis and Hyperosmolar Hyperglycemic State**

Common Factors
- *Infections:* pneumonia, urinary tract infection, sepsis, or abscess
- Omission of diabetic therapy or inadequate treatment
- New-onset diabetes mellitus
- *Preexisting illness:* cardiac, renal diseases
- *Major or acute illness:* MI, CVA, pancreatitis, trauma, surgery, renal disease
- *Other endocrine disorders:* hyperthyroidism, Cushing disease, pheochromocytoma
- Stress
- High-calorie parenteral or enteral nutrition

Medications
- Steroids (especially glucocorticoids)
- Beta-blockers
- Thiazide diuretics
- Calcium channel blockers
- Phenytoin
- Epinephrine
- Psychotropic agents, including tricyclic antidepressants
- Sympathomimetics
- Analgesics

- Cimetidine
- Calcium channel blockers
- Immunosuppressants
- Diazoxide
- Chemotherapeutic agents
- SGLT2 inhibitors
- "Social drugs" such as cocaine, ecstasy

DKA-Specific Factors
- Malfunction of insulin pump
- Insulin pump infusion set site problems (infection, disconnection, catheter kinking or migration)
- Increased insulin needs secondary to insulin-resistant states (pregnancy, puberty, before menstruation)

HHS-Specific Factors
- Decreased thirst mechanism
- Difficulty accessing fluids (e.g., nursing home resident)

CVA, Cerebrovascular accident; *DKA,* diabetic ketoacidosis; *HHS,* hyperosmolar hyperglycemic state; *MI,* myocardial infarction; *SGLT2,* sodium-glucose transport protein 2.

---

thyroid and adrenal glands must be considered, especially in unstable patients with type 1 DM.[18] In addition, the multiple endocrine changes that accompany pregnancy alter insulin needs, which escalate rapidly in the second and third trimesters.[18] Pregnant women with type 1 DM are at increased risk for DKA.[18] Signs and symptoms of DKA characteristically

develop over a short period, and patients seek medical help early because of the associated symptoms.

The incidence of recurrent DKA is higher in females and peaks in the early teenage years. The risk of recurrent DKA is also higher in patients with DM diagnosed at an early age and in those of lower socioeconomic status. The causes of recurrent

DKA are unclear but include physiological, psychosomatic, and psychosocial factors. Psychological problems complicated by eating disorders in younger patients with type 1 DM may contribute to 20% of recurrent DKA.[13]

Etiology of hyperosmolar hyperglycemic state. HHS is usually precipitated by inadequate insulin secretion or impaired action associated with rising glucose levels. It is more commonly seen in patients who have type 2 DM or no prior history of DM.[13] Most patients who develop this condition are older adults with decreased compensatory mechanisms to maintain homeostasis in hyperosmolar states. A major illness that mediates overproduction of glucose secondary to the stress response may contribute to the development of HHS. High-calorie parenteral and enteral feedings that exceed the patient's ability to metabolize glucose can induce HHS. Several medications are associated with the development of the disorder. The major etiological factors of HHS are included in Box 19.3.

Pathophysiology of Diabetic Ketoacidosis.

Fig. 19.4 details the intracellular and extracellular shifts that occur in DKA and HHS. In both disorders, high extracellular glucose levels produce an osmotic gradient between the intracellular and extracellular spaces, causing fluid to translocate out of the cells.[13] This process is called *osmotic diuresis.* When serum glucose levels exceed the renal threshold (approximately 200 mg/dL), glucose is lost through the kidneys *(glycosuria).* As glycosuria and osmotic diuresis progress, urinary losses of water, sodium, potassium, magnesium, calcium, and phosphorus occur. This cycle of osmotic diuresis causes increases in serum osmolality, further compensatory fluid shifts from the intracellular to the intravascular space, and worsening dehydration.

Typically, body water losses in DKA total 6 L.[11] The evolving hyperosmolarity further impairs insulin secretion and promotes a state of insulin resistance known as *glucose toxicity.*[18]

The glomerular filtration rate in the kidney decreases in response to the severe fluid volume deficits. Decreased glucose excretion (causing increased serum glucose levels) and hemoconcentration result. The altered neurological status frequently seen in these patients is partially the result of cellular dehydration and the hyperosmolar state.

The absolute or relative insulin deficiency that precipitates DKA causes derangement of carbohydrate, protein, and fat metabolism.[12] Protein stores are depleted through the process of gluconeogenesis in the liver. Amino acids are metabolized into glucose and nitrogen to provide energy. Without insulin, the liberated glucose cannot be used, further increasing serum blood glucose and urine glucose concentrations and worsening osmotic diuresis. As nitrogen accumulates in the peripheral tissues, blood urea nitrogen (BUN) rises. Breakdown of protein stores stimulates the shift of intracellular potassium into the extracellular serum (hyperkalemia). This additional circulating potassium may also be lost as a result of osmotic diuresis (hypokalemia). Serum electrolytes, particularly potassium, may be falsely elevated in relation to the actual intracellular level. Total body potassium deficits are common and must be considered in the overall management of DKA. Because of the fluid volume and potassium shifts, serum potassium values must be interpreted with caution in patients with DKA.[18]

The starvation state that accompanies DKA results in the breakdown of fat cells into free fatty acids.[13] The free fatty acids are released into the blood and are transported to the liver, where they are oxidized into ketone bodies (β-hydroxybutyrate) and acetoacetate. This leads to an increase in circulating ketone concentrations and further increases gluconeogenesis by the liver. Ketonuria and the accompanying rising glucose level further contribute to osmotic diuresis. The ketoacids are transported to peripheral tissues, where they are oxidized to acetone. Inadequate buffering of the excess ketone acids by circulating

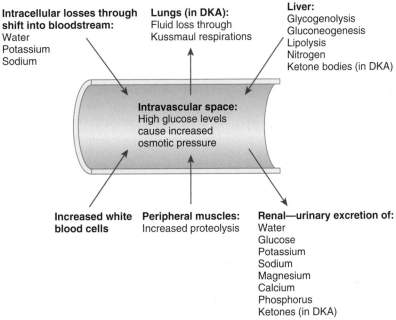

Fig. 19.4 Intracellular and extracellular shifts in hyperglycemic crises. *DKA,* Diabetic ketoacidosis.

bicarbonate results in metabolic acidosis as the ratio of carbonic acid to bicarbonate ions increases. As ketone and hydrogen ions accumulate and acidosis worsens, the respiratory system attempts to compensate for excess carbonic acid by "blowing off" carbon dioxide (CO_2), a weak acid. Kussmaul respirations, characterized by an increased rate and depth of breathing, and an acetone ("fruity") breath odor are classic clinical signs of DKA associated with this compensatory process.

In addition to ketonemia, patients with DKA may have an accumulation of lactic acid (lactic acidosis). The resulting dehydration may cause decreased perfusion to core organs, with consequent hypoxemia and worsening of the lactic acidosis. Excess lactic acid results in an increased *anion gap* (increased body acids). Sodium, potassium, chloride, and bicarbonate are responsible for maintaining a normal anion gap (<16 mEq/L). Ketone accumulation causes an increase in the anion gap greater than 16 mEq/L. To calculate the anion gap, see Box 19.4.

Many enzymatic reactions within the body function only within a limited range of pH. As the patient becomes more acidotic and enzymes become less effective, body metabolism slows. This situation promotes further ketone formation, and acidosis worsens. The stress response associated with the progressing ketoacidosis state also contributes to metabolic alterations because the liver is stimulated by hormones (glucagon, catecholamines, cortisol, and growth hormones) to metabolize protein stores. The net result is an additional increase in serum glucose, nitrogen levels, and plasma osmolality. Some of these hormones also decrease the ability of cells to use glucose for production of adenosine triphosphate (ATP) and therefore compound the problem. The alterations in central nervous system function in DKA are thought to be influenced by the combination of acidosis and severe dehydration.

In summary, cells without glucose starve and begin to use existing stores of fat and protein to provide energy for body processes (gluconeogenesis). Fats are metabolized faster than they can be stored, resulting in an accumulation of ketone acids, a byproduct of fat metabolism in the liver. Ketone acids accumulate in the bloodstream, where hydrogen ions dissociate from the ketones, resulting in a metabolic acidosis. The more acidotic the patient becomes, the less able the body is to metabolize these ketones.

Pathophysiology of Hyperosmotic Hyperglycemic State. The pathophysiology of HHS is similar to that of DKA. However, in HHS, there are significantly lower levels of free fatty acids,

resulting in a lack of ketosis but even higher levels of hyperglycemia, hyperosmolality, and severe dehydration (see Fig. 19.3). [7]

Hyperglycemia results from decreased use of glucose, increased production of glucose, or both. The hyperglycemic state causes an osmotic movement of water out of the cells, resulting in expansion of the extracellular fluid volume and intracellular dehydration. The osmotic diuresis and resultant intracellular and extracellular dehydration in HHS are typically more severe than those found in DKA because HHS usually develops insidiously over a period of weeks to months. Alterations in neurological status are common because of cellular dehydration. The typical total body water deficit is greater in HHS, approximately 9 L.[7,13] By the time these patients seek medical attention, they are profoundly dehydrated and hyperosmolar.[7] Most commonly, patients who develop HHS are older. They are also more likely to have other medical problems, such as renal insufficiency, heart failure, myocardial ischemia, and chronic lung disease, that may limit the ability of providers to aggressively treat the condition, particularly regarding fluid resuscitation.[4] The mortality rate of HHS is higher than that of DKA in older adults.

Ketoacidosis is usually not seen in patients with HHS because insulin levels in these patients are usually sufficient to prevent lipolysis and subsequent ketone formation.[7] The levels of glucose counterregulatory hormones that promote lipolysis are lower in patients with HHS than in those with DKA. However, persistence or worsening of the physiological stressor that precipitated the HHS episode may allow the hyperglycemia to progress to a state of extreme insulin deficiency. Lipolysis occurs as a consequence of the severe insulin deficit, and ketoacidosis becomes superimposed on the HHS.

Assessment

Clinical presentation. The presenting symptoms of DKA and HHS are similar (Table 19.3). Signs of DKA and HHS are due to the degree of dehydration and electrolyte imbalances. The osmotic diuresis occurring from hyperglycemia results in signs of increased thirst (polydipsia), increased urine output (polyuria), and dehydration. Increased hunger (polyphagia) may be an early sign. Signs of intravascular dehydration are common as the physiological processes continue.[7]

Hyperglycemia and ketosis both contribute to delayed gastric emptying. Vomiting can occur and further worsens total body dehydration. Patients also report symptoms of weakness and anorexia. Abdominal pain and tenderness are common presenting symptoms, particularly in DKA, and are associated with dehydration and underlying pathophysiology, such as pyelonephritis, duodenal ulcer, appendicitis, and metabolic acidosis. Pain associated with DKA usually disappears with treatment of the dehydration. Significant weight loss occurs because of the fluid losses and an inability to metabolize glucose.

Altered states of consciousness range from restlessness, confusion, and agitation to somnolence and coma. Visual disturbances, especially blurred vision, are common in hyperglycemia. Generally, altered levels of consciousness are more pronounced in patients with HHS. This is due to the severity of hyperglycemia, serum hyperosmolality, and

---

BOX 19.4	**Calculation of the Anion Gap**

The anion gap is calculated as the difference between the measured concentrations of sodium (Na^+) and potassium (K^+), the major anions, and those of chloride (Cl^-) and bicarbonate (HCO_3^-), the major cations:

$$\left(Na^+ + K^+\right) - \left(Cl^- + HCO_3^-\right)$$

The normal serum anion gap is 8 to 16 mEq/L. An elevated value indicates the accumulation of acids, such as is present in diabetic ketoacidosis.

TABLE 19.3 Manifestations of Diabetic Ketoacidosis and Hyperosmolar Hyperglycemic State

	Diabetic Ketoacidosis	Hyperosmolar Hyperglycemic State
Pathophysiology	Relative or absolute insulin deficiency resulting in cellular dehydration and volume depletion, acidosis, and protein catabolism	Insulin deficiency resulting in dehydration and hyperosmolality
Health history	History of type 1 diabetes mellitus (DM) or use of insulin Signs and symptoms of hyperglycemia before admission Can also occur in type 2 DM in severe stress	History of type 2 DM signs and symptoms of hyperglycemia before admission Occurs most frequently in older adult with preexisting renal and cardiovascular disease
Onset	Develops quickly	Develops insidiously
Clinical presentation	Flushed, dry skin Dry mucous membranes ↓ Skin turgor Tachycardia Hypotension Kussmaul respirations Acetone breath Altered level of consciousness Visual disturbances Polydipsia Nausea and vomiting Anorexia Abdominal pain	Flushed, dry skin Dry mucous membranes ↓ Skin turgor (may not be present in older adult) Tachycardia Hypotension Shallow respirations Altered level of consciousness (generally more profound and may include absent deep tendon reflexes, paresis, and positive Babinski sign)
Diagnostics	↑ Plasma glucose (average: 675 mg/dL) pH <7.30 ↓ Bicarbonate Ketosis Azotemia Electrolytes vary with state of hydration; often hyperkalemic Plasma hyperosmolality (average: 330 mOsm/kg)	↑ Plasma glucose (usually >1000 mg/dL) pH >7.30 Bicarbonate >15 mEq/L Absence of significant ketosis Azotemia Electrolytes vary with state of hydration; often hypernatremic Plasma hyperosmolality (average: 350 mOsm/kg) Hypotonic urine

electrolyte disturbances. Seizures and focal neurological signs may also be present and often lead to misdiagnosis in patients with HHS.

In DKA, ketonuria and metabolic acidosis are seen. Nausea is an early sign of DKA and is thought to be a result of retained ketones. Kussmaul respirations and an acetone breath odor are additional clinical signs of ketosis. Later in the disease process, the respiratory status of the patient may be influenced by the neurological status, precipitating impaired breathing patterns and reduced gas exchange. A decreased level of consciousness is also associated with the severe acidotic state (pH <7.15). The flushed face associated with DKA is the result of superficial vasodilation. See Lifespan Considerations box for additional information related to older adults and pregnant women.

Laboratory evaluation. Numerous diagnostic studies are used to evaluate for the presence of DKA and HHS, to rule out other diseases, and to detect complications (see Laboratory Alert box). In addition, cultures and tests are performed to determine any precipitating factors such as infection or myocardial infarction.

In DKA, an initial arterial blood gas analysis reflects metabolic acidosis (low pH and low bicarbonate level). The bicarbonate is initially low as circulating bicarbonate buffers the excess circulating hydrogen ions. The arterial partial pressure of carbon dioxide ($PaCO_2$) may be low, reflecting the respiratory system's compensatory mechanism. Acidosis is subsequently monitored by venous pH, which correlates well with arterial pH but is easier to obtain and process. The severity of DKA is determined by the pH, bicarbonate level, ketone values, and the patient's mental status.[13] Severe acidosis is associated with cardiovascular collapse, which can result in death.

In HHS, the laboratory results are similar to those in DKA but with four major differences: (1) the serum glucose concentration in HHS is usually significantly more elevated than in DKA and may exceed 1000 mg/dL; (2) plasma osmolality is higher in HHS than in DKA and is associated with the degree of dehydration; (3) acidosis is not present or is very mild in HHS compared with DKA; and (4) ketosis is usually absent or very mild in HHS compared with DKA because of the availability of basal insulin.[13] Serum electrolyte concentrations may be low, normal, or elevated and are not reliable indicators of total body stores of electrolytes or water.

Nursing and Medical Interventions. Primary interventions in the treatment of DKA and HHS include respiratory support, fluid replacement, administration of insulin to correct hyperglycemia, replacement of electrolytes, correction of acidosis in DKA, prevention of complications, and patient teaching and support (see Evidence-Based Practice box).

LIFESPAN CONSIDERATIONS

Diabetes

Older Adults

- With aging, pancreatic endocrine function declines. Fasting glucose levels trend upward with age, and glucose tolerance decreases.[19] These changes are caused by a combination of decreased insulin production and increased insulin resistance, independent of any other coexisting disease states.
- Fifty percent of adults age 65 years and older have elevated blood glucose levels and are at increased risk for diabetes (prediabetes).[4]
- More than 25% of adults older than 65 years of age have diabetes, primarily type 2 diabetes.[8]
- Older adults are more prone to develop hyperosmolar hyperglycemic state.
- Older adults have a decreased sense of thirst; therefore this sign may not be observed during hyperglycemic crises.
- The risk for lack of awareness of hypoglycemia is higher in older adults.
- Older adults with diabetes are more likely to have comorbid conditions, such as cardiac or renal disease, and to take medications that make them more reactive to electrolyte imbalances.[4,9]
- Older adults are more likely to be affected with geriatric syndromes such as cognitive dysfunction, polypharmacy, depression, and pain.[7]
- Older adults with diabetes often respond more slowly to treatments.

Pregnant Women

- Gestational diabetes mellitus (GDM) may develop during pregnancy, and it typically resolves after delivery. Unless women have an increased risk, screen for GDM between the 24th and 28th weeks of pregnancy.[3] Women who develop GDM have significant risk for type 2 diabetes later in life.
- Screen pregnant women with risk factors for type 2 diabetes (e.g., polycystic ovarian syndrome, significant obesity) at the first prenatal appointment.
- GDM is managed with blood glucose monitoring, medical nutrition therapy, and exercise. Oral agents (e.g., metformin, glyburide) and insulin therapy are added to the GDM treatment regimen if initial glucose-lowering interventions fail.[3] The risks for the neonate include macrosomia, birth trauma, neonatal hypoglycemia, and hyperbilirubinemia.[3]
- Women with pregestational type 1 or type 2 diabetes require intensive monitoring before, during, and after a pregnancy. Blood levels of glycated hemoglobin (A1c) greater than 7% at the time of conception increase the risk for early pregnancy loss and major fetal malformations, including anencephaly and congenital heart defects.[3]
- Women with a history of pregestational diabetes should seek preconception counseling, which includes interventions to optimize blood glucose, evaluate and treat chronic diabetes-related complications such as nephropathy and retinopathy, and assess for the risk of non–diabetes-related fetal and maternal risks.[18]
- Uncontrolled diabetes during pregnancy increases the risk for preeclampsia, intrauterine fetal demise, neonatal hyperbilirubinemia, and neonatal hypoglycemia.[18]
- All neonates of women who experienced diabetes during the pregnancy require intensive assessment for hypoglycemia after delivery.
- Blood glucose targets of less than 95 mg/dL fasting, less than 140 mg/dL 1 hour after meals, and less than 120 mg/dL 2 hours after meals are desired in pregnant women with diabetes.[3]
- Because many antihyperglycemic agents are contraindicated in pregnancy, prepregnancy diabetes medication regimens may require adjustment to limit fetal risks and achieve target glycemic levels. Intensive insulin therapy is indicated for management in most women with pregestational diabetes.
- The first trimester in women with pregestational type 1 diabetes is characterized by an increased risk of maternal hypoglycemia.[18]
- The influence of increasing levels of counterregulatory hormones such as growth hormone, cortisol, and glucagon causes women to become more insulin resistant during the second and third trimesters of pregnancy.[18] Insulin demands may double in the later stages of pregnancy, necessitating frequent insulin dose adjustments. These increasing insulin demands increase the risk for development of diabetic ketoacidosis (DKA).
- Women with pregestational diabetes are often given insulin infusions during labor and immediately after delivery. Women with type 1 diabetes are at an exceptionally high risk for hypoglycemia in the days and weeks after delivery because of the rapid reductions in circulating counterregulatory hormones.[18]

Respiratory support. Assessment of the airway, breathing, and circulation is always the first priority in managing life-threatening disorders. Support airway and breathing as needed through the use of oral airways and oxygen therapy. In more severe cases, the patient may be intubated and placed on ventilatory support. Prevent aspiration by elevating the head of the bed. Collaborate with the provider to determine the need for nasogastric tube suction in a patient with impaired mentation who is actively vomiting.

Fluid replacement. Dehydration may progress to hypovolemic shock by the time of admission. Immediate IV access and rehydration must be initiated. In DKA, the typical water deficit approximates 100 mL/kg, and it may be as high as 200 mL/kg in HHS.[13] Monitor for signs and symptoms of hypovolemic shock, and assess vital signs and neurological status at least every hour initially. Changes in mentation may indicate a change in fluid status. In unstable patients, monitor and record hemodynamic parameters at least every 15 minutes. Hemodynamic monitoring may be instituted to evaluate fluid requirements and to monitor the patient's response to treatment. This is particularly true for patients with HHS, who tend to be older and to have concurrent cardiovascular and renal disease. Measure intake and output hourly, and record weight daily.

Normal saline (0.9% NS) is the fluid of choice for initial fluid replacement because it best replaces extracellular fluid volume deficits. Fluid replacement usually starts with an initial bolus of 1 L of 0.9% NS. This is followed by an infusion of 10 to 15 mL/kg during the first hour if the patient is not in shock.[13,18] A rate of 20 mL/kg/h may be required if the patient shows clinical signs of shock. If the patient shows signs of hemodynamic stability, the IV infusion may be decreased to 7.5 mg/kg/h.[18] Evaluate the effectiveness of fluid replacement by assessing hemodynamic status, intake and output, laboratory measures, and the patient's general physical condition, particularly mental status. If the serum sodium level is elevated or normal, the IV fluid is changed to hypotonic saline (0.45% NS)

! LABORATORY ALERT

Pancreatic Endocrine Disorders

Serum Laboratory Test	Critical Value[a]	Significance
Glucose	≥200 mg/dL (2 h postprandial or random)	Combined with symptoms, establishes diagnosis of diabetes mellitus
	≥126 mg/dL (fasting)	
	>450 mg/dL	Suggestive of DKA; significantly higher in HHS
	<50 mg/dL	Hypoglycemia
Potassium	>6.1 mEq/L	Potential for heart blocks, bradydysrhythmias, sinus arrest, ventricular fibrillation, or asystole
	<3.0 mEq/L	Potential for ventricular dysrhythmias; muscle weakness including respiratory arrest; will further decrease with insulin administration
Sodium	>160 mEq/L	May be a result of stress and profound dehydration
	<120 mEq/L	Usually associated with disorders other than diabetes
BUN	>100 mg/dL	Values >20 mg/dL may be observed due to protein breakdown and hemoconcentration
Bicarbonate	<10 mEq/L	Decreased in DKA due to immediate compensation for acidosis
pH	<7.25	Decreased in DKA due to accumulation of nonvolatile acids
Osmolality	>320 mOsm/kg H_2O	Elevated in DKA relative to dehydration; higher in HHS
Phosphorus	<1.0 mg/dL	May result in impaired respiratory and cardiac functions; values <2.5 mg/dL are often observed and will further decrease with insulin administration
Magnesium	<0.5 mEq/L	Depleted by osmotic diuresis; may coincide with decreased potassium and calcium levels; may result in dysrhythmias
β-Hydroxybutyrate	>3.0 mg/dL	Reflects blood ketosis in DKA

[a]Critical values vary by facility and laboratory.
BUN, Blood urea nitrogen; *DKA*, diabetic ketoacidosis; *HHS*, hyperosmolar hyperglycemic state.

and is infused at a slower rate to replace intracellular fluid deficits. When the plasma glucose level approaches 200 mg/dL,[18] 5% dextrose is added to fluids to prevent hypoglycemia and assist in the resolution of ketosis.[13] The goal is to replace half of the estimated fluid deficit over the first 8 hours. The second half of the fluid deficit should be replaced during the next 16 hours of therapy so that the volume is restored in most patients within the first 24 hours of treatment.[13] Significant improvements in hyperglycemia may be seen with fluid resuscitation before initiation of insulin therapy. Hyperglycemia resolves more quickly than ketosis. IV fluids and insulin are continued until the acidosis is corrected.[18]

The goal of fluid resuscitation is normovolemia. Prevent hypervolemia, especially in patients with ischemic heart disease, heart failure, acute kidney injury, or chronic kidney disease. Prevent fluid overload from overaggressive fluid replacement by monitoring breath sounds and performing cardiovascular assessments. If available, use values from hemodynamic monitoring to guide fluid resuscitation. Signs and symptoms of fluid overload are reviewed in Box 19.5. Rapid fluid administration may also contribute to cerebral edema, a complication associated with DKA. A rapid decrease in the plasma glucose level, combined with rapid fluid administration and concurrent insulin therapy (see next section), may lead to movement of water into brain cells, resulting in brain edema, which can be fatal. Assessment of neurological status during the initial phases of fluid replacement and glucose lowering is imperative.

BOX 19.5 Signs and Symptoms of Fluid Overload

- Tachypnea
- Neck vein distension
- Tachycardia
- Crackles
- Increased pulmonary artery occlusion or right atrial pressures
- Declining level of consciousness in cerebral edema

Insulin therapy. Replacement of insulin is definitive therapy for DKA and HHS. Before starting insulin therapy, fluid replacement therapy must be underway and the serum potassium level must be greater than 3.3 mEq/L.[13] The goal is to restore normal glucose uptake by cells while preventing complications of excess insulin administration, such as hypoglycemia, hypokalemia, and hypophosphatemia. Hyperglycemic crises are commonly treated with IV insulin infusions because absorption is more predictable. An initial IV bolus of 0.1 unit/kg of regular insulin is administered, followed by a continuous infusion of 0.1 unit/kg/h. A steady decrease in serum glucose levels of 50 to 75 mg/dL/h is desired after an initial glucose drop due to rehydration.[18] Maintain the initial insulin infusion rate until the pH exceeds 7.3 and bicarbonate concentration is greater than 15 mEq/L, at which time the insulin infusion may be decreased to 0.05 unit/kg/h with a target glucose value of 100 to 150 mg/dL until acidosis is completely resolved.[18]

EVIDENCE-BASED PRACTICE

Tight Glycemic Control

Problem

Tight glycemic control in critically ill patients has been debated. Issues and outcomes of achieving glycemic control need to be identified.

Clinical Question

What are the outcomes and issues associated with tight glycemic control in critically ill patients?

Evidence

Yamada and colleagues used a systematic review and meta-analytic approach to evaluate the effect of tight glycemic control on mortality and hypoglycemic outcomes. They analyzed data from 36 randomized clinical trials and compared outcomes of various levels of glycemic control: tight (80 to <110 mg/dL), moderate (110 to <140 mg/dL), mild (140 to <180 mg/dL), and very mild (180 to 220 mg/dL). They found no reduction in mortality with tight glycemic control in critically ill patients. Severe hypoglycemia with tight control in comparison with mild or very mild control was noted.

Conclusion

Because tight glycemic control is associated with a greater risk of severe hypoglycemia, a target range of 140 to 180 mg/dL is recommended. Many IV insulin protocols used in critical care units and basal-nutrition-correction insulin protocols used in medical-surgical units have adopted these glycemic targets.

Implications for Nursing

Evolving evidence on inpatient glycemic management has resulted in a preference for basal prandial insulin protocols over traditional sliding-scale regimens. These protocols improve glycemic control and reduce treatment-related complications such as hypoglycemia. Because evidence on inpatient glycemic control is rapidly evolving and has application to many care settings, nurses must stay apprised of new research and application of these findings to practice.

Level of Evidence

A—Systematic review and meta-analysis

Reference

Yamada T, Shojima N, Noma H, et al. Glycemic control, mortality, and hypoglycemia in critically ill patients: A systematic review and network meta-analysis of randomized controlled trials. *Intensive Care Med.* 2017;43(1):1–15.

Correction of acidosis typically requires more time than normalization of blood glucose.[18] Initial insulin infusion rates of less than 0.1 unit/kg/h are typically insufficient to inhibit ketosis. Patients with mild to moderate DKA may be treated with hourly subcutaneous injections of rapid-acting insulin using a titration scale.

During the insulin infusion, monitor serum glucose levels hourly using a consistent monitoring method. While receiving an IV insulin infusion, patients are typically allowed nothing by mouth. Patients may be transitioned to subcutaneous insulin when the blood glucose is 200 mg/dL or less and at least two of the following criteria are met: (1) venous pH is greater than 7.30, (2) serum bicarbonate level is greater than 15 mEq/L, and (3) calculated anion gap is 12 mEq/L or less.[13,18] Subcutaneous insulin therapy using a basal-bolus regimen that also includes an algorithm for correction doses of rapid-acting insulin may be ordered for patients who are not receiving enteral or total parenteral nutritional support. Monitor glucose levels at least every 6 to 8 hours while the patient is receiving subcutaneous insulin. Subcutaneous insulin therapy should be initiated 1 to 2 hours before the IV insulin infusion is discontinued.[18]

In patients with HHS, insulin infusion rates may be decreased to 0.2 to 0.5 unit/kg/h when the glucose values reach 300 mg/dL.[13] Target glucose values of 200 to 300 mg/dL should be maintained until the patient's mental status improves, at which time the patient may be transitioned to subcutaneous insulin therapy.

It is important that serum glucose levels not be lowered too rapidly, not more than 35 to 90 mg/dL/h, to prevent cerebral edema, which could result in seizures and coma. Any patient who exhibits an abrupt change in level of consciousness after initiation of insulin therapy requires frequent blood glucose monitoring and institution of protective steps to prevent harm (e.g., seizure precautions). Treatment of acute cerebral edema usually involves administration of an osmotic diuretic (e.g., 20% mannitol solution).

Electrolyte management. Potassium, phosphate, chloride, and magnesium replacement may be required, especially during insulin administration. Osmotic diuresis in DKA and HHS results in total body potassium depletion ranging from 400 to 600 mEq. The potassium deficit may be greater in HHS. Insulin therapy promotes translocation of potassium into the intracellular space, resulting in a further decrease in serum potassium levels.

The need for potassium therapy is based on serum laboratory results. In the absence of renal disease, insulin replacement and monitoring begin after (1) the first liter of IV fluid has been administered, (2) the serum potassium level is greater than 3.3 mEq/L, and (3) the patient is producing urine. At that point, 20 to 30 mEq of potassium may be added to each liter of fluid administered and augmented by additional doses of intermittent potassium infusions.[13,18] Maintain serum potassium levels between 4 and 5 mEq/L during the course of therapy. In the event that a patient is admitted with hypokalemia, insulin therapy should be withheld until potassium values exceed 3.3 mEq/L.[13] Maintain the integrity of the IV site to prevent extravasation. Monitor cardiac rhythm and respiratory status during potassium administration.

Total body phosphorus levels are also depleted by osmotic diuresis, but serum phosphate levels may remain in the normal range. Insulin therapy may cause further reductions in phosphate levels. Phosphate replacement is used when there is associated respiratory or cardiac dysfunction. Potassium phosphate may be ordered to treat part of the potassium deficit in a concentration of 20 to 30 mEq/L.[13] Phosphate replacement is used with extreme caution in patients with renal failure because these patients are unable to excrete phosphate and typically have underlying hyperphosphatemia.

Treatment of acidosis. Acidosis is a hallmark feature of DKA. However, many studies have shown that treatment with sodium bicarbonate is often not beneficial and may pose increased risks of hypoglycemia, cerebral edema, cellular hypoxemia secondary to decreased uptake of oxygen by body tissues, worsening hypokalemia, and development of central nervous system acidosis.[13] Therefore sodium bicarbonate is not routinely used to treat acidosis unless the serum pH is less than 7.0. Bicarbonate replacement is used only to bring the pH up to 7.1, but not to normal levels.[4] For administration, 100 mEq/L of bicarbonate may be added to 400 mL of sterile water with 20 mEq of potassium chloride and infused at a rate of 200 mL/h until the venous pH exceeds 7.0.[13] Serum blood gas analysis is done frequently to assess for changes in pH, bicarbonate, anion gap, $PaCO_2$, and oxygenation status. Repeat infusions of the bicarbonate solution may be required every 2 hours until the pH exceeds 7.0. Once fluid and electrolyte imbalances are corrected and insulin is administered, the kidneys begin to conserve bicarbonate to restore acid-base homeostasis, and ketone formation ceases.

Patient and family education. A primary intervention to prevent DKA is patient education. Incorporate essential content into patient education: (1) manage blood glucose levels with diet, exercise, and medication; (2) monitor hemoglobin A1c levels three or four times per year to assess long-term control of blood glucose levels, changing insulin needs, and psychosocial or behavioral factors that may affect control[1]; (3) maintain a regular schedule for eating, exercise, rest, sleep, and relaxation; (4) adjust the usual diabetic control regimen for illness is known as "sick day management;" and (5) identify strategies to prevent complications. If the patient has an episode of DKA while on insulin pump therapy, reeducate the patient about pump features, insulin pump safety, management of pump failure, and troubleshooting abnormal glucose levels. Instruct patients to avoid exercise and excessive activities when blood glucose levels exceed 240 mg/dL and urine ketones are present.

Patient Outcomes. Outcomes for a patient with DKA or HHS are included with specific aspects due to hyperglycemia management in the Plan of Care for the Patient With Hyperglycemic Crisis (see also the Collaborative Plan of Care for the Critically Ill Patient in Chapter 1).

❓ CRITICAL REASONING ACTIVITY

Insulin therapy is a critical intervention in the treatment of diabetic ketoacidosis (DKA) and hyperosmolar hyperglycemic state (HHS). What crucial parameters must be monitored to ensure optimal patient outcomes?

◎ PLAN OF CARE

For the Patient with Hyperglycemic Crisis

Patient Problem
Dehydration. Risk factors include osmotic diuresis, ketosis, increased lipolysis, and vomiting.

Desired Outcomes
- Normal serum glucose levels.
- Hemodynamic stability: normal sinus rhythm, blood pressure, heart rate, right atrial pressure, and pulmonary artery occlusion pressure within normal limits.
- Urine output greater than 0.5 mL/kg/h.
- Balanced intake and output.
- Stable weight.
- Warm, dry extremities.
- Normal skin turgor.
- Moist mucous membranes.
- Serum osmolality and serum electrolyte levels (sodium, potassium, calcium, phosphorus) within normal limits.
- pH within normal limits.

Nursing Assessments/Interventions	Rationales
• Assess fluid status: 　Vital signs every hour until stable 　I&O measurements every 1-2 h 　Skin turgor, mucous membranes, thirst 　Consider insensible fluid losses 　Daily weight	• Provides clinical indications of hypovolemia and provides data for restoring cellular function.
• Initiate fluid replacement therapy: 　Monitor for signs and symptoms of fluid overload. 　Monitor effects of volume repletion.	• Corrects volume deficit and prevents or treats hypovolemic shock; neurological status should improve as electrolytes normalize.
• Monitor neurological status closely.	• Mental status changes may indicate cerebral edema if glycemic correction is too rapid.
• Administer IV insulin infusion per hospital protocol; titrate therapy hourly based on glucose levels. Provide a steady decrease in serum glucose levels; a decrease of 35-90 mg/dL/h is desired.	• Prevent cerebral edema and potentially dangerous electrolyte abnormalities.

Continued

⊚ **PLAN OF CARE—cont'd**

For the Patient with Hyperglycemic Crisis

Nursing Assessments/Interventions	**Rationales**
• Monitor glucose every hour via consistent method (serum or fingerstick capillary) during insulin infusion.	• Assess response to therapy and allow for immediate correction of glycemic abnormalities.
• Monitor for signs and symptoms of hypoglycemia.	• Hypoglycemia may occur if insulin dose exceeds patient's needs.
• Add dextrose to maintenance IV solutions once serum glucose level reaches 250 mg/dL in DKA or 300 mg/dL in HHS.	• Prevent relative hypoglycemia and a decrease in plasma osmolality that could result in cerebral edema.
• Monitor serum electrolyte levels (sodium, potassium, calcium, phosphorus), administer supplements according to protocols.	• Prevent complications of electrolyte imbalance; osmotic diuresis may result in increased excretion of potassium and hyponatremia.
• Assess causes of continuing electrolyte depletion (i.e., diuresis, vomiting, NG suction).	• Insulin therapy causes potassium and phosphate to shift to the intracellular space.
• Monitor pH.	• pH is the best indicator of acidosis and response to treatment.
	• Acidosis corrects more slowly than hyperglycemia.
	• Correction of hyperglycemia without correction of ketosis may result in recurrence of DKA.
• Administer bicarbonate only in severe acidosis (pH <7.0).	• Routine administration of bicarbonate has been associated with hypokalemia, hypoglycemia, cellular ischemia, cerebral edema, and CNS cellular acidosis.

Patient Problem

Need for Health Teaching (Patient and Family). Risk factors include the complexity of the disease process and treatment plan, as well as the health literacy of the learner.

Desired Outcomes

• Patient/family can describe the pathophysiology and causes of DKA and/or HHS; preventive interventions due to diet, exercise regimen, and medications; signs and symptoms of hypoglycemia and hyperglycemia; signs and symptoms of infections that require medical follow-up; sick day management; and emergency hypoglycemia management.

• Patient/family can identify the patient's individual glucose targets.

• Patient/family can demonstrate self-monitoring of blood glucose levels and administration of oral hypoglycemic medications and/or insulin therapy according to glucose values.

Nursing Assessments/Interventions	**Rationales**
• Assess patient/family's current diabetes self-management practices, ability to learn information, and psychomotor and sensory skills.	• Allow for individualization of patient's plan of care to match physical, psychosocial, and educational needs.
• Identify psychosocial factors that may preclude effective self-management.	• Address factors in patient education to promote self management.
• Implement a teaching program that includes information on pathophysiology and causes of DKA or HHS; diet and exercise restrictions; individualized target glucose values; signs and symptoms of hypoglycemia and hyperglycemia, including interventions; and signs and symptoms of infection and illness, including interventions.	• Prevention of acute diabetes complications primarily rests with the patient and/or family who are capable and able to follow the self-management plan and act early on significant physiological changes.
• Demonstrate methods for blood glucose monitoring.	• Regular glucose monitoring is essential for patient self-management.
• If the patient takes insulin, demonstrate administration. Review insulin pump use and abilities if used for treatment. For each skill, have the patient demonstrate abilities with repeat demonstration.	• Ensure that patient/family have the ability to perform the skills involved in at-home monitoring, insulin delivery, and problem solving due to abnormal glucose findings before discharge.
• Review administration of hypoglycemic medications and/or insulin, including dosage, frequency, action, duration, side effects, and situations in which medication may need to be adjusted.	• Patients/family require a thorough knowledge of insulin therapy to optimize treatment.
	• Failure to adjust hypoglycemic medications to match changing glycemic demands may result in acute hyperglycemia or hypoglycemia.
• Consult with clinical dietitian regarding disease-specific nutrition and diet needs.	• Assists in identifying the appropriate diet based on the patient's condition and caloric needs.
• Encourage patient to wear a form of identification for diabetes.	• Assists in prompt recognition and treatment of complications should they occur.
• Provide written materials for all content taught; provide means for the patient to get questions answered after discharge and schedule follow-up diabetes self-management education after discharge.	• Effective diabetes self-management education is a collaboration between the patient, family, and the multiprofessional team.
	• Improve glycemic control and self-management outcomes.

CNS, Central nervous system; *DKA,* diabetic ketoacidosis; *HHS,* hyperosmolar hyperglycemic state; *I&O,* intake and output; *NG,* nasogastric. Adapted from Swearingen PL, Wright JD. *All-in-One Nursing Care Planning Resource.* 5th ed. St. Louis, MO: Elsevier; 2019.

Hypoglycemia

Pathophysiology. A hypoglycemic episode is defined as a decrease in the plasma glucose level to less than 70 mg/dL; it is sometimes referred to as *insulin shock* or *insulin reaction*. Glucose production falls behind glucose use, resulting in decreased blood glucose levels. Because the brain is an obligate user of glucose, the first clinical sign of hypoglycemia is a change in mental status. A hypoglycemic event activates the sympathetic nervous system, causing a rise in counterregulatory hormones, including glucagon, epinephrine, cortisol, and growth hormone. Those at highest risk for hypoglycemia are patients taking insulin, children and pregnant women with type 1 DM, patients with autonomic diabetic neuropathy, and older adults with type 1 or type 2 DM.

Hypoglycemia unawareness, also known as hypoglycemia-associated autonomic failure, describes a diabetes-related condition in which a patient does not recognize the onset of hypoglycemic signs and symptoms.[3] In this complication, the impairment of the autonomic nervous systems results in a blunted response to critically low glucose levels (see Clinical Alert box). Patients with hypoglycemia unawareness may remain asymptomatic while experiencing extremely low blood glucose levels. Patients who have other forms of autonomic neuropathy, such as orthostasis, gastroparesis, erectile dysfunction, and cardiac autonomic neuropathy, are also at higher risk for this condition. Those at highest risk of hypoglycemia unawareness include older adults, because of their impeded stress responses, and patients with diminished mental function resulting from dementia, concurrent illness, or other factors. Patients taking beta-blockers are at risk for decreased awareness of signs of hypoglycemia because of the medication's effect on the sympathetic nervous system. The pathophysiological mechanisms associated with acute hypoglycemia and the associated central nervous system and sympathetic symptoms are reviewed in Fig. 19.5.

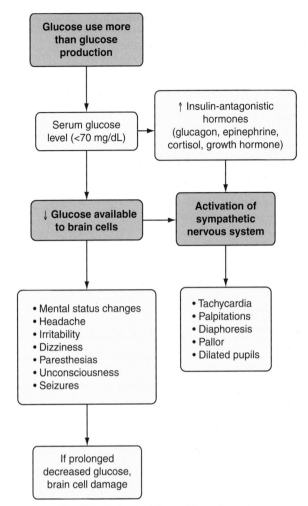

Fig. 19.5 Pathophysiology of hypoglycemia.

> **! CLINICAL ALERT**
>
> ### *Hypoglycemia Unawareness*
>
> Some patients have hypoglycemia unawareness and remain asymptomatic despite extremely low blood glucose levels. Older adult patients and those taking beta-blockers are at especially high risk.

Etiology. Closely monitor patients receiving insulin therapy for hypoglycemia in many situations. Insulin requirements may be lower because of weight loss, renal insufficiency, increase in insulin dose, new prescription or adjustment in nondiabetic medications that affect blood glucose, and rotation of insulin injection sites from a hypertrophied area to one with unimpaired absorption.

In addition, patients who use oral agents that promote production and release of endogenous insulin, such as long-acting sulfonylureas, are at risk for hypoglycemia. Amylin and agents that mimic or act on incretin hormones (exenatide and gliptins) also increase the risk for a hypoglycemic episode when they are combined with insulin or secretagogues. Other causes of hypoglycemia in the hospitalized patient include decreased caloric intake because of a missed or delayed meal or snack, nausea and vomiting, anorexia, or interrupted tube feedings or total parenteral nutrition. As a patient recovers from a stress event (e.g., infection illness, corticosteroid therapy, postpartum), the need for exogenous insulin decreases, and failure to adjust the insulin dose can precipitate hypoglycemia. Other major causes of hypoglycemia are reviewed in Box 19.6.

Both severe hypoglycemia and hypoglycemia unawareness place a patient at risk for injury secondary to a motor vehicle crash, falls, and seizures. Patients with renal impairment or liver dysfunction are at particular risk for a severe hypoglycemic episode. Delayed degradation or excretion of hypoglycemic medications potentiates or prolongs the action of many diabetes medications. The resulting increase in circulating levels of active drug, including insulin, results in erratic glucose control. Close glucose monitoring and patient and family education on prevention, recognition, and treatment of hypoglycemia is critical to promote safety in these very high-risk patients.

BOX 19.6 Causes of Hypoglycemia

Excess Insulin or Oral Hypoglycemics
- Dose of insulin or oral hypoglycemics too high
- Islet cell tumors (insulinomas)
- Liver insufficiency or failure (impaired metabolism of insulin)
- Acute kidney injury (impaired inactivation of insulin)
- Autoimmune phenomenon
- Medications that potentiate action of antidiabetic medications (propranolol, oxytetracycline, antibiotics)
- Sulfonylureas in older adult patients
- Amylin and incretin mimetic diabetes agents

Decreased Oral, Enteral, or Parenteral Intake
Underproduction of Glucose
- Heavy alcohol consumption
- Medications: aspirin, disopyramide (Norpace), haloperidol (Haldol)
- Decreased production by liver
- Hormonal causes

Too Rapid Use of Glucose
- Gastrointestinal surgery
- Extrapancreatic tumor
- Increased or strenuous exercise

Assessment

Clinical presentation. Common signs and symptoms of hypoglycemia are summarized in Table 19.4. Symptoms of hypoglycemia are categorized as (1) mild symptoms from autonomic nervous system stimulation that are characteristic of a rapid decrease in serum glucose levels, and (2) moderate symptoms reflective of an inadequate supply of glucose to neural tissues that are associated with a slower, more prolonged decline in serum glucose levels.

TABLE 19.4 Signs and Symptoms of Hypoglycemia

DECREASE IN BLOOD SUGAR	
Rapid: Activation of Sympathetic Nervous System	**Prolonged: Inadequate Glucose Supply to Neural Tissues**
Nervousness	Headache
Apprehension	Restlessness
Tachycardia	Difficulty speaking
Palpitations	Difficulty thinking
Pallor	Visual disturbances
Diaphoresis	Paresthesia
Dilated pupils	Difficulty walking
Tremors	Altered consciousness
Fatigue	Coma
General weakness	Convulsions
Headache	Change in personality
Hunger	Psychiatric reactions
	Maniacal behavior
	Catatonia
	Acute paranoia

With a rapid decrease in serum glucose levels, there is activation of the sympathetic nervous system, mediated by epinephrine release from the adrenal medulla. This compensatory fight-or-flight mechanism results in symptoms such as tachycardia; palpitations; tremors; cool, clammy skin; diaphoresis; hunger; pallor; and dilated pupils. The patient may also report feelings of apprehension, nervousness, headache, tremulousness, and general weakness.

Slower and more prolonged declines in serum glucose levels result in symptoms due to an inadequate glucose supply to neural tissues (*neuroglycopenia*). These include restlessness, difficulty in thinking and speaking, visual disturbances, and paresthesias. The patient may have profound changes in level of consciousness, seizures, or both. Personality changes and psychiatric manifestations have been reported. Prolonged hypoglycemia may lead to irreversible brain damage and coma.

Laboratory evaluation. In most patients, the confirming laboratory test for hypoglycemia is a serum or capillary blood glucose level lower than 70 mg/dL. Adults with a history of hypoglycemia unawareness, cognitively impaired elders, and older adults at high risk for falls may have higher target glucose ranges and an individualized protocol for management of lower glucose values.[3] Assess the glucose level in all high-risk patients with the aforementioned clinical signs before initiating treatment. Obtain a history of baseline values before treatment because patients who have experienced elevated glucose levels for some time may complain of hypoglycemia-like symptoms when their glucose levels are corrected to a normal range. In patients with a known history of DM, obtain a thorough history of past experiences of hypoglycemia, including patient-specific associated signs and symptoms. Identify the glucose level at which symptoms appear, which varies from patient to patient. In addition, evaluate renal function in patients with long-standing diabetes who have a new history of recurrent hypoglycemia. Decreased renal function may result in impaired clearance of insulin and erratic glucose control in patients who are taking short-acting insulins, long-acting insulins, or oral insulin secretagogues.

Patient Problems. The following problems may apply to a patient with a hypoglycemic episode:
- Potential for hypoglycemia due to excess circulating insulin in relation to available plasma glucose
- Changes in mental status due to decreased glucose delivery to the brain and nervous tissue
- Risk for seizures and falls due to altered neuronal function
- Need for health teaching due to hypoglycemia: prevention, recognition, and treatment of hypoglycemia

Nursing and Medical Interventions. After serum or capillary glucose levels have been confirmed, replace carbohydrates. The patient's neurological status and ability to swallow without aspiration determine the route to be used. Box 19.7 details a protocol for treatment of mild, moderate, and severe

BOX 19.7 Treatment of Hypoglycemia

Mild Hypoglycemia

- Patient is completely alert. Symptoms may include pallor, diaphoresis, tachycardia, palpitations, hunger, or shakiness. Blood glucose is less than 70 mg/dL. Patient is able to drink.
- *Treatment:* 15 g of carbohydrate by mouth

Moderate Hypoglycemia

- Patient is conscious, cooperative, and able to swallow safely. Symptoms may include difficulty concentrating, confusion, slurred speech, or extreme fatigue. Blood glucose is usually less than 55 mg/dL. Patient is able to drink.
- *Treatment:* 20 to 30 g of carbohydrate by mouth

Severe Hypoglycemia

- Patient is uncooperative or unconscious. Blood glucose is usually less than 54 mg/dL or patient is unable to drink
- *Treatment with IV access:* 12.5 g of 50% dextrose in water solution ($D_{50}W$)
- *Treatment without IV access:* 1 mg of glucagon subcutaneously or intramuscularly and turn patient on the side or observe to avoid potential aspiration from nausea and vomiting side effect

BOX 19.8 15/15 Rule for Hypoglycemia Management

To treat low blood glucose the 15/15 rule is usually applied. Eat 15 grams (g) of carbohydrates and then recheck your blood glucose 15 minutes later.

15 grams (g) of Carbohydrate Examples

- 4 glucose tablets[a]
- ½-1 tube of glucose gel[a]
- 4 ounces of fruit juice
- 1 Tbsp. corn syrup
- 8 ounces of milk
- 1 Tbsp. of jam, preserves, jelly, honey, or sugar

If blood glucose is still low, repeat these steps.

[a]Ask your pharmacist or healthcare team about how much is 15 grams. From US Department of Veterans Affairs. The 15-15 Rule for the Management of Low Blood Sugar. https://www.qualityandsafety.va.gov/ChoosingWiselyHealthSafetyInitiative/Files/HSI-Veteran-15-15Rule.pdf. Updated November 2017. Accessed September 2019.

hypoglycemia. Box 19.8 lists common food substances that contain at least 15 g of carbohydrate. Reassess glucose levels 15 minutes after treatment. Repeat the treatment if the blood glucose level is less than 70 mg/dL.

In the event of hypoglycemia, temporarily withhold rapid-acting and short-acting insulins. If the patient has an insulin pump, suspend the pump for moderate or severe hypoglycemia but do not remove the infusion catheter. The patient should determine whether to discontinue the infusion for mild hypoglycemia. Do not withhold longer-acting basal insulins in patients receiving subcutaneous insulin therapy who are experiencing hypoglycemia, because this will increase the risk for hyperglycemia in all patients and for DKA in patients with type 1 DM. Instruct patients to notify their diabetes care

provider if two or more events of hypoglycemia are experienced within 1 week, because the medication regimen may require adjustment.

STUDY BREAK

2. Following an assessment of the blood glucose via fingerstick, a value of 54 mg/dL was obtained on the critical care patient. What is the priority intervention using the 15/15 rule for glucose management?

A. 1 glucose tablet and monitor blood glucose again in 15 minutes

B. ¼ cup (2 ounces or 60 milliliters) of fruit juice or regular soda and repeat again in 15 minutes

C. 2 or 3 hard candies, then repeat fingerstick in 15 minutes to determine next intervention

D. 1 tablespoon (15 grams) of sugar and repeat fingerstick in 15 minutes to determine effectiveness of intervention

---

Perform neurological assessments to detect any changes in cerebral function due to hypoglycemia. Document baseline neurological status, including mental status, cranial nerve function, sensory and motor function, and deep tendon reflexes. Assess for seizure activity because there is a potential for seizure activity due to altered neuronal cellular metabolism during the hypoglycemic phase. If seizures are observed, describe the seizure event and associated symptoms. Institute seizure precautions, including padded side rails, oxygen, oral airway, bedside suction, and removal of potentially harmful objects from the environment. Neurological status is the best clinical indicator of effective treatment for hypoglycemia.

Patient and family education about hypoglycemic episodes may also be appropriate in the critically ill patient. Instruct the patient and family members on the causes, symptoms, treatment, and prevention of hypoglycemia. Explain the relationships of carbohydrate intake, actions of insulin or oral hypoglycemic agents, excessive alcohol intake, and activity changes or exercise with hypoglycemia. As needed, instruct them on the use of home blood glucose monitoring techniques, schedule, and pattern recognition. Patients at risk for severe hypoglycemia may be considered for continuous glucose monitoring units and should be prescribed a glucagon emergency kit, with family and significant regular contacts instructed in its use. Encourage the patient to wear emergency medical identification and to perform a blood glucose test before driving. If the patient is at risk for nocturnal hypoglycemia, encourage storage of glucose gel at the bedside. Childbearing women with diabetes are at very high risk for hypoglycemia after delivery as the levels of insulin-resistant hormones drop quickly. Lactating women also may be at particular risk and may be encouraged to drink milk while nursing. In addition, instruct patients on the relationship between alcohol ingestion and hypoglycemia.

❓ CRITICAL REASONING ACTIVITY

How can the hazards of hypoglycemia be prevented?

ACUTE AND RELATIVE ADRENAL INSUFFICIENCY

Etiology

Hypofunction of the adrenal gland results from either primary or secondary mechanisms that suppress secretion of cortisol, aldosterone, and androgens. Primary mechanisms, resulting in Addison's disease, are those that cause destruction of the adrenal gland itself. At least 90% of the adrenal cortex must be destroyed before clinical signs and symptoms appear. Primary disorders result in deficiencies of both glucocorticoids and mineralocorticoids. Primary adrenal insufficiency has a variety of causes, including idiopathic autoimmune destruction of the gland, infection and sepsis, hemorrhagic destruction, and granulomatous infiltration from neoplasms, amyloidosis, sarcoidosis, or hemochromatosis.

Idiopathic autoimmune destruction of the adrenal gland is the most common cause of adrenal insufficiency, accounting for 50% to 70% of cases. Autoimmune adrenal destruction may have a genetic component that leads to atrophy of the gland. Genetic adrenal disease may affect just the adrenal gland, or it may be part of a constellation of autoimmune problems, such as autoimmune polyglandular disorder.[12] Young women with spontaneous premature ovarian failure are at increased risk of developing the autoimmune form of adrenal insufficiency.[12] In addition to sepsis, HIV infection and tuberculosis are significant infectious causes of adrenal insufficiency.[12]

Secondary mechanisms that can produce adrenal insufficiency are those that decrease adrenocorticotropic hormone (ACTH) secretion; this results in deficiency of glucocorticoids alone because mineralocorticoids are not primarily dependent on ACTH secretion. Mechanisms that can produce secondary adrenal insufficiency include abrupt withdrawal of corticosteroids, pituitary

and hypothalamic disorders, and sepsis. A more detailed listing of possible causes of primary and secondary adrenal insufficiency is given in Box 19.9.

The most common cause of acute adrenal insufficiency is abrupt withdrawal from corticosteroid therapy. Long-term corticosteroid use suppresses the normal *corticotropin-releasing hormone–ACTH–adrenal feedback systems* (see Fig. 19.1) and results in adrenal suppression. It is difficult to accurately predict the degree of adrenal suppression in patients receiving exogenous glucocorticoid therapy. Longer-acting agents such as dexamethasone are more likely to produce suppression than are shorter-acting corticosteroids such as hydrocortisone. Once corticosteroid use has been tapered off, it may take several months for patients to resume normal secretion of endogenous corticosteroids. Therefore it is important to be familiar with disorders that may be treated with corticosteroids because the resulting adrenal suppression may prevent a normal stress response and may put these patients at risk of an adrenal crisis.

Other medications may also contribute to adrenal suppression. For example, administration of etomidate to facilitate endotracheal intubation is associated with significant but temporary adrenal dysfunction and increased mortality.[15]

Infection and sepsis are among the most common causes of adrenal insufficiency in the critical care setting.[12] The proinflammatory state commonly seen in critical illness is thought to produce adrenal insufficiency by suppressing the hypothalamic-pituitary-adrenal axis. Glucocorticoid resistance and suppression of feedback mechanisms are postulated to contribute to low cortisol levels commonly seen in critical illness. Sepsis and septic shock can also cause thrombotic necrosis of the adrenal gland.[12]

The concept of *relative adrenal insufficiency* has been debated for several years. The hypermetabolic state of critical illness may increase cortisol levels by as much as tenfold over baseline.[12] Patients with an inadequate physiological response to the demands of this hypermetabolic state have an increased mortality rate. The degree of response, how to best measure the response, and optimum treatment continue to be investigated.[12]

Review of Physiology

The manifestations of adrenal insufficiency result from a lack of adrenocortical secretion of glucocorticoids (primarily cortisol), mineralocorticoids (primarily aldosterone), or both. The deficiency of glucocorticoids is especially significant because their influence on the defense mechanisms of the body and its response to stress makes them essential for life.

Cortisol is normally released in response to ACTH stimulation from the anterior pituitary gland (see Fig. 19.1). ACTH is stimulated by corticotropin-releasing hormone from the hypothalamus, which is influenced by circulating cortisol levels, circadian rhythms, and stress. Circadian rhythms affect ACTH and cortisol levels, creating peak levels of cortisol in the morning and the lowest levels around midnight. This normal diurnal rhythm can be overridden by stress. During stress, plasma cortisol may increase as much as 10 times its normal level. Release of cortisol increases the blood glucose concentration by promoting glycogen breakdown and gluconeogenesis in the liver, increases lipolysis and free fatty acid production, increases

---

BOX 19.9 Causes of Adrenal Insufficiency

Primary

- *Autoimmune disease:* idiopathic and polyglandular
- *Granulomatous disease:* tuberculosis, sarcoidosis, histoplasmosis, blastomycosis
- Cancer
- *Hemorrhagic destruction:* anticoagulation, trauma, sepsis
- *Infectious:* meningococcal, staphylococcal, pneumococcal, fungal (candidiasis), cytomegalovirus
- AIDS
- *Medications:* ketoconazole, aminoglutethimide, trimethoprim, etomidate, 5-fluorouracil (suppress adrenals); phenytoin, barbiturates, rifampin (increase steroid degradation)
- Irradiation
- Adrenalectomy
- Developmental or genetic abnormality

Secondary

- Abrupt withdrawal of corticosteroids
- Pathology affecting the pituitary, such as tumors, hemorrhage, irradiation, metastatic cancer, lymphoma, leukemia, sarcoidosis
- *Systemic inflammatory states:* sepsis, vasculitis, sickle cell disease
- Postpartum pituitary hemorrhage (Sheehan syndrome)
- Trauma, especially head trauma, or surgery
- Hypothalamic disorders

BOX 19.10 Physiological Effects of Glucocorticoids (Cortisol)

- *Protein metabolism:* promotes gluconeogenesis, stimulates protein breakdown, and inhibits protein synthesis
- *Fat metabolism:* lipolysis and free fatty acid production; promotes fat deposits in face and cervical area
- *Opposes action of insulin:* glucose transport and use in cells
- *Inhibits inflammatory response:*
  - Suppresses mediator release (kinins, histamine, interleukins, prostaglandins, leukotrienes, serotonin)
  - Stabilizes cell membrane and inhibits capillary dilation
  - Formation of edema
  - Inhibits leukocyte migration and phagocytic activity
- Immunosuppression:
  - Proliferation of T lymphocytes and killer cell activity
  - Complement production and immunoglobulins
- Increases circulating erythrocytes
- *Gastrointestinal effects:* appetite; increases rate of acid and pepsin secretion in stomach
  - Increases uric acid excretion
  - Decreases serum calcium
  - Sensitizes arterioles to effects of catecholamines; maintains blood pressure
  - Increases renal glomerular filtration rate and excretion of water

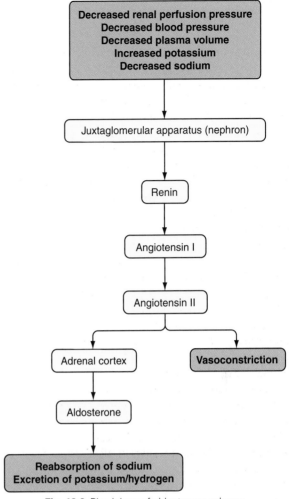

Fig. 19.6 Physiology of aldosterone release.

protein degradation, and inhibits the inflammatory and immune responses. Cortisol also increases sensitivity to catecholamines, producing vasoconstriction, hypertension, and tachycardia (Box 19.10).

Aldosterone is a mineralocorticoid synthesized in the adrenal cortex that regulates the body's electrolyte and water balance in the renal tubules. Secretion of aldosterone is regulated primarily by the renin-angiotensin-aldosterone system. Renin is an enzyme that is stored in the cells of the juxtaglomerular apparatus in the kidneys. It is released in response to stimulation of beta receptors on the surface of the juxtaglomerular apparatus. Factors that stimulate the release of renin include low plasma sodium levels, increased plasma potassium levels, decreased extracellular fluid volume, decreased blood pressure, and decreased sympathetic nerve activity. Once released, renin cleaves angiotensinogen in the plasma to form angiotensin I. Angiotensin I is then converted to angiotensin II in the lungs under the influence of angiotensin-converting enzyme. Angiotensin II stimulates the secretion of aldosterone by the adrenal cortex while causing vasoconstriction of the arterioles. Aldosterone acts in the kidneys on the ascending loop of Henle, the distal convoluted tubule, and the collecting ducts to increase sodium ion reabsorption and to increase potassium and hydrogen ion excretion. Because reabsorption of sodium creates an osmotic gradient across the renal tubular membrane, antidiuretic hormone (ADH) is activated, causing water to be reabsorbed with sodium. The physiology of aldosterone release is summarized in Fig. 19.6.

Pathophysiology

Adrenal crisis is a life-threatening absence of cortisol (glucocorticoid) and aldosterone (mineralocorticoid). A deficiency of cortisol results in decreased production of glucose, decreased metabolism of protein and fat, decreased appetite, decreased intestinal motility and digestion, decreased vascular tone, and diminished effects of catecholamines. If a patient with deficient cortisol is stressed, this deficiency can produce profound shock as a result of significant decreases in vascular tone caused by the diminished effects of catecholamines.[12]

Deficiency of aldosterone results in decreased retention of sodium and water, decreased circulating volume, and increased potassium and hydrogen ion reabsorption. These effects are seen in patients with underlying primary adrenal insufficiency but not in those with secondary adrenal insufficiency because aldosterone secretion is not primarily dependent on ACTH. A summary of the pathophysiological effects of adrenal insufficiency can be found in Fig. 19.7.

Assessment

Clinical Presentation. Adrenal crisis requires astute and rapid assessment. Box 19.11 identifies risk factors for adrenal crisis. Features of adrenal crisis are nonspecific and often attributed to other medical disorders. Signs and symptoms vary (see Fig. 19.6). Because this condition is a medical emergency, consider the diagnosis in any patient who is acutely ill with fever, vomiting, hypotension, shock, decreased serum sodium level, increased serum potassium level, or hypoglycemia (see Laboratory Alert box). Specific system disturbances are widespread. See the Lifespan Considerations box for additional information related to older adults and pregnant women.

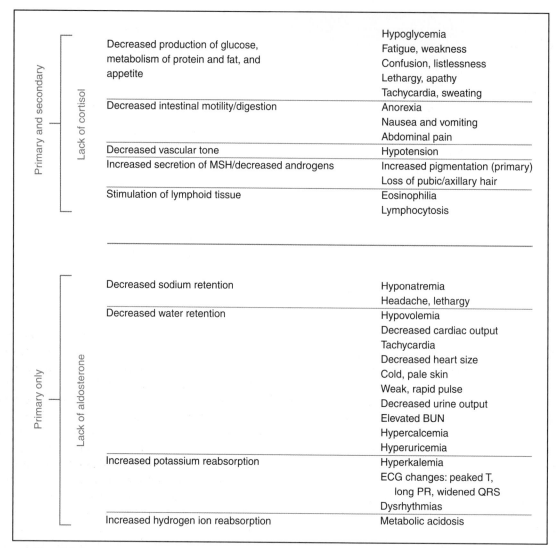

Fig. 19.7 Pathophysiological effects of adrenal insufficiency. *BUN,* Blood urea nitrogen; *ECG,* electrocardiogram; *MSH,* melanocyte-stimulating hormone.

BOX 19.11 Assessment of Risk Factors for Adrenal Crisis

Assess patients carefully for risk factors, predisposing factors, and physical findings associated with chronic adrenal insufficiency. Risk factors include the following:

- *Medication history:* steroids within the past year, phenytoin, barbiturates, rifampin
- *Illness history:* infection, cancer, autoimmune disease, diseases treated with steroids, irradiation of the head or abdomen, HIV-positive status
- *Family history:* autoimmune disease, Addison disease
- *Nutrition:* weight loss, decreased appetite
- *Miscellaneous:* fatigue, dizziness, weakness, darkening of skin, low blood glucose that does not respond to therapy, salt craving

---

LIFESPAN CONSIDERATIONS

Adrenal Disorders

Older Adults
- Use and clearance of cortisol decrease with age, resulting in increased serum cortisol levels. Cortisol secretion then decreases because feedback systems are intact, leading to lower cortisol levels in the older adult.
- The absolute level of cortisol needed to maintain homeostasis in an older adult is unknown.
- Poor nutrition and decreased stores of albumin (one of cortisol's binding proteins) may compound the decline in cortisol availability and response. This predisposes the older adult to dehydration, electrolyte imbalance, acid-base imbalance, and infection due to disorders of the adrenal cortex.[19]

Pregnant Women
- Both corticotropin (adrenocorticotropic hormone, or ACTH) and cortisol levels are elevated in pregnancy and thus can exacerbate Cushing's syndrome during pregnancy.
- Acute adrenal crisis may be precipitated by the stress of labor and delivery.[5]

Adrenal Disorders

Serum Laboratory Test	Critical Value[a]	Significance
Glucose	<50 mg/dL, male	Severe hypoglycemia
	<40 mg/dL, female	
Cortisol	No critical value specified; <10 mcg/dL considered insufficiency	In severely ill or stressed patient, indicates insufficiency
Potassium	>6.1 mEq/L	Potential for heart blocks, bradydysrhythmias, sinus arrest, ventricular fibrillation, asystole
	<3.0 mEq/L	Potential for ventricular dysrhythmias
Sodium	>160 mEq/L	May be a result of stress and dehydration
	<120 mEq/L	From lack of aldosterone
BUN	>100 mg/dL	Values >20 mg/dL may be observed due to protein breakdown and hemoconcentration
pH	<7.25	Decreased from accumulation of acids and dehydration

[a]Critical values vary by facility and laboratory.
BUN, Blood urea nitrogen.

Cardiovascular system. Cardiovascular signs and symptoms in adrenal crisis are due to hypovolemia (decreased water reabsorption), decreased vascular tone (decreased effectiveness of catecholamines), and hyperkalemia. The most common presentation of adrenal crisis in critically ill patients is hypotension refractory to fluids and requiring vasopressors. The patient may also have symptoms of decreased cardiac output; weak, rapid pulse; dysrhythmias; and cold, pale skin. Chest radiographs may show decreased heart size due to hypovolemia. Changes in the electrocardiogram may result if there is significant hyperkalemia. Hypovolemia and vascular dilation may be severe enough in crisis to cause hemodynamic collapse and shock.

Neurological system. Neurological manifestations in adrenal crisis are due to decreases in glucose levels, protein metabolism, volume and perfusion, and sodium concentrations. Patients may complain of headache, fatigue that worsens as the day progresses, and severe weakness. They may also exhibit mental confusion, listlessness, lethargy, apathy, psychoses, and emotional lability.

Gastrointestinal system. The gastrointestinal signs and symptoms in adrenal crisis are due to decreased digestive enzymes, intestinal motility, and digestion. Anorexia, nausea, vomiting, diarrhea, and vague abdominal pain are present in most patients.[12]

Genitourinary system. Diminished circulation to the kidneys from reduced circulating volume and hypotension decreases renal perfusion and glomerular filtration rate. Urine output may decline, and acute kidney injury may occur.

Laboratory Evaluation. Laboratory findings in a patient with acute adrenal crisis include hypoglycemia, hyponatremia, hyperkalemia, eosinophilia, increased BUN level, and metabolic acidosis (see Laboratory Alert box). Hypercalcemia or hyperuricemia is possible as a result of volume depletion.

The diagnosis of adrenal crisis is made by evaluating random total plasma cortisol levels.[12] The normal pattern of diurnal variation in cortisol levels is lost in the critically ill, making the timing of the test unimportant. In crisis, plasma cortisol levels are lower than 10 mcg/dL. Differentiation between primary and secondary adrenal insufficiency is accomplished by evaluating serum ACTH levels, which are elevated in primary insufficiency and normal or decreased in secondary insufficiency. Laboratory blood draws are usually collected during the morning hours.

A "normal" cortisol level in a critically ill patient actually may be abnormal and indicate an inadequate response.[16] A random total cortisol value lower than 10 mcg/dL can be life-threatening and warrants further evaluation. Cortisol levels are difficult to interpret in the context of critical illness, but guidelines recommend beginning corticosteroid replacement as soon as insufficiency is suspected.[12]

The technique for performing a cosyntropin (synthetic ACTH) stimulation is outlined in Box 19.12. The test determines baseline levels and response to stimulation. A standard dose of 250 mcg cosyntropin is given, and the expected response is an increase in cortisol level of 7 to 9 mcg/dL from the baseline. A patient whose cortisol level does not increase by this amount is deemed a nonresponder and has an increased risk of mortality.[12]

STUDY BREAK

3. A provider orders a cosyntropin test to assess adrenal status. Which of the following statements is true regarding the test?
   A. Salivary cortisol levels provide an accurate assessment of the patient's response.
   B. Dexamethasone administration does not affect cortisol values and can be administered in emergency situations.
   C. Either 1 mcg (low dose) or 100 mcg (regular dose) or cosyntropin can be administered to assess the patient's response.
   D. Following cosyntropin administration, reassess cortisol level in 15 minutes.

BOX 19.12 Cosyntropin Stimulation Test

Standard Method

- Obtain baseline serum cortisol measurement less than 30 minutes before cosyntropin administration.
- Administer cosyntropin, 250 mcg up to 750 mcg IV over a 2-minute period.
- Measure the serum cortisol level 30 and 60 minutes after cosyntropin administration.
- In emergency situations, may treat with dexamethasone (Decadron); will not interfere with cortisol levels.

Test Response

- *Expected response:* cortisol greater than 20 mcg/dL, or increase from baseline of greater than 9 mcg/dL
- *Primary aldosterone insufficiency:* a total cortisol level greater than 20 mcg/dL and/or a change from baseline of greater than 7 mcg/dL
- *Relative aldosterone insufficiency:* a change from baseline of less than 9 mcg/dL regardless of baseline level

Patient Problems

The following problems may apply to a patient with adrenal crisis based on assessment data:

- Hypovolemia due to deficiency of aldosterone hormone (mineralocorticoid) and decreased sodium and water retention
- Decreased peripheral tissue perfusion due to cortisol deficiency, resulting in decreased vascular tone and decreased effectiveness of catecholamines
- Nutrition deficit due to cortisol deficiency and resultant decreased metabolism of protein and fats, decreased appetite, and decreased intestinal motility and digestion
- Need for health teaching due to adrenal disorder: proper long-term corticosteroid management
- Low tolerance to activity due to use of endogenous protein for energy needs and loss of skeletal muscle mass as evidenced by early fatigue, weakness, and exertional dyspnea

Nursing and Medical Interventions

Many of the interventions for these patient problems are addressed in the Collaborative Plan of Care for the Critically Ill Patient (see Chapter 1). Adrenal crisis requires immediate recognition and intervention if the patient is to survive. Primary objectives in the treatment of adrenal crisis include identifying and treating the precipitating cause, replacing fluid and electrolytes, replacing hormones, and educating the patient and family. See the Evidence-Based Practice box for recommendations developed by a task force of critical care experts.

Fluid and Electrolyte Replacement. Fluid losses should be replaced with an infusion of 5% dextrose in normal saline until signs and symptoms of hypovolemia stabilize. This not only reverses the volume deficit but also provides glucose to minimize the hypoglycemia. The patient may need as much as 5 L of fluid in the first 12 to 24 hours to maintain an adequate blood pressure and urine output and to replace the fluid deficit.

Hyperkalemia frequently responds to volume expansion and glucocorticoid replacement and may require no further treatment. In fact, the patient may become hypokalemic during therapy and may require potassium replacement. The acidosis also usually corrects itself with volume expansion and glucocorticoid replacement. However, if the pH is less than 7.0 or the bicarbonate level is less than 10 mEq/L, the patient may require sodium bicarbonate.

Hormone Replacement. Initially, glucocorticoid replacement is the most important type of hormone replacement. If adrenal insufficiency has not been previously diagnosed and the patient's condition is unstable, dexamethasone phosphate (Decadron) is given until the cosyntropin test has been done. Recommended dosage varies by source; 250 mcg up to 750 mcg IV is commonly administered. This medication does not significantly cross-react with cortisol in the assay for cortisol and therefore can be administered to patients pending adrenal testing results.

EVIDENCE-BASED PRACTICE

Guidelines for Diagnosis and Management of Critical Illness–Related Corticosteroid Insufficiency in Critically Ill Patients

Corticosteroid insufficiency is common in critical illness. A multiprofessional task force representing critical care experts convened to develop evidence-based guidelines for managing critical illness–related corticosteroid insufficiency (CIRCI) in the critically ill. Recommendations were developed using a systematic approach based on rating of the evidence and were classified as strong or conditional. At least 80% of the task force members had to agree on a recommendation. The task force could not agree on a single test to reliably diagnose CIRCI; therefore consider a change in cortisol of less than 9 mcg/dL after a 250-mg cosyntropin test or a random plasma cortisol of less than 10 mcg/dL to make the diagnosis. Recommendations are as follows:

- Avoid using methods other than plasma cortisol (e.g., salivary) for diagnosis and treatment (conditional, low-quality evidence).
- Recommend the 250 mcg adrenocorticotropic hormone (ACTH) test over the 1 mcg ACTH test for diagnosis of CIRCI (conditional, low-quality evidence).

- Administer hydrocortisone less than 400 mg/day IV for 3 or more days in those with septic shock unresponsive to vasopressors (conditional, low-quality evidence).
- Do not administer corticosteroids in patients with sepsis without shock (conditional, moderate-quality evidence).
- Administer methylprednisolone 1 mg/kg/day IV in those with early moderate to severe acute respiratory distress syndrome (conditional, moderate-quality evidence).
- Avoid corticosteroids for major trauma patients (conditional, low-quality evidence).

Reference

Annane D, Pastores SM, Rochwerg B, et al. Guidelines for the diagnosis and management of critical illness–related corticosteroid insufficiency (CIRCI) in critically ill patients (Part I): Society of Critical Care Medicine (SCCM) and European Society of Intensive Care Medicine (ESICM). *Intensive Care Med.* 2017;43:1751–1763.

Hydrocortisone sodium succinate (Solu-Cortef) is the medication of choice after the diagnosis is confirmed by the cosyntropin test, because it has both glucocorticoid and mineralocorticoid activities in high doses. A bolus dose of 100 mg IV is given followed by 200 mg over 24 hours as infusion, or in divided doses every 6 hours. The higher dose is administered for 24 to 48 hours, then doses are tapered slowly to a desired maintenance dose.[12] Cortisone acetate may be given intramuscularly if the IV route is not available.

The patient can be switched to oral replacement once oral intake is resumed. At lower doses (<100 mg/day of hydrocortisone), a patient with primary adrenal insufficiency may also require mineralocorticoid replacement. Fludrocortisone, 100-200 mcg po daily, is added. A nutritional consideration, if the patient is experiencing excessive sweating or diarrhea, is to increase sodium intake to 15 mEq/day. Table 19.5 describes the medications used in the treatment of acute adrenal crisis.

Patient and Family Education. In a patient with known adrenal insufficiency and in those receiving corticosteroid therapy, adrenal crisis is preventable. Education of patients, family, and significant others is the key to prevention.

? CRITICAL REASONING ACTIVITY

In which patient population would the nurse expect to administer a cosyntropin stimulation test? What are the priority nursing interventions for educating the patient and family about the diagnostic procedure? What factors affect the interpretation of the test results?

THYROID GLAND IN CRITICAL CARE

Review of Physiology

Thyroid hormones play a role in regulating the function of all body systems. Box 19.13 lists the physiological effects of thyroid hormones. The thyroid hormones thyroxine (T_4) and triiodothyronine (T_3) are secreted by the thyroid gland under the influence of the anterior pituitary gland via secretion of thyroid-stimulating hormone (TSH, also called thyrotropin), which in turn is influenced by thyroid-releasing hormone (TRH, also called thyrotropin-releasing hormone) from the hypothalamus. Thyroid hormones are highly bound to globulin, T_4-binding prealbumin, and albumin. Only the unbound (or free) fraction of the circulating hormone is biologically

⬭ TABLE 19.5 **PHARMACOLOGY**

Medications Used to Treat Adrenal Crisis

Medication	Action/Uses	Dose/Route	Side Effects	Nursing Implications
Hydrocortisone sodium succinate (Solu-Cortef)	Antiinflammatory and immunosuppressive effects Salt-retaining (mineralocorticoid) effects in high doses Used for inflammation, adrenal insufficiency, asthma	Individualized in adrenal crisis *IV:* 100-500 mg may repeat q2-6h	Hyperglycemia Cushing's syndrome Electrolyte disorders Euphoria and other psychic symptoms Fluid retention Masking of infection Hypertension Peptic ulcers Nausea and vomiting	Institute prophylaxis against GI bleeding Be aware of multiple drug-drug interactions, especially with IV route: oral contraceptives, phenytoin, digoxin, phenobarbital, theophylline, insulin, anticoagulants, salicylates Avoid abrupt discontinuation Monitor serum glucose and electrolyte levels Watch for signs of fluid overload Observe for signs of infection (may be masked) Maintain adequate nutrition to avoid catabolic effects Provide meticulous mouth care
Dexamethasone (Decadron)	Has only glucocorticoid effects	*PO, IM, IV:* Individualized doses	Same as hydrocortisone	Same as for hydrocortisone
Fludrocortisone acetate (Florinef)	Causes sodium and water retention and increases excretion of hydrogen, potassium, and water	*PO:* 100-200 mcg/day	Increased blood volume, edema, hypertension, HF, headaches, weakness of extremities	Assess for signs of fluid overload, HF Monitor serum sodium and potassium levels Use only in conjunction with glucocorticoids Restrict sodium intake if the patient has edema or fluid overload Not used to treat acute crisis; added as glucocorticoid dose is decreased

GI, Gastrointestinal; *h,* hour; *HF,* heart failure; *IM,* intramuscular; *PO,* orally; *q,* every.
Data from Gahart BL, Nazareno AR, Ortega MQ. *Gahart's 2019 Intravenous Medications.* 35th ed. St. Louis, MO: Elsevier; 2019; Skidmore-Roth L. *Mosby's 2019 Nursing Drug Reference.* 32nd ed. St. Louis, MO: Elsevier; 2019.

BOX 19.13   Physiological Effects of Thyroid Hormones

Major Effects
- Metabolic activities of all tissues
- Rate of nutrient use and oxygen consumption for adenosine triphosphate (ATP) production
- Rate of growth
- Activities of other endocrine glands

Other Effects
- Regulate protein synthesis and catabolism
- Regulate body heat production and dissipation
- Gluconeogenesis and use of glucose
- Maintain appetite and gastrointestinal motility
- Maintain calcium metabolism
- Stimulate cholesterol synthesis
- Maintain cardiac rate, contractility, and output
- Affect respiratory rate, oxygen use, and carbon dioxide formation
- Affect red blood cell production
- Affect central nervous system affect and attention
- Produce muscle tone and vigor and provide normal skin constituents

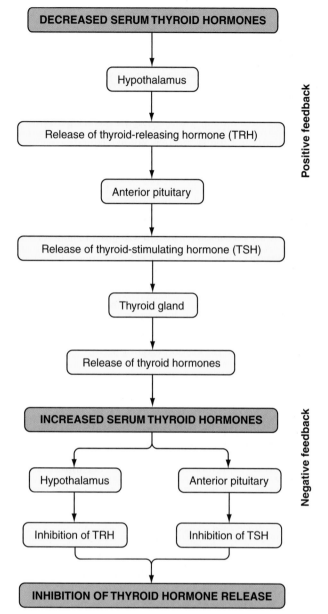

Fig. 19.8 Feedback systems for thyroid hormone regulation.

active. Regulation of these hormones occurs via positive and negative feedback mechanisms (Fig. 19.8).[15]

T_4 accounts for more than 95% of circulating thyroid hormones, but half of all thyroid activity comes from T_3. T_3 is five times more potent, acts more quickly, and enters cells more easily than T_4.[15] T_3 is derived from conversion of T_4 in nonthyroid tissue. Certain conditions and medications can block the conversion of T_4 to T_3, creating a potential thyroid imbalance. Possible causes for blocked conversion are listed in Box 19.14.

Effects of Aging

With aging, thyroid function declines. Hypothyroidism occurs in older adults, frequently with an insidious onset. The decrease in energy level; the feeling of being cold; the dry, flaky skin; and other signs are often mistakenly assumed to be part of aging but may be signs of decreased thyroid function.[15] Thyroid function should be assessed in any older adult patient through diagnostic laboratory testing. See the Lifespan Considerations box for additional information related to older adults and pregnant women.

LIFESPAN CONSIDERATIONS

Thyroid Disorders

Older Adults
- Thyroid hormone levels decrease with age because of glandular atrophy and inflammation.[19]
- Approximately 5% of older adults are affected by hypothyroidism.
- Detection of thyroid disease by assessment of signs or symptoms is more challenging in older adults. On clinical presentation, hypothyroidism can easily be confused with dementia.
- Lower amounts of thyroid medication are needed as replacement, and adjustments of dosage must be slower to prevent potentially dangerous side effects.
- Older adults are less likely to tolerate urgent treatment with liothyronine sodium.

- Older adults may not exhibit the typical signs of thyrotoxicosis. Anorexia, atrial fibrillation, apathy, and weight loss may already be present or misinterpreted.
- Goiter, hyperactive reflexes, sweating, heat intolerance, tremor, nervousness, and polydipsia are less commonly present in older adults.
- Symptoms of thyroid storm may manifest as hypomania, increasing angina, or worsening heart failure.

Pregnant Women
- Thyroid hormones are increased during pregnancy as a result of increased synthesis of thyroxine-binding globulin.[5] Free levels are unchanged.

BOX 19.14 Factors That Block Conversion of Thyroxine to Triiodothyronine

- *Severe illness:* chronic renal failure, cancer, chronic liver disease
- Trauma
- Malnutrition, fasting
- *Medications:* glucocorticoids, propranolol, propylthiouracil, amiodarone
- Radiopaque contrast media
- Acidosis

Thyroid Function in the Critically Ill

During critical illness, stress-related changes occur in thyroid hormone balance. Initially, there is a decrease in plasma T_3 levels, known as *low T3 syndrome* or *euthyroid sick syndrome.* These changes are thought to result from alterations in the peripheral metabolism of thyroid hormones, which may be an adaptation to severe illness in which the body attempts to reduce energy expenditure.[15] Generally, these changes are considered to be beneficial and do not require intervention. Within approximately 3 days, T_3 levels return to the low-normal range. In severe illness, T_3 levels may fail to normalize, and T_4 levels may also decrease.[15]

In the chronically critically ill, additional thyroid hormone changes occur. Both T_3 and T_4 levels are reduced, as is TSH secretion. The changes in chronic critical illness are not well understood but are thought to also include central neuroendocrine dysfunction.[15] Low T_4 levels may serve as a poor prognostic indicator for patient recovery.

THYROID CRISES

Thyroid disorders that have been previously diagnosed and adequately treated do not generally result in crisis states. However, if patients with thyroid disorders, especially undiagnosed thyroid disorders, are stressed either physiologically or psychologically, the results can be life-threatening. Hyperthyroidism must be explored as a causative factor in a patient with new-onset, otherwise unexplained rapid heart rates.

Etiology

Hyperthyroidism is common. The most frequent form of hyperthyroidism is *toxic diffuse goiter,* also known as *Graves' disease.*[15] It occurs most frequently in young (third or fourth decade), previously healthy women. A family history of hyperthyroidism is often present. Graves' disease is an autoimmune disease. Affected patients have abnormal thyroid-stimulating immunoglobulins that cause thyroid inflammation, diffuse enlargement, and hyperplasia of the gland.

Toxic multinodular goiter is the second most common cause of hyperthyroidism.[15] It also occurs more commonly in women, but the patients are typically older (fourth to seventh decades). Crises in patients with toxic multinodular goiter are commonly associated with heart failure or severe muscle weakness.

Hyperthyroidism also occurs secondary to exposure to radiation, interferon-alpha therapy for viral hepatitis, and other events.[15] Administration of amiodarone, a heavily iodinated compound, can result in either hyperthyroidism or hypothyroidism.[15] Other possible causes of hyperthyroidism are listed in Box 19.15.

Low levels of thyroid hormones disrupt the normal physiology of most body systems. Hypothyroidism produces a hypodynamic, hypometabolic state. *Myxedema coma* is a magnification of these disruptions initiated by some type of stressor. This condition takes months to develop and should be suspected in patients with known hypothyroidism, patients with a surgical scar on the lower neck, and those patients who are unusually sensitive to medications or narcotics.[15]

The underlying causes of myxedema coma are those that produce hypothyroidism. Most cases occur either in patients with long-standing autoimmune disease of the thyroid (Hashimoto's thyroiditis) or in patients who have received surgical or radioactive iodine treatment for Graves' disease and inadequate hormone replacement.[15]

Approximately 5% of adults have hypothyroidism as a result of a pituitary (secondary) or hypothalamic (tertiary) disorder. These and other less common causes of hypothyroidism are listed in Box 19.16.

BOX 19.15 Causes of Hyperthyroidism

Most Common
- Toxic diffuse goiter (Graves' disease)
- Toxic multinodular goiter
- Toxic uninodular goiter

Other Causes
- Triiodothyronine
- Exogenous iodine in a patient with preexisting thyroid disease: exposure to iodine load from radiographic contrast dyes, medications (amiodarone)
- Thyroiditis (transient)
- Postpartum thyroiditis
- *Medications:*
  - Nonsteroidal antiinflammatory medications
  - Salicylates
  - Tricyclic antidepressants
  - Thiazide diuretics
  - Insulin

Rare Causes
- Toxic thyroid adenoma—more common in the older adult
- Metastatic thyroid cancer
- Malignancies with circulating thyroid stimulators
- Pituitary tumors producing thyroid-stimulating hormone
- Acromegaly

Associations With Other Disorders[a]
- Pernicious anemia
- Idiopathic Addison's disease
- Myasthenia gravis
- Sarcoidosis
- Albright syndrome

[a]The presence of these disorders in a patient with thyroid crisis increases the likelihood that the patient has underlying hyperthyroidism.

BOX 19.16 Causes of Hypothyroidism

Primary Thyroid Disease
- Autoimmune (Hashimoto's thyroiditis)
- Radioactive iodine treatment of Graves' disease
- Thyroidectomy
- Congenital enzymatic defect in thyroid hormone biosynthesis
- Inhibition of thyroid hormone synthesis or release
- *Medications:*
  - Antithyroid medications
  - Iodides
  - Amiodarone
  - Lithium carbonate
  - Oral hypoglycemic agents
  - Dopamine
- Idiopathic thyroid atrophy

Secondary (Pituitary) or Tertiary (Hypothalamus) Disease
- Tumors
- Infiltrative disease (sarcoidosis)
- Hypophysectomy
- Pituitary irradiation
- Head injury
- Stroke
- Pituitary infarction

BOX 19.17 Progressive Signs of Hyperthyroidism

- *Cardiovascular:* Increased heart rate and palpitations. Hyperthyroidism may manifest as sinus tachycardia in a sleeping patient or as atrial fibrillation with a rapid ventricular response.
- *Neurological:* Increased irritability, hyperactivity, decreased attention span, and nervousness. In an older adult patient, these signs may be masked, and depression or apathy may be present.
- *Temperature intolerance:* Increased cold tolerance; heat intolerance; fever; excessive sweating; and warm, moist skin. Older patients may naturally lose their ability to shiver and may be less comfortable in the cold.
- *Respiratory:* Increased respiratory rate, weakened thoracic muscles, and decreased vital capacity are evident.
- *Gastrointestinal:* Increased appetite, decreased absorption (especially of vitamins), weight loss, and increased stools. Diarrhea is not common. Older adult patients may be constipated.
- *Musculoskeletal:* Fine tremors of tongue or eyelids, peripheral tremors with activity, and muscle wasting are noted.
- *Integumentary:* Thin, fine, and fragile hair; soft friable nails; and petechiae. Young women generally have the more classic findings. Young men may notice an increase in acne and sweating. An older adult patient with dry, atrophic skin may not have significant skin changes.
- *Hematopoietic:* Normochromic, normocytic anemia and leukocytosis may occur.
- *Ophthalmic:* Pathological features result from edema and inflammation. Physical findings may include upper lid retraction, lid lag, extraocular muscle palsies, and sight loss. Exophthalmos is found almost exclusively in Graves' disease.

Thyrotoxic Crisis (Thyroid Storm)

Pathophysiology. *Thyroid storm* occurs in untreated or inadequately treated patients with hyperthyroidism; it is rare in patients with normal thyroid gland function.[15] The crisis is often precipitated by stress due to an underlying illness, general anesthesia, surgery, or infection. It can also be associated with stroke, DKA, and trauma. Uncontrolled hyperthyroidism produces a hyperdynamic, hypermetabolic state that results in disruption of many major body functions; without treatment, death may occur within 48 hours. The specific mechanism that produces thyroid storm is unknown but includes high levels of circulating thyroid hormones, an enhanced cellular response to those hormones, and hyperactivity of the sympathetic nervous system.[15] Thyroid hormones normally increase the synthesis of enzymes that stimulate cellular mitochondria and energy production. When excess thyroid hormones are present, the increased activity of these enzymes produces excessive thermal energy and fever. It is believed that the rapidity with which hormone levels rise may be more important than the absolute levels.

Assessment

Clinical presentation. The excess thyroid hormone activity of hyperthyroidism affects the body in many ways. Box 19.17 lists progressive signs associated with hyperthyroidism. Common findings in patients with thyroid storm, their significance, and the actions nurses can take to address each of these findings are listed in Table 19.6.

Thyroid storm has an abrupt onset. The most prominent clinical features of thyroid storm are severe fever, marked tachycardia, heart failure, tremors, delirium, stupor, and coma.[15]

The patient's ability to survive thyroid storm is determined by the severity of the hyperthyroid state and the patient's general health. The severity of the hyperthyroid state is not necessarily

STUDY BREAK
4. Which of the following statements is true regarding thyroid storm?
   A. Marked tachycardia may be observed.
   B. Onset is slow.
   C. Patient often has a large goiter.
   D. Body temperature is often low.

indicated by the serum levels of thyroid hormones but rather by tissue and organ responsiveness to the hormones.[15]

Thermoregulation disturbances. Temperature regulation is lost. The patient's body temperature may be as high as 41.1°C (106°F). The increase in heat production and metabolic end products also causes the blood vessels of the skin to dilate. This enhances oxygen and nutrient delivery to the peripheral tissues and accounts for the patient's warm, moist skin.

Neurological disturbances. Thyroid hormones normally maintain alertness and attention. Excess thyroid hormones cause hypermetabolism and hyperactivity of the nervous system, resulting in agitation, delirium, psychosis, tremulousness, seizures, and coma.

Cardiovascular disturbances. Thyroid hormones play a role in maintaining cardiac rate, force of contraction, and cardiac output. The increase in metabolism and the stimulation of catecholamines produced by thyroid hormones cause a hyperdynamic heart. Contractility, heart rate, and cardiac output increase as peripheral vascular resistance decreases. These effects are magnified by the body's increased demand for oxygen and nutrients. In thyroid storm, the increased demands on the heart produce high-output heart failure and cardiovascular collapse if the crisis is not recognized and treated.

TABLE 19.6 Thyroid Crises

Clinical Concerns	Significance	Nursing Actions
Thyroid Storm		
Alterations in level of consciousness	Symptoms can be confused with other disorders (e.g., paranoia, psychosis, depression), especially in the older adult	Provide a safe environment. Assess for orientation, agitation, inattention. Control environmental influences. Implement seizure precautions.
↑ Cardiac workload due to hypermetabolic state; ↓ cardiac output	Can lead to heart failure and cardiovascular collapse	Assess for chest pain, palpitations. Monitor for cardiac dysrhythmias (e.g., atrial fibrillation or flutter) and tachycardia. Monitor blood pressure for widening pulse pressure. Auscultate for the development of an S_3 heart sound. Monitor hemodynamic status: SvO_2, SI, PAOP, RAP. Assess urine output. Evaluate response to therapy.
↑ Oxygen demand due to hypermetabolic state; ineffective breathing pattern	↑ Respiratory rate and drive can lead to fatigue and hypoventilation	Provide supplemental oxygen or mechanical ventilation as needed. Monitor respiratory rate and effort. Monitor oxygen saturation via pulse oximeter. Minimize activity.
Loss of ability to regulate with temperature	Inability to respond to fever exacerbates hypermetabolic demands	Monitor temperature and treat with acetaminophen and/or a cooling blanket as needed.
Myxedema Coma ↓ Cardiac function	Hypotension and potential for pericardial effusion	Perform ECG monitoring (look for voltage in the QRS complexes, indicating effusion). Auscultate for diminished heart sounds. Monitor blood pressure for signs of hypotension.
Muscle weakness, hypoventilation, pleural effusion; ineffective breathing	Potential for respiratory acidosis and hypoxemia	Auscultate the lungs frequently. Monitor respiratory effort (rate and depth) and pattern. Maintain I&O (probable need for fluid restriction). Monitor ABGs/pulse oximetry and CBC (for anemia). Position for optimum respiratory effort.
Alteration in level of consciousness	Ranges from difficulty concentrating to coma Seizures can occur	Assess and maintain patient safety.
Loss of ability to regulate temperature	Inability to respond to cold	Monitor temperature. Control room temperature, provide rewarming measures.

ABGs, Arterial blood gases; *CBC,* complete blood count; *ECG,* electrocardiographic; *I&O,* intake and output; *PAOP,* pulmonary artery occlusion pressure; *RAP,* right atrial pressure; *SI,* stroke index; *SvO₂,* mixed venous oxygen consumption.

Patients experience palpitations, tachycardia (out of proportion to the fever), and a widened pulse pressure. Atrial fibrillation is common. A prominent third heart sound may be heard, as well as a systolic murmur over the pulmonic area, the aortic area, or both. Occasionally, a pericardial rub may be heard. In the absence of atrial fibrillation, frequent premature atrial contractions or atrial flutter may be present. In an older adult patient with underlying heart disease, worsening of angina or severe heart failure may herald thyroid storm.

Pulmonary disturbances. Thyroid hormones affect respiratory rate and depth, oxygen use, and CO_2 formation. Tissues need more oxygen as a result of hypermetabolism. This increased need for oxygen stimulates the respiratory drive and increases the respiratory rate. However, increased protein catabolism reduces protein in respiratory muscles (diaphragm and intercostals). As a result, even with an increased respiratory rate, muscle weakness may prevent the patient from meeting the oxygen demand and may cause hypoventilation, CO_2 retention, and respiratory failure.

Gastrointestinal disturbances. Excess thyroid hormones increase metabolism and accelerate protein and fat degradation. Thyroid hormones also increase gastrointestinal motility, which may result in abdominal pain, nausea, and jaundice. Vomiting and diarrhea can occur, contributing to volume depletion during thyrotoxic crises.

Musculoskeletal disturbances. Muscle weakness and fatigue result from increased protein catabolism. Skeletal muscle changes are manifested as tremors. Thoracic muscles are weak, causing dyspnea. In thyrotoxic crises, patients are placed on bed rest to reduce metabolic demand.

Laboratory evaluation. The diagnosis of thyroid storm is made clinically. Thyroid hormone levels are elevated, but they are usually no higher than those normally found in uncomplicated hyperthyroidism. In any event, the patient must be treated before these results are available. See the Laboratory Alert box for laboratory abnormalities that may occur in thyroid storm.

Patient Problems. The following problems may apply to a patient with thyroid storm based on assessment data:

- Hyperthermia due to loss of temperature regulation, increased metabolism, increased heat production
- Risk for low cardiac output due to increased metabolic demands on the heart, extreme tachycardia, dysrhythmias, heart failure
- Changes in breathing patterns and decreased gas exchange due to muscle weakness and decreased vital capacity resulting in hypoventilation and CO_2 retention, increased oxygen need from hypermetabolism
- Inadequate nutrition due to increased requirement, increased peristalsis, decreased absorption
- Decreased mobility and inability to tolerate activity due to muscle weakness, tremors, anemia, fatigue, and extreme energy expenditure
- Need for health teaching due to thyroid disorder: disease process, therapeutic regimen, prevention of complications

Nursing and Medical Interventions. Refer to the Collaborative Plan of Care for the Critically Ill Patient (Chapter 1) for nursing interventions due to these patient problems. Thyroid storm requires immediate intervention if the patient is to survive. The primary objectives in the treatment of thyroid storm are antagonizing the peripheral effects of thyroid hormone, inhibiting thyroid hormone biosynthesis, blocking thyroid hormone release, providing supportive care, identifying and treating the precipitating cause, and providing patient and family education. Box 19.18 details the treatment of thyroid storm.

Antagonism of peripheral effects of thyroid hormones. Because it can take days or longer for treatment to affect circulating thyroid hormones, immediate action is necessary to minimize the systemic effects of thyroid storm. The mortality rate of thyroid storm has been significantly reduced since the introduction of beta-blockers to inhibit the effects of thyroid hormones. The medication used most frequently is propranolol (Inderal). Other beta-blockers, such as esmolol hydrochloride (Brevibloc) or atenolol (Tenormin), may also be used. Results are seen within minutes after IV administration and within 1 hour after oral treatment. IV effects last 3 to 4 hours. In addition, high-dose glucocorticoids are administered to block the conversion of T_4 to T_3, thereby decreasing the effects of thyroid hormone on peripheral tissues.

Inhibition of thyroid hormone biosynthesis. One of two thioamide medications may be administered to inhibit thyroid hormone biosynthesis: propylthiouracil and methimazole (Tapazole). Neither of these medications is available in IV form, but they may be given via a nasogastric or rectal tube if necessary. In high doses, propylthiouracil inhibits conversion of T_4 to T_3 in peripheral tissues and results in a more rapid reduction of circulating thyroid hormone levels. Methimazole may be used because of its longer half-life and higher potency.

The disadvantage of both propylthiouracil and methimazole is that they lack immediate effect. They do not block the release of thyroid hormones already stored in the thyroid gland, and weeks to months may be required to lower thyroid hormone levels to normal.

! LABORATORY ALERT

Thyroid Disorders

Laboratory Test	Critical Value[a]	Significance
Thyroid Storm		
T_3, free (triiodothyronine)	>0.52 ng/dL	Hyperthyroidism
T_3, resin uptake	>35% of total	
T_4 (thyroxine)	>12 mcg/dL	
TSH	<0.01 milliunits/L	
Glucose	≥ 200 mg/dL (2 h postprandial or random); >140 mg/dL (fasting)	↑ Insulin degradation
Sodium	>150 mEq/L	May be a result of stress, dehydration, and/or hypermetabolic state
BUN	>20 mg/dL	↑ Due to protein breakdown and hemoconcentration
CBC	↓ RBCs	Normocytic, normochromic anemia
	↑ WBCs	
Calcium	>10.2 mg/dL	Excess bone resorption
Myxedema Coma		
T_3, free	<0.2 mg/dL	Hypothyroidism
T_3, resin uptake	<25% of total	
T_4	<5 mcg/dL	
TSH	>25 milliunits/L	
Sodium	<130 mEq/L	
		Dilutional from increased total body water
Glucose	<50 mg/dL	Hypoglycemia due to hypermetabolic state
CBC	↓ RBCs	Anemia due to vitamin B_{12} deficiency, inadequate folate or iron absorption
Platelets	<150,000 cells/mm³	Risk for bleeding
pH	<7.35	Respiratory acidosis from hypoventilation

[a]Critical values vary by facility and laboratory.

BUN, Blood urea nitrogen; *CBC,* complete blood count; *RBCs,* red blood cells; *TSH,* thyroid-stimulating hormone (thyrotropin); *WBCs,* white blood cells.

BOX 19.18 Treatment of Thyroid Storm[a]

Antagonize Peripheral Effects of Thyroid Hormone
- Propranolol (Inderal): 1 to 3 mg IV, given 1 mg at a time IV bolus. After 2 minutes of no change, may be repeated once.
- If beta-blocker contraindicated, give reserpine 0.1 to 0.25 mg PO or guanethidine 25 to 50 mg PO every 6 to 8 hours

Inhibit Hormone Biosynthesis
- Propylthiouracil: PO loading dose of 200-400 mg q 4h for 24h until thyrotoxicosis controlled, or
- Methimazole (Tapazole): up to 60 mg PO loading dose, divided into 3 doses q 8h, then 5-15 mg PO daily.

Block Thyroid Hormone Release
Give 1 to 2 Hours After Propylthiouracil or Methimazole Loading Dose
- Saturated solution of potassium iodide (SSKI): 5 drops q 6h PO, mixed in 240 mL of water, juice, milk, or broth
- Alternatively, potassium iodide tablets: 250 mg PO tid

Supportive Therapy
- Hydrocortisone: 100 to 500 mg IV q 2-6h hours; or dexamethasone: 0.75-9 mg PO per day in divided doses q 6-12h
- Pharmacotherapy for heart failure or tachydysrhythmia
- Correct fluid and electrolyte imbalances
- Treat hyperthermia (avoid aspirin)
- High-calorie, high-protein diet

Identify and Treat Precipitating Cause

Patient and Family Education

[a]Doses are approximate and may vary based on the individual situation.
PO, Orally; *tid,* three times daily.

Blockage of thyroid hormone release. Iodide agents inhibit the release of thyroid hormones from the thyroid gland, inhibit thyroid hormone production, and decrease the vascularity and size of the thyroid gland. Serum T_4 levels decrease approximately 30% to 50% with any of these medications, with stabilization in 3 to 6 days.

Saturated solution of potassium iodide (SSKI) or Lugol's solution may be given orally or sublingually. These medications must be administered 1 to 2 hours after antithyroid medications (propylthiouracil or methimazole) to prevent the iodide from being used to synthesize more T_4. Ipodate (Oragrafin) and iopanoic acid (Telepaque) are radiographic contrast media that may be used to block thyroid hormone release. Iodide agents should be administered at least 1 hour after thioamide agents to avoid worsening of the crisis. Lithium carbonate inhibits the release of thyroid hormones but is more toxic, so it is used only in patients with an iodide allergy. Lithium carbonate is given orally or by nasogastric or rectal tube, and the dose is adjusted to maintain therapeutic serum levels. Glucocorticoids may be added to block conversion of T_4 to T_3 and may also minimize adrenal insufficiency that can accompany the crisis.[15]

Supportive care. Symptoms are aggressively treated. To manage fever, administer acetaminophen and consider applying cooling blankets or ice packs. Manage cardiac complications with prescribed pharmacotherapy. Administer oxygen to support the respiratory effort. Obtain orders for fluid replacements, and monitor hemodynamic status. Provide nutritional support. Lastly, identify and treat or remove precipitating factors.

Patient and family education. Education of patients, families, and significant others is crucial in identifying and preventing episodes of thyroid storm. Teaching varies depending on the long-term therapy chosen for each patient (e.g., medications versus radioactive iodine or surgery).

Myxedema Coma

Pathophysiology. *Myxedema coma* is the most extreme form of hypothyroidism and is life-threatening.[15] Myxedema coma in the absence of an associated stress or illness is uncommon, and infection is the most frequent stressor. The addition of stress to an already hypothyroid patient accelerates the metabolism and clearance of whatever thyroid hormone is present in the body. The patient experiences increased hormone use but decreased hormone production, which precipitates a crisis state. Common findings in patients with thyroid storm are presented with those of myxedema coma in Table 19.6.

Etiology. Myxedema coma is the end stage of improperly treated, neglected, or undiagnosed hypothyroidism.[15] It is a life-threatening emergency with a mortality rate as high as 50% despite appropriate therapy. Much of this mortality can be attributed to underlying illnesses. Most patients who develop myxedema coma are older adult women; it is rarely seen in young persons. It occurs more frequently in winter as a result of the increased stress of exposure to cold in a person who is unable to maintain body heat. Known precipitating factors include hypothermia, infection, stroke, trauma, and critical illness. Medications that may precipitate myxedema coma include those that affect the central nervous system, such as analgesics, anesthetics, barbiturates, narcotics, sedatives, tranquilizers, lithium, and amiodarone.[15] Many cases present in the winter months due to the belief that cold weather may trigger an increased risk for myxedema coma.

Assessment

Clinical presentation. Many of these patients may have had vague signs and symptoms of hypothyroidism for several years (Box 19.19). Many of the manifestations are attributable to the development of mucinous edema. This interstitial edema is the result of water retention and decreased protein. Fluid collects in soft tissues such as the face and in joints and muscles. It can also produce pericardial effusion. The clinical picture of myxedema coma varies with the rate of onset and severity. Diagnosis is based on the clinical signs and symptoms, a high index of suspicion, and a careful history and physical examination.

Cardiovascular disturbances. Cardiac function is depressed, resulting in decreases from baseline in heart rate, blood pressure, contractility, stroke volume, and cardiac output. The patient may develop a pericardial effusion, making heart tones distant. The electrocardiogram has decreased voltage because of the pericardial effusion.

- *Earliest signs:* Fatigue, weakness, muscle cramps, intolerance to cold, and weight gain.
- *Cardiovascular:* Bradycardia and hypotension.
- *Neurological:* Difficulty concentrating, slowed mentation, depression, lethargy, slow and deliberate speech, coarse and raspy voice, hearing loss, and vertigo.
- *Respiratory:* Dyspnea on exertion.
- *Gastrointestinal:* Decreased appetite, decreased peristalsis, anorexia, decreased bowel sounds, constipation, and paralytic ileus. However, the decreased metabolic rate also leads to weight gain.
- *Musculoskeletal:* Fluid in joints and muscles results in stiffness and muscle cramps.
- *Integumentary:* Dry, flaky, cool, coarse skin; dry, coarse hair; and brittle nails. The face is puffy and pallid, the tongue may be enlarged. The dorsa of the hands and feet are edematous. There may be a yellow tint to the skin from depressed hepatic conversion of carotene to vitamin A. Ecchymoses may develop from increased capillary fragility and decreased platelets.
- *Hematological:* Pernicious anemia and jaundice. Splenomegaly occurs in about 50% of patients. About 10% of patients have a decrease in neutrophils.
- *Ophthalmic:* Generalized mucinous edema in the eyelids and periorbital tissue.
- *Metabolic:* Elevated creatine phosphokinase, aspartate aminotransferase, lactate dehydrogenase, cholesterol, and triglyceride levels. Elevated cholesterol and triglyceride levels predispose persons with hypothyroidism to the development of atherosclerosis.

Pulmonary disturbances. The respiratory system responsiveness is depressed, producing hypoventilation, respiratory muscle weakness, and CO_2 retention. CO_2 narcosis may contribute to decreased mentation. As part of the picture of generalized mucinous edema and fluid retention, these patients may also develop pleural effusions or upper airway edema, further restricting their breathing.

Neurological disturbances. The low metabolic rate and resulting decreased mentation produce both psychological and physiological changes. The patient in hypothyroid crisis may present with somnolence, delirium, seizures, or coma. Personality changes such as paranoia and delusions may be evident.

Patients with hypothyroidism are unable to maintain body heat because of the decreased metabolic rate and decreased production of thermal energy. Because of this, patients may present in crisis after being stressed by exposure to cold. Hypothermia is present in 80% of patients with myxedema coma, and temperatures can be as low as 26.7°C (80°F). Patients with temperatures lower than 32°C (88.6°F) have a grave prognosis. If a patient with myxedema coma has a temperature greater than 37°C (98.6°F), underlying infection should be suspected.

Skeletal muscle disturbances. Slowed motor conduction produces decreased tendon reflexes and sluggish, awkward movements.

Laboratory evaluation. Serum T_4 and T_3 levels and resin T_3 uptake are low in patients with myxedema coma. In primary hypothyroidism, TSH levels are high. If hypothyroidism is the result of disease of the pituitary gland or hypothalamus (i.e.,

secondary or tertiary hypothyroidism), TSH levels are inappropriately normal or low. As in patients with thyroid storm, if myxedema coma is suspected, treatment should not be delayed while awaiting these results to confirm the diagnosis.

Serum sodium levels may be low as a result of impaired water excretion due to inappropriate ADH secretion and cortisol deficiency, which frequently accompany hypothyroidism. The patient should be monitored for signs and symptoms due to hyponatremia, such as weakness, muscle twitching, seizures, and coma.

Hypoglycemia is common and may be due to pituitary or hypophyseal disorders and/or adrenal insufficiency. Adrenal insufficiency may result in serum cortisol levels that are inappropriately low for stress. Laboratory manifestations of myxedema coma are summarized in Laboratory Alert: Thyroid Disorders.

Patient Problems. The following problems apply to a patient in myxedema coma based on assessment data:

- Low cardiac output due to decreased contractility, decreased heart rate, decreased stroke volume, pericardial effusion, dysrhythmias
- Decreased gas exchange due to hypoventilation, muscle weakness, decreased respiratory rate, ascites, pleural effusions
- Hypothermia due to inability of body to retain heat
- Excess fluid volume due to impaired water excretion
- Risk for injury due to edema, decreased platelet count
- Activity intolerance due to muscle weakness
- Inadequate nutrition due decreased appetite, decreased carbohydrate metabolism, hypoglycemia
- Need for health teaching due to myxedema coma: disease process, therapeutic regimen, and prevention of complications

Nursing and Medical Interventions. Myxedema coma requires immediate intervention if the patient is to survive. The primary objectives in the treatment of myxedema coma are identifying and treating the precipitating cause, providing thyroid replacement, restoring fluid and electrolyte balance, providing supportive care, and providing patient and family education. Box 19.20 details the treatment of myxedema coma. It is important to achieve physiological levels of thyroid hormone without incurring the adverse effects of excess thyroid hormones. Also refer to the Collaborative Plan of Care for the Critically Ill Patient (see Chapter 1).

Thyroid replacement. The best method of thyroid replacement is controversial. Either levothyroxine sodium (Synthroid; T_4) or liothyronine sodium (Cytomel; T_3) can be used. Levothyroxine ultimately provides the patient with both T_4 and, through peripheral conversion, T_3 replacement, whereas liothyronine sodium provides only T_3.

Levothyroxine sodium is commonly used for treatment. It has a smoother onset and a longer duration of effect. The preferred route is IV because absorption of oral or intramuscular levothyroxine is variable. The initial dose may be decreased if the patient has underlying factors such as angina, dysrhythmias, or other heart disease.

Liothyronine sodium has more pronounced metabolic effects, a more rapid onset (6 hours), and a shorter half-life (1 day) than levothyroxine. Because of liothyronine's potency, its administration may be complicated by angina, myocardial infarction, and cardiac irritability. For this reason, it is usually avoided in older adults.

The effects of levothyroxine are not as rapid as those of liothyronine, but its cardiac toxicity is lower. Serum levels of T_4 reach normal in 1 to 2 days. Levels of TSH begin to fall within 24 hours and return to normal within 10 to 14 days.

Fluid and electrolyte restoration. Thyroid replacement usually corrects hypotension or shock, but cautious volume expansion with saline also helps. Vasopressors are used with extreme caution because patients in myxedema coma are unable to respond to vasopressors until they have adequate levels of thyroid hormones available. Simultaneous administration of vasopressors and thyroid hormones is associated with myocardial irritability.

Hyponatremia usually responds to thyroid replacement and water restriction; the patient can resume water intake once thyroid hormones are replaced. If hyponatremia is severe (<120 mEq/L) or the patient is having seizures, hypertonic saline with or without a loop diuretic may be administered, but only until symptoms disappear or the sodium level is at least 120 mEq/L.

If a patient has hypoglycemia, adrenal insufficiency, or both, glucose is added to IV fluids. Glucocorticoid administration is recommended for all patients in the event that hypoadrenalism coexists with hypothyroidism. Hydrocortisone is the medication of choice for replacement. The adrenal abnormality may last for several weeks after thyroid replacement is begun, so this support is continued during that period.

Supportive care. Aggressively manage symptoms. Keep the room warm, and use passive rewarming methods to treat and prevent hypothermia. Avoid medications that depress respiration, such as narcotics. Assess and treat cardiac function. Monitor respiratory status and anticipate the need for mechanical ventilation.

Patient and family education. The education of patients, family, and significant others is critical in identifying and preventing episodes of myxedema coma.

ANTIDIURETIC HORMONE DISORDERS

Review of Physiology

The primary function of ADH is regulation of water balance and serum osmolality. ADH (also known as arginine vasopressin, or AVP) is produced in the supraoptic nuclei and paraventricular nuclei of the hypothalamus. These nuclei are positioned near the thirst center and osmoreceptors in the hypothalamus (Fig. 19.9). Once produced, ADH is stored in neurons in the posterior pituitary. Stimulation of the supraoptic and paraventricular nuclei causes release of ADH from nerve endings in the posterior pituitary. Nuclei are stimulated in several ways (Fig. 19.10). Osmoreceptors in the hypothalamus respond to changes in extracellular osmolality. Stretch receptors in the left atrium and baroreceptors in the carotid sinus and aortic arch respond to changes in circulating volume and blood pressure and stimulate the hypothalamus. Primary triggers for ADH release are increased serum osmolality, decreased blood volume (by >10%), and decreased blood pressure (5% to 10% drop). Other factors that stimulate ADH release are elevated serum sodium levels, trauma, hypoxia, pain, stress, and anxiety. Certain medications such as narcotics, barbiturates, anesthetics, and chemotherapeutic agents, also stimulate ADH release (see Fig. 19.10).

Once released, ADH acts on the renal distal tubules and collecting ducts to cause water reabsorption. In high concentrations,

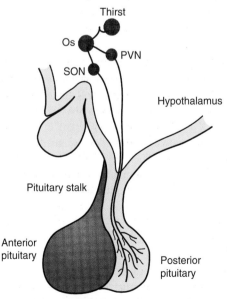

Fig. 19.9 The hypothalamic–posterior pituitary system. *Os,* Osmoreceptor; *PVN,* paraventricular nuclei; *SON,* supraoptic nuclei.

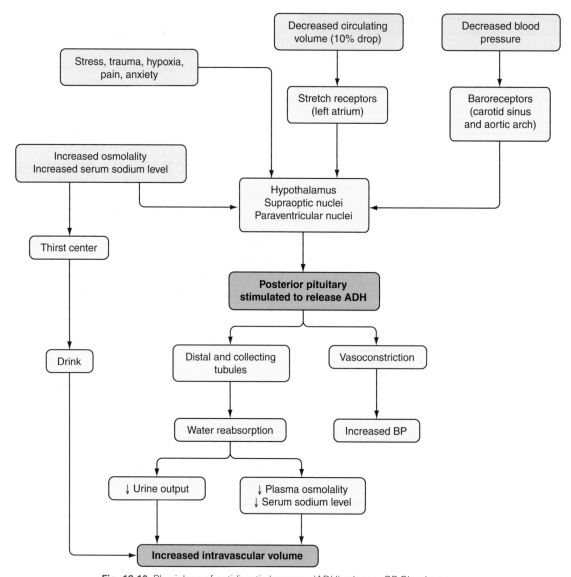

Fig. 19.10 Physiology of antidiuretic hormone (ADH) release. *BP,* Blood pressure.

ADH also acts on smooth muscles of the arterioles to produce vasoconstriction.

Two common disturbances of ADH are *diabetes insipidus* (DI) and the *syndrome of inappropriate antidiuretic hormone secretion* (SIADH). A less common disorder is cerebral salt wasting (CSW), which is similar to SIADH but with important differences. CSW is a disorder of sodium and fluid balance that occurs in patients with a neurological insult.[11] Differentiating CSW from SIADH is crucial because of opposing management strategies. Table 19.7 compares the electrolyte and fluid findings associated with DI, SIADH, and CSW.[6,11]

Diabetes Insipidus

Etiology. Various disorders produce neurogenic DI (Box 19.21), but the primary cause is traumatic injury to the posterior pituitary or hypothalamus as a result of head injury or surgery. Transient DI may be caused by trauma to the pituitary, manipulation of the pituitary stalk during surgery, or cerebral edema. Permanent DI occurs when more than 80% to 85% of hypothalamic nuclei or the proximal pituitary stalk is destroyed.

TABLE 19.7 Electrolyte and Fluid Findings in Antidiuretic Hormone Disorders

Finding	Diabetes Insipidus	SIADH	Cerebral Salt Wasting
Plasma volume	Decreased	Increased	Decreased
Serum sodium	Increased	Decreased	Decreased
Serum osmolality	Increased	Decreased	Normal or increased
Urine sodium	Normal	Increased	Increased
Urine osmolality	Decreased	Increased	Normal or increased

SIADH, Syndrome of inappropriate antidiuretic hormone secretion.

Nephrogenic DI may occur in genetically predisposed persons. It also may be acquired as a result of chronic renal disease, medications or other conditions that produce permanent kidney damage or inhibit the generation of cyclic adenosine monophosphate in the tubules.

Pathophysiology. DI results from an ADH deficiency *(neurogenic or central DI),* from ADH insensitivity *(nephrogenic DI),*

BOX 19.21 Causes of Diabetes Insipidus

Antidiuretic Hormone Deficiency (Neurogenic)
- *Idiopathic:* familial, congenital, autoimmune, genetic
- Intracranial surgery, especially in region of pituitary
- *Tumors:* craniopharyngioma, pituitary tumors, metastases to hypothalamus
- *Infections:* meningitis, encephalitis, syphilis, mycoses, toxoplasmosis
- *Granulomatous disease:* tuberculosis, sarcoidosis, histiocytosis
- Severe head trauma, anoxic encephalopathy, or any disorder that causes increased intracranial pressure

Antidiuretic Hormone Insensitivity (Nephrogenic)
- Hereditary or idiopathic
- *Renal disease:* pyelonephritis, amyloidosis, polycystic kidney disease, obstructive uropathy, transplantation
- *Multisystem disorders affecting kidneys:* multiple myeloma, sickle cell disease, cystic fibrosis
- *Metabolic disturbances:* chronic hypokalemia or hypercalcemia
- *Medications:* ethanol, phenytoin, lithium carbonate, amphotericin, methoxyflurane

Secondary Diabetes Insipidus
- Idiopathic
- Psychogenic polydipsia
- Hypothalamic disease: sarcoidosis
- Excessive IV fluid administration
- *Medication-induced disease:* anticholinergics, tricyclic antidepressants

or from excessive water intake *(secondary DI)*. Regardless of the cause, the effect is impaired renal conservation of water, resulting in polyuria (>3 L in 24 hours). As long as the thirst center remains intact and the person is able to respond to this thirst, fluid volume can be maintained. If the patient is unable to respond, severe dehydration results if fluid losses are not replaced.

Neurogenic DI occurs because of disruption of the neural pathways or structures involved in ADH production, synthesis, or release. Absent or diminished release of ADH from the posterior pituitary leads to free water loss and causes serum osmolality and serum sodium to rise. The posterior pituitary is unable to respond by increasing ADH levels; therefore the kidneys are not stimulated to reabsorb water, and excessive water loss results.

In nephrogenic DI, the kidney collecting ducts and distal tubules are unresponsive to ADH; although adequate levels of ADH may be synthesized and released, the kidneys are unable to conserve water in response to ADH. In patients with secondary DI, compulsive high-volume water consumption causes polyuria.

Assessment

Clinical presentation. Neurogenic DI usually occurs suddenly with an abrupt onset of polyuria, as much as 5 to 40 L in 24 hours. The onset of nephrogenic DI is more gradual. In both types, the urine is pale and dilute. The thirst mechanism is activated in conscious patients, and polydipsia occurs. If the patient is unable to replace the water lost by responding to thirst, signs of hypovolemia develop: hypotension, decreased skin turgor, dry mucous membranes, tachycardia, weight loss, and low right atrial and pulmonary artery occlusion pressures. Neurological signs and symptoms are seen with hypovolemia and hypernatremia.

Laboratory evaluation. The classic signs of DI are an inappropriately low urine osmolality, decreased urine specific gravity, and a high serum osmolality. Corresponding to the low urine osmolality is a decreased urine specific gravity. Serum osmolality is greater than 295 mOsm/kg, and the serum sodium level is greater than 145 mEq/L. The presence of hypokalemia or hypercalcemia suggests nephrogenic DI. Other values, such as BUN, may be elevated as a result of hemoconcentration. Further testing to differentiate neurogenic and nephrogenic DI includes water deprivation studies. However, these tests are inappropriate in the critically ill population (see Laboratory Alert box).

⚠ LABORATORY ALERT

Pituitary Disorders

Laboratory Test	Critical Value[a]	Explanation
Diabetes Insipidus		
Sodium (serum)	>145 mEq/L	Free water loss due to absent or diminished release of ADH or lack of response by the kidneys results in hemoconcentration of sodium.
Osmolality (serum)	>295 mOsm/kg	Free water loss due to absent or diminished release of ADH or lack of response by the kidneys increases serum osmolality; normal in secondary DI.
Osmolality (urine)	<100 mOsm/kg	Free water loss into urine decreases urine osmolality.
Sodium (urine)	40-200 mEq/L	Urine sodium is not affected.
Syndrome of Inappropriate Antidiuretic Hormone Secretion		
Sodium (serum)	<135 mEq/L	Free water retention due to oversecretion of ADH dilutes sodium.
Osmolality (serum)	<280 mOsm/kg	Free water retention due to oversecretion of ADH decreases osmolality.
Osmolality (urine)	>100 mOsm/kg	Lack of water excretion increases urine osmolality.
Sodium (urine)	>200 mEq/L	Sodium is excreted in an attempt to excrete excess water.
Cerebral Salt Wasting		
Sodium (serum)	<135 mEq/L	Kidneys are unable to conserve sodium.
Osmolality (serum)	>295 mOsm/kg	Kidneys are unable to conserve water.
Osmolality (urine)	<100 mOsm/kg	Free water loss into urine decreases urine osmolality.
Sodium (urine)	>200 mEq/L	Sodium wasting through renal tubules occurs.

[a]Critical values vary by facility and laboratory.
ADH, Antidiuretic hormone; *DI,* diabetes insipidus.

Patient Problems. The following problems may apply to a patient with DI:

- Decreased fluid volume due to deficient ADH, insensitivity of renal cells to ADH, polyuria, and inability to respond to thirst
- Changes in mental status due to decreased cerebral perfusion, cerebral dehydration, and hypernatremia

Nursing and Medical Interventions. The primary goals of treatment are to identify and correct the underlying cause and to restore normal fluid volume, osmolality, and electrolyte balance. Identifying the underlying cause is a necessary part of determining appropriate treatment, particularly medication therapy. Also refer to the Collaborative Plan of Care for the Critically Ill Patient (Chapter 1).

Volume replacement. Monitoring for signs and symptoms of hypovolemia is a priority. Vital signs must be recorded at least every hour, along with urine output. Hemodynamic monitoring may be instituted to evaluate fluid requirements and to monitor the patient's response to treatment. This is particularly important in older adult patients, who are likely to have concurrent cardiovascular and renal disease. Accurate intake and output and daily weights are essential. Measurement of plasma sodium and volume status assists in evaluating the patient's response to treatment.

Patients who are alert and able to respond to thirst usually drink enough water to avoid symptomatic hypovolemia. However, critically ill patients who develop DI and older adult patients with cognitive impairments are frequently unable to recognize or respond to thirst, so fluid replacement is essential.

If the patient has symptoms of hypovolemia, the volume already lost must be replaced. In addition, fluid is replaced every hour to keep up with current urine losses. Correction of hypernatremia and replacement of free water are achieved by administration of hypotonic solutions of dextrose in water. If the patient has circulatory failure, isotonic saline may be administered until hemodynamic stability and vascular volume have been restored.

Monitor the patient's neurological status frequently; alterations may indicate a change in fluid status, electrolyte status (e.g., sodium), or both. Avoid fluid overload from overly aggressive fluid replacement, particularly after hormone replacement therapy has been instituted.

Hormone replacement. Because of the decreased secretion of ADH, neurogenic DI is controlled primarily by administration of exogenous ADH preparations. These medications replace ADH and enable the kidneys to conserve water. They can be administered intravenously, intramuscularly, subcutaneously, intranasally, or orally. Injectable forms are typically more potent than the intranasal or oral forms. Absorption is more reliable through the IV route.

The drug most commonly used for management is desmopressin (DDAVP), a synthetic analog of vasopressin. Unlike aqueous vasopressin and lysine vasopressin, desmopressin is devoid of any vasoconstrictor effects and has a longer antidiuretic action (12 to 24 hours). Side effects are usually mild and include headache, nausea, and mild abdominal cramps; however, overmedication can produce water overload. Monitor the

patient for signs of dyspnea, hypertension, weight gain, hyponatremia, headache, or drowsiness.

Nephrogenic diabetes insipidus. Nephrogenic DI is treated with sodium restriction, which decreases the glomerular filtration rate and enhances fluid reabsorption. Administration of thiazide diuretics may increase tubular sensitivity to ADH.

Patient and family education. Patients who have a permanent ADH deficit require education on the following: (1) pathogenesis of DI; (2) dose, side effects, and rationale for prescribed medications; (3) parameters for notifying the provider; (4) importance of adherence to medication regimen; (5) importance of recording daily weight measurements to identify weight gain; (6) importance of wearing an identification bracelet; and (7) importance of drinking according to thirst and avoiding excessive drinking.

Syndrome of Inappropriate Antidiuretic Hormone Secretion

Etiology. Central nervous system disorders such as head injury, infection, hemorrhage, surgery, and stroke stimulate the hypothalamus or pituitary, producing excess secretion of ADH. A common cause of SIADH is ectopic production of ADH by malignant disease, especially small cell carcinoma of the lung. The malignant cells synthesize, store, and release ADH and thus place control of ADH outside the normal pituitary-hypothalamus feedback loops. Other types of malignancies known to produce SIADH include pancreatic and duodenal carcinoma, Hodgkin's lymphoma, sarcoma, and squamous cell carcinoma of the tongue.

Nonmalignant pulmonary conditions such as tuberculosis, pneumonia, lung abscess, and chronic obstructive pulmonary disease can also produce SIADH. As with malignant cells, it is believed that benign pulmonary tissue is capable of synthesizing and releasing ADH in certain disease states.

Many medications are associated with development of SIADH (Box 19.22). Of recent concern are reports of the effects of the widely prescribed selective serotonin reuptake inhibitors on ADH levels and function.[6] The mechanisms involved include increasing or potentiating the action of ADH, acting on the renal distal tubule to decrease free water excretion, or causing central release of ADH.

Pathophysiology. SIADH occurs when the body secretes excessive ADH due to plasma osmolality. This occurs when there is a failure in the negative feedback mechanism that regulates the release and inhibition of ADH. The results are inability to secrete a dilute urine, fluid retention, and dilutional hyponatremia. The primary treatment of SIADH is to restrict or withhold fluids.

Assessment

Clinical presentation. The clinical manifestations are primarily the result of water retention, hyponatremia, and hypoosmolality of the serum. The severity of the signs and symptoms is due to the rate of onset and the severity of the hyponatremia. See the Lifespan Considerations box for additional information related to older adults.

BOX 19.22 Causes of Syndrome of Inappropriate Antidiuretic Hormone

Ectopic Antidiuretic Hormone Production
- Small cell carcinoma of lung
- Cancer of prostate, pancreas, or duodenum
- Hodgkin's disease
- Sarcoma, squamous cell carcinoma of the tongue, thymoma
- *Nonmalignant pulmonary disease:* viral pneumonia, tuberculosis, chronic obstructive pulmonary disease, lung abscess

Central Nervous System Disorders
- Head trauma
- *Infections:* meningitis, encephalitis, brain abscess
- Intracranial surgery, cerebral aneurysm, brain tumor, cerebral atrophy, stroke
- Guillain-Barré syndrome, lupus erythematosus

Medications
- Angiotensin-converting enzyme inhibitors
- Amiodarone
- *Analgesics and narcotics:* morphine, fentanyl, acetaminophen
- *Antineoplastics:* vincristine, cyclophosphamide, vinblastine, cisplatin
- Barbiturates
- Carbamazepine (Tegretol) and oxcarbazepine (Trileptal)
- Ciprofloxacin
- General anesthetics
- Haloperidol (Haldol)
- Mizoribine
- Nicotine
- Nonsteroidal antiinflammatory medications
- Pentamidine
- *Serotonergic agents:* 3,4-methylenedioxymethamphetamine (MDMA; Ecstasy), selective serotonin reuptake inhibitors
- Thiazide diuretics
- Tricyclic antidepressants

Positive-Pressure Ventilation

LIFESPAN CONSIDERATIONS

Pituitary Disorders

Older Adults
- An increase in secretion of antidiuretic hormone (ADH) occurs with aging and increases the risk for dilutional hyponatremia.
- Older adults are at greater risk for the syndrome of inappropriate antidiuretic hormone secretion (SIADH) from any cause.
- Older adult patients often fail to recognize and respond to thirst and therefore are at increased risk for dehydration.[19]

Central nervous system. Manifestations such as weakness, lethargy, mental confusion, difficulty concentrating, restlessness, headache, seizures, and coma may occur in response to hyponatremia and hypoosmolality. Hypoosmolality disrupts the intracellular-extracellular osmotic gradient and causes a shift of water into brain cells, leading to cerebral edema and increased intracranial pressure. A decrease in the serum sodium level to lower than 120 mEq/L in 48 hours or less is usually associated with serious neurological symptoms and a mortality rate as high as 50%. If hyponatremia develops more slowly, the body is able to protect against cerebral edema, and the patient may remain asymptomatic even with a very low serum sodium level.

Gastrointestinal system. Congestion of the gastrointestinal tract and decreased motility occur because of hyponatremia. This is manifested by nausea and vomiting, anorexia, muscle cramps, and decreased bowel sounds.

Cardiovascular system. Water retention produces edema, increased blood pressure, and elevated central venous and pulmonary artery occlusion pressures.

Pulmonary system. Fluid overload in the pulmonary system produces increased respiratory rate, dyspnea, adventitious lung sounds, and frothy, pink sputum.

Laboratory evaluation. The hallmark of SIADH is hyponatremia and hypoosmolality in the presence of concentrated urine. A low serum osmolarity should trigger inhibition of ADH secretion, resulting in loss of water through the kidneys and dilute urine (see Laboratory Alert: Pituitary Disorders).

High urinary sodium levels (>20 mEq/L) help differentiate SIADH from other causes of hypoosmolality, hyponatremia, and volume overload (e.g., heart failure). In SIADH, renal perfusion (a major stimulus for sodium reabsorption) is usually adequate, so sodium is not conserved, resulting in urinary sodium excretion. In a disorder such as heart failure, renal perfusion is low because of decreased cardiac output triggering reabsorption of sodium.

Hemodilution may decrease other laboratory values such as BUN, creatinine, and albumin. SIADH should be suspected in a patient with evidence of hemodilution and urine that is hypertonic relative to plasma.

Patient Problems. The primary problem for the patient with SIADH is fluid overload due to water retention from excess ADH.

Nursing and Medical Interventions. The goals of therapy are to treat the underlying cause, to eliminate excess water, and to increase serum osmolality. In many instances, treatment of the underlying disorder (e.g., discontinuation of a responsible medication) is all that is needed to return the patient's condition to normal. Also refer to the Collaborative Plan of Care for the Critically Ill Patient (Chapter 1).

Fluid balance. In mild to moderate cases (serum sodium level, 125 to 135 mEq/L), fluid intake is restricted to 800 to 1000 mL/day, with liberal dietary salt and protein intake. Evaluate the patient's response by monitoring serum sodium levels, serum osmolality, and weight loss for a gradual return to baseline.

In severe, symptomatic cases (coma, seizures, serum sodium level <110 mEq/L), small amounts of hypertonic (1.5% to 3%) saline may be administered, following rigorous guidelines and with careful monitoring (Box 19.23). Correction of the serum sodium level must be done slowly—no more than 12 mEq within the first 24 hours. Administering hypertonic saline too rapidly, correcting the serum sodium level too rapidly, or both, can result in central pontine myelinolysis, a severe neurological syndrome that can lead to permanent brain damage or death.[11] The risk of heart failure is also significant. A diuretic such as furosemide may be given during hypertonic saline administration to promote diuresis and free water clearance. Treatments for chronic or resistant SIADH are listed in Box 19.24.

BOX 19.23 Nursing Considerations for Administration of 3% Sodium Chloride

- Administer via central rather than peripheral access.
- Administer via pump only.
- Rate should not exceed 50 mL/h.
- Monitor serum sodium levels every 4 hours; hold infusion if serum sodium level exceeds 155 mEq/L.
- Wean solution rather than stopping abruptly.
- Monitor level of responsiveness for evidence of decline (could indicate cerebral edema or worsening hyponatremia).
- Monitor lungs sounds for crackles indicating pulmonary edema.
- Monitor intake and output every hour.

BOX 19.24 Treatments for Chronic or Resistant Syndrome of Inappropriate Antidiuretic Hormone Secretion[a]

- Water restriction of 800 to 1000 mL/day.
- Administration of loop diuretics in conjunction with increased salt and potassium intake is the safest method for treating chronic hyponatremia. The diuretic prevents urine concentration, and the increased salt and potassium intake increases water output by increasing delivery of solutes to the kidney.

[a]Doses are approximate and may vary based on the individual situation. *ADH*, Antidiuretic hormone; *PO*, orally.

Nursing. Prevention of SIADH may not be possible, but early detection and treatment may prevent more serious sequelae from occurring. Be aware of the populations at risk, and monitor at-risk patients for clinical signs of alterations.

Closely monitor fluid and electrolyte balance. Weigh the patient daily. Hourly, record intake and output and measure the urine specific gravity. Fluid overload may occur from hypervolemia or from too rapid administration of hypertonic saline. Monitor for fluid overload by assessing for tachycardia, increased blood pressure, increased hemodynamic pressures, full bounding pulses, and distended neck veins. Monitor respiratory function for signs of tachypnea, labored respirations, shortness of breath, or fine crackles. Regularly monitor potassium and magnesium levels for the need to replace diuresis-induced losses.

Adherence to fluid restriction is critical but difficult for patients. Ensure that the patient and family understand the importance of the restriction and that they are included in planning types and timing of fluids. Encourage patients to choose fluids high in sodium content, such as milk, tomato juice, and beef or chicken broth. To relieve some of the discomfort caused by fluid restriction, provide frequent mouth care, oral rinses without swallowing, chilled beverages, and hard candy.

Assess the patient's neurological status to monitor the effects of treatment and to identify complications. Observe the patient for subtle changes that may indicate water intoxication, such as fatigue, weakness, headache, or changes in level of conscious-

ness. Strict adherence to rates of administration of hypertonic (3%) saline solutions and measurement of serial serum sodium levels are essential to prevent neurological sequelae. Institute seizure precautions if the patient's sodium level decreases to less than 120 mEq/L.

Patient and family education. Some patients with SIADH may need long-term treatment, ongoing monitoring, or both. These patients and their families require instruction on the following: (1) early signs and symptoms to report to the healthcare provider—weight gain, lethargy, weakness, nausea, and mental status changes; (2) the significance of adherence to fluid restriction; (3) dose, side effects, and rationale for prescribed medications; and (4) the importance of daily weights.

Cerebral Salt Wasting

Etiology. Patients with any type of serious brain insult may develop CSW. Brain trauma, subarachnoid hemorrhage and other types of stroke, and meningitis are associated with development of CSW.[6,11]

Pathophysiology. The exact pathophysiology of CSW is unknown. A defect in renal sodium transport has been suggested,[6] and a change from cerebral salt wasting to renal salt wasting has been suggested as a more accurate term. Natriuretic peptides, which are commonly released in severe brain injury, and impaired aldosterone have been implicated as factors in defective renal sodium transport. However, research has produced conflicting data.

Assessment

Clinical presentation. The findings associated with CSW are due to hypovolemia and hyponatremia. Signs of hypovolemia include decreased skin turgor, dry mucous membranes, tachycardia, weight loss, and hypotension. Signs of hyponatremia include weakness, lethargy, mental confusion, difficulty concentrating, restlessness, headache, seizures, and coma. Neurological signs and symptoms are seen with both hypovolemia and hyponatremia.

Laboratory evaluation. An increased serum osmolality, decreased serum sodium, and increased urine sodium characterize CSW. Hemoconcentration may increase other laboratory values such as BUN, creatinine, and albumin (see Laboratory Alert: Pituitary Disorders).

Patient Problems. The primary problem that may apply to a patient with CSW is low fluid volume and risk for dehydration due to lack of renal sodium retention and diuresis.

Nursing and Medical Interventions. The primary goal of treatment is to simultaneously restore both sodium and fluid volume. Replacing fluids without sodium may worsen the hyponatremia, resulting in life-threatening consequences. Both isotonic saline and hypertonic (1.5% to 3%) saline are used. Isotonic saline is administered to replace volume at a rate that matches urine output, and hypertonic saline is given so that sodium levels increase at a rate of no more than

12 mEq/h. Oral or IV fludrocortisone, 100-200 mcg daily, may be given to increase sodium retention in the renal tubules. Refer to the Collaborative Plan of Care for the Critically Ill Patient (Chapter 1).

 CRITICAL REASONING ACTIVITY

In a patient with neurological injury, how do laboratory values help to differentiate diabetes insipidus (DI), syndrome of inappropriate antidiuretic hormone secretion (SIADH), and cerebral salt wasting (CSW)?

CASE STUDY

Mr. F., a 68-year-old man, is admitted to the critical care unit from the emergency department with respiratory failure and hypotension. His history is significant for type 2 diabetes mellitus, steroid-dependent chronic obstructive pulmonary disease, peripheral vascular disease, and cigarette and alcohol abuse. His medications at home include glipizide, prednisone, and a metered-dose inhaler with albuterol and ipratropium (Combivent). In the emergency department he received a single dose of ceftriaxone and etomidate for intubation.

On examination he is intubated, on pressure-controlled ventilation, and receiving normal saline at 200 mL/h and dopamine at 8 mcg/kg/min. His blood pressure is 86/50 mm Hg; heart rate, 126 beats/min; oxygen saturation, 88%; and temperature, 39.6°C. His cardiac rhythm shows sinus tachycardia and nonspecific ST-T wave changes. Arterial blood gas values are as follows: pH, 7.21; PaO_2, 83 mm Hg; $PaCO_2$, 50 mm Hg; and bicarbonate, 12 mEq/L. Other laboratory values are as follows: serum glucose, 308 mg/dL; serum creatinine, 2.1 mg/dL; and white blood cell count, 19,000/mm³.

Questions

1. What disease state do you suspect this patient is experiencing and why?
2. What potential endocrine complications do you anticipate?
3. What further laboratory studies would you want? What results do you anticipate?
4. What treatment goals and strategies do you anticipate?
5. In providing patient and family education and support, what issues need to be addressed immediately and which can be delayed?

REFERENCES

1. American Diabetes Association. Classification and diagnosis of diabetes mellitus. *Diab Care*. 2019;42(Suppl 1):S13–S28.
2. American Diabetes Association. Diabetes care in the hospital, nursing home, and skilled nursing facility. *Diab Care*. 2019;42(Suppl 1):S173–S181.
3. American Diabetes Association. Standards of medical care in diabetes. *Diab Care*. 2019;42(Suppl 1):S187–S193.
4. American Diabetes Association. Older adults. *Diab Care*. 2019;42 (Suppl 1):S139–S147.
5. Baldisseri MR. Cardiovascular and endocrinologic changes associated with pregnancy. In: Vincent JL, Abraham E, Moore FA, et al., eds. *Textbook of Critical Care*. 7th ed. Philadelphia, PA: Elsevier; 2017:988–993.e1.
6. Brimioulle S. Diabetes insipidus. In: Vincent JL, Abraham E, Moore FA, et al., eds. *Textbook of Critical Care*. 7th ed. Philadelphia, PA: Elsevier; 2017:1043–1045.e1.
7. Burand CF, Young LA, American Diabetes Association. *Medical Management of Type 2 Diabetes*. 7th ed. Alexandria, VA: Helm Publishing; 2019.
8. Centers for Disease Control and Prevention. *National Diabetes Statistics Report: Estimates of Diabetes and Its Burden on the United States, 2018*. Atlanta, GA: US Department of Health and Human Services, Centers for Disease Control and Prevention; 2018.
9. Cornell S, Halstenson C, Miller DK. *The Art and Science of Diabetes Self-Management: Education Desk Reference*. 4th ed. Chicago, IL: American Association of Diabetes Educators; 2017.
10. Drasnin B. *Managing Diabetes and Hyperglycemia in the Hospital Setting*. Alexandria, VA: American Diabetes Association; 2016:123.
11. Fried E, Weissman C. Water metabolism. In: Vincent JL, Abraham E, Moore FA, et al., eds. *Textbook of Critical Care*. 7th ed. Philadelphia, PA: Elsevier; 2017:743–750.e1.
12. Gerlach H. Adrenal insufficiency. In: Vincent JL, Abraham E, Moore FA, et al., eds. *Textbook of Critical Care*. 7th ed. Philadelphia, PA: Elsevier; 2017:1024–1033.e2.
13. Gosmanov AR, Gosmanova EO, Kitabchi AE. Hyperglycemic crises: Diabetic ketoacidosis (DKA) and hyperglycemic hyperosmolar state (HHS). In: Feingold KR, Anawalt B, Boyce A, et al., eds. *Endotext* [Internet]. South Dartmouth, MA: MDText.com, Inc.; 2018. https://www.ncbi.nlm.nih.gov/books/NBK279052/
14. Griesdale DEG, de Souza RJ, van Dam RM, et al. Intensive insulin therapy and mortality among critically ill patients: A meta-analysis including NICE-SUGAR study data. *Can Med Assoc J*. 2009; 180:821–827.
15. Leung AM, Farwell AP. Thyroid disorders. In: Vincent JL, Abraham E, Moore FA, et al., eds. *Textbook of Critical Care*. 7th ed. Philadelphia, PA: Elsevier; 2017:1034–1042.e2.
16. Mesotten D, Ven Den Berghe G. Hyperglycemia and blood glucose control. In: Vincent JL, Abraham E, Moore FA, et al. *Textbook of Critical Care*. 7th ed. Philadelphia, PA: Elsevier; 2017:1018–1023.e2.
17. NICE-SUGAR Study Investigators. Intensive versus conventional glucose control in critically ill patients. *N Engl J Med*. 2009:360:1283–1297.
18. Wang CCL, Shah AC, American Diabetes Association. *Medical Management of Type 1 Diabetes*. 7th ed. Alexandria, VA: Helm Publishing; 2017.
19. Winton MB. Endocrine function. In: Meiner SE, Yeager JJ. *Gerontologic Nursing*. 6th ed. St. Louis, MO: Elsevier; 2019:521–571.
20. World Health Organization. 10 Facts About Diabetes. http://www.who.int/features/factfiles/diabetes/en/. Published 2016. Accessed June 19, 2019.

Trauma and Surgical Management

Linda Staubli, MSN, RN, CCRN-K, ACCNS-AG
Mary Beth Flynn Makic, PhD, RN, CCNS, CCRN-K, FAAN, FNAP, FCNS

Many additional resources, including self-assessment exercises, are located on the Evolve companion website at http://evolve.elsevier.com/Sole/.
- Animations
- Clinical Skills: Critical Care Collections
- Student Review Questions
- Video Clips

INTRODUCTION

Trauma is defined as an injury or wound to a living tissue caused by external force.[64] Traumatic injury typically includes unintentional injuries and violence-related injuries.[23] Every year an estimated 27 million emergency department (ED) visits are attributed to traumatic injury and 2.8 million people are hospitalized due to injuries.[23]

Injury and violence affect everyone, regardless of age, race, or economic status. Unintentional injury is the third leading cause of death in the United States, predominantly claiming the lives of young individuals.[22,24] Only heart disease and cancer result in a higher death rate. The four major mechanisms of injury, accounting for 73.3% of all injury deaths, are poisoning (e.g., prescription or illegal drug overdose), motor vehicle traffic events, firearms, and falls.[22,24,27,29]

An overarching goal in trauma care is prevention. However, when traumatic injuries occur, the priority is early and aggressive intervention to save life and limb. This chapter provides a review of trauma systems, the trauma team concept, the systematic and standardized approach to trauma care, and phases of trauma care. Because the nature of traumatic events usually requires surgical interventions, the postsurgical management of the trauma patient is discussed. Special populations, common traumatic injuries, and mass casualty incident response are also described.

Trauma Demographics

Motor vehicle crashes (MVCs) are the leading cause of death in the United States, with more than 100 people dying every day and more than 2.5 million drivers and passengers treated in EDs each year as the result of a MVCs.[25] Trauma is frequently referred to as a disease of the young because injury is the leading cause of death in persons ages 1 to 44 years in the United States.[23] MVCs are the leading cause of death for persons 15 to 24 years of age.[22,24] Approximately six teens ages 16 to 19 years die in MVCs in the United States every day. Although people ages 15 to 19 years represent only 6.5% of the US population, they account for 8.4% ($13.6 billion) of the total costs of MVC injuries.[27] Fortunately, MVC injuries are preventable, and proven strategies can improve the safety of young drivers on the road.[25]

A peak in trauma-related injuries also occurs between the ages of 25 and 44 years, in which poisoning from prescription or illegal drugs is the leading cause of unintentional deaths; MVCs are the next highest cause in this age group.[24,30] In 2016 the age-adjusted rate of drug overdose deaths was more than three times the rate in 1999, with increases in death rate as high as 18% per year.[26] Adults ages 25 to 54 years had the highest rates of drug overdose deaths at around 35 per 100,000.[26]

Unintentional injuries and deaths also peak in the population 65 years of age and older and consist of injuries related to falls.[24] Males are more likely than females to experience traumatic injury.[24]

Trauma is a major healthcare and economic concern because of the loss of life, the societal burden in terms of lost productivity and increased disability of injured persons, and the consumption of healthcare resources. Economic factors associated with traumatic injury include both direct and indirect costs. Direct costs are related to the actual expense of treatment and rehabilitative care. Indirect costs are associated with lost work, physical and psychological disability (temporary and permanent), and lost productivity. Traumatic injuries and violence have been estimated to cost more than $600 billion in medical care and lost productivity each year.[23] A recent study assessed these costs to be as high as $1.8 trillion when applying an injury cost model to include an estimated value of lost quality of life.[93] Almost 10% ($168 billion) of total US medical expenditures is attributable to injury care costs.[35]

Injury is a potentially preventable public health problem of enormous magnitude, whether measured by years of productive life lost, prolonged or permanent disability, or financial cost. Advocates of organized trauma systems identify prevention as an essential component of a structured approach to trauma care. Once a trauma injury happens, an organized and structured approach to trauma care has repeatedly demonstrated improved outcomes with decreased patient morbidity and mortality.[2-4,69] Nurses play an essential role in the care of the patient after traumatic injury, from prevention to resuscitation through rehabilitation.

SYSTEMS APPROACH TO TRAUMA CARE

Trauma System

Trauma systems are effective in reducing morbidity and mortality of severely injured individuals by providing care to all injured patients in an organized, coordinated manner across geographical areas and the continuum of care.[3,4,20,42] Optimal trauma care requires a systematic approach that is coordinated along the entire continuum of injury care, including injury prevention, prehospital advanced life-support interventions, rapid transport, acute hospital care with evidence-based trauma protocols

and resources to care for injured patients, rehabilitation, and reassimilation of the injured individual into the community (Fig. 20.1).[3,83] This model of a trauma system expands care from single centers to multiple facilities. Specifically, a network of regional and state trauma systems allows for the best possible care to be delivered for the type and severity of traumatic injury by matching the patient's medical needs to the level of trauma hospital with the necessary resources. The goal of every trauma system is to match the needs of injured patients to the capabilities of the trauma center.[2] Therefore a trauma system includes a combination of levels of designated trauma centers with other acute care facilities. Levels of trauma centers distinguish a difference in resources available within the specific hospital.[2]

Levels of Trauma Care. Formal categorization of trauma care facilities, based on resources and capabilities to meet the needs of an injured patient, is essential to provide optimal care. The American College of Surgeons (ACS) has established the process for categorizing hospitals as Levels I, II, III, or IV based on minimum standards at each level.[4] The organization also conducts on-site reviews of hospitals seeking trauma designation

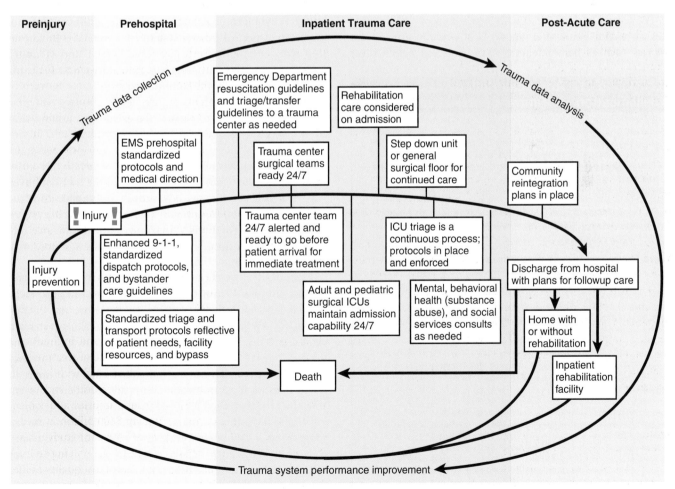

Fig. 20.1 A preplanned trauma care continuum. *EMS,* Emergency medical services; *ICU,* intensive care unit. (From US Department of Health and Human Services [HHS], Health Resources and Services Administration. *Model Trauma System Planning and Evaluation.* Rockville, MD: HHS; 2006. http://www.facs.org/quality-programs/trauma/tsepc/resources.)

and provides consultations with hospitals, communities, and states regarding trauma centers.[4] A current list of hospitals with verified trauma centers is published on the ACS website (http://www.facs.org/trauma/verified.html).

The ACS trauma system identifies four levels of trauma care: Levels I, II, III, and IV (Table 20.1).[3] Hospitals of all designations collaborate to develop transfer agreements and treatment protocols that maximize patient survival. All states with an identified trauma system are divided into regions, each with an identified lead trauma hospital. The lead hospital is usually the Level I trauma center and has the additional responsibility of engaging other regional trauma centers, acute care facilities, and emergency medical services (EMS) in a systemwide approach to continually enhance trauma care services.[2-4]

Trauma Continuum. Death caused by traumatic injury is historically described as having a trimodal distribution, implying that death due to injury occurs in one of three peaks. The first peak, labeled as *immediate death*, occurs within seconds to minutes from the time of injury. These patients are declared dead at the scene or shortly after arrival in an ED. Death is caused by severe injuries, such as apnea from severe brain or high spinal cord injury or massive hemorrhage.[2] Only trauma prevention will decrease deaths that occur in the first peak.

The second peak is labeled *early death*. It occurs within minutes to several hours after injury. Death results from severe injuries such as hemopneumothorax, ruptured spleen, liver laceration, pelvic fracture, or other multiple injuries associated with significant blood loss. The first hour of emergent care, called the "golden hour," focuses on rapid assessment, resuscitation, and treatment of life-threatening injuries.

The third peak, *late death,* occurs several days to weeks after the initial injury. It is most often the result of sepsis, acute respiratory distress syndrome (ARDS), increased intracranial pressure (ICP), and multiple organ dysfunction syndrome (MODS).

Since the seminal publication of a trimodal distribution of trauma deaths, the development of trauma systems has altered the distribution of deaths to a bimodal or unimodal pattern with an overall reduction in trauma mortality.[2,47,73] Specifically, late deaths accounted for approximately 20% of all trauma deaths in the 1970s, and now only 9% of deaths are attributed to late deaths.[46] This shifting distribution of death supports the central concept of trauma systems: matching patients' severity of injury to the available resources for optimal care at a designated trauma center. Special resources, including early surgical management of injuries, are needed to decrease the morbidity and mortality of severely injured patients; therefore the most critically injured patients should be cared for in higher-level trauma centers to maximize patient outcomes.[2,5,6]

Injury Prevention. Traumatic injury prevention is the most important aspect of trauma system effectiveness.[32] In partnership with community organizations, Level I and II trauma centers must implement programs that address one of the major causes of injury in the community.[6]

Injury prevention occurs at three levels. *Primary prevention* involves interventions to prevent the event (e.g., driving safety classes, speed limits, campaigns against drinking and driving, fall prevention interventions, domestic violence prevention campaigns, drug awareness campaigns). *Secondary prevention* entails strategies to minimize the impact of the traumatic event (e.g., seat belt use, airbags, advances in automobile construction, car seats, helmets, antibullying hotlines). *Tertiary prevention* refers to interventions to maximize patient outcomes after a traumatic event through emergency response systems, medical care, and rehabilitation.

Historically, traumatic events were considered accidents or events that resulted from human error, fate, or bad luck. Today, it is understood that injuries and violence are not random events.[34,87] An individual's knowledge, risk-taking behaviors, beliefs, and decisions to engage in certain activities influence the outcomes of actions. The word *accident* conveys a message of randomness in which an individual cannot prevent the event. Because most traumatic events are considered preventable, this word has been removed from discussion of traumatic injuries such as those sustained in MVCs. Changing the language—*motor vehicle crash* instead of *motor vehicle accident*—conveys the message that efforts can be implemented to prevent MVCs and that additional behaviors, such as wearing a seat belt, may minimize their impact.

Nurses are role models for trauma prevention within their families and communities and through political involvement. Simple efforts include writing letters to local and national policy

TABLE 20.1 American College of Surgeons Classification of Trauma Center Level

Level	
Level I	• Provides comprehensive trauma care • Serves as a regional resource center to provide leadership in education, outreach, and systems planning • Admits at least 1200 trauma patients annually or has at least 240 admissions with an Injury Severity Score (ISS) >15 • Provides 24-hour in-house availability of an attending surgeon, who will be in the emergency department on patient arrival or within 15 min for the highest level of activation • Conducts trauma research
Level II	• Provides comprehensive trauma care as a supplement to a Level I center • Meets the same attending surgeon expectations for care as a Level I center
Level III	• Provides immediate emergency care and stabilization of a patient before transfer to a higher level of care • Provides continuous general surgical coverage with a maximum response time of 30 min after patient arrival in the emergency department • Serves a community that does not have immediate access to a Level I or II center
Level IV	• Provides advanced trauma life support before transfer to higher-level trauma center • Has a primary goal of resuscitation and stabilization of the patient and arrangement for immediate transfer to a higher level of care

Modified from American College of Surgeons, Committee on Trauma. *Resources for Optimal Care of the Injured Patient, 2014.* Chicago, IL: American College of Surgeons, Committee on Trauma; 2014.

makers encouraging changes in laws and enforcement of public policies favoring injury prevention, such as helmet and seat belt laws, laws regarding driving under the influence of drugs or alcohol, laws limiting access to firearms, and support programs to end domestic violence and bullying. Involvement in injury and violence prevention programs includes supporting community and national coalition networks for prevention, such as Mothers Against Drunk Drivers and antibullying campaigns.[82] Nurses collaborate with trauma prevention coordinators to provide ongoing injury prevention education to patients and families.[86,90]

Trauma Team Concept. The term *trauma team,* similar to a code team, refers to healthcare professionals who respond immediately to and participate in the initial resuscitation and stabilization of the trauma patient. Box 20.1 lists the composition of a typical trauma team. Trauma care begins in the field when the EMS team responds to an event. Trauma systems work with EMS teams to create protocols that maximize treatment in the field. Once a patient has been stabilized in the field, the EMS team communicates with the hospital en route and the hospital acute care trauma team is activated. Essential to the team approach is ensuring that each team member is preassigned and understands the specific responsibilities inherent in a particular team role. The *trauma surgeon* is ultimately responsible for the activities of the trauma team and acts as the team leader in establishing rapid assessment, resuscitation, stabilization, and intervention priorities. Other team members, such as ED physicians, consultants (e.g., orthopedic surgeons, neurosurgeons, otolaryngologists, thoracic surgeons, ophthalmologists, plastic surgeons), nurses, pharmacists, respiratory therapists, social workers, chaplains, and interventional radiologists, all have specific responsibilities. Each member of the trauma team is vital to meeting the needs of a patient with multiple traumas.

> **! CLINICAL ALERT**
>
> Evidence suggests that healthcare professionals who engage in stress reduction, mindfulness techniques (e.g., meditation, self-awareness skills, journaling), and regular exercise are more resilient when faced with difficult work situations such as trauma-emergency response situations.[33,63,80]

BOX 20.1 Multiprofessional Trauma Team

- Emergency medical services (EMS) response team
- Trauma surgeon (team leader)
- Emergency physician
- Anesthesiologist
- Trauma nurse team leader (coordinates and directs nursing care)
- Trauma resuscitation nurse (hangs IV fluids, blood, and medications; assists physicians)
- Trauma scribe (records all interventions on the trauma flowsheet)
- Pharmacist
- Respiratory therapist
- Laboratory phlebotomist
- Radiology technologist
- Social worker or pastoral services provider
- Hospital security officer
- Physician specialists (neurosurgeon, orthopedic surgeon, urological surgeon)

MECHANISMS OF INJURY

Injury and death result from both unintentional events and deliberate actions such as violent aggression or suicide. The term *mechanism of injury* refers to how a traumatic event occurred, the injuring agent, and information about the type and amount of energy exchanged during the event. Knowledge of the mechanism of injury assists the trauma team in early identification and management of injuries that may not be apparent on initial assessment.[2,3,59] Understanding the mechanism of traumatic injury provides insight into the transfer of energy to the body guiding the assessment and interventions to minimize the chance of missing injuries that are more subtle (e.g., organ contusions). Questions regarding mechanisms of injury are directed to the patient (if applicable), prehospital care providers, law enforcement personnel, or bystanders in an attempt to reenact the scene of the trauma (Box 20.2).

Personal and environmental risk factors include patient age, gender, race, alcohol or substance abuse, geography, and temporal variation. The term *temporal variation* describes the pattern and timing of the trauma. For example, injuries and violent deaths occur most frequently on weekends, and unintentional injuries occur most often during recreational activities. Injury may also occur when patients are deficient in oxygen, as with drowning or suffocation, or in response to cold, leading to frostbite.

The transfer of energy causes traumatic injury. Energy may be kinetic (e.g., crashes, falls, blast injuries, penetrating injuries), thermal, electrical, chemical, or radiant. *Kinetic energy* is defined as mass multiplied by velocity squared. Therefore the greater the mass and velocity (speed), the more significant the displacement of *kinetic energy* to body structures, resulting in more severe injury. The effects of the energy released and the resultant injuries depend on the force of impact, the duration of impact, the body part involved, the injuring agent, and the presence of associated risk factors.[59]

Injury patterns resulting from energy exchange are further described as blunt, penetrating, and blast injuries. The incidence of blunt trauma is usually greater in rural and suburban areas, whereas penetrating trauma occurs more frequently in inner-city urban neighborhoods. Blast injuries include construction site explosions, fireworks, and terrorist attacks.[47,60]

BOX 20.2 Questions to Ask to Determine Mechanism of Injury and Potential Complications

- Was the patient wearing a seat belt?
- Was the airbag deployed?
- What was the speed of the vehicle on impact?
- Where was the patient located in the car? Driver? Passenger? Front seat or back seat?
- Was the patient wearing a helmet (e.g., for a bicycle, motorcycle, or snow sporting crash)?
- What type of weapon was used (e.g., length of knife, type and caliber of gun)?
- How far did the patient fall (or how far was the patient thrown by the impact)?
- How long was the patient in the field before emergency medical services (EMS) arrived?
- Was there a death in the vehicle or at the event?

Blunt Trauma

Blunt trauma is the most common mechanism of injury.[59] It most often results from MVCs, but it also occurs from motorcycle crashes, assaults with blunt objects, falls from heights, sports-related activities, and pedestrians struck by a motor vehicle. The severity of injury varies. Blunt trauma may be caused by accelerating, decelerating, shearing, crushing, and compressing forces. Vehicular injury often results from a mechanism of acceleration-deceleration forces. The vehicle and the body accelerate and travel at an identified speed. In normal circumstances, the vehicle and body slow to a motionless state concurrently. However, when a vehicle stops abruptly, the body continues to travel forward until it comes in contact with a stationary object such as the dashboard, windshield, or steering column. Injury occurs in the presence of rapid deceleration, when the movement ceases and contents within the body continue to travel within an enclosed space or compartment. An example of this occurs when a passenger's head strikes the windshield after the automobile collides with a cement barrier. The brain tissue strikes the cranium and is thrown back against the opposite side of the cranial vault, with a resulting coup-contrecoup injury. Fig. 20.2 shows potential sites of injury to an unrestrained passenger and driver as a result of blunt trauma.

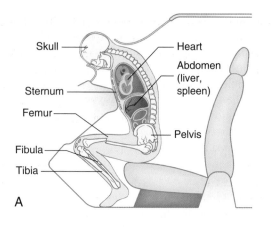

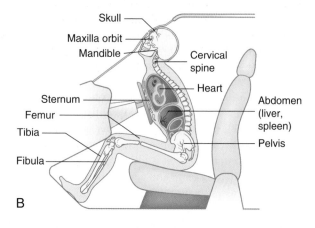

⁇ CRITICAL REASONING ACTIVITY

A patient presents to the trauma center after a motor vehicle crash en route to an antique automobile event. The patient was restrained by his seat belt; however, he was driving an antique car that did not have airbags. He was awake at the scene, but his level of consciousness quickly declined during transport by emergency medical services (EMS). Initial assessment revealed a 6-cm scalp laceration, a right closed femur fracture, four broken ribs, and possible cardiac and pulmonary contusions. What additional prehospital information would be helpful in anticipating care for this patient? Considering the mechanism and patterns of the injuries, what are the immediate nursing management priorities for this patient?

Body tissues and structures respond to kinetic energy in different ways. Low-density porous tissues and structures, such as the lungs, tolerate energy transference and often experience little damage because of their elasticity. Conversely, organs such as the heart, spleen, and liver are less resilient because of their high-density tissue and decreased ability to release energy without resultant tissue damage.[50] These types of organs often present with lacerations, contusions, or rupture. The severity of injury resulting from a blunt force is contingent on the duration of energy exposure, the body organ involved, and the underlying structures.

Blunt trauma requires expert clinical judgment to assess and diagnose actual and potential injuries, as organ injury from blunt trauma may not be immediately visible. Knowledge of the mechanism of injury and the adverse effects of blunt force is important.

Penetrating Trauma

Penetrating trauma results from impalement of the body by foreign objects (e.g., knives, bullets, debris). Penetrating injuries are more easily diagnosed and treated than blunt

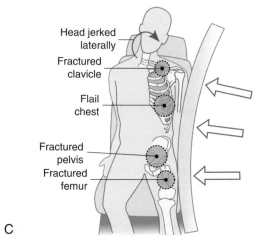

Fig. 20.2 Potential sites of blunt trauma injury to an unrestrained passenger and driver in a motor vehicle crash. **A,** Unrestrained passenger in front seat. **B,** Unrestrained driver. **C,** Lateral impact collision. (From Herm RL. Biomechanics and mechanism of injury. In: Cohen SS, ed. *Trauma Nursing Secrets.* Philadelphia, PA: Hanley & Belfus; 2003.)

force injuries because of the obvious signs of injury. Stab wounds are low-velocity injuries; the velocity is equal only to the speed with which the object was thrust into the body. The direct path of injury occurs when the impaled object contacts underlying vessels and tissues. Important considerations in a stabbing are the length and width of the impaling object and the presence of vital organs in the area of the stab wound. Gender differences are seen and may provide information on the trajectory of the injury. Women tend to stab with a downward thrust, whereas male assailants use an upward force.

Ballistic trauma is categorized as either medium- or high-velocity injuries. Medium-velocity weapons are handguns and some rifles. High-velocity weapons are assault weapons and hunting rifles.[75] High-velocity injuries result in greater dissipation of the kinetic energy and more significant bodily injury. The velocity and type of bullet (missile) influence the transfer of energy creating tissue injury. As the missile penetrates the tissues, vessels are stretched and compressed, creating tissue damage (referred to as a *cavitation*). Depending on the range, the distance from the weapon to the point of bodily impact, and the velocity of the missile, the cavitation may be as great as 30 times the diameter of the bullet. As bullets travel through the body, damage to surrounding tissues and organs may occur. Knowledge of the type of bullet (e.g., size, round versus hollow point, shotgun pellet) influences the assessment as to the type of internal tissue damage that may have occurred.

Assessment of the penetrating injuries from a gunshot involves examination of the entrance and exit wounds. The entrance wound is usually smaller than the exit wound; however, forensic experts, rather than the trauma team, determine the direction of the bullet's path.[75] Penetrating injuries are monitored closely for subsequent complications, including organ damage, hemorrhage, and infection.

Blast Injuries

Blast injuries are forms of blunt and penetrating trauma. Energy exchanged from the blast causes tissue and organ damage. Penetrating injury may occur as a result of debris entering the body. Blast injuries are classified as primary, secondary, tertiary, or quaternary.[56,60,68] The *primary* explosive blast generates shock waves that change air pressure, and tissue damage results from the pressure waves passing through the body. Initially after an explosion, there is a rapid increase in positive pressure for a short period, followed by a longer period of negative pressure. The increase in positive pressure injures gas-containing organs. The tympanic membrane ruptures, and stomach, bowel, lungs, and brain may show evidence of contusion, acute edema, or rupture. Intraocular hemorrhage and intestinal rupture may occur from the first shock wave after an explosion. *Secondary* injuries occur as increased negative pressure from the shock wave causes debris to impale the body, creating organ and tissue damage. *Tertiary* blast injuries result as the body is thrown or propelled by the force of the explosion, resulting in blunt tissue trauma including closed head injuries, fractures, and visceral organ injury. *Quaternary* blast injuries occur as a result of chemical, thermal, and biological exposures.[56,60,68]

Disaster and Mass Casualty Management. A disaster is a sudden event in which local EMS, hospitals, and community resources are overwhelmed by the demands placed on them. Disasters can be caused by fire, weather (e.g., earthquake, hurricane, floods, tornado), explosions, terrorist activity, radiation or chemical spills, epidemic outbreaks, and human error (e.g., plane crash, mass-transit or multicar crash). Disaster planning and management response have long been considered a primary responsibility of trauma systems in conjunction with community municipalities. However, each disaster is unique, placing tremendous strain on communities to minimize mortality, injury, and destruction of property.[11,40,72,84]

Disasters are classified by the number of victims involved or the extent of resources required to provide assistance.[11,72] Disasters may also be classified as institutional based (internal), occurring within a hospital and rendering the center partially or totally inoperable, or community based (external), including any natural or humanmade situation that overwhelms a community's ability to respond with existing resources. Disasters also vary in terms of resource demand, depending on whether any warning was available before the event. For example, with impending weather disasters (e.g., hurricane), medical personnel can prepare a tentative plan for response, but some disasters (e.g., tornado, plane crash, industrial explosion) do not allow for preparation.

Several principles of disaster management and care for individuals injured in a mass casualty incident (MCI) exist. Initially, the local EMS system notifies the area hospitals of the disaster. Level I trauma centers take the lead in responding and preparing to care for the most severely injured patients. Effective field triage is vital in determining how patients are transported to local hospitals and trauma centers.

Command control centers and communication stations are established at the event site whenever possible and maintain contact with the lead hospital to facilitate efficient transport of patients.[43,81,84] Effective, consistent, and accurate communication of the activities at the disaster site and effective management of the severity and volume of incoming victims at the hospitals are critical to successful disaster and MCI management.[11,43,78]

Hospitals have well-developed disaster plans (e.g., for weather-related emergencies, bombings, MCIs) that outline specific healthcare provider responses during an event. These plans describe the roles and responsibilities of all healthcare providers, including administrators and security personnel. All personnel are required to be familiar with the disaster response policy.

Hospitals maintain and activate disaster phone call lists. When a disaster occurs, a coordinated effort within each hospital activates this phone list or texting system to contact all the people on the list. Individuals are informed when and where to respond to help with the disaster management. Both human resources and medical supplies are assessed, and healthcare personnel are frequently rotated to minimize fatigue. Maximal treatment is provided to the victims; however, supplies are judiciously used to avoid running out of essential items. Victims are triaged based on the severity of their injuries. Many mass casualty triage classification schemes exist. A system frequently used to identify patient needs is a color-coding system based on the type of care needed: (1) red indicates emergent, life-threatening injuries; (2) yellow means urgent major injuries requiring care within 1 hour; (3) green indicates nonurgent injuries that the patient can self-treat; and (4) black signifies that the patient is dead or near death.[11,47]

Patients receive treatment based on the assessment of their chance for survival matched to the resources available for medical intervention. Often injuries include blast, crush, burns, penetrating, and traumatic amputations injuries.[84] Matching resources to the trauma patient's needs is necessary to reduce morbidity and mortality.

Disasters cause significant psychological stress both during the event and after the situation has been stabilized.[33,80,81] Too often, the psychological well-being of the healthcare provider is not acknowledged after a disaster event. Current standards encourage debriefing of healthcare providers soon after an event to address the psychological stress on the individual and the team.[33,80] Debriefing frequently occurs as a group discussion session involving all healthcare team members who participated in the disaster response; however, individual and ongoing psychological interventions may be necessary.[80]

EMERGENCY CARE PHASE: TRIAGE

Prehospital Care and Transport

The ultimate goal of any EMS system is to get the patient to the right level of hospital care in the shortest span of time to optimize patient outcomes without duplicating services.[19,49] Rapid assessment in the field by EMS with immediate patient transport to an appropriate trauma center reduces morbidity and mortality.[19] Once EMS personnel arrive at the scene of an incident, they direct the situation and prepare the patient for transport. The time from injury to definitive care is a determinant of survival, particularly for those with major internal hemorrhage.[2,5,19,36,49] Treatment of life-threatening problems is provided at the scene, with careful attention given to the *airway* with cervical spine immobilization, *breathing,* and *circulation* (ABCs). Interventions include establishing an airway, providing ventilation, applying pressure to control hemorrhage, immobilizing the complete spine, and stabilizing fractures.[2,6,36] Additional life-saving prehospital interventions may include maintaining spinal precautions, placing occlusive dressings on open chest wounds, and performing needle thoracotomy to relieve tension pneumothorax.

Large-caliber IV or intraosseous (IO) access and administration of crystalloid solution (e.g., Lactated Ringer's solution) to restore blood volume and maintain systemic arterial blood pressure is often initiated.[39,92] Administration of IV fluids depends on the mechanism of injury. Large-volume resuscitation is avoided because aggressive over-resuscitation can precipitate complications such as inflammatory organ injury (e.g., ARDS, MODS), abdominal compartment syndrome, and worsening coagulopathy.[49,88,92] Fluid resuscitation is guided by vital signs and assessment of end-organ perfusion (i.e., goal-directed resuscitation). Studies have explored the use of hypertonic IV fluids for resuscitation to effectively restore circulating volume without increasing ICP; however, evidence remains controversial regarding support for fluid resuscitation in trauma.[53] Aggressive resuscitation with normal saline can result in hyperchloremic metabolic acidosis.[88,92] Until the cause of hemorrhage is addressed in hemorrhagic shock, fluid resuscitation may be initiated to treat hypotension (60 to 80 mL/kg/h for a systolic blood pressure of 80 to 90 mm Hg), or delayed resuscitation may be desired. Fluid resuscitation that raises the blood pressure to normotensive or higher may disrupt tenuous early clots.[18,88]

Ground or air transport is appropriate to move the patient from the scene of the injury to the trauma center. Considerations in the choice of transport include travel time, terrain, availability of air and ground units, capabilities of transport personnel, and weather conditions. Once the decision is made to transport a patient to a trauma center, the trauma team is notified. In most trauma centers, the initial resuscitation and stabilization of the trauma patient occur in a designated resuscitation area, usually within the ED. Optimally, the trauma team responds before the patient's arrival and begins preparations based on the report of the patient's injuries and clinical status. Trauma patients in unstable condition may be admitted directly to the operating room for resuscitation and immediate surgical intervention.

Trauma Triage. Triage of an injured patient to the appropriate trauma center based on assessment and established protocols is an essential component of a successful trauma system. *Triage* means sorting the patients to determine which patients need specialized care for actual or potential injuries. Triage decisions are often made by EMS personnel based on knowledge of the mechanisms of injury and rapid assessment of the patient's clinical status. Medical direction of this process occurs through voice communication and medical review of triage decisions.

Trauma is classified as minor or major depending on the severity of injury. *Minor trauma* refers to a single-system injury that does not pose a threat to life or limb and can be appropriately treated in a basic emergency center. *Major trauma* refers to serious multiple-system injuries that require immediate intervention to prevent disability, loss of limb, or death. In some regions, an injury scoring system is used to objectively measure and convey the severity of injury an individual has sustained. Several scoring systems are used for this purpose.[55] The Abbreviated Injury Scale (AIS) divides the body into six regions and applies a severity score from 1 to 6 for each injury. The scores from the three most severely injured body regions are squared and added together to arrive at the Injury Severity Score (ISS). The risk for mortality increases with a higher ISS. An AIS score of 1 indicates minor injury, and a score of 6 indicates an unsurvivable injury (see https://www.aci.health.nsw.gov.au/get-involved/institute-of-trauma-and-injury-management/Data/injury-scoring/injury_severity_score).

Another scoring system that is used to objectively evaluate a patient's severity of neurological injury is the Glasgow Coma Scale (GCS). The lower the GCS score, based on three assessment parameters, the more severe the neurological injury, suggesting the need for emergent transport to a trauma center (see Chapter 14).

The development of and adherence to established triage criteria are essential for maintaining an effective system of optimal care for the trauma patient. Triage decisions are based on abnormal findings in the patient's physiological functions, the mechanism of injury, the severity of injury, the anatomical area of injury, or evidence of risk factors such as age and preexisting disease.[55,66,74] Prehospital personnel may elect to transport the patient to a trauma center in the absence of accepted triage criteria. This decision is most often based on visualization of the trauma incident and the patient's clinical condition.

Hospital triage. Information obtained during the prehospital phase provides data to ensure a coordinated, life-saving approach in the management of trauma patients. Most traumatic events are considered "scoop and run" situations with short transport times to the closest appropriate trauma center; other patients may arrive at the hospital by private car. Triage continues after the patient arrives at the hospital to identify those patients who need immediate treatment as well as to match available resources with treatment needs based on injury mechanism and severity. Procedures exist within hospitals to activate the trauma team, including the operating room team for emergent surgical interventions.

EDs in trauma centers designate resuscitation rooms in a central location to facilitate a rapid initial assessment, stabilization, and determination of the immediate medical needs of the patient. The resuscitation room must always be in a state of readiness for the next trauma patient. Equipment needed for management of the airway with cervical spine immobilization, breathing, circulatory support, and hemorrhage control must be immediately available and easily accessible.

Preparation. Standard Precautions are used when preparing for a trauma patient. The risk of coming in contact with body fluids in severely injured patients is high. The ACS recommends face mask, eye protection, water-impervious gown, and gloves as minimum precautions and protection for all healthcare providers when coming in contact with body fluids.[2]

EMERGENCY CARE PHASE: RESUSCITATION

Initial Patient Assessment

Patient survival after a serious traumatic event depends on a rapid and systematic assessment in conjunction with immediate resuscitative interventions. Priorities of care are based on the patient's clinical presentation, physical assessment, history of the traumatic event (mechanism of injury), and knowledge of any preexisting disease. Critical components of care that take immediate precedence include management of airway patency, ventilation, hemorrhage control, and stabilization of fractures. A systematic approach, using primary and secondary surveys, is implemented so that life-threatening emergencies are evaluated and addressed as a priority.

Primary and Secondary Surveys

The assessment begins with a primary survey and resuscitation adjuncts. The *primary* survey is the most crucial assessment tool in trauma care. This rapid, 1- to 2-minute evaluation is designed to identify life-threatening injuries accurately, establish priorities, and provide simultaneous therapeutic interventions. An **ABCDEFG** mnemonic is used to guide the *primary survey:* **A**irway with cervical spine immobilization, **B**reathing and ventilation, **C**irculation with hemorrhage control, **D**isability or assessment of neurological status, **E**xposure with environmental considerations, **F**ull set of

vital signs and family presence, and **G**et resuscitation adjuncts.[2,47] Life-threatening conditions are identified, and management is instituted simultaneously (Table 20.2).

The *secondary survey* is initiated after all actual or potential life-threatening injuries have been addressed and resuscitative efforts have been initiated. It is a methodical approach to obtain a patient and event history (**H**) and a head-to-toe assessment of the patient (**I**). Assess each region of the body to minimize the potential for missing an injury or failing to grasp the significance of an injury. Assessment techniques of inspection, palpation, percussion, and auscultation are used to identify all injuries, including inspection of posterior surfaces (Table 20.3).[47]

Information about actual and potential injuries is noted and used to establish diagnostic and treatment priorities. Radiological and ultrasound studies are completed according to a standardized trauma protocol or an assessment of suspected injuries. The sequence of diagnostic procedures is influenced by the patient's level of consciousness and hemodynamic stability, the mechanism of injury, and the identified injuries. As data are obtained, the team leader determines the need for consultation with specialty physicians such as neurosurgeons or orthopedic surgeons. Supportive interventions such as management of pain and anxiety, splinting of extremities, wound care, and administration of tetanus prophylaxis and antibiotics are completed. The primary and secondary surveys are repeated frequently to identify change in the patient's status, indicating the need for additional intervention.[2] As initial life-threatening injuries are managed, other equally life-threatening problems and less severe injuries may become apparent, which can significantly affect the patient's prognosis.[2,47]

From the time of initial injury until the patient is stabilized in the ED or operating room, the trauma team resuscitates the patient. *Resuscitation* in trauma refers to reestablishing an effective circulatory volume and a stable hemodynamic status in the patient and is a central component of the primary and secondary surveys. The ABCDEFG of emergency care continues, and life-threatening injuries (e.g., pneumothorax, cardiac tamponade) are treated emergently. Each of these interventions is discussed in detail in the following sections.

> **STUDY BREAK**
> 1. The key purpose of the primary survey is to:
>   A. Identify and treat all potential injuries
>   B. Obtain a thorough head-to-toe examination of the patient
>   C. Quickly identify and treat the greatest life-threatening emergencies
>   D. Identify the need for additional consultation teams and resources

Establish Airway Patency and Restrict Cervical Spine Motion

Every trauma patient has the potential for an ineffective airway, whether it occurs at the time of injury or develops during resuscitation. A patient may lose airway patency for many reasons, including obstruction, structural impairments, and an inability to protect the airway associated with a change in level of consciousness. The tongue, because of posterior displacement, is the most common cause of airway obstruction. Other causes of

TABLE 20.2 Primary Survey: ABCDEFG

Assessment	Observations Indicating Impairment	Simultaneous Management
A = Airway • Open and patent • Maintain cervical spine immobilization • Patency of artificial airway (if present)	Shallow, noisy breathing Stridor Central cyanosis Nasal flaring Accessory muscle use Inability to speak Drooling Anxiety Decreased level of consciousness (GCS score ≤8) Trauma to face, mouth, or neck Evidence of inhalation injury Debris or foreign matter in mouth or pharynx	Suction the airway Use jaw-thrust maneuver to open the airway while maintaining cervical spine stabilization Consider a definitive airway (nasal or oral airway, endotracheal intubation)
B = Breathing • Presence and effectiveness	Asymmetrical chest movement Absent, decreased, or unequal breath sounds Open chest wounds Blunt chest injury Dyspnea Central cyanosis Respiratory rate <8-10 or >40 breaths/min Accessory muscle use Anxiety Altered mental status Tracheal shift	Administer oxygen at 15 L/min via non-rebreather device Consider a definitive airway (nasal or oral airway, endotracheal intubation) See Table 20.4
C = Circulation • Presence of major pulses • Presence of external hemorrhage	Weak, thready pulse HR >120 beats/min Pallor Systolic BP <90 mm Hg MAP <65 mm Hg Obvious external hemorrhage Decreased level of consciousness	Apply direct pressure to site of bleeding Consider a pelvic binder for an unstable pelvic fracture Insert two large-caliber peripheral IV catheters Initiate infusions of warmed isotonic crystalloid solution Consider blood administration
D = Disability • Gross neurological status • Pupil size, equality, and reactivity to light • Spontaneous movements or moves to command	GCS score ≤13 Agitation Lack of spontaneous movement Posturing Lack of sensation in extremities	Consider need for CT Consider alcohol level and/or toxicology screening Consider ABG for evaluation of hypoxia and glucose level for assessment of hypoglycemia
E = Expose patient with environmental control	Presence of soft tissue injury, crepitus, deformities, edema	Preserve clothing in paper bag for use as evidence Maintain body temperature by covering the patient with warm blankets, covering the patient's head, using warmed IV fluids, and increasing the room ambient temperature
F = Full set of vital signs and family presence		Obtain full set of vital signs (BP, HR, respiratory rate, temperature) Obtain oxygen saturation via pulse oximetry Identify family; provide updates; facilitate visitation with patient
G = Get resuscitation adjuncts (LMNOP) • L—Laboratory studies (lactic acid, ABG, type and crossmatch)	Lactic acid levels >2.2-4 mmol/L reflect poor tissue perfusion Base deficit less than −6 may indicate poor perfusion and tissue hypoxia	Obtain blood and urine for laboratory studies
• M—Monitor cardiac rhythm	Dysrhythmias may indicate blunt cardiac trauma or electrolyte abnormalities PEA may indicate cardiac tamponade, tension pneumothorax, or significant hypovolemia	Connect patient to cardiac monitor

TABLE 20.2 Primary Survey: ABCDEFG—cont'd

Assessment	Observations Indicating Impairment	Simultaneous Management
• N—Nasogastric or orogastric tube		Insert nasogastric or orogastric tube, indwelling urinary catheter
• O—Oxygen and ventilation assessment		
• P—Pain assessment and management and psychosocial support		Provide pain management Provide appropriate spiritual and psychosocial support

ABG, Arterial blood gas; *BP,* blood pressure; *CT,* computed tomography; *GCS,* Glasgow Coma Scale; *HR,* heart rate; *MAP,* mean arterial pressure; *PEA,* pulseless electrical activity.
Modified from Gurney D. *Trauma Nursing Core Course (TNCC): Provider Manual.* 7th ed. Des Plaines, IL: Emergency Nurses Association; 2014.

TABLE 20.3 Secondary Survey: HI

Survey Activities	Actions	Inspection	Palpation	Auscultation
H = History 1. History of event: MIST • M—Mechanism of injury • I—Injuries sustained • S—Signs and symptoms in the field • T—Treatment in the field 2. Patient history: SAMPLE • S—Symptoms • A—Allergies • M—Medications • P—Past medical history • L—Last oral intake • E—Events and environmental factors **Head-to-toe Assessment**	Perform head-to-toe assessment Obtain information on allergies, current medications, past illnesses, pregnancies, last meal	*Head/face:* Inspect for wounds, ecchymosis, deformities, drainage, pupillary reaction, unusual drainage from ears or nose *Neck:* Inspect for wounds, ecchymosis, deformities, distended neck veins *Chest:* Inspect for breathing rate and depth, wounds, deformities, ecchymosis, use of accessory muscles, paradoxical movement *Abdomen:* Inspect for wounds, distension, ecchymosis, scars *Pelvis/perineum:* Inspect for wounds, deformities, ecchymosis, priapism, blood at the urinary meatus or in the perineal area *Extremities:* Inspect for ecchymosis, movement, wounds, deformities	*Head/face:* Palpate for tenderness, crepitus, deformities *Neck:* Palpate for tenderness, crepitus, deformities, tracheal position *Chest:* Palpate for tenderness, crepitus, subcutaneous emphysema, deformities *Abdomen:* Palpate all four quadrants for tenderness, rigidity, guarding, masses, femoral pulses *Pelvis/perineum:* Palpate the pelvis and anal sphincter tone *Extremities:* Palpate for pulses, skin temperature, sensation, tenderness, deformities, crepitus	*Chest:* Auscultate breath and heart sounds *Abdomen:* Auscultate bowel sounds; observe for passing flatulence
I = Inspect Posterior Surfaces	Maintain cervical spine stabilization Log roll patient using three hospital personnel	Inspect posterior surfaces for wounds, deformities, and ecchymosis	Palpate posterior surfaces for deformities and pain Assist physician with the rectal examination, if not previously completed	

Modified from Gurney D. *Trauma Nursing Core Course (TNCC): Provider Manual.* 7th ed. Des Plaines, IL: Emergency Nurses Association; 2014.

obstruction include foreign debris (blood or vomitus) and anatomical obstructions due to maxillofacial fractures. Direct injuries to the throat or neck can structurally impair the airway. Patients with an altered sensorium or high spinal cord injury may not be able to protect their airway.

Maintaining the patient's airway with simultaneous cervical spine protection is an important initial intervention.[2,47] Suspect a cervical spine injury in any patient with multisystem trauma until radiographic studies and clinical evaluation determine otherwise. Until a cervical spinal injury has been cleared, manually stabilize the cervical spine by holding the head and neck in alignment or restrict cervical spine motion with a cervical collar when establishing the patient's airway.

If the patient is able to communicate verbally, the airway is not likely to be in immediate jeopardy; however, repeated assessment of airway patency is necessary.[2,47] If a patient is unable to open his or her mouth, does not follow commands, or is

unresponsive, use a jaw-thrust maneuver to open and assess the airway. Clear the airway of any foreign material such as blood, vomitus, bone fragments, or teeth by gentle suction with a tonsillar tip catheter. Nasopharyngeal and oropharyngeal airways are the simplest artificial airway adjuncts used in patients with spontaneous respirations and adequate ventilatory effort. Both devices help prevent posterior displacement of the tongue. Do not insert an oropharyngeal airway in a conscious patient because it may induce gagging, vomiting, and aspiration; if an artificial airway is needed, a nasopharyngeal airway is better tolerated (see Chapter 10).

A definitive airway may be required for a patient who presents with apnea, a GCS score of 8 or less, or an inability to protect the airway. Examples of definitive airways include endotracheal intubation and surgical cricothyroidotomy. Endotracheal intubation is the definitive nonsurgical airway management technique. Oral intubation is often preferred, but nasotracheal intubation is acceptable depending on circumstances and injury. Nasotracheal intubation is contraindicated if there are signs of facial, frontal sinus, basilar skull, or cribriform plate fractures.[2,47] Evidence of nasal fracture, raccoon eyes (bilateral ecchymosis in the periorbital region), Battle's sign (postauricular ecchymosis), and possible cerebrospinal fluid (CSF) leaks (rhinorrhea or otorrhea) are all signs of these injuries.[2] During intubation, precautions to restrict cervical spine movement are followed. Refer to Chapter 10 for intubation procedures. Rapid sequence intubation (sequential administration of a sedative or anesthetic and a neuromuscular blocking agent) may be used to facilitate the procedure.

In rare circumstances, it may be difficult to intubate the patient. If endotracheal intubation is not feasible or has failed, an alternative airway device, such as a laryngeal mask airway (LMA) or laryngeal tube airway (LTA), may be used until a definitive airway can be placed.[2] Another option is performing a cricothyroidotomy, a surgical intervention, to establish an effective airway. Conditions that may require cricothyroidotomy include maxillofacial trauma, laryngeal fractures, severe oropharyngeal hemorrhage, or an inability to place an endotracheal tube through the vocal cords.[2,47]

Maintain Effective Breathing

Assess the patient frequently for sensorium, spontaneous breathing, respiratory rate and effort, heart rate and rhythm, breath sounds, symmetrical rise and fall of the chest, contusions or abrasions, temperature, tracheal position, and jugular venous distension. When spontaneous breathing is present but ineffective, consider the presence of a life-threatening condition if any of the following are present: altered mental status; central cyanosis; asymmetrical expansion of the chest wall; use of accessory muscles, abdominal muscles, or both; paradoxical movement of the chest wall during inspiration and expiration; diminished or absent breath sounds; tracheal shift from midline position; decreasing oxygen saturation via pulse oximetry; or distended jugular veins. Interventions to restore normal breathing patterns are directed toward the specific injury or underlying cause of respiratory distress, with the goal of improving ventilation and oxygenation. Provide supplemental oxygen with ventilatory assistance (if applicable), position for effective ventilation, and evaluate interventions. Ineffective breathing patterns may be the result of certain traumatic injuries. These injuries and specific interventions are listed in Table 20.4 and discussed throughout this chapter. Arterial blood gas analysis and diagnostic studies including chest radiography and computed tomography (CT) imaging may be completed to assist in determining the effectiveness of specific interventions.

Impaired oxygenation follows airway obstruction as the most crucial problem following traumatic injury. Impaired gas exchange can result from ineffective ventilation, an inability to exchange gases at the alveoli, or both. Possible causes include a decrease in inspired air, retained secretions, lung collapse or compression, atelectasis, or accumulation of blood in the thoracic cavity. Assess any patient who presents with multiple systemic injuries, hemorrhagic shock, chest trauma, and/or central nervous system trauma for impaired gas exchange.

TABLE 20.4 Specific Interventions for Ineffective Breathing Patterns

Etiology	Interventions
Decreased level of consciousness	Position the patient's head at midline with the head of the bed elevated Anticipate a computed tomography scan Implement interventions to prevent aspiration Prepare for intubation and mechanical ventilation
Spinal cord injury	Avoid hyperextension or rotation of the patient's neck Observe ventilatory effort and use of accessory muscles Maintain complete spinal immobilization Prepare for application of cervical traction tongs or a halo device Monitor motor and sensory function Monitor for signs of distributive (neurogenic) shock
Pneumothorax	Provide supplemental oxygen Prepare for chest tube insertion on affected side
Tension pneumothorax	Prepare for decompression by needle thoracotomy with a 14-gauge needle in the second intercostal space at the midclavicular line on affected side Prepare for chest tube insertion on affected side
Open chest wound	Seal the wound with an occlusive dressing and tape on three sides Prepare for chest tube insertion on affected side
Massive hemothorax	Establish two 14- or 16-gauge peripheral IV catheters for crystalloid infusion Obtain blood for type and crossmatch Prepare for chest tube insertion on affected side Administer blood or blood products as ordered Anticipate and prepare for emergency open thoracotomy
Pulmonary contusion	Prepare for early endotracheal intubation and mechanical ventilation
Flail chest	Prepare for early endotracheal intubation and mechanical ventilation Administer analgesics as ordered

These conditions have the potential to affect the patient's volume status and oxygen-carrying capacity, interfere with the mechanics of ventilation, or interrupt the autonomic control of respirations. The nurse must be prepared to assist with endotracheal intubation and subsequent mechanical ventilation, needle thoracostomy, chest tube insertion, and restoration of circulating blood volume at any time during the resuscitation phase of care. Because conditions that compromise breathing may not manifest during the first assessment of airway or breathing, ongoing airway assessment is a nursing priority.

STUDY BREAK

2. Which three elements are commonly referred to as the "trauma triad of death?" (Select all that apply.)
   A. Hypothermia
   B. Acidosis
   C. Hypotension
   D. Tachycardia
   E. Coagulopathy

Maintain Circulation

The most common cause of impaired cardiac output and circulation after traumatic injury is hypovolemic shock from acute blood loss. Causes may be external (hemorrhage) or internal (hemothorax, hemoperitoneum, solid organ injury, long bone or massive pelvic fractures). Initial management of actively bleeding patients includes hemorrhage control by applying pressure or a tourniquet to control bleeding, replacing circulatory volume with blood products, and surgery focused on hemorrhage control (damage control surgery) rather than definitive surgical management.[48] In the face of hypovolemic shock from hemorrhage, early, rapid surgical intervention is life-saving and limb-saving.[2,48]

The management of hypovolemic shock focuses on finding and eliminating the cause of the bleeding and concomitant support of the patient's circulatory system with IV fluids and blood products (see Chapter 12). It is often difficult to assess blood loss, especially with internal hemorrhage from blunt trauma. Furthermore, when blood volume decreases, the sympathetic nervous system compensatory mechanisms in the body respond through tachycardia, narrowing pulse pressure, tachypnea, vasoconstriction, and decreased urine output. Signs and symptoms of hypovolemic shock may not be obvious until the patient is in a later stage of hypovolemic shock.[2,48] It is estimated that signs of hypotension may not be clinically obvious until a patient has lost more than 30% to 40% of blood volume.[2] Continually assesses the patient for subtle changes in vital signs and end-organ function. Initiate hemorrhage control and fluid resuscitation when early signs and symptoms of blood loss are apparent or suspected rather than waiting for overt signs associated with a decreasing blood pressure.[2,48]

Perform Diagnostic Testing

Diagnostic testing is completed early in the resuscitative phase to determine injuries and potential sources of bleeding. Potential injuries to the chest, pelvis, and abdomen and suspected extremity fractures are assessed. Diagnostic studies include CT, radiography, *focused assessment with sonography for trauma (FAST)*, and *extended FAST (E-FAST)*. FAST is an ultrasound assessment that provides a rapid, noninvasive means of diagnosing accumulation of blood or free fluid in the peritoneal cavity or pericardial sac.[2,8,61,66,76] E-FAST simply extends the ultrasound examination to evaluate possible injuries in the chest, looking for hemothorax and pneumothorax. In the context of traumatic injury, free fluid identified on the FAST examination is usually due to hemorrhage. If free fluid or hemorrhage is found, a CT scan may be obtained and/or surgical interventions initiated.[2,8,61] An echocardiogram, a 12-lead electrocardiogram (ECG), and continuous ECG with ST segment monitoring may also be ordered to evaluate cardiac function, especially if the patient is showing signs of diminished cardiac output, if thoracic injury is present, or if the patient has a history of cardiovascular disease.

Pelvic fractures can be a hidden cause of hemorrhage because the retroperitoneum can be a site for significant blood loss. In the patient with blunt force trauma and an unidentifiable cause of hypotension, radiographic evaluation and a pelvic examination are critical to identify an unstable pelvic fracture as a source of injury and bleeding. Apply a pelvic binder or sheet to stabilize the injury and minimize further bleeding.

STUDY BREAK

3. A construction worker is admitted after falling approximately 15 feet from scaffolding. What diagnostic intervention does the nurse anticipate in the care of this trauma patient to evaluate sources of potential bleeding?
   A. FAST or E-FAST
   B. Complete metabolic laboratory test panel
   C. Chest radiograph
   D. Urinalysis

Perform Fluid Resuscitation

Venous access and infusion of volume are required for optimal fluid resuscitation in the trauma patient with hypovolemic shock. Insert at least two large-caliber peripheral IV catheters. The preferred sites are the forearm or antecubital veins.[2,47] If peripheral access cannot be obtained, IO needles may be used for temporary access through bone in the sternum, leg (tibia), or arm (humerus) if the patient's injuries do not interfere with the procedure.[2,47,48,57] (Fig. 20.3). IO access should not be performed in an extremity with a known or suspected fracture.[2] The IO access may be placed in the field by EMS personnel or in the ED. Resuscitation fluids, medications, and blood products can be administered through an IO device.[2,47,48,57] Potential complications with IO access include pain on instillation of fluids, extravasation of fluids, and compartment syndrome.

A central venous catheter (single-lumen or multiple-lumen) may be necessary because of peripheral vasoconstriction and venous collapse. It may be beneficial as a resuscitation monitoring tool and for rapid administration of large volumes of fluid.

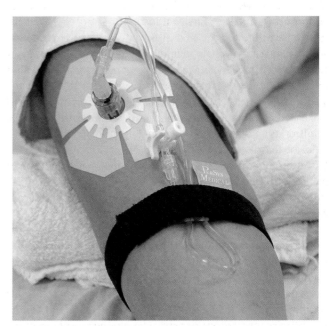

Fig. 20.3 Tibial insertion of an intraosseous (IO) device that is taped in place with IV extension attached to the needle for instillation of fluids and medications. (Courtesy Waismed, Ltd., Houston, TX.)

A pulmonary artery catheter is not usually helpful in the emergency care phase of trauma management, but one may be inserted in the critical care unit to evaluate the response to fluid resuscitation and cardiac function (see Chapter 8).

As a general rule, venous access is achieved rapidly with the largest-bore catheter possible to initiate early fluid resuscitation. Immediate management of severely injured trauma patients focuses on replacing lost intravascular volume with fluids and blood and treating coagulopathy.[2] The provision of fluids and blood products is contingent on obtaining adequate vascular access to the patient's venous system.

Appropriate initiation, timing, and choice of fluid used for resuscitation are pivotal in affecting patient outcomes. Under-resuscitation results in worsening tissue ischemia, shock, and death, whereas over-resuscitation causes life-threatening complications such as abdominal compartment syndrome and ARDS. Therefore continual assessment of fluid volume status is critical throughout resuscitation. Warmed isotonic crystalloid fluids (e.g., Lactated Ringer's solution, normal saline) are the first-line fluids used for trauma resuscitation.[2,47] Lactated Ringer's solution is the preferred crystalloid fluid over normal saline, as it favors a lower incidence of adverse kidney events and mortality.[79] Because large volumes of crystalloid, especially normal saline, are associated with poor patient outcomes by worsening acidosis and coagulopathy, current practice focuses on determining which type of fluid resuscitation is best during this phase.[2,37] Patients who have hypotension secondary to blood loss are resuscitated with blood products for "hemostatic resuscitation" or "damage control resuscitation."[45,49] Patients with massive hemorrhage lose clotting factors as well as red blood cells and plasma. To effectively stop bleeding, packed red blood cells (PRBCs), fresh frozen plasma (FFP), and platelets must be replaced. Coagulation factors are present in FFP and platelets, and to minimize coagulopathies, it is critical that PRBCs, FFP, and platelets are all administered as part of resuscitation. To support this practice, massive transfusion protocols have been developed with the intention of getting all blood components to the patient in a timely manner. Type-specific blood may be administered, but in the event of life-threatening blood loss, unmatched type-specific or type O (universal donor) blood may be prescribed. Crossmatched type-specific blood should be instituted as soon as it is available. Massive transfusion often requires more than 10 units of blood products within 24 hours or more than 4 units in 1 hour.[2,47,49]

A thromboelastography (TEG) or rotational thromboelastometry (ROTEM) test evaluates whole blood coagulation and assists the clinician in identifying whether a patient has normal hemostasis or a coagulopathy. If available, it may be used to monitor coagulation and guide blood product administration during massive transfusion.[2] The results of the test are displayed in a unique tracing as well as discrete values. If a coagulopathy is identified, the TEG results are used to identify the specific product used for treatment, including FFP, cryoprecipitate, or an antifibrinolytic or thrombolytic medication. TEG supports individualized resuscitation of trauma patients by tailoring massive transfusion to the dynamic biology of individual hemostasis.[45] Trials have demonstrated that TEG-directed resuscitation

EVIDENCE-BASED PRACTICE

The Pragmatic Randomized Optimal Platelet and Plasma Ratios (PROPPR) Clinical Trial

Problem
Severely injured trauma patients experiencing hemorrhagic shock require massive transfusion. Damage control resuscitation is defined as rapid hemorrhage control through early administration of blood products in a balanced ratio of 1:1:1 for units of red blood cells, plasma, and platelets, respectively. This ratio is the closest approximation to whole blood. Damage control resuscitation prevents coagulopathy and minimizes crystalloid fluid administration and secondary complications associated with third-spacing.

Clinical Question
Which is the most effective and safe method of transfusing patients with severe trauma and major bleeding, using a 1:1:1 ratio of red blood cells, plasma, and platelets compared to a 1:1:2 ratio?

Evidence
Severely injured trauma patients were randomized to receive blood products in a ratio of 1:1:1 (338 patients) or 1:1:2 (342 patients). All patients were cared for in Level I trauma centers and were predicted to require massive transfusion based on their severity of injury. The primary outcomes measured were 24-hour and 30-day all-cause mortality, time to hemostasis, blood product volumes transfused, complications, incidence of surgical procedures, and patient functional status. No statistically significant differences were detected in patient mortality at 24 hours or 30 days between the two transfusion ratios. However, patients in the 1:1:1 transfusion group achieved hemostasis faster, and fewer died of exsanguination (86% versus 78%, $P = 0.006$). Posttransfusion complications were similar in both groups.

Implications for Nursing
Before this study, massive transfusion for patients with severe trauma and major bleeding was guided by tradition; no empirical evidence was available to guide blood product ratios for damage control resuscitation. The results of this study support administration of blood products in a 1:1:1 ratio, which is closest to the composition of whole blood, enhancing earlier achievement of hemostasis and improving patient survival. Anticipating the need to rapidly transfuse plasma, platelets, and red blood cells in equal ratios in the care of acutely ill, hemorrhaging trauma patients is important to patient survival.

Level of Evidence
B—Multisite randomized controlled trial

Reference
Holcomb JB, Tiley BC, Baraniuk S, et al. Transfusion of plasma, platelets, and red blood cells in a 1:1:1 vs a 1:1:2 ratio and mortality in patients with severe trauma: The PROPPR randomized clinical trial. *JAMA*. 2015;313(5):471–482.

improves survival after injury and promotes appropriate use of hemostatic blood products.[45]

Three patterns of response to initial fluid administration are used to determine further therapeutic and diagnostic decisions[2]:
- *Rapid responders* react quickly and remain hemodynamically stable after administration of the initial fluid bolus. Fluids are then slowed to maintenance rates.
- *Transient responders* improve in response to the initial fluid bolus but begin to show deterioration in perfusion when fluids are slowed to maintenance rates. This finding indicates ongoing blood loss or inadequate resuscitation. Continued fluid administration and blood transfusion are needed. If

the patient continues to respond in a transient manner, the patient is probably bleeding and requires rapid surgical intervention.

- *Minimal or nonresponders* fail to respond to crystalloid and blood administration in the ED, and surgical intervention is needed immediately to control hemorrhage.

Monitor the patient's response to the initial fluid administration by assessing urine output (goal: 0.5 mL/kg/h in the adult), level of consciousness, heart rate, blood pressure, pulse pressure, and laboratory indices (e.g., serum lactate level, base deficit). The goal is to provide adequate fluid resuscitation to prevent tissue hypoxemia. Specific markers of tissue oxygenation and consumption such as mixed venous oxygen saturation (SvO_2) may also be used to evaluate the effectiveness of fluid resuscitation. Also monitor for hypothermia, electrolyte imbalances, dilutional coagulopathies, and consequences of excessive third-spacing of fluids.[47]

Dilutional coagulopathy and *third-spacing* may occur with excessive IV fluid resuscitation and extensive blood loss.[37] During states of hypoperfusion and acidosis, inflammation occurs and vessels become more permeable to fluid and molecules. With aggressive fluid resuscitation, this change in permeability allows movement of fluid from the intravascular space into the interstitial spaces (third-spacing). Hypovolemia occurs in the intravascular space, and patients require a larger volume of fluid replacement, creating a vicious cycle. As more IV fluids are given to support systemic circulation, fluids continue to migrate into the interstitial space, causing excessive edema and predisposing the patient to additional complications such as abdominal compartment syndrome, ARDS, acute kidney injury, and MODS. More than 75% of crystalloid solution diffuses into the interstitial space within 30 minutes of administration. This deficit results in the need for additional fluids to maintain hemodynamic stability, causing a cascade of negative effects, including excessive tissue edema, hemodilution, and increased coagulopathy.[37] Banked blood products have high levels of citrate, which may induce transient hypocalcemia. Decreased serum calcium levels may lead to ineffective coagulation because calcium is a necessary cofactor in the coagulation cascade. Further inhibition of the clotting cascade is observed when platelet dysfunction develops secondary to hypothermia or metabolic acidosis. Management focuses on improving perfusion to the body tissues, increasing the patient's body temperature, and administering clotting factors (FFP, cryoprecipitate, and platelets). Monitor the hemoglobin level, hematocrit value, plasma fibrinogen level, platelet count, prothrombin time (PT), and partial thromboplastin time (PTT). TEG and/or ROTEM can be helpful in determining the clotting deficiency and appropriate blood components to correct the deficiency.[2]

Assess for Neurological Disabilities

Assess for neurological disabilities by evaluating the patient's level of consciousness, pupillary size and reaction, and spontaneous and reflexive spinal movements. The GCS is the standard method for evaluating level of consciousness in the injured patient (see Chapter 14).[47] Accurate GCS assessment is limited in patients who are intubated or unable to respond to the verbal component of the exam.[47] Consider possible neurological injuries based on the history of the injury (e.g., ejection from motor vehicle, fall, diving accident). Perform a complete sensory and motor neurological examination to identify the presence and level of spinal cord injury.

Use of recreational drugs and/or alcohol by the patient can mask neurological responsiveness, resulting in misleading findings. Hypotension, hypoventilation, and hypoglycemia can also alter the neurological examination. Hypotension decreases cerebral perfusion; therefore consider the patient's response to interventions and the degree of tissue ischemia during the neurological examination. If an effective neurological examination cannot be conducted, management is based on knowledge of the traumatic event and the current neurological response. Management priorities focus on the premise that changes in level of consciousness are the result of the traumatic injury until proven otherwise. The key to neurological assessments is trending the results to detect improvement or deterioration and notifying the physician for prompt intervention (see Chapter 14).

Exposure and Environmental Considerations

Standard practice in trauma management is to remove all clothing and expose the patient to allow for full body visualization and identification of all injuries. However, exposure decreases body temperature, and preventing hypothermia by

---

> ⚠ **LABORATORY ALERT**

Laboratory Test	Normal Range	Critical Value[a]	Significance
Lactic acid (lactate)	0.6-2.2 mmol/L or 5-20 mg/dL (venous) 0.3-0.8 mmol/L or 4-7 mg/dL (arterial)	>4 mmol/L	• Lactate is a by-product of anaerobic metabolism that results from inadequate tissue perfusion • It is a marker for cellular hypoxia in hypovolemic/hemorrhagic shock • Lactate levels >2.2 to 4.0 mmol/L indicate widespread tissue hypoperfusion and insufficient resuscitation; and is an independent predictor of mortality in trauma patients[9,47]
Base deficit/excess	−2 to + 2 mEq/L	−3 mEq/L +3 mEq/L	• Base deficit/excess represents the number of buffering anions in the blood • A negative value (base deficit) indicates metabolic acidosis (e.g., lactic acidosis) • A positive value (base excess) indicates metabolic alkalosis or a compensatory response to respiratory acidosis

[a]Critical values vary by facility and laboratory.
From Pagana K, Pagana T. *Mosby's Manual of Diagnostic and Laboratory Tests.* 6th ed. St. Louis, MO: Elsevier; 2018.

maintaining body temperature is a critical nursing priority. Hypothermia, defined as a core body temperature less than 35°C (95°F), is caused by a combination of accelerated heat loss and decreased heat production and is associated with poor outcomes.[2,47,54] Patients, and especially older persons, are more susceptible to hypothermia after severe injury, excessive blood loss, alcohol use, and massive fluid resuscitation. Body temperature continues to fall after clothing removal, contact with wet linens, and surgical exposure of body cavities during the initial assessment. Prolonged exposure to hypothermia is associated with the development of myocardial dysfunction, coagulopathies, reduced perfusion, dysrhythmias (bradycardia and atrial or ventricular fibrillation), and decreased metabolic rate.

The combination of hypothermia, hypotension, and acidosis is commonly referred to as trauma's lethal triad of death.[2,54] Even mild hypothermia in a trauma patient can result in devastating physiological consequences that affect the coagulation system, ultimately resulting in worsening hemorrhage and adverse patient outcomes. Minimize the negative effects of hypothermia by covering the patient with warm blankets, administering warmed IV fluids, warming the room, covering the patient's head, and using convection air blankets. Suggested techniques for rewarming are listed in Table 20.5.

Full Set of Vitals and Family Presence

A full set of vital signs, including heart rate and rhythm, blood pressure, respiratory rate, pulse oximetry, and temperature, is monitored and trended to assess the effectiveness of resuscitation. Facilitate family presence during this part of the primary assessment.[1,38,47]

Get Resuscitation Adjuncts

Specific adjuncts are crucial to continue to assess and manage elements in the primary assessment (LMNOP): Laboratory studies, Monitoring, Nasogastric or orogastric tube consideration, Oxygenation and ventilation, and Pain and psychosocial management.[47] Laboratory studies, including lactate and base deficit, reflect the effectiveness of cellular perfusion, the adequacy of ventilation, and the success of fluid resuscitation

(circulation). As a result of hypovolemia and hypoxemia, metabolic acidosis occurs secondary to a shift from aerobic to anaerobic metabolism and the production of lactic acid. Increases in lactate level and base deficit are accompanied by a decrease in tissue perfusion with increased morbidity and mortality.[47,51,74] Insertion of a nasogastric or orogastric tube provides a route to decompress the stomach, preventing emesis and aspiration, and allows optimal inflation of the lungs. Capnography monitoring provides immediate information about the patient's ventilation and perfusion status. Appropriate pain management and psychosocial support for the patient and family are important aspects of trauma care.[47]

Secondary Survey

The secondary survey begins after resuscitative efforts have been initiated and vital functions have been stabilized in the primary survey. The secondary survey includes obtaining history of the patient and the event, a head-to-toe assessment, and inspection of the posterior surfaces (HI). The SAMPLE pneumonic is used to obtain important aspects of the patient and event history: Symptoms associated with the injury, Allergies and tetanus status, Medications currently used, Past medical and surgical history, Last oral intake, and Events and Environmental factors related to the injury.

If the patient is responsive, eliciting symptoms is helpful to identify areas of pain and otherwise unrecognized injuries. For example, the trauma team might have identified a significant burn during the primary survey, and the patient might complain of pain in a nonburned area. This can identify need for additional assessment and radiological imaging to rule out a fracture that might not have been recognized. When obtaining information regarding current medication use, identify medications that affect initial management, including anticoagulants and beta-blockers. Coagulopathy contributes to worsening hemorrhage and worse outcomes and may be reversed with other pharmaceutical agents or blood products in the resuscitation phase of trauma care. Warfarin may be emergently reversed using IV vitamin K and 4-factor prothrombin complex concentrate (PCC) to reduce bleeding prior to surgery or other interventions.[91] Medical or comorbid factors that place the injured patient at greater risk for complications include older age and pregnancy greater than 20 weeks.[47]

Event and environmental considerations are related to the location and circumstances of the traumatic event. Environmental considerations are important in farming accidents, impalement with machinery or contaminated industrial equipment, exposure to contaminated water, or wound contamination with soil and road dirt. Initial attempts to cleanse the wound are not priorities in the emergency care phase of trauma management; however, once the patient is stabilized, the wounds are cleansed and debrided, and appropriate antibiotics are initiated.

During the head-to-toe assessment and inspection of posterior surfaces, identify all injuries using a systematic evaluation moving from the patient's head to the lower extremities and posterior surface.[47] Inspection, auscultation, palpation, and percussion is used. To inspect the posterior surfaces, maintain cervical spine mobilization using additional team members to

TABLE 20.5 Rewarming Strategies

Type	Interventions
Passive external	Removal of wet clothing Warm room Decreased airflow over patient Blankets Head coverings
Active external	Radiant lights Fluid-filled warming blankets Convection air blankets
Active internal	Warmed gases to respiratory tract Warmed IV fluids, including blood Body cavity irrigation (peritoneal, mediastinal, pleural, gastric) Continuous arteriovenous rewarming Cardiopulmonary bypass

assist with logrolling the patient to maintain vertebral column alignment of the torso, hips, and lower extremities. If possible, avoid turning the patient on an injured extremity. While inspecting for lacerations, abrasions, puncture wounds, deformity, and tenderness along the vertebral column, a provider also assesses rectal tone to assess for neurological disabilities.

Obtain information regarding the event to rule out nonaccidental trauma in pediatrics, older adult abuse, and intimate partner violence. Each state has regulations regarding reporting such events.

STUDY BREAK

4. Which laboratory value indicates that the patient is under-resuscitated?
   A. Potassium (K^+) of 6.1 mEq/L
   B. Calcium (Ca^{++}) of 8.0 mg/dL
   C. Hematocrit (Hct) of 28.2%
   D. Lactate of 5 mmol/L

ASSESSMENT AND MANAGEMENT OF SPECIFIC INJURIES

This section discusses common traumatic injuries, which may be diagnosed and managed in the emergency care phase or in the subsequent critical care phase. Rapid assessment, resuscitation, and damage control surgery to minimize bleeding in the emergency care phase, coupled with definitive surgical interventions in the critical care phase, has decreased mortality.[2,12] However, not all injuries require surgical intervention. Ongoing assessment, management of specific organ injuries, and an awareness of the patient's response to the stress of the injury are vital during the resuscitative and critical care phase of trauma care.

Head Injuries

Lacerations to the scalp often result in significant bleeding. These wounds are cleansed, debrided, and sutured. Fractures of the skull may be linear, basilar, closed depressed, open depressed, or comminuted. Underlying brain injury may occur with skull fractures. Basilar skull fractures are located at the base of the cranium and potentially involve the five bones that form the skull base. The diagnosis is based on the presence of cerebrospinal fluid in the nose (rhinorrhea), in the ears (otorrhea), or both; ecchymosis over the mastoid area (Battle's sign); or hemotympanum (blood in the middle ear). Raccoon eyes or periorbital ecchymoses are present after a basilar skull fracture (see Chapter 14).

Traumatic brain injury (TBI) contributes to about 30% of all injury deaths.[28] Falls are the leading cause of TBI, accounting for almost 50% of all TBI-related ED visits, hospitalizations, and deaths in the United States. Nearly 4 in 5 (79%) TBIs are associated with falls in adults ages 65 years and older, and they are a leading cause of death.[28] After falls, being struck by or against an object (including intentional self-harm) and MVCs are common causes of TBI.[28]

Patients who sustain TBIs may develop postconcussive syndrome days to months after the head injury. Assessment findings include persistent headache, memory and judgment impairment, dizziness and nausea, and attention deficits. If the symptoms persist, these patients may require ongoing evaluation, treatment, and extended rehabilitation before they are able to return to their previous level of activities.[47]

Injuries to the head may result from blunt or penetrating trauma. Primary head injury from blunt trauma typically occurs in the presence of acceleration, deceleration, or rotational forces. Injury may be focal or diffuse. Secondary head injury refers to systemic changes (hypotension, hypoxia, anemia, hyperthermia) or intracranial changes (edema, intracranial hypertension, seizures) that result in alterations in the nervous system tissue.[10] Patients with secondary injury often have poor outcomes, including death. Ensure adequate blood pressure to meet cerebral perfusion; maximize ventilation and oxygenation through effective airway management; maintain the head in a midline position to enhance cerebral blood flow; administer analgesics and sedatives to address pain, agitation, and increased ICP; conduct frequent neurological assessments; and provide nutrition.[10] Goals for blood pressure focus on interventions to maintain a cerebral perfusion pressure (equal to the mean arterial pressure minus ICP) greater than 60 mm Hg. A cerebral perfusion pressure less than 60 mm Hg has been associated with poor patient outcomes.[47]

Spinal Cord Injury

Spinal cord injury (SCI) is a major neurological disability that is assessed early in the emergent phase of traumatic injury (see Chapter 14). Mechanisms of injury that may result in SCI include hyperflexion, hyperextension, axial loading, rotation, and penetrating trauma. Secondary injury can occur from progressive cell damage to the spinal cord due to the inflammatory response, hemorrhage, hypoperfusion, and hypoxemia.[2,47] The initial treatment of a patient with suspected SCI includes the ABCs of resuscitation, spine immobilization, and prevention of further injury through surgical stabilization of the spine. A complete sensory and motor neurological examination is performed during the disability assessment of the primary survey, and radiographic studies of the cervical spine are considered. A spinal CT scan may be performed to rule out occult injury. It is important to determine the approximate level of the SCI because higher cervical spine injuries may result in loss of phrenic nerve innervations, compromising the patient's ability to breathe spontaneously.

SCI causes a loss of sympathetic output, resulting in distributive shock with hypotension and bradycardia. Blood pressure may respond to IV fluids, but vasopressor medications are often required to compensate for the loss of sympathetic innervation and resultant vasodilation. The patient with a SCI presents complex challenges for the trauma team as they attempt to minimize loss of function associated with the injury. Proactive, aggressive, and comprehensive care is necessary to help the patient achieve optimal functional outcomes.

Thoracic Injuries

The thoracic region contains vital organs such as the heart, great vessels, and lungs. It is considered a critical region because injuries to the thoracic organs and structures can quickly become life-threatening. FAST and E-FAST are typically the first-line diagnostic tools used in the emergent evaluation of a patient presenting with thoracic injury, providing essential information for the immediate management of the trauma patient.[2,61,76]

Blunt Cardiac Injury, Cardiac Contusion, and Cardiac Tamponade. Blunt cardiac injury encompasses a wide range of clinical manifestations, from asymptomatic cardiac contusion to cardiac tamponade and cardiac rupture. Blunt cardiac trauma is most often a consequence of an MVC, a fall, or any mechanism of injury involving decelerating forces with direct thoracic or chest impact.[2,47]

Blunt trauma to the chest is the most frequent cause of cardiac contusion.[50] The force of the traumatic event bruises the heart muscle and can compromise effective heart functioning and cause dysrhythmias.[2,50] In the event of significant anterior chest trauma, obtain a 12-lead ECG and serum levels of cardiac isoenzymes and troponin to rule out ischemia or infarction. If conduction abnormalities are identified, ongoing monitoring for symptomatic cardiac dysrhythmias via continuous monitoring of the ECG is indicated for 24 hours.[2] With severe cardiac contusion injuries, inotropic medications are occasionally needed to support myocardial function.

Cardiac tamponade is a life-threatening condition caused by rapid accumulation of fluid (usually blood) in the pericardial sac. Cardiac tamponade may be caused by penetrating or blunt trauma to the chest.[2,47] It should also be suspected in any patient with chest and multisystem injuries who presents in shock and does not respond to aggressive fluid resuscitation. As the intrapericardial pressure increases, cardiac output is impaired because of decreased venous return. The development of pulsus paradoxus may occur, with a decrease in systolic blood pressure during spontaneous inspiration. Blood, if unable to flow into the right side of the heart, causes increased right atrial pressure and distended neck veins. Classic signs of cardiac tamponade are hypotension, muffled or distant heart sounds, and elevated venous pressure (Beck's triad). Beck's triad may not be present until late in the development of tamponade. ECG changes may include multiple premature ventricular contractions (PVCs), atrial fibrillation, bundle branch block and ST segment changes, or indications of a myocardial infarction.[2] FAST exam can facilitate early diagnosis of cardiac tamponade. Cardiac tamponade is treated by *pericardiocentesis* (needle aspiration of the pericardial sac) followed by a thoracotomy.[2,47,50] Pericardiocentesis is performed by the physician; a needle is used to aspirate blood from the pericardial sac. Removal of as little as 15 to 20 mL of blood may dramatically improve blood pressure. Anticipate and obtain equipment for an emergency thoracotomy in the event of cardiac arrest during the pericardiocentesis.

Aortic Disruption. Aortic disruption is produced by blunt trauma to the chest and frequently results in death at the scene of the traumatic event. Rapid deceleration forces produced by a head-on MVC, ejection, or fall can cause shearing forces and dissection of the aorta. The proximal descending aorta is at greatest risk, with injuries ranging from complete transection to hematomas. Although this injury has a high mortality, early diagnosis can prevent tearing of the innermost layer, exsanguination, and death.

Specific signs of traumatic aortic disruption are frequently absent but may include greater muscle strength in upper extremities compared to lower extremities or paraplegia.[2,47] Chest radiography and/or CT may demonstrate a widened mediastinum, tracheal deviation to the right, depressed left mainstem bronchus, first and second rib fractures, and left hemothorax.[2,47] The diagnosis is confirmed by angiography if available. Definitive, emergent surgical resection and repair are necessary with this injury.

Pneumothorax, Tension Pneumothorax, and Open Pneumothorax. Pneumothorax occurs when air escapes from the injured lung into the pleural space, altering the negative intrapleural pressure and resulting in a partial or complete collapse of the lung.[8,61] The patient presents with respiratory distress, tachypnea, tachycardia, diminished or absent breath sounds on the injured side, and chest pain.[47] Pneumothorax may be confirmed by chest radiography or E-FAST. Treatment focuses on providing supplemental oxygen and chest tube placement to evacuate the pleural air and reexpand the lung.[47]

Tension pneumothorax is a rapidly fatal emergency that is easily resolved with early recognition and intervention. It occurs when an injury to the chest allows air to enter the pleural cavity without a route for escape. With each inspiration, additional air accumulates in the pleural space, increasing intrathoracic pressure and leading to lung collapse. The increased pressure causes compression of the heart and great vessels toward the unaffected side, as evidenced by mediastinal shift and distended neck veins. The resulting decreased cardiac output and alterations in gas exchange are manifested by anxiety, severe respiratory distress, absence of breath sounds on the affected side, hypotension, distended neck veins, and tracheal deviation away from the side of injury (see Fig. 20.4). Cyanosis is a late manifestation of this life-threatening clinical situation. The diagnosis of tension pneumothorax is based on the patient's clinical presentation. Never delay treatment to confirm the diagnosis by radiography.[2] Immediate decompression of the intrathoracic pressure is accomplished by *needle thoracentesis* followed by definitive treatment with a chest tube.[2,47]

Open pneumothorax is associated with penetrating chest trauma that allows air to pass in and out of the pleural space. In addition to the signs and symptoms of a pneumothorax, subcutaneous emphysema may also be present. Management of the open chest wound is accomplished with a nonporous dressing taped securely on three sides.[47] The fourth side is left open to allow for exhalation of air from within the pleural cavity. If the dressing becomes completely occlusive on all sides, a tension pneumothorax may occur.[47]

Hemothorax. Hemothorax is a collection of blood in the pleural space; it results from injuries to the heart, the great vessels, or the pulmonary parenchyma. Bleeding can be moderate (from intercostal vessels) or massive (from the aorta or subclavian or pulmonary vessels). Decreased breath sounds, dullness to percussion on the affected side, hypotension, and

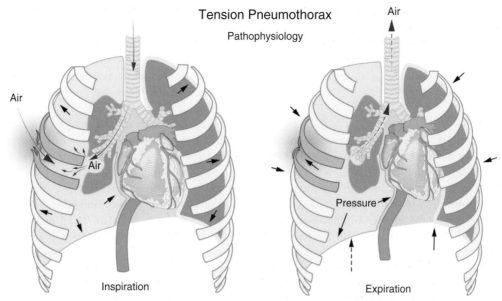

Fig. 20.4 Tension pneumothorax. Following a chest injury air enters the pleural cavity on inspiration and, without a route to escape, pressure increases compressing the heart and great vessels to the uneffected side (mediastinal shift). (Reprinted with permission, Cleveland Clinic Center for Medical Art & Photography ©2015-2019. All rights reserved.)

respiratory distress may be seen.[2,47] Placement of a chest tube facilitates removal of blood from the pleural space with resolution of ventilation and gas exchange abnormalities. Nursing interventions include managing the chest tube, closely observing the amount of blood drained from the pleural space, and monitoring the patient's hemodynamic response.

Pulmonary Contusion. Pulmonary contusion occurs as a result of rapid deceleration, blunt impact, or blast forces to the chest. A contusion develops when capillary blood leaks into the lung parenchyma, resulting in inflammation and edema. The contusion may be localized or diffuse. The degree of respiratory distress develops gradually, with worsening severity of oxygenation and ventilation as the edema progresses.[47] It is commonly seen with other thoracic injuries such as rib fractures and is one of the most common causes of death after chest injury.[2,77] It is often difficult to detect because the initial chest radiographic study may be normal and is frequently only seen on CT scan with other injuries.[77] The clinical presentation includes worsening dyspnea, ineffective cough, hypoxia, chest wall abrasions, and chest pain. Interventions focus on providing supplemental oxygen and possibly mechanical ventilation. Administer fluids cautiously to avoid further lung edema.[47,77] Provide adequate pain relief with IV narcotics to optimize lung expansion and respiratory effort and to prevent complications, including atelectasis, pneumonia, and ARDS.

Rib Fractures and Flail Chest. Rib fractures are the injury most commonly associated with chest trauma.[2,47] Rib fractures may lead to significant respiratory dysfunction and may indicate a serious injury to organs and structures below and near the rib cage. A high-impact force is needed to fracture the clavicle and first rib with the risk of associated injuries of the head, neck, spinal cord, and great vessels.[2] Assess

for hemodynamic instability, which may indicate the presence of major vessel injury such as aortic disruption or injury to the subclavian artery.[2,47] Injury to the liver, spleen, or kidney may accompany fractures of the lower ribs. The diagnosis of rib fractures is frequently made after a chest radiographic study. However, there are situations in which rib fractures are not visualized on chest radiographs and the diagnosis is made through clinical assessment.

The management of rib fractures depends on the number of ribs fractured, the degree of underlying injury, and the age of the patient. Assess the patient's ventilation and oxygenation and provide effective pain management. Provide education on coughing and deep-breathing exercises, the benefits of early ambulation, and pain management. Effective pain management enables the patient to maximally participate in pulmonary exercises and improves outcomes in patients with rib fractures.[2,47]

A *flail chest* is frequently defined as fractures of three or more adjacent ribs in two or more places, creating a free-floating segment of the rib cage. The flail segment results in paradoxical chest movement; the chest contracts inward with inhalation and expands outward with exhalation. Normal respiratory mechanics depend on a rigid chest wall to generate negative intrathoracic pressure for effective ventilation. The uncoordinated chest movement in flail chest impairs the ability of the body to generate effective changes in intrathoracic pressure for ventilation. The clinical presentation includes paradoxical chest movement, increased work of breathing, tachypnea, and eventually signs and symptoms of hypoxemia. Management frequently involves endotracheal intubation and mechanical ventilation with adequate pain control, which may include epidural analgesia or a regional block.[2,47] Internal surgical fixation of rib fractures may be used in some patients. Position the patient to enhance ventilation and oxygenation and provide frequent pulmonary care to prevent pneumonia.

❓ CRITICAL REASONING ACTIVITY

If a patient experiences thoracic trauma, what laboratory analysis is anticipated and why? Why is cardiac monitoring and/or a 12-lead electrocardiogram (ECG) prescribed?

Abdominal Injuries

Abdominal injuries are often difficult to diagnose. A normal initial examination does not necessarily rule out intraabdominal injury. The classic sign of abdominal injury is pain. However, pain cannot be used as an assessment tool if the patient has an altered sensorium, drug intoxication, or SCI with impaired sensation. Injuries to the intraabdominal organs can cause significant bleeding and uncontrolled hemorrhage. The peritoneum can accommodate a significant blood volume and abdominal distension might not be apparent until several liters of blood are in the peritoneal cavity.[13] Since hemodynamic instability from intraabdominal injuries arises from major hemorrhage, immediate management is focused on resuscitation with early use of blood products until definitive hemostasis can be achieved, usually through surgical intervention. In unstable patients who are unresponsive, or transient responders to resuscitation, resuscitative endovascular balloon occlusion of the aorta (REBOA) may be considered.[13,14] A specially trained physician inserts a REBOA catheter through the femoral artery and inflates a balloon on the catheter in the distal thoracic aorta or the distal abdominal aorta to achieve aortic occlusion. This temporizing measure increases systolic blood pressure and allows patient transport to an operating room for damage control surgery.[13,14] Document the procedure as well as balloon inflation and/or deflation time.

The liver is the most commonly injured abdominal organ by blunt or penetrating trauma.[2,47] The patient may present with a history of right lower thoracic trauma, fractured lower right ribs, right upper quadrant ecchymosis, right upper quadrant tenderness, and hypotension. The diagnosis is confirmed with the use of FAST and/or abdominal CT. The degree of liver injury is graded on a scale of I to VI, with I representing a nonexpanding subcapsular hematoma and VI signifying hepatic avulsion. Angiographic embolization or surgical management is indicated for patients with high-grade liver injuries and signs of hemodynamic instability, in which there is expansion of the hemorrhage, a large laceration, or complete avulsion of the liver from its vascular supply.[47,65] Hemodynamically stable patients with a liver injury are managed nonoperatively with frequent monitoring (regular abdominal assessment and serial hemoglobin and hematocrit measurements).[2,47]

Splenic injury occurs most often as a result of blunt trauma to the abdomen, penetrating trauma to the left upper quadrant of the abdomen, or fracture of the anterior left lower ribs. The patient may present with left upper quadrant tenderness, peritoneal irritation, referred pain to the left shoulder (Kehr's sign), and hypotension or signs of hypovolemic shock. An encapsulated hemorrhage of the spleen produces no immediate signs of bleeding. The diagnosis is confirmed by using the same tests as for liver injuries. Management of splenic injury is similar to that of liver injuries. Close monitoring of the patient is vital. Assess the patient's hemodynamic status and assess the abdomen for guarding, rebound tenderness, rigidity, or distension. Operative intervention is often necessary after severe splenic injuries, and the spleen may rupture days to weeks after the initial injury. A ruptured spleen is a life-threatening event that requires immediate surgical intervention. Every effort is made to preserve splenic tissue because of its role in immune function. Patients who have undergone splenectomy are susceptible to infections, and administration of the pneumococcal, *Haemophilus influenzae* type b (Hib), meningococcal, and other vaccines are strongly recommended.[16]

Injuries to the stomach, small bowel, and large bowel are most frequently the consequence of penetrating trauma from gunshot wounds. Blast injuries can also cause injury to these hollow organs. Gastric and bowel injury is suspected based on the mechanism of injury, and surgical intervention is usually required. Postoperative complications include infection and difficulty maintaining nutrition.

Blunt trauma to the abdomen may also injure the kidneys; however, usually only one kidney is affected. The patient may present with costovertebral tenderness, microscopic or gross hematuria, bruising or ecchymosis over the 11th and 12th ribs, hemorrhage, and/or shock.[47] Diagnostic studies include FAST, CT, angiography, IV pyelography, and cystoscopy. For minor injuries, management focuses on hydration and monitoring of kidney function, which includes adequacy of urine output; urinalysis; hematuria; blood urea nitrogen, creatinine, and electrolyte levels; and a complete blood count. Management of major and critical kidney injuries focuses on surgical intervention, including control of bleeding, repair of the injury, or nephrectomy. Postsurgical complications include refractory hypertension, hemorrhage, fistula formation, and infection.

Blunt trauma causing disruption of the pelvic structure is a challenging clinical problem because of the large vascular supply, nervous system pathways, location of urological structures, and articulation of the hip joint within the pelvic ring. Treatment of pelvic injuries often requires the expertise of many specialties (e.g., orthopedics, general surgery, neurosurgery, urology). Pelvic injuries occur most frequently in high-deceleration MVCs, pedestrian-vehicle impacts, and falls.

The mortality rate from pelvic injuries is estimated at 5% to 30% and up to 50% in patients with open pelvic fractures.[2] Mortality is primarily related to hemorrhage and hemodynamic instability. Primary interventions focus on pelvic stabilization and aggressive fluid resuscitation to ensure adequate tissue perfusion. Initially, pelvic stabilization can be accomplished by tying a large sheet or pelvic binder around the patient's hips at the level of the greater trochanter to control the bleeding.[2-4,13,14] Early definitive treatment is accomplished through surgical repair in the operating room, although interventional radiology procedures that use embolization or coil techniques may also be used to stop the bleeding. Surgical repair may be required for internal or external fixation of complex pelvic fractures.

LIFESPAN CONSIDERATIONS

Older Adults

- Falls are the most frequent cause of injury for the elderly population and the leading cause of injury-related deaths in individuals older than 65 years of age.[30] Falls result in fractures of the hips, arms, hands, legs, feet, pelvis, ribs, and vertebrae.
- Three factors contribute to a higher morbidity and mortality in this population: comorbidities, diminished physiological reserve, and age-related physiological changes.[6,7]
- Physiological changes associated with aging and reduced physiological reserves predispose older adults to serious injury, prolonged recovery, and increased mortality. Older adults with poor functional status and multiple comorbidities have worse outcomes after trauma.[24]
- Approximately 75% of people ages 65 years and older have multiple chronic conditions that require ongoing medical attention or limit activities of daily living.[29] Individuals with chronic hypertension may appear to have a normal blood pressure when in fact they are hypotensive. An older adult who is taking beta-blockers and a calcium channel blocker may have a blunted hemodynamic response to trauma.[24] Therefore slight changes in heart rate or blood pressure may signify unrecognized injury.
- Knowledge of current medications, specifically anticoagulants, steroids, cardiac medications (e.g., beta-blockers, calcium channel blockers), and nonsteroidal antiinflammatory drugs (NSAIDs), is important because they may increase the risk of injury and the risk of complications.
- The Beers Medication List is updated by the American Geriatric Society and provides information on medications and potential adverse reactions in the older adult.[7]

Pregnant Women

- Risk factors for additional injuries associated with the pregnant state include Rh exposure, placental abruption, uterine rupture, preterm labor, and fetal compromise.[52]
- Advanced stages of pregnancy increase a pregnant patient's risk for failure to maintain a patent airway and challenge pulmonary mechanics (e.g., ventilation effort); therefore continuously monitor oxygenation and ventilation.[52] Administer supplemental oxygen by a nasal cannula, mask, or mechanical ventilation (if indicated) due to the marked increases in basal oxygen consumption.[52]
- The pregnant patient experiences significant changes in fluid volume status, which may make it harder to detect blood loss. The pregnant trauma patient may lose up to 40% of circulating volume before there is an appreciable drop in blood pressure.[2,47]
- Compression of the vena cava by the uterus can cause a significant reduction in cardiac output. The gravid uterus is moved off the inferior vena cava to increase venous return and cardiac output in the acutely injured pregnant woman.[2,47,52] This can be achieved by manual displacement of the uterus or left lateral tilt while maintaining spinal precautions.
- Consult obstetrical and neonatal specialists (providers and nurses) to evaluate the patient and fetus.
- Evaluate for traumatic injury associated with domestic violence.

on whether the patient is bleeding or has a high probability of bleeding due to unavailable or ineffective clotting factors. The presence of abnormal values indicates the need for more aggressive resuscitation or blood component therapy.

Ongoing Care

Ongoing patient care priorities evolve from the patient's diagnosis and the surgical procedure. Careful attention is given to anticipating potential problems and intervening when actual problems are identified. Perform a comprehensive reassessment every 4 hours to identify changes in the patient's status, prepare for additional diagnostic procedures, and intervene appropriately. Evaluate the patient continuously for alterations in oxygenation, ventilation, acid-base balance, perfusion, metabolic status, and hemodynamic status and for signs and symptoms of infection. Potential complications include infections (pneumonia and urinary tract infections), ARDS, and DVT.[71]

Optimal nutritional support is considered an integral component of care of the critically injured patient. Nutritional needs of the patient are addressed early in the postoperative phase (within 24 to 48 hours) to assist with healing and meeting the body's needs related to an elevated metabolic demand. The route of administration (oral, enteral, or parenteral), type of nutritional replacement, and rate of administration depend on the severity of illness or injury and the expected recovery period. In critically ill patients who are unable to maintain intake, enteral nutrition initiated within 24 to 48 hours is associated with a reduction in mortality and infectious morbidity.[62] Obtain a nutritional consultation to evaluate the metabolic needs of the patient and determine the optimal feeding formula and rate of administration (see Chapter 7).

Ensure that the patient has pharmacological prophylaxis for VTE and stress ulceration and an aggressive protocol for mobilization. Immobility places a patient at increased risk of developing VTE, pneumonia, pressure ulcers, urostasis, and delirium. Strategies to prevent complications of immobility include frequent turning, offloading pressure on bony prominences with pillows, frequent skin assessments, application of moisture barriers to skin to prevent maceration from feces or leaking drainage devices, coughing and deep-breathing exercises, early extubation, urinary catheter care and early removal of the catheter, and early ambulation.

Patients with multisystem injuries are at high risk for myriad complications associated with the overwhelming stressors of the injury, prolonged immobility, and consequences of inadequate tissue perfusion. Even with optimal care, the stressors and overwhelming inflammatory responses to injury influence the risk of secondary complications. These include respiratory impairment (abdominal compartment syndrome, acute lung injury, ARDS, pneumonia), infection (catheter infection, sepsis), acute kidney injury, high nutritional demands, and MODS. A full discussion of these secondary complications can be found in other chapters within this text.

SPECIAL CONSIDERATIONS AND POPULATIONS

Alcohol and Drug Use

Many injuries have alcohol and drug use as a contributing factor. Most trauma patients who have a high blood alcohol concentration on admission meet criteria that indicate an alcohol problem. Because of the high incidence of traumatic events involving the use of alcohol and drugs, trauma prevention cannot be successful unless these concerns are addressed. Screening and brief intervention for alcohol use is required of all trauma centers.[3,31]

Evidence-based programs are available to guide intervention programs and provide tools to address alcohol and drug problems in patients during an acute hospital admission. These include the Screening, Brief Intervention, and Referral to Treatment (SBIRT) services provided by Medicare and Medicaid.[31] Trauma centers need to have alcohol and drug intervention programs that can be implemented at the time of admission and maintained throughout the hospitalization by appropriately trained staff. Brief interventions initiated during hospitalization affect the high correlation of alcohol and/or illicit drug use and serious traumatic injury by decreasing the incidence of trauma recidivism.[31]

Drug use and abuse impair a patient's cognitive processes and create physiological stress. Multiple categories of drugs may be used by the trauma patient, ranging from inhalant intoxicants to hallucinogens, designer drugs (e.g., Ecstasy, ketamine), cocaine, methamphetamine, cannabis, and prescription opioids. Drug use, especially drug overdose, causes significant physiological stressors. After addressing the traumatic injury, the physiological consequences of the drug and subsequent drug withdrawal must be addressed. Nursing care of the trauma patient with an alcohol or drug addiction provides both a challenge and an opportunity. Because addiction is associated with physiological dependence, serious or life-threatening withdrawal may occur when the patient no longer consumes these agents. Closely monitor the patient's physiological status during withdrawal. Implement protocols to address withdrawal by providing preemptive treatment. Common signs and symptoms include increased agitation, anxiety, auditory and visual hallucinations, disorientation, headache, nausea and vomiting, paroxysmal diaphoresis, and tremors (Box 20.3). Assess the time of the patient's last use of the drug or alcohol to plan treatment strategies. As patients experience withdrawal, medications may be ordered to ease the physiological and behavioral symptoms. Assess the patient hourly, especially in the presence of worsening anxiety, hallucinations, and other symptoms, to ensure patient safety. Someone may be designated to sit with the patient at all times during acute drug or alcohol withdrawal. Implement drug and alcohol prevention interventions before discharge from the hospital.

BOX 20.3   Signs and Symptoms of Alcohol Withdrawal

- Irritability, anxiety, agitation, and/or confusion
- Hallucinations and delusions
- Insomnia
- Tremors
- Nausea, vomiting, and diarrhea
- Diaphoresis
- Tachycardia and hypertension
- Fever
- Seizures

Abuse of Vulnerable Populations and Intimate Partner Violence

Vulnerable populations (children, mentally and/or physically dysfunctional adults, and older adult patients who cannot care for themselves) are at risk for abuse. Many states have mandatory reporting laws for reported or suspected abuse in these vulnerable populations. When abuse is suspected, the nurse must follow the hospital's reporting processes and provide emotional support to the patient.

Intimate partner violence, also called domestic or dating violence, can be physical, sexual, or psychological. Several questionnaires are available to screen for intimate partner violence: Humiliation, Afraid, Rape, Kick (HARK); Hurt/Insult/Threaten/Scream (HITS); Extended Hurt/Insult/Threaten/Scream (E-HITS); Partner Violence Screen (PVS); and Woman Abuse Screening Tool (WAST). Intimate partner violence is not restricted to heterosexual couples. Individuals who identify as lesbian, gay, bisexual, transgender, and queer or questioning (LGBTQ) also experience intimate partner violence, as well as other types of violence, and may not seek help or disclose the mechanism of injury.[17] Lack of understanding of the problem, stigma, and system inequalities are potential barriers to LGBTQ survivors seeking and receiving help.[17]

Family and Patient Coping

Traumatic injury is frequently unexpected and is a potentially devastating event, producing physical, psychological, and emotional stress for the patient and family. The event leaves the patient and family feeling overwhelmed, vulnerable, and often ill-prepared to cope with ramifications of the injury. The traumatic event often creates a crisis within the patient's family unit. Critical decisions for the patient frequently must be made in seconds by family members. The trauma team can assist the patient and family in crisis by helping them establish a consistent communication process between the healthcare team and the family. Explore the patient's and family's perception of the event, support systems, and coping mechanisms. Involve the social worker early to assist the patient and family with coping and decision making. Coordinate a family conference early in the emergency care phase and frequently during the critical care phase to assist with communication and understanding of the patient's and family's expectations for care and to enhance the decision-making and coping skills of the patient and family.

Posttraumatic stress disorder (PTSD) and acute stress disorder (ASD) are trauma- and stressor-related psychiatric disorders that can occur after experiencing or witnessing events involving physical injury, death, or other threats to physical integrity.[67] Symptoms of trauma- and stressor-related disorders include reexperiencing the traumatic event and avoidance of trauma-related stimuli. If the patient exhibits symptoms of ASD or PTSD during screening, obtain consultations and provide resources such as the Trauma Survivors Network support group and crisis intervention call-in lines.

REHABILITATION PHASE

The final phase of trauma care encompasses rehabilitation of the patient. The initiation of the rehabilitative process begins the moment the patient is admitted to the trauma center. Prevention of complications that prolong hospitalization and delay rehabilitation is imperative. Early involvement of physical medicine and rehabilitation personnel is vital to achieve positive functional patient outcomes. Early in this phase of trauma care, a case manager or discharge planner evaluates the patient for the need for extensive rehabilitation at a specialty center. An individualized plan is developed for each patient based on physical injuries and rehabilitation potential, patient and family preferences, and insurance coverage.

Nursing interventions in the critical care phase influence the patient's rehabilitative needs. For example, focus on positioning the immobile patient to prevent foot drop. This intervention facilitates ambulation during recovery. Apply splints to injured extremities to improve functionality. Provide emotional support to both the patient and the family as the patient convalesces through the critical care phase and begins more independent activities. Prepare them for the rehabilitation phase of trauma recovery.

Transition of the patient into rehabilitation is both an exciting and a frightening time for the patient and family. The patient has relied on the nursing staff for encouragement and support at a critical time in the patient's life. Transfer to another center brings with it uncertainty in new relationships, as well as excitement, because rehabilitation is the last step before returning to the patient's home.

 QSEN EXEMPLAR

Quality Improvement; Patient Safety

A nurse notices that essential life-saving equipment (e.g., manual resuscitation bag, oxygen flow meter, Lactated Ringer's solution, suture material) are often missing from the trauma room designated for admission of patients with traumatic injury. The lack of essential equipment in the room causes delays in care as team members leave the room to obtain necessary supplies and increases the tension of the team during the acute admission. On exploring the reasons for missing items, the nurse discovers that there is no checklist for what is considered essential equipment for the trauma room. The nurse surveys the trauma team (providers, nurses, technicians, support staff, laboratory personnel) to understand what equipment each healthcare professional deems essential to provide initial care to the trauma patient. After developing the list of items to be stocked in the trauma room, the nurse approaches the unit leadership to ask for a trauma cart so that the equipment needed could be more easily stocked and stored in the trauma room. The nurse agrees to track the efficiency in care resulting from moving to a trauma cart, as reported by all members of the trauma team.

CASE STUDY

Mr. M., a 27-year-old male, was dropped off in the emergency department (ED) with a gunshot wound to his right chest. He was awake on arrival, but his level of consciousness quickly declined as the trauma team transported him to the resuscitation room. Once in the resuscitation room, Mr. M. became unresponsive with a weak pulse. Vital signs were as follows: sinus tachycardic with heart rate 125 beats/min; blood pressure, 72/48 mm Hg; respiratory rate, 8 breaths/min; oxygen saturation (SpO_2), 75%; and temperature, 35.8°C. The patient was immediately intubated to secure his airway and placed on the ventilator at 100% fraction of inspired oxygen (FiO_2). Two large-bore peripheral IV catheters were placed, and resuscitation was started with normal saline at 500 mL/h. The focused assessment with sonography for trauma (FAST) examination was positive for free fluid in the abdomen. The patient's blood was typed and crossmatched, and the massive transfusion protocol was initiated at a ratio of 1:1:1 (packed red blood cells, fresh frozen plasma, and platelets). The patient was transported to the operating room for damage-control surgery. A thoracotomy was performed, and the site of hemorrhage was located; the bullet had lacerated the descending aorta. The aorta was repaired, chest tubes were placed, and the patient was transported to the critical care unit in critical condition.

Upon arrival to the unit, the critical care nurses performed a rapid and systematic primary and secondary survey. The airway remained secure via the endotracheal tube, the patient was tolerating mechanical ventilation, and his bilateral lung sounds were clear. He had equal chest rise and fall, and his oxygen saturation was 95%. Circulation assessment revealed weak pulses, his color was pale, heart rate was sinus tachycardia at 150 beats/min, blood pressure was 90/60 mm Hg, respiratory rate was 18 breaths/min, and temperature was 35.9°C. Fluid resuscitation with Lactated Ringer's solution was continued. The patient was not responsive to verbal commands or moving any extremities, and his pupils were 2 mm and reactive to light. During the head-to-toe assessment and inspection of posterior surfaces of the secondary survey, a small wound was discovered in the midline posterior aspect of his cervical spine, consistent with a penetrating injury. No other injuries were discovered.

Laboratory results were as follows:

Hemoglobin	7.2 g/dL
Hematocrit	22.3%
White blood cell count	16,000 cells/microliter
Platelet count	200,000/microliter
Potassium	5.5 mEq/L
Other electrolyte levels	Unremarkable
Arterial Blood Gas Results	
pH	7.19
Partial pressure of arterial oxygen (PaO_2)	160 mm Hg
Partial pressure of arterial carbon dioxide ($PaCO_2$)	42 mm Hg
Bicarbonate (HCO_3^-)	18 mEq/L
Base deficit	−14
Lactate	8 mmol/L

Aggressive fluid resuscitation continued as the patient was transported for computed tomography to evaluate his head and spine for additional injuries. The ED contacted his family, who were in the waiting room of the critical care unit.

Questions

1. What are the priority interventions on arrival of the patient in the ED based on his vital signs?
2. What additional procedures do you anticipate in the emergent evaluation and treatment of this patient considering the mechanism of injury?
3. Why is it important to administer platelets and fresh frozen plasma along with packed red blood cells to a patient who requires a massive blood transfusion?
4. What is your interpretation of the laboratory results? What interventions do you anticipate based on these results?
5. How does hypothermia affect the care of the postoperative patient? What are nursing interventions to address hypothermia?
6. What are the needs of the family?

REFERENCES

1. American Association of Critical Care Nurses. Family presence during resuscitation and invasive procedures. *Crit Care Nurse.* 2016;36(1):E11–E14.

2. American College of Surgeons, Committee on Trauma. *Advanced Trauma Life Support: Student Course Manual.* 10th ed. Chicago, IL: American College of Surgeons, Committee on Trauma; 2018.

3. American College of Surgeons, Committee on Trauma. Regional trauma systems: Optimal elements, integration, and assessment. In: American College of Surgeons, Committee on Trauma. *Resources for Optimal Care of the Injured Patient, 2014.* Chicago, IL: American College of Surgeons, Committee on Trauma; 2014:8–15.

4. American College of Surgeons, Committee on Trauma. Part I: A Brief History of Trauma Systems. https://www.facs.org/quality-programs/trauma/tqp/systems-programs/trauma-series/part-i. Accessed April 23, 2019.

5. American College of Surgeons, Committee on Trauma. ACS TQIP Best Practices in the Management of Orthopedic Trauma. https://www.facs.org/~/media/files/quality%20programs/trauma/tqip/tqip%20bpgs%20in%20the%20management%20of%20orthopaedic%20traumafinal.ashx. Accessed April 23, 2019.

6. American College of Surgeons, Committee on Trauma. ACS TQIP Geriatric Trauma Management Guidelines. https://www.facs.org/~/media/files/quality%20programs/trauma/tqip/geriatric%20guide%20tqip.ashx. Accessed April 23, 2019.

7. 2019 American Geriatrics Society Beers Criteria® Update Expert Panel. American Geriatrics Society 2019 updated AGS Beers criteria® for potentially inappropriate medication use in older adults. *J Am Geriatr Soc.* 2019;67(4):674–694.

8. Baugher KM, Euerie BD, Sommerkamp SK, et al. Image quality evaluation of a portable handheld ultrasound machine for the focused assessment with sonography for trauma examination. *Am J Emerg Med.* 2014;32:383–391.

9. Baxter J, Cranfield K, Clark G, et al. Do lactate levels in the emergency department predict outcome in adult trauma patients? A systematic review. *J Trauma Acute Care Surg.* 2016;81(3):555–566.

10. Bay EH, Chartier KS. Chronic morbidities after traumatic brain injury: An update for the advanced practice nurse. *J Neurosci Nurs.* 2014;46(3):142–152.

11. Benson M, Koenig KL, Schultz CH. Disaster triage: START, then SAVE, a new method of dynamic triage for victims of a catastrophic earthquake. *Prehosp Disaster Med.* 1996;11(2):117–124.

12. Benz D, Balogh Z. Damage control surgery: Current state and future directions. *Curr Opin Crit Care.* 2017;23(6):491–497.

13. Brenner M, Bulger EM, Perina DG, et al. Joint statement from the American College of Surgeons Committee on Trauma (ACS COT) and the American College of Emergency Physicians (ACEP) regarding the clinical use of Resuscitative Endovascular Balloon Occlusion of the Aorta (REBOA). *Trauma Surg Acute Care Open.* 2018;3(1):e000154.

14. Brenner M, Hicks C. Major abdominal trauma: Critical decisions and new frontiers in management. *Emerg Med Clin North Am.* 2018;36(1):149–160.

15. Brill J, Badiee J, Zander A, et al. The rate of deep vein thrombosis doubles in trauma patients with hypercoagulable thromboelastography. *J Trauma Acute Care Surg.* 2017;83(3):413–419.

16. Bonanni P, Grazzini M, Niccolai G, et al. Recommended vaccinations for asplenic and hyposplenic adult patients. *Hum Vaccin Immunother.* 2016;13(2):359–368.

17. Calton JM, Cattaneo LB, Gebhard KT. Barriers to help seeking for lesbian, gay, bisexual, transgender, and queer survivors of intimate partner violence. *Trauma Violence Abuse.* 2016;17(5):585–600.

18. Cannon J, Khan MA, Raja AS, et al. Damage control resuscitation in patients with severe traumatic hemorrhage: A practice management guideline from the Eastern Association for the Surgery of Trauma. *J Trauma Acute Care Surg.* 2017;82(3):605–617.

19. Ceilsa DJ, Kerwin AJ, Tepass JJ. Trauma systems, triage, and transport. In: More EE, Feliciano DV, Mattox KL, eds. *Trauma.* 8th ed. New York, NY: McGraw-Hill Education; 2017:49–70.

20. Celso B, Tepas J, Langland-Orban B, et al. A systematic review and meta-analysis comparing outcome of severely injured patients treated in trauma centers following the establishment of trauma systems. *J Trauma.* 2006;60(2):371–378.

21. Chavez LO, Leon M, Einav S, Varon J. Beyond muscle destruction: A systematic review of rhabdomyolysis for clinical practice. *Crit Care.* 2016;20(1):135.

22. Centers for Disease Control and Prevention. Injury Prevention and Control: Fatal Injury Data. https://www.cdc.gov/injury/wisqars/fatal.html. Published January 18, 2019. Accessed April 23, 2019.

23. Centers for Disease Control and Prevention. Injury Prevention and Control: Key Data and Statistics. https://www.cdc.gov/injury/wisqars/overview/key_data.html. Published May 8, 2017. Accessed April 23, 2019.

24. Centers for Disease Control and Prevention. Leading Cause of Death Reports, 1981–2017. https://webappa.cdc.gov/sasweb/ncipc/leadcause.html. Published January 18, 2019. Accessed April 23, 2019.

25. Centers for Disease Control and Prevention. Motor Vehicle Safety: Cost Data and Prevention Policies. https://www.cdc.gov/motorvehiclesafety/costs/index.html. Published May 31, 2017. Accessed April 23, 2019.

26. Centers for Disease Control and Prevention, National Center for Health Statistics. Drug Overdose Deaths in the United States, 1999–2016. https://www.cdc.gov/nchs/products/databriefs/db294.htm. Published December 21, 2017. Accessed April 23, 2019.

27. Centers for Disease Control and Prevention. Teen Drivers: Get the Facts. http://www.cdc.gov/motorvehiclesafety/teen_drivers/teendrivers_factsheet.html. Accessed April 23, 2019.

28. Centers for Disease Control and Prevention. Traumatic Brain Injury & Concussion. https://www.cdc.gov/traumaticbraininjury/get_the_facts.html. Published February 25, 2019. Accessed April 23, 2019.

29. Centers for Disease Control and Prevention, National Center for Chronic Disease Prevention and Health Promotion. Multiple Chronic Conditions. https://www.cdc.gov/chronicdisease/about/multiple-chronic.htm. Published August 14, 2018. Accessed April 23, 2019.

30. Centers for Disease Control and Prevention, WISQARS. Injury Prevention and Control: Ten Leading Causes of Death and Injury. https://www.cdc.gov/injury/wisqars/LeadingCauses.html. Published February 7, 2019. Accessed April 23, 2019.

31. Centers for Medicare & Medicaid Services. Screening, Brief Intervention, Referral to Treatment (SBIRT) Services. https://www.cms.gov/Outreach-and-Education/Medicare-Learning-Network-MLN/MLNProducts/downloads/SBIRT_Factsheet_ICN904084.pdf. Published March 2017. Accessed April 23, 2019.

32. Crandall M, Zarzaur B, Tinkoff G. American Association for the Surgery of Trauma Prevention Committee topical overview: National trauma data bank, geographic information systems, and teaching injury prevention. *Am J Surg.* 2013;206(5):709–713.

33. Crowe L. Tips on building resilience and improving well-being. *Emerg Nurse.* 2017;24(10):14–15.

34. Della Rocca GJ, Dunbar RP, Burgess AR, et al. Opportunities for knowledge translation in the decade of road traffic safety. *J Orthop Trauma*. 2014;28(6):S18–S21.

35. Dieleman JL, Baral R, Birger M, et al. U.S. Spending on Personal Health Care and Public Health, 1996–2013. *JAMA*. 2016;316(24): 2627–2646.

36. Dutton RP. Management of traumatic haemorrhage: The US perspective. *Anaesthesia*. 2015;70(Suppl 1):108–127.

37. Eick B, Denke N. Resuscitative strategies in the trauma patient: The past, the present, and the future. *J Trauma Nurs*. 2018;25(4): 254–263.

38. Emergency Nurses Association. Clinical Practice Guideline: Family Presence During Invasive Procedures and Resuscitation. https:// www.ena.org/docs/default-source/resource-library/practice-resources/cpg/familypresencecpg3eaabb7cf0414584ac2291fe-ba3be481.pdf?sfvrsn=9c167fc6_16. Published 2017. Accessed April 23, 2019.

39. Engels PT, Passos E, Beckett AN, et al. IV access in bleeding trauma patients: A performance review. *Injury*. 2014;45(1):77–82.

40. Federal Emergency Management Agency. National Preparedness System. https://www.fema.gov/national-preparedness-system. Published January 29, 2019. Accessed April 23, 2019.

41. Fukumoto LE, Fukumoto KD. Fat embolism syndrome. *Nurs Clin North Am*. 2018;53(3):335–347.

42. Gabbe B, Simpson P, Sutherland A, et al. Improved functional outcomes for major trauma patients in a regionalized, inclusive trauma system. *Ann Surg*. 2012;255(6):1009–1015.

43. Glow SD, Colucci JV, Allington DR, et al. Managing multiple casualty incidents: A rural medical preparedness training assessment. *Prehosp Disaster Med*. 2013;28(4):334–341.

44. Godat LN, Kobayashi L, Chang DC, et al. Can we ever stop worrying about venous thromboembolism after trauma? *J Trauma Acute Care Surg*. 2015;78(3):475–481.

45. Gonzalez E, Moore E, Moore H, et al. Goal-directed hemostatic resuscitation of trauma-induced coagulopathy: A pragmatic randomized clinical trial comparing a viscoelastic assay to conventional coagulation assays. *Ann Surg*. 2017;263(6):1051–1059.

46. Gunst M, Ghaemmaghami V, Gruszecki A, et al. Changing epidemiology of trauma deaths leads to a bimodal distribution. *Proc (Baylor Univ Med Cent)*. 2010;23(4):349–354.

47. Gurney D. *Trauma Nursing Core Course (TNCC): Provider Manual*. 7th ed. Des Plaines, IL: Emergency Nurses Association; 2014.

48. Harris T, Davenport R, Mak M, et al. The evolving science of trauma resuscitation. *Emerg Med Clin North Am*. 2018;36(1):85–106.

49. Holcomb JB, Tiley BC, Barainuk S, et al. Transfusion of plasma, platelets, and red blood cells in a 1:1:1 vs a 1:1:2 ratio and mortality in patients with severe trauma: The PROPPR randomized clinical trial. *JAMA*. 2015;313(5):471–482.

50. Huis in 't Veld MA, Craft CA, Hood RE. Blunt cardiac trauma review. *Cardiol Clin*. 2018;36(1):183–191.

51. Ibrahim I, Chor WP, Chue KM, et al. Is arterial base deficit still a useful prognostic marker in trauma? A systematic review. *Am J Emerg Med*. 2016;34(3):626–635.

52. Jain V, Chari R, Maslovitz S. Guidelines for the management of a pregnant trauma patient. *J Obstet Gynaecol Can*. 2015;37(6):553–574.

53. Joseph B, Aziz H, Snell M, et al. The physiological effects of hyperosmolar resuscitation: 5% vs 3% hypertonic saline. *Am J Surg*. 2014;208:697–702.

54. Keane M. Triad of death: The importance of temperature monitoring in trauma patients. *Emerg Nurse*. 2016;24(5):19–23.

55. Lecky F, Woodford M, Edwards A, et al. Trauma scoring systems and databases. *Br J Anaesth*. 2014;113(2):286–294.

56. Lesperance RN, Nunez TC. Blast injury impact on brain and internal organs. *Crit Care Nurs Clin N Am*. 2015;27(2):277–287.

57. Lewis P, Wright C. Saving the critically injured trauma patient: A retrospective analysis of 1000 uses of intraosseous access. *Emerg Med J*. 2015;32:463–467.

58. Postoperative care. Lippincott Procedures. http://procedures.lww.com/lnp/vie.do?pld=2958613. Published December 18, 2018. Accessed April 23, 2019.

59. Marr AB, Stuke LE, Greiffenstein P. Kinematics. In: More EE, Feliciano DV, Mattox KL, eds. *Trauma*. 8th ed. New York, NY: McGraw-Hill Education; 2017.

60. Mathews ZR, Koyfman A. Blast injuries. *J Emerg Med*. 2015;49(4):573–587.

61. Matsushima K, Khor D, Berona K, et al. Double jeopardy in penetrating trauma: Get FAST, get it right. *World J Surg*. 2018;42(1):99–106.

62. McClave S, Taylor B, Martindale R, et al. Guidelines for the provision and assessment of nutrition support therapy in the adult critically ill patient: Society of Critical Care Medicine (SCCM) and American Society for Parenteral and Enteral Nutrition (A.S.P.E.N.). *JPEN J Parenter Enteral Nutr*. 2016;40(2):159–211.

63. Mealer M, Conrad D, Evans J, et al. Feasibility and acceptability of a resilience training program for intensive care unit nurses. *Am J Crit Care*. 2014;23(6):e97–e105.

64. Merriam-Webster Dictionary Online. 2019. Trauma. https://www.merriam-webster.com/dictionary/trauma. Published 2019. Accessed April 23, 2019.

65. Mutschler A, Nienaber U, Brockamp T, et al. A critical reappraisal of the ATLS classification of hypovolaemic shock: Does it really reflect clinical reality? *Resuscitation*. 2013;84:309–313.

66. Nadler R, Convertino VA, Gendler S, et al. The value of noninvasive measurement of the compensatory reserve index in monitoring and triage of patients experiencing minimal blood loss. *Shock*. 2014;42(2):93–98.

67. Ophuis RH, Olij BF, Polinder S, Haagsma JA. Prevalence of posttraumatic stress disorder, acute stress disorder and depression following violence related injury treated at the emergency department: A systematic review. *BMC Psychiatry*. 2018;18(1):311.

68. Owens C, Garner J. Intra-abdominal injury from extra-peritoneal ballistic trauma. *Injury*. 2014;45:655–658.

69. Porter A, Karim S, Bowman SM, et al. Impact of a statewide trauma system on the triage, transfer, and inpatient mortality of injured patients. *J Trauma Acute Care Surg*. 2018;84(5): 771–779.

70. Prevaldi C, Paolillo C, Locatelli C, et al. Management of traumatic wounds in the emergency department: Position paper from the Academy of Emergency Medicine and Care (AcEMC) and the World Society of Emergency Surgery (WSES). *World J Emerg Surg*. 2016;11:30.

71. Prin M, Li G. Complications and in-hospital mortality in trauma patients treated in intensive care units in the United States, 2013. *Inj Epidemiol*. 2016;3(1):18.

72. Pucher PH, Batrick N, Taylor D, et al. Virtual-world hospital simulation for real-world disaster response: Design and validation of a virtual reality simulator for mass casualty incident management. *J Trauma Acute Care Surg*. 2014;77(2):315–321.

73. Rauf R, von Matthey F, Croenlein M, et al. Changes in the temporal distribution of in-hospital mortality in severely injured patients: An analysis of the TraumaRegister DGU. *PLoS One*. 2019;14(2):e0212095.

74. Raux M, Vivien B, Tortier JP, et al. Severity assessment in trauma patient. *Ann Fr Anesth Reanim*. 2013;32:472–476.

75. Rhee P, Moore E, Bellal J, et al. Gunshot wounds: A review of ballistics, bullets, weapons, and myths. *J Trauma Acute Care Surg.* 2016;80(6):853–867.

76. Richards J, McGahan J. Focused assessment with sonography in trauma (FAST) in 2017: What radiologists can learn. *Radiology.* 2017;283(1):30–48.

77. Rodriguez R, Friedman B, Langdorf M. Pulmonary contusion in the pan-scan era. *Injury.* 2016;47(5):1031–1034.

78. Schultz CH, Koenig KL, Whiteside M, et al. Development of national standardized hazard disaster core competencies for acute care physicians, nurses, and EMS professionals. *Ann Emerg Med.* 2012;59(3):196–208.

79. Semler MW, Self WH, Wanderer JP, et al. Balanced crystalloids versus saline in critically ill adults. *N Engl J Med.* 2018;378(9): 829–839.

80. Shonin E, VanGordon W, Griffiths MD. Mindfulness-based interventions: Towards mindful clinical integration. *Front Psychol.* 2013;4:1–4.

81. Timbie JW, Ringel JS, Fox S, et al. Systematic review of strategies to manage and allocate scarce resources during mass casualty events. *Ann Emerg Med.* 2013;61(6):677–689.

82. US Department of Health and Human Services. Get Help Now. http://www.stopbullying.gov/get-help-now/. Published September 8, 2017. Accessed April 23, 2019.

83. US Department of Health and Human Services, Health Resources and Services. Administration: Model Trauma System Planning and Evaluation. https://www.facs.org/~/media/files/quality%20programs/trauma/tsepc/pdfs/hrsa%20mtspe.ashx. Published 2006. Accessed April 23, 2019.

84. VandenBerg SL, Davidson SB. Preparation for mass casualty incidents. *Crit Care Nurs Clin N Am.* 2015;27(2):157–166.

85. Via AG, Oliva F, Spoliti M, Maffulli N. Acute compartment syndrome. *Muscles Ligaments Tendons J.* 2015;5(1):18–22.

86. Violano P, Weston I, Tinkoff G. Approach to a standardized injury prevention coordinator training curriculum. *J Trauma Nurs.* 2016;23(6):343–346.

87. Waller JA. Reflections on a half century of injury control. *Am J Public Health.* 1994;84(4):664–670.

88. West N, Dawes R. Trauma resuscitation and the damage control approach. *Surgery (Oxford).* 2015;33(9):430–436

89. Wheeler DS, Sheets AM, Ryckman FC. Improving transitions of care between the operating room and intensive care unit. *Transl Pediatr.* 2018;7(4):299–307.

90. Wilson FA, Stimpson JP, Pagan JA. Fatal crashes from drivers testing positive for drugs in the U.S. 1993–2010. *Public Health Rep.* 2014;39:342–350.

91. Wong H, Lovett N, Curry N, et al. Antithrombotics in trauma: Management strategies in the older patients. *J Blood Med.* 2017;8:165–174.

92. Yitzhak A, Glick Y, Benov A, et al. The need for optimized crystalloid-based resuscitation. *J Trauma Acute Care Surg.* 2017;82(6 Suppl 1):S66–S69.

93. Zonfrillo MR, Spicer RS, Lawrence BA, Miller TR. Incidence and costs of injuries to children and adults in the United States. *Inj Epidemiol.* 2018;5(1):37.

Burns

Sarah Taylor, MSN, RN, ACNS-BC

Many additional resources, including self-assessment exercises, are located on the Evolve companion website at http://evolve.elsevier.com/Sole/.
- Animations
- Clinical Skills: Critical Care Collections
- Student Review Questions
- Video Clips

INTRODUCTION

There is no greater challenge in critical care nursing than caring for a severely burned patient. Approximately once every minute, someone in the United States sustains a burn injury that is serious enough to require treatment.[5] Burn injuries result in an estimated 486,000 hospital emergency department (ED) visits and 45,000 acute hospital admissions each year in the United States.[6] Although injury prevention efforts have resulted in a reduction of burn injuries, such injuries constitute a major worldwide health problem, with low-socioeconomic populations being disproportionately at highest risk for injury.[3,6,25,37] Initial management of the seriously injured burn patient dramatically affects the patient's long-term outcome. Ideally, burn patients are treated in hospitals with special capabilities for managing extensive burn injuries. Despite the nationwide network of burn center facilities, most patients are first seen in a community hospital, making it crucial that the multiprofessional team has the knowledge and skills necessary to provide initial resuscitative care to burn-injured patients.

Burn injuries lead to significant economic and social consequences, as well as marked morbidity and mortality. Historically, burn injuries have been one of the most lethal forms of trauma. However, application of research-based advances in fluid resuscitation, early excision and closure of the wound, tissue healing and engineering, metabolic and respiratory support, microbial surveillance, and infection prevention have dramatically improved survival and recovery from burn injury.[1,30] Despite improvements, morbidity and mortality remain significant in patients with inhalation injuries, burns on greater than 50% of total body surface area (TBSA), and advancing age.[6] Knowledge of the physiological changes and the potential complications associated with burn injuries prepares the critical care nurse to care for these complex patients and to optimize outcomes.

REVIEW OF ANATOMY AND PHYSIOLOGY OF THE SKIN

The skin, also called the integumentary system, is the largest organ of the body. It is a vital organ because of its many functions, including provision of a protective barrier against infection and injury, regulation of fluid loss, thermoregulatory (or body heat) control, synthesis of vitamin D, sensory contact with the environment, and determination of identity and cosmetic appearance. The skin is composed of two layers, the *epidermis* and the *dermis,* with an underlying *subcutaneous* fat tissue layer that binds the dermis to organs and tissues of the body (Fig. 21.1). The *epidermis* is the outermost and thinnest skin layer. The *dermis* is considerably thicker and contains collagen and elastic fibers, blood and lymph vessels, sweat glands, hair follicles, sebaceous glands, and sensory fibers for the detection of pain, pressure, touch, and temperature. The underlying subcutaneous tissue is a layer of connective tissue and fat deposits. When an extensive amount or depth of skin is damaged from burn injury, alterations of these multiple physiological functions place the patient at risk for complications.

MECHANISMS AND ETIOLOGY OF INJURY

Burn injuries are classified into three types: thermal, chemical, and electrical. Approximately 90% of burn injuries are thermally induced (e.g., flame, scald, contact). Chemical and electrical burns account for the remaining 10% of the injuries.[4,6] These types of injuries can also occur with inhalation injury, which is observed in 2% to 14% of patients admitted to burn centers. Inhalation injury often occurs in combination with substantial skin injury, which significantly increases the risk of death.[4] In addition to standard management, chemical and electrical burns require special initial management and ongoing assessment, as discussed later in the chapter.

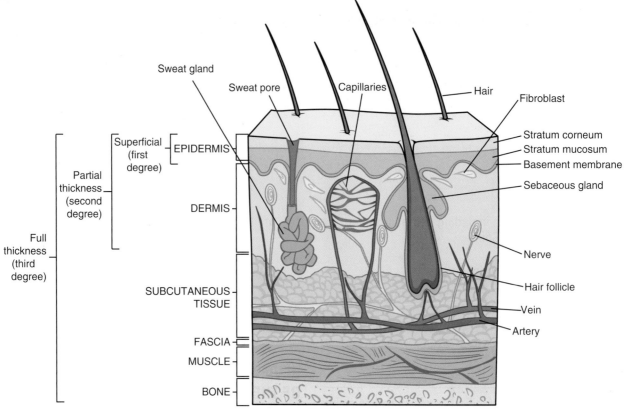

Fig. 21.1 Anatomy of the skin.

Males, averaging 20 to 29 years old, make up almost 71% of the patients admitted to burn centers.[6] Children younger than 5 years of age account for approximately 17% of burn center admissions, primarily from scalding injuries.[6] Flame or fire is the primary cause of burns for all other ages. The overwhelming majority (74%) of burn injuries occur in the home.[6] Burn injuries occur at a disproportionate rate among nonwhite minorities and those of lower socioeconomic status.[6] It is important to consider how these epidemiological factors potentially affect the treatment and recovery of patients.

Thermal Injury: Flame, Scald, and Contact

Thermal injury is caused when the skin comes in contact with a source of sufficient temperature to cause cell injury by coagulation. This can occur from flame (e.g., house fires, ignition of clothing, explosion of gases), scalding liquids (e.g., water, cooking oil, grease), steam (e.g., car radiators, cooking pots, industrial equipment), or direct contact with a heat source (e.g., space heater, metal, glass fireplace doors). Children and the elderly are at greatest risk for thermal injury because of their thinner skin and decreased agility in moving to avoid harm.

Approximately 41% of burn injuries are from flame, 34% from scalds, and 9% from contact.[6] The severity of injury is related to the heat intensity and the duration of contact. For example, a heat source of less than 40°C (104°F) does not cause a burn regardless of the length of exposure, but exposure to a temperature of 60°C (140°F) causes *full-thickness* tissue destruction (third-degree burn) in as little as 3 to 5 seconds.[4] This fact poses an injury prevention issue because 140°F is a common setting for home water heaters despite recommendations that temperature be set at 49°C (120°F) or just below the medium setting.[6]

Chemical Injury

Chemical burns are caused by contact, inhalation of fumes, ingestion, or injection. Although chemical injuries account for only a small percentage of admissions to burn centers, they can be severe and can have both local and systemic effects. The severity of injury is related to the type, volume, duration of contact, and concentration of the agent. Tissue damage from chemical burns continues until the chemical is completely removed or neutralized. Chemical agents are found in every home and workplace, so the potential for injury from exposure is great. The US Occupational Safety and Health Administration requires that employees receive educational training on hazardous materials in the workplace and that Material Safety Data Sheets (MSDSs) be posted in work areas. MSDSs list information on chemicals in the workplace, including composition, side effects, and potential for systemic toxicity. The Joint Commission also monitors compliance with this regulation.

Three categories of chemical agents exist: alkalis, acids, and organic compounds. Alkalis (also known as bases) commonly encountered in the home and industrial environments include oven cleaners, lye, wet cement, and fertilizers. Burns caused by alkalis are more severe than those caused by acids because alkalis loosen tissue through protein denaturation and liquefaction necrosis, allowing the chemical to diffuse deeply into the tissue. Alkalis also bind to tissue proteins and make it more difficult to stop the burning process.

Acids are found in many household and industrial products, such as bathroom cleansers, rust removers, and pool chemicals. The depth of burn injury from acids (except hydrofluoric acid) tends to be limited because acids cause tissue coagulation necrosis and protein precipitation. In contrast, hydrofluoric acid is potentially lethal even with small exposures because it causes hypocalcemia by rapidly binding to free calcium in the blood.

Organic compounds such as phenols and petroleum products (e.g., gasoline, kerosene, chemical disinfectants) can produce cutaneous burns and can be absorbed with resulting systemic effects. Phenols cause severe coagulation necrosis of dermal proteins and produce a layer of thick, nonviable burn tissue called *eschar*.[4] Petroleum products such as gasoline promote cell membrane injury and dissolution of lipids with resulting skin necrosis. The systemic effects of petroleum products include central nervous system (CNS) depression, hypothermia, hypotension, pulmonary edema, and intravascular hemolysis, which can be severe or even fatal. Chemical pneumonitis and bronchitis may occur from inhalation of toxic fumes. Other complications observed with exposure to petroleum products include hepatic and renal failure as well as sudden death.[4]

Natural disasters, industrial accidents, warfare, terrorist attacks, and mass casualty incidents can produce burn injuries from chemical or thermal exposure.[4] A mass casualty event with significant burn and inhalation injuries can quickly exceed local resources, and critical care nurses must be prepared for such a situation.[4] Disaster management is discussed further in Chapter 20.

Electrical Injury

Electrical injury is caused by contact with varied electrical sources such as household or industrial current, car batteries, electrosurgical devices, high-tension electrical lines, and lightning. Electrical injuries are frequently work related.[6] Electricity flows by either alternating current (AC), as in most home and commercial applications, or direct current (DC), as in lightning and car batteries. Although AC and DC are both dangerous, AC has the greater probability of producing cardiopulmonary arrest by ventricular fibrillation. The AC causes tetanic muscle contraction that may "lock" the patient to the source of electricity and cause respiratory muscle paralysis. Electrical injuries are arbitrarily classified as high voltage (>1000 V) or low voltage (≤1000 V).[4]

In electrical burns, tissue damage occurs during the process of converting electrical energy to heat. The resulting dissipation of heat energy is often greatest at the points of contact (entry and exit), which are frequently on the extremities. Several factors affect the extent of injury: type and pathway of the current, duration of contact, environmental conditions, body tissue resistance, and cross-sectional area of the body involved. Therefore electrical injury wounds are extremely variable in presentation. At the point of contact, either a small burn or a crater-like "blowout" wound may be observed. Because electricity follows the path of least resistance, the low resistance of nerve tissue was theorized to have the highest risk of damage or degeneration. Now, the density and high resistance of bone tissue is thought to generate the most heat, which is dissipated, damaging adjacent deep muscle tissue.[4] *Electroporation*, a significant increase in the conductivity and permeability of cell membranes, also contributes to extensive tissue damage.[4] Both of these processes cause deep tissue necrosis beneath viable and more superficial tissue. On initial presentation, the wound may appear minimal or superficial, but several days or weeks later it can manifest as an extensive, deep wound with neurological impairment.

Inhalation Injury

Lung injury caused by inhalation of smoke, chemical toxins, and products of incomplete combustion is associated with increased mortality (e.g., up to 19 times greater risk of death than burns without inhalation injury).[6] Inhalation injury is classified as (1) systemic injury caused by exposure to toxic gases (e.g., carbon monoxide, cyanide), (2) supraglottic injury (i.e., above the glottis), and (3) subglottic injury (i.e., below the glottis), or a combination of these.[4,9] Table 21.1 summarizes the pathology of each type of injury. A universally accepted standardized inhalation injury severity scoring system does not currently exist. Diagnosis is based on injury history, clinical signs, and bronchoscopy findings. Inhalation injury stimulates an airway inflammatory response with physiological changes in biochemical mediators and cells, which often results in lung damage.[29] Inhalation injury typically warrants admission to a critical care unit, even if there are no cutaneous surface burns.

Carbon Monoxide and Cyanide Poisoning.
Carbon monoxide poisoning is the most frequent cause of death at the injury scene.[4] Carbon monoxide is released when organic compounds, such as wood or coal, are burned. It has an affinity for

TABLE 21.1	Types and Pathology of Inhalation Injury	
Type of Injury	**Pathology**
Systemic: Injury caused by exposure to toxic gases	Carbon monoxide poisoning: Carbon monoxide binds to hemoglobin molecules more rapidly than oxygen molecules do; tissue hypoxia results
	Cyanide poisoning: Cyanide binds to respiratory enzymes in the mitochondria, inhibiting cellular metabolism and use of oxygen
Supraglottic: Inhalation injury above the glottis	Most often a thermal injury; heat absorption and damage occur mostly in the pharynx and larynx; may cause airway obstruction from edema
Subglottic: Inhalation injury below the glottis	Usually a chemical injury that produces impaired ciliary activity, erythema, hypersecretion, edema, ulceration of mucosa, increased blood flow, and spasm of bronchi and/or bronchioles

TABLE 21.2 Carboxyhemoglobin

Carboxyhemoglobin Level[a]	Clinical Presentation
<10% to 15%	No symptoms, or mimic changes in visual acuity and headache
15% to 40%	Central nervous system dysfunction: restlessness, confusion, impaired dexterity, headache, dizziness, nausea and vomiting
40% to 60%	Loss of consciousness, tachycardia, tachypnea, seizures, cherry red or cyanotic skin
>60%	Coma; death generally ensues

[a]Percentage of hemoglobin molecules bound with carbon monoxide.

hemoglobin that is 200 times greater than that of oxygen.[4] When carbon monoxide is inhaled, it binds to hemoglobin to form *carboxyhemoglobin* (COHgb) and prevents red blood cells from transporting oxygen to body tissues, leading to systemic hypoxia. Carbon monoxide poisoning is difficult to detect because it may not manifest with significant clinical findings. Although the oxygen content of blood is reduced, the amount of oxygen dissolved in the plasma (PaO_2) is unaffected by carbon monoxide poisoning. Blood gas analysis and oxygen saturation measured by pulse oximetry are usually normal except for an elevated COHgb level.[6] Therefore the COHgb levels are measured and reported as the percentage of hemoglobin molecules that are bound with carbon monoxide. Levels lower than 10% to 15% are found in mild carbon monoxide poisoning and are commonly associated with heavy smoking and continual exposure to dense traffic pollution (Table 21.2). CNS dysfunction of varying degrees (e.g., restlessness, confusion) manifests at levels of 15% to 40%. Loss of consciousness occurs at COHgb levels of 40% to 60%, and death typically occurs when the COHgb level exceeds 60%.

Cyanide poisoning occurs from inhalation of smoke byproducts. Combustion of household synthetics (e.g., carpeting, plastics, vinyl flooring, upholstered furniture, window coverings) is the primary source of exposure.[4,7,11] Cyanide impedes cellular respiration and oxygen use by binding with the aa3-type cytochrome *c* oxidase, which is present in high concentrations in the mitochondria. This action inhibits cell metabolism and adenosine triphosphate (ATP) production, resulting in a shift from aerobic to anaerobic metabolism. The state of anaerobic metabolism depletes cellular ATP and leads to lactic acidosis and cell death.[7,11] The clinical symptoms of cyanide poisoning mimic those of carbon monoxide poisoning, and both may be present simultaneously.

Injury Above the Glottis. Inhalation injury above the glottis, also referred to as upper airway injury, is caused by breathing in heat or noxious chemicals that are produced during the burning process. The nose, mouth, and throat dissipate the heat and prevent damage to lower airways, but the patient is still at high risk for airway obstruction due to edema resulting from upper airway thermal injury. Airway obstruction clinically manifests as hoarseness, dry cough, labored or rapid breathing, difficulty swallowing, or stridor.

Injury Below the Glottis. Injury below the glottis is almost always caused by breathing noxious chemical byproducts of burning materials and smoke. Extensive damage to alveoli and

impaired pulmonary functioning result from the injury (see Table 21.1 and the Clinical Alert box). A hallmark sign is *carbonaceous sputum* (soot or carbon particles in secretions). Tracheal and bronchial or bronchiolar constriction and spasms with resulting wheezing can occur within minutes to several hours after injury.[4] Acute respiratory failure and acute respiratory distress syndrome (ARDS) may develop within the first few days. Respiratory tract mucosal sloughing may occur within 4 to 5 days. Chest radiographs obtained on admission are often normal. Later studies may reveal reduced lung expansion, atelectasis, and diffuse lung edema or infiltrates. Fiberoptic bronchoscopy may be indicated to provide a definitive diagnosis.[29]

> ### ❗ CLINICAL ALERT
> #### *Clinical Indicators of Inhalation Injury*
>
> - History of exposure in confined or enclosed space
> - Facial burns
> - Singed nasal hairs
> - Presence of soot around mouth and nose and in sputum (carbonaceous sputum)
> - Signs of hypoxemia (tachycardia, dysrhythmias, agitation, confusion, lethargy, loss of consciousness)
> - Abnormal breath sounds
> - Signs of respiratory difficulty (change in respiratory rate, use of accessory muscles, flaring nostrils, intercostal or sternal retractions, stridor, hoarseness, difficulty swallowing)
> - Elevated carboxyhemoglobin levels
> - Abnormal arterial blood gas values

BURN CLASSIFICATION AND SEVERITY

Burn injury severity is determined by the type of injury, wound characteristics (depth, extent, body part burned), concomitant injuries, patient age, and preexisting health status. Accurate classification and assessment of injury severity enable appropriate triage and transfer of patients to a burn center.

Depth of Injury

Burn depth predicts wound care treatment requirements, determines the need for skin grafting, and affects scarring, cosmetic, and functional outcomes. Burn injuries are often classified as first, second, or third degree. However, the terms *superficial, partial-thickness,* and *full-thickness* burns more closely correlate with the pathophysiology of burn injury and the level of skin layer involvement (see Fig. 21.1). Accurate depth assessment is difficult to determine initially because progressive edema formation and compromised wound blood flow during the first 48 to 72 hours after injury may increase the definitive burn depth.[19]

Superficial burns involve only the first layer of skin or the epidermis (hence called first-degree injury) and typically heal in 3 to 5 days without treatment. Superficial burn injuries are not included in burn size (extent of injury) calculations used for fluid resuscitation requirements because they only cause erythema and do not involve the dermis. *Partial-thickness* burns involve injury to the second skin layer or dermal layer (hence a second-degree injury), and are further subdivided into superficial and deep classifications. *Superficial partial-thickness* burn injuries that involve the epidermis and a limited portion of the dermis heal by growth of undamaged basal cells within 7 to 10 days. *Deep partial-thickness* burns involve destruction of the epidermis and most of the dermis. Although such wounds may heal spontaneously within 2 to 4 weeks, they are typically excised and grafted to reduce healing time and hospitalization and achieve better functional and cosmetic results. Destruction of all layers of the skin down to or past the subcutaneous fat, fascia, muscles, or bone is defined as a *full-thickness* injury (i.e., third-degree injury; sometimes called fourth-degree when muscle and bone are involved). This creates a thick, leathery, nonelastic, coagulated layer of dead, necrotic tissue called *eschar*. The nerves are destroyed, resulting in a painless wound. These injuries always require skin grafting for permanent wound closure. Table 21.3 describes the characteristics of superficial, partial-thickness, and full-thickness burn injuries.

Differentiating partial-thickness from full-thickness injuries is initially difficult because burn wounds mature or progress within the first few days. The three zones of thermal injury explain this phenomenon (Fig. 21.2) by illustrating the relationship between depth and extent of injury and viability of damaged tissue. The outermost area of minimal cell injury is called the *zone of hyperemia*. It has early spontaneous recovery and is similar to a superficial burn. The *zone of coagulation* at the core of the wound contains the greatest area of tissue necrosis. It is the site of irreversible skin death and is similar to a full-thickness burn. Surrounding this area is a *zone of stasis*, where vascular damage and reduced blood flow occur. Secondary insults such as inadequate resuscitation, edema, infection, or poor nutrition result in conversion of this potentially salvageable area to full-thickness skin destruction with irreversible tissue *necrosis* or death.

In cutting-edge research, topical nanoemulsion therapy has shown promise as a novel intervention targeted at halting tissue destruction and burn depth conversion in the zone of stasis.[16] Nanoemulsions are tiny nanometer-size (i.e., one billionth of a meter), broad-spectrum antimicrobial oil-in-water droplets that are mixed in a high-energy state and stabilized with surfactants. When nanoemulsions are topically applied to the wound, both the active antimicrobial ingredients and the high-energy release destabilize the microbe membrane, resulting in pathogen cell death. Nanoemulsions are selectively toxic to pathogens but are not irritating to skin or mucous membranes. In burn injury, nanoemulsion therapy attenuates the wound inflammatory response, wound progression, bacterial growth, and infection.[16]

STUDY BREAK

1. A superficial partial-thickness (second-degree) burn is characterized by:
   A. Charred gray skin or black skin
   B. Blistered skin with pink or moist base
   C. White waxy and dry skin
   D. Reddened skin without blisters

Extent of Injury

The extent of injury or size of a burn is expressed as a percentage of *total body surface area* (%TBSA). Accurate calculation of the extent of injury is essential for assessing burn severity and for estimating fluid resuscitation requirements. The *rule of nines* is the quickest method to initially calculate %TBSA. This technique divides the TBSA into areas representing 9% or multiples of 9% (Fig. 21.3). The %TBSA that is burned is estimated by summing all areas of partial- and full-thickness burns (superficial burns are not included). The nurse can use the size of the patient's palm (including fingers) to calculate injury extent of irregular or scattered small burns; the patient's palm represents 1% of the TBSA.[4] The rule of nines varies between children and adults because children have a proportionally larger head compared with adults.

TABLE 21.3 **Depth of Burn Injury**			
Degree of Injury	**Morphology**	**Healing Time**	**Wound Characteristics**
Superficial (first-degree)	Destruction of epidermis only	3-5 days	Pink or red, dry, painful
Superficial partial-thickness (second-degree)	Destruction of epidermis and some dermis	7-10 days	Moist, pink or mottled red; very painful; blisters; blanches briskly with pressure
Deep partial-thickness (second-degree)	Destruction of epidermis and most of dermis; some skin appendages remain	2-4 weeks	Pale, mottled, pearly red/white; moist or somewhat dry; typically less painful; blanching decreased and prolonged; difficult to distinguish from full-thickness injury
Full-thickness (third-degree)	Destruction of epidermis, dermis, and underlying subcutaneous tissue	Does not heal; requires skin grafting	Thick, leathery eschar; dry; white, cherry-red, or brown-black; painless; does not blanch with pressure; thrombosed blood vessels
Full-thickness (fourth-degree)	Involves underlying fat, fascia, muscle, tendon, and/or bone	Does not heal; may require amputation or extensive debridement	Black, charred, thick, leathery eschar may be present; bone, tendon, or muscle may be visible

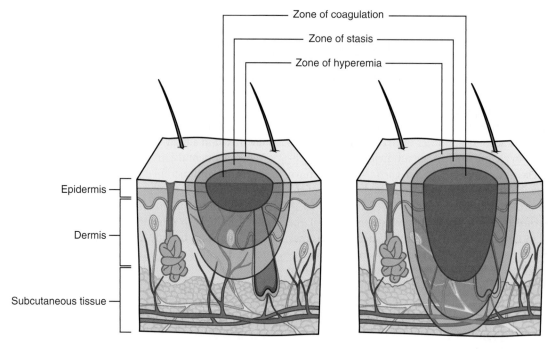

Fig. 21.2 Zones of thermal injury.

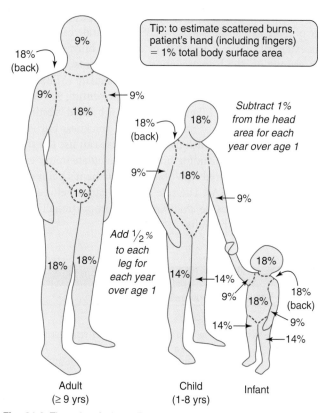

Fig. 21.3 The rule of nines. For example, the calculation for an adult with superficial burns to the face and partial-thickness burns to the lower half of the right arm, entire left arm, and chest is 4.5% (lower right arm) + 9% (entire left arm) + 9% (chest or upper anterior trunk), for a total of 22.5% total body surface area (TBSA). (Superficial burns to the face are not included in the %TBSA calculation.) (Courtesy University of Michigan Trauma Burn Center, Ann Arbor, MI.)

The *Lund and Browder chart* (Fig. 21.4), provides a more accurate determination of the extent of burn injury by correlating body surface area with age-related proportions. Although it has traditionally been used in paper format, the calculations are embedded in some electronic medical record systems. Mobile, three-dimensional computer modeling technology may also facilitate more reliable and accurate %TBSA calculations.[17]

STUDY BREAK

2. The palmar surface, including the fingers, of the patient's hand represents what percent of his or her total body surface area?
   A. 12%
   B. 1%
   C. 3%
   D. 5%

PHYSIOLOGICAL RESPONSES TO BURN INJURY

The body responds to major burn injuries with significant hemodynamic, metabolic, and immunological effects that occur locally and systemically as a result of cellular damage (Table 21.4). The magnitude and duration of the systemic response and the degree of physiological changes are proportional to the %TBSA injured. Direct thermal damage to blood vessels causes intravascular coagulation, with arterial and venous blood flow ceasing in the wound injury area. The damaged and ischemic cells release *mediators,* endogenously produced substances that initiate a protective inflammatory response. Mediators such as histamine, prostaglandins, bradykinins, catecholamines, and cytokines are

Burn Estimate and Diagram

Age vs. Area

Area	Birth 1 yr	1–4 yr	5–9 yr	10–14 yr	15 yr	Adult	2°	3°	Total	Donor Areas
Head	19	17	13	11	9	7				
Neck	2	2	2	2	2	2				
Ant. Trunk	13	13	13	13	13	13				
Post. Trunk	13	13	13	13	13	13				
R. Buttock	2 ½	2 ½	2 ½	2 ½	2 ½	2 ½				
L. Buttock	2 ½	2 ½	2 ½	2 ½	2 ½	2 ½				
Genitalia	1	1	1	1	1	1				
R. U. Arm	4	4	4	4	4	4				
L. U. Arm	4	4	4	4	4	4				
R. L. Arm	3	3	3	3	3	3				
L. L. Arm	3	3	3	3	3	3				
R. Hand	2 ½	2 ½	2 ½	2 ½	2 ½	2 ½				
L. Hand	2 ½	2 ½	2 ½	2 ½	2 ½	2 ½				
R. Thigh	5 ½	6 ½	8	8 ½	9	9 ½				
L. Thigh	5 ½	6 ½	8	8 ½	9	9 ½				
R. Leg	5	5	5 ½	6	6 ½	7				
L. Leg	5	5	5 ½	6	6 ½	7				
R. Foot	3 ½	3 ½	3 ½	3 ½	3 ½	3 ½				
L. Foot	3 ½	3 ½	3 ½	3 ½	3 ½	3 ½				
						Total				

Burn Diagram

Age _____

Sex _____

Weight _____

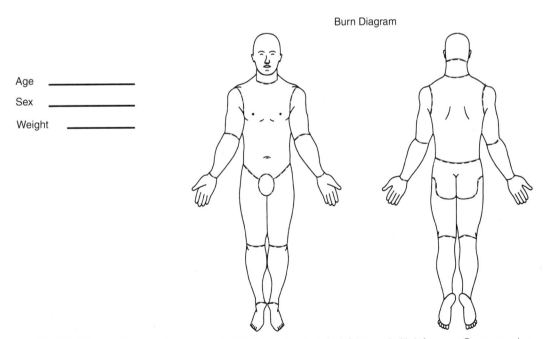

Fig. 21.4 Burn estimate and diagrams. *Ant*, Anterior; *L*, left; *L. L.*, left lower; *L. U.*, left upper; *Post*, posterior; *R*, right; *R. L.*, right lower; *R. U.*, right upper.

TABLE 21.4 **Pathophysiology: Local and Systemic Responses to a Major Burn Injury**

System	Response
Neurological	↓ LOC from inhalation injury, carbon monoxide or cyanide poisoning, concomitant trauma, polysubstance use, and/or hypoglycemia Massive stress response with activation of sympathetic nervous system ↑ Catecholamine release
Respiratory	↑ O_2 demand from ↑ oxygen consumption Tissue damage from direct heat, edema, or inhaled noxious chemicals Release of vasoconstrictive substances ↓ O_2 tension and lung compliance Transient pulmonary hypertension Hypoxemia If inhalation injury present (see Tables 21.1 and 21.2), ↑ mortality above expected for %TBSA burn Acid-base disturbances
Gastrointestinal	↓ GI blood flow Oral medications and fluids not absorbed Increased risk of ileus Stress or Curling's ulcer (if no prophylaxis)

Integumentary: Skin/tissue/cells	Direct heat-induced tissue damage or ischemia and cell lysis
	Stimulation of inflammatory response (can be massive)
	Extensive edema in burned and unburned areas (maximum effect about 18-36 h after burn)
	↓ Tissue perfusion and ↑ potential tissue necrosis
	Cellular dysfunction
	  • ↓ Cell transmembrane potential
	  • Cell edema
	Loss of skin barrier
	Loss of thermoregulation (↓ ability to regulate temperature)
	↑ Evaporative H_2O loss

Immunological	Release of multiple mediators, cellular enzymes, and vasoactive substances Activation of complement system Overstimulation of suppressor T cells ↓ T helper cell, T killer cell, and polymorphonuclear leukocyte activity Impaired immune function or response: ↑ risk of opportunistic infections until burn wound closes Leukocyte sequestration

Resuscitation and late effects	With adequate fluid resuscitation, in 24-36 h:
	  • Cell transmembrane potential and capillary wall integrity restored
	  • CO returns to normal or ↑
	  • Diuresis
	  • ↓ Edema (cell and tissue)
	Without adequate resuscitation:
	  • Multiorgan dysfunction due to ↓ perfusion
	  • Reperfusion oxidation injury with returned blood flow
	Biphasic initial hypofunction, then hyperfunction pattern of all systems
	Normal CO and organ function returns when burn wounds are closed (healed or are covered)
	Hypermetabolic state may continue for months to 3 years

Cardiac	↑ Myocardial depressant cytokines (TNF and interleukins) with ↓ cardiac function ↓ Cardiac contractility Tachycardia ↓ CO (leads to ↑ SVR and resulting ↑ afterload) ↓ Blood pressure ↑ SVR (due to catecholamine-induced peripheral vasoconstriction) leads to redistribution of blood flow to priority organs
Renal	↓ Renal blood flow ↓ Glomerular filtration rate ↓ Urine output or oliguria Hemoglobin or myoglobin in urine (especially with electrical injury from cell lysis or rhabdomyolysis) ↑ Risk of acute kidney injury related to inadequate fluid resuscitation

TABLE 21.4   Pathophysiology: Local and Systemic Responses to a Major Burn Injury—cont'd

Vascular	Heat-induced hemolysis, cell lysis, and endothelial injury
	↑ Capillary permeability or "leak"
	• Shift of protein, fluid, and electrolytes from intravascular to extravascular (interstitial) space
	• Third-spacing
	• Oncotic pressure effects
	• ↑ Edema
	Serum electrolyte imbalances
	• Hyperkalemia or hypokalemia
	• Hyponatremia or hypernatremia
	↓ Circulating blood volume (up to 50%) and "burn shock"
	Hypovolemia
	↑ Concentration of red blood cells with ↑ hematocrit and ↑ blood viscosity (hyperviscosity)
Metabolic	Stress response and ↑ catecholamine release triggers adrenal corticoid hormones
	↑ Catabolism or hypermetabolism (100%-200% above basal rates)
	• ↑ Corticosteroid levels, hyperglycemia, and poor wound healing
	• Protein wasting and weight or muscle mass loss
	• Bone demineralization
	• Degree of response depends on %TBSA, age, sex, nutritional status, and preexisting medical conditions
	Acid-base disturbances

CO, Cardiac output; *GI*, gastrointestinal; *H₂O*, water; *LOC*, level of consciousness; *O₂*, oxygen; *SVR*, systemic vascular resistance; *TBSA*, total body surface area; *TNF*, tumor necrosis factor.

stimulated and released, causing vasoactive, cellular, and cardiovascular effects. Gaps between endothelial cells in vessel wall membranes develop, making vessel walls porous or "leaky." This *increased capillary membrane permeability* allows a significant shift of protein molecules, fluid, and electrolytes from the *intravascular space* (inside the blood vessels) into the *interstitium* (the space between cells and the vascular system) in a process also referred to as *third-spacing* (Fig. 21.5). There is rapid and dramatic edema formation. Cellular swelling also occurs as the result of a decrease in cell transmembrane potential and a shift of extracellular sodium and water into the cell.[13] The leakage of proteins into the interstitium dramatically lowers the intravascular *oncotic pressure*, which draws even more intravascular fluid into the interstitium and contributes to the development of edema and *burn shock* (shock from intravascular volume loss, created by the sudden fluid and solute shifts that occur immediately after a burn injury). In burns greater than 20% TBSA, the increased capillary permeability and edema formation process occurs not only locally at the site of burn injury but also systemically in distant unburned tissues and organs.[4,9] Edema is further exacerbated as lymph drainage flow is obstructed due to either direct damage of lymphatic vessels or blockage by serum proteins that have leaked into the interstitium. Edema is a natural inflammatory response to injury that aids transport of white blood cells to the site of injury for bacterial digestion; however, the extent and rate of edema formation associated with a major burn injury far exceed the intended beneficial inflammatory effect.[14] Following burn injury, edema expands until it reaches a maximum at approximately 24 hours after injury, and reabsorption and resolution begin 1 to 2 days after a burn injury.[14]

Intravascular fluid volume lost into the interstitium causes the unique phenomenon of burn shock. *Burn shock* is a combination of *distributive* and *hypovolemic shock*. There is a distributive component because third-spacing greatly expands the area in which total body fluid is contained to include the intravascular space plus the intracellular and interstitial spaces. The hypovolemic component is caused by massive loss of intravascular fluid due to increased vessel membrane permeability and evaporative losses through the open wounds. Burn shock ensues when the plasma or intravascular volume becomes insufficient to maintain circulatory support and adequate preload, causing cardiac output to decrease and impairing tissue perfusion. Fluid resuscitation is crucial to replace intravascular fluid losses and restore preload deficits.

In summary, significant burn injuries trigger local and systemic responses involving many complex mechanisms and cascades of physiological events that stress all body systems. The magnitude of the physiological response produces dramatic shifts in intravascular fluid, mediator activation, exaggerated inflammatory cascade reaction, and extensive edema formation. The specific organ system responses are summarized in the following sections and in Table 21.4.

❓ CRITICAL REASONING ACTIVITY

Explain why patients with burns need extensive fluid resuscitation even though they are extremely edematous.

Cardiovascular Response

Loss of intravascular volume after a major burn injury produces a decrease in cardiac output and oxygen delivery to the body tissues. The sympathetic nervous system activates as a compensatory mechanism, with the release of catecholamines causing tachycardia and vasoconstriction to maintain arterial blood pressure. Alterations in tissue and multiorgan perfusion occur when the blood flow redistributes early in the postburn period to perfuse essential organs such as the heart and brain. Early after a burn injury, cardiac dysfunction develops and exerts a negative inotropic effect on myocardial

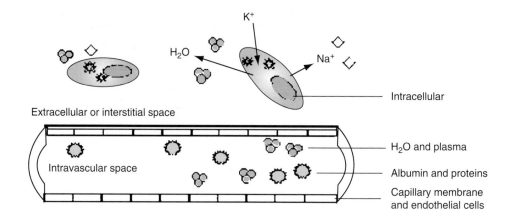

NORMAL PHYSIOLOGY BEFORE BURN INJURY
Intact capillary wall membranes keep large protein molecules within the blood vessels or intravascular space. This maintains normal protein oncotic pressure and retains intravascular fluid volume.

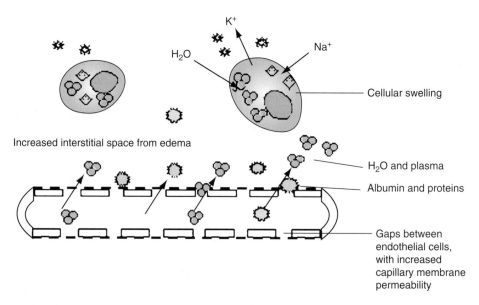

PHYSIOLOGICAL CHANGES FOLLOWING BURN INJURY
Gaps develop between endothelial cells, causing increased capillary membrane permeability. Intravascular proteins and fluids flow into the interstitium in a process called third-spacing and produce tissue edema. Loss of intravascular proteins decreases intravascular oncotic pressure, pulls additional fluid into the interstitium, and reduces intravascular fluid volume. Decreased cell transmembrane potential shifts sodium into the cells, drawing in water and producing cellular swelling and further tissue edema.

Fig. 21.5 Burn edema and shock development. H_2O, Water; K^+, potassium; Na^+, sodium.

tissues. The magnitude of myocardial depression exceeds that which would be explained by intravascular fluid volume loss.[6,18,20,27] The exact mechanism is unknown; however, secretion of inflammatory cytokine mediators, such as tumor necrosis factor and interleukins, within the myocardium and systemic activation of the complement system with production of anaphylatoxins are implicated as major contributors to contractile dysfunction.[20,27] Cardiac instability in burn patients is further exacerbated by under-resuscitation (hypovolemia), over-resuscitation (hypervolemia), or increased afterload. Impaired cardiac function improves approximately 24 to 30 hours after injury.[4,9] Initial postburn fluid resuscitation aids in restoring normal cardiac output and perfusion to tissues.

Immune System Response

The loss of skin from a burn injury destroys the body's primary barrier to microorganisms. Tissue damage invokes simultaneous activation of all inflammatory response cascades, including the complement, fibrinolytic, clotting, and kinin systems. The end result of this inflammatory response is overstimulation of suppressor T cells and depression of the activities of other components such as helper T cells, killer T cells, and polymorphonuclear leukocytes. Immunosuppression interferes with the ability of the patient's host defense mechanisms to fight invading microorganisms, increasing the risk for developing infection and sepsis.

Pulmonary Response

Release of vasoconstrictive mediator substances causes an initial transient pulmonary hypertension associated with a decreased oxygen tension and lung compliance. This occurs in the absence of lung injury and edema.[9,15] Inhalation injury complicates the pulmonary response; the pathology of inhalation injury is described in Table 21.1.

Renal Response

The renal circulation is sensitive to decreasing cardiac output. Hypoperfusion and a decreased glomerular filtration rate signal the nephrons to initiate the renin-angiotensin-aldosterone cascade. Sodium and water are retained to preserve intravascular fluid in an attempt to increase cardiac preload. Oliguria occurs, and urine becomes more concentrated. If fluid resuscitation is inadequate, acute kidney injury can develop. With effective resuscitation and improved renal perfusion, diuresis occurs approximately 48 hours after injury.

Gastrointestinal Response

The inflammatory response and hypovolemia after a major burn injury trigger the gastrointestinal (GI) circulation to undergo compensatory vasoconstriction and redistribution of blood flow to preserve perfusion to the brain and heart. The resulting ischemia of the stomach and duodenal mucosa places burn patients at high risk of developing a duodenal ulcer, called a *stress ulcer* or *Curling's ulcer*. Initiation of peptic ulcer prophylaxis reduces the risk of developing a stress ulcer. GI motility or peristalsis is also decreased, resulting in *paralytic ileus*. The ileus clinically manifests as gastric distension, nausea, or vomiting and decreased bowel sounds.

Metabolic Response

Two phases of metabolic dysfunction occur after a major burn injury. First, organ function decreases, followed by a second phase of a hypermetabolic and hyperfunctional response of all systems. Hypermetabolism begins as resuscitation is completed and is one of the most significant and persistent alterations observed after burn injury. The postburn hypermetabolic response is greater than that seen in any other forms of trauma.[1,18] Patients with severe burns have metabolic rates that are 100% to 200% above their basal rates, with some degree of elevation continuing for 1 to 3 years after injury.[1,18] The rapid metabolic rate is caused by the secretion of inflammatory response mediators or catabolic hormones such as catecholamines, cortisol, and glucagon in an effort to support gluconeogenesis, tissue remodeling, and repair.[1,2,36,39] The hypermetabolic state produces a catabolic effect on the body, with skeletal muscle breakdown, decreased protein synthesis, increased glucose use, and rapid depletion of glycogen stores.[1,20,36,39] The amount of protein wasting and weight loss that occurs is affected by several factors, including %TBSA burned, age, sex, preburn nutritional status, comorbidities, medical conditions, exercise, and nutrient intake.

PHASES OF BURN CARE ASSESSMENT AND COLLABORATIVE INTERVENTIONS

Assessment and management of the burn-injured patient consist of three phases of care: resuscitative, acute, and rehabilitative. The *resuscitative phase* or emergency phase begins at the time of injury and continues for approximately 48 hours until the massive fluid and protein shifts have stabilized. The primary focus of assessment and intervention is on maintenance of the ABCs (airway, breathing, and circulation) and prevention of burn shock. The resuscitative phase spans care in the prehospital setting, care in the ED, and transfer to and care at a burn center. The *acute phase* begins with the onset of diuresis at approximately 48 to 72 hours after injury and continues until wound closure occurs. This phase typically occurs in a burn center and may last for weeks or months. Nursing care focuses on the promotion of wound healing, the prevention of infections and complications, and the provision of psychosocial support. Although the critical care nurse is rarely involved in the *rehabilitative phase*, the care given in the first two phases is instrumental in achieving optimal rehabilitative outcomes. The primary goals in the rehabilitative phase are to improve function and range of motion (ROM), to minimize scarring and contractures, and to restore the patient's ability to return to preburn family, social, and career roles.

Critical care activities usually occur in the resuscitative and acute phases. In both of these phases, patient assessment and management are prioritized and follow the primary and secondary surveys described in the Advanced Burn Life Support Course.[4] Pain control, wound management, infection prevention, special considerations for unique burn injuries, and psychosocial concerns are important issues throughout all phases of burn care. See the Plan of Care for Acute Care and Resuscitative Phases of Major Burn Injury for more information. These care plans include only burn-specific interventions not otherwise shown in the Collaborative Plan of Care for the Critically Ill Patient (Chapter 1).

Resuscitative Phase: Prehospital

Primary Survey. Prehospital personnel are the first healthcare providers to arrive at the scene of injury. The patient's likelihood of survival is greatly affected by the care rendered during the first few hours after a significant burn injury. The priorities of prehospital care and management are to extricate the patient safely, stop the burning process, identify life-threatening injuries, and minimize time on the scene by rapidly transporting the patient to an appropriate care facility. As with any other type of trauma,

◎ PLAN OF CARE

Acute Care and Resuscitative Phases of Major Burn Injury

Patient Problem

Potential for Insufficient Airway Clearance and Decreased Gas Exchange. Risk factors include tracheal or interstitial edema, inhalation injury, or circumferential torso eschar.

Desired Outcomes

- PaO_2 greater than 90 mm Hg; $PaCO_2$ less than 45 mm Hg; SaO_2 greater than 95%; COHgb less than 10%.
- Respiration rate 16 to 20 breaths/min and unlabored; chest wall excursion symmetrical and adequate.
- On teaching, the patient demonstrates an effective cough.
- After interventions, the patient's airway is free of excessive secretions and adventitious breath sounds.

Assessments/Interventions	Rationales
• Assess respiratory rate, depth, and rhythm every hour; monitor COHgb.	• Assess early warning signs of impending respiratory difficulties.
• Ensure that the patient performs deep-breathing with coughing exercises at least every 2 hours.	• Clear the airway of secretions.
• If patient is not intubated, assess for stridor, hoarseness, use of accessory muscles, and wheezing every hour.	• Identify airway edema and need for immediate intubation or airway control.
• Administer 100% humidified oxygen as ordered.	• Expedite elimination of carbon monoxide to prevent or treat hypoxemia; decrease viscosity of secretions.
• Evaluate need for chest escharotomy during fluid resuscitation.	• Improve ventilation and oxygenation by alleviating constricted chest wall movement.
• Elevate HOB.	• Decrease edema of face, neck, and mouth.
• Alternate periods of increased activity (e.g., wound care, ROM, therapy activities, mobility) with periods of rest to avoid fatigue.	• Prevents atelectasis and promotes oxygenation.

Patient Problem

Dehydration. Risk factors include fluid shifts into the interstitium and evaporative loss of fluids from the injured skin.

Desired Outcomes

- Heart rate 60 to 100 beats/min.
- Blood pressure 90 mm Hg or higher (adequate in relation to pulse and urine output).
- Pulse pressure variation (PPV) less than 12% (if greater than 12%, patient requires fluid resuscitation).
- Hemodynamic parameters at upper ends of normal range.
- Sensorium clear.
- Optimal tissue perfusion.
- Nonburned skin warm and pink.
- Urine output 0.5 mL/kg/h (1.5 mL/kg/h in electrical injury).
- Weight gain based on volume of fluids given in first 48 hours followed by diuresis over next 3 to 5 days.
- Serum laboratory values WNL; specific gravity normal except during diuresis; urine negative for glucose and ketones.

Assessments/Interventions	Rationales
• Monitor vital signs and urine output every hour until stable; evaluate mental status every hour for at least 48 hours.	• Assess perfusion and oxygenation status.
• Titrate calculated fluid requirements in first 48 hours to maintain urinary output and hemodynamic stability.	• Restore intravascular volume.
• Record daily weight and hourly I&O; evaluate trends.	• Urine output closely reflects renal perfusion and overall tissue perfusion status.
• Monitor serum electrolytes, hematocrit, hemoglobin, serum glucose, BUN, and serum creatinine levels at least twice daily for first 48 hours and then as required by patient status.	• Evaluate fluid loss and replacement.
	• Evaluate need for electrolyte and fluid replacement associated with large fluid and protein shifts.

Patient Problem

Hypothermia. Risk factors include loss of skin and/or external cooling.

Desired Outcome

- Rectal or core temperature 37° to 38°C (98.6° to 101.3°F).

Assessments/Interventions	Rationales
• Monitor and document rectal or core temperature every 1-2 hours.	• Evaluate body temperature status.
• Assess for shivering.	• After a major thermal injury, routine methods of heat conservation are inadequate.
• Minimize skin exposure; maintain environmental temperatures.	• Prevent evaporative and conductive losses.
• For temperatures <37°C (98.6°F), institute rewarming measures.	• Prevent complications of wound progression related to vasoconstriction.

◎ PLAN OF CARE—cont'd

Acute Care and Resuscitative Phases of Major Burn Injury

Patient Problem

Decreased Peripheral Tissue Perfusion. Risk factors include hypovolemia or impaired vascular circulation in extremities with circumferential deep partial- or full-thickness burns.

Desired Outcomes

- Peripheral pulses present and strong.
- Warm extremities.
- Absence of compartment syndrome.

Assessments/Interventions	Rationales
• Assess peripheral pulses, color, and temperature every hour for 72 hours; notify physician of changes in pulses, capillary refill, color, temperature, or pain sensation.	• Assess peripheral perfusion and the need for escharotomy.
• Elevate upper extremities with IV poles or on pillows; elevate lower extremities on pillows.	• Decrease edema formation.
• Assist with escharotomy or fasciotomy in circumferential burns to an extremity.	• Escharotomy or fasciotomy allows for edema expansion and permits peripheral perfusion.

Patient Problem

Acute Pain. Risk factors include burn trauma and medical-surgical interventions.

Desired Outcome

- Using the appropriate pain scale, pain is either reduced or at an acceptable level within 1 to 2 hours.
- Patient participates in wound care and ROM and therapy activities.

Assessments/Interventions	Rationales
• Administer IV analgesic and/or anxiolytic medications during critical care phases.	• Facilitate pain relief and anxiety. • IM and oral medications are not consistently absorbed, especially during early post-burn fluid shifts and ileus.
• Medicate patient before wound care, dressing changes, bathing, ROM, therapy, and major procedures as needed.	• Assist patient to perform at higher level of function. • Exposed nerve endings increase pain.
• Explore use of nonpharmacological pain management strategies (e.g., guided imagery, virtual games, music) as adjuncts to pharmacological pain management strategies.	• Provide optimal pain relief and provide the patient with control over pain treatment options.

Patient Problem

Potential for Delayed Wound Healing and Risk for Infection. Risk factors include loss of skin, impaired immune response, and invasive therapies.

Desired Outcomes

- Absence of inflamed burn wound margins.
- No evidence of burn wound, donor site, or invasive catheter site infection.
- Autograft or allograft skin is adherent to healthy tissue.

Assessments/Interventions	Rationales
• Monitor burn wound healing, including presence of exudate and/or odor.	• Facilitate early detection of developing infection.
• Use appropriate protective isolation; provide meticulous wound care with antimicrobial topical agents as ordered; clip or shave hair (except eyebrows) 1 inch around burn wounds.	• Decrease exposure to pathogens; hair is a medium for microorganism growth; proper hand washing and use of protective barriers decrease contamination. • Reduce scarring.
• Obtain wound cultures as ordered.	• Determine infection source and specific invading microorganism to guide topical or systemic antimicrobial therapy.

Patient Problem

Weight Loss. Risk factors include increased metabolic demands secondary to physiological stress and wound healing.

Desired Outcomes

- Normal intake of food within restrictions, as indicated.
- Evidence of weight maintenance or gain.

Assessments/Interventions	Rationales
• Place nasogastric tube for gastric decompression if burns >20% TBSA.	• Prevent nausea, emesis, and aspiration.
• Administer medications for stress ulcer prophylaxis.	• Prevent stress ulcer development.

Continued

⊚ PLAN OF CARE—cont'd

Acute Care and Resuscitative Phases of Major Burn Injury

Assessments/Interventions	Rationales
• Consult dietitian. Initiate enteral feeding and evaluate tolerance; provide high-calorie or protein supplements; record all oral intake and count calories.	• Caloric or protein intake must be adequate to maintain positive nitrogen balance and promote healing.
• Schedule interventions and activities to avoid interrupting feeding times.	• Pain, fatigue, and sedation interfere with the desire to eat.

Patient Problem

Decreased Mobility. Risk factors include burn injury, therapeutic splinting, immobilization requirements after skin graft, and/or contractures.

Desired Outcomes

- The patient verbalizes understanding of the use of analgesics and adjunctive methods to decrease pain.
- The patient uses mobility aids safely if required.
- Demonstrates ability to care for burn wounds.
- No evidence of permanent decreased joint function.
- Vocation resumed with burn-associated limitation adaptations, or adjustment to new vocation.

Assessments/Interventions	Rationales
• Perform active and passive ROM of extremities every 2 hours while patient is awake.	• Prevent burn wound contractures and loss of joint movement or function.
• Increase activity as tolerated.	
• Reinforce importance of maintaining proper joint alignment with splints and antideformity positioning.	
• Elevate burned extremities.	• Decreases edema and promotes ROM and mobility.
• Provide pain relief measures before self-care activities, ROM therapy, OT/PT therapies.	• Facilitate mobility and assists patient to perform at a higher level of function.

Patient Problem

Decreased Ability to Cope. Risk factors include acute stress of critical burn injury and potential life-threatening crisis.

Desired Outcomes

- Before hospital discharge, the patient verbalizes feelings, identifies strengths and coping behaviors, and does not demonstrate ineffective coping behaviors.
- Patient and family coping is realistic for phase of hospitalization and the family's processes at pre-crisis level.

Assessments/Interventions	Rationale
• Consult social worker for assistance in discharge planning and psychosocial assessment issues; consult psychiatric services for inadequate coping skills or substance abuse treatment; promote use of group support sessions.	• Provide expert consultation and intervention; assist patient and family in understanding experiences and reactions after burn injury and methods of dealing with trauma.
• Encourage patient and family to identify previous methods of coping.	• Identify known strategies that promote stress management.

BUN, Blood urea nitrogen; *COHgb,* carboxyhemoglobin; *HOB,* head of bed; *I&O,* intake and output; *IM,* intramuscular; *OT/PT,* occupational therapy/physical therapy; *PaCO₂*, partial pressure of carbon dioxide; *PaO₂*, partial pressure of oxygen; *ROM,* range of motion; *SaO₂*, oxygen saturation; *TBSA,* total body surface area; *WNL,* within normal limits.

Adapted from Swearingen PL, Wright JD. *All-in-One Nursing Care Planning Resource.* 5th ed. St. Louis, MO: Elsevier; 2019.

---

the primary survey is used to provide a fast, systematic assessment that prioritizes evaluation of the patient's airway, breathing, and circulatory status (Fig. 21.6).

Stop the burning process. The first priority of patient care is to stop the burning process by removing the patient from the source of burning while preventing further injury.[4] Extinguish flame burns by rolling the patient on the ground, smothering the flames with a blanket or other cover, or dousing the flames with water. Never apply ice or cold water to the wounds because further tissue damage may occur as a result of vasoconstriction and hypothermia. Remove jewelry quickly because metal retains heat and can cause continued burning. Treat scald, tar, and asphalt burns by immediately removing saturated clothing, rinsing with cool water if available, or both. Do not attempt to remove adherent tar or clothing (clothing that is burned into and stuck to the

skin) at the scene because this can cause increased tissue damage and bleeding. Treat electrical injuries with prompt removal of the patient from the electrical source while protecting the rescuer. Ensure that the source of electricity is no longer in contact with the patient or is turned off before attempting rescue. The burning process of chemical injuries continues for as long as the chemical is in contact with the skin; immediately remove all clothing and institute water lavage (unless contraindicated) before and during transport. Brush powdered chemicals off of clothing and skin first, before performing lavage. Apply copious amounts of clean water lavage. If the chemical is in or near the eyes, remove contact lenses (if present) and irrigate the eyes with saline or clean water. Prevent cross-contamination of the opposite eye during lavage by irrigating in the direction from inner to outer canthus. Do not use neutralizing agents on chemical burns, as heat is produced

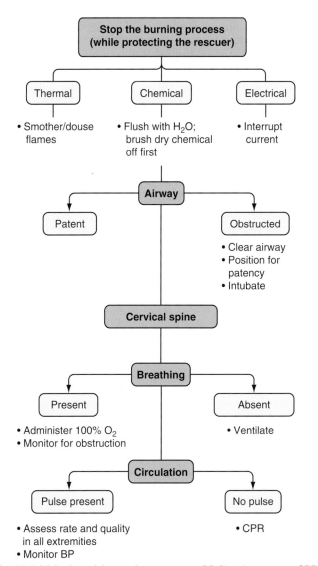

Fig. 21.6 Major burn injury: primary survey. *BP,* Blood pressure; *CPR,* cardiopulmonary resuscitation; *H₂O,* water; *O₂,* oxygen.

Flowchart content:

Stop the burning process (while protecting the rescuer)

- Thermal
  - • Smother/douse flames
- Chemical
  - • Flush with H_2O; brush dry chemical off first
- Electrical
  - • Interrupt current

Airway
- Patent
- Obstructed
  - • Clear airway
  - • Position for patency
  - • Intubate

Cervical spine

Breathing
- Present
  - • Administer 100% O_2
  - • Monitor for obstruction
- Absent
  - • Ventilate

Circulation
- Pulse present
  - • Assess rate and quality in all extremities
  - • Monitor BP
- No pulse
  - • CPR

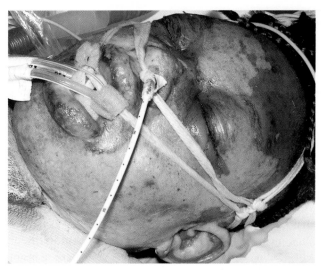

Fig. 21.7 Facial edema. (Courtesy University of Michigan Trauma Burn Center, Ann Arbor, MI.)

when such agents come into contact with chemicals, further increasing the depth of injury. Wear protective barrier garments such as plastic gowns, gloves, goggles, and a face shield to prevent exposure during initial treatment and lavage of chemical injuries.

Airway (with cervical spine precautions). Any suspicion of inhalation injury requires immediate intervention for airway control while maintaining cervical spine immobilization precautions, if indicated. Refer to Clinical Alert: Clinical Indicators of Inhalation Injury earlier in the chapter. Respiratory stridor indicates airway obstruction and mandates immediate endotracheal intubation at the scene. Patients with severe facial burns are prophylactically intubated because delayed endotracheal intubation can be difficult or impossible as edema develops (Fig. 21.7).

Breathing. All patients with suspected smoke inhalation are treated at the scene with 100% humidified oxygen delivered by non-rebreather mask or endotracheal tube. Administration of 100% oxygen reduces the half-life of carbon monoxide to 45 to 60 minutes compared with 4 hours in room air. Monitor for clinical signs of decreasing oxygenation, such as changes in

respiratory rate or neurological status. Pulse oximetry may not be accurate in acute inhalation injuries because the pulse oximeter cannot distinguish between carbon monoxide and oxygen attached to the hemoglobin. Consider and treat cyanide poisoning in patients involved in closed-space fires (see Clinical Alert box).

! CLINICAL ALERT

Cyanide Toxicity

Clinical indicators of cyanide toxicity:
- Patient involved in a closed-space fire
- Unexplained hypotension
- Unexplained hypoxemia
- Lactic acidosis (>10 mmol/L)

STUDY BREAK

3. Appropriate initial management of a patient with a documented inhalation injury includes:
   A. Fluid restriction to minimize lung injury
   B. Colloid infusion to decrease extravascular lung water
   C. Prophylactic antibiotics to decrease the incidence of pneumonia
   D. 100% humidified oxygen to decrease carboxyhemoglobin levels

---

Circulation. Remove all clothing and jewelry to prevent constriction and ischemia of the distal extremities secondary to edema formation. Insert two large-bore (≥16-gauge or larger) IV catheters, preferably through nonburned tissue, and infuse Lactated Ringer's solution (LR) at 500 mL/h (adults) until fluid requirements are calculated based on the %TBSA.[4] Monitor closely for signs of hypovolemia such as changes in level of consciousness, rapid or thready pulses, decreased blood pressure, or narrowing pulse pressure. Burn injuries rarely result in hypovolemic shock in the early prehospital phase. Consequently, suspect associated internal or external injuries if evidence of shock is present.

Heat loss occurs rapidly in a major burn injury because the protective covering of skin is lost. Cover the patient with a clean, dry sheet and blankets to prevent hypothermia and further wound contamination.

Secondary Survey. Perform a brief secondary survey in the prehospital setting so as not to delay transport to a hospital. A rapid head-to-toe assessment is completed to rule out any additional trauma as part of the secondary survey (Fig. 21.8). In patients with an injury mechanism suggestive of spinal injury, apply standard precautions (cervical collar, immobilization, log rolling before transport).

Often the patient is most alert during this initial period. Obtain an accurate history of the events that led to the burn injury, including the time of injury, the source of burns, and events leading to the injury. Also obtain a brief medical history, including allergies, current medical problems and medications

taken, past surgical procedures and/or trauma, time of last meal, and history of tetanus immunization.[4]

In preparation for transport, a short-acting IV opioid such as morphine sulfate may be administered for pain relief. Intramuscular medications are not given during the resuscitative phase because perfusion of edematous tissues is poor and produces sporadic narcotic absorption. The patient receives nothing by mouth before or during transport to prevent vomiting and aspiration.

Resuscitative Phase: Emergency Department and Critical Care Burn Center

The burn patient is transferred from the injury scene to either a community hospital ED or a burn center. See the recommendations for referral to a burn center in the Clinical Alert box. Management goals at either facility continue to be restoration and maintenance of the ABCs and prevention of burn shock.

Transfer to a Burn Center. Patients with a major burn injury require complex care and the expertise of a specially trained multiprofessional team. Burn team members include nurses, physicians and surgeons (general, plastic and reconstructive, and critical care), occupational and physical therapists, dietitians, respiratory therapists, infection prevention specialists, pharmacists, social workers, psychiatrists, psychologists, chaplains, injury prevention educators, and physician specialists (rehabilitation, neurosurgeons) as indicated. Burn centers provide resources to improve burn patient care and outcome, including a dedicated trained staff, prehospital and community education, injury prevention, and research. Hospitals without a burn center may not have the personnel or supplies necessary for specialized burn care.

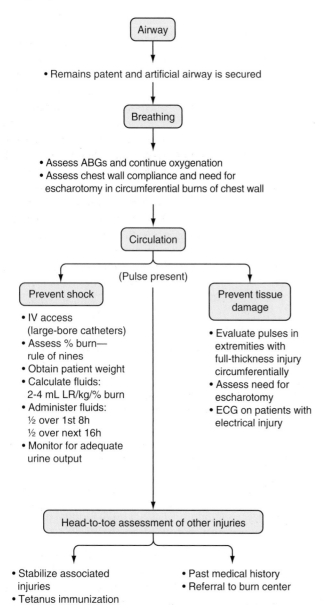

Fig. 21.8 Major burn injury: secondary survey. *ABG,* Arterial blood gas; *ECG,* electrocardiogram; *LR,* Lactated Ringer's solution.

? CRITICAL REASONING ACTIVITY

Why is multiprofessional team care of the burn-injured patient important? Who is involved?

! CLINICAL ALERT

Guidelines for Burn Center Referral[4]

- Partial-thickness burns 10% of total body surface area (TBSA)
- Full-thickness burns
- Burns involving the face, hands, feet, genitalia, perineum, or major joints
- Chemical burns
- Electrical burns
- Inhalation injury
- Preexisting medical disorders
- Associated trauma
- Hospital without qualified personnel or equipment to care for burn-injured children
- Patients requiring special social, emotional, or rehabilitative intervention

When considering transfer to a burn center, the referring physician directly contacts the burn center physician. The burn center and referring physicians collaborate on the mode of transportation (ground ambulance or air) and the treatment necessary to stabilize the patient for transport.[4] Transport is optimally done early in the postburn period, during the resuscitative phase, based on guidelines provided by the receiving burn center. A standardized transfer form is used to summarize information on a burn patient's status to ensure continuity of care between facilities.[4]

Primary Survey. On arrival at either the ED or the burn center, assess the patient using a systematic approach such as the ABCDE (airway, breathing, circulation, disability, and exposure) primary survey. Once the patient arrives in the critical care burn unit, perform a thorough primary and secondary assessment.

Airway. Airway management issues related to tracheal edema may occur early or may not be apparent until after fluid resuscitation is initiated. Frequently monitor patients with suspected inhalation injuries who are not already intubated for hoarseness, stridor, or wheezing. Massive edema formation is an anticipated response to fluid resuscitation in an extensively burned patient. Anticipate assisting with early intubation of patients with severe facial burns. The presence of other symptoms suggestive of inhalation injury (see Clinical Alert: Clinical Indicators of Inhalation Injury earlier in the chapter) necessitates early intubation to maintain adequate oxygenation and perfusion. A fiberoptic bronchoscopy may be performed to confirm the presence of inhalation injury. If the patient is already intubated, assess for accurate tube position. Securely tie (not tape) the endotracheal tube in place to prevent accidental extubation, but prevent the ties from placing pressure on burned ears (see Fig. 21.7). Protecting the artificial airway is critical because it may be impossible to reintubate the patient after massive edema and airway obstruction have developed, necessitating an emergency cricothyroidotomy or tracheostomy. Elevate the head of the patient's bed to reduce facial and airway edema.

Breathing. Assess for impaired gas exchange related to carbon monoxide poisoning, cyanide poisoning, or inhalation injury. Evaluate breath sounds, characteristics of respirations, work of breathing, sputum color and consistency, and symmetry of chest wall expansion. Measure arterial blood gases on all intubated patients and COHgb if inhalation injury is suspected. Administer humidified 100% oxygen via face mask or endotracheal tube until COHgb levels are determined. Once COHgb levels normalize (<10%), wean oxygen as tolerated. The goal is a PaO_2 greater than 90 mm Hg and an oxygen saturation (SaO_2) greater than 95%.

In suspected cyanide poisoning (see Clinical Alert: Cyanide Toxicity earlier in the chapter), continue treatment with 100% oxygen. Empirical treatment with an antidote, hydroxocobalamin, is also indicated.[7,9,11] Red discoloration of urine and body fluids is an expected side effect of hydroxocobalamin therapy and may interfere with some clinical laboratory evaluations.

Patients with circumferential full-thickness burns of the thorax may demonstrate inadequate ventilatory effort due to edema and restrictive eschar inhibiting chest wall expansion. Early signs of inadequate ventilatory effort may include increased peak inspiratory pressure and decreased tidal volumes. Clinically, patients with a pneumothorax, hemothorax, or tension pneumothorax present in similar ways, so these differential

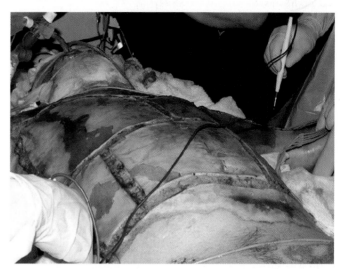

Fig. 21.9 Escharotomy. (Courtesy University of Michigan Trauma Burn Center, Ann Arbor, MI.)

diagnoses are ruled out first. Consider the need for a chest wall escharotomy (Fig. 21.9) if these differential diagnoses have been ruled out and the patient continues to show signs of inadequate ventilation. In this situation, an immediate chest wall *escharotomy* is indicated to facilitate breathing. An escharotomy is an incision performed at the bedside (or in the operating room) through a full-thickness burn to reduce constriction caused by the tight, nonelastic band of eschar. This relieves pressure, restores ventilation, and improves blood flow. Local anesthesia is not required because the full-thickness burn eschar is painless.

Perform ongoing assessment of breath sounds, arterial blood gases, and ventilatory status. Provide aggressive pulmonary-focused interventions to patients with inhalation injury. New critical care positioning beds and percussive technology improve pulmonary function in patients with limited mobility or pulmonary injury. Turn patients every 2 hours to promote skin integrity and facilitate secretion movement. In addition, encourage coughing, deep breathing, and suctioning as needed for patients with inhalation injury to optimize pulmonary function.[29] Early mobility is also encouraged. Continuously monitor pulse oximetry and end-tidal carbon dioxide as appropriate. Lung-protective ventilation strategies are used in intubated patients with inhalation injury, such as lower tidal volumes (6 mL/kg of ideal body weight) and plateau pressures lower than 30 mm Hg.[9,38] Consider implementing prone positioning, which has been shown to increase oxygenation.[9] Research also suggests that administration of nebulization therapy with aerosolized heparin, β_2-adrenergic agonist agents (albuterol, terbutaline), and N-acetylcysteine (Mucomyst) may be beneficial treatment adjuncts to open airways and reduce inflammatory response effects.[29]

Circulation

Fluid resuscitation. Fluid resuscitation is a critical intervention for burn management. To estimate fluid resuscitation requirements, assess the depth and extent of injury. Estimate fluid resuscitation requirements according to body weight in kilograms, the %TBSA burned, and the patient's age. IV fluid resuscitation is instituted in patients with burns greater than

20% TBSA. These patients have more diffuse capillary leak and greater intravascular fluid loss. Patients with smaller %TBSA burns may be resuscitated with oral hydration.

The *Parkland formula* is one of the most widely used burn resuscitation fluid formulas. It approximates fluid replacement requirements by calculating the amount of LR to infuse during the first 24 hours after injury at 4 mL/kg per %TBSA.[9,13] Half of the calculated amount is given over the first 8 hours after injury, and the remaining half is given over the next 16 hours. The American Burn Association recommends using a modified version of the Parkland formula, called the *Advanced Burn Life Support (ABLS) fluid resuscitation formula*.[4] Fluid requirements for those with high-voltage electrical injuries are higher during the initial 48 hours after the burn. Many units use the ABLS formula for the first 24 hours and the Parkland formula during the second 24 hours, as shown in Box 21.1.

Two large-bore (16-gauge or larger) peripheral IV catheters are inserted. If an unburned location is not available, place the IV catheters through burned skin. Central venous catheters are commonly inserted in patients with major burns to facilitate and accommodate large IV fluid infusion requirements and to monitor resuscitation end points. LR is the preferred initial IV fluid for burn resuscitation.[4,9] It is a crystalloid solution with an osmolality and electrolyte composition similar to normal body fluids. It does not contain dextrose, which can cause a misleadingly high urine output due to glycosuria and osmotic diuresis. It contains lactate, which helps buffer the metabolic acidosis associated with hypoperfusion and burn shock. LR does not provide any intravascular protein replacement to increase intravascular oncotic pressure. In the presence of increased capillary membrane permeability, the intravascular retention of LR is only about 25% of the infused volume, necessitating large fluid volume infusions to maintain circulating blood volume.[26] Normal saline (0.9%) is not used because of its high sodium and chloride concentrations, which can cause detrimental hyperchloremic acidosis.

Fluid requirements calculated by the ABLS fluid resuscitation formula serve only as a guide for estimating initial fluid needs. Patients react differently to burn injury and may require varying amounts of IV fluid to support perfusion. Several factors affect fluid requirements: age, depth of burn, concurrent inhalation injury, preexisting disease or comorbidities, delay in treatment of burn injury, use of methamphetamine or other polysubstances, and associated injuries. Patients with inhalation injuries typically require larger-volume fluid resuscitation, and those with electrical injuries require larger fluid resuscitation volumes to prevent acute tubular necrosis by clearing the renal tubules from precipitating myoglobin caused by skeletal muscle damage or *rhabdomyolysis* (see discussion later in this chapter and in Chapter 20). Because evaporative fluid losses continue until burn wounds are closed, either with a temporary covering (e.g., homograft, xenograft) or with permanent split-thickness skin grafts, these losses are calculated as a part of the total daily maintenance fluid replacement formula. Accurately calculate fluid intake and output by also weighing saturated bed pads, linens, and dressings.

Increased crystalloid infusion alone is incapable of restoring cardiac preload in burn shock and can cause complications such as compartment syndrome from fluid overload. Colloids, such as albumin, that contain proteins are sometimes used in burn resuscitation to increase intravascular oncotic pressure. The increase in intravascular oncotic pressure pulls fluid from the interstitium back into the circulating intravascular volume, thereby reducing edema and combating burn shock. However, during increased permeability, colloids leak into the interstitium and contribute to further intravascular fluid loss. Historically, colloids administration was avoided within the first 12 hours after burn injury, when capillary permeability is at its highest level.[26,32] However, current evidence indicates that administering albumin within the first 12 hours after burn shock resuscitation may reduce mortality and compartment syndrome, enhance intravascular volume preservation, decrease overall edema formation, and reduce fluid resuscitation requirements.[9,12,32] Other alternative fluids and augmenting agents, such as high-dose antioxidant vitamin C, are being explored to ameliorate the inflammatory response, reduce resuscitation fluid requirements, and decrease edema.[35] Blood purification methods, including plasma exchange, continuous venovenous hemofiltration, and absorbing membranes, have been used recently to eliminate proinflammatory cytokines during the initial resuscitation. This technology has been shown to regulate cytokine homeostasis, modulate inflammatory reactions, and decrease myoglobin.[27]

During the second 24 hours after burn injury, when capillary permeability has decreased, a fluid formula such as the Parkland

---

BOX 21.1   Burn Fluid Resuscitation Formulas

During First 24 Hours

Administer Fluid According to ABLS Resuscitation Formula[4]

- *Adults:* LR, 2 mL/kg/%TBSA[a]
- *Adults with high-voltage electrical injuries:* LR, 4 mL/kg/%TBSA[a]
- *Children 13 years old and younger and weighing 10 to 30 kg:* LR, 3 mL/kg/%TBSA[a]
- *Infants weighing less than 10 kg:* D_5LR, 3 mL/kg/%TBSA[a]

Give half over the first 8 hours after injury and the remaining half over the next 16 hours.

Titrate fluids to maintain urine output of 0.5 mL/kg/h, or 30 to 50 mL/h in adults, and 1 mL/kg/h in children weighing less than 30 kg.

Example: For an adult weighing 75 kg with a 55% TBSA burn injury:

- 2 mL LR × 75 kg × 55% TBSA = 8250 mL of LR infused over 24 hours
- First 8 hours after burn injury: 4125 mL of LR infused over 8 hours, or 515.6 mL/h
- Next 16 hours after burn injury: 4125 mL of LR infused over 16 hours, or 257.8 mL/h

During Second 24 Hours

Administer Fluid According to the Parkland Formula[9]

- Dextrose in water, plus potassium to maintain normal electrolyte balance
- Colloid-containing fluid equal to 20% to 60% of calculated plasma volume, or an infusion rate of approximately 0.35 to 0.5 mL/kg/%TBSA

[a]%TBSA, Percentage of TBSA with second- or third-degree burns. *ABLS*, Advanced Burn Life Support; D_5LR, dextrose in 5% Lactated Ringer's solution; *LR*, Lactated Ringer's solution; *TBSA*, total body surface area.

formula (see Box 21.1), which incorporates colloids, dextrose, and electrolyte replacement, may be used. Hypertonic dextrose solutions and colloids increase oncotic pressure, which helps pull third-spaced fluid from the interstitium back into the circulatory system. Potassium is added to IV fluids to replace potassium losses in the urine.

STUDY BREAK

4. Initial fluid resuscitation requirements are calculated based on the following parameters:

A. Age, total body surface area burned, patient weight, and cause of burn injury

B. Injury mechanism (flame or nonflame), total body surface area burned, and patient weight

C. Total body surface area burned, patient weight, and the presence of inhalation injury

D. Age category (adult or child), patient temperature, and total body surface area burned

---

End point monitoring. The goal of burn resuscitation is to maintain tissue perfusion and organ function while preventing the complications of inadequate or excessive fluid therapy.[4,9] Resuscitation fluid infusion rates are titrated to physiological end points, including urine output, blood pressure, and hemodynamic parameters such as cardiac preload, systemic vascular resistance, and stroke volume.[4,12] Insert a urinary catheter to evaluate resuscitation adequacy. Adjust IV infusion rates to ensure a urinary output greater than 0.5 mL/kg/h (i.e., 30 to 50 mL/h) in adults.[4] Other resuscitation end points, such as pulse pressure variation and stroke volume variation, may be used to identify early failing resuscitation despite adequate urine output. These additional resuscitation end points may reduce the amount of crystalloid resuscitation needed, reducing complications of overresuscitation.[12] During the resuscitation phase, adjust IV administration rates based on resuscitation end points rather than administration of fluid boluses to reduce third-spacing and burn edema.[4]

Peripheral circulation. Special attention is given to full-thickness burns of the extremities that are *circumferential* (completely surrounding a body part). Pressure from bands of eschar or from edema that develops as resuscitation proceeds may impair blood flow to underlying and distal tissue. Elevate extremities to reduce edema. Perform active or passive ROM exercises every hour for 5 minutes to increase venous return and minimize edema. Assess pain, sensation, and peripheral pulses every hour, especially in circumferential burns of the extremities, to confirm adequate circulation. Use an ultrasonic flow meter (Doppler) to auscultate radial, palmar, digital, and/or pedal pulses. Closely monitor for signs of developing extremity *compartment syndrome* (see Clinical Alert box). Compartment syndrome occurs when tissue pressure in the fascial compartments of extremities increases, compressing and occluding blood vessels and nerves. Absent distal pulses and poor capillary refill are not reliable in diagnosing compartment syndrome because they are often late signs.

If signs and symptoms of extremity compartment syndrome are present, prepare for an escharotomy to relieve pressure and restore circulation. If decreased perfusion is not quickly detected, ischemia and necrosis with loss of the limb may occur. A *fasciotomy* (incision through fascia) may be indicated for deep electrical burns or severe muscle damage to restore blood flow. Escharotomy and fasciotomy sites are treated with a topical antimicrobial agent and closely monitored for bleeding. Cautery, silver nitrate sticks, or sutures may be indicated to stop continued bleeding.

⚠ CLINICAL ALERT

Clinical Indicators of Extremity Compartment Syndrome

- Presence of circumferential deep partial- or full-thickness extremity burns
- Electrical injury
- Pain: increasing, greater than expected, or out of proportion to the injury
- Increasing edema: muscle compartments tense on palpation or asymmetrical in size
- Altered sensation (e.g., tingling, numbness)
- Late signs (often associated with pending limb necrosis or loss): pallor, poor capillary refill, and absent distal pulses

---

Secondary Survey. The secondary survey includes a head-to-toe assessment, a complete history and physical examination, reassessment of interventions implemented during the primary survey, and vital signs. If associated trauma is suspected, continue spinal immobilization precautions until spinal injury has been ruled out. Convey the patient's medical and injury event history to the medical team. Assess indices of essential organ function to evaluate adequacy of burn shock resuscitation and to prevent complications. Monitor blood pressure, heart rate, cardiac rhythm, respiration quality and rate, temperature, peripheral pulse presence and quality, and urinary output at least hourly. In addition, consider evaluating urine specific gravity, urine glucose and ketone levels, every 2 to 4 hours. Because of the increased risk for gastric ulcers in the burn population, gastric pH is often assessed regularly. If GI bleeding is suspected, tests for occult blood may also be done. Weigh the patient on admission and daily thereafter. Closely monitor pain levels and perform interventions to adequately control pain. Document all parameters for analysis of trends. Assessment, early detection, and intervention in the resuscitative phase to prevent problems in the various body systems are discussed in the following sections.

Cardiovascular system. Historically, a mean arterial pressure greater than 70 mm Hg and absence of tachycardia (heart rate <120 beats/min) have been standard assessments of adequate burn shock resuscitation.[4] However, the cardiovascular response of the patient to burn injury warrants special consideration. Metabolic changes occur hours after burn injury and often cause elevated baseline heart rates of 100 to 120 beats/min. Assess for associated trauma if hypotension is noted in the immediate postburn period. Compensatory mechanisms prevent hypotension until significant intravascular volume losses have occurred; therefore decreasing blood pressure is a late sign of inadequate perfusion. Both arterial and noninvasive cuff pressure readings may be altered by peripheral tissue edema or by catecholamine- and mediator-induced arteriospasm. Changes in heart rate and blood pressure may also be masked or may occur secondary to pain, anxiety, or fear. Consider the entire patient and assess trends in vital signs, hemodynamics, and symptom changes rather than focusing on any single value.

The routine insertion of pulmonary artery catheters is not universally supported; however, patients with significant cardiopulmonary disease, elderly patients with burn injury, and those who have unexplained large resuscitation fluid volume requirements may benefit from more intensive monitoring.[4] A low right atrial pressure and low pulmonary artery occlusion pressure indicate hypovolemia and require intervention. Assess trends in cardiac output variables and oxygen transport variables to trend data to guide burn shock resuscitation.

Local thermal injury, venous stasis, hypercoagulability, and immobility place the burn patient at risk for developing deep vein thrombosis (DVT) and/or pulmonary embolism (PE), known collectively as venous thromboembolism (VTE). Clinical findings indicative of DVT may be absent or may be obscured by extremity burn wound pain, edema, or erythema. As many as 25% of burn patients develop a VTE, with obese patients having as much as a 43% risk.[28] Recommendations for VTE prophylaxis vary. Recent data suggest that patients who are appropriately anticoagulated according to anti-Xa levels with enoxaparin have fewer VTE events.[28] Based on best evidence, burn patients should receive mechanical VTE prophylaxis (e.g., sequential compression devices, early mobility) and/or medications (e.g., enoxaparin). Inferior vena cava (IVC) filters are not recommended but may be beneficial in high-risk patient populations.[28] Because traditional signs of VTE may be absent, closely monitor the burn patient for sudden respiratory deterioration, which may indicate PE.

Neurological system. Severely injured burn patients are initially awake, alert, and oriented; therefore closely monitor the patient's sensorium. If a burn patient initially presents with a decreased level of consciousness (LOC), suspect other injuries or causes (e.g., head injury, carbon monoxide or cyanide poisoning, drug overdose, alcohol intoxication). Evaluate the patient's sensorium hourly; increased agitation or confusion or a continued decreased LOC may be an indication of hypovolemia, hypoxemia, or both. Elevate the head of bed 30 degrees to prevent facial swelling during fluid resuscitation unless contraindicated.

Renal system. Urine output closely reflects renal perfusion, which is sensitive to decreasing cardiac output and developing shock. Urinary output is the quickest and most reliable indicator of adequate fluid resuscitation. Titrate calculated fluid requirements according to hourly urine output during resuscitation. Closely monitor urine output, color, and concentration, as oliguria occurs if fluid resuscitation is inadequate.

Gastrointestinal system. Monitor the GI system for problems such as ileus or Curling's ulcer. Assess for the presence of abdominal distension, gastric pH, characteristics of gastric secretions, and the presence of GI bleeding. Because patients with burns greater than 20% TBSA may develop an ileus, insert a nasogastric tube and connect it to low suction to prevent vomiting and reduce the risk of aspiration. Most burn patients require

nutritional support in the form of nutritional supplements and/or enteral feeding via the small bowel. Ensure that stress ulcer prophylaxis is ordered. Monitor tolerance to feedings.

Intraabdominal hypertension (IAH) is a serious complication caused by circumferential torso eschar, bowel edema from aggressive fluid resuscitation, and/or the burn inflammatory response. Increased crystalloid infusion rates during burn resuscitation contributes to IAH.[23] IAH is defined as intraabdominal pressure (IAP) of at least 12 mm Hg; it causes compression of intraabdominal contents and leads to renal, gut, and hepatic ischemia.[23] If not treated by trunk escharotomies, diuresis, gastric decompression, body repositioning, and/or sedation and chemical paralytics, IAH can progress to abdominal compartment syndrome (ACS) or death. The definition of *ACS* (see Clinical Alert box) is the presence of sustained IAP greater than 20 mm Hg, with or without abdominal perfusion pressure (APP = MAP − IAP) less than 60 mm Hg, and associated new organ system dysfunction or failure.[23]

> **! CLINICAL ALERT**
>
> *Clinical Indicators of Abdominal Compartment Syndrome*
>
> - Poor abdominal wall compliance (e.g., circumferential full-thickness burns of the torso or trunk)
> - Increasing IAH, not resolved by chest or torso escharotomy, repositioning, gastric decompression, sedation, or other interventions
> - Decreased urine output despite increased fluid administration
> - Increasing lactate concentration greater than 2.2 mEq/L
> - Distended abdomen with an IAP greater than 20 mm Hg
> - Increased ventilator requirements (e.g., increased FiO_2, increased peak airway pressure, increased PEEP)

FiO_2, Fraction of inspired oxygen; *IAH,* intraabdominal hypertension; *IAP,* intraabdominal pressure; *PEEP,* positive end-expiratory pressure.

To facilitate early detection of IAH, perform serial IAP measurements using bladder pressure monitoring on patients with greater than 40% TBSA burned, those with 20% TBSA burned and concomitant inhalation injury, and those requiring fluid resuscitation volumes greater than expected.[23] Do not rely on the appearance of physical symptoms to diagnose IAH and ACS; doing so delays necessary interventions and increases the likelihood of adverse outcome.[23] ACS is a life-threatening complication that mandates immediate decompression by laparotomy; otherwise, multiple organ dysfunction and death quickly ensue. Percutaneous drainage of peritoneal fluid may precede formal laparotomy as long as the patient is monitored closely, and laparotomy is immediately instituted if the patient continues to deteriorate. The resulting "open abdomen" laparotomy wound is treated with topical dressings or a vacuum-assisted device (see later discussion) and carefully assessed to prevent infectious complications until definitive operative closure can occur. Early abdominal fascial closure, or at least performed during the same hospitalization, is recommended.[23]

Integumentary system. Burn wounds place the patient at risk of tetanus; therefore administer tetanus toxoid–containing vaccine (e.g., Tdap, Td, or DTaP) if more than 5 years have elapsed since the last dose or if the patient's immunization history is unknown.[4]

During the resuscitation phase, the patient is at risk of developing hypothermia due to loss of the protective skin layer and administration of large amounts of room-temperature fluids. Closely monitor the patient's temperature. Implement measures to minimize loss of body heat, including limiting skin exposure and covering the patient with clean, dry sheets and blankets; using fluid or blood warmers for IV fluid infusion; increasing room temperature; closing room doors to prevent air drafts; and using external heat lamps, warming blankets, or radiant heat shields.

Blood and electrolytes. Measure serum electrolyte levels on admission and with changes in the patient's status. Serum sodium levels typically approach the concentration of sodium in the resuscitation fluid being administered. Monitor serum potassium, as values may be elevated from the release of potassium from injured tissue; conversely values may be low secondary to losses in the urine from fluid resuscitation. Blood urea nitrogen (BUN) levels may also increase when excessive protein catabolism occurs, and hyperglycemia may occur as a result of catecholamine release. Evaluate arterial blood gas values and serum lactate levels frequently because metabolic acidosis and elevated lactate can indicate inadequate tissue perfusion (see Laboratory Alert box).

Acute Care Phase: Critical Care Burn Center

With successful resuscitation, burn shock typically stabilizes approximately 48 to 72 hours after injury, and the acute phase of burn care begins. Implement interventions to promote wound healing, prevent complications, and improve function of the various body systems.

Respiratory System. Continue assessment for signs of respiratory compromise and pneumonia. Inhalation injury and ventilator management increase the risk for pneumonia.[6,18,31] Tachypnea, abnormal breath sounds, fever, increased white blood cell count, purulent secretions, and infiltrations on chest radiographs indicate developing pneumonia. Refer to Chapters 10 and 15 for nursing interventions. Collaborate with respiratory therapy personnel to perform spontaneous awakening trials and breathing trials to promote early extubation.[31]

✳ QSEN EXEMPLAR

Quality Improvement

A nurse in the burn clinic notices that patients returning to clinic after critical care unit hospital discharge were having a difficult time with activities of daily living. Specifically, the patients could not tie their shoes or brush their hair if they had sustained hand burns. When exploring the reasons that this may be occurring, the nurse discovers that there is no standard hand range of motion (ROM) exercises for the bedside critical care unit nurse to perform. The clinic nurse collaborates with physical and occupational therapy to understand the role and amount of therapy a patient in the critical care unit requires. The clinic nurse also works with the critical care unit nurses to understand their role in mobility of the burn patient in the critical care unit. With the help of physical and occupational therapy, a list of upper body ROM exercises, including specifics for the hand, is developed for the critical care unit bedside nurses to perform outside of the standard therapy sessions. The clinic nurse agrees to track patients' upper extremity, specifically hand, ROM when they return for clinic visits and share the findings with the entire burn team at the monthly quality meeting.

❗ LABORATORY ALERT

Alterations Seen During Acute Care Management of the Adult Burned Patient

Laboratory Test	Normal Range	Critical Value[a]	Significance
Carboxyhemoglobin	Nonsmoker: <3% Smoker: ≤10%	>20%	Present in carbon monoxide poisoning
Hematocrit	Male: 42%-52% Female: 37%-47%	<21% >65%	↑ In hypovolemia; ↓ as third-spaced fluid reenters the intravascular compartment or with concomitant traumatic injury
Serum lactate	Venous blood: 0.6-2.2 mmol/L Arterial blood: 0.3-0.8 mmol/L	>4.0 mmol/L	↑ In metabolic acidosis; should ↓ if fluid resuscitation is adequate
Potassium	3.5-5.0 mEq/L	<3.0 mEq/L >8 mEq/L	↑ Related to tissue damage; assess for cardiac dysrhythmias. Value may ↓ as potassium reenters cells
Sodium	136-145 mEq/L	<120 mEq/L >160 mEq/L	Levels approach the sodium concentration of fluids being administered. May ↑ with inadequate fluid replacement or ↓ with diuresis
Blood urea nitrogen	10-20 mg/dL	>100 mg/dL	May ↑ from catabolism or hypovolemia; monitor nutrition and volume status. May be higher in older adults
Platelets	150,000-400,000/mm³ (150-400 × 10⁹ SI units)	<20,000 or >1 million/mm³	↓ In large %TBSA burns, hypothermia-induced bleeding disorders, or infection
White blood cell count	5000-10,000/mm³ (5-10 × 10⁹ SI units)	<2,000 or >40,000/mm³	Transient ↓ from use of topical silver sulfadiazine; ↑ with infection

[a]Critical values vary by facility and laboratory.
%TBSA, Percentage of total body surface area.
From Pagana K, Pagana T. _Mosby's Manual of Diagnostic and Laboratory Tests._ 6th ed. St. Louis, MO: Elsevier; 2018.

Cardiovascular System. As capillary permeability stabilizes, IV fluid requirements decrease. Patients receive maintenance IV fluid infusions that match their overall fluid output. Monitor daily weight, intake, and output. Increased fluid resuscitation requirements after debridement and grafting operations are often required because the inflammatory response is triggered by the surgical intervention. Continue frequent monitoring of vital signs.

Neurological System. Perform ongoing assessment for changes in neurological status, which may indicate hypoxemia, hypoperfusion, or sepsis.

Renal System. Continue hourly urine output assessment. Postburn diuresis starts approximately 48 to 72 hours after injury. Urine output ranging from 100 to 600 mL/h is commonly observed. After postburn diuresis, urinary output should correlate with intake of IV and oral fluids. In the absence of diabetes, glycosuria may indicate an early sign of sepsis.

Gastrointestinal System. Continue assessment of GI function. Monitor the patient for the development of a stress ulcer. Assess enteral feeding tolerance. Nutritional considerations are a treatment priority and are discussed later in this chapter.

Integumentary System. The burn wound becomes the major focus of the acute phase of burn recovery. Continue monitoring for burn wound healing, burn wound depth conversion, and signs of infection. Isolation may be implemented (see Evidence-Based Practice box).

Blood and Electrolytes. Although fluid and protein shifts stabilize during the acute care phase, blood and electrolyte abnormalities related to other processes may be observed. Hemodilution with an associated decreased hematocrit may result from reentry of fluid into the intravascular compartment and from loss of red blood cells destroyed at the burn injury site. Hyponatremia from diuresis may occur, but it usually resolves within 1 week after onset. Inadequate replacement of evaporative water loss may produce hypernatremia. Hypokalemia may develop as potassium reenters the cells. Electrolyte shifts also affect the ability to maintain a proper acid-base balance and may cause metabolic acidosis. Hypoproteinemia and negative nitrogen balance may occur from an increase in metabolic rate and insufficient nutrition. Leukopenia may develop from administration of the topical antimicrobial agent silver sulfadiazine. Infection and excessive carbohydrate loading contribute to hyperglycemia. In addition, an increase in white blood cell count, prolonged coagulation times, and a decreased platelet count may result from infection or sepsis.

SPECIAL CONSIDERATIONS AND AREAS OF CONCERN

Burns of the face, ears, eyes, hands, feet, major joints, genitalia, and perineum pose distinct concerns because they contribute to overall burn injury severity and require unique management.

EVIDENCE-BASED PRACTICE

Decreasing the Incidence of Hospital-Acquired Infections in the Burn Unit

Problem

Burn patients are susceptible to various types of infections due to compromised skin integrity. Skin is the body's primary protection against infections. As the size of a wound increases, the immunological function of the patient decreases, which places him or her at a higher risk of infection. Common infections in these patients include pneumonia, blood stream infections, urinary tract infections, and wound infections. Many of the infections that develop contain multidrug-resistant organisms due to the patient's long hospital length of stay. Without new antibiotics to treat these infections, patient morbidity and mortality can increase.

Clinical Question

Does the implementation of protective isolation precautions in the burn unit decrease the incidence of hospital-acquired infections?

Evidence

A systematic review and meta-analysis were conducted to understand the relationship between protective isolation precautions and hospital-acquired infections in the burn unit. The literature review focused on articles written in English only, burn patients of all ages, all percentages of total body surface area burn sizes, and only patients in a burn unit. The analysis concluded:
1. Protective isolation includes strict hand hygiene and glove use; the use of masks, gowns, and sterile gloves during wound care; and single-patient isolation rooms.
2. A significant reduction in colonization and infection rates was seen through the implementation of protective precautions.
3. The use of protective isolation precautions for burn patients in daily practice was recommended.

Implications for Nursing

This study demonstrated that the use of protective isolation precautions—including strict hand hygiene with glove use; the use of masks, gowns, and sterile gloves during wound care; and the use of single-patient rooms—decreased the rate of hospital-acquired infections and colonization of bacteria in burn patients. The studies reviewed were lower quality before/after studies; however, due to the ethical nature of creating a randomized, placebo-controlled, double blind study for isolation practices in burn patients, higher level studies for review are not available. Consider implementation of protective isolation precautions in burn units.

Level of Evidence

A—Meta-analysis

Reference

Raes K, Blot K, Vogelaers D, et al. Protective isolation precautions for the prevention of nosocomial colonization and infection in burn patients: A systematic review and meta-analysis. *Intensive Crit Care Nurs.* 2017;42:22–29.

Burns of the Face

Suspect inhalation injury with any head or neck burns. Associated facial edema may lead to a compromised airway. Closely monitor the patient's respiratory status. Elevate the head of the bed to facilitate ventilation and edema reabsorption. Take special care during cleansing of facial burns to prevent excessive bleeding and damage to new tissue growth. Shave all hair (except for eyebrows) from the wound each day. Once the wound is cleaned and debrided, apply a topical antimicrobial agent according to unit protocol. Because of the rich blood supply in the face, partial-thickness burns usually heal quickly as long as infection is prevented. Perform regular oral hygiene.

Burns of the Ears

The ears are especially prone to inflammation and infection of the cartilage (chondritis), which leads to complete loss of ear cartilage. Ear burns are treated with a topical antimicrobial agent. Mafenide acetate (Sulfamylon) is the agent of choice because of its ability to penetrate the cartilage. Prevent mechanical pressure on the ears from dressings or other external sources (e.g., tube ties, pillows) because the pressure impairs blood flow and contributes to the development of chondritis. Use cloth ties to secure tubes to the face and frequently monitor them to ensure that pressure is not placed on top of the ears. Do not use pillows to support the head. Instead, use a foam donut with a hole for the ear to rest in while the patient is in a lateral position.

Burns of the Eyes

Immediate examination of the eyes is necessary on arrival to the hospital because eyelid edema forms rapidly. Eyelid edema can cause the cornea to become exposed as the eyelid retracts. Remove contact lenses if present. A thorough examination by an ophthalmologist is mandatory for serious injuries. The eyes are stained with fluorescein to rule out corneal injury and then irrigated with copious amounts of physiological saline if injury is confirmed. Frequently apply ophthalmic ointment or artificial tears to protect the cornea and conjunctiva from drying. Carefully observe eyelashes because they may invert and scratch the cornea.

Burns of the Hands, Feet, or Major Joints

Extensive burns of the hands and feet can cause permanent disability, necessitating a long convalescence. After prioritizing life-sustaining interventions, it is important to preserve limbs and function. Elevate burned hands above the level of the heart on slings or wedges to reduce edema formation. Individually wrap fingers and toes during dressing changes with gauze, bandages, or biological products to keep digits separated to prevent *webbing* (growing together of skin between burned body parts). Occupational and physical therapists are involved in the patient's plan of care from the day of admission to address and evaluate function and mobility parameters. Although ROM exercises can be painful or tiring, they should be initiated as soon as possible after injury and performed frequently throughout each day. Active ROM exercises prevent muscle atrophy, reduce the shortening of ligaments, prevent joint contracture formation, and decrease edema. If patients are unable to move their extremities actively, perform passive ROM exercises.

Burn wounds over joints are prone to scar tissue contractures that limit ROM. The position of comfort is the position of contracture and deformity development. Therefore splinting and antideformity positioning (e.g., extension of knees and elbows, extension and supination of wrists, abduction of hips and shoulders) are required to maintain function and prevent deformities of the affected part. When the patient is ambulating or sitting, apply a compression bandage over burn wounds of the feet and legs to prevent venous stasis and pooling of blood. Venous pooling delays wound healing, contributes to autograft loss, and increases the risk of VTE. Remove the elastic bandage when the feet are elevated. When establishing a plan of care, remember that patients with bilateral burned hands are dependent on others to assist in meeting their physical needs.

> ### ❓ CRITICAL REASONING ACTIVITY
>
> What interventions can be used in the critical care unit to promote early rehabilitation of a patient with a burn injury?

Burns of the Genitalia and Perineum

Patients with perineal burns often require hospitalization for monitoring of urinary tract obstruction. An indwelling urinary catheter is indicated until the surrounding wounds are healed or grafted. Meticulous wound care is essential because of the high risk of urine or fecal contamination and resulting risk of infection. Shave perineal hair over wound areas. Because scrotal edema is common, elevate the scrotum on towels or foam.

Electrical Injury

Cardiopulmonary arrest is a common complication of high-voltage electrical injury. Other severe complications related to electrical injury are summarized in Box 21.2. Hypoxemia may occur secondary to tetanic contractions and resulting paralysis of the respiratory muscles. Oxygen and endotracheal intubation with mechanical ventilation are implemented as indicated. Evaluate patients for spinal fractures from tetanic contractions or from falls during the injury event. Ensure spinal precautions until injury is ruled out. Closely monitor all patients with electrical injury for cardiac dysrhythmias. If present, provide continuous cardiac monitoring or serial electrocardiographic evaluations for at least 24 hours after injury. Tea-colored urine indicates the presence of hemochromogens (myoglobin) released as a result of severe deep tissue damage in a process called *rhabdomyolysis*. To prevent kidney injury, urinary output is maintained at greater

> ### BOX 21.2   Manifestations and Complications of Electrical Injury
>
> - Cardiac dysrhythmias or cardiopulmonary arrest
> - Hypoxia secondary to tetanic contractions and paralysis of the respiratory muscles
> - Deep tissue necrosis
> - Compartment syndrome of extremities
> - Long bone or vertebral fractures from tetanic muscle contractions
> - Rhabdomyolysis and acute kidney injury
> - Acute cataract formation
> - Neurological deficits such as spinal cord paralysis, traumatic brain injury, peripheral neuropathy, seizures, deafness, neuropathic pain, and motor and sensory deficits

than 1 mL/kg/h (75 to 100 mL/h) in adults until the urine becomes clear.[6] Resuscitation fluid volumes larger than predicted by the ABLS fluid resuscitation formula are often required to achieve this high urine output. Routine alkalization of the urine is not indicated. Closely monitor affected extremities for the development of compartment syndrome (see Clinical Alert: Clinical Indicators of Extremity Compartment Syndrome earlier in the chapter). Amputations can occur with the initial electrical contact or may be surgically required later in nonviable limbs.

Chemical Injury

Treatment of chemical injuries focuses on stopping the burning process while maintaining the safety of the burn team. The burn team must wear protective gear such as plastic gowns, gloves, masks, and goggles during decontamination. Decontamination is also required if burn injury is suspected to be from illegal drug manufacturing, such as methamphetamine. Illegal production often involves toxic and corrosive chemicals. During decontamination for all chemical exposures, immediately remove the patient's clothing. Brush off dry chemicals and continuously flush the area exposed to chemicals with water for at least 30 minutes. Question the patient and significant others to identify the specific chemical agent involved. Some chemicals such as alkalis require even longer lavage, which can be quite uncomfortable for the patient. Control pain and minimize heat loss caused by continual irrigation. Closely monitor the patient for signs of systemic chemical absorption.

Current Trends in Burn Injury Epidemiology

Injury resulting from illegal drug manufacturing is a challenging issue in burn care; examples include "cooking" methamphetamine (meth) in clandestine "laboratories" and extracting butane hash oil to make concentrated marijuana.[4] Despite legislative changes to restrict access to production components, use of in-vehicle mobile meth laboratories involving the manufacturing of smaller quantities has proliferated. When injury occurs, both thermal and chemical burns result. These cases are associated with more extensive %TBSA injury and inhalation injuries, requiring longer mechanical ventilation and longer length of stay.[4] Clinicians caring for these patients are at risk for chemical exposure if patients are not properly decontaminated. In most meth-related injuries, patients test positive for other illegal substances as well, making pain management challenging.[4] Suspect potential drug manufacturing–related injuries when observing burns to the face and hands, signs of agitation and substance withdrawal, lack of family visitors, presence of suspicious non-family visitors, or a vague or inconsistent injury history.

A rise in use of home medical oxygen therapy also poses unique challenges. Despite the high risk, many patients choose to continue smoking while using home oxygen, resulting in flash or flame burns and explosions. The incidence of burns involving home oxygen has quadrupled in the past decade.[8] These patients are three to five times more likely to have respiratory failure requiring mechanical ventilation, leading to increased mortality.[8] To address this challenging issue, multiprofessional team members must collaborate on patient and family home safety education and smoking cessation treatment for patients on home oxygen therapy.

Injuries from electronic cigarettes are also on the rise. Injuries occur from exploding batteries or contact from an overheating device.[21] The burn caused from an electronic cigarette can be particularly concerning, as it involves a flame or contact burn from the device exploding as well as a chemical burn from the lithium battery, which produces lithium hydroxide.[21] This is a growing problem, and it creates an opportunity for injury prevention experts.

Abuse and Neglect

Burns are a prevalent form of abuse and can result either from an active intent to injure or from neglect. Vulnerable populations such as children, the elderly, disabled persons, and mentally impaired persons are at increased risk of abuse and neglect. Critical care nurses play a key role in recognizing and identifying potential abuse or neglect cases because they spend the most time interfacing with the patient and significant others. Elicit the history of the story and circumstances surrounding the injury event, meticulously and accurately document the wound appearance and the pattern of injury (including use of photographs), and observe the interactions between the patient and caregivers or family. Question the injured individual privately and separately from the family caregiver. The reported injury history should correlate with physical findings. Discrepancies between reported accounts of the injury event and physical assessment findings indicate a potential abuse or neglect situation. The presence of other injuries (e.g., associated bruising, fractures, abrasions, other trauma) and the distribution and characteristics of the burn wound also provide key information on the true cause of the burn injury. For example, a scald burn with a clear demarcation or symmetrical wound pattern on the extremities without splash mark burns indicates an intentional immersion injury instead of an accidental scald (Fig. 21.10). Lack of witnesses to the injury event, blaming of others, and delay in seeking care are also indicators of potential abuse situations. It is mandatory to report all potential or suspected abuse cases to the appropriate authorities as governed by state laws. The patient is hospitalized until social workers and protective services have investigated the home environment to determine whether the patient will be safe upon discharge.

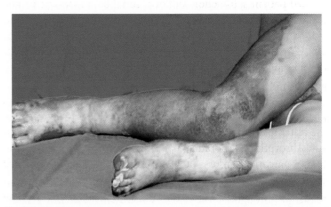

Fig. 21.10 Abuse by hot water immersion. The thigh burn wound edges have a clear demarcation line (are in a straight line), and there are no splash marks. The caregivers delayed seeking medical treatment for the patient's burns until 3 days after injury (notice the dry, crusty appearance of the wounds). The patient also had a forearm fracture and multiple bruises. (Courtesy University of Michigan Trauma Burn Center, Ann Arbor, MI.)

Describe an injury history and physical assessment findings that might lead you to suspect that a burn was caused by abuse.

PAIN CONTROL

Pain is a tormenting consequence of burn injury and is not limited to the period immediately after the injury; it is a major factor throughout the wound healing process. Pain experienced during the acute phase of recovery consists of a constant *background* or *resting pain* and shorter peaks of excruciating pain *(procedural* or *breakthrough pain)* often associated with activity and therapeutic procedures.[9,34,37] Many aspects of burn treatment produce pain, including dressing changes, debridement, surgical intervention, splints, application of topical antimicrobial agents, and physical and occupational therapy. Proactive pain management is thus important.

Adequately treating a burn patient's pain is a challenge. Altered pharmacokinetics secondary to changes in volume distribution and hypermetabolism is associated with burn injury. Bulky dressings, positioning, electrical injury, and neuropathies from direct thermal injury affect pain control.[37] Burn patients commonly have histories of mental illness, acute stress disorder, regular alcohol consumption, or polysubstance use that further compounds pain management and leads to opioid tolerance.[34,37] Because of the unexpected, sudden, traumatic nature of sustaining a burn injury and then enduring the ongoing trauma of necessary painful treatments, many patients experience acute stress disorder (ASD) or posttraumatic stress disorder (PTSD).[9]

Quantities of analgesics required by burn patients often exceed those of standard dosing guidelines.[9,37] Follow specific institutional policies regarding what constitutes pain management (versus conscious sedation) and appropriate patient monitoring. Inaccurate assessment of a patient's pain or fear of addiction can lead to undermedicating the patient. Inadequate pain control is associated with long-term negative patient outcomes such as development of mental health disorders, decreased compliance with care plans and ROM therapies, and increased incidence of chronic pain.[9,34] To successfully control a patient's pain and to achieve increased patient satisfaction, perform serial pain assessments and involve the patient in creating an individualized analgesic treatment plan.[34] Frequently reassess pain levels before, during, and after all procedures and treatments. Serve as the patient's advocate by ensuring that pain medications are administered by appropriate delivery methods and in adequate dosages.

Opioids are the analgesics most commonly used to treat burn pain. Subcutaneous or intramuscular injections are ineffective in the resuscitative phase because of impaired circulation in soft tissue. Absorption is sporadic, increasing the risk of undermedication or narcotic overdose. IV opioid administration is the route of choice. For patients requiring mechanical ventilation, consider using a continuous IV infusion of opioids to maintain a consistent level of analgesia. Involve patients in pain management and explore the use of patient-controlled analgesia (PCA), which facilitates pain relief and reduces feelings of helplessness. Administer analgesic medications by the oral or enteral tube route once the patient is hemodynamically stable. Although pain is reduced when wounds are covered with temporary dressings or skin grafts, frequent surgical and wound care procedures produce episodes of pain until permanent wound closure or healing is completed. Itching that occurs during the healing process also contributes to the patient's overall discomfort.

Burn care and treatment experiences produce anxiety, which further exacerbates pain.[9,34,37] The ideal pain management regimen incorporates treatment of both pain and anxiety. Fear and a loss of control over their lives and schedules increase patients' anxiety. Provide frequent and repeated explanations of care plans, interventions, and procedures at a level appropriate for the patient's age and development. Encourage patients to participate as much as possible in their wound care, medication administration, feeding, and exercise therapy. Anxiolytics are commonly administered in the acute care phase as an essential element of pain management interventions. Virtual reality technology and techniques such as relaxation, massage, hypnosis, distraction, and guided imagery also serve as useful adjuncts for reducing anxiety and enhancing pain relief.

INFECTION PREVENTION

Prevention of infection is an important nursing intervention in burn patient care. Burn patients have a high risk of infection related to disruption of normal skin integrity and altered immune response. When the skin's natural mechanical barrier protection is lost, susceptibility to infection increases. In addition, other host defense mechanisms are impaired, and immunosuppression develops. Although great strides in management have been made, the incidence of infection is higher in burn patients than in other patient groups and remains a predominant determinant of outcome.[6,18,31] The outbreak of infection with multidrug-resistant organisms is an ongoing issue in burn centers worldwide and contributes to an increased risk of sepsis.[36] Concomitant inhalation injury places the burn patient at particularly high risk of developing pneumonia, which further increases the mortality rate.[6] Invasive monitoring and the presence of indwelling urinary catheters, IV catheters, and endotracheal tubes also are potential sources of infection.

Since the inflammatory response is a common mechanism in burns, the American Burn Association consensus panel adapted sepsis definitions that are more applicable to the unique pathophysiological state of patients with burn injury.[18] The hypermetabolic state unique to burn patients can increase baseline temperatures to about 38.5°C (101.3°F), thus making presence of a low-grade fever (without other symptoms) an inaccurate indication of infection.[18,36]

The goals of infection prevention in burn care include preserving existing immune defenses, preventing transmission of exogenous organisms, and controlling the transfer of endogenous organisms (normal flora) to sites at increased risk for infection. In addition to Standard Precautions, specific interventions for infection prevention are listed in Box 21.3.

What specific strategies and interventions can the critical care nurse use to reduce the incidence of infection in burn patients?

BOX 21.3 Strategies for Infection Prevention for Burn Injuries

- Provide aseptic management of the wound and the environment, including effective decontamination of equipment and hydrotherapy rooms
- Use topical antibacterial agents
- Properly care for invasive catheters with special consideration to IV catheters placed through or near burn wounds where occlusive dressings will not adhere
- Provide aggressive wound management with close monitoring for changes in wound appearance
- Prevent infection from multidrug-resistant organisms through prudent and microbial-guided use of systemic antibiotics
- Provide adequate nutrition
- Closely monitor laboratory values and clinical signs of infection
- Facilitate early wound closure to restore the protective barrier of skin
- Prohibit live plants and flowers

WOUND MANAGEMENT

Although burn wound care protocols and procedures vary among burn centers, the underlying goals of wound care are the same: removal of nonviable tissue to promote epithelialization and prompt coverage via skin grafts when necessary. Perform interventions to attain these goals such as wound cleansing, debridement, topical antimicrobial and/or biological/biosynthetic dressing therapy, and definitive surgical wound closure.

Wound Care

Meticulous wound care is essential to prevent infection and promote healing of the burn wound. Wound care is typically completed once or twice a day, depending on the healing status of the wound, the dressing or topical agents used, and the number of postoperative days since grafting. Before initiating wound care, explain the procedure and encourage patient participation as appropriate. Administer analgesics (and sedatives or anxiolytic agents if indicated) before starting the procedure. Cleanse all wounds with a mild soap or surgical disinfectant, then rinse with warm tap water. Do not "soak" or tub-bathe the patient in water because immersion creates a significant potential for cross-contamination of wounds. Instead, allow water to flow over the wounds and immediately drain away. This regimen is best accomplished in a shower or hydrotherapy stretcher, but bed baths may be used for hemodynamically unstable patients. Remove all previously applied topical agents, necrotic tissue, exudate, and fibrous debris from the wound to expose healthy tissue, control bacterial proliferation, and promote healing. Debride loose eschar and wound debris with washcloths or gauze sponges, scissors, and forceps. Avoid mechanical trauma and damage from aggressive cleansing of newly formed epithelial skin buds or healing granulation tissue. Clip or shave hair in and immediately surrounding the wound bed (except eyebrows) to eliminate a medium for bacterial growth and to facilitate wound assessment. Closely inspect all wounds and carefully document wound location, size, color, texture, and drainage. Note any changes in appearance or developing signs of infection. Closely monitor the patient's core body temperature. During wound care, maintain the room temperature at a minimum of 85° to 90°F to prevent chilling and excessive body heat loss.

Topical Agents and Dressings

One of the most rapidly changing aspects of burn care is the development of novel tissue engineering techniques for wound treatment. Numerous new topical agents and biosynthetic dressings are available, with many others in development. These new products have broader, longer-lasting antimicrobial actions; interact with wound growth factors and collagen fibers to accelerate healing and to stop the zone of stasis from expanding; help fill in defects; and may reduce scarring. All of these actions positively affect outcomes by reducing infection, shortening healing time, preventing wound conversion to full-thickness depth, decreasing pain (due to less frequent dressing changes), and improving long-term cosmetic appearance and scarring. After each hydrotherapy session, cover the unhealed or unexcised burn wound with an antimicrobial topical agent, a dressing, or both. Table 21.5 describes various agents that are commonly used in the United States and their related nursing considerations. The multitude of ever-evolving available agents and dressings precludes a complete listing. Many agents are also used in nonburn, chronic, or surgical wounds. The selection of an agent and dressing is determined by wound depth, anatomical location, frequency of wound visualization desired, and presence and type of microorganisms identified. The ideal antimicrobial agent demonstrates long-lasting, broad-spectrum activity against microorganisms with a low risk of developing resistance; penetrates eschar; and has limited adverse effects. The burn center physician orders the antimicrobial agent, as well as the frequency and method of application.

Advances in wound dressing development and skin substitutes provide many new options in coverage for major burns. Temporary wound coverings or dressings are classified as either *biological* or *biosynthetic* (a combination of biological and synthetic properties). Table 21.6 describes common types and uses for biological and biosynthetic coverings. Biological or biosynthetic dressings are used as temporary wound coverings for freshly excised (surgically debrided) burn wounds until autograft skin is available; examples include allograft, xenograft, Integra, and AlloDerm. Biological or biosynthetic wound coverings are used as dressings for partial-thickness burns, meshed autograft skin, or donor sites to promote healing; examples include allograft, xenograft TransCyte, BioBrane, and OrCel. Temporary wound coverings have the added benefits of controlling heat and fluid loss, decreasing infection risk, stimulating the healing process, and increasing patient comfort.

Enzymatic agents such as collagenase, papain/urea, or sutilains are sometimes used for debridement of smaller necrotic tissue areas on deep partial- and full-thickness burns. Topical enzymatic agents are proteolytic enzyme ointments that act as potent digestants of nonviable protein matter or necrotic tissue but are harmless to viable tissue. Enzymatic agents do not have antimicrobial properties; therefore closely monitor wounds for infection.

Burn wounds are treated by either an open or a closed method. The decision of which method to use depends on the location, size, and depth of the burn and on specific burn center protocols. Each method has advantages and disadvantages.

TABLE 21.5 Topical Antimicrobial Agents for Burn Wound Management

Agent	Indications	Nursing Considerations
Clotrimazole cream or nystatin (Mycostatin)	Fungal colonization of wounds	Apply 1-2 times daily. Use with an antibacterial topical agent. May cause skin irritation.
Mafenide acetate (Sulfamylon)	Active against most gram-positive, gram-negative, and *Pseudomonas* pathogens; agent of choice for ear burns; penetrates thick eschar and ear cartilage	Apply 1-2 times daily. Strong carbonic anhydrase inhibitor, can cause metabolic acidosis; monitor respiratory rate, electrolyte values, and ABGs. Hydroscopic (draws water out of tissue) and can be painful for 15-60 min after application. Slows eschar separation. Assess for sulfa allergy before use.
Silver-coated dressings (Acticoat, Aquacel Ag, Mepilex Ag, Silverlon, Tegaderm Ag)	Silver-coated, flexible, nonadhesive wound dressings with or without absorptive layer; as long as dressing is moist, provides continuous release of silver ions for 3-14 days (depending on product); effective broad-spectrum coverage for numerous pathogens (gram-negative/gram-positive bacteria, antibiotic-resistant bacteria, yeast, mold); alternative for patients allergic to sulfa medications	Apply new dressing every 1-7 days to moist open wound with (1) wound exudate maintaining silver activation until drainage stops or wound heals or (2) rewetting with sterile water every 4-6 h to keep dressing moist (not wet). Use sterile water to moisten dressings; saline renders silver ions ineffective. A decrease in number of required dressing changes increases patient comfort and cost-effectiveness. Aquacel Ag and Mepilex Ag do not require wetting.
Silver nitrate	Effective against wide spectrum of common wound pathogens; acts on surface microorganisms only; poor eschar penetration; alternative for patients allergic to sulfa medications	Apply 0.5% solution to wet dressing 2-3 times daily; rewet every 2 h to keep moist. Hypotonic solution causes electrolyte leaching; monitor serum electrolyte levels and replace according to protocol. Must be kept in light-resistant container. Causes staining; protect equipment and floors with plastic.
Silver sulfadiazine (SSD, Silvadene)	Active against wide spectrum of gram-negative, gram-positive, and *Candida albicans* pathogens; acts only on cell wall and membrane; does not penetrate thick eschar	Apply 1-2 times daily. Wrap wounds or leave as open dressing. Can cause leukopenia; monitor white blood cell count. Assess for sulfa allergy before use.

ABGs, Arterial blood gases.

TABLE 21.6 Biological and Biosynthetic Dressings

Type of Dressing	Definition
Biological Dressings	**Temporary Wound Cover From Human or Animal Tissue**
Allograft (homograft)	Graft of skin transplanted from another human, living or cadaver
Xenograft (heterograft)	Graft of skin (usually pigskin) transplanted between different species
Biosynthetic Dressings	**Wound Cover From Biological and Synthetic Materials**
Epidermal Replacements (Epicel, Epidex, MySkin)	Commercially manufactured cultured epidermal autografts (CEAs) from autologous keratinocytes (via skin biopsy) and murine fibroblasts delivered on a silicone or gauze layer
Dermal Substitutes	
AlloDerm	Transplantable tissue consisting of human cryopreserved allogeneic dermis from which the epidermal cells, fibroblasts, and endothelial cells targeted for immune response have been removed
Integra	Dressing system composed of two layers: (1) dermal layer of animal collagen and glycosaminoglycan that interfaces with wound and functions as dermal matrix for cellular growth and collagen synthesis; (2) temporary outer synthetic epidermal layer of Silastic that acts as a barrier to water loss and bacteria. Dermal layer biodegrades within months as new wound collagen matrix is synthesized. Silastic layer is removed in 14-21 days and replaced with thin autograft
TransCyte	Temporary dressing composed of outer polymer membrane and nylon mesh seeded with human neonatal fibroblasts and porcine collagen; matrix contains proteins and growth factors but no viable cells because of cryopreservation
Bilayer Dermo-Epidermal Substitutes (Apligraf, OrCel)	Consist of an outer epidermal layer of cultured allogeneic (from another human) neonatal keratinocytes and a bottom dermal layer matrix embedded with neonatal fibroblasts and bovine collagen; the matrix's viable or living cells secrete growth factors and cytokines to promote healing

With the *open method,* the burn wounds are left open to air after application of the antimicrobial agent. Superficial burns of the face or perineum are commonly treated with the open method by applying a topical antimicrobial agent such as bacitracin. The open method provides increased wound visualization and more opportunities for observation, eliminates dressing supplies, and improves joint mobility that is otherwise limited by the presence of restrictive dressings. The open method has some disadvantages. It allows direct contact between the wound and the environment. The topical antimicrobial agent may rub off on clothing, bedding, or equipment. The open method increases wound exposure time and the risk of hypothermia.

With the *closed method,* a gauze dressing is placed over the agent that was applied directly to the wound, or the wound is covered with gauze dressings saturated with a topical antimicrobial agent. The closed method is commonly used on full-thickness burns treated with silver sulfadiazine and new grafts. The closed method reduces heat loss and pain or sensitivity from wound exposure, and it assists in protecting wounds from external mechanical trauma. The dressings applied may also assist with debridement. However, the closed method requires a dressing change to assess the wound, and the presence of dressings may impair ROM.

Negative pressure wound therapy (NPWT) or vacuum-assisted closure (VAC) devices can be used for grafts, partial-thickness burns, and deep surgical wounds (as seen in nonburn necrotizing soft tissue infections or post-ACS decompression). NPWT consists of a sponge and suction tubing placed on the wound bed and covered with an occlusive dressing (Fig. 21.11). The device creates a negative-pressure dressing to decompress edematous interstitial spaces and increase local perfusion; help draw wound edges closed uniformly; remove wound fluid; and provide a closed, moist wound healing environment. NPWT also allows the collection and quantification of wound drainage. NPWT has been associated with increased granulation tissue formation and earlier epithelialization, removal of wound exudate, lower wound bacterial counts, reduction in large wound defects, and a reduction in graft loss due to reduced edema and preservation of blood flow.[10,22]

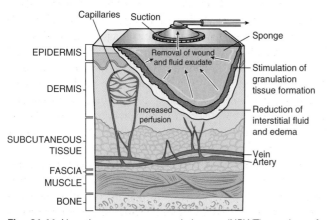

Fig. 21.11 Negative pressure wound therapy (NPWT) consists of a negative-pressure dressing to decompress edematous interstitial spaces; increase wound perfusion; remove wound exudate fluid; stimulate granulation tissue growth; and provide a closed, moist wound healing environment.

Surgical Excision and Grafting

The depth of the injury determines whether a burn will heal or require skin grafting. Superficial (first-degree) and partial-thickness (second-degree) burns heal because the necessary elements to generate new skin remain. Full-thickness burns are nonvascular, and all dermal appendages have been destroyed. Full-thickness burns require skin grafting to achieve wound closure. Deep partial-thickness burns are also commonly grafted to decrease the risk of infection by achieving earlier wound closure and to minimize scarring and improve cosmetic appearance. *Excision* is surgical debridement by scalpel or electrocautery to remove *necrotic* (dead) tissue until a layer of healthy, well-vascularized tissue is exposed. *Skin grafting* is placing skin on the excised burn wound (Fig. 21.12A). Several types of skin can be used for skin grafting, including *autograft* (the patient's own skin, which is transferred to a new location on the body), *allograft* (skin from another human, such as cadaver skin; also called homograft), and *xenograft* (skin from another animal, such as pigskin). Autografts are the only permanent type of skin grafting (Table 21.7). Allografts and xenografts are temporary biological dressings (see Table 21.6). With autografts, a partial-thickness wound called a *donor site* is created, where skin is excised (harvested) or removed from the patient with a tool called a *dermatome.*

Excision and grafting are performed in the operating room and are typically initiated within the first week after burn injury. Early excision within the first 1 to 3 days has been associated with decreased mortality and morbidity.[20,36] Advantages reported include modulation of the hypermetabolic response, reduced infection and wound colonization rates, increased graft take, and decreased length of hospitalization.[20,36]

Depending on the size of the burn and the presence of infection, sequential or repeated surgical debridement and grafting may be required. In major burns it is often not possible to graft all full-thickness wound areas initially, either because of the patient's hemodynamic instability from the size and severity of burned areas or because of a lack of donor sites to provide adequate coverage. Priority areas for autograft skin application include the face, the hands, the feet, and over joints. In addition, other temporary and permanent synthetic products have been developed to substitute for a person's own skin (see Table 21.6). These products allow early burn wound coverage while delaying autografting until previously used donor sites have healed and can be excised (harvested) again.

Autograft skin is applied as meshed grafts or as sheet grafts. *Sheet* (nonmeshed) grafts are often used on the face and hands for better cosmetic results. Meshed grafts are commonly used elsewhere on the body (see Fig. 21.12B). A meshed graft is created by using a device, called a skin graft mesher, which places multiple tiny slits or holes in the piece of skin that was harvested from the donor site. The wider the graft's mesh, the larger the area that can be covered with the autograft skin. However, wider-mesh grafts also contribute to more scarring and a less cosmetically pleasing appearance (see Fig. 21.12C). Table 21.7 summarizes the types of skin autografts used, along with nursing care requirements. Graft sites are splinted as indicated to prevent movement and shearing of the grafts until adherence

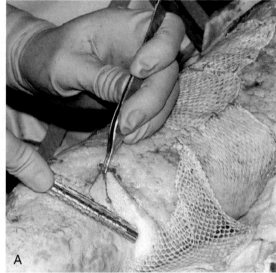

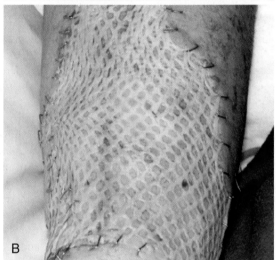

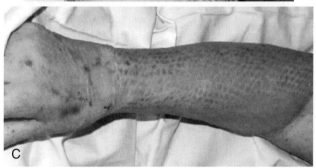

Fig. 21.12 Excision and autografting. **A,** Surgical debridement (excision) with meshed autograft placement in the operating room. **B,** Meshed autograft on postoperative day 2. **C,** Comparison of sheet autograft (on hand) and meshed autograft (on forearm) 3 weeks postoperatively. Use of meshed autograft allows larger body surface area coverage but also typically leads to more scarring and a less cosmetically pleasing appearance. (Courtesy University of Michigan Trauma Burn Center, Ann Arbor, MI.)

occurs. Elevate extremities to prevent pooling of blood and edema, which can lead to increased pressure and graft loss.

Many types of dressings can be used on donor sites (Table 21.8), but the product chosen must promote healing of the donor site within 7 to 10 days. Donor sites can be reused or harvested again

once healed. When patient donor sites are limited because of the severity of the burn injury, cultured epidermal autograft (CEA) can be used to provide coverage for a major burn injury. With CEA, a skin biopsy is obtained from the patient and is sent to a laboratory where keratinocytes are cultured and grown. The process takes about 3 weeks and results in small pieces of skin. These fragile pieces of skin are surgically applied to a clean, excised burn wound. The disadvantage of CEA is its extreme fragility, which is partly the result of the lack of a durable dermis. To overcome these shortcomings, researchers are actively investigating novel approaches in tissue engineering, such as developing different types of epidermal substitutes, incorporating CEA with a dermal layer to increase durability, constructing biologically active dermo-epidermal replacements, integrating stem cells, and using topical nanoemulsion technology.[16,20,30] Burn centers vary in their protocols for treating grafted areas and donor sites. Apply basic wound care principles, with infection prevention always being the primary goal. Although the critical care nurse may not actually develop the wound treatment plan, input and involvement by all burn team experts is essential for positive patient outcomes. Use of a standard wound treatment documentation method facilitates day-to-day team communication of care requirements.

Inherent in all wound care management is the necessity to improve and maintain function. Consult occupational and physical therapists on the day of admission to develop a treatment plan. Often the position of comfort for the patient is one that leads to dysfunction or deformity. Prevent future complications by using specialized splints, antideformity positioning, and exercises throughout the acute burn care phase. Continually reinforce the need for splinting or positioning and monitor for compliance.

NUTRITIONAL CONSIDERATIONS

Adequate nutrition plays an important role in the survival of extensively burned patients. A major burn injury produces a stress-induced hypermetabolic-catabolic response greater than any other disease process or injury. Skeletal muscle is the major protein store in the body. Postburn hypermetabolism leads to deleterious consequences, including significant skeletal muscle breakdown with protein degradation, weight loss, marked delays in wound healing, skin graft loss, impaired immunological responsiveness, sepsis, physiological exhaustion, or even death if adequate nutrition is not provided and an anabolic or positive nitrogen balance is not achieved.[1,18,20] Muscle weakness and atrophy also contribute to prolonged mechanical ventilation, delayed ambulation, impaired activities of daily living, and extended acute rehabilitation.

Institute nutritional therapy immediately after the burn injury to meet energy demands, maintain host defense mechanisms, replenish body protein stores, and curtail progressive loss of lean body mass. Collaborate with the patient, the registered dietitian, and the physician to coordinate a nutritional plan. If the patient is able to tolerate an oral diet, institute a high-calorie, high-protein diet with supplements and perform daily calorie counts to monitor dietary intake. If oral intake is

TABLE 21.7 **Autograft Skin: Nursing Implications**

Type of Autograft	Definition	Nursing Implications
Split-thickness *sheet* graft	Sheet of skin composed of epidermis and a variable portion of dermis harvested at a predetermined thickness. Sheet is kept intact (not meshed) to improve cosmetic appearance; often used on face and hands.	Immobilize grafted area. Evacuate pockets of serous or serosanguineous fluid by needle aspiration or rolling of the fluid with cotton tip applicator toward the skin edges; if fluid is not evacuated, graft adherence is compromised.
Split-thickness *meshed* graft	Split-thickness sheet graft that is mesh-cut to expand the graft 1.5 to 9 times its original size before being placed on a recipient bed of granulation tissue; used to cover large surface areas.	Cover graft with layers of fine and coarse mesh gauze to prevent shearing, wrap with absorbent gauze, and splint for immobilization. Keep dressings moist (not saturated) to promote epithelialization of meshed skin interstices. Perform first dressing change within 3-5 days.
Full-thickness graft	Sheet of skin is harvested down to subcutaneous tissue (all layers of skin); typically used for eyelids or later reconstructive procedures.	Requires same care as a sheet skin graft.
Cultured epidermal autograft (CEA)	Autologous epidermal keratinocytes derived from skin biopsy of patient are grown in a laboratory using tissue culture techniques (takes ~3 wk). Epidermal layer replacement only. Typically used with extensive percent total body surface area burns when limited donor sites are available.	Perform daily dressing changes of outer gauze for 7-10 days (underlying coarse mesh and petroleum jelly gauze layers are not disturbed); outer dressing must remain dry. Many topical antimicrobial agents are toxic to CEA skin and should not come into contact with graft dressings. Remove petroleum jelly gauze when it becomes loose (7-10 days), and begin gentle range-of-motion exercises. Use moist saline dressings until graft is well adherent (typically 21 days).

TABLE 21.8 **Donor Site Dressings**

Dressing	Description
BioBrane	Bilaminate dressing composed of nylon mesh embedded with a collagen derivative and an outer silicone membrane; permeable to wound drainage and topical antimicrobial agents; peels away as wound heals
Calcium alginate dressings	Hydrophilic, flexible dressings in which alginate fibers convert to a gel when activated by wound exudates (Algicell, Algisite M, Kaltostat, Sorbsan, Tegaderm HG, and others); change dressing within 7 days or more frequently if there is a large amount of drainage
DuoDerm	Hydrocolloid dressing that adheres by interacting and bonding with skin moisture
Fine mesh gauze	Cotton gauze placed directly on wound; a crust or "scab" is formed as gauze dries and wound epithelialization occurs under the dressing; gauze peels away as wound heals
N-Terface	Translucent, nonabsorbent, and nonreactive surface material used between the burn wound and outer dressing
Op-Site	Thin, elastic film that is occlusive, waterproof, and permeable to air and moisture vapor; fluid under dressing may need to be evacuated
Vigilon	Colloidal suspension on a polyethylene mesh that provides a moist environment; permeable to air and water vapor
Silver-coated dressings	Silver-coated, flexible dressings (with or without absorptive layer) that provide continuous release of silver ions for 3-14 days while dressing is moist (Acticoat, Aquacel AG, Mepilex AG, Silverlon, Tegaderm AG, and others)
Xeroform	Fine mesh gauze containing 3% bismuth tribromophenate in a petrolatum blend; promotes healing as with other mesh gauze dressings

not tolerated or caloric intake is insufficient, begin enteral tube feeding. Early enteral feeding, within the first 24 hours after burn injury, decreases the production of catabolic hormones, improves nitrogen balance, reduces the wound infection rate, maintains gut integrity, lowers the incidence of diarrhea, and decreases hospital stay.[1,20,39] The small bowel (rather than the stomach) is the preferred location for tube placement so that enteral feedings can be continued during wound care requiring conscious sedation and/or surgical operative procedures.

Ongoing research efforts target the use of beta-blockade, anabolic hormones, and other medications to ameliorate the hypermetabolic-catabolic response to burn injury.[1,20,39] Although studies have focused more on pediatric burn patients, the administration of beta-blockers has been found to reduce fatal outcome, catabolism, and wound healing time.[1,36]

A landmark prospective, randomized, blinded, multicenter trial demonstrated that treatment of burn patients with oxandrolone, an anabolic hormone, significantly decreased hospital length of stay.[39] Additional research is required to determine the exact cause of this reduction, but the currently proposed contributing factors are normalization of metabolism, decreased inflammation, improved organ function, increased strength, and/or improved wound healing.[1,20,39] It is advocated to treat all patients with greater than 20% TBSA burns with oxandrolone while monitoring levels of hepatic transaminases.[33,39] Refer to Chapter 7 for additional nutrition information.

CRITICAL REASONING ACTIVITY

What strategies might the critical care nurse use to meet the high caloric needs of burn patients who can take foods by mouth?

PSYCHOSOCIAL CONSIDERATIONS

As improvements in critical care protocols and technologies have increased survival from burn injury, quality of life and psychosocial considerations become priorities in treatment plans. Burns are one of the most complex and psychologically devastating injuries to patients and their families. Not only is there a very real threat to survival, but also psychological and physical pain, fear of disfigurement, and uncertainty of long-term effects of the injury on the future can precipitate a crisis for the patient and family. During the acute and rehabilitative phases, the patient may exhibit stages of psychological adaptation (Box 21.4). A patient may not manifest every stage, but support and therapy must be provided for any patient and family experiencing major burn injury.

To facilitate a person's emotional adjustment to burn injury, consider the complex interaction of preinjury personality, extent of injury, social support systems, cultural factors, and home environment.[3] For example, many burn injuries are the

---

BOX 21.4   Stages of Postburn Psychological Adaptation

Survival Anxiety
Often manifested by anxiety, shock, fear, grieving, anger, mood swings, feelings of helplessness, lack of concentration, easy startle response, tearfulness, social withdrawal, and inappropriate behavior or outbursts. Repeat instructions and give the patient time to verbalize concerns and fears. Increased reports of pain are frequently associated with high levels of anxiety.

Search for Meaning
Patient repeatedly recounts events leading to the injury and tries to determine a logical explanation that is emotionally acceptable. Listen actively, participate in the discussions, provide support, and avoid judging the patient's reasoning.

Investment in Recuperation and Treatment Plan
Patient is cooperative with the treatment plan, motivated to be independent, and takes pride in small accomplishments. Educate the patient on discharge goals and involve both patient and family in planning an increased self-care program. Provide the patient with much praise and verbal encouragement.

Investment in Rehabilitation
As self-confidence increases, patient is focused on achieving as much preburn function as possible. Depression may occur as new losses in function are realized. This phase usually occurs after hospital discharge, when the patient is undergoing outpatient rehabilitation. Although staff support is typically limited in this phase, provide praise, support, and continued information as possible.

Reintegration of Identity
Patient accepts losses and recognizes that changes have occurred. Adaptation is completed, and staff involvement is terminated.

Modified from Blakeney PE, Rosenburg L, Rosenburn M, Fauerbach JA. Psychosocial recovery and reintegration of patients with burn injuries. In: Herndon DN, ed. *Total Burn Care*. 3rd ed. Philadelphia, PA: Saunders Elsevier; 2007.

BOX 21.5   Support Programs for Patients With Burn Injuries and Their Families

- The Phoenix Society for Burn Survivors, a national organization that provides tools and support networks to assist survivors and families in their journey of healing: http://www.phoenix-society.org
- Peer support, such as Survivors Offering Assistance in Recovery (SOAR): http://www.phoenix-society.org/phoenix-soar
- The Model Systems Knowledge Translation Center, which provides evidence-based resources for those living with burn injuries: http://www.msktc.org/burn
- Burn units at local hospitals
- Burn survivor retreats and camps
- School reintegration programs, such as "The Journey Back" and R.E.A.C.H. (Return to Education and Continued Healing)

---

result of poor supervision, abuse, suicide attempts, assaults, illegal activities, safety code violations, arson, or military involvement. The patient may be dealing with loss of loved ones in the fire, injury event flashbacks, loss of home and belongings, job or financial concerns, societal repercussions, or fear of assailants. The patient may also be facing legal consequences. Preinjury psychiatric disorders and alcohol and substance abuse frequently exist in the burn patient population.[3,34,37] Closely assess the patient's and family's support systems, coping mechanisms, and potential for developing ASD and PTSD. Inadequate coping is demonstrated by changes in behavior, anxiety, agitation, manipulation, regression, acting out, psychosis or hallucinations, apathy, sleep disturbances, or depression. The most beneficial interventions are based on individual assessments and incorporate cultural traditions. Assistance will likely be required from hospital support personnel such as chaplains, clinical nurse specialists, child life specialists, psychiatrists, psychologists, and social workers. As the patient is transferred from the critical care unit, maintain support mechanisms and continuity of care; psychosocial recovery can take months, years, or a lifetime. Several integrative support programs are available to positively facilitate a burn survivor's return to society, family, work, and school (Box 21.5). Help promote hope and alleviate anxiety by informing patients and families of these support resources in the immediate acute postinjury phase.

If a burn injury is not survivable, support the patient and family members, participate in withdrawal-of-treatment discussions, and provide palliative and end-of-life care until death.

❓ CRITICAL REASONING ACTIVITY

Many patients with burn injuries must be treated at institutions far from home. What approaches can be used to meet the psychosocial needs of these patients and their families?

LIFESPAN CONSIDERATIONS

Many unique pathophysiological, physical, and cognitive changes occur across the lifespan, and their impact affects burn injury, treatment, and outcomes (see Lifespan Considerations box). Regardless of age, a patient's physical and mental health greatly affect critical care management and outcome.[4,6]

Despite improved survival rates, advanced age, especially in combination with deeper burns or inhalation injury, is a major determinant of mortality after thermal injury.[6,20,31] Carefully consider the decision to proceed with resuscitation in elderly patients with large burns and concomitant inhalation injury. Guidance from advance directives, next of kin, and/or the designated healthcare surrogate is also vital to this decision-making process. Preexisting dementia exacerbated by injury and medications has major implications for an elderly patient's ability to participate in rehabilitation to regain function and independence. Aggressive burn treatment that promotes extension of life must be balanced with quality of life, including comfort, dignity, and patient wishes if known. Poor outcomes after burn injury highlight the importance of prevention of these injuries in the elderly.

NONBURN INJURIES

The expertise of the burn team in providing excellent wound and critical care has led to burn center admissions of patients with various other severe exfoliative and necrotizing skin disorders, such as toxic epidermal necrolysis (TEN), staphylococcal scalded skin syndrome (SSSS), and necrotizing fasciitis. These conditions create a clinical wound picture similar to that of a burn wound and require similar patient management and wound care. Management of these conditions in a burn center is associated with a marked increase in survival.[31,40]

Severe Exfoliative Disorders

TEN, Stevens-Johnson syndrome (SJS), and erythema multiforme (EM) are conditions in which the body sloughs its epidermal layer. The exact pathophysiological mechanism remains unclear, but the sloughing is thought to result from a direct toxic effect, a genetic susceptibility, and/or an immune-mediated response to a causative agent.[40] The primary clinical

---

LIFESPAN CONSIDERATIONS

Older Adults

- Older adults have thinner dermal layers, resulting in deeper burn injuries at lower temperatures or with shorter exposure times.[4]
- Older adults have reduced physiological reserves and capacity to respond to the significant metabolic stressors, hemodynamic demands, and inflammatory challenges after a burn injury. Preexisting cardiovascular, renal, and pulmonary diseases lead to challenges in fluid resuscitation, repeat hospitalizations, and increased morbidity and mortality.[4,12]
- Diminished manual dexterity, reaction time, senses, vision, hearing, balance, mobility, and judgment render the older adults more vulnerable to burn injuries. Many older adults live alone, and they are often physically or mentally incapable of responding appropriately to an emergency.
- Advanced hemodynamic monitoring may help guide fluid administration.
- Age-related decline in immune system functioning contributes to increased susceptibility to infection.
- Frail older adults are at higher risk for hypothermia. Small muscle mass decreases the ability to generate heat by shivering.
- Factors contributing to the burn injury (e.g., dangers in the home environment, abuse, supervision or caregiving assistance, syncope, medication side effects) must be addressed before elderly patients are discharged.

---

finding is a positive *Nikolsky sign,* elucidated by applying lateral pressure to the skin surface with resultant sloughing of the epidermis. Diagnosis of this related continuum of disorders is based on the skin biopsy histopathology (separation at the epidermal-dermal junction) and the extent of involvement of dermal detachment. EM is characterized by less than 10% TBSA affected, with peripheral distribution of lesions. Patients with SJS also have less than 10% TBSA affected, but lesions are widespread. If SJS occurs with TEN, lesions appear on 10% to 30% of TBSA. TEN is characterized by involvement of more than 30% TBSA, and lesions are extensive and widespread.[40]

Toxic Epidermal Necrolysis

TEN is the most extensive form of severe exfoliative disorder. It is associated with a mortality rate of 25% to 50%, compared with only 1% to 5% for SJS.[40] The most common cause of TEN is a drug reaction, particularly from antibiotics, especially sulfa drugs, phenobarbital, allopurinol, phenytoin, and nonsteroidal antiinflammatory drugs. In some cases, a definitive etiology is never identified.[40] Patients initially have fever and flu-like symptoms, with erythema and blisters developing within 24 to 96 hours. As large bullae develop, the skin and mucous membranes slough, resulting in a significant and painful partial-thickness injury. TEN is also associated with mucosal wound involvement of conjunctival, oral, GI tract, and/or urogenital areas.[40] Immune suppression occurs and contributes to life-threatening infection-related complications such as sepsis and pneumonia. Primary treatment includes immediate discontinuation of the potential offending drug. Although anticonvulsants and antibiotics are the most common causes, suspect any medication initiated in the past 3 to 4 weeks.[40] Optimal wound treatment consists of early coverage of cutaneous wounds with silver-based or biological dressings. Severe exfoliative disorders typically require intensive critical care management to provide fluid resuscitation and nutritional support. Corticosteroids should not be given.[40] Low-sucrose IV immune globulin administration may be beneficial in modulating the causative inflammatory response.[40] Provide supportive care and prevent infection; otherwise, wounds can easily progress to full-thickness depth. Long-term follow-up with the burn team is important to monitor for the development of commonly reported ophthalmic, skin, nail, and vulvovaginal complications and to address continued issues in health-related quality of life.[40]

Staphylococcal Scalded Skin Syndrome

SSSS occurs primarily in young children and often manifests with a clinical picture similar to that of TEN. SSSS is caused by a reaction to a staphylococcal toxin, with intraepidermal splitting (unlike the epidermal-dermal separation seen in TEN) resulting in skin sloughing. Differential diagnosis is critical because the treatment for SSSS involves antibiotics, which can exacerbate TEN. Diagnosis is made by microscopic examination of the denuded skin to determine the level of skin separation. SSSS is limited to superficial epidermal involvement and does not affect the mucous membranes. SSSS is best treated with antibiotic therapy and wound care management.

Necrotizing Soft Tissue Infections

Necrotizing soft tissue infections (NSTIs) are a group of rapidly invasive infections that include diagnoses such as necrotizing fasciitis, gas gangrene, hemolytic streptococcal gangrene, Fournier gangrene (NSTI specifically involving the perineum and scrotum), and necrotizing cellulitis. NSTIs occur more frequently in middle-aged adults and are associated with high mortality rates, especially if treatment is delayed or sepsis develops.[10] NSTIs are caused by polymicrobial organisms, including at least one anaerobic species in combination with one or more facultative anaerobic species, often introduced from minor skin disruptions such as insect bites or cuts that lead to widespread tissue and muscle necrosis. Diabetes mellitus, obesity, immune suppression, end-stage renal failure, IV drug use, smoking, recent surgery, and hypertension are some of the risk factors for NSTI.[10] NSTIs typically have a subtle initial presentation of a localized, painful edematous area with increasing erythema and induration. Crepitus, necrosis, and anesthesia are infrequently seen and are late signs. The pain is severe and out of proportion to cutaneous findings. Because of the rapidly progressive infectious nature of NSTIs, patients can quickly become critically ill with observed high rates of sepsis and septic shock.[10,18] Early diagnosis, prompt and aggressive surgical excision, appropriate wound care, and empirical broad-spectrum antibiotic therapy are essential for a positive outcome.

DISCHARGE PLANNING

Discharge planning for critically ill burned patients and for those who have sustained a nonburn injury begins on the day of admission. Assessments are made regarding patient survival, the potential or actual short-term or long-term functional disabilities secondary to the injury, the financial resources available, the family roles and expectations, and the psychological support systems. Educate both the patient and the family to prepare for transfer from the critical care unit and eventual discharge from the hospital. Be aware that preexisting learning disabilities or new cognitive deficits caused by the injury can affect a patient's understanding.[37] Patients and families who are returning home must understand how to manage their physical requirements and care for their psychological and social needs. Nurses play an important role in multiprofessional team discharge planning by providing patient and family education and evaluating the need for additional resources to meet the patient's long-term rehabilitative and home care requirements.

BURN PREVENTION

The overwhelming majority of burns and fire-related injuries are preventable. Typically, injuries do not occur from random events or "accidents" but rather predominantly from predictable incidents. If people are not aware of potential risks, they do not take appropriate precautions to prevent an injury from occurring. Alcohol and substance abuse contribute to high-risk behavior; screening and brief intervention are effective in reducing alcohol intake and repeat injuries in the burn patient population (see Chapter 20). Successful prevention efforts

consider the targeted population and focus on interventions involving education (i.e., changing behavior), engineering or environment (i.e., modifications in safety designs), or enforcement (i.e., laws or safety regulations). Critical care nurses have an active and vital role in teaching prevention concepts and in promoting safety legislation to assist in reducing fires and burn injuries.[24,25] The incidence of burn injuries has been successfully decreased with widespread public safety education and government-mandated regulations regarding industrial environments, building codes, products, and home safety (e.g., child-resistant lighters, preset water heater temperature, self-extinguishing cigarettes, fire sprinklers, mandatory smoke alarms).[5,24,25] The National Fire Protection Association provides multiple resources for preventing burn injuries (https://www.nfpa.org/Public-Education).

CASE STUDY

Mrs. J. is a 75-year-old woman who sustained a thermal burn injury in a house fire. She was smoking a cigarette in bed while receiving home medical oxygen therapy. She was trapped in the bedroom for approximately 15 minutes before being rescued by firefighters. No smoke alarms were noted.

Questions

1. Once Mrs. J. is removed from the fire, what priorities are essential in her initial management?
2. Mrs. J. weighs 65 kg. She has burned an estimated 30% of her body. What is her estimated fluid requirement during the first 24 hours?
3. Given Mrs. J.'s age and past medical history, what are important assessments during aggressive fluid resuscitation?
4. Mrs. J. has circumferential, white, leathery burn wounds on both arms. What type of burn wound does she have? What assessments should be performed? What type of surgical treatment and wound care should be expected during the resuscitative phase and later in the acute care phase?
5. Considering the circumstances surrounding Mrs. J.'s injury, what issues will need to be addressed before her discharge from the hospital?

REFERENCES

1. Abdullahi A, Jeschke MG. Nutrition and anabolic pharmacotherapies in the care of burn patients. *Nutr Clin Pract.* 2014;29(5):621–630.
2. Ahrns KS. Trends in burn resuscitation: Shifting the focus from fluids to adequate endpoint monitoring, edema control, and adjuvant therapies. *Crit Care Nurs Clin North Am.* 2004;16(1):75–98.
3. Ahrns-Klas KS, Wahl WL, Hemmila MR, et al. Do burn centers provide juvenile firesetter intervention?. *J Burn Care Res.* 2012;33(2):272–278.
4. American Burn Association. *Advanced Burn Life Support Course: Provider's Manual.* Chicago, IL: American Burn Association; 2016.
5. American Burn Association. *Burn Incident and Treatment in the United States.* Chicago, IL: American Burn Association; 2016.
6. American Burn Association. *National Burn Repository 2017: Report of Data From 2008–2017.* Chicago, IL: American Burn Association; 2017.
7. Anseeuw K, Delvau N, Burillo-Putze G, et al. Cyanide poisoning by fire smoke inhalation: A European expert consensus. *Eur J Emerg Med.* 2013;20(1):2–9.

8. Assimacopoulos EM, Heard J, Liao J, et al. The national incidence and resource utilization of burn injuries sustained while smoking on home oxygen therapy (HOT). *J Burn Care Res*. 2016;37(1):25–31.

9. Bittner EA, Shank E, Woodson L, et al. Acute and perioperative care of the burn-injured patient. *Anesthesiology*. 2015;122(2):448–464.

10. Bonne SL, Kadri SS. Evaluation and management of necrotizing soft tissue infections. *Infec Dis Clin N Am*. 2017;31:497–511.

11. Borron S, Baud F, Barriot P, et al. Prospective study of hydroxocobalamin for acute cyanide poisoning in smoke inhalation. *Ann Emerg Med*. 2007;49(6):794–801.

12. Cartotto R, Greenhalgh DG, Cancio C. Burn state of the science: Fluid resuscitation. *J Burn Care Res*. 2017;38(3):e596–e604.

13. Cope D, Moore FD. The redistribution of body water in the fluid therapy of the burn patient. *Ann Surg*. 1947;126(6):1010–1045.

14. Demling RH, Mazess RB, Witt RM, et al. The study of burn wound edema using dichromatic absorptiometry. *J Trauma*. 1978;18(2):124–128.

15. Demling RH, Wong C, Jin LJ, et al. Early lung dysfunction after major burns: Role of edema and vasoactive mediators. *J Trauma*. 1985;25(10):959–966.

16. Dolgachev VA, Ciotti SM, Eisma R, et al. Nanoemulsion therapy for burn wounds is effective as a topical antimicrobial against gram negative and gram positive bacteria. *J Burn Care Res*. 2016;37(2):e104–e114.

17. Goldberg H, Klaff J, Spjut A, et al. A mobile app for measuring the surface area of a burn in three dimensions: Comparison to the Lund and Browder assessment. *J Burn Care Res*. 2014;35(6):480–483.

18. Greenhalgh DG, Saffle JR, Holmes JH 4th, et al. American Burn Association consensus conference on burn sepsis and infection group: American Burn Association consensus conference to define sepsis and infection in burns. *J Burn Care Res*. 2007;28(6):776–790.

19. Jaskille AD, Ramella-Roman JC, Shupp JW, et al. Critical review of burn depth assessment techniques: Part II. Review of laser doppler technology. *J Burn Care Res*. 2010;31(1):151–157.

20. Jeschke MG, Herndon DN. Burns in children: Standard and new treatments. *Lancet*. 2014;383(9923):1168–1178.

21. Jones CD, Ho W, Gunn E, et al. E-cigarette burn injuries: Comprehensive review and management guidelines proposal. *Burns*. 2019;45(4):763–771.

22. Kantak NA, Mistry R, Halvorson EG. A review of negative-pressure wound therapy in the management of burn wounds. *Burns*. 2016;42:1623–1633.

23. Kirkpatrick AW, Roberts DJ, De Waele J, et al. Intra-abdominal hypertension and the abdominal compartment syndrome: Updated consensus definitions and clinical practice guidelines from the world society of the abdominal compartment syndrome. *Intensive Care Med*. 2013;39(7):1190–1206.

24. Klas KS, Smith SJ, Matherly AF, et al. Multicenter assessment of burn team injury prevention knowledge. *J Burn Care Res*. 2015;36(3):434–439.

25. Klas KS, Vlahos PG, McCully MJ, et al. School-based prevention program associated with increased short- and long-term retention of safety knowledge. *J Burn Care Res*. 2015;36(3):376–393.

26. Lawrence A, Faraklas I, Watkins H, et al. Colloid administration normalizes resuscitation ratio and ameliorates "fluid creep." *J Burn Care Res*. 2010;31(1):40–47.

27. Linden K, Stewart IJ, Kreyer SF, et al. Extracorporeal blood purification in burns: A review. *Burns*. 2014;40(6):1071–1078.

28. Meizoso JP, Ray JJ, Allen CJ, et al. Hypercoagulability and venous thromboembolism in burn patients. *Semin Thromb Hemost*. 2015;41(1):43–48.

29. Miller AC, Elamin EM, Suffredini AF. Inhaled anticoagulation regimens for the treatment of smoke inhalation–associated acute lung injury: A systematic review. *Crit Care Med*. 2014;24(2):413–419.

30. Nyame TT, Chiang HA, Orgill DP. Clinical applications of skin substitutes. *Surg Clin North Am*. 2014;94(4):839–850.

31. Palmieri TL. Infection prevention: Unique aspects of burn units. *Surg Infect*. 2019;20(2):111–114.

32. Park SH, Hemmila MR, Wahl WL. Early albumin use improves mortality in difficult to resuscitate burn patients. *J Trauma Acute Care Surg*. 2012;73(5):1294–1297.

33. Real DS, Reis RP, Piccolo MS, et al. Oxandrolone use in adult burn patients: Systematic review and meta-analysis. *Acta Cir Bras*. 2014;29(Suppl 3):68–76.

34. Retrouvey H, Shahrokhi S. Pain and the thermally injured patient: A review of current therapies. *J Burn Care Res*. 2015;36(2):315–323.

35. Rizzo JA, Rowan MP, Driscoll IR, et al. Vitamin C in burn resuscitation. *Crit Care Clin*. 2016;32:539–546.

36. Snell JA, Loh NH, Mahambrey T, et al. Clinical review: The critical care management of the burn patient. *Crit Care*. 2013;17(5):241.

37. Stoddard FJ Jr, Ryan CM, Schneider JC. Physical and psychiatric recovery from burns. *Surg Clin North Am*. 2014;94(4):863–878.

38. Villar J, Kacmarek RM, Perez-Mendez L, et al. A high positive end-expiratory pressure, low tidal volume ventilatory strategy improves outcome in persistent acute respiratory distress syndrome: A randomized, controlled trial. *Crit Care Med*. 2006;34(5):1311–1318.

39. Wolf SE, Edelman LS, Kemalyan N, et al. Effects of oxandrolone on outcome measures in the severely burned: A multicenter prospective randomized double-blind trial. *J Burn Care Res*. 2006;27(2):131–139.

40. Woolum JA, Bailey AM, Baum RA, et al. A review of the management of Stevens-Johnson syndrome and toxic epidermal necrolysis. *Adv Emerg Nurs J*. 2019;41(1):56–64.

CHAPTER 1

1. A. Part of the American Association of Critical-Care Nurses' mission is: "Acute and critical care nurses rely on AACN for expert knowledge and the influence to fulfill their promise to patients and their families."
2. D. CCRN® is a specialty certification for nurses who provide the majority of their direct care to acutely ill or critically ill adult patients. Certification affirms eligibility to take the examination and successful testing.
3. B. Crew resource management is psychological training used in the airline industry to assist crew members in avoiding or mitigating threats by developing, communicating, and implementing an action plan after identifying potential and existing threats.
4. C. The AACN defines a healthy work environment as integrating the following six standards to achieve improved patient, nurse, and family outcomes: skilled communication, true collaboration, appropriate staffing, meaningful recognition, effective decision making, and authentic leadership.

CHAPTER 2

1. B. Perceptual disturbances may occur secondary to frequent vital signs and procedures, noise, and an unfamiliar environment.
2. C. Even if patients are sedated or unconscious, it is important to remember that many patients can still hear, understand, and respond emotionally to what is being said.
3. D. The three problems reported most often by survivors of a critical illness experience are disability and weakness, psychiatric pathologies, and cognitive dysfunction. Collectively, these symptoms are deemed post-intensive care syndrome, or PICS.
4. C. If a patient, especially an older adult, is severely ill with a prolonged length of stay, he or she is at greater risk for more complications. This affects the patient's health-related quality of life, as many patients do not return to their baseline health status.

CHAPTER 3

1. D. Options A, B, and C are all components of the ANA Code of Ethics.
2. A. The principle of autonomy refers to the patient's right to make his or her own choices.
3. D. POLST is a medical order that complements an advance directive.
4. D. This is an example of the doctrine of double effect. It is ethically acceptable for a nurse to titrate medication to relieve suffering even if the medication causes the patient to stop breathing.

CHAPTER 4

1. B. Financial or payor status never affects whether aggressive medical care is continued, as this would be unethical and illegal (i.e., it would violate the Emergency Medical Treatment and Labor Act).
2. B. Palliative care is not merely focused on withdrawal of care but includes improving the quality of life for patients and individuals with life-threatening or serious illness.

CHAPTER 5

1. A. First-person consent, such as consent on a driver's license, provides consent for organ donation in the event of death.
2. D. An increased-risk donor is defined as one who, according to medical and social history, has a documented risk of disease transmission.
3. B. Most programs prefer that there be no history of smoking, diabetes, dyslipidemia, or hypertension. Low LDL levels are desirable.

CHAPTER 6

1. A. The nociceptive pain is divided into somatic and visceral. Visceral pain is diffuse and poorly localized, and often referred.
2. B. Activation of the SNS results in tachycardia and hypertension, which leads to increased myocardial oxygen demand.
3. A. In nonverbal patients, observe behaviors using either the Behavioral Pain Scale (BPS) or the Critical-Care Pain Observation Tool (CPOT). Both tools demonstrate the greatest validity and reliability for monitoring pain in noncommunicative patients.
4. D. Two of the most frequently used and validated instruments are the Confusion Assessment Method for the ICU (CAM-ICU) and the Intensive Care Delirium Screening Checklist (ICDSC).

CHAPTER 7

1. A. It is appropriate to begin EN as long as the the patient is hemodynamically stable, GI tract is intact, has enteral access, and is not experiencing extreme nausea and/or vomiting.
2. C. Abdominal distention and pain are indicative of a potential gastrointestinal (GI) obstruction or some other process that may affect the patient's motility and ability to absorb nutrition through the GI tract.
3. C. Based on the guidelines, TPN should be avoided in the first 7 days of admission in low-risk patients or if the patient is unable to meet at least 60% of energy and protein requirements after 7 to 10 days of enteral nutrition (EN).

CHAPTER 8

1. C. The R-R interval shortens, reducing ventricular filling time (this occurs during ventricular diastole) and also reducing coronary artery perfusion (which also occurs during ventricular diastole).
2. C. Not visualizing any P waves rules out sinus rhythm, sinus arrhythmia, and premature atrial contractions, as all three of these rhythms contain P waves. The term *sinus* means that there is a P wave. In addition, the term *atrial* connotates that there is likely to be a P wave. Therefore the most likely correct answer is junctional rhythm.
3. B. The patient is symptomatic, evidenced by his complaint of feeling lightheaded and low blood pressure. Emergency interventions include administering adenosine, so anticipating the need to assist with this intervention is the first priority.

CHAPTER 9

1. B. An increased RAP is synonymous with too much fluid; thus the best treatment is to decrease fluid by administering diuretics ordered by a provider.
2. A. The distal tip of the pulmonary artery catheter is positioned to obtain pulmonary artery pressures. These pressures reflect left ventricular function.
3. D. A positive response to fluids has been observed when the PPV is 10% or higher in most patients who are in normal sinus rhythm, are intubated on mechanical ventilation without spontaneous respirations, and have no alterations in chest wall compliance.

CHAPTER 10

1. C. Objective verification of correct placement of the endotracheal tube (ETT) in the trachea (versus incorrect placement in the esophagus) is imperative and is performed through clinical assessment and confirmation devices. Clinical assessment includes auscultating the epigastrium and lung fields and observing for bilateral chest expansion. Devices to confirm ETT placement include either a handheld or a disposable end-tidal carbon dioxide ($ETCO_2$) detector or a bulb aspiration device (esophageal detector device).
2. C. Pressure support ventilation is a weaning method that provides inspiratory support to overcome resistance to gas flow through ventilator circuit and artificial airway.
3. B. Noninvasive ventilation (NIV) is indicated for the treatment of acute exacerbations of chronic obstructive pulmonary disease (COPD) and respiratory failure associated with pneumonia. The other patients have contraindications for NIV (i.e., hemodynamic instability, high risk for aspiration secondary to copious secretions, active ST elevation myocardial infarction [STEMI]).

CHAPTER 11

1. A. Rapid response teams (RRTs) have been implemented to address changes in a patient's clinical condition *before* a cardiac or respiratory arrest occurs.

2. C. Symptomatic bradycardia occurs when the heart rhythm is slow enough to cause hemodynamic compromise and poor perfusion with signs and symptoms such as hypotension, diaphoresis, chest pain, shortness of breath, decreased level of consciousness, and syncope. The cause of these signs and symptoms is related to the decreased cardiac output associated with the decreased heart rate.
3. B. Epinephrine is indicated for the restoration of cardiac electrical activity in an arrest. In addition, epinephrine increases automaticity and the force of contraction, an effect that makes the heart more susceptible to successful defibrillation. Epinephrine is used to treat VF or pulseless VT that is unresponsive to initial defibrillation, asystole, and PEA.
4. D. Hypothermia should be initiated as soon as possible after resuscitation. Attainment of a temperature below 34°C within 3.5 hours of return of spontaneous circulation (ROSC) may be beneficial. After 24 hours of cooling, rewarming proceeds slowly (0.25°C/h to 0.5°C/h) to prevent sudden vasodilation, hypotension, and shock.

CHAPTER 12

1. B. Shock begins when the cardiovascular system fails to function properly because of an alteration in at least one of the four essential circulatory components: blood volume, myocardial contractility, blood flow, or vascular resistance. Capillary refill is not one of these components.
2. A. Glucocorticoids and mineralocorticoids are released by the anterior pituitary gland in response to the reduction in blood pressure that occurs during the compensatory stage of shock. Mineralocorticoids act on the renal tubules, causing the reabsorption of sodium and water, resulting in an increased intravascular volume and blood pressure.
3. C. In neurogenic shock, there is an interruption of impulse transmission or a blockage of sympathetic outflow that results in vasodilation, inhibition of baroreceptor response, and impaired thermoregulation. These reactions result in hypotension, bradycardia, and warm, dry skin.

CHAPTER 13

1. B. After blood has been oxygenated in the lungs, newly oxygenated blood flows from the pulmonary vein to the left atrium.
2. D. P stands for Provocation. Q stands for Quality, R for Region and Radiation, S for Severity, and T for Timing and Treatment.
3. D. The LVEF is the percentage of blood ejected from the left ventricle during systole, normally 55% to 60%.
4. B. Variant, or Prinzmetal's, angina is caused by coronary artery spasms. It often occurs at rest and without other precipitating factors. The electrocardiogram (ECG) shows a marked ST elevation (usually seen only in acute myocardial infarction [AMI]) during the episode.
5. B. Placement of bare metal stents or drug-eluting stents is common during angioplasty to maintain patency of the vessel.

6. C. HFrEF refers to heart failure with reduced ejection fraction.

CHAPTER 14

1. A. The hypothalamus, not the brainstem, is responsible for temperature control.
2. D. The Babinski reflex is present at birth as a normal reflex and disappears as the nervous system matures. The appearance of the Babinski reflex in an adult is a pathological reflex.
3. B. Head elevation to 30 degrees facilitates mechanisms that control intracranial pressure.
4. D. To determine potential eligibility for thrombolytic therapy within 3 hours of stroke, time of symptom onset must be clearly identified.
5. A. The patient should be placed on droplet precautions.
6. C. Neurogenic shock is characterized by hypotension, bradycardia, and hypothermia.

CHAPTER 15

1. D. All of the above are components of the Berlin definition of ARDS. In particular, the PaO_2/FiO_2 ratio determines the severity of ARDS.
2. B. Lower tidal volumes are an evidence-based method for preventing ventilator-induced lung injury.
3. D. All of the above are methods for treating ARF in COPD. Early treatment with noninvasive ventilation has been found to decrease mortality. Bronchodilators can decrease airway resistance, and corticosteroids can decrease inflammation and edema, improving lung function.
4. C. Components of the ventilator bundle to prevent VAP include HOB elevation to at least 30 degrees, daily awakening ("sedation vacation") with assessment of need for continuing mechanical ventilation, prophylaxis for stress ulcers and DVT, and regular antiseptic oral care to include chlorhexidine.
5. E. All of these are acquired risks for the development of DVT.

CHAPTER 16

1. B. Glomerular filtration rate occurs as the result of a pressure gradient, which requires the mean arterial pressure to be 60 mm Hg or greater. As the mean arterial pressure decreases, so does the glomerular filtration rate.
2. D. Both the proximal and distal tubules reabsorb bicarbonate to regulate the acid-base balance.
3. A. Decreased urine output, or oliguria, is defined as a reduction to less than 0.5 mL/kg/h and generally reflects a decrease in the glomerular filtration rate.
4. D. Creatine clearance, after correcting for age, represents kidney function. Reductions in creatine clearance can indicate a decline in kidney function, which may affect medication dosing.
5. C. Although calcium chloride has no effect on serum potassium, it is effective in managing life-threatening hyperkalemia by stabilizing the cardiac cell membrane. An almost immediate effect will be noted on the electrocardiogram (ECG), reducing the patient's risk for a cardiac arrhythmia and death.
6. C. Through the process of convection, CVVH slowly removes fluids and solutes to provide fluid, electrolyte, and acid-base balance.

CHAPTER 17

1. B. The band neutrophils are referred to as immature neutrophils. A *shift to the left* happens with an increased number of bands or band neutrophils.
2. B. Thrombocytopenia is defined as a quantitative deficiency of platelets, specifically a platelet count of less than 150,000/mm^3. The best treatment option for this condition is infusion of platelets.
3. D. Gram-negative bacterial infection is one of the listed "infections" to cause DIC. In addition, abruptio placentae is one of the obstetrical causes of DIC. Transfusion reactions are an identified case of hematological disorders that cause DIC. Acute renal failure is not a likely cause of DIC. See Table 17.12 for reference.

CHAPTER 18

1. B. Albumin maintains blood oncotic pressure and prevents plasma loss from the capillaries.
2. C. Assessment of pain assists in identifying potential problems. Assessment of the usual diet provides information on intake that may contribute to constipation, such as low fiber intake.
3. A. The first-line treatment for *H. pylori* infection consists of triple therapy with a proton pump inhibitor (PPI; e.g., esomeprazole, omeprazole, pantoprazole, rabeprazole) plus the antibiotics amoxicillin and clarithromycin.
4. D. Esophageal varices are a late sign of liver disease associated with portal hypertension.

CHAPTER 19

1. C. The situation of two elevated findings greater than 300 mg/dL in a 12-hour period is the priority to ensure that safe and quality care is administered to this patient in a timely manner.
2. D. Options for the 15/15 rule include the following: 3 glucose tablets; ½ cup (4 ounces or 120 milliliters) of fruit juice or regular soda; 6 or 7 hard candies; 1 tablespoon (15 grams) of sugar. Choosing any one of these appropriate doses of the sugar replacement is acceptable. Once glucose is given, fingerstick glucose is reassessed in 15 minutes to evaluate effectiveness.
3. B. Patients may need emergency treatment. Dexamethasone can be given and does not interfere with the results of the test.
4. A. Marked tachycardia is commonly noted in thyroid storm secondary to the increase in metabolism and the stimulation of catecholamines produced by excess thyroid hormones.

CHAPTER 20

1. C. The primary survey encourages continual evaluation for uncontrolled hemorrhage and life-threatening conditions, which require immediate intervention through the ABCDEFG mnemonic.

2. A, B, E. The "trauma triad of death" is a vicious cycle that occurs in the severely injured patient. The patient can lose the ability to autoregulate temperature due to the injuries or hypovolemic shock, which causes hypothermia. Acidosis occurs secondary to hypothermia, lactic acid production during hypovolemic shock, and/or over-resuscitation with unbalanced crystalloids. Coagulopathy occurs secondary to the aforementioned hypothermia and acidosis but is worsened via consumption of coagulation factors and potential dilution from over-resuscitation with crystalloids.

3. A. The focused assessment with sonography for trauma (FAST) or extended FAST (E-FAST) exams are typically the first-line diagnostic tools used for the emergent evaluation of a patient presenting with traumatic injuries.

4. D. An elevated lactate indicates that the patient's cellular perfusion is poor and anaerobic metabolism is still occurring. Adequate ventilation and successful fluid resuscitation lead to a decrease in lactate levels.

5. B. A patient who is developing compartment syndrome typically complains of an increasing throbbing pain disproportionate to the injury. Attempts to reduce the pain with narcotic administration do not relieve the pain.

CHAPTER 21

1. B. Superficial partial-thickness burns are wounds that are moist, pink or mottled red, and very painful and that blanch briskly with pressure. Blisters are characteristic of a superficial partial-thickness burn.

2. B. Using the rule of nines, the palmar surface, including the fingers, of the patient's hand represents 1% of his or her total body surface area.

3. D. Humidified 100% oxygen via face mask or endotracheal tube is administered in the patient with an inhalation injury until carboxyhemoglobin (COHgb) levels are determined. Once COHgb levels normalize (<10%), wean oxygen as tolerated.

4. A. During the first 24 hours, age, total body surface area burned, patient weight, and cause of burn injury are used to guide fluid resuscitation.

Page numbers followed by "*f*" indicate figures, "*b*" indicate boxes, and "*t*" indicate tables.

607

SPECIAL FEATURES